KT-528-418

BM

CLINICAL
GYNECOLOGIC
ONCOLOGY

NINTH EDITION

CLINICAL GYNECOLOGIC ONCOLOGY

PHILIP J. DISAIA, MD
The Dorothy Marsh Chair in Reproductive Biology
Professor, Department of Obstetrics and Gynecology
University of California, Irvine College of Medicine
Irvine, California
UCI Medical Center
Orange, California

WILLIAM T. CREASMAN, MD
Distinguished University Professor
Department of Obstetrics and Gynecology
Medical University of South Carolina
Charleston, South Carolina

ROBERT S. MANNEL, MD
Professor
Division of Gynecologic Oncology
Stephenson Cancer Center
University of Oklahoma Health Sciences Center
Oklahoma City, Oklahoma

D. SCOTT MCMEEKIN, MD (†)
Presbyterian Foundation Presidential Professor
University of Oklahoma Health Sciences Center
Oklahoma City, Oklahoma

DAVID G. MUTCH, MD
Ira C. and Judith Gall Professor of Obstetrics and
  Gynecology
Department of Obstetrics and Gynecology
Vice Chair of Gynecology
Washington University School of Medicine
St. Louis, Missouri

†Deceased.

ELSEVIER

ELSEVIER

1600 John F. Kennedy Blvd.
Ste 1800
Philadelphia, PA 19103-2899

CLINICAL GYNECOLOGIC ONCOLOGY, NINTH EDITION　　　　ISBN: 978-0-323-40067-1

Previous editions copyrighted 2012, 2007, 2002, 1997, 1993, 1989, 1984, 1981.

Library of Congress Cataloging-in-Publication Data

Names: Di Saia, Philip J., 1937- editor. | Creasman, William T., 1934- editor. | Mannel, Robert S., editor. | McMeekin, Scott, editor. | Mutch, David G., editor.
Title: Clinical gynecologic oncology / [edited by] Philip J. DiSaia, William T. Creasman, Robert S. Mannel, Scott McMeekin, David G. Mutch.
Description: 9th edition. | Philadelphia, PA : Elsevier, [2018] | Includes bibliographical references and index.
Identifiers: LCCN 2016049213 | ISBN 9780323400671 (pbk. : alk. paper) | ISBN 9780323443166 (eBook)
Subjects: | MESH: Genital Neoplasms, Female
Classification: LCC RC280.G5 | NLM WP 145 | DDC 616.99/465–dc23 LC record available at https://lccn.loc.gov/2016049213

Executive Content Strategist: Kate Dimock
Director, Content Development: Rebecca Gruliow
Publishing Services Manager: Deepthi Unni
Senior Project Manager: Beula Christopher
Designer: Julia Dummitt
Marketing Manager: Michele Milano

Printed in Canada

Last digit is the print number:　9　8　7　6　5　4　3　2　1

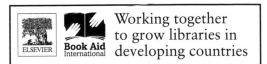

Working together
to grow libraries in
developing countries

www.elsevier.com • www.bookaid.org

We dedicate this book in memory of our friend, colleague, and co-editor, Dr. Scott McMeekin, who recently lost his own battle with cancer at 51 years of age. Readers of this book are undoubtedly familiar with his name because he authored more than 100 publications in the field of gynecologic oncology, and his expertise in uterine cancer placed him at the forefront of defining the standard of care for the management of this disease. His dedication to helping women with gynecologic cancers was only surpassed by his dedication to his wife Cathy; their children Charlotte, Jackson, and Remy; and his loving parents, Donald and Charlene. Although we will benefit from his scientific contributions for years to come, we will all miss his presence.

CONTRIBUTORS

Sheri A. Babb, MS, CGC
Genetic Counselor, Department of Obstetrics and Gynecology, Division of Gynecologic Oncology, Washington University School of Medicine, St. Louis, Missouri

Floor J. Backes, MD
Assistant Professor, Division of Gynecologic Oncology, James Cancer Hospital, Ohio State University Comprehensive Cancer Center, Columbus, Ohio
Role of Minimally Invasive Surgery in Gynecologic Malignancies

Emma L. Barber, MD
Clinical Fellow, Department of Obstetrics and Gynecology, Division of Gynecologic Oncology, University of North Carolina, Chapel Hill, North Carolina
Gestational Trophoblastic Disease

Wendy R. Brewster, MD, PhD
Director Center for Women's Health Research, Professor, Department of Obstetrics and Gynecology, Division of Gynecologic Oncology University of North Carolina, Chapel Hill, North Carolina
Epidemiology and Commonly Used Statistical Terms and Analysis of Clinical Studies

Dana M. Chase, MD
Assistant Professor, Creighton University School of Medicine, University of Arizona College of Medicine at St. Joseph's Hospital and Medical Center, Phoenix, Arizona
Palliative Care and Quality of Life

Christina S. Chu, MD
Associate Professor, Division of Gynecologic Oncology, Department of Surgical Oncology, Fox Chase Cancer Center, Philadelphia, Pennsylvania
Basic Principles of Chemotherapy

Daniel L. Clarke-Pearson, MD
Robert A. Ross Professor of Obstetrics and Gynecology, University of North Carolina, Chapel Hill, North Carolina
Complications of Disease and Therapy

David E. Cohn, MD
Professor, Division of Gynecologic Oncology, James Cancer Hospital, Ohio State University Comprehensive Cancer Center, Columbus, Ohio
Role of Minimally Invasive Surgery in Gynecologic Malignancies

Robert L. Coleman, MD
Professor, Department of Gynecologic Oncology and Reproductive Medicine, University of Texas, MD Anderson Cancer Center, Houston, Texas
Invasive Cancer of the Vagina; Targeted Therapy and Molecular Genetics

Larry J. Copeland, MD
Professor and William Greenville Pace III and Joann Norris Collins-Pace Chair, Department of Obstetrics and Gynecology, James Cancer Hospital, The Ohio State University, Columbus, Ohio
Epithelial Ovarian Cancer

Patricia A. Cronin, MD
Breast Service, Department of Surgery, Memorial Sloan Kettering Cancer Center, New York, New York
Breast Diseases

William T. Creasman, MD
Distinguished University Professor, Department of Obstetrics and Gynecology, Medical University of South Carolina, Charleston, South Carolina
Adenocarcinoma of the Uterine Corpus; Sarcoma of the Uterus

Philip J. Di Saia, MD
The Dorothy J. Marsh Chair in Reproductive Biology; Director, Division of Gynecologic Oncology; Professor, Department of Obstetrics and Gynecology, University of California–Irvine College of Medicine, Orange, California
The Adnexal Mass; Genes and Cancer: Genetic Counseling and Clinical Management

Kemi M. Doll, MD, MSCR
Assistant Professor, Department of Obstetrics and Gynecology, University of Washington, Seattle, Washington
Complications of Disease and Therapy

Eric L. Eisenhauer, MD
Associate Professor, Department of Obstetrics and Gynecology, Director, Division of Gynecologic Oncology, University of Cincinnati College of Medicine, Cincinnati, Ohio
Epithelial Ovarian Cancer

Jeffrey M. Fowler, MD
Professor, Division of Gynecologic Oncology, James Cancer Hospital, Ohio State University Comprehensive Cancer Center, Columbus, Ohio
Role of Minimally Invasive Surgery in Gynecologic Malignancies

Mary L. Gemignani, MD
Associate Attending Surgeon, Department of Surgery/Breast Service, Memorial Sloan-Kettering Cancer Center, New York, New York
Breast Diseases

Camille C. Gunderson, MD
Assistant Professor, Gynecologic Oncology, Stephenson Cancer Center, University of Oklahoma, Oklahoma City, Oklahoma
The Adnexal Mass

Chad A. Hamilton, MD
Director, Division of Gynecologic Oncology, Walter Reed National Military Medical Center, Bethesda, Maryland
Germ Cell, Stromal, and Other Ovarian Tumors, Fallopian Tube Cancer

Thomas J. Herzog, MD
Deputy Director, University of Cincinnati Cancer Institute, Vice Chair of Quality and Safety; Paul and Carolyn Flory Professor, Department of Ob Gyn, University of Cincinnati, Cincinnati, Ohio
Invasive Cancer of the Vulva

Erica R. Hope, MD
Walter Reed National Military Medical Center, Division of Gynecologic Oncology, Bethesda, Maryland
Fallopian Tube Cancer

Marilyn Huang, MD
Assistant Professor, Division of Gynecologic Oncology, Sylvester Comprehensive Cancer Center/University of Miami/Miller School of Medicine, Miami, Florida
Invasive Cancer of the Vagina

Lisa M. Landrum, MD, PhD
Assistant Professor of Obstetrics and
Gynecology, University of Oklahoma
Health Sciences Center, Oklahoma City,
Oklahoma
*Endometrial Hyperplasia, Estrogen Therapy,
and the Prevention of Endometrial Cancer*

Robert S. Mannel, MD
Professor, Division of Gynecologic
Oncology, Stephenson Cancer Center,
University of Oklahoma Health Sciences
Center, Oklahoma City, Oklahoma
*The Adnexal Mass; Role of Minimally
Invasive Surgery in Gynecologic
Malignancies*

Charlotte S. Marcus, MD
Attending Physician, Division of
Gynecologic Oncology, Walter Reed
National Military Medical Center,
Bethesda, Maryland
*Germ Cell, Stromal, and Other Ovarian
Tumors*

L. Stewart Massad, MD
Division of Gynecologic Oncology,
Department of Obstetrics and
Gynecology, Washington University
School of Medicine, St. Louis, Missouri
Preinvasive Disease of the Cervix

Cara A. Mathews, MD
Assistant Professor, Gynecologic Oncology,
Department of Obstetrics and
Gynecology, Women and Infants'
Hospital, Warren Alpert Medical School
of Brown University, Providence, Rhode
Island
*Preinvasive Disease of the Vagina and Vulva
and Related Disorders*

G. Larry Maxwell, MD
Chairman, Department of Obstetrics and
Gynecology, Inova Fairfax Hospital;
Assistant Director, Inova Schar Cancer
Institute; Co-P.I., DOD Gynecologic
Cancer Translational Research Center of
Excellence; Professor, Virginia
Commonwealth University School of
Medicine, Falls Church, Virginia
Fallopian Tube Cancer

D. Scott McMeekin, MD(†)
Presbyterian Foundation Presidential
Professor, University of Oklahoma
Health Sciences Center, Oklahoma City,
Oklahoma
The Adnexal Mass; Sarcoma of the Uterus

David Scott Miller, MD, FACOG, FACS
Amy and Vernon E. Faulconer Distinguished
Chair in Medical Science, Director and
Dallas Foundation Chair in Gynecologic
Oncology, Professor of Obstetrics and
Gynecology, University of Texas
Southwestern Medical Center, Dallas,
Texas
Adenocarcinoma of the Uterine Corpus

Bradley J. Monk, MD
Professor, Creighton University School of
Medicine, University of Arizona College
of Medicine at St. Joseph's Hospital and
Medical Center, Phoenix, Arizona
*Invasive Cervical Cancer; Palliative Care and
Quality of Life, Palliative Care and
Quality of Life*

David G. Mutch, MD
Judith and Ira Gall Professor of Gynecologic
Oncology; Vice Chair of Gynecology,
Washington University School of
Medicine, St. Louis, Missouri
*Genes and Cancer: Genetic Counseling and
Clinical Management; Appendix A
Staging; Appendix B Modified from
Common Terminology Criteria for Adverse
Events (Common Terminology Criteria for
Adverse Events); Appendix C Blood
Component Therapy; Appendix D
Suggested Recommendations for Routine
Cancer Screening; Appendix E Nutritional
Therapy*

Emily R. Penick, MD
Fellow, Division of Gynecologic Oncology,
Walter Reed National Military Medical
Center, Bethesda, Maryland
*Germ Cell, Stromal, and Other Ovarian
Tumors*

Stephen C. Rubin, MD
Professor and Chief, Division of
Gynecologic Oncology, Department of
Surgical Oncology, Fox Chase Cancer
Center, Philadelphia, Pennsylvania
Basic Principles of Chemotherapy

Ritu Salani, MD
Associate Professor, Department of
Obstetrics and Gynecology, James
Cancer Hospital, The Ohio State
University, Columbus, Ohio
Epithelial Ovarian Cancer

Brian M. Slomovitz, MD, MS, FACOG
Sylvester Professor of Obstetrics and
Gynecology and Human Genetics, Chief,
Division of Gynecologic Oncology,
Sylvester Comprehensive Cancer Center,
Miller school of Medicine of the
University of Miami, Miami, Florida
Invasive Cancer of the Vagina

Anil K. Sood, MD
Professor and Director, Ovarian Cancer
Research, Department of Gynecologic
Oncology and Reproductive Medicine,
The University of Texas, MD Anderson
Cancer Center, Houston, Texas
Targeted Therapy and Molecular Genetics

John T. Soper, MD
Professor, Department of Obstetrics and
Gynecology, Division of Gynecologic
Oncology, University of North Carolina
School of Medicine, Chapel Hill, North
Carolina
Gestational Trophoblastic Disease

Krishnansu S. Tewari, MD
Associate Professor, University of
California–Irvine College of Medicine,
Division of Gynecologic Oncology,
Orange, California
*Cancer in Pregnancy; Invasive Cervical
Cancer*

Joan L. Walker, MD
Professor of Gynecologic Oncology,
Department of Obstetrics and
Gynecology, University of Oklahoma
Health Sciences Center, Oklahoma City,
Oklahoma
*Endometrial Hyperplasia, Estrogen Therapy,
and the Prevention of Endometrial
Cancer; Preinvasive Disease of the Vagina
and Vulva and Related Disorders*

Lari B. Wenzel, PhD
Professor, Department of Medicine and
Public Health, Associate Director,
Population Science and Cancer Control,
University of California, Irvine,
California
Palliative Care and Quality of Life

Shannon N. Westin, MD, MPH
Associate Professor, Department of
Gynecologic Oncology and Reproductive
Medicine, University of Texas MD
Anderson Cancer Center, Houston, Texas
Targeted Therapy and Molecular Genetics

†Deceased.

Siu-Fun Wong, PharmD, FASHP, FCSHP
Associate Dean of Assessment and
    Scholarship, Professor, Chapman
    University School of Pharmacy, Irvine,
    California; Volunteer Clinical Professor
    of Medicine, University of California-
    Irvine, Irvine, California
Palliative Care and Quality of Life

Catheryn M. Yashar, MD, FACR, FACRO
University of California, San Diego, Moores
    Cancer Center, Radiation Oncology, La
    Jolla, California
Basic Principles in Gynecologic Radiotherapy

Rosemary E. Zuna, MD
Associate Professor of Pathology, Pathology
    Department, University of Oklahoma
    Health Sciences Center, Oklahoma City,
    Oklahoma
*Endometrial Hyperplasia, Estrogen Therapy,
    and the Prevention of Endometrial Cancer*

The first eight editions of *Clinical Gynecologic Oncology* were stimulated by a recognized need for a readable text on gynecologic cancer and related subjects addressed primarily to the community physician, resident, and other students involved with these patients. The practical aspects of the clinical presentation and management of these problems were heavily emphasized in these editions, and we have continued that style in this text. As in every other textbook, the authors interjected their own biases on many topics, especially in areas where more than one approach to management has been used. On the other hand, most major topics are treated in depth and supplemented with ample references to current literature so that the text can provide a comprehensive resource for study by the resident, fellow, or student of gynecologic oncology and serve as a source for review material.

We continued the practice of placing an outline on the first page of each chapter as a guide to the content for that section. We added "bullet" points to the chapters of this edition to emphasize important areas. Readers will notice that we have included topics not discussed in the former editions and expanded areas previously introduced. Some of these areas include new guidelines for managing dying patients; current management and reporting guidelines for cervical and vulvar cancer; current management and reporting guidelines for breast cancer; expanded discussion on the basic principles of genetic alterations in cancer; techniques for laparoscopic surgery in treatment of gynecologic cancers; and new information on breast, cervical, and colon cancer screenings and detection. The seventh edition contained, for the first time, color photographs of key gross and microscopic specimens for readers' review; we have continued that in this edition. In addition, Drs. Di Saia and Creasman have handed the reigns over to the three associate editors. We have included several new authors. Much more information is included to make the text as practical as possible for the practicing gynecologist. In addition, key points are highlighted for easy review.

Fortunately, many of the gynecologic malignancies have a high "cure" rate. This relatively impressive success rate with gynecologic cancers can be attributed in great part to the development of diagnostic techniques that can identify precancerous conditions, the ability to apply highly effective therapeutic modalities that are more restrictive elsewhere in the body, a better understanding of the disease spread patterns, and the development of more sophisticated and effective treatment in cancers that previously had very poor prognoses. As a result, today a patient with a gynecologic cancer may look toward more successful treatment and longer survival than at any other time. This optimism should be realistically transferred to the patient and her family. Patient denial must be tolerated until the patient decides that a frank conversation is desired. When the prognosis is discussed, some element of hope should always be introduced within the limits of reality and possibility.

The physician must be prepared to treat the malignancy in light of today's knowledge and to deal with the patient and her family in a compassionate and honest manner. Patients with gynecologic cancer need to feel that their physicians are confident and goal oriented. Although, unfortunately, gynecologic cancers will cause the demise of some individuals, it is hoped that the information collected in this book will help to increase the survival rate of these patients by bringing current practical knowledge to the attention of the primary care and specialized physician.

Our ideas are only intellectual instruments which we use to break into phenomena; we must change them when they have served their purpose, as we change a blunt lancet that we have used long enough.

—*Claude Bernard (1813-1878)*

Some patients, though conscious that their condition is perilous, recover their health simply through their contentment with the goodness of their physician.

—*Hippocrates (440-370 bc)*

Philip J. Di Saia, MD
William T. Creasman, MD
Robert S. Mannel, MD
D. Scott McMeekin, MD
David G. Mutch, MD

ACKNOWLEDGMENTS

We wish to acknowledge the advice given and contributions made by several colleagues, including Michael A. Bidus, Wendy R. Brewster, Dana Chase, Christina S. Chu, Daniel L. Clarke-Pearson, Robert L. Coleman, Larry J. Copeland, Eric Eisenhauer, Jeffrey Fowler, Mary L. Gemignani, Emily M. Ko, Robert S. Mannel, Cara Mathews, D. Scott McMeekin, David Miller, Bradley J. Monk, David G. Mutch, G. Scott Rose, Stephen C. Rubin, Ritu Salani , Jeanne Schilder, Brian M. Slomovitz, John T. Soper, Frederick B. Stehman, Krishnansu S. Tewari, Joan Walker, Lari B. Wenzel, Siu-Fun Wong, Catheryn Yashar, and Rosemary E. Zuna. We give special thanks to Lucy DiGiuseppe and, especially, Lisa Kozik for their diligent administrative support in preparing the manuscript and to David F. Baker, Carol Beckerman, Richard Crippen, Susan Stokskopf, and David Wyer for their excellent and creative contributions to many of the illustrations created for this book.

We are grateful to the sincere and diligent efforts of Kate Dimock, Rebecca Gruliow, Teresa McBryan, Ashley Miner, and Beula Christopher from Elsevier in bringing this book to fruition. Through their deliberate illumination and clearing of our path, this material has traversed the far distance from mere concept to a compelling reference book.

Drs. Mannel, McMeekin, and Mutch would like to acknowledge and thank Drs. DiSaia and Creasman for their continuous and tireless mentorship throughout our careers. They have served as role models in our professional and personal lives.

CONTENTS

Preinvasive Disease of the Cervix

L. Stewart Massad, MD

OUTLINE

KEY POINTS

1. Human papillomavirus (HPV) persistent expression is required for progression to cancer.
2. HPV vaccination has the potential to eradicate cervical cancer.
3. Cervical cancer screening now relies heavily on HPV testing.
4. mRNA expression is as sensitive but more specific than DNA testing.
5. Screening guidelines have changed dramatically with the use of contesting and increased intervals between screenings.

Cervical cancer was once the most common cancer in women. It is among the most preventable cancers, and it has become rare among women who engage in cervical cancer prevention programs. Nevertheless, with some 100,000 preinvasive lesions diagnosed in the United States annually, it remains a substantial threat. After tremendous gains following introduction of cytology screening half a century ago, cervical cancer rates continue to fall by about 1% annually. Careful compliance with evidence-based guidelines remains critical to sustaining progress. Effective programs reflect organized public health efforts encompassing patient and clinician education, vaccination against causative types of human papillomavirus (HPV), cytology and HPV screening, colposcopy triage for abnormal screening test results, and destruction of the at-risk cervical transformation zone for women with cancer precursors.

NATURAL HISTORY

Essentially all cervical cancers arise from persistent genital HPV infections (Fig. 1.1). The International Agency for Research on Cancer has designated as carcinogenic 12 HPV types: HPV-16, -18, -31, -33, -35, -39, -45, -51, -52, -56, -58, and -59. As described by Halec and associates, another eight types have been designated as possibly or probably carcinogenic: HPV–26, -53, -66, -67, -68, -70, -73, and -82. Almost 200 HPV types have been identified. A new genotype is based on DNA sequencing. A new type must share less than 90% DNA homology in the L1, E6, and E7 compared with known HPV types.

HPV-16 is the most oncogenic, accounting for more than 50% of cervical cancers. HPV-18 is found in 10% of cervical cancers and plays a particularly important role in adenocarcinogenesis. Types 31, 33, and 45 each account for around 5% of cancers. The other types are less oncogenic but have been reported in large typing studies of cervical cancers. HPV-18 and related HPV-45 are linked to cancers found at a younger age.

HPV infection leads to cancer through multiple pathways, but interaction of the HPV E6 and E7 gene products with p53 and pRb are critical: By inactivating or activating degradation of their targets, E6 and E7 eliminate genetic surveillance and allow unchecked cell cycling, leading to accumulation of mutations and eventual invasive cancer. HPV-16 E6 and E7 bind their targets with greater affinity than other HPV types; this may

FIGURE 1.1 **A,** Koilocytotic cells with intranuclear virions (×6900). **B,** Human papillomavirus particles. Note the intranuclear crystalline array ("honeycomb") arrangement of virions (×20,500). See the *insert* (×80,000). (Courtesy of Alex Ferenczy, MD, Montreal, Canada.)

FIGURE 1.2 A cervical intraepithelial neoplasia lesion with multiple mitotic figures.

partly explain its greater oncogenicity. Persistent infections lead to cancer in steps: Initial infection into basal epithelial cells leads to establishment of a ring chromosome from which carcinogenic proteins are elaborated while virion production occurs in maturing epithelium. Disruption of the ring, often at the HPV E2 regulatory region, allows integration of E6 and E7 sequence into the host genome. The accumulation of mutations leads to nuclear changes visible cytologically as a high-grade squamous intraepithelial lesion (HSIL) and histologically as high-grade cervical intraepithelial neoplasia (CIN) (Fig. 1.2) is apparent histologically. Selection for invasiveness and metastasis through additional mutation and through gene methylation results in evolution to cancer. Multitype infections do not appear to increase cancer risk, and when multitype infections include HPV-16, most lesions are caused by HPV-16. Extant HPV infections do not appear to predispose to or protect from infection by unrelated types.

Vertical transmission of HPV from mother to infant has been documented in the Finnish HPV Family Study but does not appear to result in cervical infection, with genital HPV in only 1.5% of infants after 2 years; fathers' HPV infections did not increase infant HPV risk. Although lifetime abstinence protects against genital HPV infection, nonpenetrative sexual behaviors may transmit the virus, and male exposures modulate female risk. For example, spouses of men who engaged in sex with prostitutes were at higher risk for cervical cancer than those of men who did not, and cervical cancer risk is higher among women whose husbands had more sexual partners. Women who report recent sex only with women are also at risk, though their risk may be marginally lower than that of heterosexual women. Condom use is not fully protective against HPV infection because condoms fail to cover wide areas of genital skin, though it speeds clearance of HPV infections. Male circumcision also reduces but does not eliminate HPV and cancer risks. For these reasons, all women with prior sexual experience, including those who have not been sexually active for years, remain at risk for cervical cancer and merit screening until they have multiple negative test results.

Despite the high frequency of HPV infection, most women infected with carcinogenic HPV, including those with HPV-16, do not develop cervical cancer. Instead, most infections are cleared immunologically. HPV is an intraepithelial virus, and clearance appears to require recognition of infection by cell-mediated immune cells. Roughly half of new infections are cleared within 6 months, with half of the remainder cleared by the end of the first year after infection. Clearance is associated with greater density of CD8+ cells and lower density of

T-regulatory cells in underlying stroma. Cervical treatment speeds clearance and reduces risk for posttreatment acquisition of new HPV infections. The type distribution of HPV infection after hysterectomy shows that HPV-16 and HPV-18 have a greater predilection for cervical rather than vaginal epithelium, with HPV types of lesser oncogenicity dominating in the posthysterectomy vagina.

HPV persistence is required for progression of infection to cancer, and women who clear their infections are at low risk. New infections in older women typically do not progress to preinvasive disease or cancer, and women who clear carcinogenic HPV infections have low risk for reappearance with subsequent high-grade CIN. These findings have important implications for termination of screening. Nevertheless, aging appears to result in immune senescence, with many HPV infections in older women attributable to reactivation of previously acquired by latent infections. Oral contraceptive use reduces clearance.

Although determinants of HPV persistence and progression of HPV infection to invasive cancer are poorly understood, several risk factors are known. HPV infection of a cervix undergoing active metaplasia increases risk, as reflected by the epidemiologic observations that early onset of first intercourse is associated with cancer. Smoking is linked to both CIN and cervical cancer. Benzopyrenes have been identified in cervical mucus, and the interaction of tobacco carcinogens with carcinogenic HPV increases risk substantially. Smoking also reduces immune-mediated HPV clearance. Cervical adenocarcinoma and adenocarcinoma in situ (AIS) have been linked to oral contraceptive use. Deficiencies in nutrients such as folate have been linked to cervical oncogenesis but are uncommon among US women. Variants of common HPV types that segregate by ethnicity and polymorphisms in genes related to HPV immune recognition or HPV protein products also modulate HPV persistence and carcinogenic progression. Perhaps most important, lack of screening is a high risk factor for progression of HPV infection to precancer and cancer: Whereas appropriately screened women with multiple risk factors are at relatively low risk, women with few risk factors who are not screened are at higher risk.

Immune factors play a clear role in the clearance or persistence of HPV-related cervical lesions, but the nature of immune defects is poorly understood. Fukuda and associates showed that lesions that persist have fewer Langerhans cells and helper T cells than lesions that are cleared, and tobacco smoking also lowers Langerhans and helper T-cell numbers. In contrast, Molling and associates showed that, although natural killer cells are decreased, regulatory T-cell numbers are increased in women with persistent HPV-16. Immunosuppression related to coinfection with the human immunodeficiency virus (HIV-1) illustrates the importance of immunity in the typical control of HPV. Women with HIV have much higher rates of HPV infection, including multitype infections. HPV clearance rates are lower, although most women do clear their HPV infections if observed long enough, especially if immune reserve as measured by CD4 lymphocyte count remains above 200/cmm. Although most HPV infections in HIV-seropositive women are cleared to

such low levels of viral expression that they become nondetectable even with sensitive assays, reactivation appears to occur. This is apparent in cohort studies as the reappearance of previously cleared infections in women who deny sexual activity, often because of illness. Risks in other immunosuppressed states appear to be similar.

HPV infection predicts risk for subsequent high-grade CIN, even among cytologically normal women. In most cases, persistent HPV infections result first in cytologically detectable abnormalities and then in colposcopically visible lesions that grow laterally before developing into invasive cancers. The 10-year risk of high-grade CIN after a single detected HPV infection exceeds 10%.

As developed by Richart through observational studies of the cervix using cytology and colpomicroscopy, a diagnosis of CIN was based on progressively severe nuclear aneuploidy, abnormal mitotic figures, and loss of epithelial maturation. Initially considered a progressive lesion, CIN was thought to begin as a small lesion with atypia near the basement membrane of the cervical transformation zone, gradually increasing in size and becoming less differentiated with an increasing proportion of the epithelium taken up by atypical cells until a full-thickness carcinoma in situ developed and then became invasive. Given this concept of progression from low-grade to high-grade disease to cancer, lesions of all grades were treated. When progression does occur, however, it appears to require years. The median age of sexual debut in the United States is around 17 years of age, and HPV acquisition commonly follows, but the peak age of cervical cancer diagnosis lags by some 3 decades. This long transition time allows for even moderately sensitive screening tests to identify persistent lesions for treatment before invasive cancer develops (Table 1.1).

Gradually, the regressive nature of most low- and midgrade lesions became apparent. Low-grade lesions, including warts and CIN1, are histologic expressions of HPV infection. Greenberg and associates found that of 163 women with CIN1 after low-grade cytology followed for a median of 36 months, 49% regressed, 43% persisted, and only 8% progressed to CIN3. In the Atypical Squamous Cells of Undetermined Significance/ Low Grade Squamous Intraepithelial Lesion Triage Study (ALTS), a large randomized trial of management options for women with borderline cytology results conducted under the auspices of the US National Cancer Institute (NCI), 2-year risk for CIN3 were 10% among women with CIN1. As reported by Castle and coworkers, after controlling for HPV genotype, with HPV-16–associated CIN1 progressing to CIN3 in 19% of cases, biopsy-proven CIN1 was not a risk factor for progression. These risk estimates may be substantially higher for women with prior high-grade cytology.

TABLE 1.1 Transition Time of Cervical Intraepithelial Neoplasia

Stages	Mean Years
Normal to mild to moderate dysplasia	1.62
Normal to moderate to severe dysplasia	2.2
Normal to carcinoma in situ	4.51

Higher grades of dysplasia appear to represent clonal lesions arising from single-type HPV infections. Although women may harbor multiple HPV types in the genital tract, most multitype infections are associated with multifocal lesions. Moscicki and her team showed that 63% of adolescents and young women with CIN2 resolved lesions without treatment within 2 years; subsequent clearance was minimal, rising only to 68% after an additional year. McAllum and colleagues showed a similar 62% regression after only 8 months of observation for women with CIN2 younger than 25 years of age. No patients in either study progressed to cancer during observation. In both studies, identified CIN2 likely represented recent HPV infections. Regression rates are lower in older women, at least in part because lesions detected later may have been persistent for years, and lesions that have evolved mechanisms to evade host immune-mediated clearance are likely to continue to persist. Castle and coworkers compared CIN2 rates in the immediate colposcopy and cytology surveillance arms of the ALTS. They found that over 2 years, some 40% of CIN2 regressed. Trimble and colleagues showed that HPV-16–associated lesions are less likely to resolve. Their finding of associations with human leukocyte antigen (HLA) alleles and regression support a role for HLA-restricted HPV-specific immune responses in determining clearance.

Untreated, CIN3 poses considerable risk of progression to invasive cancer. This was best shown in a study of New Zealand women with CIN3 who were diagnosed between 1955 and 1976 and were observed. Among 143 women reported by McCredie and coworkers, managed only by punch or wedge biopsy, 31 progressed to cancer of the cervix or vagina after 30 years. Risk rose to 59% in 92 women with persistent disease after 2 years of observation. These findings show both that treatment of CIN3 is mandatory regardless of age or other factors but also that not all CIN3 lesions will inevitably progress to cancer.

Treated CIN3 continues to pose a risk of progression to cancer. Women in the New Zealand study whose treatment appeared adequate by current standards faced only 0.7% cancer risk after 30 years. Studies from Scandinavian countries with integrated health systems can link databases on procedures and subsequent cancers and provide accurate long-term results with minimal loss to follow-up. Strander and associates showed that risk for cervical cancer rose significantly in previously treated women after age 50 years, with standardized incidence ratios compared with untreated women ranging from 3 to 5. Vaginal cancer risks were elevated across all ages, although the absolute risk of vaginal cancer was low. Kalliala and colleagues in Finland confirmed this long-term increased risk and also found an increased risk for nongenital smoking-related cancers. Jakobsson and coworkers found that in addition to cervical cancer, women treated for CIN faced higher mortality rates from circulatory system, alcohol-related, and traumatic death, consistent with the demographic and behavioral factors linked to CIN.

EPIDEMIOLOGY

More than 80% of sexually active individuals acquire genital HPV infections. Some 20 million Americans and 630 million persons worldwide are infected with HPV. In the United States, about 6.2 million people will acquire a new infection annually. Prevalence rates are highest among women in their late teens and early 20s, declining with age. Risk factors for HPV acquisition include smoking, oral contraceptive use, and new male partners.

Among high-risk HPV types, HPV-53 is most common, detected in 5.8% of US women ages 14 to 59 years screened in the National Health and Nutrition Examination Survey (NHANES) in 2003 to 2006. This was followed by HPV-16 (4.7%), HPV-51 (4.1%), HPV-52 (3.6%), and HPV-66 (3.4%). HP-V18 was present in only 1.8% of screened women. In NHANES, demographic risk factors for prevalent HPV infection included younger age, peaking at ages 20 to 24 years; non-Hispanic black ethnicity; unmarried; never educated beyond high school; and living below the poverty line. Behavioral risk factors included reporting ever having sex, first intercourse before age 16 years, greater numbers of lifetime partners, and number of partners in the past year. HPV type distributions vary across continents.

HPV infection determines subsequent risk for precancer. Among women enrolled in a Portland health maintenance organization who had HPV-16, the 10-year risk for CIN3, AIS, or cancer was more than 15% after HPV-16 infection, almost 15% after HPV-18, less than 3% after other oncogenic HPV infections, and less than 1% after a negative HPV test result.

In the United States more than 400,000 cases of CIN are identified annually, at a cost of approximately $570 million. Of these, Flagg and colleagues estimate about 100,000 are true precancers. The annual incidence of high-grade CIN is some 6 to 10 times higher than cervical cancer incidence. Preinvasive lesions begin to appear some 2 years after infection. Cancer risk is quite low soon after infection: Despite a high prevalence of HPV detection among sexually active teens, cervical cancer incidence is only about 1 in 1,000,000 before 20 years of age. Among women who develop high-grade CIN, only 30% to 50% will develop cancer over years of observation.

Although demographic and behavioral risk factors cannot be used to target evaluation or therapy, clear risks for CIN and cervical cancer have been identified. The international Collaboration of Epidemiological Studies of Cervical Cancer reviewed evidence for various risk factors for cervical cancer and carcinoma in situ, although their studies were not linked to HPV data. They found that oral contraceptive use raised the risk for cervical disease by 1.9-fold for every 5 years of use. First intercourse before 15 years of age was associated with twice the risk of cervical cancer found in women with first intercourse after 23 years of age, and having more than five lifetime sexual partners carried more than double the cervical cancer risk of lifetime monogamy. Lesser but still significant increases in risk were associated with number of pregnancies and earlier age at first term pregnancy. Both squamous cancers and adenocarcinomas share epidemiologic risk factors, except that smoking is linked only to the former.

The role of family history in determining cervical cancer risk. Dissociating genetic components of familial risk from cultural ones is difficult, as sexual attitudes and behaviors, reproductive patterns, and smoking are often linked to family.

Zelmanowicz and associates assessed the role of family history in cohorts of women prospectively studied in Costa Rica and the United States. A family history of cervical cancer in a first-degree relative tripled the risk for CIN3 or squamous cervical cancer. The effect persisted after controlling for HPV exposure. No effect of family history on adenocarcinoma risk was seen. Although several genome-wide association studies (GWASs) have identified a range of genetic variants in candidate pathways that might contribute to cervical oncogenesis, Chen and colleagues in a large Chinese GWAS found that only HLA and major histocompatibility class I polypeptide-related sequence A genes were identified as candidate risk genes across several populations.

Lower socioeconomic status (SES) and minority ethnicity are also linked to CIN and cervical cancer risk in the United States, although distinguishing cultural contributions to cervical cancer risk, such as a sense of fatalism, distrust of the medical care system providing screening services, and lack of health education about the benefits of screening, are difficult to distinguish from biologic risks related to ethnicity and SES, such as genetic predisposition, toxin exposure, and micronutrient deficiencies.

HUMAN PAPILLOMAVIRUS VACCINATION

Because HPV is the cause of essentially all cervical cancer, HPV vaccination has the potential to eliminate cervical cancer. However, the US experience with HPV vaccination has shown that several barriers will limit achievement of this goal.

Intramuscular delivery of synthetic HPV L1 capsid antigens results in humor immunity; current vaccines are created in protein synthesis using cell culture systems; because no actual live or killed virions are used, HPV vaccines cannot cause HPV-related cancer. Despite early concerns that humoral immunity would be insufficient to prevent infection, vaccine efficacy appears to approach 100%. However, currently available vaccines are prophylactic: They must be delivered before HPV exposure and do not appear to reduce risk in untreated women with established target-type HPV infections. This is reflected in the epidemiology of vaccine effectiveness, which declines with age, number of prior sexual partners, and prior abnormal cytology. These findings mean that, although vaccination is effective for type-specific HPV naïve women through 45 years of age, population effectiveness is too low to justify widespread use of vaccines beyond the upper age limit in vaccine trials, which extended to 26 years of age. Within trials, effectiveness declined with age, and the American Cancer Society has reiterated its guidance that HPV vaccination extend only through 18 years of age.

Three HPV vaccines are available. US clinicians have favored the quadrivalent HPV vaccine, which protects against HPV-16 and -18, which together account for almost 70% of all cervical cancers, as well as HPV-6 and -11, which are the most common causes of genital warts. The benefit of cervical cancer prevention, which might take decades to become manifest, is augmented by its ability to prevent genital warts, a concern for many young women. The bivalent HPV vaccine protects against only HPV-16 and -18 and is less commonly used in the United States. It may have superior antigenicity and may have some cross-protection against HPV types related to HPV-16 and -18. Most recently, a nonavalent vaccine has been introduced, which is effective against the same types as the quadrivalent vaccine and also includes coverage against HPV types 31, 33, 45, 52, and 58; enhanced coverage should prevent 90% of all cervical cancers.

Because HPV vaccines are prophylactic, population-based vaccination should begin before first sexual intercourse. Because some 5% of US 13-year-old girls are sexually active, the target age for HPV vaccination is the ages of 11 to 12 years. However, vaccination can be initiated at 9 years of age in populations in which sexual debut may occur earlier. Three injections over 6 months are recommended for all vaccines, although schedules vary. Some data suggest that two injections or even one may be sufficient, at least for adolescents, but shortened vaccination schedules have not been approved by the US Food and Drug Administration (FDA). Because teen sexual activity is unpredictable, delaying vaccination until girls are more mature risks missing the vaccination window for many. Nevertheless, many sexually active young women show no evidence of infection by target HPV types, and "catch-up" vaccination should be considered. Testing of cervicovaginal secretions and serum antibody testing are both insensitive for detecting prior HPV vaccination and are not recommended before a decision about HPV vaccination.

Several countries have instituted organized vaccination programs, either mandatory or using a school-based opt-in mechanism with high uptake. Countries that used quadrivalent vaccine have documented a dramatic decrease in genital warts among teens but not older women, and abnormal cytology rates have also fallen in the youngest women.

In the United States, vaccination rates are suboptimal, with barely one-third of girls in target populations having received all three injections. Regrettably, despite the potential for vaccination to eliminate the disparately high risk of cervical cancer among women of minority ethnicity and lower SES, uptake has been lowest in these groups, potentially widening cancer disparities in future years. Nevertheless, decreases in HPV-16 and -18 in the pool of sexually active young women have been documented, suggesting that less than ideal vaccination rates may nevertheless eventually yield population effectiveness.

Vaccine risks appear tolerable. Common side effects include fever, rash, injection site pain, nausea, headache, and dizziness. Anaphylactic and vagal reactions may be fatal, so vaccination should only be administered in sites with ability to manage anaphylaxis and fainting. Despite initial concerns, HPV vaccination status does not enter into young women's decisions to initiate sex. Vaccination is contraindicated for pregnant women, although no congenital anomalies or adverse pregnancy outcomes have been linked to HPV vaccination; the vaccine series may begin after delivery. Interruption of vaccination does not appear to require reinitiation of the three-shot series.

The duration of vaccine effectiveness is unclear, but antibody levels remain elevated for several years after vaccination. Booster doses are not recommended at this time. However, revaccination with nonavalent vaccine may provide additional benefit and should be considered for women younger than 26 years of age who previously completed bivalent or quadrivalent vaccines, especially those who have not initiated sexual activity and so are at low risk for having acquired HPV.

A history of HPV vaccination does not alter screening recommendations for US women. This is because many women of screening age were not vaccinated before initiating intercourse, so vaccine effectiveness is unclear. There is no central US vaccine registry, and identifying vaccinated women by self-report may be inaccurate. No HPV vaccine covers all carcinogenic HPV types, so women vaccinated before first intercourse remain at risk for infection and cancer due to nonvaccine types. However, for women known to have been vaccinated against HPV-16 and -18 before first intercourse, and so at much lower risk for disease, deferring screening initiation until age 25 years and screening with HPV testing alone at 5-year intervals is rational.

SCREENING

The goal of any cancer prevention program is the reduction of morbidity and mortality through intervention before symptom onset. The current mechanism to achieve this goal is the identification and destruction of high-grade CIN lesions that are presumed precancers. Many novices and some experienced clinicians mistake the mechanism for the goal. However, identification of apparent precancers in women with comorbidities that will be fatal in the medium term, before progression to symptomatic cancer, is not helpful. High-grade CIN in young women may resolve spontaneously and in some cases may be observed to avoid the sequelae of treatment. On the other hand, some women without identified high-grade CIN face cancer risks similar to those of women with high-grade CIN and merit destructive cervical therapy.

Classically, screening has relied on Papanicolaou cytology testing followed by colposcopic assessment of women with Pap abnormalities, directed biopsy of the worst colposcopic lesion, and treatment of biopsy proven high-grade lesions. Papanicolaou testing is relatively insensitive: A single Pap test may be negative in almost half of women with high-grade CIN. However, progression from HPV infection to cancer usually requires several years, allowing for multiple rounds of screening, with greater sensitivity than single tests.

Cytology is the interpretation of all the mutations, methylations, and other genetic modifications that alter the nuclear and cytoplasmic appearance of cells. As such, it is infinitely graded. To be clinically useful, these changes must be aggregated into categories that reflect a common natural history. Papanicolaou developed a five-class grading system, from normal to invasive cancer, with atypia, dysplasia, and carcinoma in situ between. Modified systems were developed, and alternatives were proposed. To unify terminology, the NCI convened a consensus meeting that developed the 1988 terminology known as the Bethesda System for cervicovaginal cytologic diagnosis. With the most recent update in 2001, this classification system identifies cytology as satisfactory or unsatisfactory, includes

TABLE 1.2   **Bethesda 2001 Classification**

1. Negative for intraepithelial lesion or malignancy
   a. Organisms may be identified
   b. Other nonneoplastic findings may be noted
      (1) Inflammation
      (2) Radiation changes
      (3) Atrophy
   c. Glandular cells status after hysterectomy
   d. Atrophy
2. Epithelial cell abnormalities
   a. Squamous cells
      (1) Atypical squamous cells (ASC)
      (2) Of undetermined significance (ASC-US)
      (3) Cannot exclude high-grade squamous intraepithelial lesion (ASC-H)
      (4) Low-grade squamous intraepithelial lesions (LSIL)
      (5) Human papillomavirus (HPV), cervical intraepithelial neoplasia (CIN) 1
      (6) HSIL (CIN2, CIN3)
      (7) Squamous cell carcinoma
   b. Glandular cell
      (1) Atypical glandular cells (AGC)—specify origin
      (2) Atypical glandular cells favor neoplastic—specify origin
      (3) Endocervical adenocarcinoma in situ (AIS)
      (4) Adenocarcinoma

nonneoplastic changes, and divides epithelial cell abnormalities into squamous and glandular changes of varying degrees of severity (Table 1.2). Distinguishing squamous from glandular abnormalities is critical because glandular abnormalities carry much higher risk for high-grade CIN, including squamous dysplasias, as well as endometrial cancer and cervical adenocarcinoma and AIS. Squamous changes related to HPV are termed "squamous intraepithelial lesions (SILs)" because some lesser changes do not reflect dysplasia or neoplasia, only cytomorphologic changes of HPV infection. Indeterminate lesions are termed "atypical squamous cells (ASC)," and these are subdivided into ASC "of undetermined significance (ASC-US)," which carries a low risk of associated high-grade CIN, or "cannot exclude high-grade SIL (ASC-H)," which is a more ominous finding that requires immediate colposcopy (see later discussion). An online atlas allows pathologists to standardize findings and interpretations against national norms (http://nih.techriver.net). The 2001 update provided the basis for subsequent consensus conferences that provided risk-based management guidelines.

Traditional Pap smears were collected by smearing samples across a glass slide and applying fixative followed by staining with a Papanicolaou stain. Today most cytology tests in the United States are conducted using liquid-based assays. In these tests, cells are collected and suspended in preservative solution and then transferred to a slide. Liquid-based cytology results in an even dispersion of cells, and techniques are available that allow for elimination of red and white blood cells, but the "tumor diathesis" of pus and necrosis that allowed identification of cancer is lost, as are the "microbiopsies" that allowed interpretation of epithelial fragments. Liquid-based cytology was marketed as more sensitive than conventional Pap smears. However, a meta-analysis by Arbyn and colleagues showed that, although liquid-based cytology yields more abnormalities, including high-grade SILs, it is not superior to conventional smears in cancer prevention. It remains preferred in the United States because it allows for molecular triage of equivocal results using HPV and other assays. Interpretation is still done visually, although some centers use automated imaging and pattern recognition software to eliminate the least abnormal slides. Cytotechnologists perform initial assessment, with slides containing abnormal findings and a proportion of normal slides read by cytopathologists.

The effectiveness of screening has not been demonstrated in randomized trials, but population studies have shown unequivocal benefits. Papanicolaou and Traut propounded the concept of screening in 1941. An NCI study by Erickson and associates assessed cytology screening by vaginal aspiration for 108,000 women in Shelby County, Tennessee. They showed a high yield of unsuspected high-grade CIN and early cancer at the first screen, with a substantial reduction in invasive lesions in the second screen. Gustafsson and associates reviewed data from 17 cancer registries and showed marked effects, especially in Scandinavian countries. Eddy assessed the impact of screening on cervical cancer incidence and death. Without screening, a 20-year-old average-risk woman faces a 2.5% risk of cancer and a 1.2% risk of cancer death. Triennial screening between ages 20 and 75 years reduces risk to less than 0.4% and 0.1%. Annual screening improves effectiveness but by less than 5% of these low rates, with substantial increase in cost.

Initially, screening was opportunistic: Women had screening when they presented for care, usually at annual visits. Opportunistic screening remains the norm in the United States, although screening intervals have lengthened; some electronic medical records prompt clinicians when screening is due; and some health care organizations have developed standards, rewards, and reminders. Several countries with centralized medical care systems have developed organized screening, with coordinated identification, invitation, and management of women due for screening. Serraino and colleagues showed that the move from opportunistic to organized screening in Italy resulted in a decline in cervical cancer incidence and a downstaging of incident cervical cancers after an increase in precursor detection. Quinn and coworkers found that institution a national call/recall system with incentive payments to general practitioners in Britain instituted in 1988 increased screening coverage to 85% of the target population, increased detection of high-grade CIN, and reduced mortality in women younger than age 55 years.

Cytology-based screening has several weaknesses. Most fundamentally, the process of screening, triage, and treatment is cumbersome, and noncompliance at any point renders it ineffective. Cytology results are reported in ways that can be confusing, and efficient, effective management may require integration of current results with prior abnormalities. Multiple studies have shown that most women who develop cervical cancer in developed countries, especially those presenting at advanced stages, are inadequately screened. Sung and associates studied incident cancers in a US prepaid health plan. They reported that 53% were nonadherent to screening, 28% had false-negative Pap tests, 4% had inadequate follow-up after an abnormal Pap test result, and the rest either developed cancer despite appropriate investigations or were unclassified. Kinney and associates in the same US health maintenance organization found that 60% of cervical cancer patients were inadequately screened. Deeper exploration of the records of long-standing plan members with inadequate screening showed that 70% had missed opportunities for screening in primary care clinics.

In addition, cytology-based screening performs poorly in younger women. Sasieni and colleagues from Britain showed that cervical screening in women ages 20 to 24 years had little impact on actual cancer risk until those women reached 30 years of age, but screening older women results in an immediate benefit. Because younger women have low rates of cervical cancer incidence and death but high rates of HPV infection, abnormal cytology, and CIN destined to regress, the benefits of early initiation of screening may be difficult to balance against potential harms. Cytology preferentially detects squamous cell carcinomas, and the impact of cytology screening on adenocarcinoma incidence has been muted.

The harms of excessive screening are more difficult to quantify. These include stigmatization, unfounded fear of cancer, and interventions without cancer prevention benefit. Sharp and associates showed that depression, distress, and anxiety occurred in 15% to 30% of women in the months after reporting of marginal cytology abnormalities. The costs, pain, and inconvenience of testing, triage, and treatment of abnormalities destined to regress with no impact on cancer morbidity or mortality must outweigh nonexistent benefits, though prospectively identifying these lesions in individuals is problematic.

Essentially all cervical cancer is caused by HPV. Castle and colleagues have shown that women who test HPV negative remain at low risk for precancer and cancer for more than a decade. Incorporation of HPV testing into screening has allowed for longer screening intervals. The development of HPV assays has allowed the development of protocols for HPV testing as a primary screening test in combination screening with cytology (co-testing) and as a triage test for women with borderline cytology results. Only high-risk HPV types have a role in screening; because low-risk types essentially play no role in screening and identification of HPV infection in the absence of visible genital warts causes stigmatization without impacting care, testing for low-risk types is contraindicated. HPV genotyping assays for types 16 and 18 identifies women at higher risk. The disadvantage of HPV testing is poor specificity, with up to 30% of young women testing positive in some studies. Because all commercially available HPV tests have a detection threshold designed to balance sensitivity and specificity, a negative test result does not absolutely exclude HPV infection, and prior cytologic or histologic abnormalities may mandate close follow-up or even treatment despite absence of detectable HPV. The performance characteristics of HPV assays that have not been FDA approved are unknown, and these tests should not be used in the absence of peer-reviewed literature describing their sensitivity and specificity against histologically defined precancer in large screening populations. HPV tests also should not be collected in media whose effects of test performance have not been evaluated by the FDA.

Although only one HPV assay was approved in the United States for primary screening at the time of writing, four assays were approved for risk stratification for women with ASC-US cytology and for screening in conjunction with Pap testing. Comparative trials are few. Cuzick et al. studied six HPV assays, some of which are available only in Europe. They found that an mRNA test had similar sensitivity but greater specificity than DNA tests.

Beyond these weaknesses, screening has potential harms. Identification of HPV infection, abnormal cytology, and cervical cancer precursors is not without consequences, including anxiety, relationship disruption after diagnosis of a sexually transmitted infection, the inconvenience and cost of accelerated follow-up visits, and the pain of repeated examinations. Treatment of precursor lesions also carries risks, including bleeding, infection, and injury to adjacent organs. Some studies have suggested that destructive cervical treatments increase the risk for preterm delivery and pregnancy loss. US studies have failed to replicate these results in women after cervical loop electrosurgical excision procedure (LEEP). Women with cervical dysplasias are at higher risk for pregnancy loss that those who do not, perhaps because of common risk factors, including smoking, nutritional deficiencies, and lower SES, and these confounding factors may account for differences. However, there may be a threshold effect for treatment, and women with deep or repeated excisional procedures may be at higher risk for pregnancy loss. Shorter screening intervals with increasingly sensitive tests will reduce cancer risk, but benefits decline toward an irreducible asymptote, but harms and costs climb.

After the utility of screening is accepted, societies, women at risk, and clinicians must decide when to initiate screening, which screening tests to use, how often to screen, and when toward the end of life the identification of asymptomatic disease ceases to be beneficial. With all choices, sensitivity and specificity must be balanced. Earlier screening starts with more sensitive tests at shorter intervals until later in life will decrease cancer incidence and mortality, but costs and harms from diagnosing lesions that would never have progressed to cancer will increase. In developed societies, guidelines for screening have been developed by experts assessing evidence for benefit and harm and deciding how these can best be balanced. **In the United States, the most cited guidelines were released in 2012 guidelines by the US Preventive Services Task Force (USPSTF) and a consensus conference sponsored the American Cancer Society (ACS), the American Society for Colposcopy and Cervical Pathology (ASCCP), and the American Society for Clinical Pathology (ASCP)** (Table 1.3). The two guidelines were developed from a common evidence assessment and reached similar conclusions. In both sets, screening is recommended to begin at 21 years of age, continuing at 3-year intervals until 65 years of age, when screening should stop if the patient is adequately screened and has no history or prior high-grade CIN. Screening also should stop at the time of total hysterectomy for

TABLE 1.3   Comparison of Current US Cervical Cancer Screening Guidelines

	USPSTF	ACS/ASCCP/ASCP
When to start?	Age 21 years	Age 21 years
How often?	Pap tests every 3 years Co-tests every 5 years at ages 30–64	Pap tests every 3 years at ages 21–29 years Co-tests every 5 years at ages 30–64 years preferred Pap tests every 3 years remain an option
When to stop?	Age 65 years if adequate prior screens	Age 65 years if the patient has had three negative Pap tests or two negative co-tests After hysterectomy for benign disease

ACS, American Cancer Society; *ASCCP,* American Society for Colposcopy and Cervical Pathology; *ASCP,* American Society for Clinical Pathology; *USPSTF,* US Preventive Services Task Force.

indications other than high-grade CIN or cervical cancer. The ACS/ASCCP/ASCP guidelines contain a preference for screening using combination cytology and HPV testing beginning at 30 years of age; the USPSTF considered co-testing between 30 and 65 years of age to be acceptable but did not find evidence sufficiently compelling to prefer it. Table 1.3 compares the two guidelines.

The rationale for initiating screening at 21 years of age is founded on the low risk of cervical cancer in teens: with only one to two cases per 1,000,000 women, few cancers will be missed by a later screening start. HPV infections are common in sexually active young women, and the specificity of screening in that population is suboptimal. Although CIN2 and CIN3 are more common, most HPV infections, abnormal cytology test results, CIN1 and CIN2 in young women will regress with time. Harms from screening appear to outweigh benefits. As girls who were vaccinated before their first intercourse reach the age of screening initiation, population risk for cancer and precancer will decline. Future US screening guidelines may recommend initiation at 25 years of age. Although some societies and clinicians retain 18 years of age for screening initiation, many societies with organized programs defer screening until age 25 years, and some delay screening until 30 years of age.

Consensus conferences and professional societies in the United States have established 3-year cytology screening as providing optimal balance between benefits and harms. Because HPV testing is more sensitive than cytology, adding an HPV test to cytology should provide greater reassurance against missed disease and so lead to longer screening intervals. Dillner and colleagues have shown that a 5-year Pap/HPV co-testing interval provides superior negative predictive value against precancer than 3-year cytology testing, with a risk that is similar to 1-year cytology testing intervals (Fig. 1.3). Intervals should be based on documented cytology results; Boyce and others have shown that women's ability to recall prior screening is flawed. Centers

FIGURE 1.3 Incidence of cervical intraepithelial neoplasia (CIN) 3 or worse across time after negative screening test results. Five-year risk after a negative human papillomavirus (HPV) test of cytology/HPV co-test approximates risk 1 year after negative cytology. (From Dillner J, Rebolj M, Birembaut P, et al.; Joint European Cohort Study. Long term predictive values of cytology and human papillomavirus testing in cervical cancer screening: joint European cohort study. *BMJ* 2008;337:a1754.)

for Disease Control and Prevention (CDC) researchers have shown that despite guidelines, US clinicians continue to screen women at short intervals.

The risk for cervical cancer in adequately screened women after 65 years of age becomes negligible. Prior HPV infection that has been cleared without development of high-grade CIN does not appear to increase risk substantially. New HPV infections may be acquired after 65 years of age despite prior negative screening, but in the absence of active metaplasia, these are unlikely to progress to cancer for years and so are unlikely to result in morbidity or mortality, but evaluation and treatment of atrophic postmenopausal women is technically difficult and painful. Vaginal cancer risks are low after hysterectomy for benign disease; too low to justify screening. Women with high-grade CIN remain at risk for cervical and vaginal cancer despite treatment, including hysterectomy, and evaluation until comorbidity suggests a short residual lifespan remains indicated. **Women at low risk for disease during their remaining lifespans should not be screened. This is most apparent for women with illnesses that will be fatal in the medium term: The discomfort and risks of screening and treatment of identified precursors are not justified when the woman is unlikely to survive long enough to develop symptomatic cervical cancer.** Similarly, cervical and vaginal cancer risk in the absence of a cervix is functionally zero. After hysterectomy for CIN, screening appears justified based on risk for coexistent vaginal intraepithelial neoplasia and vaginal cancer, and post-treatment surveillance for recurrent cervical cancer treated with hysterectomy is recommended. Women who reach 65 years of age after multiple negative cytology results, including three in the previous decade and two in the previous 5 years, are at low risk for cervical cancer, as are women with two negative HPV–cytology co-test results, including one in the previous 5 years. These women can stop undergoing screening. Women without

adequate prior screening should continue undergoing screening until they meet these criteria. Although older women can acquire new HPV infections, they are not undergoing active metaplasia, and transition time to cancer appears to be decades long, as in younger women, so few are likely to survive to develop cancer. For this reason, acquisition of new sexual partners by women who have otherwise met criteria for stopping should not be a consideration for continuing screening.

In 2014, the Food and Drug Administration approved HPV testing as a primary screening test for cervical cancer. Approval was granted only for the cobas HPV test (Roche). At a consensus meeting sponsored by the Society of Gynecologic Oncologists and ASCCP, Huh and fellow consensus meeting delegates developed guidelines to inform clinicians and women at risk on strategies to incorporate primary screening into practice. When used according to an algorithm (Fig. 1.4) that appears to optimize disease detection while minimizing colposcopy, HPV testing is more sensitive that Pap testing when initiated at 25 years of age. Screening intervals for primary HPV testing are controversial. Huh and coauthors recommended that screening be no more often than every 3 years, language that reflected disagreement about 3-year versus 5-year testing intervals. The pivotal trial for the cobas HPV test did not extend beyond 3 years, so performance data are unknown. However, other HPV tests with similar sensitivity and specificity have been tested, and a 5-year interval seems to provide sensitivity superior to 3-year cytology screening while allowing more time for transient lesions to regress.

Few predictors of high-grade CIN have been identified that would allow clinicians to focus more intensive screening efforts on high-risk groups. Boardman and colleagues found that smokers faced a higher risk of CIN2 or worse than nonsmokers, but the odds ratio of 1.6 did not provide sufficient discrimination to allow observation of nonsmokers. Fundamentally, cytology and HPV testing are powerful tools for identifying risk, and the low positive predictive value of borderline cytology grades can be refined by triage using HPV testing or genotyping. Women with abnormal cytology or high-risk HPV infections merit further assessment regardless of demographic or behavioral risks.

CORE PRINCIPLES FOR MANAGING ABNORMAL SCREENING TEST RESULTS

In 2007, Castle and colleagues at the US NCI proposed that management of abnormal cervical cancer screening tests should be based on the associated risk for significant disease. Cancer mortality would be the ideal risk outcome for comparison across tests, but it is too uncommon in screened populations and its frequency is determined by downstream interventions after most tests. Katki and associates proposed instead that risk after various test results and combinations should be benchmarked to CIN3 or worse (CIN3+, including CIN3, AIS, and cancer). Because some lesions are present but inapparent initially because women fail to present for assessment or lesions are clinically too small for detection, the optimal benchmark endorsed by a 2012 consensus conference is 5-year risk for

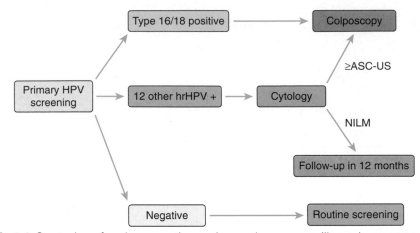

FIGURE 1.4 Strategies for incorporating primary human papillomavirus screening into practice. *ASC-US,* Atypical squamous cells undetermined significance; *hrHPV,* high risk human papillomavirus; *NILM,* negative for intraepithelial lesion or malignancy.

CIN3+. Using this benchmark, clinicians can use similar management strategies for women with similar levels of risk, without regard to how risk was determined. Conventionally, risk was defined by cytology and colposcopy findings. More recently, HPV testing allowed recalibration of risk, especially for women with borderline findings such as ASC-US. HPV genotyping for types 16 and 18 further defines risk categories. On the horizon are other molecular tests whose results will modify risk stratification and management, such as spectroscopic analysis and molecular testing for p16^{ink4a}, the Ki-67 proliferation marker, and others.

Determining optimal management for each test or combination can be confusing. In an ideal world, comparative trials would define which triage tests were optimal. Unfortunately, few comparative trials have been undertaken. National health budgets across the developed world are increasingly constrained. Industry lacks incentive to fund trials that might find their products inferior. With the proliferation of screening tests, management options become increasingly complex because algorithms must incorporate all options clinicians might select. In fact, current management guidelines have been criticized as too complex for even experts to master. Fortunately, computerized decision tools have eliminated the need for clinicians to memorize cervical cancer prevention strategies. Electronic medical record platforms can be programmed to generate reminders when women come due for screening. Online algorithm sets are available. Smartphone apps allow entry of patient information and lead clinicians to relevant algorithms. Clinicians still must understand the limits of algorithm-based management, especially the impact of prior abnormalities on subsequent emergence of disease.

To address these concerns, Katki and colleagues analyzed data from more than 1 million women screened by the Kaiser Permanente of Northern California health care system to define 5-year CIN3+ risk after various tests and test combinations. At the base of management options is the 5-year follow-up for women who test negative in Pap/HPV co-testing; these women have a 5-year CIN3+ risk of less than 0.01%. Women screened

with cytology alone are followed at 3-year intervals when their test results are negative, with a 5-year CIN3+ risk of less than 0.1%. One-year retesting is standard for women with a positive test result for HPV but negative cytology, with a risk less than 5%. The consensus threshold for colposcopy in the United States is a low-grade SIL result, with 5-year CIN3+ risk of just above 5%; lesser results are triaged by serial testing or triage tests. The threshold for treatment is CIN2, although not all women with CIN2 require treatment, and few studies have assessed use of other test results except high-grade SIL cytology as a treatment indication.

Traditionally, colposcopy was used as the triage modality to identify women with high-grade CIN for treatment. Colposcopy is the magnified stereoscopic visualization of the cervix under intense illumination. Magnification ranges from 3× to 30×. A green filter over the light source accentuates vascular patterns and lesion margins. Although colposcopy without staining has been advocated to maximize visualization of cancer, most colposcopic assessments are augmented by the application of vital stains such as 3% to 5% acetic acid and Lugol's iodine solution.

In colposcopy, the cervical transformation zone is assessed. The transformation zone is that area of the cervix and vagina initially covered by columnar epithelium that has undergone metaplasia to squamous epithelium. A range of terms are used to describe colposcopic findings (Table 1.4 and Figs. 1.5 to 1.8). The procedure for colposcopy is inspection of the cervix without stains and then cleansing of the cervix with an application of 3% to 5% acetic acid for at least 90 seconds. This removes mucus and debris and accentuates vascular and epithelial patterns. Most cervical lesions stain white with acetic acid (acetowhitening).

Because earlier lesions have been targeted via the inclusion of low-grade SIL, HPV+ ASC-US, persistent HPV infection, and HPV-16/-18 infection as thresholds for colposcopy, colposcopy is being done for women with smaller and less apparent lesions. The accuracy of colposcopy has been questioned, and now multiple colposcopic biopsies are recommended. HPV vaccination

TABLE 1.4   Abnormal Colposcopic Findings

Atypical transformation zone
Keratosis
Acetowhite epithelium
Punctation
Mosaicism
Atypical vessels
Suspect frank invasive carcinoma
Unsatisfactory colposcopic findings

FIGURE 1.6 White epithelium at the cervical os (a colposcopic view).

FIGURE 1.5 A, Squamocolumnar junction (transformation zone). B, Large transformation zone.

promises to reduce cervical cancer risk in coming decades but more immediately will reduce the prevalence of high-grade lesions. This in turn will reduce the specificity of screening tests and lower the sensitivity of colposcopy. Opportunities for further changes to screening and management strategies will follow, especially longer screening intervals, more HPV-based assessment, more intermediate triage tests before colposcopy, and a move toward immediate treatment without colposcopy for women at highest risk.

Immunocompromised women are screened under management guidelines defined by the CDC. Women with HIV are screened according to the guidelines for the prevention and treatment of opportunistic infections in HIV-infected adolescents and adults from the CDC. Under these guidelines, women should be screened with cytology alone twice within a year of

FIGURE 1.7 A punctation pattern is seen clearly above a mosaic structure (a colposcopic view).

FIGURE 1.8 A large anterior lip lesion with white epithelium punctation and mosaic patterns.

sexual activity, if previously HIV infected, or within 1 year of HIV diagnosis, regardless of age, followed by lifetime annual cytology. These guidelines were in review at the time of publication and may change.

Diethylstilbestrol- (DES-) exposed women continue Pap testing annually for life; evidence on HPV–cytology co-testing for DES-exposed women is insufficient to recommend for or against it.

MANAGING ABNORMAL CERVICAL CANCER SCREENING TEST RESULTS

Since 2001, the ASCCP has led three consensus development conferences to define standard guidelines for management of US women with abnormal cervical cancer screening test results and CIN or AIS. Conferences were cosponsored by numerous professional societies, with collaboration from the American Cancer Society, federal agencies, and other stakeholder groups. The most recent conference, in 2012, used risk estimates developed by Katki and colleagues to define management.

Clinicians should keep in mind that guidelines are for women with abnormal screening tests; for women with symptoms such as abnormal bleeding or pain or abnormal examination findings such as contact bleeding, cervical friability, or cervical enlargement, biopsy may be indicated regardless of cytology or HPV results. In addition, guidelines do not cover all potential permutations of screening test, colposcopy, and

biopsy results, especially accumulated abnormalities across years. Prior abnormal results raise risk for CIN3+ associated with subsequent abnormalities: Management does not "reset" after each test. For example, risk is higher after two cytology reports read as ASC-US than after only one, and ASC-US cytology after prior treatment for CIN3 is more ominous than a first ASC-US report; in both of these cases, colposcopy is indicated.

Managing Abnormal Results in Young Women

Cervical cancer risk is low among women 21 to 24 years of age, but high-risk HPV infections can be found in more than 20%. Most CIN1 and many CIN2 lesions in this age group will regress without intervention. CIN3 is unlikely to progress to cancer in the short run if missed. Treatment of intermediate-risk lesions may impact future pregnancies. For these reasons, women in this age group are managed less aggressively than older women. For women in this age group, most abnormal cytology results reflect HPV infection; HPV testing should not be ordered, and if obtained, results should not modify management.

In addition, because of concern about impact on subsequent pregnancies, women with biopsies read as CIN2, CIN2,3, or HSIL can be observed, provided colposcopy is satisfactory. There is no specific age range for observational management of these lesions, and a decision to treat or follow these lesions depends on a discussion between the woman and her clinician, balancing the potential risk to future pregnancies against the risk of progression to cancer during observation; both risks appear to be low.

Unsatisfactory Cytology

When cytology is unsatisfactory for evaluation, it must be repeated. The only exception is when the test was not indicated, as in an adolescent younger than 21 years of age, after hysterectomy for a benign condition, or in women older than 65 years of age with adequate prior screening. Some studies have suggested that rates of abnormality might be increased immediately after sampling, but a large US trial failed to validate this, suggesting that immediate resampling is acceptable. For women with atrophy, a short course of vaginal estrogen may improve sample cellularity. Women with obscuring inflammation should be assessed for specific infections and treated for any that might be identified; empiric vaginal antibiotic therapy does not appear beneficial. Samples that are unsatisfactory because of obscuring blood raise concern for cancer. When repeated samples are unsatisfactory, colposcopy should be considered.

Pap-Negative, Human Papillomavirus–Positive Women (Fig. 1.9)

Identification of a carcinogenic HPV type carries substantial risk for CIN3+, but the 5-year risk does not reach the 5% threshold for colposcopy. A positive HPV result is most often encountered in HPV–cytology co-testing for women ages 30 to 65 years.

Women with a positive HPV test but negative concurrent cytology may be managed in one of two ways. They can be reassessed with repeat HPV–cytology co-testing in 1 year, allowing

Management of women age ≥30 years who are cytology negative but HPV positive

FIGURE 1.9 Management of women age 30 years or older who are cytology negative but human papillomavirus positive (HPV). *ASC,* Atypical squamous cells; *ASCCP,* American Society for Colposcopy and Cervical Pathology. (From Massad SL, Einstein MH, Huh WK, et al. 2012 Updated consensus guidelines for the management of abnormal cervical cancer screening tests and cancer precursors. *J Low Genit Tract Dis* 2013;17(5 suppl 1):S1-S27, © 2013 American Society for Colposcopy and Cervical Pathology.)

time for HPV regression; if either test result is abnormal, then colposcopy is indicated. Disadvantages to this approach include losing the advantage of HPV testing for early detection of cytology-negative cancers and the inability to assess whether persistent HPV positivity results from persistence of the same HPV type or clearance of the original type followed by reinfection with a second type, with low risk for CIN3+ unless the new infection becomes persistent. Alternatively, women can be triaged immediately using a genotyping test for HPV-16 or -18; women positive for either type should have colposcopy, but those with negative results should have co-testing repeated in 1 year, with colposcopy only if either test result is abnormal.

Atypical Squamous Cells of Undetermined Significance (Fig. 1.10)

Risk of CIN3+ among women with ASC-US cytology is insufficient to justify immediate colposcopy, at about 3%. ASC-US results are common. Triage using HPV testing on the liquid-based cytology sample appears to be cost effective and minimizes delay and loss to follow-up. If HPV testing is positive for high-risk types, then colposcopy is indicated. A negative HPV result in the context of ASC-US indicates a low risk of CIN3+, though the risk is higher than among women with negative co-testing; 3-year co-testing is recommended.

HPV genotyping distinguishes between higher risk women with HPV-16/-18 and lower risk women negative for HPV-16/-18, but for all HPV-positive women, 5-year CIN3+ risk approximates or exceeds the threshold for colposcopy. Because management is not changed by results, HPV genotyping is not recommended for triage of ASC-US cytology.

Where HPV testing is not available and follow-up is reliable, ASC-US cytology results can be triaged using a repeat Pap test in 1 year with colposcopy if persistently abnormal and return to routine 3-year Pap testing if negative.

For women 21 to 24 years of age, ASC-US cytology results should be followed with annual rather than triennial Pap testing. Colposcopy is not indicated unless ASC-US or low-grade squamous intraepithelial lesion (LSIL) cytology results persist for 2 years or unless cytology returns ASC-H, HSIL, or AGC.

Low-Grade Squamous Intraepithelial Lesion (Fig. 1.11)

Low-grade squamous intraepithelial lesion is the paradigmatic threshold for colposcopy in the United States. With few exceptions (pregnancy, age 21–24 years, HPV-negative result), women with LSIL cytology should be managed with colposcopy. When HPV co-testing is available women with HPV-LSIL should have repeat co-testing in 1 year, with colposcopy if HPV positive or with persistent abnormal cytology. LSIL triage may be considered in postmenopausal women, given their lower background risk for HPV.

Atypical Squamous Cells, Cannot Exclude HSIL

Women with a cytology report of "atypical squamous cells, cannot exclude high-grade squamous intraepithelial lesion" have a 5-year risk of CIN3+ similar to that of women with HSIL cytology, although their immediate risk of CIN3+ is lower. All women with ASC-H should undergo colposcopy, regardless of HPV result. In contrast to young women with ASC-US, women

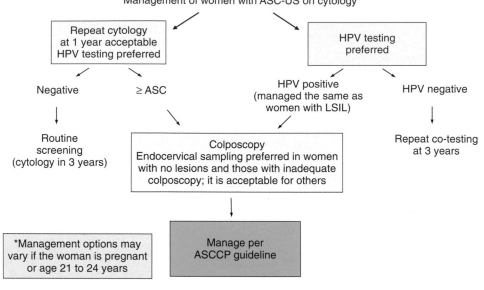

FIGURE 1.10 Management of women with atypical squamous cells of undetermined significance (ASC-US) on cytology. *ASCCP,* American Society for Colposcopy and Cervical Pathology; *HPV,* human papillomavirus; *LSIL,* low-grade squamous intraepithelial lesion. (From Massad SL, Einstein MH, Huh WK, et al. 2012 Updated consensus guidelines for the management of abnormal cervical cancer screening tests and cancer precursors. *J Low Genit Tract Dis* 2013;17(5 suppl 1):S1-S27, © 2013 American Society for Colposcopy and Cervical Pathology.)

FIGURE 1.11 Management of women with low-grade squamous intraepithelial lesions (LSILs). *CIN,* Cervical intraepithelial neoplasia; *HPV,* human papillomavirus. (From Massad SL, Einstein MH, Huh WK, et al. 2012 Updated consensus guidelines for the management of abnormal cervical cancer screening tests and cancer precursors. *J Low Genit Tract Dis* 2013;17(5 suppl 1):S1-S27, © 2013 American Society for Colposcopy and Cervical Pathology.)

21 to 24 years of age need colposcopy after ASC-H cytology, as do pregnant women.

High-Grade Squamous Intraepithelial Lesion

CIN2+ is found in some 60% of women with HSIL cytology, and some 2% will have cancer at colposcopy. This substantial risk justifies aggressive management. In many settings, especially for women in clinics with high rates of loss to follow-up and for women who have completed childbearing, immediate loop excision is an efficient approach to management. Immediate excision is unacceptable for women up to 24 years of age because of their low near-term risk for cancer and the likelihood that CIN2 and CIN2,3, but not CIN3, will regress. HPV results modulate risk, but even women with HPV-HSIL face a 30% 5-year risk for CIN3+. For this reason, colposcopy is required regardless of HPV result, and triage of HSIL cytology using HPV testing is unacceptable. Observation with repeat cytology is similarly unacceptable.

Atypical Glandular Cells

Despite its name, AGC cytology is more often associated with squamous than glandular lesions. The risk of CIN3, AIS, or cancer (CIN3+) after a Pap test read as AGC is almost 10%, and risk for cancer is 3%. Squamous and glandular lesions can coexist, and identification of CIN does not rule out adenocarcinoma. Many associated cancers are of endometrial origin and would be HPV negative; endometrial lesions are more common in older women and in women with such risk factors as obesity, unexplained bleeding, and anovulation. Thorough evaluation is needed regardless of HPV test results.

Women with AGC cytology need colposcopy with endocervical sampling and biopsies of any acetowhite cervical lesion. Endometrial sampling is needed if the patient is older than 35 years of age or if endometrial cancer risk factors are present. For women with AGC subcategorized as "atypical endometrial cells," evaluation can be truncated: Initial endometrial biopsy and endocervical curettage are needed, with colposcopy only if no endometrial pathology is found. In contrast to ASC-US, triage of AGC results with HPV testing or serial cytology testing is inappropriate. Management of AGC in women 21 to 24 years of age is identical to that of older women. Pregnant women with AGC cytology results need colposcopy, but endocervical curettage and endometrial sampling are contraindicated.

Endometrial Cells in Older Women

Among postmenopausal women, a finding of benign endometrial cells on cytology is associated with a 5% risk of clinically important pathology, including cancer. However, endometrial cells appear to have no association with disease in premenopausal women, and no further evaluation is needed for them. For postmenopausal women with endometrial cells on cytology, endometrial assessment is indicated using either endometrial sampling or imaging of endometrial thickness.

POSTCOLPOSCOPY MANAGEMENT

Managing Women With No Lesion or CIN1 at Colposcopy (Fig. 1.12)

A colposcopic biopsy result of no lesion or CIN1 does not exclude the presence of a higher grade lesion in an unsampled area of the cervix. Risk for subsequent CIN3+ depends on patient age and the prior abnormality. Risk is lower for women with what ASCCP terms "lesser abnormalities" than for women with ASC-H, HSIL, or AGC. Lesser abnormalities include negative cytology with either HPV-16 or repeated HPV positivity, ASC-US, or LSIL.

For women with lesser abnormalities and no lesion or only CIN1 on colposcopy, observation with serial co-testing is indicated. If a first co-test result is negative, repeat testing is indicated 3 years later. If all test results are negative, then routine screening is appropriate. If any test result is abnormal, repeat colposcopy is required. This can become burdensome. Treatment of CIN1 is acceptable once disease has persisted for 2 years, although continuing observation is also acceptable if fertility is a concern. Treatment of persistent HPV-positive tests or persistent ASC-US/LSIL cytology in the absence of a cervical lesion is not indicated because many of these women will have vaginal lesions. This includes topical therapies such as trichloroacetic acid. Hysterectomy is never indicated for CIN1 or abnormal cytology.

For women 21 to 24 years of age with no lesion or CIN1 after ASC-US or LSIL, observation with repeat cytology annually is indicated. Repeat colposcopy is only needed if cytology progresses to ASC-H, HSIL, or AGC, or if cytology remains borderline abnormal for 2 years. After a negative result, routine screening at 3 years is indicated. HPV testing and co-testing are not indicated in this age groups. For pregnant women with no lesion or CIN1 after lesser abnormalities during pregnancy, colposcopy should be deferred until postpartum.

When colposcopy reveals no lesion or CIN1 after ASC-H or HSIL cytology, risk for CIN3+ is much higher, and more aggressive management is indicated. ASCCP guidelines lump together ASC-H and HSIL, but diagnostic excision is more often indicated after HSIL; observation with annual co-testing is more appropriate after ASC-H, although either management strategies can be used after either result, according to clinical risk profiling. Observation is limited to women with satisfactory colposcopy and negative endocervical sampling; CIN1 in endocervical curettings is managed like CIN1 on cervical biopsy. If observation is elected, repeat colposcopy and biopsies are indicated after a positive HPV test or any grade of abnormal cytology. Women with persistent HSIL despite negative colposcopy should have a diagnostic excision procedure.

For women 21 to 24 years of age with no lesion or CIN1 after ASC-H or HSIL, diagnostic excision is indicated if colposcopy is unsatisfactory. When colposcopy is satisfactory in visualizing the entire squamocolumnar junction, either treatment or observation is indicated. Observation entails colposcopy and cytology every 6 months until two test result are negative, when routine screening can resume. If HSIL cytology persists,

Management of women with no lesion or biopsy-confirmed CIN1
preceded by "lesser abnormalities"*†

FIGURE 1.12 Management of women with no lesion or biopsy-confirmed grade 1 cervical intraepithelial neoplasia (CIN1) preceded by "lesser abnormalities." *ASCCP*, American Society for Colposcopy and Cervical Pathology; *ASC-US*, atypical squamous cells undetermined significance; *CIN*, cervical intraepithelial neoplasia; *ECC*, endocervical curettage; *HPV*, human papillomavirus; *LSIL*, low-grade squamous intraepithelial lesion. (From Massad SL, Einstein MH, Huh WK, et al. 2012 Updated consensus guidelines for the management of abnormal cervical cancer screening tests and cancer precursors. *J Low Genit Tract Dis* 2013;17(5 suppl 1):S1-S27, © 2013 American Society for Colposcopy and Cervical Pathology.)

treatment is indicated. For pregnant women with no lesion or only CIN1 after ASC-H or HSIL, colposcopy should be repeated post partum: The short-term cancer risk is low, and no other intervention is needed during pregnancy

When no lesion or CIN1 is found after AGC cytology, annual co-testing is indicated, with colposcopy for any abnormality; after two negative co-test results, risk declines, and 3-year co-testing intervals are appropriate. Colposcopy is needed if any result is abnormal. Hysterectomy is unacceptable as primary therapy for any grade of CIN, although after prior excision, hysterectomy may be indicated if lesions recur or persist and repeat diagnostic excision is not feasible.

Managing Women With CIN2 or CIN3 (Fig. 1.13)

A colposcopic biopsy of CIN2 is the threshold for treatment. CIN2 is an intermediate lesion: Many represent transient but exuberant HPV infection, and half or more resolve without therapy. Some progress to CIN3 and cancer. Because compliance with follow-up cannot be assured, treatment is recommended. Testing biopsy specimens for the presence of block staining for p16[ink4a] can identify CIN2 lesions at risk for progression and can be used as a test for triage. All lesions read as CIN3 should be treated regardless of the patient's age or desire for future childbearing, because there is no margin for progression, and some will harbor undiagnosed cancer; ongoing pregnancy is the main exception to this standard. Biopsies read as high grade or CIN2,3 can be managed expectantly

or with immediate treatment, depending on patient risk and preferences.

Observation is an acceptable option for women who after counseling consider risk to future pregnancies from treatment to outweigh cancer risk from observation. There is no specific age threshold: A 21-year-old woman who has had a tubal ligation should be treated, but a 43-year-old woman undergoing infertility treatment after a diagnosis of incompetent cervix might prefer to be observed. Observation is only acceptable when the entire lesion and squamocolumnar junction is observed colposcopically. Observation consists of colposcopy and cytology at 6-month intervals until the lesion resolves, as evidenced by regression of colposcopic abnormalities and normalization of cytology. After that occurs, women should be followed with a co-test 1 year later and then 3 additional years later before returning to routine screening; if either the Pap test or HPV test result is abnormal in follow-up, then colposcopy and biopsies should be repeated.

Women with a diagnosis of AIS on colposcopic biopsy should be managed with diagnostic excision to exclude associated invasive cancer. The excision should be done to produce a single specimen; traditionally, this has involved knife conization, but needle, straight wire, or loop conization is acceptable if thermal artifact is minimized. If the margins of the excision specimen are involved or uninterpretable, then reexcision or hysterectomy is required. Women with negative margins at diagnostic excision face a 10% risk of persistent AIS and a lesser

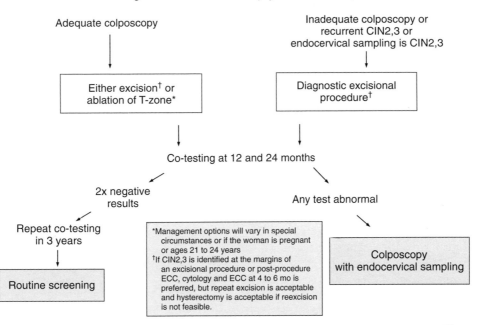

Management of women with biopsy-confirmed CIN2,3*

FIGURE 1.13 Management of women with biopsy-confirmed grade 2 and 3 cervical intraepithelial neoplasia (CIN2,3). (From Massad SL, Einstein MH, Huh WK, et al. 2012 Updated consensus guidelines for the management of abnormal cervical cancer screening tests and cancer precursors. *J Low Genit Tract Dis* 2013;17(5 suppl 1):S1-S27, © 2013 American Society for Colposcopy and Cervical Pathology.)

risk of invasive cancer, as shown by Costa and colleagues. This risk justifies hysterectomy when childbearing is complete. However, the risk is considered acceptable for women who wish to preserve fertility, although careful monitoring is recommended using colposcopy and co-testing 6 months after the diagnostic excision procedure, with co-testing in follow-up at 1- to 3-year intervals.

TREATMENT OF CERVICAL DISEASE

Although Trimble and colleagues have shown that a therapeutic vaccine can achieve almost 50% efficacy in the elimination of CIN2/3, 90% cure rates for CIN2+ still require destructive therapies. In the United States, ablational therapies include cryotherapy and laser ablation. Excision can be accomplished with an electrosurgical wire loop or needle or with a scalpel.

Cervical ablation results in the elimination of lesional tissue without rendering a specimen for pathologic analysis. For this reason, many gynecologists consider outpatient loop excision a preferred approach. However, randomized trials showed similar failure rates for excision and ablation. This suggests that as long as invasive cancer is microinvasive, with little risk for metastasis, the method of destruction is irrelevant. Nevertheless, using ablational therapies for cervical disease requires careful attention to well-defined exclusion criteria. Ablation cannot be undertaken unless the entire squamocolumnar junction, including all lesional tissue, is visible colposcopically. Ablation of such an unsatisfactory transformation zone risks missing

invasive cancer within the endocervix that then progresses undetected. A corollary to this is that ablation should not be attempted when disease extends into the endocervix above the depth that can be ablated. Thus, although manipulation may allow visualization of the squamocolumnar junction deep in the endocervical canal, ablation would remain inappropriate. Other criteria that must be met before proceeding with ablation include concordance of high-grade cytology with colposcopy and histology findings; an endocervical curettage specimen showing no dysplasia or only CIN1; and suspicion of invasive cancer by cytology, colposcopy, or biopsy.

Cryotherapy is performed using nitrous oxide, a delivery gun, and various sizes of metal probes designed to cover the transformation zone of the cervix. Figge and Creasman described use of a freeze–thaw–freeze technique with good success rates, but regardless of the use of double- or single-freeze approaches, identifying the development of at least a 5-mm "ice ball" or zone of freezing lateral to the cryotherapy probe is essential to achieving deep thermal destruction. One standard approach is outlined in Table 1.5. Advantages of cryotherapy include relatively low cost and low risk for injury. Disadvantages include a copious discharge from cervical tissues suffering from sublethal thermal injury and lack of a surgical specimen.

Cervical laser ablation involves the use of carbon dioxide laser energy to destroy abnormal cervical tissue. When optimally used, the laser energy is delivered at a power density of 750 to 1250 W/cm². This results in flash boiling of impacted cells, and

TABLE 1.5   Cryosurgery Technique
1. N$_2$O or CO$_2$
2. K-Y Jelly on probe
3. Double-freeze
a. 4- to 5-mm ice ball
b. Thaw
c. 4- to 5-mm ice ball

energy is dissipated from the operating field through the smoke plume without causing deeper tissue injury. Lower power density may create the illusion of greater control of tissue destruction, but it requires longer beam application, with greater hidden, delayed coagulation injury to underlying stroma. As with all therapies, laser should be used to ablate the entire at-risk transformation zone. CIN can involve the metaplastic epithelium of cervical glands, which extend some 5 mm into the cervical stroma; for this reason, ablation should be carried to a depth of about 7 mm and should encompass all lesional tissue. If the lesion extends onto the vagina, ablation is carried only to 1 to 2 mm in depth. As described by Stanhope and associates, laser therapy can result in persistent CIN risk of less than 90%. Advantages include precision in application, allowing extension of therapy to lesions that involve the vagina, and rapid recovery from injury. Disadvantages include the need for an expensive laser generator that requires frequent maintenance. Unskilled use of laser energy can result in immediate and delayed injury.

Most US gynecologists treat cervical precancers by excision with electrosurgical loops, termed LEEP or large loop excision of the transformation zone (LLETZ). The entire transformation zone is excised using loops with diameters of 1.5 to 2.5 cm. Excision should extend to the deepest glands, or 7 to 8 mm. For women with disease extending into the endocervical canal and those with inadequate colposcopy, either using deeper loops or a second endocervical pass, colloquially termed a "top-hat" excision for the appearance of the stacked specimen that results; this endocervical excision must encompass the lateral extent of endocervical glands, so 6 to 8 mm from the endocervical surface. For most women, LEEP can be done in an office setting under local anesthesia. Epinephrine is injected with the local anesthetic to minimize blood loss. The injection should be subepithelial rather than stromal, and a paracervical block does not provide the same hemostatic benefit of intracervical injection. Although an operating suite it not required, office LEEP should be done in a setting that includes equipment for suturing and response to anaphylactic reactions. Colposcopic visualization allows optimal tailoring of the excision. Hemostasis is achieved with a combination of fulguration using ball electrodes and application of Monsel's paste. Delayed bleeding should occur in fewer than 5% of cases but is a known complication of the procedure. Obese women and those with anatomic variations or anxiety that prevents optimal cervical visualization in the office may require general anesthesia. Advantages to LEEP include the availability of a surgical specimen with minimal thermal artifact at margins and the ability to adapt excision to the extent of lesions and metaplasia. Disadvantages include risk

FIGURE 1.14 Cone biopsy for endocervical disease. Limits of the lesion were not seen colposcopically.

FIGURE 1.15 Cone biopsy for cervical intraepithelial neoplasia of the exocervix. Limits of the lesion were identified colposcopically

of surgical injury and hemorrhage and the need for careful operator technique.

Some lesions require intact diagnostic specimens to exclude invasive cancer and assess margins. These include in situ adenocarcinomas and microinvasive cancers. Traditionally, these lesions have been treated with knife conization (Figs. 1.14 and 1.15), which results in an optimal diagnostic specimen while treating in situ and microinvasive lesions for women who wish to retain fertility. As LEEP has become pervasive in training programs, knife conization skills may be disappearing. Needle or straight wire electrosurgical conization has been developed as an alternative, allowing similar adaptation of excision while minimizing blood loss and tissue injury.

MANAGING ABNORMAL RESULTS DURING PREGNANCY

The goal of cervical cancer prevention measures during pregnancy is to identify cervical cancer so malignant lesions can be monitored closely for progression or treated. The risk is remote for cancer developing during pregnancy in women who have CIN, including CIN3. ASC-US and LSIL cytology results do not require colposcopy until postpartum, even if associated with HPV infection, although colposcopy is acceptable. Wetta and colleagues found no cancers and few high-grade lesions among 625 pregnant women with these borderline cytology results. For women with ASC-H, HSIL, or AGC cytology results, colposcopy is indicated. Because of the vascularity of the pregnant cervix, often only one biopsy can be obtained; mini-Tischler forceps should be used and immediate direct pressure applied to the biopsy site. Clinicians without experience with colposcopy during pregnancy should consider referral to a center with expertise because pregnancy will cause colposcopic abnormalities. Biopsy should be done for lesions that appear high grade because limiting biopsy to malignant-appearing lesions results in missed cancers. Women with CIN2+ may be followed with postpartum colposcopy and repeat biopsy or with serial colposcopy during pregnancy, with repeat biopsy only if the colposcopic impression worsens. Conization is indicated only when cancer is suspected by examination, cytology is read as showing malignant cells, or colposcopy or biopsy shows possible invasion. When performed, complete excision of the transformation zone is not needed because the goal is to determine if a deeply invasive cancer is present, not to definitively treat the cervix. Limited excision using an electrosurgical loop with blended current in a controlled operating room setting that allows for cervical suturing may be considered.

FUTURE DIRECTIONS

In developed countries with effective HPV vaccination programs, HPV-16 and HPV-18 are being eliminated from the circulating pool of HPV types. This will have profound implications for cervical cancer prevention. In fact, the introduction of nonavalent vaccination promises to reduce cervical cancer incidence to a rate too low to justify screening. The transition to such a welcome development over the coming decades will create opportunities and controversies as the scientific community adapts to the disappearance of what was once the most common cancer killer of women. Whether this promising future is attained in the United States, with its opportunistic approach to vaccination, remains to be measured.

As HPV-16 prevalence falls among at-risk women as vaccinated girls age, the prevalence of CIN3+ will decline. This will result in a lower incidence of abnormal Pap test results and more abnormalities that occur will reflect transient HPV infections or benign cytologic changes: As disease prevalence falls, the positive predictive value of an abnormality should decline. This should drive a shift away from cytology as a primary screening test. Primary HPV testing should replace cytology. Although cytology may be retained as a triage test for women with HPV types other than 16 or 18, as described by Huh and colleagues, other tests may prove superior, either because of greater predictive accuracy or because they can be automated.

Risk-based guidelines will need to become flexible as risk becomes dynamic. Vaccinated women are likely to face much lower risk than unvaccinated women, and epidemiologic studies suggest that vaccination will result in age-specific declines in HPV-16/-18 and CIN3+ prevalence as sexual segregation by age results in herd immunity for younger women. As vaccinated age cohorts mature, the optimal age for initiation of screening will rise. As more CIN2+ identified by colposcopy reflects infection by HPV types other than HPV-16/-18, with lower oncogenic potential, observation for immune-mediated regression may become preferred over treatment. Integrating this change into practice will be difficult because by the time age-based changes in risk are observed, published, reviewed, and integrated into new guidelines, women will have grown older yet retained immunity. This welcome challenge will structure coming debates on cervical cancer for decades to come.

For the bibliography list, log onto www.expertconsult.com ⟨http://www.expertconsult.com⟩.

Preinvasive Disease of the Vagina and Vulva and Related Disorders

Cara A. Mathews, MD, Joan L. Walker, MD

KEY POINTS

1. Lichen sclerosis is associated with vulvar cancer.
2. Treatment of vaginal intraepithelial neoplasia III is laser vaporization.
3. Wide local excision is the treatment of choice for vulvar intraepithelial neoplasia III.
4. Imiquimod treatment is a potentially noninvasive treatment of vulvar dysplasia.

EMBRYOLOGY

At approximately 12 to 14 weeks of gestation, the simple columnar epithelium that lines the vaginal portion of the uterovaginal canal begins to undergo transformation into stratified Müllerian epithelium. This transformation proceeds cranially until it reaches the columnar epithelium of the future endocervical canal. The vagina, which is lined initially by simple columnar epithelium of Müllerian origin, acquires stratified Müllerian epithelium. The vaginal plate advances in a caudocranial direction, obliterating the existing vaginal lumen. By caudal cavitation of the vaginal plate, a new lumen is formed, and the stratified Müllerian epithelium is replaced by a stratified squamous epithelium, probably from a urogenital sinus origin. Local proliferation of the vaginal plate in the region of the cervicovaginal junction produces the circumferential enlargement of the vagina known as the vaginal fornices, which surround the vaginal part of the cervix.

The administration of diethylstilbestrol (DES) through the 18th week of gestation can apparently result in the disruption of the transformation of columnar epithelium of Müllerian origin to the stratified squamous successor (Fig. 2.1). This retention of Müllerian epithelium gives rise to adenosis. Adenosis may exist in many forms: glandular cells in place of the normal squamous lining of the vagina, glandular cells hidden beneath an intact squamous lining, or mixed squamous metaplasia when new squamous cells attempt to replace glandular cells.

Vaginal adenosis has been observed in patients without a history of DES exposure but rarely to a clinically significant degree. Adenosis is more common in patients whose mothers began DES treatment early in pregnancy and is not observed if DES administration began after 18 weeks of gestation. At least 20% of women exposed to DES show an anatomic deformity of the upper vagina and cervix; transverse vaginal and cervical ridges, cervical collars, vaginal hoods, and cockscomb cervices have all been described. The transverse ridges and anatomic deformities found in one-fifth of women exposed to DES make it difficult to ascertain the boundaries of the vagina and cervix. The cervical eversion causes the cervix grossly to have a red appearance. This coloration is caused by the numerous normal-appearing blood vessels in the submucosa. With a colposcope and application of 3% acetic acid solution, numerous papillae ("grapes") of columnar epithelium are observed, similar to those seen in the native columnar epithelium of the endocervix. The hood (Fig. 2.2) is a fold of mucous membrane surrounding the portio of the cervix; it often disappears if the portio is pulled down with a tenaculum or is displaced by the speculum. The cockscomb is an atypical peaked appearance of the anterior lip of the cervix, and vaginal ridges are protruding circumferential bands in the upper vagina that may hide the cervix. A pseudopolyp formation (see Fig. 2.2) has been described that occurs

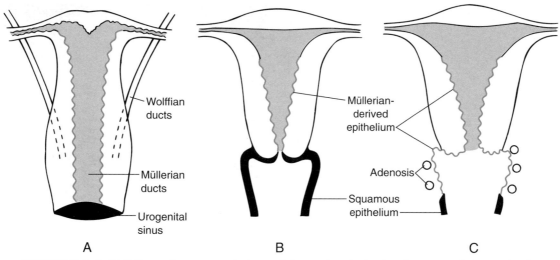

FIGURE 2.1 **A–C,** Schematic representations of the embryologic development of the vagina in unexposed (**A**) and diethylstilbestrol-exposed (**B** and **C**) women. (From Stillman RJ. In utero exposure to diethylstilbestrol: adverse effects on the reproductive tract and reproductive performance in male and female offspring. *Am J Obstet Gynecol* 1982;142(7):905.)

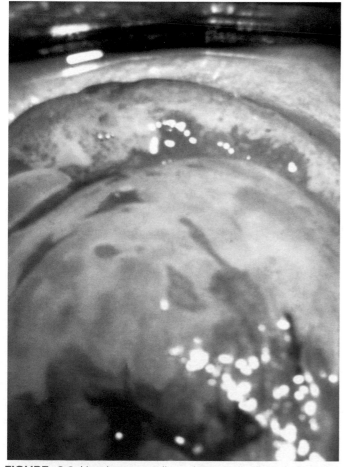

FIGURE 2.2 Hood surrounding the small diethylstilbestrol-exposed cervix, which is completely covered by columnar epithelium (pseudopolyp).

when the portio of the cervix is small and protrudes through a wide cervical hood.

The occurrence of vaginal adenosis among young women without in utero DES exposure implies that an event in embryonic development is responsible. The development of the Müllerian system depends on and follows formation of the Wolffian, or mesonephric, system. The emergence of the Müllerian system as the dominant structure appears unaffected by intrauterine exposure to DES when studied in animal systems. However, it is apparent that steroidal and nonsteroidal estrogens, when administered during the proper stage of vaginal embryogenesis in mice, can permanently prevent the transformation of Müllerian epithelium into the adult type of vaginal epithelium, thus creating a situation like adenosis. The colposcopic and histologic features of vaginal adenosis strongly support the concept of persistent, untransformed Müllerian columnar epithelia in the vagina as the explanation of adenosis.

EXAMINATION AND TREATMENT OF FEMALES EXPOSED TO DIETHYLSTILBESTROL

Essentially no DES has been prescribed to pregnant women since 1971, when the US Food and Drug Administration issued an alert regarding the risk of vaginal clear cell adenocarcinoma for females exposed in utero. The youngest women with in utero exposure were born in 1972, and many previously important clinical topics have become less relevant in everyday practice. The associated congenital anomalies and teenage cancers, for example, are no longer being diagnosed. However, an understanding of the disease process remains essential in order to care for this cohort of women as they age. Additionally, the evolution and understanding of DES is of great historical importance with many implications and lessons for today's practice.

Approximately 60% of women with in utero DES exposure have vaginal adenosis, cervical-like epithelium in the vagina, which appears red and granular. This is a benign condition that does not require treatment unless symptomatic, and it will generally resolve on its own over time. The premenopausal risk of clear cell adenocarcinoma is approximately 40 times higher among women with in utero DES exposure compared with those without the exposure. In unexposed women, clear cell adenocarcinoma occurs almost exclusively in menopause; in women with in utero exposure, most cases are diagnosed during the late teens and 20s. The oldest reported patient with DES-associated clear cell adenocarcinoma was diagnosed at 51 years. Overall, the incidence of clear cell adenocarcinoma is low in women with in utero exposure (≈1.5 cases/1000 women), but the risk is significantly higher than among unexposed women. The etiology of clear cell adenocarcinoma is unclear, and evolution of adenosis to cancer has never been directly proven, only suspected. Because of an increased risk of clear cell adenocarcinoma of the cervix and vagina and an increased risk of cervical intraepithelial neoplasia (CIN), annual examinations with Pap cytology testing are recommended for the entire lifetime of women with in utero DES exposure. No increased association has been observed between DES and squamous cell cervical cancer.

All DES-exposed females should have an annual gynecologic examination with cytology screening (Table 2.1). Cytology should include separate sampling of the cervix and upper vagina. If suspicious lesions are present, colposcopy and directed biopsies should be performed regardless of the cytology results. If delineations of the vagina, cervix, and endocervix are difficult, Lugol's solution may be helpful in detecting abnormal areas. Colposcopic examination of these patients is hindered by the abnormal patterns seen with squamous metaplasia (Fig. 2.3), which can be confused with neoplastic lesions. Histologic confirmation is essential before any treatment is undertaken. Marked mosaic (Fig. 2.4) and punctation patterns that normally herald intraepithelial neoplasia are commonly seen in the vagina of DES-exposed women as a result of widespread metaplasia. The purpose of regular examination is to permit

FIGURE 2.3 A, Area of white epithelium of squamous metaplasia. **B,** Histologic section of the area in *A* showing metaplasia to the left partially covering the adenosis (columnar epithelium) to the right.

FIGURE 2.4 Heavy mosaic pattern (histologically proven metaplasia) in a hood surrounding the cervix of an offspring exposed to diethylstilbestrol.

TABLE 2.1   **Examination of the Female Offspring Exposed to Diethylstilbestrol**
1. Inspect the introitus and hymen to assess the patency of the vagina.
2. Palpate the vaginal membrane with the index finger (especially noting non–Lugol-staining areas), noting areas of induration or exophytic lesions, which should be considered for biopsy.
3. Perform a speculum examination with the largest speculum that can be comfortably inserted (virginal-type speculums are often necessary). Adenosis usually appears red and granular (strawberry surface).
4. Obtain cytologic specimens from the cervical os and the walls of the upper third of the vagina.
5. Perform a colposcopic examination or Lugol staining on the initial visit.
6. Do a biopsy of indurated or exophytic areas and colposcopically abnormal areas with a dysplastic Papanicolaou smear.
7. Perform a bimanual rectovaginal examination.

detection of adenocarcinoma and squamous neoplasia during the earliest stages of development. Although many therapies have been attempted, no recommended treatment plan for vaginal adenosis exists. In most cases, the area of adenosis is physiologically transformed into squamous epithelium during varying periods of observation, and no therapy is necessary.

NONNEOPLASTIC EPITHELIAL DISORDERS OF THE VULVA

Nonneoplastic epithelial disorders of the vulvar skin and mucosa are frequently seen in clinical practice. Diagnosis is difficult without a biopsy to provide a histologic result, and multiple changes in terminology over the past 25 years add confusion to clinical management. The most recent classification guidelines were published in 2007 by the International Society for the Study of Vulvovaginal Disease (ISSVD) (Table 2.2). The lichenoid pattern subset includes two chronic diseases, lichen sclerosus and lichen planus, which are relevant to this review because of the association of those two diseases with vulvar cancer. Lichen simplex chronicus is not included in the lichenoid subset; it is classified in the acanthotic pattern subset. This is appropriate from an oncology viewpoint because lichen simplex chronicus is not associated with invasive cancer. With similar presenting symptoms and a hyperkeratotic appearance,

however, lichen simplex chronicus can be difficult to discriminate from lichen sclerosus and lichen planus on examination (Table 2.3).

Lichen Simplex Chronicus

Lichen simplex chronicus presents in girls and women of all ages, but it is more common in the reproductive and postmenopausal years. Lichen simplex chronicus is a chronic eczematous condition, and most women with this condition also have a history of atopic dermatitis. Pruritus is the most common symptom, and over time, scratching leads to epithelial thickening and hyperkeratosis. The status of the skin usually relates to the amount of scratching. Exacerbating agents may include heat, moisture, sanitary or incontinence pads, and topical agents. Lichen simplex chronicus may be seen in conjunction with other processes such as *Candida* infections or lichen sclerosus; these primary diseases must be treated in order to treat the pruritus leading to scratching and hyperkeratosis.

The locations most often involved on the vulva include the labia majora, interlabial folds, outer aspects of the labia minor, and clitoris. Changes can also extend to the lateral surfaces of the labia majora or beyond. Areas of lichen simplex chronicus are often localized, elevated, and well-delineated, but they may be extensive and poorly defined. The appearance of lesions may vary greatly even in the same patient. The vulva often appears dusky red when the degree of hyperkeratosis is slight and may appear thickened and leathery when hyperkeratosis persists. At other times, well-defined white patches may be seen, or a combination of red and white areas may be observed in different locations. Thickening, fissures, and excoriations require careful evaluation because carcinoma may be exhibited by these same features. For this reason, biopsy is essential in ascertaining the correct diagnosis.

Biopsy reveals a variable increase in the thickness of the horny layer (hyperkeratosis) and irregular thickening of the

TABLE 2.2 **2006 World Congress International Society for the Study of Vulvovaginal Disease (Classification of Vulvar Dermatoses)**	
Pathologic Subset	**Clinical Correlate**
Spongiotic pattern	Atopic dermatitis
	Allergic contact dermatitis
	Irritant contact dermatitis
Acanthotic pattern	Psoriasis
	Lichen simplex chronicus
	Primary (idiopathic)
	Secondary (superimposed on other vulvar disease)
Lichenoid pattern	Lichen sclerosus
	Lichen planus
Dermal homogenization/sclerosis pattern	Lichen sclerosus
Vesiculobullous pattern	Pemphigoid, cicatricial type
	Linear IgA disease
Acantholytic pattern	Hailey-Hailey disease
	Darier disease
	Papular genitocrural acantholysis
Granulomatous pattern	Crohn's disease
	Melkersson-Rosenthal syndrome
Vasculopathic pattern	Aphthous ulcers
	Behçet disease
	Plasma cell vulvitis

TABLE 2.3 **Other Dermatoses**			
Disorder	**Lesion**	**Genital**	**Other Locations**
Seborrheic dermatitis	Erythema with mild scale oval plaques	Mild scaling; also "inverse type"	Central face, neck, scalp, chest, back
Psoriasis	Annular scaly plaques that bleed easily	Red plaques with gray-white scale	Scalp, elbows, knees, sacrum
Tinea	Annular plaques with central clearing	Common	Skinfolds or single "ringworm" lesion
Lichen simplex chronicus	Lichenified plaques, some dermatitic	Scrotum or labia majora	Nape of the neck, ankle, forearm, antecubital and popliteal fossae
Lichen planus	Flat-topped lilac papules and plaques	White network, erosive vaginitis	Volar wrists, shins, buccal mucosa

FIGURE 2.5 Progression from early (**A**) to late (**B**) lichen sclerosus, with characteristic loss of labial architecture. (Courtesy Dr. Lori Boardman, MD, ScM, University of Central Florida College of Medicine.)

malpighian layer (acanthosis). This latter process produces a thickened epithelium and lengthening and distortion of the rete pegs. Parakeratosis may also be present. The granular layer of the epithelium is usually prominent. An inflammatory reaction is often present within the dermis with varying numbers of lymphocytes and plasma cells.

Lichen Sclerosus

Lichen sclerosus represents a specific disease found in genital and nongenital sites. The vulva is the most common lesion site in women. The age distribution of the disease is bimodal with peaks during the premenarchal and postmenopausal years, but the highest incidence is among postmenopausal women. Although the overall incidence and prevalence are unknown, Leibovitz and colleagues reported the prevalence among elderly women in a nursing home setting as 1 in 30. The mean age in this population was 82 years, 88% were wheelchair users, and 86% were incontinent (Figs. 2.5 and 2.6).

Over time, pruritus occurs with essentially all lesions, leading to scratching, which can develop into ecchymosis and ulceration. Symptoms evolve to include burning, tearing, and dyspareunia. Studies have suggested that the epithelium in lichen sclerosus is metabolically active and nonatrophic. A chronic inflammatory, lymphocyte-mediated dermatosis is present. The etiology of the disease is poorly understood, but autoimmune mechanisms appear to be involved.

The microscopic features of lichen sclerosus include hyperkeratosis, epithelial thickening with flattening of the rete pegs, cytoplasmic vacuolization of the basal layer of cells, and follicular plugging. Beneath the epidermis is a zone of homogenized, pink-staining, collagenous-appearing tissue that is relatively acellular. Edema is occasionally seen in this area. Elastic fibers are absent. Immediately below this zone lies a band of inflammatory cells that is consistent with lymphocytes and some

FIGURE 2.6 Lichen sclerosus with stenosis of the introitus, fissuring in the posterior fourchette, and perianal involvement producing the "keyhole appearance." (Courtesy of Dr. Lori Boardman, MD, ScM, University of Central Florida College of Medicine.)

plasma cells. Lichen sclerosus is often associated with foci of both hyperplastic epithelium and thin epithelium. Lichen simplex chronicus has been found in 27% to 35% of women with lichen sclerosus after microscopic study of vulvar specimens, likely secondary to pruritus and scratching.

In a well-developed classic lesion, the skin of the vulva is crinkled ("cigarette paper") and thinned, or appears parchment-like. The process often extends around the anal region in a figure-of-8 or keyhole configuration, and 30% of women have perianal lesions. At other times, the changes are localized, especially in the periclitoral area or the perineum. Clitoral involvement is usually associated with edema of the foreskin, which may obscure the glans clitoris. Phimosis of the clitoris is often seen late in the course of the disease. As the disease progresses, there is loss of architecture of the normal external genitalia. The labia minora may completely disappear as a result of atrophy. Synechiae often develop between the edges of the skin in these locations, causing pain and limited physical activity. Fissures also develop in the natural folds of the skin and especially in the posterior fourchette. The introitus may become so strictured or stenosed that intercourse is impossible. The vaginal mucosa is generally spared in this disease, which is helpful in discriminating between lichen sclerosus and lichen planus. In a study by Dalziel, 44 women with lichen sclerosus were evaluated for sexual dysfunction. Apareunia was experienced by 19 of the women at some point. Dyspareunia and decreased frequency of intercourse were noted by 80%, and orgasm was altered and relationships were affected in half. Local steroids improved sexual function in two-thirds of these patients.

Lichen sclerosus is a risk factor for invasive vulvar cancer, likely as a result of chronic inflammation and sclerosis. In untreated populations, approximately 5% of patients with lichen sclerosus also have intraepithelial neoplasia. Wallace followed 290 women with lichen sclerosus for an average of 12.5 years and found that 4% (n = 12) developed vulvar cancer. Carlson et al. reported that 4.5% of patients with lichen sclerosus developed vulvar cancer over a mean of 10 years. In treated populations, however, the risk may be lower. Cooper and associates treated 233 women in a vulvar teaching clinic over a 10-year period; 89% of the cohort received superpotent steroid treatment. Invasive vulvar cancer developed in 3% (n = 7), and vaginal intraepithelial neoplasia (VAIN) developed in 2% (n = 4). Jones and colleagues reported one case of cancer from a vulvar clinic treating 213 girls and women older than age 8 years. Renaud-Vilmer et al. reported results from an urban dermatology clinic caring for 83 girls and women with no prior treatment of vulvar lichen sclerosus. Invasive cancer was present at the time of presentation in 7% (n = 6) and developed in 2% (n = 2); in those who developed cancer, one did not return for follow-up, and one did not use the prescribed treatment. In a cohort followed prospectively with repeat vulvar examinations at the University of Florence by Carli and associates, two cases of invasive cancer and one case of vulvar intraepithelial neoplasia (VIN) developed among 211 women with treated lichen sclerosus. All three cases occurred after more than 3 years of follow-up in the cohort.

The absolute incidence of vulvar cancer is low in women with lichen sclerosus, but 50% to 70% of squamous cell vulvar cancers occur in a background of lichen sclerosus. Currently, there is no diagnostic tool to differentiate between lichen sclerosus that will remain benign versus lichen sclerosus that will evolve into squamous cell carcinoma (SCC). Two biomarkers,

p53 and monoclonal antibody MIB1, have shown promise in retrospective tissues studies, but further testing is necessary. The standard of care for cancer screening in this population remains serial examination with directed biopsies for new, evolving, or suspicious lesions, teaching self-examination with a mirror, and having self-reporting to a physician when lesions change visibly and to palpation.

Lichen Planus

Lichen planus is a distinct dermatologic disease that may affect the oral mucosa, esophageal mucosa, skin, scalp, nails, and eyes in addition to the vulva. Approximately 1% of the population likely develops lichen planus; 25% to 50% of women with lichen planus are believed to have vulvar symptoms. Both vulvovaginal-gingival syndrome and penile-gingival syndrome have been described. The disease appears to be a cell-mediated immune disorder causing chronic inflammation. Similar to lichen sclerosus, symptoms are most common in postmenopausal women in their 50s and 60s; usually include pruritus; and can evolve as the disease progresses to include burning, pain, and dyspareunia. Labial agglutination and loss of architecture of the labia and clitoris may occur. The vaginal mucosa is frequently involved, as opposed to lichen sclerosus, which rarely involves the vagina (Fig. 2.7).

The relationship between lichen planus and vulvar cancer is not as well-established as the association between lichen sclerosus and cancer. Small studies have suggested an increased risk of vulvar cancer, and subjects with oral lichen planus may also

FIGURE 2.7 Erosive lichen planus. (Courtesy of Dr. Lori Boardman, MD, ScM, University of Central Florida College of Medicine.)

have an increased risk of oral cancer. In the early 1990s, case reports by Franck and Young, Lewis and Harrington, and Dwyer and colleagues reported incidences of vulvar SCC in subjects with lichen planus and within erosive lichen planus lesions. In a review of 113 patients with erosive vulvar lichen planus followed by Kennedy and colleagues over an 8-year period, one woman developed vulvar cancer. Of interest, two women in this cohort with oral lichen planus were subsequently diagnosed with oral or esophageal cancer, and two additional women were diagnosed with cervical adenocarcinoma in situ and rectal adenocarcinoma. Similar findings were reported by Cooper and associates. Of 114 women with erosive vulvar lichen planus, seven developed VIN, one developed oral SCC, two developed anogenital SCCs of the labium minora and perianal area.

Diagnosis and Treatment

Biopsies are critical to appropriate management; before any treatment is given on a long-term basis, biopsies should be performed from representative areas to ensure the correct diagnosis. (The exception for biopsy is the pediatric population, which will not be discussed here.) Biopsies should be focused at sites of fissuring, ulceration, induration, and thick plaques. Patient education regarding hygienic measures for keeping the vulva clean and dry is important; any soaps, perfumes, deodorizers, or other contact irritants should be avoided. A thorough history should be taken to evaluate possible causes of vulvar pruritus. After lesions with malignant potential have been ruled out, local measures for control of symptoms, primarily pruritus, can be instituted (Table 2.4). Additionally, infectious vaginitis should be ruled out with a saline wet preparation, potassium hydroxide (KOH) wet preparation, and yeast culture to evaluate for atypical yeast that may be missed on plain microscopy.

Lichen Simplex Chronicus

Therapy for lichen simplex chronicus is treatment of the underlying cause of irritation and pruritus. All offending environmental agents should be avoided, including wipes, lubricants, sanitary and incontinence pads, detergents, perfumes, and soaps. A thorough history is often necessary to identify possible sources of irritation. Any underlying vaginitis also requires treatment. For isolated lichen simplex chronicus, a topical steroid ointment such as triamcinolone 0.1% or hydrocortisone 2.5% can be applied daily (after bathing to help seal in moisture) until symptoms are improved, generally in 3 to 4 weeks. If symptoms are particularly severe or a course of low-dose steroids is insufficient, a trial of higher dose steroid ointment is

acceptable. Pruritus is often most severe at night, and short-term use of a pharmacologic sleep aid may be necessary. Lichen simplex chronicus should resolve with removal of the offending agent and treatment; if symptoms persist or recur, repeat biopsies and the diagnosis should be reconsidered.

Lichen Sclerosus

Lichen sclerosus is a chronic condition with no curative treatment; the goal is symptom control. The standard treatment for lichen sclerosus is a topical corticosteroid. Typical regimens begin with a superpotent steroid ointment (ie, clobetasol propionate ointment 0.05%) used nightly until resolution of symptoms (usually 8–12 weeks). Because of the chronicity of lichen sclerosus, maintenance therapy is necessary after initial treatment; application one to three times per week is usually sufficient. Many women stop treatment when their symptoms improve and then present again months later with recurrent symptoms. Therapy can be reinitiated at treatment levels for 6 to 12 weeks, and emphasis given to maintenance therapy. Theoretically, long-term use of topical steroids may result in striae and thinning of the dermis, but this is infrequently observed in patients with lichen sclerosus. Topical testosterone is no longer the treatment of choice for lichen sclerosus.

A prospective randomized study by Bracco and associates evaluated 79 patients with lichen sclerosus using four different treatment regimens: a 3-month course of testosterone (2%), progesterone (2%), clobetasol propionate (0.05%), and a cream base preparation. Patients experienced greater relief of symptoms with clobetasol (75%) than with testosterone (20%) or other preparations (10%). Clobetasol therapy was the only treatment in which the gross and histologic evaluation of patients improved after treatment. Recurrences after stopping the steroid occurred, but symptoms were relieved when therapy was resumed. Clobetasol was also more effective than testosterone in the randomized trial performed by Bornstein and colleagues, with a significant improvement in long-term relief experience by clobetasol users. Lorenz and colleagues reported 77% had complete remission of symptoms with clobetasol therapy but again noted that maintenance therapy was needed after baseline treatment. In the cohort followed by Cooper and associates discussed previously, 65% were symptom free, 31% had a partial response, and 5% has a poor response after steroid use. Improvement was also seen on physical examination; 23% had total resolution, 69% had partial resolution (improvement in purpura, hyperkeratosis, fissures, and erosions but no change in color and texture), 6% had minor resolution, and 2% had no improvement. Renaud-Vilmer and colleagues noted a different response rate by age group in women treated with 0.05% clobetasol propionate ointment. Complete remission, defined as complete resolution of symptoms, normalization of physical examination, and histologic regression of lichen sclerosus, was observed in 72% of women younger than age 50 years, 23% of women between 50 and 70 years, and 0% in women older than 70 years. Relapse was 84% at 4 years but was not associated with subject age.

Occasionally, vulvar pruritus is so persistent that it cannot be relieved by topical measures. Topical treatment may also fail

TABLE 2.4 **Vulvar Nonneoplastic Epithelial Disorders**	
Disorder	**Treatment**
Lichen sclerosus	Topical high-potency steroid ointment
Lichen planus	Topical high-potency steroid ointment
Lichen simplex chronicus	Topical corticosteroid after evaluation and removal of offending environmental agents and treatment of concurrent vaginitis, lichen sclerosus, or lichen planus

if significant hyperkeratosis is present. In such cases, intradermal and lesional injection of steroids has been reported to be effective. If lesions persist and symptoms do not improve after a course of superpotent topical steroids, biopsies should be repeated to confirm the initial diagnosis. It is again critical to rule out cancer and VIN to ensure appropriate treatment. Other regimens have been reported for lichen sclerosus recalcitrant to corticosteroids. Specifically, tacrolimus and photodynamic therapy may have some efficacy, but further trials are necessary.

Lichen Planus

Lichen planus is similarly treated with complete evaluation, patient education, and topical steroids. Additionally, the physical examination should exclude the presence of lichen planus on the skin, scalp, nail beds, and oral mucosa. If systemic disease is present, consultation with a dermatologist is useful. Treatment of vulvar lesions should begin with an ultrapotent steroid ointment (ie, clobetasol propionate ointment 0.05%) applied nightly for 6 to 8 weeks. If symptoms improve, the frequency of application can be reduced to two to three times weekly for 4 to 8 additional weeks. Cooper and associates reported that in a cohort of 114 women followed and treated for lichen planus, 71% of those treated with ultrapotent topical corticosteroids experienced relief of symptoms with treatment. On examination, 50% experienced healing of erosions, but no patients had resolution of scarring. When lichen planus symptoms are in a prolonged remission, the lowest effective dose is used for maintenance therapy, which may involve less frequent administration and a lower potency steroid. Similar to lichen sclerosus, symptoms will return if maintenance therapy is not used.

Lichen planus does appear more resistant to therapy than lichen sclerosus. In a small series of women with vulvar lichen planus that was nonresponsive to other treatments, Byrd and colleagues at the Mayo Clinic reported that 15 of 16 subjects experienced symptomatic relief after a course of topical tacrolimus. The mean response time was 4 weeks, and six subjects experienced mild irritation, burning, or tingling that resolved with persistent use. Tacrolimus therapy was less successful in the subjects followed by Cooper and associates, who were nonresponsive to topical steroid treatment. Of seven patients treated, two had complete symptomatic relief, three had some relief, and two had no improvement in symptoms.

INTRAEPITHELIAL NEOPLASIA OF THE VAGINA

Clinical Profile

The incidence of VAIN is not well described. The first report was by Graham and Meigs in 1952. They reported three patients with carcinoma of the vagina, two intraepithelial and one invasive, that were discovered 6, 7, and 10 years, respectively, after total hysterectomy for CIS (carcinoma in situ) of the cervix. Carcinoma in situ is a historical diagnosis, equivalent to the modern diagnosis of HSIL or CIN2/3. The most recent analysis of the incidence of VAIN in the United States, published in 1977, reported 0.2 to 0.3 cases per 100,000 women. Data published by Joura and colleagues from a large vaccine trial give

a more recent estimate: The incidence of high-grade VAIN in the placebo group—women from 24 countries between 16 and 26 years of age who were followed for a mean of 36 months—was 21 cases in 9087 subjects. There may be multiple reasons for the higher incidence observed in the vaccine trial such as a true rise in incidence since 1977 similar to the increase seen for VIN, a higher rate of diagnosis because the women were being followed with serial examinations, or a different population from a more heterogeneous international setting. VAIN has many of the same risk factors associated with CIN, including smoking, earlier age at first intercourse, increased number of sexual partners, and HPV infection.

CIN of the vagina is much less common than that of the cervix or vulva. For the year 2015, the American Cancer Society estimated that 4080 cases of invasive cancer of the vagina would be diagnosed in the United States. Although the incidence of vaginal cancer has increased over the past several years, it remains rare. Because of the low prevalence of the disease, routine screening for VAIN and vaginal cancer is not recommended. After hysterectomy for benign disease, the incidence of VAIN is extraordinarily low, and guidelines from the American College of Obstetricians and Gynecology (ACOG) and the American Society for Colposcopy and Cervical Pathology (ASCCP) do not support Pap testing in this population. These guidelines were written in part based on evidence from Pearce and colleagues, Noller and Stokes-Lampard and colleagues showing that a huge number of women would undergo unnecessary cytology screening and colposcopy in order to diagnose a rare outcome. The exceptions to this guideline include women who have a history of in utero DES exposure, are immunosuppressed, or have a history of cervical or vulvar dysplasia. Many women have accepted historical guidelines recommending annual Pap testing and may require counseling and patient education to accept these new guidelines. Rare, unfortunate cases of VAIN or invasive cancer will occasionally be diagnosed in women who have undergone hysterectomy for benign disease, but these exceptional cases cannot drive screening guidelines. Additionally, because VAIN and vaginal cancer are strongly associated with HPV infection, the HPV vaccination should drive a decrease in the number of these cases in the future.

Patients with VAIN tend to have either an antecedent or coexistent neoplasia in the lower genital tract. This is the usual situation in at least half to two-thirds of all patients with VAIN. In patients who have been treated for disease in the cervix or vulva, VAIN can appear many years later, necessitating long-term follow-up. First van der Linde, then Gusberg and Marshall, and later Parker indicated that 2%, 1.9%, and 0.9% of patients, respectively, had vaginal recurrences after hysterectomy for a similar lesion in the cervix. More recently, Schockaert and associates were able to follow 94 women who had hysterectomies and concurrently carried a diagnosis of CIN II, CIN III, or FIGO stage Ia1 cervical cancer. In a median interval of 35 months, 7.4% ($n = 7$) developed VAIN II+ (vaginal intraepithelial neoplasia II or greater), including two vaginal cancers. Ferguson and Maclure reported positive cytologic findings in 151 (20.3%) of 633 previously treated patients. This large group included invasive and in situ cancers of the cervix, which were treated by irradiation or hysterectomy. The long-term recurrence rate for CIS of the vagina is uncertain, but it is sufficient to merit continued careful follow-up.

Vaginal intraepithelial neoplasia and invasive cancer are both associated with HPV. HPV positivity rates reported in the literature range from 82% to 94% for VAIN and 60% to 75% for vaginal cancer, and HPV-16 and -18 account for the majority of HPV positivity. In early reports, vaccination appears to be effective at preventing HPV-16– and HPV-18–associated vaginal lesions in women who receive the vaccination before HPV exposure. HPV mapping has shown identical DNA integration loci between primary lesions of cervical dysplasia and later dysplastic lesions of the vagina and vulva, indicating that later disease may result from monoclonal lesions from the primary cervical dysplasia. Vaginal dysplasia appears to mimic cervical dysplasia with a high prevalence of HPV infection, as opposed to vulvar dysplasia, which displays inconsistent associations.

Isolated lesions can usually be recognized colposcopically (Fig. 2.8). The most frequent finding is acetowhite epithelium; mosaicism and punctuation can also be present, and some authors have described a "pink blush" appearance or a slightly granular texture. The diagnosis is confirmed by biopsy. The extent of the lesion can be evaluated with the colposcope or with Lugol's solution. Almost all lesions are asymptomatic, although a patient will occasionally have discharge or postcoital staining. An abnormal Pap smear result usually initiates the diagnostic survey. In almost all series, the upper third of the

vagina is most frequently involved (as is the case with the invasive variety), and the posterior wall of the vagina appears more susceptible.

Diagnosis

Patients with an abnormal Pap test result who do not have a cervix or patients with an abnormal Pap test result and no cervical abnormality visualized should undergo a careful examination of the vaginal epithelium. Colposcopic examination of the vagina can be difficult to perform. The largest possible speculum should be used and repositioned frequently to allow inspection of all surfaces. Colposcopic findings are similar to those described for the cervix. Each of the four walls should be examined from the apex to the introitus as separate and sequential steps. Small biopsy specimens are taken with a Tischler or Kevorkian–Younge alligator-jaw forceps. Sometimes a sterilized skin-hook for traction at the biopsy site may be helpful. Most patients can tolerate these biopsies without local anesthesia, but the anticipated pain from the biopsies versus pain from a local anesthetic injection should be considered. Lugol's solution is often helpful in delineating lesions of the vagina. Normal vaginal epithelium is stained brown, but dysplastic lesions with abnormal glycogen levels remain pale. In postmenopausal patients, local use of estrogen creams for several weeks helps to highlight the abnormal areas for identification by colposcopy.

The majority of VAIN is multifocal; even if a lesion is identified, one must search the entire vagina for coexisting, multiple lesions. Lesions are more common in the upper third of the vagina, but disease-free skip areas may be encountered with additional VAIN in the lower vagina. In hard-to-locate lesions, selective cytologic methods, such as obtaining Pap smears from different locations in the vagina, can often pinpoint the area of abnormality so that attention can be paid specifically to the area of highest suspicion.

Management

Local excision of the involved area has been the mainstay of therapy. In many cases, a single isolated lesion can be removed easily in the office with biopsy forceps. If larger areas are involved, an upper colpectomy may be necessary if the lesion is to be removed by surgery. A dilute pitressin solution or lidocaine with epinephrine can be injected submucosally at the beginning of the procedure and will greatly facilitate the vaginectomy.

As in CIN, outpatient modalities of therapy have been investigated for VAIN. Many patients have been treated historically with 5-fluorouracil (5-FU), but toxicity generally makes this a less desirable option, particularly in women who are sexually active. However, studies by Petrilli and associates and Caglar and colleagues indicate that this modality can be effective. One of the problems with 5-FU is the selection of the best mode of application, dosage, and length of treatment. Several techniques have been suggested with equivalent results. One-quarter applicator of 5% 5-FU cream is inserted high in the vagina each night after the patient is in bed. The patient can be instructed to coat the vulva and introitus with white petroleum because the cream leaks out during sleep. A small tampon or cotton ball at the introitus is also helpful to prevent leakage. Because of irritation

FIGURE 2.8 Carcinoma in situ of the vagina (colposcopic view).

to the vagina and perineum, the cream should be removed by douching with warm water the next morning. This is done every night for 5 to 8 days followed by a 10- to 14-day rest period, and then the application cycle is repeated. This usually allows an adequate treatment time without having the patient experience the tremendous local reaction that can occur with prolonged use. Treatment can be repeated if it is not successful after the first cycle. Weekly insertions of 5-FU cream, approximately 1.5 g (one-third of an applicator), deep into the vagina once per week at bedtime for 10 consecutive weeks has also been shown to be efficacious. Placement of cotton balls at the introitus and application of a petroleum barrier on the perineum and vaginal introitus help prevent 5-FU contamination of the perineum with resultant skin irritation. Douching the next morning, which is advocated by some, is unnecessary with the weekly instillation. Patient compliance is likely higher and toxicity less with the second approach.

Dungar and Wilkinson noted an interesting finding in the vagina after 5-FU therapy, and it has been confirmed by others. After treatment, a red area suggestive of a lack of squamous epithelium may be present. They found that this represented columnar epithelium consistent with a metaplastic process in which squamous epithelium is replaced with columnar epithelium. They called this finding "acquired vaginal adenosis." These changes are usually found in the upper third of the vagina but may extend into the middle third. The columnar epithelium was of a low cuboidal or mucus-secreting endocervical type. In some cases, squamous epithelium was noted overlying the glandular elements. Marked superficial chronic inflammation was also present. This has also been noted in the vagina after laser therapy.

Cryosurgery has largely fallen out of favor in the treatment of VAIN, and laser therapy is preferred as an ablative technique. To give guidance about the depth of vaginal destruction required by the laser, Benedet and associates evaluated 56 patients who ranged from 22 to 84 years of age. Measurement of the epithelium was performed on involved and uninvolved tissue. The involved epithelium had a mean thickness of 0.46 mm (range, 0.1–1.4 mm). Uninvolved tissue was thinner and had a mean thickness of 0.28 mm. No statistical difference was seen in the thickness of the involved epithelium in the premenopausal and postmenopausal patients; however, the uninvolved epithelium was thinner in the postmenopausal patients compared with the premenopausal patients (0.25 vs. 0.37 mm). Based on this study, the authors believed that destruction of 1 to 1.5 mm would only destroy the epithelium without damaging underlying structures.

Over a 6-year period, Townsend and associates treated 36 patients from two large referral hospitals with a CO_2 laser. In 92% of the patients, the lesions were completely removed by the laser without significant side effects. Almost one-fourth of the patients, however, required more than one treatment session. Krebs treated 22 patients with topical 5-FU and 37 patients with laser therapy. The success rate was similar for the two treatments. Pain and bleeding have been the main complications but appear to be minimal. Healing is excellent, and impaired sexual function has not been a problem. The optimal technique of

laser therapy for vaginal lesions has yet to be determined; whereas some investigators suggest removing only the identified lesions, others advocate treating the entire vagina to avoid missing other lesions. A thorough diagnostic investigation of the vagina to rule out invasive cancer can be difficult, but it is obviously mandatory. Evidence from vaginectomy series shows that invasive cancer may be present concurrently with VAIN. In the 105 patients with VAIN II or VAIN III treated with vaginectomy by Indermaur and colleagues, 12% ($n = 13$) had invasive cancer on final pathology, and 22% ($n = 23$) had negative findings. Multifocal lesions, particularly posthysterectomy, with deep vaginal angles may be difficult to treat with the laser. Small skin hooks and dental mirrors can be used as adjuncts to successful laser therapy.

More recently, experience with 5% imiquimod cream in the management of VAIN has been reported. In a study by Buck and Guth, 56 women with VAIN (mostly low grade) were treated with 0.25 g of the cream placed in the vagina once weekly for 3 weeks. Of 42 women available for follow-up, 36 (86%) were clear of VAIN on colposcopic evaluation 1 week or later after the last treatment. Five patients' disease required two treatment cycles, and one needed three treatment cycles before clearing of their lesions. Vulvar or vestibular excoriation was reported in only two individuals. No vaginal ulcerations were noted.

Ultrasonic surgical aspiration has been successfully used by Robinson, von Gruenigen and colleagues, and Matsuo and colleagues, but the technique is not widely practiced. Some have advocated surface irradiation using an intravaginal applicator, but adverse effects may be severe and include vaginal stenosis, urinary symptoms, and vaginal ulceration. Additionally, vaginal stenosis can make follow-up extremely difficult. Total vaginectomy, with vaginal reconstruction using a split-thickness skin graft, should be reserved for the patient who has failed more conservative therapy because there appears to be no recurrence benefit from the more invasive procedure.

Treated VAIN often recurs, regardless of the treatment method, and there is no clear standard of treatment. In a retrospective series of 121 women treated for VAIN between 1989 and 2000 by Dodge and colleagues, 33% of subjects experienced recurrence of VAIN, and 2% progressed to invasive cancer; multifocal lesions were more likely to recur. When stratified by treatment type, VAIN recurred in 0% ($n = 0$ of 13) of those treated with partial vaginectomy, 38% ($n = 16$ of 42) of those treated with laser, and 59% ($n = 13$ of 22) of those treated with 5-FU. However, Indermaur and colleagues noted a higher rate of recurrence in their cohort of patients treated with vaginectomy. Of 52 patients available for follow-up who received vaginectomy as treatment for VAIN II or VAIN III, six patients recurred at a mean of 24 months, and one was diagnosed with invasive cancer. Sillman and associates reported on 94 patients with VAIN who were treated by various methods. The remission rate was high, but 5% of the cases progressed to invasive disease despite close follow-up.

Incomplete excision of sufficient vaginal cuff with hysterectomy for CIS of the cervix with involvement of the fornices may explain an early recurrence. The finding of CIS in the vaginal cuff area in less than 1 year after hysterectomy makes this explanation likely. Therefore, it is important to perform a preoperative evaluation of the upper vagina by Schiller tests or colposcopy at the time of hysterectomy for CIS of the cervix. This allows the surgeon to determine accurately how much of the upper vagina has to be removed. It is also apparent that both CIS and dysplasia may develop in the vagina as primary lesions without an association with a similar process on the cervix or vulva. Still other preinvasive lesions of the vagina may appear after irradiation therapy for invasive carcinoma of the cervix. Data from MD Anderson suggest that these postradiation lesions are premalignant and can progress to invasive cancer if they are not treated. Without therapy, approximately 25% of the patients in this series progressed to the invasive state over varying periods of follow-up. Local therapy must be executed with care because of the previous irradiation.

VULVAR INTRAEPITHELIAL NEOPLASIA

Clinical Profile

Many pathologists still identify intraepithelial lesions of the vulva as VIN I, VIN II, and VIN III, but terminology has recently changed. In 2004, the ISSVD clarified the VIN classification system (Table 2.5), and in 2012, a consensus group was cosponsored by the College of American Pathologists and the American Society for Colposcopy and Cervical Pathology to further clarify terminology (Lower Anogenital Squamous Terminology [LAST]) among HPV-associated lesions of the lower genital tract, including the cervix, vagina, vulva, and anus.

The ISSVD eliminated the previous term "VIN I" because there was no evidence that it was a precancerous lesion. The term "VIN" now refers only to lesions previously classified as VIN II or VIN III. In the current system, there is no discrimination between VIN II and III, and the two previously distinct classifications are consolidated as "VIN." Many pathology laboratories still include the older VIN I, II, and III terminology in parentheses for clarity.

Two distinct subtypes of VIN exist: the usual type and the differentiated type. The two subtypes are different in epidemiology, morphology, and their association with vulvar cancer (Table 2.6). Whereas the differentiated type may also be called simplex VIN, the usual type may be called warty, basaloid, or undifferentiated VIN. In comparison with the usual type, the differentiated type tends to occur in older women, be

unifocal and unicentric, be found at the edge of vulvar SCC and in the setting of lichen sclerosus or planus, and be less associated with HPV. Usual type VIN, with warty and basaloid subtypes, is found in younger women, has a strong association with cigarette smoking, is often multifocal, is less frequently found in conjunction with squamous cell cancer, and is usually associated with HPV. Although there is an association between VIN and vulvar cancer, the relationship is less clear than the known progression from CIN to invasive cervical squamous carcinoma.

The LAST Project attempted to unify terminology referring to HPV associated-intraepithelial neoplasia of the lower genital tract. The recommended terminology for all cervical, vaginal, vulvar, and anal lesions is "low-grade" or "high-grade" squamous intraepithelial lesion (SIL) based on a combination of cell morphology and p16 immunostaining. Unfortunately, vulvar intraepithelial lesions are not as strongly associated with HPV as cervical lesions, so these guidelines would only be applicable to usual type VIN as differentiated VIN is normally p16 negative and p53 positive. Additionally, VIN I was eliminated by the ISSVD in 2004, so all currently diagnosed HPV-associated VIN should by definition be HSIL vulvar intraepithelial lesions. As clinical pathology practice continues to catch up to new guidelines, it is important to understand all of the terminology used recently and to talk to the pathologist before making meaningful clinical decisions if there is any doubt about terminology being used.

According to a Surveillance, Epidemiology, and End Results (SEER) data analysis by Judson and colleagues, whereas the incidence of vulvar CIS increased 411% between 1973 and 2000, the rates of invasive vulvar cancer rose only 20%. Several hypotheses regarding the changing incidence of VIN exist: increased physician awareness and evaluation of vulvar disease, increased prevalence of smoking among women, and increased HPV prevalence. Women with a history of preinvasive cervical disease or cervical cancer are at increased risk of preinvasive

---

TABLE 2.5 **2003 International Society for the Study of Vulvovaginal Disease (Classification of Vulvar Intraepithelial Neoplasia (VIN)***

A. VIN, usual type
   1. Warty type
   2. Basaloid type
   3. Mixed (warty or basaloid) type
B. VIN, differentiated type

*The previous classifications of VIN II and VIN III were consolidated as VIN, and the previous classification of VIN I was eliminated.

TABLE 2.6 **Vulvar Intraepithelial Neoplasia Histologic Subtypes and Associations**

	Usual (Warty-Basaloid, Undifferentiated)	Differentiated (Simplex)
Age	Premenopausal women (30s–40s)	Postmenopausal women (65 years)
Overall %VIN	≈95	≈5
HPV associated	Yes	No
HPV type	16	N/A
Risk factors	Smoking, immunosuppression	None identified
Distribution	Multifocal	Unifocal, unicentric
Background histology	Lichen sclerosus	
Progression to	Warty, basaloid squamous cell cancer	Keratinizing squamous cell cancer
	Invasive cancer	(Rare)

NA, Not applicable.

vulvar dysplasia. HPV is a risk factor for vulvar disease, but the progression from HPV infection to precancer to invasive cancer is poorly understood. In contrast to cervical cancer, which has a peak age in dysplasia incidence followed by a peak age in invasive cancer (after a lag period), there is no similar time course established in vulvar cancer. In fact, the peak incidence of VIN occurs during the mid-40s followed by a declining incidence, but the incidence of invasive vulvar cancer continues to increase and never stabilizes, reaching approximately 13 in 100,000 women by the age of 80 years.

Case reports definitively document the development of invasive squamous cell cancers in VIN usual type lesions in patients followed prospectively. In a review of more than 3300 patients with VIN III, van Seters identified occult invasive cancer in 3.2% of subjects at the time of excision, and an additional 3.3% developed cancer during follow-up. Chafe and associates noted that 19% of women who were thoroughly evaluated and thought to have VIN actually had invasive cancer on the vulvectomy specimen. Kagie and associates reported on 66 women with invasive vulvar SCC; 39 (62%) had synchronous VIN. In other cases, it appears that invasive lesions may arise de novo rather than from precursor VIN lesions, but this may be from a misdiagnosis of differentiated VIN previously diagnosed as lichen sclerosus. In a population of 405 women followed for VIN II and III in New Zealand between 1962 and 2003, 2% of cases recurred as invasive cancer at a median time of 2.4 years, and 1.8% of cases recurred as invasive cancer in new fields at a median time of 13.5 years. Additionally, 11.6% of biopsy-proven VIN regressed before treatment (mean age, 24.6 years). If observation is considered in young women with small lesions and usual type histology, frequent examinations with directed biopsies are necessary. Barbero and colleagues noted three of 55 patients treated with VIN whose conditions progressed to carcinoma in 14 months to 15 years. These three patients ranged in age from 58 to 74 years. In the New Zealand cohort, there were 10 cancers diagnosed in untreated patients; Jones and McLean have previously reported on five of the cases diagnosed between 1970 and 1974, and an additional five cases were diagnosed between 1983 and 1992. The median interval between VIN and invasive cancer was 3.9 years (range, 1.1–7.3 years).

HPV is strongly associated with VIN usual type, but it is less commonly associated with VIN differentiated type. There is a wide variation in the reported presence of HPV in VIN because of the changing terminology and classification of VIN and the improved sensitivity of recent HPV testing. The usual type comprises the majority of VIN, so a high prevalence of HPV positivity would be expected in studies that do not differentiate between the two histologies. In more recently published literature, HPV is present in 61% to 100% of VIN. HPV-16 appears to be the most common type, accounting for as high as 91% of infection in some series. The prevalence of HPV infection in VIN and vulvar cancer decreases with age, probably reflecting a change in the underlying histology. The efficacy of HPV vaccines in preventing vulvar dysplasia and cancer will be determined not only by the vaccine properties but also by the prevalence of HPV-related vulvar disease in the population. For example, the HPV VVAP (Vulvar, Vaginal, and Penile) study group published

an analysis of HPV contribution to VIN and invasive cancers worldwide. In their sample, whereas approximately 89% of VIN was associated with HPV positivity, 25% of invasive cancer was HPV positive, and HPV-16 was the most common type, accounting for 72.5%. Among geographic regions, however, HPV was more likely in cases from North America.

In initial publications from the vaccine studies, there does appear to be efficacy against VIN. Joura and colleagues report on the vaccine efficacy in reducing specifically HPV-16– or HPV-18–related VIN with a mean duration of follow-up of 36 months. Among subjects who remained HPV negative while receiving the vaccination series, the vaccine was 100% efficacious; zero cases were diagnosed in 7811 vaccinated women, and eight cases were diagnosed in 7785 women who received placebo. Among subjects who were HPV negative at the time of the first injection but did not necessarily remain HPV negative for the duration of the vaccination series, the vaccine was 95% efficacious; one case was diagnosed in 8757 vaccinated women, and 20 cases were diagnosed in 8774 women who received placebo. An analysis was also performed on the incidence of VIN, regardless of HPV association, among all subjects, HPV naïve and HPV exposed at the time of vaccination, and the rate of VIN II/III was reduced by half in the vaccinated group, but there did not appear to be any benefit for those who were HPV exposed at the time of vaccination.

One recent study by Kenter and colleagues tested a synthetic long-peptide vaccine as treatment for VIN in women with HPV-16–positive VIN using a series of three or four vaccinations. Among 19 patients examined on 12-month follow-up, nine had a complete clinical response, and this was maintained at 24 months. This suggests a potential treatment role for vaccines in addition to prevention.

Diagnosis

The disease is asymptomatic in more than 50% of cases. In the remainder of cases, the predominant symptom is pruritus. The presence of a distinct mass, bleeding, or discharge strongly suggests invasive cancer. The most productive diagnostic technique is careful inspection of the vulva in bright light during a routine pelvic examination followed by biopsies of suspicious lesions. A handheld lens or colposcope can be very helpful, especially after application of 5% acetic acid to the skin and introitus.

Careful inspection of the vulva during routine gynecologic examinations is essential; this remains the most likely diagnostic technique. The milder forms of VIN first appear clinically as pale areas that vary in density. More severe forms are seen as papules or macules, coalescent or discrete, or single or multiple. Lesions on the cutaneous surface of the vulva usually appear as lichenified or hyperkeratotic plaques or white epithelium (Figs. 2.9 and 2.10). By contrast, lesions of mucous membranes are usually macular and pink or red. Vulvar lesions are hyperpigmented in 10% to 15% of patients (Fig. 2.11). These lesions range from mahogany to dark brown, and they stand out sharply when observed solely with the naked eye.

The entire vulva, perineum, and perianal area must be evaluated for multifocal lesions. It is not uncommon to find

FIGURE 2.9 Multiple white lesions *(arrows)* of the vulva caused by vulvar intraepithelial neoplasia.

FIGURE 2.10 Histologic section of carcinoma in situ of the vulva.

FIGURE 2.11 Pseudopigmented lesions of vulvar carcinoma in situ.

intraepithelial lesions on hemorrhoid tags or more superiorly in the gluteal cleft. The use of acetic acid is helpful in identifying subtle lesions. In contrast to the mucous membrane of the cervix, the keratinized epithelium of the vulva requires application of acetic acid for 5 minutes or longer before many lesions become apparent. Placement of soaked cotton balls or sponges on the vulva for several minutes before examination is effective. After a lesion has been diagnosed, colposcopic examination of the entire vulva and perianal area should follow to rule out multifocal disease. A handheld magnifying glass can also be used, which allows greater viewing area at one time compared with the colposcope. In general, whereas multifocal lesions are more common in premenopausal patients, postmenopausal patients have a higher rate of unifocal disease.

Some investigators prefer to use toluidine blue to identify vulvar lesions. A 1% aqueous solution of the dye is applied to the external genital area. After drying for 2 to 3 minutes, the region is then washed with 1% to 2% acetic acid solution. Suspicious foci of increased nuclear activity become deeply stained (royal blue); normal skin accepts little or none of the dye. Hyperkeratotic lesions, even though neoplastic, are only lightly stained, but benign excoriations are often brilliant, an observation that accounts for the high false-positive and false-negative rates.

The diagnosis of VIN can be subtle. To avoid delay, the physician must exercise a high degree of suspicion. Vulvar biopsy should be performed on any suspicious lesion. It is best accomplished under local anesthesia (lidocaine or bupivacaine) with a Keyes dermatologic punch (4- to 6-mm size). This instrument allows removal of an adequate tissue sample and orientation for future sectioning. The biopsy site can be made hemostatic with silver nitrate, Monsel's, a stitch, or a piece of absorbable gelatin powder (eg, Gelfoam) cut with the Keyes punch; this is positioned in the skin defect and kept in place with a small dressing for at least 24 hours. Adequate biopsy specimens can also be obtained with a sharp alligator-jaw instrument if one has proper traction on the skin. The problem with ordinary knife "shave" biopsies is that only superficial epithelium can be reached. If this technique is used, one must be careful to get full-thickness skin to adipose tissue for adequate sampling of deeper layers.

Pigmented Lesions

Pigmented lesions of the vulva are usually intraepithelial, with the exception of melanoma. Pigmented lesions account for approximately 10% of all vulvar disease. The most common pigmented lesion is a lentigo, which is a concentration of melanocytes in the basal layer of cells. It can have the clinical appearance of a freckle, although it is more commonly confused with a nevus. The borders are fuzzy, but it is not a raised lesion. A lentigo is benign, and the diagnosis is usually made by inspection with magnification. If there is any doubt, a biopsy should always be performed.

Intraepithelial neoplasia of the vulva may appear as a pigmented lesion. Friedrich found that CIS of the vulva was more frequent in pigmented lesions than in nevi. Characteristic raised, hyperkeratotic pigmented lesions are suggestive of CIS and should be biopsied.

Bowenoid papulosis is a variant of a pigmented lesion noted by dermatologists for some time. These are small pigmented papules that develop and spread rapidly. According to dermatologists, these papules often regress spontaneously. Histologically, at least on the vulva, these are SCCs in situ. These lesions have been reported to have an aneuploid DNA pattern. Many authorities have not found bowenoid papulosis of the vulva to spontaneously regress. Regardless of the clinical characteristics, if VIN is present histologically, the physician should treat the patient accordingly.

The management of nevi can be conservative. A nevus can often be detected only microscopically. Unfortunately, a simple nevus and an early melanoma cannot be differentiated on clinical evaluation. Excisional biopsy of these raised, smooth, pigmented areas can be done easily in the physician's office. If the nevus changes in color, size, and shape, it should be removed for diagnostic purposes. After a nevus is removed, no further therapy is needed regardless of whether it is a compound, intradermal, or junctional type.

Management

Surgical excision has been the mainstay of therapy for VIN, although laser is a frequently used technique, especially for multifocal lesions, and medical management with immune modulators has gained recent prominence. An important advantage of surgical excision is that complete histologic assessment is performed; lesions with early invasion can thus be found. Most localized lesions are managed effectively by wide local excision with end-to-end approximation of the defect. The vulvar skin and mucous membrane are usually very elastic, and cosmetic results are satisfactory after uncomplicated healing. There are inadequate data to evaluate the best surgical ablative techniques, but studies are ongoing.

Excision

Wide local excision is the most commonly performed treatment of VIN. The goal of VIN surgery is to obtain a 5-mm disease-free margin. Margin status and histology results are available on final pathology results, which is a benefit of the excisional procedure. Modesitt and associates reported that recurrences were three times higher (46% vs. 17%) when margins were positive for residual VIN II and III. In the New Zealand study discussed earlier, 50% of those with positive margins versus 15% of those with negative margins required further treatment. Hillemanns and colleagues showed an overall recurrence rate of 43% in subjects retrospectively analyzed who had been heterogeneously treated with laser, photodynamic therapy, excision,

or vulvectomy. No patients recurred in the vulvectomy group ($n = 8$). In the natural history review by van Seters and colleagues, 1921 patients were surgically treated. Recurrence was noted in 19% after vulvectomy, 18% after partial vulvectomy, and 22% after local excision. Recurrences were significantly lower after free surgical margins (17%) than after positive surgical margins (47%). Progression to invasive disease occurred in 58 patients, 52% of the time after vulvectomy, and 48% of the time after local excision. In this retrospective review, the surgical approach was likely selected based on individual patient characteristics so that patients considered at higher risk for invasive cancer may have more frequently received vulvectomy. However, there is no definitive evidence or randomized controlled trial (RCT) to show that vulvectomy is associated with better outcomes and the morbidity associated with the procedure is much greater. Wide local excision is the accepted excisional procedure for VIN.

In the series by Modesitt and colleagues, 17 of 73 subjects were diagnosed with invasive cancer at the time of treatment for VIN III. Similarly, 16 of 78 patients undergoing surgical excision for VIN III had invasive cancer in the report by Husseinzadeh and Recinto. To avoid returning to the operating room for deeper reexcision and lymph node dissection, biopsies must be liberally performed preoperatively. Multiple biopsies may be required. Adequate postoperative follow-up with repeat biopsy for any suspicious lesions is also essential.

Occasionally, a skinning vulvectomy is indicated. With multicentric lesions (Fig. 2.12), the involved skin can be excised and substituted with a split-thickness skin graft taken from the buttocks or inner aspect of the thigh. This skinning vulvectomy and skin graft procedure was introduced by Rutledge and Sinclair in 1968 (Fig. 2.13). Its purpose was to replace the skin at risk in the

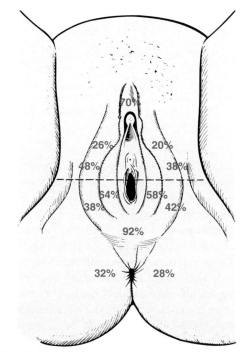

FIGURE 2.12 Plot of lesion locations in 36 patients treated for multifocal carcinoma in situ of the vulva.

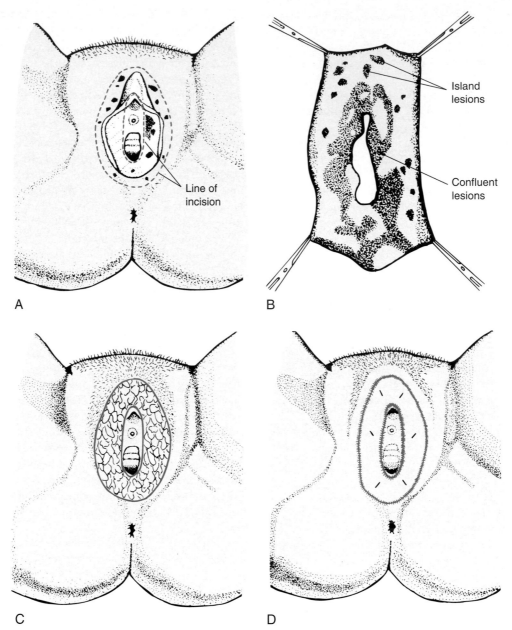

FIGURE 2.13 Skinning vulvectomy and skin graft. **A,** Excise all areas of involvement en bloc. **B,** Lesions may be isolated or confluent. **C,** Preserve all subcutaneous tissue as the graft bed. **D,** Suture the skin graft to the graft bed.

vulvar site with ectopic epidermis from a donor site. In more than 100 patients treated, the authors reported no complaints of dyspareunia or diminished sexual responsiveness. The benefits of the skinning vulvectomy and skin graft procedure are preservation of the subcutaneous tissue of the vulva and a better cosmetic and functional result (Fig. 2.14). In previous editions of this text, Creasman reported a modification of the procedure with preservation of the clitoris, in which any lesions on the glans are scraped off with a scalpel blade, and the epithelium of the glans regenerates without loss of sensation. In older adult patient, simple vulvectomy may be preferred because the skinning vulvectomy and skin graft operation requires prolonged bedrest (6–7 days) to allow the split-thickness graft to adhere to the graft bed. Thus, the potential for morbidity is

increased. The patient's wishes concerning cosmetic results and sexual function, however, must be taken into account regardless of the person's age.

Laser

Ablative therapy is an alternative to excision. The disadvantage of ablative therapy is that a necrotic ulcer on the vulva may result, and wound healing may be slow. Complete healing may take up to 3 months. The treated area is often very painful for much of that time. Many consider laser therapy the treatment of choice in the management of VIN, particularly for those who have multifocal disease. Townsend and colleagues treated 33 patients with laser therapy and reported success in 31 (94%), but 14 patients required two or more treatments, and two

FIGURE 2.14 Excellent cosmetic results are present after superficial vulvectomy and skin graft for vulvar intraepithelial neoplasia.

TABLE 2.7	CO₂ Laser Vaporization of the Vulva
Instrument	CO₂ laser, colposcopic, micromanipulator
Power density	600–1000 W/cm²
Depth of destruction	Nonhairy areas <1 mm
Hairy areas	>3 mm
Lateral margins	"Brush"
Anesthesia	General, local
Analgesia	Significant postlaser pain: narcotics

thickness of the epithelium was 0.52 mm (range, 0.1–1.9 mm). In patients with hair follicles involved with VIN, the mean depth of involvement was 1.9 mm (range, 1–3.4 mm). Only 19 patients had appendiceal involvement. Age did not seem to affect the thickness of involved epithelium. Multifocal lesions were present in 64% of all patients. The most common sites were the labia minora, posterior fourchette, and perineum. Based on this study, the authors believe that 1-mm destruction of non–hair-bearing epithelium is adequate treatment. If skin appendages are involved, 2.5 to 3 mm is required (Fig. 2.15). When performing excision, the burn level does not need to be carried to the level of the subcutaneous fat. Also, the carbon from the surgical site can be wiped during the procedure to be certain that the shiny white lower dermis is preserved. Reid has defined surgical planes in the vulva as a guide to laser therapy. The first plane is the surface epithelium only, which includes the basement membrane. Opalescent cell debris is noted through the heat char. Healing is rapid, with good cosmetic results. The second plane involves the dermal papillae, with necrosis extending to the deep papillary area. The appearance is a homogeneous yellow color that resembles a chamois cloth. Again, healing is rapid with good cosmesis. The third plane affects the upper and midreticular area, where the pilosebaceous ducts are located. Some hypertrophy may appear in this area during the healing process. The fourth plane affects the deep reticular area, and "sand grains" can be visualized. Healing is slow and usually occurs by granulation from the sides. Skin grafting may be required. Destruction to the third plane is adequate for hair-bearing tissue; plane one to two is the depth needed for non–hair-bearing skin.

After laser therapy, the vulva is covered with Silvadene. Sitz baths, topical lidocaine, and rinsing of the vulva with water after urination and defecation are important. A hair dryer is then used to dry the area. Repeat application of steroids is used after each washing and drying. A local anesthetic can be applied for mild to moderate pain control. Oral pain medication, including narcotics, may be necessary. The most severe pain is usually evident 3 to 4 days after the laser therapy. Laser therapy is particularly effective around the areas where excision can lead to external sphincter weakening.

Cavitational Ultrasonic Surgical Aspirator

A cavitational ultrasonic surgical aspirator (CUSA) is a less frequently used ablative option. In a randomized prospective

patients required five laser treatments. The results published by Baggish and Dorsey were similar; 32 of 35 patients were believed to have been cured from their disease, 26 of 35 patients required three or more treatments, and two women had six treatments. In the review article of the 253 patients treated with laser, 23% recurred.

Only a small portion of the vulva can be treated on an outpatient basis. Patients require general anesthesia if large areas of the vulva are treated at one time. Pain, which is severe in some patients, is the main complication with laser therapy. Bleeding and infection have also been reported. The cosmetic results appear to be excellent. It appears that laser therapy can be an acceptable treatment modality, but patients must be carefully evaluated before treatment to rule out invasive carcinoma (Table 2.7). Greater expertise with the laser is required for this therapy than is needed for cervical vaporization. The depth of destruction must be controlled. Too deep a wound can result in long-term ulcers, which may take some time to heal and cause considerable discomfort. Benedet and colleagues evaluated 165 women with VIN. Of the 122 patients with VIN III, the mean

First plane

Second plane

Sweat glands

Pilosebaceous duct

Third plane

Epidermis

Papillary dermis

Reticular dermis

Hair follicle

Fat

FIGURE 2.15 "Planes" for therapy for vulvar intraepithelial neoplasia using a laser.

trial, von Gruenigen and associates compared outcomes from laser ablation versus CUSA. Recurrence was similar in both arms (25% overall), but subjects treated with CUSA had less postoperative pain and less scarring. Other adverse events, including infection, dysuria, adhesions, and discharge, were similar between both groups.

Imiquimod

Imiquimod 5% cream is an immune response modifier with indirect antiviral and antitumor properties. It activates macrophages and dendritic cells to release interferon-α and other cytokines that provoke an antigen-specific immune response. Imiquimod cream was first shown to be effective and safe in the treatment of HPV-associated genital warts and was subsequently evaluated and has shown great promise in the treatment of VIN. In a phase II trial completed by Le and colleagues, 33 patients with VIN were treated for 16 weeks with 5% imiquimod application; six additional subjects were unable to complete the study. At 20 weeks, 21 of 33 subjects had complete response (complete disappearance of the visible lesion and histologic regression), nine of 33 had a partial response (50% decrease from baseline measurement), and three had stable lesions. In a randomized, double-blinded controlled trial, Mathieson and associates treated 21 subjects with 5% imiquimod and 10 with placebo. There was a complete response in 17 of 21 subjects in the treatment group (complete histologic regression) and in none of the 10 subjects in the placebo group. Because of side effects, the dose was reduced in 14 of 21 women in the treatment group. Van Seters and colleagues report similar results but also include 12-month follow-up from their RCT. In 26 subjects

treated with imiquimod, histologic and virologic regression was seen in 15 and 14 subjects, respectively. In the 26 subjects who received placebo, histologic and virologic regression was seen in one and two subjects, respectively. Progression to invasive disease occurred in one subject in the treatment arm (who initially had a weak, partial response with imiquimod) and two subjects in the placebo arm. Treatment was reduced to once-weekly application in five women receiving imiquimod because of severe inflammation. Investigator-reported side effects, including erythema, erosion, vesiculation, and edema, were significantly worse in the treatment group than in the placebo group. At 20 weeks and 12 months, however, self-reported pruritus and pain were significantly better in the treatment group than in the placebo group. In a recent study of women randomized to surgical excision alone versus surgical excision followed by imiquimod, there was no difference in recurrence between groups (45% and 48%, respectively), but recurrence was more common in women with multifocal disease. Cidofovir, an antiviral agent with activity against HPV, has also been reported as treatment for VIN. In an RCT (n = 180) comparing imiquimod and cidofovir, 46% of patients in each treatment group achieved a complete clinical response at the 6-week posttreatment visit. However, grade 3 or higher toxicities were more significant in the imiquimod group (46%) compared with the cidofovir group (37%) with grade 3 vulvar pain reported in 2% of cidofovir users and 1% of imiquimod users.

One of the obvious benefits of medical therapy is avoidance of disfiguring surgery. Randomized trials show promise in its use as a primary therapy for VIN, and it has been relatively well tolerated, but dose reductions have been necessary in all trials for a considerable number of subjects. The trials previously mentioned varied in application frequency from once per week to three times per week when tolerated. Because some of the main benefits are quality-of-life related, it will be important to evaluate the side effects and complications of imiquimod versus excisional procedures. Even in women who did not receive a complete response, a partial response was observed in many. Reduction in lesion size may be another potential application of the therapy, particularly if disease is present in a multifocal, clitoral, or sphincter distribution. Another important question for future trials is whether immune modulators have any effect on non–HPV-associated VIN; it is possible that the treatment varies depending on the origin and differentiation. Because the ISSVD classification has now changed, future trials should specifically evaluate efficacy in usual type VIN versus differentiated type VIN.

After initial diagnosis and treatment, American College of Obstetrics and Gynecology guidelines recommend repeat visualization of the vulva at 6 months and 12 months and annually thereafter. An increased risk of recurrence has previously been associated with increasing lesion size, positive margins, smoking history, and multifocal disease.

In summary, it is important to remember that these lesions often develop in young women who remain asymptomatic. Women should be taught vulvar self-examination to identify early lesions. Physical examination performed by a physician will likely become inadvertently less frequent as Pap screening guidelines continue to evolve, and self-examination may become more important in the future. Postmenopausal women should be instructed in the importance of annual vulvar examinations, even if Pap screening is not required. The goal of earlier diagnosis and intervention is more successful therapy that is also less radical. Early diagnosis depends on careful vulvar examination under a bright light at regular intervals. Biopsy must be done on any suspicious lesions, and if the histologic report confirms intraepithelial neoplasia, an examination for multicentric foci should follow. The therapy of choice depends on the extent of disease, the location of the lesions, and the personal desires of the patient.

For the bibliography list, log onto www.expertconsult.com ⟨http://www.expertconsult.com⟩

Invasive Cervical Cancer

Krishnansu S. Tewari, MD, Bradley J. Monk, MD

KEY POINTS

1. Conservative management of early staged cervical cancer in young women should be considered if childbearing is important to that patient.
2. In many developing countries, cervical cancer is the leading cause of cancer death in young women.
3. Adenocarcinoma of the cervix is increasing in frequency.
4. Positron emission tomography is a very sensitive method for detecting the extent of cervical cancer.
5. Adjuvant chemotherapy using cisplatin and concomitant radiation therapy is the standard of care for locally advanced cervical cancer.

GENERAL OBSERVATIONS

Anatomy

The cervix (Latin for "neck") is a narrow, cylindrical segment of the uterus; it enters the vagina through the anterior vaginal wall and lies, in most cases, at a right angle to it. In the average patient, the cervix measures 2 to 4 cm in length and is contiguous with the inferior aspect of the uterine corpus. The point of juncture of the uterus and the cervix is known as the isthmus; this area is marked by slight constriction of the lumen. Anteriorly, the cervix is separated from the bladder by fatty tissue and is connected laterally to the broad ligament and parametrium (through which it obtains its blood supply). The lower intravaginal portion of the cervix, a free segment that projects into the vault of the vagina, is covered with mucous membrane. The cervix opens into the vaginal cavity through the external os. The cervical canal extends from the anatomic external os to the internal os, where it joins the uterine cavity. The histologic internal os is where there is a transition from endocervical to endometrial glands. **The intravaginal portion of the cervix (portio vaginalis, exocervix) is covered with stratified squamous epithelium that is essentially identical to the epithelium of the vagina. The endocervical mucosa is arranged in branching folds (plicae palmatae) and is lined by cylindrical, columnar epithelium.** The stroma of the cervix consists of connective tissue with stratified muscle fibers and elastic tissue. The elastic tissue is found primarily around the walls of the larger blood vessels.

The stratified squamous epithelium of the portio vaginalis is composed of several layers that are conventionally described as basal, parabasal, intermediate, and superficial. The basal layer consists of a single row of cells and rests on a thin basement membrane. This is the layer in which active mitosis occurs. The parabasal and intermediate layers together constitute the prickle-cell layer, which is analogous to the same layer in the epidermis. The superficial layer varies in thickness, depending on the degree of estrogen stimulation. It consists primarily of flattened cells that show an increasing degree of cytoplasmic acidophilia toward the surface. The thickness and the glycogen content of the epithelium increase after estrogen stimulation and account for the therapeutic effect of estrogens in atrophic vaginitis. The staining of glycogen in the normal epithelium of the portio vaginalis is the basis of the Schiller test.

Epidemiologic Studies
Clinical Profile
In the United States, the mortality from cervical cancer in 1945 was 15 of 100,000 women. This had declined to approximately 4.6 of 100,000 by 1986 and 3.4 of 100,000 by 1991. It is unclear whether the mortality rate from cervical cancer is falling as a result of cervical cytologic screening and intervention at the in situ stage or whether cervical screening has caused an increase in the proportion of early-stage cancer at diagnosis and registration. After therapy for invasive disease, adequate follow-up is the key to early detection of a recurrence (Table 3.1). The yield of examinations such as intravenous pyelography (IVP), computed tomography (CT) scan, and chest radiograph in patients with initial early disease (stages I–IIa) is so low that many have discontinued their routine use.

West studied the age of registration and the age of death of women with cervical cancer in South Wales. He found that the observed age at death was very close to 59 years regardless of stage and age at diagnosis. Although the 5-year survival rate of women with localized (early-stage) cervical cancer was much higher than that of women with nonlocalized (late-stage)

cancer, the women with localized cancer tended to be younger than those with advanced cancer. Calculations of expected age at death of the whole population suggest that more than half the advantage in survival rate shown by women with early-stage cancers is a result of the diagnosis of the former in younger women.

Christopherson and colleagues reported that the percentage of patients diagnosed as having stage I disease increased by 78% in the population studied from 1953 to 1965. The increase was most remarkable in younger women. The authors concluded that the major problem in cervical cancer control was the screening of older women. Older women had higher incidence rates; the percentage with stage I disease also decreased with each decade, reaching a low of 15% for those 70 years of age and older. These older women with cervical cancer are rarely screened and contribute heavily to the death rate. The initial advanced stage contributes to the patient population with advanced recurrent cervical cancer. These patients, therefore, deserve very close posttreatment observation in an effort to detect a recurrence in its earliest possible form.

In 2011, there were 12,710 new cases of invasive cervical cancer and 4290 deaths from this disease in the United States. **In fact, for the past decade, the annual incidence and mortality rates due to cervical cancer have been approximately 12,000 and 4,000, respectively.** It is particularly distressing that more than one-third of women diagnosed will die from a disease that is largely preventable by vaccination and screening. There is no other human malignancy for which we have identified the causative agent, have successfully implemented excellent screening programs, and now have efficacious and tolerable prophylactic vaccination available (Fig. 3.2). Oncogenic subtypes of the human papillomavirus (HPV) have been identified as the etiologic cause of cervical neoplasia (Fig. 3.1). The power, consistency, and specificity of the association between subclinical HPV infection and cervical neoplasia raise the strong possibility that this relationship is causal. The biologic plausibility of this is supported by evidence that this sexually transmitted oncogenic virus often produces persistent asymptomatic infection of metaplastic epithelium in the cervical transformation zone.

Epidemiologic surveillance studies performed in the United States during the past 2 decades have documented decreased incidence rates for invasive cervical cancer. Ethnic and racial disparities, however, still exist. In a Surveillance, Epidemiology and End Results (SEER) analysis of 13 US cancer registries containing cases from 1992 to 2003, Hispanic whites had the highest incidence rate of cervical cancer overall (24 per 100,000), squamous cell carcinoma (SCC) (18 per 100,000), and adenocarcinoma (5 per 10,000). Non-Hispanic whites had the lowest rates of cervical cancer overall (11 per 100,000) and SCC (7 per 100,000), and African Americans had the lowest rate of adenocarcinoma (2 per 100,000). In a recent study using data obtained from the Cancer in North America (CINA) deluxe 1995 to 2004 database created by the North American Association of Central Cancer Registries (NAACCR), African American and Hispanic US populations continue to have the highest rates of invasive cervical cancer compared with non-Hispanic whites. Variations

TABLE 3.1 Proposed Schedule for Interval Evaluation of Cervical Cancer after Radiotherapy or Surgery (Asymptomatic Patient*)

Year	Frequency	Examination
1	3 months	Pelvic examination, Pap smear
	6 months	Chest radiography, CBC, BUN, creatinine
	1 year	IVP or CT scan with contrast
2	4 months	Pelvic examination, Pap smear
	1 year	Chest radiography, CBC, BUN, creatinine, IVP or CT scan with contrast
3–5	6 months	Pelvic examination, Pap smear

*Symptomatic patients should have appropriate examination where indicated.
BUN, Blood urea nitrogen; CBC, complete blood count; CT, computed tomography; IVP, intravenous pyelogram; Pap, Papanicolaou.

FIGURE 3.1 Human papillomavirus genome. (From microbiologybytes.com.)

FIGURE 3.2 Human papillomavirus prophylactic vaccine. (From www.cancer.gov.)

in screening utilization and socioeconomic status are thought to account for the majority of the racial/ethnic disparities.

In November 2014, the nine-valent, HPV9 (providing protection against HPV-6, -11, -16, -18, -31, -33, -45, -52, and -58), was approved by the US Food and Drug Administration (FDA) for the same indications as HPV-4 (ie, GARDASIL).

MICROINVASIVE CARCINOMA OF THE CERVIX

The diagnosis and management of microinvasive carcinoma of the cervix remains controversial. The evolution and sometimes revolution concerning the diagnosis and management have occurred since Mestwerdt, in 1947, observed that invasive cervical cancer diagnosed only microscopically could be cured by nonradical surgery. During the past 3 decades, definitions and treatment plans have changed dramatically. It is hoped that most of these changes had occurred as new data became available and that changes were therefore logical. Much of the confusion can be related to the fact that the Federation of International Gynecologists and Obstetricians (FIGO) has changed the criteria for early-stage invasive carcinoma of the cervix since 1960. These changes were made as additional information in regard to this disease process became available. Other influences, however, also contributed to the confusion. Over the years, as many as 20 different definitions have been proposed, and as many as 27 terms have been applied to this entity. The recommended therapy has also changed, going from radical surgery with any invasion to being more conservative with various depths of invasion.

In 1971, FIGO designated stage Ia carcinoma of the cervix as cases of preclinical carcinoma. In 1973, the Society of Gynecologic Oncologists (SGO) accepted the following statement concerning the definition of microinvasive carcinoma of the cervix:

1. Cases of intraepithelial carcinoma with questionable invasion should be regarded as intraepithelial carcinoma; and
2. A microinvasive lesion should be defined as one in which a neoplastic epithelium invaded the stroma in one or more places to the depth of less than 3 mm below the base of the epithelium and in which lymphatic or vascular involvement is not demonstrated.

In 1985, for the first time, FIGO attempted to quantify the histologic definition of stage Ia carcinoma of the cervix. Stage Ia was defined as the earliest form of invasion in which minute foci of invasion are visible only microscopically. Stage Ia2 is a macroscopically measurable microcarcinoma that should not exceed 5 mm in depth and 7 mm in width. Vascular space involvement, either venous or lymphatic, should not alter staging. This definition has been criticized for several reasons. Although the upper limits of invasion for depth and width were stated, upper limits for measurement for stage Ia1 were not defined. It was therefore difficult to quantify patients in the two subgroups. Other areas of criticism were aimed at the fact that the FIGO definition could not be used as a guide for treatment, and the definition covered patients with vascular lymphatic channel involvement. These variations illustrate the problem with a specific definition.

TABLE 3.2 Stage 1a Cancer of the Cervix

Stage	Description
Ia	Cancer invasion identified only microscopically. All gross lesions, even with superficial invasion, are stage Ib cancers. Measured stromal invasion with maximum depth of 5 mm and no wider than 7 mm*
Ia1	Measured invasion of stroma up to 3 mm
Ia2	Measured invasion of stroma of 3–5 mm and no wider than 7 mm

*The depth of invasion should not be larger than 5 mm taken from the base of the epithelium, either surface or glandular, from which it originates. Vascular space involvement, either venous or lymphatic, should not alter the staging.

In 1994, FIGO, in an attempt to better qualify the definition of microinvasive carcinoma of the cervix, adopted the following definition for microinvasive carcinoma of the cervix (Table 3.2). Stage Ia1 cancers are those with stromal invasion up to 3 mm in depth and no greater than 7 mm. Stage Ia2 are when invasion is present at 3 to 5 mm in depth and no greater than 7 mm. Lymphatic vascular space involvement does not exclude a patient from this definition. The recurrence rate of patients in these two substages is probably no more than 1% to 2%. Survival of stage Ia1 approaches 99%, and stage Ia2 survival approaches 97% to 98%. This new definition allows further evaluation of what might be appropriate therapy for the different substages, particularly stage Ia2 cancers.

Vascular space involvement was not excluded from the FIGO definition for several reasons. Pathologists disagree with regard to the reproducibility of this entity. At least in one study, the number of slides prepared from the cervix depended on the incidence of capillary-like space involvement. Shrinkage artifact can lead to an overdiagnosis, and verification has been suggested with special staining to verify true capillary-like space involvement. In one study in which immunoperoxidase staining with Ulex Europaeus agglutinin 1 lectin (UEAI) was used, 10 of 32 cases of vascular space involvement were excluded in which involvement was initially thought to exist. In a combined study of 1004 patients at three reference centers, Burghardt and colleagues observed that the frequency with which angiolymphatic space involvement was detected ranged from 9% in Munich to 23% in Erlangen and finally up to 43% in Graz.

As greater experience is obtained, the tendency has been toward conservative management involving conization of the cervix if fertility preservation is desired or simple hysterectomy for superficial invasion (0–3 mm) and even in some patients with 3–5 mm of invasion. In 1978, Lohe reported on 285 patients with early stromal invasion and 134 patients with microcarcinoma. He defined early stromal invasion as only isolated, variably shaped projections with true signs of infiltration present, whereas microcarcinomas' true confluent carcinomatosis masses were present. Tumor length and depth were 10 mm and 5 mm. He stated that the three-dimensional definition of the size of the tumor is essential to the microscopic diagnosis of early stromal invasion and of microcarcinoma. In his series, 72% with early stromal invasion and 41% with microcarcinoma were treated with conservative surgery (conization or simple hysterectomy). After long-term follow-up, no patients with early stromal invasion died. Three patients with microcarcinomas have recurred and died. In a larger collected series of 435 patients with microcarcinoma, 24 (5.5%) had a recurrence of disease. Using his criteria, Lohe predicted <1% incidence of lymph node metastasis in microcarcinoma and essentially none in early stromal invasion. Boyce and colleagues have reported a large series with both "microscopic foci" of invasion (360 cases) and "occult invasion" (390 cases). Most (283) of the patients with microscopic foci invasion were treated with simple hysterectomy and only 14 with conization. After 5–15 years of follow-up, only one patient died of the disease. Most (262) of the patients with occult invasion received irradiation therapy. Most of these lesions were greater than 5 mm in depth, and all were characterized by confluent masses of neoplastic cells. Twenty-four of the 390 patients with occult invasion died of the disease in 5 years. Benedet and colleagues reported on 180 patients with microinvasion and occult invasive squamous cell carcinoma of the cervix who were examined by colposcopy during a 10-year period. Colposcopy led to the correct management in 90% of patients with occult invasive carcinoma and in 84% of patients with microinvasive cancer. Colposcopy appeared to be less sensitive in detecting microinvasive lesions than in detecting occult carcinoma. Atypical vessels indicative of early invasive cancer are often subtle and difficult to identify. They are best visualized when the cervix has been bathed in normal saline. In many cases, acetic acid can cover atypical vessels by enhancing white epithelium that obscures the vessels. Östör in Australia has made an extensive review on this subject of the literature published since 1976. As a pathologist, he has critically reviewed many of the parameters that have historically been suggested as important prognostic factors.

0–3 mm Invasion

Östör identified 3683 patients from the literature with <1 mm of invasion. Four patients had lymph node metastasis. With the incidence of lymph node metastasis in this group being essentially 0, it appears that lymphadenectomy has no place in this group of patients. There were 17 invasive recurrences and 16 cancer-related deaths. In several cases that resulted in death, patients refused further therapy or follow-up. Therefore, the death rate in this group of patients appears to be <0.1%, invasive recurrences were approximately 0.4% (Table 3.3).

Östör identified 1324 patients who had invasion of 1–3 mm. Of these, 333 definitely had lymphadenectomies with seven nodal metastases. At least two of these probably had >3 mm of stromal invasion. The incidence based on these figures suggests that lymph node metastasis would be approximately 1%. There were 26 invasive recurrences and 6 deaths. Some of these patients probably had >3 mm of invasion and also included some patients with "microinvasive adenocarcinoma". In a review of reports over the last 15 years, most of which occurred within the last decade, Creasman and colleagues identified 1704 patients who had an invasion of 0–3 mm and 17 (1%) recurred. Only three (0.17%) died of their cancer. These recurrences were in patients with squamous lesions.

The management of early invasive lesions (0–3 mm of invasion, Fig. 3.3A–C) has generally been agreed on by the gynecologic oncology community. **Patients with FIGO stage Ia1 and SGO criteria for microinvasion could be treated conservatively with simple hysterectomy, or if continued fertility is desired conization only, provided surgical margins are free of cancer.** Most of the data in the literature concerning patients with 0–3 mm of invasion are based on conservative therapy, although some patients have had lymphadenectomies. From collected series, it would, therefore, appear that the role of vascular space involvement in this group of patients does not predict lymph node metastasis or recurrence. Although still in dispute, a growing number of investigators apparently do not use capillary-like space involvement as an exclusion criterion for this stage.

3–5 mm Invasion

Östör identified 674 patients in this category of which 221 definitely had lymphadenectomies, 6% had nodal metastasis. If most or all of the other patients had lymphadenectomy, which is possible, and the results of all of the nodes were negative, the figure would be close to 2%. Twentyfive (4%) patients developed an invasive recurrence, and 13 (2%) died of their disease. Twenty-three percent of the patients were said to have had capillary-like space involvement. Creasman identified from the literature 264 patients with 3–5 mm invasion who had lymphadenectomy in which vascular space involvement was specifically evaluated. In patients with vascular space involvement, 2 of 83 (2.4%) and 7 of 181 (3.8%) without vascular space involvement had lymph node metastasis. In the literature, 488 patients with 3–5 mm were identified and 15 (3%) developed a recurrence with 9 (1.8%) dying of cancer deaths. The recurrence and death rates in patients with 3–5 mm approaches

TABLE 3.3   Lymph Node Metastases, Recurrences and Deaths in Stage Ia Carcinoma of the Cervix

Invasion Depth (mm)	No. of Patients	Invasion Recurrence	Died of Cancer	No. With CLSI	No. With Positive Nodes
0–3	5007	35 (0.7%)	10 (0.2%)	182 (3.6%)	8/666 (1.2%)
3–5	674	25 (4%)	13 (2%)	124 (18.4%)	14/221 (6.3%)

CLSI, capillary-like space involvement.
Modified from Östör AG: Pandora's Box or Ariodne's Thread? Definition and prognostic significance of microinvasion into uterine cervix. Ann Pathol, 105, 1995.

FIGURE 3.3 *A,* Microinvasion (stage Ia1) of squamous cell carcinoma of the cervix. Invasion of less than 1 mm, no confluency or vascular space involvement; true microinvasion. *B,* Microcarcinoma with less than 3 mm of invasion but with vascular space involvement. *C,* Microcarcinoma "spray" type with less than 1 mm of invasion.

those with 0–3 mm invasion. Most, but not all, of patients treated for 3–5 mm invasion were managed with radical hysterectomy and pelvic lymphadenectomy. However, there are patients in this category who have been managed only with conization. In the 3–5 mm range, vascular space status does not appear to correlate with lymph node metastasis. There is limited experience with patients with these clinical lesions, but patients with limited invasion of 3–5 mm have a much greater incidence of lymph node metastasis (7%), which should be treated as a stage Ib cancer.

The data on patients with 3–5 mm invasion still remain fairly limited. With a very low incidence of lymph node metastasis (2–3%), it seems reasonable to evaluate the role of more conservative therapy in this group of patients. This may be done after consultation with the pathologist and gynecologic oncologist. If one is concerned about the 3% incidence of lymph node metastasis, these nodes can be evaluated with laparoscopy or retroperitoneal lymphadenectomy. If there is no evidence of extrauterine disease via these procedures, simple hysterectomy or even conization may be reasonable treatments. Twenty years ago, it was not unusual for investigators to suggest radical hysterectomy and pelvic lymphadenectomy for any degree of stromal invasion. With increased experience, more conservative therapy was found to be just as efficacious as radical therapy. It appears that we are now in the same arena for 3–5 mm today as we were for 0–3 mm two decades ago. Although vascular space involvement does not appear to predict lymph node metastasis with 3–5 mm invasion, anecdotal reports in the literature have suggested that recurrences are higher in patients with capillary-like space involvement but with no metastasis in the lymph nodes.

It may be of significance that with progressively greater depth of stromal invasion, there is an increased risk of angiolymphatic space involvement. In point of fact, Fuller et al from the Memorial Sloan-Kettering Cancer Center detected a linear relationship between depth of cervical stromal invasion and the presence of angiolymphatic invasion. Although vascular space involvement was predictive of recurrence to the same degree it was predictive of nodal metastases, when stratified for the latter, vascular invasion lost its adverse prognostic effects. Östör noted in his review that 496 (14%) of 3597 patients who had capillarylike space involvement did not have an invasive recurrence. Morice et al retrospectively studied the clinicopathologic features of 193 patients who underwent radical surgery and lymphadenectomy for early stage cervical carcinoma, and found that both lymphovascular and nodal status were prognostic factors upon multivariate analysis. It was noteworthy that among a subgroup of 89 patients with a small tumor (<2 cm) and absence of nodal or isthmic involvement, that the overall survival was significantly correlated with the presence of lymphovascular space involvement. Recently, in an analysis of 93 patients who had undergone resection of early stage lesions, Memarzadeh et al demonstrated that the presence of lymphovascular space invasion in the parametria was an independent predictor of metastases in the pelvic ($P < 0.001$) and para-aortic ($P < 0.05$) lymphatic chains, an altogether not surprising finding. Hopefully, the role of lymphovascular space involvement will be further clarified and possibly even resolved in the future as more data are accumulated.

The Gynecologic Oncology Group (GOG) reported 50 patients with 3–5 mm invasion in the conization specimen. All underwent a radical hysterectomy and pelvic lymphadenectomy. The uterine specimen showed no evidence of residual disease. There were 23% with lymphatic space involvement (LSI), but none of the patients had positive nodes and there have been no recurrences. (Note that the term LSI is used interchangeably with vascular space involvement [VSI].)

In a report from Japan, 402 patients were identified with 0–5 mm invasion. These authors noted that 72 (18%), although had depth of invasion satisfying the FIGO definition, had >7 mm of horizontal spread. As the depth of invasion increased, there was a greater possibility that horizontal spread was >7 mm (6% stage Ia1 and 61% for stage Ia2). Lymph node metastasis was 1.4% for true Ia1 and 3.4% for Ia2 cancers. For those with >7 mm spread, lymph node metastasis was 7.4%. LSI was 18% in those >7 mm compared to 3.6% if <7 mm. Four patients had a recurrence, but three recurrences occurred in those with >7 mm lateral spread. Other authors have noted recurrences and deaths in patients with 0–5 mm invasion; however, when lateral spread was evaluated, it was >7 mm. Tumor volume is an important prediction for metastasis, recurrence, and cancer-related deaths. Now that there are quantifiable perimeters for stage Ia cancers, more precise data can be evaluated with regard to risk and appropriate therapy for stage Ia2 can be considered.

Conservative management for stage Ia2 carcinoma of the cervix does not seem unreasonable in light of the fact that some investigators have suggested that conservative therapy might be feasible for patients with "small stage Ib" cervical cancers. Girardi and colleagues from Graz reported on a series of 69 patients with small stage Ib carcinomas of the cervix. Treatment consisted of conization or simple hysterectomy in 27, radical hysterectomy with lymphadenectomy in 25, radical vaginal hysterectomy in 13, and conization followed by radiotherapy in 4. No patient developed a recurrence during the ensuing 2–35 years. Two of the 25 patients with lymphadenectomy had one positive lymph node each. This study comes from a group of investigators who over the years have meticulously evaluated pathologic specimens and traditionally have been surgically aggressive. Östör reviewed the literature since 1976 with regard to conization as definitive therapy for stage Ia cancers. He identified 655 patients with 0–5 mm invasion treated with conization, which resulted in 12 invasive recurrences and one death.

CLINICAL PROFILE OF INVASIVE CANCER

A substantial and well-publicized screening program is needed to make the public and the profession more aware of cervical cancer as the possible cause of even minimal gynecologic symptoms. All public education should emphasize the prevention and cure of cancer, and a more optimistic attitude would help motivate patients and physicians to seek appropriate action. The need for early diagnosis rests on the incontrovertible fact that definite cure, in actuarial terms, is readily achieved

when cervical cancer is minimal—but almost impossible if the tumor is given time to grow and spread to the pelvic wall or into adjacent structures such as the bladder and rectum. The gradient of percentage curability from early invasive cancer to late, grossly invasive disease is such a steep one that even a moderate reduction in tumor size could not fail to create a substantial improvement in curability. It is true, of course, as with other cancers, that some carcinomas of the cervix grow more rapidly than others. The basis for this difference in growth rate is still beyond our knowledge, but it is not beyond our capability to prevent unnecessary growing time. Even the relatively slow-growing malignancy, if given enough time, will become incurable, and the most rapid-growing tumor, if diagnosed while of still moderate dimension, is definitely curable. The earlier that most tumors are detected and treated, the better will be the chance of cure. A Pap smear from a patient with early invasive SCC illustrates a typical multinucleated "tadpole" cell (Fig. 3.4). Cytology and colposcopy are valuable tools in the eradication of cervical cancer. Every opportunity should be taken to disseminate modern concepts of cancer control to schools of nursing and other paramedical organizations because there is still a need for a more coordinated effort in these fields. The burden should not be left with physicians alone. The frequency with which invasive cervical cancer occurs in the United States is unknown, but the best incidence data indicate a rate of approximately 8 to 10 per 100,000/year (Fig. 3.5). The incidence and mortality rates in the United States have been slowly declining (Fig. 3.6). The occurrence of cervical cancer is apparently less frequent in Norway and Sweden than in the United States. However, in the underdeveloped areas of the world, the frequency of cervical cancer is more noteworthy, relative to the overall cancer problem, especially compared with that in the United States (see Table 3.2) and Western Europe.

In many South American and Asian countries, cervical cancer accounts for the largest percentage of cancer deaths in women. One wonders whether nutritional deficiencies in these underdeveloped nations play a role in the etiology of cervical cancer. Orr and colleagues reported that abnormal vitamin levels were more commonly present in patients with cervical cancer. When compared with control values, levels of plasma

FIGURE 3.4 Multinucleated "tadpole" cell–early invasive squamous cell carcinoma.

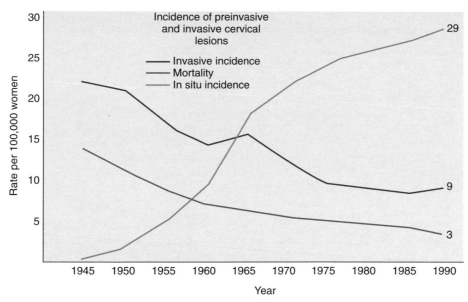

FIGURE 3.5 American Cancer Society data for 1991. Cervical cancer incidence and mortality.

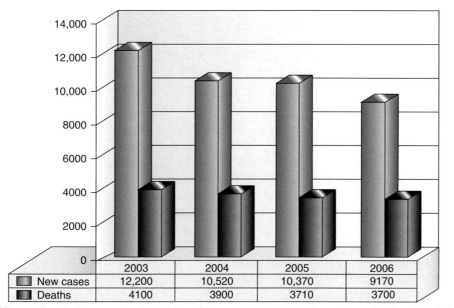

	2003	2004	2005	2006
New cases	12,200	10,520	10,370	9170
Deaths	4100	3900	3710	3700

FIGURE 3.6 Cervical cancer in the United States: 2003–2006. (From Jermal, Siegel R, Ward E, et al. Cancer statistics, 2006. *CA Cancer J Clin* 2006;56:106.)

folate, beta-carotene, and vitamin C were significantly lower in patients with cervical cancer. Personal cigarette smoking and exposure to passive smoke as risk factors for cervical carcinoma have been examined in case-control studies. Personal cigarette smoking increases the risk of cervical cancer after adjustment for age, educational level, church attendance, and sexual activity. The adjusted risk estimate associated with being a current smoker was 3.42; for having smoked for 5 or more pack-years, it was 2.81; and for having smoked at least 100 lifetime cigarettes, it was 2.21. The adjusted risk estimate associated with passive smoke exposure for 3 hours or more per day was 2.96. This study, reported by Slattery and colleagues in 1989, has been reinforced by others, confirming a strong association of smoking and increased risk of SCC of the cervix.

Some studies suggest that cancer of the cervix is more frequent among oral contraceptive users; however, these studies may be influenced by confounding factors such as early onset of sexual activity after puberty, multiple sexual partners, and previous history of sexually transmitted diseases. Ursin and colleagues reported a twofold greater risk of adenocarcinoma of the cervix, especially among those who used oral contraceptives for 12 years or more.

Because of the cervix's sensitivity to hormonal influences, it may be considered biologically plausible that oral contraceptives could induce or promote cervical carcinoma. Piver reviewed a large number of early investigations of this issue and failed to show a consistent association. Moreover, these data are based on exposure to oral contraceptive preparations that contained

TABLE 3.4	Histologic Classification of Cervical Cancer	

Epithelial Tumors

Nonglandular	Glandular	Other, Including Mixed
Squamous cell carcinoma	Adenocarcinoma, usual endocervical type	Adenosquamous
Verrucous carcinoma	Mucinous adenocarcinoma	Glassy cell carcinoma
Warty (condylomatous) carcinoma	Endometrioid adenocarcinoma	Mucoepidermoid carcinoma
Papillary squamotransitional carcinoma	Well-differentiated villoglandular adenocarcinoma	Adenoid cystic carcinoma
Lymphoepithelial-like carcinoma	Adenoma malignum (minimal deviation)	Adenoid basal carcinoma
Sarcomatoid carcinoma	Intestinal-like adenocarcinoma	Small cell carcinoma
	Signet ring cell adenocarcinoma	Classical carcinoid tumor
	Colloid adenocarcinoma	Gestational choriocarcinoma
	Clear cell adenocarcinoma	
	Serous papillary adenocarcinoma	
	Mesonephric adenocarcinoma	

Nonepithelial Tumors

Mesenchymal Tumors	Germ Cell Tumors	Miscellaneous
Carcinosarcoma	Mature teratoma	Melanoma
Leiomyosarcoma	Immature teratoma	Lymphoma
Epithelioid leiomyosarcoma	Yolk sac tumor	Primitive neuroectodermal tumor
Extrauterine endometrial stromal sarcoma	Nongestational choriocarcinoma	
Adenosarcoma		
Embryonal rhabdomyosarcoma		
Granulocytic sarcoma (chloroma)		

From Tewari KS, Monk BJ, Tumors of the cervix. In: Raghavan D, Brecher ML, Johnson DH, et al, eds. *Textbook of Uncommon Cancer*, ed 3. Hoboken, NJ, 2006, John Wiley & Sons, Ltd.

high doses of estrogen and progestin and are no longer available.

In most large series, approximately 75% to 80% of malignant lesions of the cervix are squamous cell, but other lesions are possible (Table 3.4). Most information regarding etiology and epidemiology is pertinent only to the more common squamous cell lesions.

The greatest risk for cervical cancer is not ever having a Pap test or obtaining one infrequently. Everywhere in the world where the incidence of cervical cancer and its death rates have decreased, an active screening program is present. The older patients have a higher incidence of cervical cancer, at least in the United States, and these women have the most infrequent Pap smear screening.

Symptoms

A typical patient with clinically obvious cervical cancer is a multiparous woman between 45 and 55 years who married and delivered her first child at an early age, usually before 20 years of age. Probably the first symptom of early cancer of the cervix is a thin, watery, blood-tinged vaginal discharge that frequently goes unrecognized by the patient. The classic symptom is intermittent, painless metrorrhagia or spotting only postcoitally or after douching, although this is not the most common symptom. As the malignancy enlarges, the bleeding episodes become heavier and more frequent, and they last longer. The patient may also describe what seems to her to be an increase in the amount and duration of her regular menstrual flow;

ultimately, the bleeding becomes continuous. In postmenopausal women, the bleeding is more likely to prompt early medical attention.

Late symptoms or indicators of more advanced disease include the development of pain referred to the flank or leg, which is usually secondary to the involvement of the ureters, pelvic wall, or sciatic nerve routes. Many patients complain of dysuria, hematuria, rectal bleeding, or obstipation resulting from bladder or rectal invasion. Distant metastasis and persistent edema of one or both lower extremities as a result of lymphatic and venous blockage by extensive pelvic wall disease are late manifestations of primary disease and frequent manifestations of recurrent disease. Massive hemorrhage and development of uremia with profound inanition may also occur and occasionally be the initial presenting symptom.

Gross Appearance

The gross clinical appearance of carcinoma of the cervix varies considerably and depends on the regional mode of involvement and the nature of the particular lesion's growth pattern. Three categories of gross lesions have traditionally been described. The most common is the exophytic lesion, which usually arises on the ectocervix and often grows to form a large, friable, polypoid mass that can bleed profusely. These exophytic lesions sometimes arise within the endocervical canal and distend the cervix and the endocervical canal, creating the so-called barrel-shaped lesion. A second type of cervical carcinoma is created by an infiltrating tumor that tends to show little visible ulceration or exophytic mass but is initially seen as a stone-hard cervix that regresses slowly with radiation therapy. A third category of lesion is the ulcerative tumor (Fig. 3.7), which usually erodes a portion of the cervix, often replacing the cervix and a portion of the upper vaginal vault with a large crater associated with local infection and seropurulent discharge.

Routes of Spread

The main routes of spread of carcinoma of the cervix are as follows:

1. Into the vaginal mucosa, extending microscopically down beyond visible or palpable disease
2. Into the myometrium of the lower uterine segment and corpus, particularly with lesions originating in the endocervix
3. Into the paracervical lymphatics and from there to the most commonly involved lymph nodes (ie, the obturator, hypogastric, and external iliac nodes)
4. Direct extension into adjacent structures or parametria, which may reach to the obturator fascia and the wall of the true pelvis. Extension of the disease to involve the bladder or rectum can result, with or without the occurrence of a vesicovaginal or rectovaginal fistula.

The prevalence of lymph node disease correlated well with the stage of the malignancy in several anatomic studies. Lymph node involvement in stage I is between 15% and 20%; in stage II, it is between 25% and 40%; and in stage III, it is assumed that at least 50% have positive nodes. Variations are sometimes seen with different material. The best study of lymph node involvement in cervical cancer was done by Henriksen (Fig. 3.8). The nodal groups described by Henriksen follow.

Primary Group

1. The parametrial nodes, which are the small lymph nodes traversing the parametria
2. The paracervical or ureteral nodes, located above the uterine artery where it crosses the ureter
3. The obturator or hypogastric nodes surrounding the obturator vessels and nerves
4. The hypogastric nodes, which course along the hypogastric vein near its junction with the external iliac vein
5. The external iliac nodes, which are a group of six to eight nodes that tend to be uniformly larger than the nodes of the other iliac groups
6. The sacral nodes, which were originally included in the secondary group

Secondary Group

1. The common iliac nodes
2. The inguinal nodes, which consist of the deep and superficial femoral lymph nodes
3. The periaortic nodes

In his autopsy studies, Henriksen plotted the percentage of nodal involvement for treated and untreated patients (Figs. 3.9 and 3.10). Distribution is, as one would expect, with a greater number of involved nodes found in the region of the cervix than in distant metastases. Although the series was an autopsy study, Henriksen found that only 27% had metastasis above the aortic chain. Cervical cancer kills by local extension, with ureteral obstruction in a high percentage of patients.

In 1980, the Gynecologic Oncology Group (GOG) reported the results of a series of 545 patients with cancer of the cervix who were surgically staged within their institutions. This study was prompted because traditional ports of radiation therapy were destined to treatment failure when the disease extended to the periaortic nodes (Fig. 3.11). They found periaortic node involvement in 18.2% of patients with stage IIa disease and up to 33.3% in patients with stage IVa disease. Piver correlated the size of the cervical lesion with the incidence of lymph node metastasis in stage I disease (Table 3.5).

When clinical staging was compared with surgical staging, inaccuracies were found of the magnitude of a 22.9% misstaged occurrence in stage IIb disease and a 64.4% misstaged occurrence in stage IIIb disease. These data raise the question of whether knowing that disease has spread to the periaortic area enables the clinician to institute therapeutic modalities that can

FIGURE 3.7 Ulcerative squamous cell carcinoma of the cervix.

TABLE 3.5 Size of Cervical Lesion and Lymph Node Metastasis in Stage Ib Cervical Cancer

Site (cm)	Patients	Patients With Metastasis	Patients (%)
≤1	22	4	18.1
2-3	72	16	22.1
4-5	45	16	35.5
≥6	6	3	50
Total	**145**	**39**	**26.9**

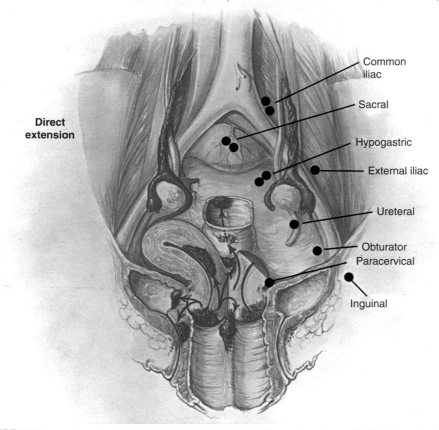

FIGURE 3.8 Lymph node chains draining the cervix. (From Henriksen E. The lymphatic spread of carcinoma of the cervix and of the body of the uterus; a study of 420 necropsies. *Am J Obstet Gynecol* 1949;58:924-942.)

FIGURE 3.9 Percentage involvement of draining lymph nodes in treated patients with cervical cancer. (From Henriksen E. The lymphatic spread of carcinoma of the cervix and of the body of the uterus; a study of 420 necropsies. *Am J Obstet Gynecol* 1949;58:924-942.)

FIGURE 3.10 Percentage involvement of draining lymph nodes in untreated patients with cervical cancer. (From Henriksen E. The lymphatic spread of carcinoma of the cervix and of the body of the uterus; a study of 420 necropsies. *Am J Obstet Gynecol* 1949;58:924-942.)

FIGURE 3.11 A computed tomography scan of the abdomen illustrating very enlarged periaortic nodes that have eroded a portion of the vertebral bone on the right.

TABLE 3.6 Percentage Increase of Pelvic and Periaortic Node Metastasis by Clinical Stage

Clinical Stage	Positive Pelvic Nodes	Positive Periaortic Nodes
I	15.4	6.3
II	28.6	16.5
III	47.0	8.6

result in increased salvage. In other words, does the treatment of patients with spread of disease beyond the pelvis result in more cures? Berman and colleagues, reporting the GOG experience with staging laparotomy, indicated that 20% of 436 patients (stages IIb–IVa) were found to have metastatic disease to periaortic nodes. He also reported that 25% of these patients, or 5% of those surgically staged, demonstrated a 3-year, disease-free survival. Most of the patients with known periaortic node involvement received extended postoperative field irradiation.

Cumulative results from many studies utilizing lymphadenectomy in the surgical staging of cervix cancer have shown increased frequency of positive pelvic nodes, as shown in Table 3.6.

GLANDULAR TUMORS OF THE CERVIX

Approximately 75% to 80% of cervical cancers are SCCs, and most of the remaining cases are adenocarcinomas. There appears to be an increase in the frequency of cervical adenocarcinomas, but this may be a result of the decrease in the incidence of invasive squamous cell lesions. With respect to histopathology, a SEER population study conducted on cases registered from 1973 to 2002 noted increasing numbers of adenocarcinomas despite a general decline, suggesting the inefficiency of conventional screening for these tumors. Adenocarcinoma arises from the endocervical mucous-producing gland cells, and because of its origin within the cervix, it may be present for a

considerable time before it becomes clinically evident. These lesions are characteristically bulky neoplasms that expand the cervical canal and create the so-called barrel-shaped lesions of the cervix. The spread pattern of these lesions is similar to that of SCC, with direct extension accompanied by metastases to regional pelvic nodes as the primary routes of dissemination. Local recurrence is more common in these lesions, and this has resulted in the commonly held belief that they are more radioresistant than are their squamous counterpart. It seems more likely, however, that the bulky, expansive nature of these endocervical lesions, rather than a differential in radiosensitivity, accounts for the local recurrence. Two controversial issues continue with regard to management of adenocarcinoma of the cervix. First, does this cell type carry a worse prognosis than squamous or adenosquamous cell types? Second, for early-stage disease, which therapy (radical surgery, radiation, or combined treatment) is superior?

Most studies suggest no difference in survival when adenocarcinomas are compared with SCCs after correction for stage. The 1998 FIGO Annual Report, which reported more than 10,000 SCCs and 1138 adenocarcinomas using multivariant analysis, noted no difference in survival in stage I cancers. In a study by Chen and associates of 302 adenocarcinomas, it was noted that in early stages, multivariant analysis noted better survival in patients treated with radical surgery compared with those treated with radiation therapy.

Kjorstad and Bond investigated the metastatic potential and patterns of dissemination in 150 patients with stage Ib adenocarcinoma of the cervix treated from 1956 to 1977. All patients were treated with a combination of intracavitary radium followed by radical hysterectomy with pelvic lymph node dissection. The incidence of pelvic metastases and distant recurrences and the survival rates were the same as those given in previously published reports for SCC treated in the same manner. In one respect, the adenocarcinomas showed a significant difference from the squamous cell cancers. The incidence of residual tumor in the hysterectomy specimens after intracavitary treatment was much higher (30% vs. 11%). Kjorstad and Bond considered this a strong argument for surgical treatment of patients with early stages of adenocarcinoma of the cervix.

Moberg and colleagues reported on 251 patients at Radiumhemmet in Stockholm with adenocarcinoma of the uterine cervix. The 5-year survival rate was compared with that in the total of cervical epithelial malignancies, and the rate was lower in the adenocarcinoma cases, with respective crude 5-year survival rates of 84%, 50%, and 9% in stages I, II, and III, respectively. Combined treatment consisting of two intracavitary radium treatments with an interval of 3 weeks followed by a radical hysterectomy with pelvic lymphadenectomy done within 3 months gave improved 5-year survival in a nonrandomized series. Prempree and colleagues also suggested combined therapy for stage II lesions or for those larger than 4 cm.

A large series of 367 cases of adenocarcinoma of the cervix was reported by Eifel and associates. Their conclusions were that the central control of adenocarcinomas with radiation therapy is comparable to that achieved for SCCs of comparable bulk. They found no evidence that combined treatment (radiation therapy plus hysterectomy) improved local regional control or survival. In their study, radiation therapy alone was as effective a treatment for most patients with stage I disease. They noted, as others have, that patients with bulky stage I (>6 cm), stage II, or stage III disease, particularly with poorly differentiated lesions or evidence of nodal spread, had a very high rate of extrapelvic disease spread.

Eifel reported the results of 160 patients with adenocarcinoma of the cervix. Of these patients, 84 were treated with radiation therapy alone; 20 were treated with external and intracavitary radiation followed by hysterectomy, and 56 were treated with radical hysterectomy. Survival was strongly correlated with tumor size and grade. There was a 90% survival rate for lesions smaller than 3 cm. After 5 years, 45% of the patients treated with radical hysterectomy had a recurrence. These recurrences were strongly correlated with lymph or vascular space invasion, poorly differentiated lesions, and larger tumor size.

Chen and associates from Taiwan reviewed 3678 cases of cervical cancer treated between 1977 and 1994, of which 302 (8.5%) were adenocarcinoma. A higher proportion of cases with adenocarcinoma were of the lower stages and in the younger patient even within a given stage. Survival was better in all stages in patients with squamous compared with adenocarcinoma (81% vs. 76% in stage I, $P = 0.0039$). When surgery was primary therapy, there was no difference in survival in stage I (83% vs. 80.3% survival of squamous and adenocarcinoma, respectively). Survival with radiation therapy noted 71% vs. 49%, respectively ($P = 0.0039$), in stage I. Survival decreased as age increased within a given stage.

The MD Anderson Hospital group compared 1538 patients with SCC with 229 patients with adenocarcinoma, all stage Ib and treated with radiation. In patients with tumors larger than 4 cm, multivariate analysis confirmed that patients with adenocarcinoma had a significantly poorer survival than did those with SCC (59% vs. 73%). In a study by the GOG, 813 stage Ia2 and Ib cancers were evaluated. All were treated with radical hysterectomy. There were 645 squamous, 104 adenocarcinoma, and 64 adenosquamous cancers. Radiation was given postoperatively to 16% squamous, 13% adenocarcinomas, and 20% of adenosquamous patients. After adjusting for multiple risk factors, survival was worst for adenosquamous cancer compared with squamous and adenocarcinoma (71.8%, 82.1%, and 88%, respectively). A similar finding was noted in a study from Taiwan in which 134 stage Ib or II cervical adenocarcinomas or adenosquamous cancers were compared with 757 similarly staged squamous carcinomas treated with radical hysterectomy. The overall survival (OS) rate was 72.2% for the former compared with 81.2% for the SCCs. The histology was an independent prognostic factor for recurrence-free survival and OS.

STAGING

The staging of cancer of the cervix is a clinical appraisal, preferably confirmed with the patient under anesthesia; it cannot be changed later if findings at operation or subsequent treatment reveal further advancement of the disease.

International Federation of Gynecology and Obstetrics

International classification of cancer of the cervix according to FIGO was recently revised in 2009 (Fig. 3.12):

Stage	Description
0	Carcinoma in situ, intraepithelial carcinoma
I	The carcinoma is strictly confined to the cervix (extension to the corpus should be disregarded)
Ia	Invasive cancer identified only microscopically; all gross lesions, even with superficial invasion, are stage Ib cancers. Invasion is limited to measured stromal invasion with maximum depth of 5 mm and no wider than 7 mm
Ia1	Measured invasion of stroma no greater than 3 mm in depth and no wider than 7 mm
Ia2	Measured invasion of stroma greater than 3 mm and no greater than 5 mm and no wider than 7 mm

The depth of invasion should not be more than 5 mm taken from the base of the epithelium, surface or glandular, from which it originates. Vascular space involvement, venous or lymphatic, should not alter the staging.

Stage	Description
Ib	Clinical lesions confined to the cervix or preclinical lesions greater than stage Ia
Ib1	Clinical lesions no greater than 4 cm
Ib2	Clinical lesions greater than 4 cm
II	Involvement of the vagina but not the lower third, or infiltration of the parametria but not out to the sidewall
IIa	Involvement of the vagina but no evidence of parametrial involvement
IIa1	Clinically visible lesion no greater than 4 cm in greatest dimension
IIa2	Clinically visible lesion greater than 4 cm in greatest dimension
IIb	Infiltration of the parametria but not out to the sidewall
III	Involvement of the lower third of the vagina or extension to the pelvic sidewall; all cases with a hydronephrosis or nonfunctioning kidney should be included unless they are known to be attributable to other causes
IIIa	Involvement of the lower third of the vagina but not out to the pelvic sidewall if the parametria are involved
IIIb	Extension onto the pelvic sidewall or hydronephrosis or nonfunctional kidney
IV	Extension outside the reproductive tract
IVa	Involvement of the mucosa of the bladder or rectum
IVb	Distant metastasis or disease outside the true pelvis

In 2013, using the revised FIGO 2009 staging, Wagner et al. investigated the impact of size within FIGO stages I to IIIB using the 1988 to 2008 SEER Program database. The investigators evaluated a total of 18,649 cases and reported that the

FIGURE 3.12 A–J, Federation of International Gynecologists and Obstetricians stagings and classification of cancer of the cervix. See staging in Appendix A.

Continued

hazard ratios (HRs) were significantly worse for larger tumors on both univariate and multivariate modeling. The prognostic significance of the size subdivisions of 2 cm and 4 cm for stage 1, 4 cm for stage IIB, and 4 cm and 6 cm for stage IIIB were also maintained. These findings were believed to validate the changes to the FIGO system made in 2009.

The clinical evaluation of patients with cervical cancer is outlined in Table 3.7. **The following diagnostic aids are acceptable for determining a staging classification: physical examination, routine radiographs, colposcopy, cystoscopy, proctosigmoidoscopy, IVP, and barium studies of the lower colon and rectum. Other examinations, such as lymphography,** CT scans, magnetic resonance imaging (MRI) examinations, arteriography, venography, laparoscopy, and hysteroscopy, are not recommended for staging because they are not uniformly available from institution to institution. It is important to emphasize that staging is a method of communicating between one institution and another. Probably more important, however, is that staging is a means of evaluating the treatment plans used within one institution. For these reasons, the method of staging

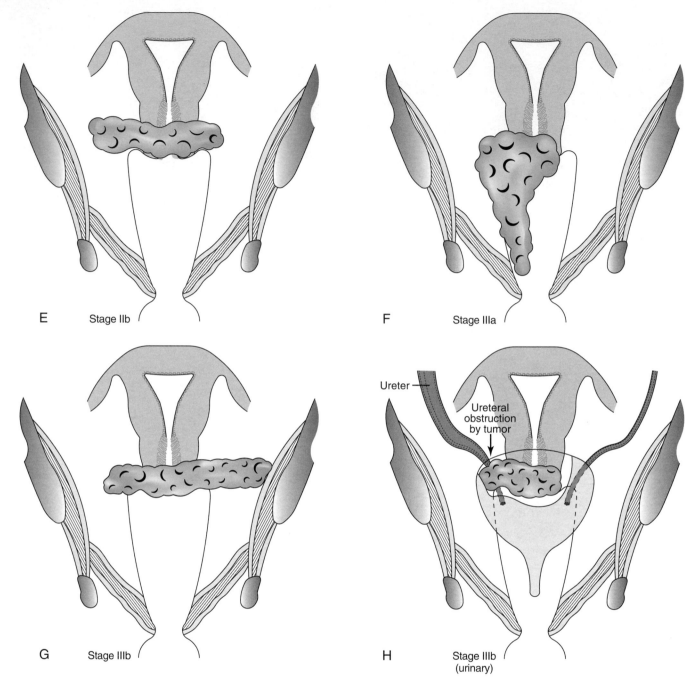

E   Stage IIb

F   Stage IIIa

Ureter —

Ureteral obstruction by tumor

G   Stage IIIb

H   Stage IIIb (urinary)

FIGURE 3.12, cont'd

should remain fairly constant. Staging does not define the treatment plan, and therapy can be tailored to the architecture of the malignancy in each patient.

Positron Emission Tomography

In 2005, the Centers for Medicare & Medicaid Services implemented coverage for 18-fluorodeoxyglucose positron emission tomography (FDG-PET) for patients with newly diagnosed and locally advanced cervical cancer undergoing pretreatment staging who have no extrapelvic metastases on conventional imaging studies (Fig. 3.13). It should be noted that all imaging modalities are more specific than sensitive in detecting nodal metastases. **The pooled sensitivity of PET in detecting pelvic nodal metastases in patients with untreated cervical cancer approaches 80% compared with MRI (≈70%) or CT (≈48%).** It is important to recognize that the available studies are limited by low numbers of patients and wide confidence intervals (CIs).

Grosu and colleagues from Munich analyzed the results of clinical studies on the integration of PET in target volume definition for lung, head and neck, GU, and brain tumors. FDG-PET had a significant impact on gross tumor volume and planning target volume delineation in lung cancer and was able to detect lymph node involvement and differentiate malignant tissue from atelectasis. In high-grade gliomas and

Stage IVa

I

J   Stage IVb

FIGURE 3.12, cont'd

TABLE 3.7	Clinical Evaluation of Patients With Newly Diagnosed Cervical Cancer	
History	**Review of Systems**	**General Physical Examination**
Risk factors (STDs, smoking, OCPs, HIV), prior abnormal Pap tests, previous dysplasia and treatment	Abnormal vaginal bleeding or discharge; pelvic pain, flank pain, sciatica, hematuria, rectal bleeding, anorexia, weight loss, bone pain	Peripheral lymphadenopathy
Evaluation	Common procedures (FIGO)	Alternative procedures
Invasive cancer	Cervical biopsy	Histologic diagnosis required
	Endocervical curettage	
	Cervical conization	
Tumor size; involvement of the vagina, bladder, rectum and parametria	Pelvic examination under anesthesia	MRI pelvis preferred over CT
Anemia	Complete blood count	—
Renal failure	Serum chemistries	—
Hematuria	Urinalysis	—
Bladder involvement	Cystoscopy with biopsy and urine cytology	CT, MRI pelvis
Rectal infiltration	Proctoscopy with biopsy	CT, MRI pelvis; barium enema
Hydronephrosis	IVP	Renal ultrasonography; CT abdomen
Pulmonary metastases	Chest radiography	CT chest; PET scan
Retroperitoneal lymphadenopathy	—	Lymphangiogram, CT, MRI, PET scan

CT, Computed tomography; *FIGO,* Federation of International Gynecologists and Obstetricians; *HIV,* human immunodeficiency virus; *IVP,* intravenous pyelography; *MRI,* magnetic resonance imaging; *OCP,* oral contraceptive pill; *PET,* positron emission tomography; *STD,* sexually transmitted disease.

meningiomas, methionine PET helped to differentiate tumor from normal tissue. Furthermore, the investigators suggest that FDG-PET seems to be particularly valuable in lymph node status definition in cervical cancer. With limited experience, several commentators have noted that FDG-PET may be superior to CT and MRI not only in the detection of lymph node metastases but also in the detection of unknown primary cancer and in the differentiation of viable tumor tissue after treatment. The accurate delineation of gross tumor volume suggests the potential for sparing of normal tissue. The imaging of hypoxia, cell proliferation, angiogenesis, apoptosis, and gene expression by new PET tracers such as choline and acetate may lead to the identification of different areas of a biologically heterogeneous tumor mass that can be individually targeted

FIGURE 3.13 Positron emission tomography. (From http://www.radassociates.com.)

TABLE 3.8 Sensitivity of FDG-PET for Lymph Node Staging in Locally Advanced Disease

	n	FIGO Stages	Imaging Modality	Lymph Nodes	Sensitivity
Sugawara et al.	21	IB-IVA	PET vs. CT	Overall	0.86 (PET)
					0.57 (CT)
Rose et al.	32	IIB-IVA	PET	PALN	0.75
				PELN	1.00
Yildirim et al.	16	IIB-IVA	PET	PALN	0.5
Grigsby et al.	152	IB-IV	PET	Overall	0.67
Narayan et al.	7	IB-IVB	PET	PELN	0.80
Yeh et al.	42	IB-IVA	PET	PALN	0.83
Lin et al.	50	IB-IVA	PET	PALN	0.86
Yen et al.	135	IB2-IVB + recurrence	PET	PELN	0.88
				PALN	0.95
Choi et al.	22	IB-IVA	PET-CT	PELN	0.77
Amit et al.	75	I-IV	PET-CT	PELN	0.60
Loft et al.	119	IB1-IVA	PET-CT	PELN	0.96
				PALN	1.00

CT, Computed tomography; *FDG,* 18-fluorodeoxyglucose; *PALN,* para-aortic lymph nodes; *PELN,* pelvic lymph nodes; *PET,* positron emission tomography.
Adapted from Magne N, Chargari C, Vicenzi L, et al. New trends in the evaluation and treatment of cervix cancer: the role of FDG-PET. *Cancer Treat Rev* 2008;34:67-6811.

using intensity-modulated radiotherapy (IMRT). In addition, a biologic dose distribution can be generated permitting dose painting.

A 2007 meta-analysis of 41 studies was undertaken to compare the diagnostic performances of CT, MRI, and PET or PET/CT in patients for detection of metastatic lymph nodes in patients with cervical cancer. Whereas PET or PET/CT showed the highest pooled sensitivity (82%) and specificity (95%), CT showed 50% and 92% and MRI showed 56% and 91%, respectively (Table 3.8). In a recent investigation of 83 women with FIGO stages IB1 to IIIB cervical cancer, F-18 fluorodeoxyglucose-avid pelvic lymph nodes (SUVPLN) was found to be a prognostic biomarker, predicting treatment response, pelvic recurrence risk, and disease-specific survival. Finally, a prospective validation study conducted between 2000 and 2009 enrolled 560 women who underwent pretreatment FDG-PET lymph node staging. Overall, 47% of patients had lymph node involvement by FDG-PET at diagnosis and within a stage, patients with PET-positive lymph nodes had significantly worse disease-specific survival than those with PET-negative lymph nodes ($P<0.001$). The HRs for disease recurrence increased incrementally based on the most distant level of nodal disease: pelvic, 2.4 (95% confidence interval [CI], 1.63, 3.52); paraaortic, 5.88 (95% CI 3.8, 9.90); and supraclavicular, 30.27 (95% CI, 16.56, 55.34).

Vanderperre et al. recently compared surgical staging with PET-CT, PET, and CT imaging of the paraortic lymph nodes in patients with locally advanced disease (ie, FIGO IB2-IVA). The 204 patients studied were divided into the following four groups: positive surgical staging with negative paraaortic imaging ($n = 16$), negative surgical staging ($n = 172$), positive imaging without surgical staging ($n = 20$), and negative imaging without surgical staging ($n = 128$). OS rates at 2 years (median follow-up 31 months) were 40%, 83%, 58%, and 69%, respectively ($P <0.001$ for positive surgical staging and positive imaging without surgical staging vs. the other two groups). The authors noted that despite negative imaging, aortic nodal metastases were present among 8% of patients who underwent surgical staging, with OS being significantly influenced by the presence of paraaortic metastases.

Surgical Staging

Findings uncovered by fusion PET-CT or conventional MR and CT examinations can be used in the planning of therapy but should not influence the initial clinical staging of the lesion. Unfortunately, clinical staging is only of rough value in prognosis because disease distribution and extent are often included under one stage subheading. Clinical staging is enhanced with the liberal use of rectovaginal examinations (Fig. 3.14) in that this type of pelvic examination allows more complete palpation of the parametria and cul-de-sac. The role of surgical assessment of lymph nodes with extraperitoneal, laparoscopic, or robotic lymphadenectomy is expanding. **The ability to perform pelvic and paraaortic lymphadenectomy provides prognostic information, improves direction of radiation therapy (ie, extended-field radiation with positive paraaortic nodes) and**

FIGURE 3.14 Technique of rectovaginal examination.

FIGURE 3.15 Pelvic diagram. The *dashed line* indicates the radiation field and the position of the uterus and cervix within the field. The *bold line* indicates the J incision path relative to the field and to the major vessels.

may offer a therapeutic effect particularly in grossly involved lymph nodes. To date, no prospective data on surgical staging of cancers of the cervix exist to indicate a survival advantage to this approach.

Some gynecologic oncologists believe that limited staging procedures are warranted on patients with advanced-stage cervical cancer to place patients on institutional or national group protocols. The status of paraaortic nodes should be known before treatment is initiated in such cases to plan appropriate modalities, such as the extent of the radiation field or concomitant chemotherapy. An extraperitoneal approach for removal of the periaortic nodes is preferred by many clinicians in an effort to reduce morbidity from the procedure. More advanced lesions have been investigated with a retroperitoneal lymphadenectomy to determine the extent of disease before planning radiotherapy fields (Fig. 3.15). Fig. 3.16 illustrates one such approach. With the increased use of PET, it is expected that the indications for surgical staging in cervical cancer will decrease.

TREATMENT OF EARLY-STAGE DISEASE

After the diagnosis of invasive cervical cancer is established, the question is how to best treat the patient. Proposed management algorithms for early-stage disease, locally advanced malignancy, and disseminated tumors appear in Fig. 3.17. Specific therapeutic measures are usually governed by the age and general health of the patient, by the extent of the cancer, and by the presence and nature of any complicating abnormalities. It is thus essential to carry out a complete and careful investigation of the patient (see Table 3.7), and then a joint decision regarding treatment should be made by the radiotherapist and gynecologic oncologist. The choice of treatment demands clinical judgment, but apart from the occasional patient for whom only symptomatic treatment may be best, this choice lies between surgery and

radiotherapy (almost always given with cisplatin chemotherapy). In most institutions, the initial method of treatment for locally advanced disease is chemoradiation, both intracavitary and external radiographic therapy. **The controversy between surgery and radiotherapy has existed for decades and essentially surrounds the treatment of stage I and stage IIa cervical cancer** (see Fig. 3.17). For the most part, most patients with stages more advanced than stage I and stage IIa are treated with combination cisplatin and radiotherapy (see Fig. 3.17). The 5-year survival figures from two large series, one treated with radiotherapy alone and the other with surgery, are included here. Currie reported the results of 552 radical operations for cancer of the cervix:

Stage	Patients
Preinvasive carcinoma in situ	555 cases (99.9%)
Stage I	189 cases (86.3%)
Stage IIa	103 cases (75%)
Stage IIb	78 cases (58.9%)
Other stages	41 cases (34.1%)

Some of these patients with positive nodes received postoperative radiotherapy.

In 1981, Zander and colleagues reported results of a 20-year cooperative study from Germany of 1092 patients with stages Ib and II cancer of the cervix treated with radical hysterectomy of the Meigs type and bilateral pelvic lymphadenopathy. Of the 1092 patients, 50.6% had surgery only, with a 5-year survival rate of 84.5% in stage Ib and 71.1% in stage II (most were stage IIa). This correlates well with the figures reported by Currie and Falk. The rest of the patients reported by Zander received postoperative whole-pelvis irradiation therapy. No significant difference could be observed in the survival rates of patients

A

B

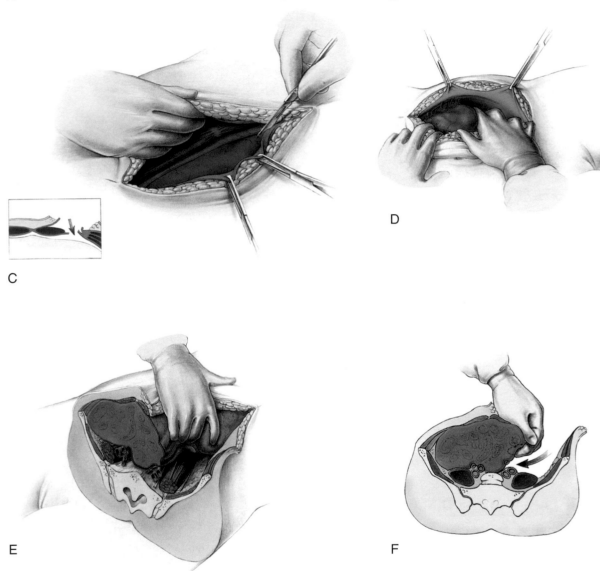

C

D

E

F

FIGURE 3.16 **A,** Path of incision. First measurement of 2 to 3 cm (two finger widths) above the pubic symphysis; second measurement 2 to 3 cm medial to the anterior superior iliac spine. A diagonal line connects these points. A vertical line is drawn superiorly to 3 to 4 cm above the level of the umbilicus. The incision begins at the lateral margin of the rectus muscle. **B,** Division of the external sheath of the rectus and a cross-section. After the initial incision through the skin, the lateral margin of the sheath is divided with a Bovie along the length of the muscle. On cross-section, an *arrow* points to the ideal point of separation. **C,** Division of the internal sheath of the rectus and a cross-section. The rectus muscle is mobilized medially. The internal sheath is divided carefully to preserve the underlying exposed peritoneum. **D,** Blunt dissection with a hand following the plane of the peritoneum and separating it from the transversalis fascia. **E,** Blunt dissection: perspective cross-section. Dissection along the peritoneum until contact is made with the left ureter. The ureter is preserved with the peritoneum and is mobilized medially as dissection continues. The psoas muscle and the common iliac vessels are exposed. **F,** A cross-section. Proper pathway of dissection along the peritoneum over the psoas.

G

H

I

J

FIGURE 3.16, cont'd G, Cross-section of deep dissection. Exposure of the left and right common iliac vessels underneath the peritoneum at about the level of L5 to S1. Avoid damage to the inferior mesenteric artery. **H,** Lymphadenectomy begins along the left common iliac vessels. After medial and superior retraction of the mesentery and beginning about the bifurcation of internal and external iliac vessels, lymph nodes are removed along the length of the left common iliac to the junction with the aorta. **I,** Obturator nodes. Lateral mobilization of the external iliac vessels with a vein retractor. The obturator nerve is identified, and nodes are removed. **J,** The right common iliac. The right common and paraaortic lymph nodes are clipped and removed. The diagram shows deep access to the right common iliac nodes.

Fertility preservation		Standard therapy
Cone biopsy	**FIGO stage IA1 SCCA (no LVSI) or AIS**	Extrafascial hysterectomy
Cone biopsy Laparoscopic lymphadenectomy	**FIGO stage IA1 with LVSI**	Extrafascial hysterectomy ± lymphadenectomy
Radical trachelectomy with lymphadenectomy (vaginal, robotic assisted, laparoscopic, abdominal)	**FIGO stage IA2 or occult IB1**	Modified radical hysterectomy with lymphadenectomy (robotic, laparoscopic, open); tailored adjuvant therapy
Radical trachelectomy with lymphadenectomy as outlined above for FIGO IB1 ≤2 cm	**FIGO IB1-IIA**	Radical hysterectomy with lymphadenectomy (robotic assisted or laparoscopic for stage IB1); tailored adjuvant therapy

A

FIGURE 3.17 A and B, Algorithm for therapy.

undergoing only surgery compared with those of patients undergoing adjuvant postoperative radiation. In fact, in 199 patients with lymph node involvement, the difference in survival rates of those undergoing only surgery and those undergoing additional postoperative radiation therapy was statistically insignificant.

Landoni and colleagues from the University of Milan conducted a prospective randomized trial in 243 patients comparing class II versus class III radical hysterectomy in stage IB to IIA cervical cancer. Although mean blood loss and transfusions were similar for both arms, mean operative time and late urologic morbidity were significantly lower in patients who underwent class II radical hysterectomy. The use of adjuvant radiotherapy was similar in both arms (54%, 55%). **The recurrence rate (24%, 26%) and overall disease-free survival (75%, 73%) was not significantly different between the arms.** Multivariate analysis confirmed that survival did not depend on the type of operation. This rare phase III surgical trial in early-stage cervical cancer has served as the platform from which our (non–phase III) experience in less radical surgery for early-stage disease is based (eg, radical trachelectomy and cervical conization for fertility preservation in the setting of invasive disease). In general, in the early stages, comparable survival rates result from both treatment techniques. The advantage of radiotherapy is that it is applicable to almost all patients, but radical surgery of necessity excludes certain patients who are medically

inoperable. The possible occurrence of immediate serious morbidity must be kept in mind when this treatment plan is selected. In many institutions, surgery for stage I and stage IIa disease is reserved for young patients in whom preservation of ovarian function is desired and improved vaginal preservation is expected. The modern operative mortality rate and the postoperative ureterovaginal fistula rate both have been reported to be less than 1%, making an objective decision for therapy even more difficult. Other reasons given for the selection of radical surgery over radiation include cervical cancer in pregnancy, concomitant inflammatory disease of the bowel, previous irradiation therapy for other disease, presence of pelvic inflammatory disease or an adnexal neoplasm along with the malignancy, and patient preference. Among the disadvantages of radiation therapy, one must consider the permanent injury to the tissues of the normal organ bed of the neoplasm and the possibility of second malignancies developing in this bed.

Radical Abdominal Hysterectomy With Lymphadenectomy

The use of radical hysterectomy in the United States was initiated by Joe V. Meigs at Harvard University in 1944, and shortly thereafter, the radical hysterectomy with pelvic lymphadenopathy was adopted by many clinics in the United States because of dissatisfaction with the limitations of radiotherapy. Some had found that many lesions were not radiosensitive, and some

FIGURE 3.17, cont'd

patients had metastatic disease in regional lymph nodes that were alleged to be radioresistant. Radiation injuries had been reported, and one of the overriding points in favor of surgery was that gynecologists were surgeons rather than radiotherapists and thus felt more comfortable with this treatment. At the time of the popularization of this procedure, modern techniques of surgery, anesthesia, antibiotics, and electrolyte balance had emerged, reducing the enormous morbidity that once attended major operative procedures in the abdomen.

Radical hysterectomy is a procedure that must be performed by a skilled technician with sufficient experience to make the morbidity acceptable (1%–5%). The procedure involves removal of the uterus, the upper 25% of the vagina, the entire uterosacral and uterovesical ligaments (Fig. 3.18), and all of the parametrium on each side, along with pelvic node dissection encompassing the four major pelvic lymph node chains: ureteral, obturator, hypogastric, and iliac. Metastatic lesions to the ovaries are rare, and preservation of these structures is acceptable, especially in young women with small lesions. The procedure is complex because the tissues removed are in close

proximity to many vital structures such as the bowel, bladder, ureters (Figs. 3.19 and 3.20), and great vessels of the pelvis. The object of the dissection is to preserve the bladder, rectum, and ureters without injury but to remove as much of the remaining tissue of the pelvis as is feasible.

There is no doubt that in stage I and in the more restricted stage II cases, surgical removal of the disease is feasible. The addition of pelvic lymphadenectomy to the operative procedure caused considerable controversy in the early part of the century. Wertheim removed nodes only if they were enlarged and then not systematically. He believed that when accessible regional nodes were involved, the inaccessible distant nodes were also involved, and removal of suspicious nodes was more for prognostic than therapeutic value. He thought that node involvement was a measure of the lethal quality of the tumor and not merely a mechanical extension of the disease. The operative procedure popularized by Meigs included meticulous pelvic lymphadenectomy. Meigs demonstrated a 42% 5-year survival rate in another series of patients with positive nodes. Lymphadenectomy is now an established part of the operative

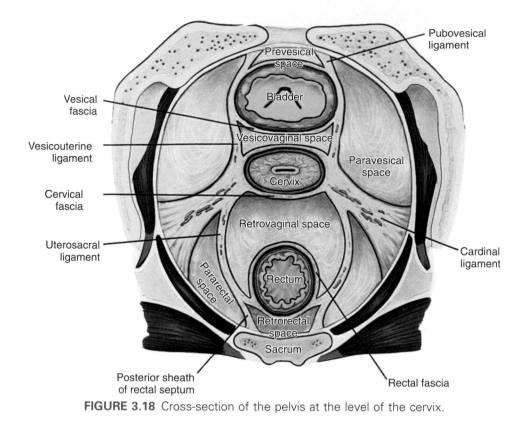

FIGURE 3.18 Cross-section of the pelvis at the level of the cervix.

procedure for any patient with disease greater than stage Ia1. There has been some interest in combining a radical vaginal operation with a retroperitoneal lymphadenectomy, and the results reported by Mitra, Navratil and Kastner, and McCall are surprisingly good. The survival rate in patients with negative nodes is usually in the range of 90% or more.

Rutledge and colleagues devised a system of rating radicality of hysterectomy (Table 3.9) used in treating women with cervical cancer at the MD Anderson Hospital. He suggested that the term "radical hysterectomy" is not adequate to record and communicate the different amounts of therapy attempted and the subsequent risk of complications when different surgeons report their results. These authors believed that describing the technical features of five operations enabled them to evaluate more accurately their results and provided a better understanding of the need to tailor each patient's treatment by using an operation that was adequate but not excessive.

The goal of the class I hysterectomy was to ensure removal of all cervical tissue. Reflection and retraction of the ureters laterally without actual dissection from the ureteral bed allows one to clamp the adjacent paracervical tissue without cutting into the side of the cervical tissue itself. Class I operations are advocated primarily for in situ and true microinvasive carcinomas of the cervix. A class I procedure is also performed after preoperative radiation in adenocarcinoma of the cervix or after preoperative radiation in the so-called barrel-shaped endocervical SCC. The operation described is essentially the extrafascial hysterectomy used routinely at the MD Anderson Hospital.

TABLE 3.9 Rutledge's Classification of Extended Hysterectomy

Class	Description	Indication
I	Extrafascial hysterectomy; pubocervical ligament is incised, allowing lateral deflection of the ureter	CIN, early stromal invasion
II	Removal of the medial half of the cardinal and uterosacral ligaments; upper third of the vagina removed	Microcarcinoma postirradiation
III	Removal of the entire cardinal and uterosacral ligaments; upper third of the vagina removed	Stages Ib and IIa lesions
IV	Removal of all periureteral tissue, superior vesical artery, and three fourths of the vagina when preservation of the bladder is still possible	Anteriorly occurring central recurrences
V	Removal of portions of the distal ureter and bladder	Central recurrent cancer involving portions of the distal ureter or bladder

CIN, Cervical intraepithelial neoplasia.
From Piver MS, Rutledge FN, Smith PJ. Five classes of extended hysterectomy for women with cervical cancer. *Obstet Gynecol* 1974;44:265-272. Reprinted with permission from The American College of Obstetricians and Gynecologists.

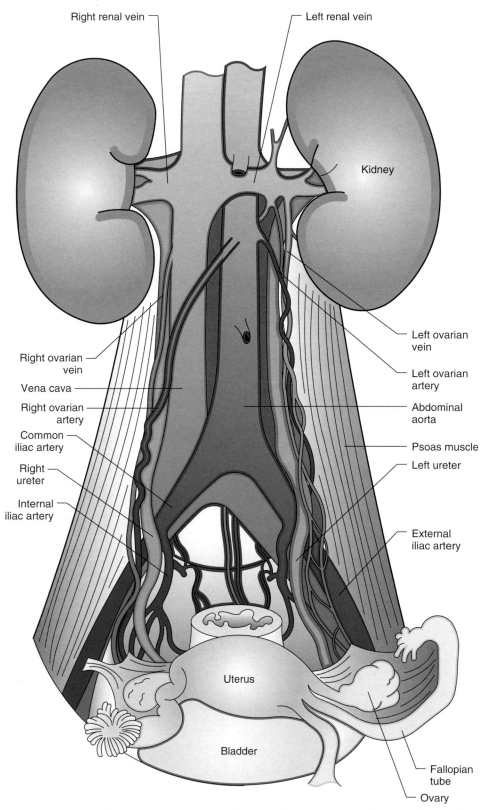

FIGURE 3.19 The retroperitoneal anatomy of the pelvis and lower abdomen illustrating the course of the ureters.

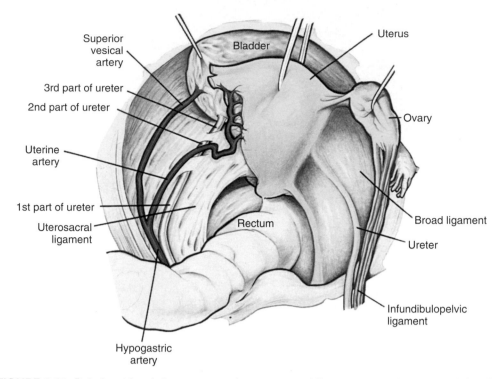

FIGURE 3.20 Relationship of the ureter to the uterosacral ligaments, uterine artery, infundibulopelvic ligament, and uterus.

Class II extended hysterectomy is described as a modified radical hysterectomy. **The purpose of the class II hysterectomy is to remove more paracervical tissue** (Fig. 3.21) **while still preserving most of the blood supply to the distal ureters and bladder.** The ureters are freed from their paracervical position but are not dissected out of the pubovesical ligament. The uterine artery is ligated just medial to the ureter as it lies in "the tunnel," ensuring preservation of the distal ureteral supply. The uterosacral ligaments are transected midway between the uterus and their sacral attachments (Fig. 3.22). The medial halves of both cardinal ligaments are removed, as is the upper 25% of the vagina. A pelvic lymphadenectomy is usually performed with a class II hysterectomy. A class II operation is reported to be suitable for the following conditions:

1. Microinvasive carcinomas in which the depth of invasion is considered greater than early stromal invasion
2. Small postirradiation recurrences limited to the cervix.

The class III procedure is a wide radical excision of the parametrial and paravaginal tissues in addition to the removal of the pelvic lymphatic tissue. The uterine artery is ligated at its origin on the internal iliac artery. In the dissection of the ureter from the pubovesical ligament (between the lower end of the ureter and the superior vesical artery), care is taken to preserve the ligament, maintaining some additional blood supply to the distal ureter. The hazard of fistula formation is decreased by preservation of the superior vesical artery along with a portion of the associated pubovesical ligament. The uterosacral ligaments are resected at the pelvic sidewall. The upper 25% of the vagina is removed (Fig. 3.23), and a pelvic lymphadenectomy is routinely performed. This operation is primarily for patients with stage I or IIa carcinoma of the cervix with or without preservation of ovarian function.

FIGURE 3.21 *Broken lines* identify the point of transection of the cardinal ligaments in class II and class III radical hysterectomy. (Courtesy of Gregorio Delgado, MD.)

FIGURE 3.22 *Broken lines* identify the point of transection of the uterosacral ligaments in class II and class III radical hysterectomy. (Courtesy of Gregorio Delgado, MD.)

FIGURE 3.23 *Broken lines* illustrate the level of vaginal removal of class II and class III radical hysterectomy. (Courtesy of Gregorio Delgado, MD.)

The aim of the class IV radical hysterectomy is complete removal of all periureteral tissue; a more extensive excision of the paravaginal tissues; and, when indicated, excision of the internal iliac vessels along an involved portion of the medial pelvic wall tissue. This differs from the class III operation in three respects:

1. The ureter is completely dissected from the pubovesical ligament

2. The superior vesical artery is sacrificed
3. 50% of the vagina is removed.

This procedure is used primarily for more extensive anteriorly occurring central recurrences when preservation of the bladder is seemingly still possible. Extension of the dissection laterally is needed when the disease has focally involved the medial parametrium. Sacrificing blood vessels to the bladder is unfavorable because the risk of fistula formation increases significantly. In most cases, these patients are more appropriately treated with an anterior exenteration.

The purpose of the class V hysterectomy is to remove a central recurrent cancer involving portions of the distal ureter or bladder. It differs from a class IV operation because the disease involves a portion of the distal ureter, bladder, or both, which is removed with the disease. A reimplantation of the ureter into the bladder, often as a ureteroneocystostomy, is then performed. This procedure has a rare application to a small, specifically located recurrence when exenteration is considered unnecessary or has been refused by the patient.

The modified Rutledge classification of extended hysterectomies has considerable practical value. It again underlines the necessity for the surgeon to tailor the operative procedure to the disease extent. A stage Ia2 lesion does not need an operative procedure that is as radical as the procedure for a large IIa lesion. This is particularly pertinent in the decision between a class II and class III radical hysterectomy. In many countries, the class II radical hysterectomy (called a modified radical hysterectomy) is combined with a bilateral pelvic lymphadenectomy as standard therapy for early-stage cervical cancer. Indeed, the class III type of radical hysterectomy is a phenomenon of particular prevalence in the Western hemisphere and Asia because of the dual influences of Meigs and Okabayashi. The class III, or Meigs–Okabayashi procedure, is a derivative of the Halstedian principle that a lesion should be removed en bloc with its draining lymphatics; thus, the class III radical hysterectomy calls for removal of all the parametria at the pelvic sidewall and transection of the uterosacral ligaments at the sacrum. Advocates of the modified radical hysterectomy or class II procedure with pelvic lymphadenectomy for stages I and IIa lesions suggest that the intervening lymphatics are not at risk in an early cancer of the cervix. Indeed, spread from the primary lesion to the draining pelvic wall nodes probably occurs as an embolic phenomenon. One virtually never finds a tumor in lymphatics except surrounding the primary lesions. However, it is prudent for the pathologist to take several sections of the most distal portion of the parametria following a class III radical hysterectomy for stage I or IIa cervical cancer in an effort to determine the presence or absence of malignant cells in lymphatics distant from the primary lesion. In the presence of a bulky central lesion, the need for an adequate surgical margin of resection often mandates a more extensive procedure than the typical class II radical hysterectomy. However, preservation of any portion of the lateral parametria appears to be associated with a greatly diminished incidence of bladder atony. Forney reported on 22 women extensively studied after undergoing radical hysterectomy; in 11 women, the cardinal ligaments had been divided completely, and in the other 11, the inferior 1 to

2 cm of these ligaments had been spared. Satisfactory voiding occurred significantly earlier (20 vs. 51 days) in women who had undergone an incomplete transection. In a similar manner, preservation of a portion of the uterosacral ligaments appears to be associated with fewer complaints of postoperative obstipation. Undoubtedly, the preserved tissue contains intact nerve tracts, which avoid the extensive denervation associated with the typical class III type or radical hysterectomy.

Complications

Acute complications of radical hysterectomy include pelvic hemorrhage, urinary tract injury, injury to the genitofemoral or obturator nerves, deep venous thrombosis (DVT), and pulmonary embolism. Although hemorrhage requiring transfusion of blood products is a risk of any radical hysterectomy, this complication may occur more frequently when this procedure is performed in obese patients. Soisson and colleagues reported on 43 women undergoing radical hysterectomy for early-stage cervical cancer. All patients had a body weight at least 25% greater than their ideal weight. Survival was not compromised, and the incidence of serious complications was not increased in obese patients compared with a control group. The operative technique is more difficult; the procedure lasts longer, and surgery is associated with greater blood loss.

Pulmonary embolism is the one complication most likely to cause death in the period surrounding the operative therapy of cervical cancer. This must be kept in mind at all times, and particular care must be exercised during and after surgery to avoid this devastating complication. The operative period is the most dangerous period for the formation of a thrombus in the leg or pelvic veins. Care should be taken to ensure that a constriction of veins in the leg does not occur during the operative procedure, and careful dissection of the pelvic veins should lead to minimal thrombus formation in those structures. Because of the risk of pulmonary embolism and DVT, prophylactic heparin or pneumatic compression boots (or both) are strongly recommended.

Chronic complications after radical hysterectomy include urinary dysfunction, lymphocyst formation, lymphedema, extensive abdominal scarring, fistula formation (vesicovaginal and rectovaginal), compromised sexual function, and loss of fertility. All of these complications are preventable, and the incidence is decreasing steadily (Table 3.10). With highly successful

surgical treatment programs in place for early-stage disease, quality of life (QoL) among survivors becomes important.

The major complication after radical surgery for invasive cancer of the cervix is postoperative bladder dysfunction. Reports in the literature by Seski and Carenza and Nobili and Giacobini suggest that bladder dysfunction is a direct result of injury to the sensory and motor nerve supply to the detrusor muscle of the bladder. The more radical the surgery, the greater will be the extent of damage and the more likely postoperative bladder dysfunction will result.

This dysfunction is usually manifested in the patient by a loss of the sense of urgency to void and an inability to empty the bladder completely without the Credé maneuver. Although most patients learn to compensate for the sensory and motor loss and return to near-normal function, patients occasionally need to be taught intermittent self-catheterization, or long periods of constant bladder drainage may be necessary postoperatively. Sophisticated urodynamic studies have shown that a residual hypertonicity in the bladder detrusor muscle and urethral sphincter mechanism sometimes produces dysuria and stress incontinence. Treatment is symptomatic, with near-total recovery in most patients. Limitation of the extent and radicality of surgery, especially in patients with early lesions, can minimize this morbidity. Bandy and colleagues reported on the long-term effects on bladder function after radical hysterectomy (class III) with and without postoperative radiation. In his study, the necessity for bladder drainage of 30 or more days after surgery in 30% of patients was associated with significantly worse long-term residual and other bladder dysfunction. Adjunctive pelvic radiation was associated with significantly more contracted and unstable bladder. In a study reported from Greece of stage Ib cancers, 68 had a Rutledge type III, and 50 had a type II radical hysterectomy. Age, grade, bulky tumor, and lymph node metastasis were similar in the two groups. Postoperative radiation was given to 31% of type III and 64% of type II hysterectomies. Major complications, mainly voiding problems, were significantly more common in those treated with type III hysterectomy; however, the disease-free survival was better in the class III hysterectomy (86.5% vs. 76.5%, $P < 0.05$). This study would suggest type III surgery is better than type II plus radiation.

Ureteral fistulas are now infrequent (0%–3%), primarily as a result of the improvement in techniques, such as avoiding excessive damage to the structure itself and preserving alternate routes of blood supply. With respect to lymphocyst formation, two studies testing the hypothesis that avoiding reperitonealization of the pelvic peritoneum obviates the need for such drainage have been reported; both studies suggest that drainage is not necessary if the peritoneum is left open over the surgical site. Ligation of the lymphatics entering the obturator fossa under the external iliac vein helps reduce the flow of lymph into this area, where lymphocyst formation is prevalent. Lymphocysts, if present, rarely cause injury and are usually reabsorbed if given enough time. Choo and colleagues reported that cysts smaller than 4 to 5 cm usually resolve within 2 months and that only observation is necessary. Surgical intervention is necessary when there is some evidence of a significant ureteral

TABLE 3.10 **Complications of Radical Hysterectomy With Approximate Incidences**	
Complication	**Patients (%)**
Vesicovaginal fistula	1
Ureterovaginal fistula	2
Severe bladder atony	4
Bowel obstruction (requiring surgery)	1
Lymphocyst (requiring drainage)	3
Thrombophlebitis	2
Pulmonary embolus	1

obstruction. During laparotomy, the surgeon should unroof the lymphocyst and prevent re-formation by suturing a tongue of omentum into the cavity (internal marsupialization). Percutaneous aspiration of the cyst, which is often associated with subsequent infection, should be used cautiously.

Preservation of ovarian function is often desirable for patients who must undergo a surgical procedure for invasive cancer of the cervix. Often, after a careful histologic examination of the operative specimen, including the pelvic lymph nodes, a postoperative recommendation for pelvic radiation is indicated. Standard pelvic placement of preserved ovaries will result in postirradiation ovarian failure; therefore, a procedure for transposition of the ovaries to an extrapelvic site (Fig. 3.24) has been devised. Shielding during postoperative pelvic irradiation is possible with the ovaries so placed. The ovaries receive some radiation but not usually enough to prevent continued steroid production. A word of caution has been interjected by Mann and others regarding the rare occurrence of occult metastases to the ovary in patients with adenocarcinoma of the cervix. The two largest studies suggest that the incidence is between 0.6% and 1.3%. Most patients with metastatic disease in the ovary are postmenopausal or have had gross adnexal pathology or positive pelvic lymph nodes. These guidelines can be helpful in identifying patients for whom preservation of ovarian tissue is unwise. The incidence of occult metastasis to the ovary from SCC of the cervix (stages I and IIa) is so rare that preservation of ovarian tissue does not carry the same concerns. Lateral ovarian transposition will be discussed further in the following section on fertility preservation.

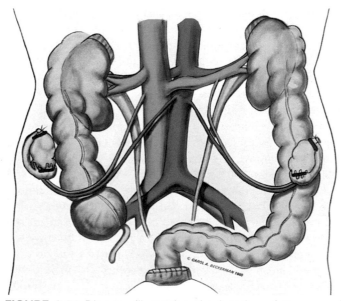

FIGURE 3.24 Diagram illustrating the location of transposed adnexae to a nonpelvic site where they can be spared from postoperative pelvic irradiation. (From DiSaia PJ. Surgical aspects of cervical carcinoma. *Cancer* 1981;48:548. Copyright 1981 American Cancer Society. Reprinted by permission of Wiley-Liss, Inc., a subsidiary of John Wiley.)

Indications for Postoperative Adjuvant Therapy

Table 3.11 contains data sets from two randomized studies that have established the role for adjuvant therapy after radical surgery based on intermediate and high-risk surgicopathologic factors. In a GOG study (protocol 92) of 277 patients with intermediate risk factors, stage Ib cancers were randomized to radical hysterectomy with or without postoperative irradiation. Of these patients, 137 were randomly assigned to radiation therapy, and 140 were not given further treatment. Based on a previous GOG study, intermediate risk was defined as greater than one-third of stromal invasion, lymph space involvement, and large clinical tumor diameter. (Note that the term *lymph space involvement* is used interchangeably with *vascular space involvement.*) All patients had negative lymph nodes. Four combinations of the risk factors were developed. Tumor size varied to greater than 4 cm. Although the two arms were equal with regard to the four combinations, in which group(s) the recurrences occurred is not stated. Using a one-tail test, there is a greater recurrence-free survival for the combined group (84.6% compared with 72.1%). OS was not significant; 11%

TABLE 3.11 When to Use Adjuvant Therapy After Radical Hysterectomy

Randomized Trial of Adjuvant Pelvic Radiotherapy for FIGO Stage IB

	n	Recurrence (%)	RR[†]
GOG 92*			
Adjuvant pelvic RT	137	n = 21 (15)	0.53, P = 0.008
No further therapy	140	n = 39 (28)	

Randomized Trial of Synchronous Adjuvant Radiation Therapy and Chemotherapy for FIGO Stage IA2–IIA

	n	Projected PFS (%)	Projected OS (%)
GOG 109/SWOG 8797/ RTOG 91-12[‡]			
Adjuvant pelvic RT + CT	127	80 HR 2.01, P = 0.003	81 HR 1.96, P = 0.007
Adjuvant pelvic RT alone	116	63	71

*All patients underwent radical hysterectomy and lymphadenectomy, followed by randomization based on intermediate surgicopathologic risk factors (ie, depth of stromal invasion, tumor size, presence of angiolymphatic space involvement).
†Reduction in the relative risk of recurrence.
‡All patients underwent radical hysterectomy and lymphadenectomy followed by randomization based on high surgicopathologic risk factors (ie, metastatic tumor to the lymph nodes, parametria, or vaginal margin).
FIGO, Federation of International Gynecologists and Obstetricians; *GOG*, Gynecologic Oncology Group; *OS*, overall survival; *PFS*, progression-free survival; *RR*, relative risk; *RT*, radiation therapy; *RTOG*, Radiation Therapy Oncology Group; *SWOG*, Southwestern Oncology Group.
GOG-92 data from Sedlis A, Bundy BN, Rotman MZ, et al. A randomized trial of pelvic radiation therapy versus no further therapy in selected patients with stage IB carcinoma of the cervix after radical hysterectomy and pelvic lymphadenectomy: A Gynecologic Oncology Group Study. *Gynecol Oncol* 1999;73:177-183; GOG 109/SWOG 8797/RTOG 91-12 data from Peters WA 3rd, Liu PY, Barrett RJ 2nd et al. Concurrent chemotherapy and pelvic radiation therapy compared with pelvic radiation therapy alone as adjuvant therapy after radical surgery in high-risk early-stage cancer of the cervix. *J Clin Oncol* 2000;18:1606-1613.

died of cancer compared with 18% of the radical hysterectomy-only group. There was a 10% noncompliance rate in the radiation group. These authors are able to apply this information to clinical practice because more than 90% of patients would be treated without benefit with regard to survival. Data were presented with an intent-to-treat evaluation (see Table 3.11).

Patients with positive pelvic nodes usually receive postoperative whole-pelvis irradiation and chemotherapy (see Table 3.11). Peters and colleagues randomized 268 patients with FIGO stage Ia2, Ib, and IIa carcinoma of the cervix, initially treated with radical hysterectomy and pelvic lymphadenectomy and found to have positive pelvic lymph nodes or positive margins or microscopic involvement of the parametrium, to receive either pelvic radiation therapy alone or concurrent chemoirradiation. Among the 243 patients who were accessible, progression-free survival (PFS) and OS were significantly improved in the patients receiving chemotherapy. The projected PFS at 4 years was 63% with pelvic radiation therapy alone and 80% with concurrent chemoirradiation (HR, 2.01; $P = 0.003$). The projected OS rate at 4 years was 71% with pelvic radiation therapy alone and 81% with concurrent chemoirradiation (HR, 1.96; $P = 0.007$). The combined therapy arm had more frequent grade III and IV4 hematologic and gastrointestinal (GI) toxicity. **This landmark intergroup study of the GOG (protocol 109), the Southwest Oncology Group (protocol 8797), and the Radiation Therapy Oncology Group (protocol 91–12) was one of five randomized trials to be published between 1999 and 2000 attesting to the value of radiosensitizing chemotherapy in the management of cervical cancer (discussed further later).**

Prognostic factors have been evaluated by several authors in patients with early-stage disease who have been treated surgically. In a study by Francke and associates, 105 patients with stage Ib were treated with radical hysterectomy and had negative lymph nodes. Only LSI showed significant correlation with local failure. There were 32 patients with SCC and positive LSI, 17 received postoperative radiation with 0 of 17 recurrences, and 4 of 15 (27%) treated with surgery only developed recurrence. The OS rate at 5 years was 96% in those treated with radiation and 93.3% in those with LSI not treated with radiation. Stockler and colleagues evaluated 194 patients with stage Ib and IIa who were treated with radical hysterectomy and had negative nodes. Nuclear grade 2 or 3 ($P = 0.02$) and small cell squamous histology ($P = 0.001$) were each associated with a fourfold increase in risk of recurrence, but LSI ($P = 0.02$), age younger than 36 years ($P = 0.03$), and either tumor size greater than 28 mm ($P = 0.03$) or surgical clearance less than 5 mm ($P = 0.02$) was associated with a 2.5-fold increase in risk of recurrence. Survival data were not given. Delgado, in reporting a GOG study of 645 women with stage Ib squamous carcinoma, including 100 patients with positive nodes, found depth of invasion, tumor size, and lymph space involvement to be important risk factors for recurrence in multivariate analysis. The group from Boston evaluated 171 patients with lymph node–negative stage Ib and IIa cervical cancer treated primarily with surgery. A total of 116 (68%) patients were treated with surgery only, and 55 (32%) received radiation. Overall, 28

patients (16%) developed recurrent disease with no difference in the two treatment groups. After correction for other factors, patients with LSI who received radiation were less likely to develop recurrence than similar patients treated with surgery only ($P = 0.04$); however, OS was similar in the two groups. In a study from Gateshead, United Kingdom, 527 patients with stage Ib to IIb cervical cancer treated with radical hysterectomy were evaluated. There were 102 (19.3%) with lymph node metastasis. In those with lymph node metastasis, histologic differentiation ($P = 0.009$), and metastatic extent ($P = 0.045$) were the only independent prognostic factors for risk of cervical cancer deaths.

Shibata and colleagues evaluated adjuvant chemoradiation in 37 patients who had undergone radical hysterectomy with pelvic lymphadenectomy. In addition to accepted high-risk surgicopathologic criteria (eg, positive pelvic lymph nodes or positive surgical margins), the investigators also included the presence of lymphovascular space involvement (LVSI) as part of their inclusion criteria for protocol eligibility. Adjuvant chemotherapy consisted of cisplatin (70 mg/m^2 on day 1) and 5-fluoracil (5-FU) (700 mg/m^2/per day on days 1–4) every 4 weeks for a total of three cycles. Pelvic radiotherapy was started concurrently with the first cycle of chemotherapy and administered to a dose of 45 Gy in 25 fractions. The incidence of grade III/IV toxicities included neutropenia (24.3%), nausea and vomiting (8.1%), and diarrhea (18.9%). The 5-year PFS was 89.2%. Both the GOG and the Korean GOG have emphasized the importance of further improvement of outcomes of women found to have high-intermediate surgicopathologic risk factors (eg, large tumor diameter, deep stromal invasion, LVSI) after radical surgery for early-stage disease. A prospective, randomized trial involving adjuvant pelvic radiotherapy versus adjuvant single agent weekly cisplatin-based chemoradiation has recently been designed through collaboration of both cooperative groups.

The optimal adjuvant therapy for patients found to have high-risk surgicopathologic factors has not yet been determined. Specifically, the role of adjuvant chemotherapy in place of or in addition to adjuvant chemoradiation has been the subject of much debate. Takeshima and colleagues treated 65 consecutive patients with FIGO stage IB to IIA cervical carcinoma with adjuvant chemotherapy after radical hysterectomy and pelvic lymphadenectomy. Patients with intermediate-risk factors (stromal invasion >50%; $n = 30$) and those with high-risk factors (positive surgical margin, parametrial invasion, or lymph node involvement; $n = 35$) were treated with bleomycin, vincristine, mitomycin, and cisplatin (three cycles for intermediate-risk cases and five cycles for high-risk cases). Chemotherapy was well tolerated with no significant adverse effects and no cases of severe bleomycin-related pulmonary toxicity. The 5-year disease-free survival was 93.3% for the intermediate-risk group and 85.7% for the high-risk group. All patients with SCCs in the intermediate-risk group and 89.3% of high-risk patients with SCC remained disease free. Despite the absence of adjuvant pelvic radiotherapy, local-regional recurrence occurred in 3.3% of the intermediate-risk group and in 8.6% of the high-risk group. A randomized trial comparing adjuvant chemoradiation with and without continued systemic "consolidation" platinum-based and taxane-based chemotherapy is being considered by the GOG for patients found to have high-risk surgicopathologic factors after radical surgery.

To summarize, the recommendation for postoperative adjuvant therapy (pelvic radiotherapy with or without radiosensitizing chemotherapy) after radical hysterectomy is based on high-intermediate risk surgicopathologic factors (ie, tumor diameter, depth of stromal invasion, and presence of LVSI) and high-risk surgicopathologic factors (ie, presence of tumor at the vaginal margin, in the parametria, or in the lymph nodes). The major research questions center around limiting the toxicity of chemoradiation, continued intravenous systemic therapy, and the triage of patients with locally advanced resectable lesions (ie, IB2-IIA) to primary chemoradiation versus potentially trimodality therapy (ie, radical surgery followed by adjuvant chemoradiation).

Sexual Function

The subject of sexual function after therapy for cervical cancer is often ignored. Many patients never regain pretreatment sexual function. Patients treated with full pelvic irradiation therapy (ie, external-beam and vaginal brachytherapy) experience decreased sexual function resulting from vaginal stricture formation with obliteration and premature ovarian failure (see forthcoming discussion). Andersen studied the sexual behavior, the level of sexual responsiveness, and the presence of sexual dysfunction of 41 women with uterine cancer compared with a matched group of healthy women. The two groups were similar until the onset of signs of disease, which sometimes occurred long before diagnosis, at which time the patients with cancer began experiencing significant sexual dysfunction. Sexual morbidity therefore begins actually in the prediagnosis period for many patients. Seibel reported on 46 patients who were interviewed more than 1 year after treatment for carcinoma of the cervix to establish the effects of radiation therapy and of surgical therapy on sexual feelings and performance. The patients who were irradiated experienced statistically significant decreases in sexual enjoyment, opportunity, and sexual dreams. The surgically treated group had no significant change in sexual function after treatment. Both groups experienced a change in self-image but did not believe that their partners or families viewed them differently. Myths about cancer and the actual effects of pelvic irradiation were found to have disrupted the sexual marital relationships of many women. Therapeutic programs with counseling and vaginal rehabilitation with the use of estrogen vaginal creams and possibly the use of dilators may be beneficial. Although radical hysterectomy offers an enhanced functional outcome, the procedure does not always leave sexual function undisturbed, with orgasmic problems and dyspareunia resulting from reduced vaginal size having been reported.

Nerve-Sparing Radical Hysterectomy

Lin and colleagues evaluated urodynamic function in 20 women with cervical cancer who underwent radical hysterectomy. Urodynamic parameters measured preoperatively and postoperatively included bladder voiding and bladder storage functions, both of which were found to be significantly impaired in all 20 cases after surgery. Surgical damage to the pelvic autonomic nerves is likely to be responsible for not only subsequent impaired bladder function but also in defecation problems and sexual dysfunction. The development of a nerve-sparing procedure that does not compromise the radicality of the operation is highly desirable.

Trimbos and colleagues introduced elements of the Japanese nerve-sparing technique in their Dutch population, citing that in various Japanese oncology centers, it had been recognized that the anatomy of the pelvic autonomic nerve plexus permits a systematic surgical approach to preserve these structures. The investigators first identified and preserved the hypogastric nerve in a loose tissue sheath underneath the ureter and lateral to the uterosacral ligament; next, the inferior hypogastric plexus in the parametrium is lateralized and avoided during parametrial transection; finally, the most distal part of the inferior hypogastric plexus is preserved during the dissection of the posterior part of the vesicouterine ligament. Trimbos and colleagues concluded that the procedure is feasible and safe and deserves further consideration.

An updated series was presented by Maas and colleagues, who observed that the incidence of urinary dysfunction appears to be very low after nerve sparing. These findings have been supported by an Italian series of 23 patients reported by Raspagliesi and colleagues and by two recent Japanese papers for which urodynamic data were recorded for 27 patients. In the study by Sakuragi and colleagues, none of 22 patients for whom the nerve-sparing procedure was performed had urinary dysfunction, compared with three of the five patients for whom the procedure could not be performed.

Nerve-sparing radical hysterectomy is an attractive approach because of improved urogenital, anorectal, and sexual functions. The sympathetic fibers that innervate the uterus, vagina, urinary bladder, and rectum come from T11 to L2 and form the superior hypogastric plexus. The parasympathetic fibers come from S2 to S4 at the pelvic wall as the pelvic splanchnic nerve. These fibers merge and form the inferior hypogastric plexus and branch to innervate the uterus and the urinary bladder. Professor Fujii from the Kyoto University Gynecology Group has gone to great lengths to provide a step-by-step anatomic identification of the nerve-sparing radical hysterectomy (Table 3.12). The first step in the nerve-sparing procedure involves isolation and separation of the deep uterine vein from the pelvic splanchnic nerve (Fig. 3.25). This is then followed by isolation and separation of the hypogastric nerve. Ultimately, the bladder branch from the inferior hypogastric plexus is identified running parallel to the blood vessels in the paracolpium, and the uterine branch from the inferior hypogastric plexus is separated and divided (Fig. 3.26). This procedure can be accomplished only through meticulous division of the posterior leaf of the vesicouterine ligament. Through separation of the inferior vesical vein in this ligament, the bladder branch from the inferior hypogastric plexus can be identified and preserved.

van den Tillaart and colleagues evaluated the feasibility, safety, and local recurrence rate in 122 patients with FIGO stage

IA to IIA lesions and compared them with 124 patients who underwent non–nerve-sparing surgery. Unilateral or bilateral sparing of nerves was possible in 80% of cases in the nerve-sparing group. Operative time and blood loss were less in the nerve-sparing group, but the postoperative courses were similar. The local recurrence rates were not significantly different at

2 years of follow-up. Nerve-sparing surgery was not a significant prognostic factor for local recurrence in univariate and multivariate regression analyses. Neuronavigation systems and robotic-assisted nerve-sparing techniques continue to be under investigation along with the incorporation of the nerve-sparing procedure to radical trachelectomy for fertility preservation.

From 2003 to 2005, Roh et al. randomly assigned 92 women with FIGO stage IA2 to IIA disease to conventional radical hysterectomy or nerve-sparing surgery. The patients were well-balanced in clinicopathologic characteristics, and among 86 patients included in final analysis, the frequency of long-term urinary symptoms was higher in the conventional surgery group, with significant deterioration of volume of residual urine and bladder compliance at 12 months. There were no significant differences observed in the 10-year disease-free survival between groups.

In 2009, Querleu and Morrow proposed a new classification system for radical hysterectomy that continues to gain acceptance, particularly in Europe. In this new scheme, four main categories are described according to the extent of removal of the paracervix, using only the ureter, internal iliac vessels, and pelvic wall as reliable landmarks. The new system also incorporates nerve-preservation techniques and paracervical lymphadenectomy in subcategory assignments. In class A, the cervix is removed completely with minimal removal of the paracervix; in class B, the paracervix is removed to the level of the ureter. In class C, the entire paracervix is removed at the pelvic sidewall, and class D describes various exenterative procedures. Class C1 allows for preservation of the autonomic nerves, class D1 includes removal of the vascular parietal system, and class D2 requires removal of muscle and fascia at the lateral pelvic wall.

Cibula et al. have approached the new classification scheme by Querleu and Morrow by developing it further into a

TABLE 3.12   Comparison of Nerve-Sparing Radical Hysterectomy With Traditional Radical Hysterectomy

	Nerve-Sparing Radical Hysterectomy	Traditional Radical Hysterectomy	*P* Value
FIGO stage IB1	10	8	ns
FIGO stage IB2	0	1	
FIGO stage IIA	0	1	
Mean operative time (min)	197	155.5	0.05
Median lymph nodes removed (*n*)	17.8	15.7	NS
Hospital stay (days)	7.6	8.4	NS
Postvoid residual urine volume >50 mL (days)	3.5	9.1	0.00078
Mean decrease in hgb concentration (g%)	1.7	2.5	ns
Complications	1 (blood transfusion)	0	ns

FIGO, Federation of International Gynecologists and Obstetricians; *hgb,* hemoglobin; *NS,* not specified.
Modified from Skret-Magierlo J, Naróg M, Kruczek A, et al. Radical hysterectomy during the transition period from traditional to nerve-sparing technique. *Gynecol Oncol* 2010;116:502-505.

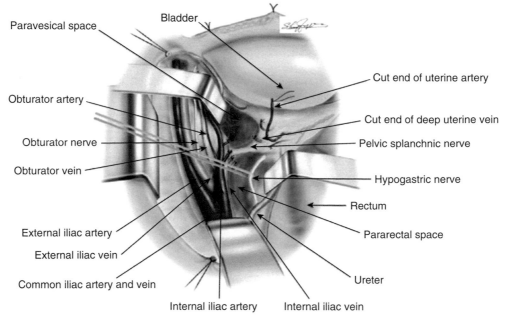

FIGURE 3.25 Nerve sparing. (From Fujii S. An atomic identification of nerve-sparing radical hysterectomy: a step-by-step procedure. *Gynecol Oncol* 2008;111(2 suppl):S33-S41.)

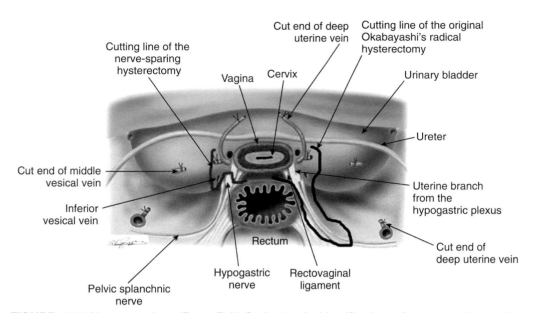

FIGURE 3.26 Nerve sparing. (From Fujii S. Anatomic identification of nerve-sparing radical hysterectomy: a step-by-step procedure. *Gynecol Oncol* 2008;111(2 suppl):S33-S41.)

FIGURE 3.27 Sentinel node. (A from Niikura H, Okamura C, Akahira J, et al. Sentinel lymph node detection in early cervical cancer with combination 99mTc phytate and patent blue. *Gynecol Oncol* 2004;94(2):528-532. B from Gil-Moreno A, Díaz-Feijoo B, Roca I, et al. Total laparoscopic radical hysterectomy with intraoperative sentinel node identification in patients with early invasive cervical cancer. *Gynecol Oncol* 2005;96(1):187-193.)

three-dimensional (3D) model using the standard anatomic landmarks for definition of resection margins in longitudinal and transverse dimensions. In their 2011 manuscript, figures included photographs of the resulting 3D anatomic template that presents the parametrial resection in three dimensions along with the nerve-sparing procedure. The investigators intent is to increase adoption of the new classification scheme within the oncologic community and to enhance harmonization of clinical practice as it pertains to radical hysterectomy.

Sentinel Lymph Node Identification

Although the risk of nodal metastases is low in women with small, early cancers (ie, FIGO Ia2 and Ib1 lesions), the need for bilateral pelvic lymphadenectomies must still be emphasized. Controversy has centered on the existence and ability to identify sentinel lymph nodes (SLNs) in cervical cancer.

The rationale for identifying an SLN in cervical cancer is to avoid full pelvic lymphadenectomies, which can result in lymphocyst formation and lower-extremity lymphedema, especially when adjuvant pelvic radiotherapy is given. Two techniques for sentinel node identification are available. An injection is performed around the tumor using either a blue dye or an isotopic colloid. Ideally, the two techniques are used concomitantly in patients with early-stage lesions (Fig. 3.27).

Dargent and Enria reported the results on 70 consecutive patients. Failure in identification of the SLN occurred in 14 of the 139 attempted dissections. One SLN was detected in 121 dissections, and two SLNs were detected in four dissections. The investigators carried out a systematic pelvic lymphadenectomy after removal of the SN. A metastatic involvement of the SLN was put in evidence in 19 of the 129 retrieved SLNs. The other regional lymph nodes were involved in 13 cases and not involved

TABLE 3.13 Studies on Sentinel Node Detection in Cervical Cancer

Reference	Patients (n)	Technique	Detection Rate (%)	Metastases Sentinel Node (%)	False-Negative (%)
Frumovitz et al.	831	R/B	89.8	20.5	8.2
Bats et al.	71	R/B	87.3	25.8	11
Altgassen et al.	590	R/B	88.6	15.7	22.6
Diaz-Feijoo et al.	50	R/B	100	Unknown	0
Kara et al.	32	R/B	100	28.1	0
Fader et al.	38	R/B	92.1	15.7	16.7
Van de Lande et al.	58	R/B	96.6	21.4	0
Pluta et al.	60	R/B	100	8.3	0

B, Blue dye; *R,* radioactive tracer.
Modified from Oonk MHM, van de Nieuwenhof HP, de Hullu JA, et al. The role of sentinel node biopsy in gynecological cancer: a review. *Curr Opin Oncol* 2009; 21:425-432.

TABLE 3.14 Literature Review of Total Laparoscopic Radical Hysterectomy With Lymphadenectomy

Authors	Patients (n)	BMI	OR Time (min)	EBL (mL)	Hospital Stay (days)	Transfusion	Pelvic Lymph Nodes
Spirtos et al.	78	≤35	205	225	2.9	1	34
Ramirez et al.	20	26	332.5	200	1	1	13
Gil Moreno et al.	27	26	285	400	5	2	19.1
Abu-Rustum et al.	19	23.1	371	301	4.5	1	25.5
Pomel et al.	50	21.5	258	200	7.5	1	13.22
Nezhat et al.	7	—	293	143	3.2	—	27.8
Puntambekar	248	—	92	165	3	—	18
Frumovitz	35	28.1	344	319	2	6	14
Malzoni et al.	77	27	186	57	4	0	23

BMI, Body mass index; *OR,* odds ratio.
Modified from Malzoni M, Tinelli R, Cosentino F, et al. Laparoscopic radical hysterectomy with lymphadenectomy in patients with early cervical cancer: our instruments and technique. *Surg Oncol* 2009;18:289-297.

in six cases. In the 110 cases in which the SLN was not involved, all of the other regional nodes were free from metastasis.

Table 3.13 contains studies on SLN detection in cervical cancer from 2007 to 2010. Most studies were performed with a combination of blue dye and a radioactive tracer with detection rates ranging from 87.3% to 100%. False-negative rates have ranged from 0% to 22.6%. Darlin and colleagues noted that the technique appears to be an accurate method for identifying lymph node metastases in cervical cancer patients with tumors that are 2 cm or smaller. The investigators recommend that in the case of a unilateral SLN only, a complete lymphadenectomy should be performed on the radionegative side. Although a randomized clinical trial to assess the equivalency of SLN mapping will not be feasible because a sample size of more than 1800 patients will be required to evaluate a decrease in recurrence rate from 15% to 10%, the GOG is prospectively studying the utility of lymphatic mapping and SLN identification in patients with early-stage cervical cancer (GOG protocol 206).

Laparoscopic Radical Hysterectomy With Lymphadenectomy

Advantages of minimally invasive surgery include magnification for improved visualization, decreased blood loss, shorter hospitalization, more rapid recovery to full function, less adhesion formation, improved cosmesis, and decreased wound complications (eg, infection, hernia formation). A type III Wertheim–Meigs radical hysterectomy with bilateral pelvic and aortocaval lymphadenectomies can be accomplished via operative laparoscopy and has been reported by several centers (Table 3.14, Fig. 3.28). Malzoni and colleagues published a series of 77 patients, 60 of whom underwent a class III operation and 17 who underwent a class II operation. The median body mass index (BMI) was 27 kg/m2 (range, 19–35 kg/m²). Mean operative time was 186 minutes, median blood loss was 57 mL (range, 30–90 mL), and the median hospital stay was 4 days (range, 3–7 days). Chen and colleagues performed 290 laparoscopic radical hysterectomies with lymphadenectomy. The median blood loss was 230 mL (range, 50–1200 mL), and the mean operative time was 162 minutes (range, 110–350 minutes). Positive lymph nodes were detected in 27.1%, and surgical margins were clear in all patients. Postoperative complications occurred in 10.8% and included ureterovaginal fistula ($n = 5$), vesicovaginal fistula ($n = 4$), ureterostenosis ($n = 3$), DVT ($n = 9$), lymphocyst ($n = 4$), lymphedema ($n = 5$), and trocar insertion site metastasis ($n = 1$). Recurrent disease occurred in 16.3% ($n = 48$) at a median follow-up of 36.5 months.

Single-site laparoscopic surgery platforms have been developed and are being evaluated in gynecologic oncology centers.

FIGURE 3.28 A, Laparoscopic radical hysterectomy. B, Placement of 5 mm to 12 mm laparoscopic ports. 5-12, either 5 mm diameter ports up to 12 mm diameter ports. (A: From Frumovitz M, Ramirez PT. Total laparoscopic radical hysterectomy: surgical technique and instrumentation. *Gynecol Oncol* 2007;104(1 suppl):13-6. B: From Abu-Rustum NR, Gemignani ML, Moore K, et al. Total laparoscopic radical hysterectomy with pelvic lymphadenectomy using the argon-beam coagulator: pilot data and comparison to laparotomy. *Gynecol Oncol* 2003;91:402.)

Reports of this technique using the multichannel single-incision laparoscopic surgery port for laparoscopic cases or a single channel Gelport for robotic-assisted cases on the da Vinci Surgical System in the performance of radical hysterectomy with lymphadenectomy using articulating endoscopes and articulating instrumentation are forthcoming.

Robotic-Assisted Laparoscopic Radical Hysterectomy With Lymphadenectomy

Worldwide adoption of a minimally invasive surgical approach for radical hysterectomy with lymphadenectomy using standard laparoscopic techniques has been slow because of technical difficulties, long surgeon learning curve, and long operative time in many cases. The counterintuitive hand movements, two-dimensional visualization, and limited degrees of instrument motion within the body in addition to ergonomic difficulty and tremor amplification constitute additional obstacles. **The development of the robotic-assisted laparoscopic technique using the da Vinci Surgical System has allowed for high-definition 3D visualization, instruments that increase surgical accuracy by mimicking the complex movements of the human hand, enhanced dexterity with tremor abolition, and faster suturing** (Fig. 3.29). In both laboratory drills and in clinical settings, robotic-assisted laparoscopic techniques appear to require a shorter learning curve.

During the preceding 5 years, reports of robotic-assisted laparoscopic radical hysterectomy with lymphadenectomy has started appearing in the literature (Table 3.15). Maggioni and colleagues compared the surgical outcome of robotic radical hysterectomy (*n* = 40) with that of radical abdominal hysterectomy (*n* = 40 historic cases). The two groups did not differ significantly in BMI, stage, histology, or intraoperative complications. The median age did differ significantly (44 years in the robotic cohort vs. 49 years in the historic group; *P* = 0.035). The mean operative time was significantly shorter for the laparotomy group (mean, 200 minutes vs. 272 minutes; *P* = 0.0001), but the

FIGURE 3.29 Robotic port placement (Da Vinci Surgical System). (From Shafer A, Boggess JF. Robotic-assisted endometrial cancer staging and radical hysterectomy with the da Vinci surgical system. *Gynecol Oncol* 2008;111(1 suppl):S18-23.)

mean blood loss was statistically significant in favor of the robotic group (78 mL vs. 222 mL; *P* <0.0001). A higher number of pelvic lymph nodes was removed via laparotomy (mean, 26 nodes vs. 20 nodes; *P* <0.05). The mean length of stay was significantly shorter for the robotic group. There were no significant differences in terms of postoperative complications between the two groups.

Finally, Cantrell and colleagues reported their 3-year experience involving 63 patients who underwent successful robotic-assisted laparoscopic type III radical hysterectomy. There was one intraoperative complication (asystole after induction) and two postoperative complications (intensive care unit admission for cardiac evaluation and reoperation for vaginal cuff dehiscence). Thirty-two percent of patients received adjuvant therapy. At a median follow-up period of 12.2 months, there has been recurrence and death of one patient, resulting in a 94% PFS and OS. These survival outcomes did not differ significantly from those of a historic cohort at the investigators' institution.

TABLE 3.15   Case-Matched Analysis of Robotic Radical Hysterectomy With Lymphadenectomy Compared With Laparoscopy and Laparotomy

	Robotic (n = 32)	Laparoscopic (n = 17)	Laparotomy (n = 14)	P Value
IA2	—	2 (11.8%)	—	NS
IB1	29 (90.6%)	14 (82.4%)	13 (92.9%)	NS
IB2	3 (9.4%)	1 (5.9%)	1 (7.1%)	NS
BMI (mean)	29.7	28.1	29.5	NS
Operative time (mean)	2.4 hr	2.2 hr	1.9 hr	0.05 (robotic vs. laparotomy)
EBL (mean)	130 cm^3	209.4 cm^3	621.4 cm^3	0.009 (robotic vs. laparoscopy); <0.0001 (robotic vs. laparotomy)
Total nodes (mean)	32.4	18.6	25.7	<0.001 (robotic vs. laparoscopy); <0.05 (robotic vs. laparotomy)
Positive margins	5 (15.6%)	3 (17.7%)	3 (21.4%)	ns

EBL, NS, not specified.
Modified from Estape R, Lambrou N, Diaz R, et al. A case matched analysis of robotic radical hysterectomy with lymphadenectomy compared with laparoscopy and laparotomy. *Gynecol Oncol* 2009;113:357-361.

Robotic-assisted techniques for the management of early-stage cervical carcinoma appear to be feasible, but continued evaluation of oncologic outcomes and a cost–benefit analysis is still needed. Important complications that also require careful evaluation and scrutiny are those that may be specific to robotic techniques, including adverse effects associated with prolongation of steep Trendelenburg position, herniation at 8-mm port sites, vaginal cuff dehiscence, freezing of the robotic arms intraoperatively, and consequences of collisions. In addition, there has been a report of an 8-mm robotic port-site metastasis in a patient who underwent robotic-assisted laparoscopic radical hysterectomy and bilateral pelvic lymphadenectomy for a node-negative FIGO stage IB1 adenocarcinoma of the cervix.

A systematic review and meta-analysis of robotic radical hysterectomy for early-stage disease was recently performed by Shazly et al. Using MEDLINE, EMBASE, and SCOPUS from the time of database inception through February 2015, 26 nonrandomized studies enrolling 4013 women were identified. Robotic radical hysterectomy was associated with significantly less blood loss and blood transfusion, lower febrile morbidity, shorter hospital stay, and decreased wound-related complications compared with abdominal radical hysterectomy. Compared with laparoscopic radical hysterectomy, robotic radial hysterectomy was associated with comparable intra- and postoperative outcomes.

Fertility-Preserving Surgery for Early-Stage Tumors

For patients with microinvasive cervical carcinoma, management depends on the depth of invasion, and select patients may undergo conservative treatment with either cervical conization (FIGO Ia1) or radical trachelectomy with lymphadenectomy (FIGO Ia1 with LVSI, FIGO Ia2, and FIGO Ia adenocarcinoma) (see Fig. 3.17). In addition, patients with FIGO stage Ib lesions smaller than 2 cm with limited endocervical involvement and no pathologic evidence of lymph node metastases may be candidates for radical trachelectomy. In patients who are selected for conservative therapy, there should be no clinical evidence of impaired fertility and a strong desire for future childbearing. In addition, close surveillance should be instituted with scheduled Pap testing, colposcopic evaluation, and endocervical curettage.

Cervical Conization for Adenocarcinoma in Situ and Microinvasive Carcinoma

There has been a movement during the past decade to seriously explore fertility-sparing surgery for patients with adenocarcinoma in situ (AIS) and microinvasive carcinomas. **For many patients with AIS, local excision appears to be sufficient treatment provided ectocervical and endocervical margins are clear and patient compliance with follow-up is demonstrable.** It would appear that cold knife, CO_2 laser, and large loop excision of the transformation zone (LLETZ) conization procedures produce acceptable results; however, these approaches should be reserved for highly selected patients (Table 3.16). Patients with margin involvement should be considered for repeat excisional biopsy. A 2009 meta-analysis composed of 33 studies indicated a recurrence rate for AIS of 2.6% for negative margins and 19.4% for positive margins (odds ratio [OR], 2.48; 95% CI 1.05, 1.622; P <0.001). Invasive adenocarcinoma was more commonly associated with positive margins (5.2%) compared with negative margins (0.1%).

In a study of 85 patients with FIGO stage IA1 SCC treated by electrosurgical conization and cold conization to preserve fertility, there was one recurrence (1.2%) at a median follow-up of 81 months. In a second report containing 75 patients with FIGO stage IA1 SCC, there were no recurrences among the 53 women who underwent conization followed by hysterectomy nor in the 22 who underwent conization alone. As in the case with AIS and microinvasive SCC, conservative fertility-preserving therapy may be considered for select cases of microinvasive adenocarcinoma, although this remains controversial. It would seem that for FIGO stage IA1 adenocarcinomas, conization is safe. When LVSI is present, laparoscopic pelvic lymphadenectomy seems advisable. In summary, for highly selected patients with early-stage disease seen in consultation with a gynecologic oncologist, cold knife cervical conization is a reasonable alternative to preserve fertility provided compliance with follow-up

TABLE 3.16 Conization for Microinvasive Adenocarcinoma of the Cervix

Author	Depth ≤ 3.0 mm	Recurrences	Depth 3.1–5.0 mm	Recurrences
Schorge et al.	5	0	—	—
McHale et al.	4	0	—	—
Webb	20	Not specified	18	Not specified
Smith	31	1	29	1
Ceballos et al.	1	0	—	—
Poynor et al.	2	0	1	0
Bisseling et al.	16	0	2	0
Total	**79**	**1**	**50**	**1**

Modified from Bisseling KC, Bekkers RL, Rome RM, Quinn MA. Treatment of microinvasive adenocarcinoma of the uterine cervix: a retrospective study and review of the literature. *Gynecol Oncol* 2007;107:424-430.

is not problematic and pathology review has excluded highly aggressive histologic subtypes (eg, neuroendocrine tumors).

Vaginal Radical Trachelectomy With Laparoscopic Lymphadenectomy

Radical trachelectomy involves removing all or most of the cervix along with the bilateral parametria and upper vagina. This procedure allows for preservation of the uterus for childbearing and can be performed vaginally, abdominally, or through a minimally invasive approach (ie, straight-stick laparoscopy or robotic-assisted laparoscopy). Of note, patients with stage Ia2 disease have a 6.3% risk of nodal metastases, so treatment must include a formal pelvic lymphadenectomy.

In 1987, Dargent designed a fertility-preserving operation for stage Ia2 and some Ib1 lesions. A variant of the classical Shauta operation of vaginal radical hysterectomy, the vaginal radical trachelectomy (VRT) is performed in conjunction with bilateral laparoscopic lymphadenectomies. The VRT is performed with division of the uterus underneath the isthmus, and at the completion of the procedure, the uterus is sutured to the vagina. Oncologically, the technique is satisfying because a wide margin around the lesion is obtained containing the parametria and the upper vagina but leaving the body of the uterus in situ.

Plante and colleagues collected more than 600 reports of the vaginal technique from the past decade's literature, including 115 of her own. Oncologic outcomes have been satisfactory with an overall recurrence rate of 4.5% and death rate from disease of 2.5% (Table 3.17). Risk factors for recurrence include lesions 2 cm or larger (29% vs. 1%) and the presence of LVSI (12% vs. 2%). Adenocarcinomas and adenosquamous carcinomas are not clearly associated with an increased risk of recurrence. Patients with neuroendocrine tumors should probably not be offered fertility-sparing surgery. Approximately 10% to 12% of patients selected for VRT are found to have more extensive endocervical disease at the time of surgery or positive nodes on frozen section, leading to abandoning the procedure in favor of adjuvant therapy or completion radical hysterectomy.

Plante and colleagues also tabulated obstetric outcomes for 256 patients (Table 3.18). Approximately 62% of pregnancies after VRT will reach the third trimester, of which 65% will reach term. The preterm delivery rate is in the range of 28%, but only 12% will end with significant prematurity (<32 weeks) in which

TABLE 3.17 Oncologic Outcomes After Vaginal Radical Trachelectomy

Author	Patients (n)	Median Follow-Up (mo)	Recurrence Rate (%)	Death (%)
Marchiole	118	95	7 (6)	5 (4)
Plante	115	74	4 (3)	2 (2)
Shepherd	112	45	3 (3)	2 (2)
Hertel	100	29	3 (3)	2 (2)
Covens et al.	93	30	7 (7.5)	4 (4)
Sonoda	36	21	1 (3)	0
Burnett et al.	19	21	2 (10.5)	?
Schlearth	10	48	0	0
Total	**603**		**27 (4.5)**	**15 (2.5)**

From Plante M. Vaginal radical trachelectomy: an update. *Gynecol Oncol* 2008;111:S105-S110.

most neonatal morbidity occurs. Overall, 40% of all pregnancies can be expected to culminate with the birth of a healthy newborn at term.

Abdominal approaches to radical trachelectomy may include nerve-sparing, laparoscopic, or robotic-assisted techniques. Potential benefits of the abdominal approach for radical trachelectomy include wider parametrial resection, possible lower intraoperative complication rates, and techniques familiar to most gynecologic oncologists (Fig. 3.30). Cibula and colleagues reviewed the more than 100 reported cases of abdominal radical trachelectomy (ART) in 2008 and then updated their own experience with the abdominal approach in 2009. Specific indications for the abdominal approach have included clear cell carcinoma of the upper vagina, clear cell cervical carcinoma in pediatric patients, cervical cancer in patients with distorted vaginal anatomy, cancer in the cervical stump after subtotal hysterectomy, bulky exophytic cervical cancer, extent and location of cervical cancer that requires increased radicality of parametrial resection (type III), and cervical cancer in the first half of pregnancy. In total, nine live births have been reported, of which at least two were premature deliveries.

Einstein and colleagues compared surgical and pathologic outcomes for 43 adult patients with FIGO stage IB1 lesions who

TABLE 3.18 Obstetrical Outcomes After Vaginal Radical Trachelectomy

Author	Pregnancies	TAB, Ectopic (%)	First-Trimester Loss (%)	Second-Trimester Loss (%)	Third-Trimester Deliveries (%)	Deliveries <32 wk (%)	Deliveries 33–36.6 wk (%)	Deliveries >37 wk (%)	Currently Pregnant
Plante	87	4 (5)	17 (20)	3 (4)	58 (66)	3 (5)	8 (14)	47 (81)	5 (5)
Mathevet	56	5 (9)	9 (16)	8 (14)	34 (61)	2 (6)	3 (9)	29 (85)	0
Shepherd	55	3 (5)	14 (25)	7 (13)	28 (51)	8 (29)	12 (43)	8 (29)	3 (5)
Bernardini et al	22	0	3 (14)	1 (4)	18 (82)	3 (17)	3 (17)	12 (67)	0
Hertel	18	2 (11)	1 (5)	0	12 (67)	—	—	—	3 (16)
Sonoda	11	0	3 (27)	0	4 (36)	0	0	4 (100)	4 (36)
Burnett et al	3	0	0	1	2	1	0	1	0
Schlearth	4	0	0	2	2	1	0	1	0
Total	**256**	**14 (5)**	**47 (18)**	**22 (8.6)**	**158 (62)**	**18 (12)**	**26 (16)**	**102 (65)**	**15 (6)**

From Plante M. Vaginal radical trachelectomy: an update. *Gynecol Oncol* 2008;111:S105-S110.

FIGURE 3.30 Vaginal radical trachelectomy. (From Einstein MH, Park KJ, Sonoda Y, et al. Radical vaginal versus abdominal trachelectomy for stage IB1 cervical cancer: a comparison of surgical and pathologic outcomes. *Gynecol Oncol* 2009;112: 73-77.)

TABLE 3.19 Pathologic Results of the Unfixed Trachelectomy Specimens With Bilateral Parametrial Measurements by the Pathologist

	VRT (*n* = 28)	ART (*n* = 15)	*P* Value
Median gross length (cm)	1.45 (0.73–1.63)	3.97 (2.7–5.36)	0.01
Median histologic length (cm)	1.07 (0.89–1.25)	1.51 (1.36–1.77)	≤0.0001
Patients with parametrial lymph nodes detected	0 (0%)	8 (57.3%)	0.0002

ART, Abdominal radical trachelectomy; *VRT*, vaginal radical trachelectomy.
From Einstein MH, Park KJ, Sonoda Y, et al. Radical vaginal versus abdominal trachelectomy for stage IB1 cervical cancer: a comparison of surgical and pathologic outcomes. *Gynecol Oncol* 2009;112:73-77.

underwent VRT (*n* = 28) or ART (*n* = 15) (Table 3.19). The median measured parametrial length in the VRT group was 1.45 cm compared with 3.97 cm in the ART group (*P* <0.0001). Parametrial nodes were only detected in the ART specimens (*n* = 8, 57.3%). There was no difference in histologic subtypes, LVSI, or median total regional lymph nodes removed in the two groups. Median blood loss was greater but not clinically significant in the ART group, and the median operating time was less in the ART group. The two groups did not differ significantly in the overall complication rate. The investigators concluded that the abdominal approach allows for wider parametrial resection, including contiguous parametrial nodes.

Minimally invasive approaches (ie, laparoscopic and robot assisted) to radical trachelectomy were recently studied retrospectively by Vieira et al. One hundred patients from four institutions were identified with early-stage disease and treated via an open approach (*n* = 58) or a minimally invasive approach

(*n* = 42). There were no differences in clinicopathologic factors between the two groups, including BMI, histology, FIGO stage, or the presence of lymphovascular space invasion. Intraoperative and postoperative complications did not differ significantly between the two groups. Although the pregnancy rate was higher in the open surgery group (51% vs. 28% *P* = 0.018), the authors note that median follow-up was shorter in the minimally invasive surgery group (25 vs. 66 months). As expected, minimally invasive approaches were associated with less blood loss and shorter hospital stays.

By allowing for the preservation of the body of the uterus and thereby the potential for reproductive function, the radical trachelectomy emerges as a true breakthrough in the management of young women with early-stage cervical cancer (Fig. 3.31). It is currently the fertility-sparing procedure with the most available data supporting its use. Although these results are encouraging, there is lack of level I evidence (ie, randomized controlled trials [RCTs]) comparing safety and survival rates between conservative and radical methods. Therefore, these techniques should be used by fully trained operators. In our opinion, the technique can be considered in conjunction with laparoscopic transperitoneal lymphadenectomy in patients who strongly desire future fertility and harbor a stage Ia1 lesion with LVSI, an Ia2 lesion, or an Ib1 tumor less than 2 cm in diameter.

FIGURE 3.31 Abdominal radical trachelectomy. (From Einstein MH, Park KJ, Sonoda Y, et al. Radical vaginal versus abdominal trachelectomy for stage IB1 cervical cancer: a comparison of surgical and pathologic outcomes. *Gynecol Oncol* 2009;112: 73-77.)

For patients with FIGO stage IB tumors larger than 2 cm, VRT is not recommended because of unacceptable recurrence rates. There are no clear consensus guidelines regarding the safety of abdominal radical trachelectomy, laparoscopic radical trachelectomy, or robotic radical trachelectomy for such patients. One option is to administer neoadjuvant chemotherapy to reduce tumor size. In a recent literature review by Pareja et al., different approaches to radical trachelectomy were analyzed, and the outcome measures appear in the table below:

	ART >2 cm (%)	ART All Sizes (%)	NACT Followed by Surgery (%)	VRT (%)	VRT >2 cm (%)
Pregnancy	—	16.2	30.7	24	—
Recurrence	6	3.8	7.6	4.2	17

ART, Abdominal radical trachelectomy; *NACT,* neoadjuvant chemotherapy; *VRT,* vaginal radical trachelectomy.

Lateral Ovarian Transposition

As described previously, young patients with FIGO stage I to IIa cervical carcinoma who are considered to be at high risk for requiring adjuvant pelvic irradiation (with or without radiosensitizing chemotherapy) should have the ovaries transposed to the paracolic gutters at the time of radical abdominal hysterectomy. The infundibulopelvic ligament is mobilized, and two large metallic clips should be placed in an "X" formation across the mesosalpinges to assist in radiographic localization during radiation treatment planning. Patients with locally advanced carcinomas (ie, FIGO stage Ib2 to IVa) who will receive primary chemoirradiation can undergo lateral ovarian transposition via laparoscopy in anticipation of therapy. **The incidence of ovarian failure following transposition ranges from 28% to 50% when pelvic irradiation is used.** There is a tendency to become postmenopausal if the scatter radiation dose at the transposed ovaries is greater than 300 cGy. This scatter radiation dose does not appear to depend on the distance the ovaries are placed from the linea innominata. The risk of premature ovarian failure when adjuvant radiation therapy is not required is approximately 5% in patients who have undergone lateral ovarian transposition. The risk of developing symptomatic ovarian cysts appears to be approximately 5%.

Husseinzadeh and colleagues performed lateral ovarian transposition in 22 patients with invasive cervical cancer, 15 of whom received whole pelvic external radiation therapy. Nine patients also received one or two intracavitary insertions. Ovarian function was measured by the serum gonadotropins, follicle-stimulating hormone (FSH), and luteinizing hormone (LH). Five patients developed postmenopausal symptoms. Ovarian function was preserved in seven patients, all of whom received an average dose of 250 cGy to the ovaries via external radiation and intracavitary insertion(s). FSH values ranged from 3.3 to 38.8 mIU mL-1 (mean, 17.7 mIU mL-1).

TREATMENT OF LOCALLY ADVANCED DISEASE

Radiotherapy

Over the past century, radiotherapy has emerged as a notable alternative to radical surgery, primarily because of improvements in technique. The number of radiation-resistant lesions was discovered to be small, and skilled radiologists limit radiation injury, especially with the moderate dosages used for early disease. Much evidence has been presented that proves that radiotherapy can destroy disease in lymph nodes and in the primary lesion. Over the past 2 decades, radical hysterectomy has been reserved in many institutions for patients who are relatively young, lean, and in otherwise good health. In other areas of the United States, radiotherapy or surgery is used alone when the alternative modality is not available. The relative safety of both treatment modalities and the high curability for stages I and IIa lesions give physicians and patients a true option for therapy.

Radiotherapy for cancer of the cervix was begun in 1903 in New York by Margaret Cleaves. In 1913, Abbe was able to report an 8-year cure. The Stockholm method was established in 1914, the Paris method in 1919, and the Manchester method in 1938. Radium was the first element used; it has always been the most important element in radiotherapy of this lesion. External irradiation was used to treat the lymphatic drainage areas in the pelvis lateral to the cervix and the paracervical tissues.

Successful radiation therapy depends on the following:
1. Greater sensitivity of the cancer cell, compared with the cells of the normal tissue bed, to ionizing radiation
2. Greater ability of normal tissue to recuperate after irradiation
3. A patient in reasonably good physical condition.

The maximal effect of ionizing radiation on cancer is obtained in the presence of a good and intact circulation and adequate cellular oxygenation. Preparation of the patient for a radical course of irradiation therapy should be as careful as the preparation for radical surgery. The patient's general condition should be as well maintained as possible with a diet high in proteins, vitamins, and calories. Excessive blood loss should be controlled, and hemoglobin should be maintained well above 10 g.

Some consideration must be given to the tolerance of normal tissues of the pelvis, which are likely to receive relatively high doses during the course of treatment of cervical malignancy.

The vaginal mucosa in the area of the vault tolerates between 20,000 and 25,000 cGy. The rectovaginal septum is said to tolerate approximately 6000 cGy over 4 to 6 weeks without difficulty. **The bladder mucosa can accept a maximal dose of 7000 cGy. The colon and rectum will tolerate approximately 5000 to 6000 cGy, but small bowel loops are less tolerant and are said to accept a maximal dose of between 4000 and 4200 cGy.** This pertains to small bowel loops within the pelvis; the tolerance of the small bowel when the entire abdomen is irradiated is limited to 2500 cGy. One of the basic principles of radiotherapy is implied here: The normal tissue tolerance of any organ is inversely related to the volume of the organ receiving irradiation. External irradiation and intracavitary radium therapy must be used in various combinations (Table 3.20). Treatment plans must be tailored to each patient and her particular lesion. The size and distribution of the cancer, not the stage, should be treated. Success in curing cancer of the cervix depends on the ability of the therapy team to evaluate the lesion (and the

geometry of the pelvis) during treatment and then make indicated changes in therapy as necessary. Intracavitary radium therapy is ideally suited to the treatment of early tumors because of the accessibility of the portio of the cervix and the cervical canal. It is possible to place radium or cesium in close proximity to the lesion and thus deliver surface doses that approximate 15,000 to 20,000 cGy. In addition, normal cervical and vaginal tissue has a particularly high tolerance to irradiation. One therefore has an ideal situation for the treatment of cancer because there are accessible lesions that lie in a bed of normal tissue (cervix and vagina) that is highly radioresistant.

Intensity-Modulated Whole Pelvic Radiotherapy

Traditional external-beam radiotherapy is based on field limits determined by bony landmarks, resulting in generous amounts of healthy tissue being encompassed by large treatment volumes. However, the margins of oncologic security are large, so target motion and the gross tumor volume (GTV) have a negligible impact. With increasing adoption of conformal treatment and attendant steep dose gradients, both the GTV and clinical target volume (CTV) must be precisely defined.

Using variable intensity across the face of the radiation beam to shape isodoses, (IMRT delivers a high tumor dose with minimization of radiation exposure to healthy tissue. Dosimetric advantages can be exploited using a combination of 3D planning and variable radiation intensity in each field. Reductions of both acute and chronic GI and genitourinary (GU) toxicity have been trumpeted among the dosimetric advantages of IMRT and some evidence suggesting that IMRT can spare bone marrow.

Uncertainty exists when considering IMRT for the management of locally advanced cervical cancer, including delineation of the required margins and what the acceptable degree of homogeneity is for the target. Importantly, given the large volume of hematopoietically active marrow in the pelvis and lower lumbar spine, in their review, Fernandez-Otz and Crook propose specific planning constraints be required, including use of a contouring atlas for pelvic volumes as currently used in current Radiation Therapy Oncology Group protocols (now part of NRG Oncology).

Radiation Therapy Oncology Group (RTOG) protocol 0418 established the current role of IMRT in gynecologic cancers to be relegated to the postoperative (ie, adjuvant) setting. The unacceptable toxicity of dose escalation to the pelvis and para-aortic regions using conventional radiotherapy has been prohibitive. However, with IMRT, simultaneous boosts to the target or affected lymph nodes results in an improvement of the therapeutic ratio and the added advantage of shortening the treatment time. Because of cervical-utero movement, the use of IMRT in the setting of the intact cervix requires continued investigation. RTOG protocols require a full bladder and empty rectum to minimize movement, but cervical tumor regression during treatment is also an issue, with a median volume reduction of 46% being reported in the literature. For this reason, Fernandez-Otz and Crook suggest that IMRT should be replanned during the final third of treatment to take advantage of the shrinking GTV.

TABLE 3.20   Suggested Therapy for Cervical Cancer

| | Whole Pelvis | | |
Stage	Radiation Dose (cGy)	Brachytherapy (mg/hr)	Surgery
Ia1 true microinvasive	—	—	Extrafascial hysterectomy
Ia2	2000 (2000 parametrial)	8000 (two applications)	Radical hysterectomy with bilateral pelvic lymphadenectomy as an option
Ib	4000	6000 (two applications)	
IIb	4000–5000*	5000–6000 (two applications)	Consider pelvic exenteration for tumor persistence
IIIa	5000–6000*	2000–3000 or interstitial implant	—
IIIb	5000–6000*	4000 (one application), 5000 (two applications)†	—
IVa	6000	4000 (one application), 5000 (two applications)†	—
IVb	500–1000 pulse two to four times 1 wk apart	Palliative	—

*Patients with larger lesions or poor vaginal geometry merit the higher dose of external radiation.

†Two applications are suggested after whole-pelvis radiation with larger lesions or when the first application has less than optimum dosimetry.

Ly et al. developed dose-volume histograms of the target volume in a comparison of conventional radiotherapy, 3D conformal radiotherapy, and IMRT for cervical cancer. They reported that the planning target volume dose of the IMRT was significantly higher than the other two modalities and that when more than 30 Gy was administered in IMRT, organs at risk including the small intestine, rectum, bladder, and bone marrow received reduced volumes of radiations. To date, however, there are no head-to-head randomized phase III trials comparing IMRT with conventional radiotherapy in the primary treatment of locally advanced cervical cancer.

Radium and Cesium Therapy

Radium is the isotope that has been used traditionally in the treatment of cancer of the cervix. Its greatest value is that its half-life is approximately 1620 years; therefore, it provides a very stable, durable element for therapy. In recent years, both cesium and cobalt have been used for intracavitary therapy. Cesium has a half-life of 30 years; with the current technology, cesium provides an adequate substitute for radium. Four major technologies for the application of radium in the treatment of cervical cancer continue to be favored among gynecologists. Of these technologies, three are intracavitary techniques using specially designed applicators, and the fourth technique involves the application of radium in the form of needles directly into the tumor. The variations among the three techniques of intracavitary brachytherapy are found in the Stockholm, Paris, and Manchester schools of treatment (Fig. 3.32). The differences are mainly found in the number and length of time of applications, the size and placement of the vaginal colpostats, and radium loading. In the United States, the tendency has been to use fixed radium applicators with the intrauterine tandem and vaginal colpostats originally attached to each other. Over the past 3 decades, a flexible afterloading system, Fletcher-Suit, has gained increasing popularity because it provides flexibility and the safety of afterloading techniques.

The Paris method originally used a daily insertion of 66.66 mg of radium divided equally between the uterus and the vagina. The radium remained in place for 12 to 14 hours, and the period of treatment varied from 5 to 7 days. An essential feature of the Paris method, and a part of the modification of this technique, is the vaginal colpostat, which consists of two hollow corks that serve as radium containers joined together by a steel spring that separates them into the lateral vaginal wall.

The Stockholm technique uses a tandem in the uterine cavity surrounded by a square radium plaque applied to the vaginal wall and portio vaginalis of the cervix. No radium is placed in the lower cervical canal, and vaginal sources are used to cover the cervical lesion. The uterine tandem and vaginal plaque are immobilized by packing and left in place for 12 to 36 hours. Two or three identical applications are made at weekly intervals.

The Manchester system is designed to yield constant isodose patterns regardless of the size of the uterus and vagina. The source placed in the neighborhood of the cervical canal is considered the unit strength. The remaining sources in the corpus and vagina are applied as multiples of this unit and are selected and arranged to produce equivalent isodose curves in each case and an optimal dose at preselected points in the pelvis. The applicator is shaped to allow an isodose curve that delivers radiation to the cervix in a uniform amount. The Fletcher-Suit system (Fig. 3.33) previously mentioned is a variation of the Manchester technique.

An effort is made in the two radium insertions to administer approximately 7000 cGy to the paracervical tissues as the total of the dose from both external and intracavitary irradiation. The isodose distribution around a Manchester system is pear shaped (Fig. 3.34). The maximal total dose delivered by the two radium insertions is a function of the total dose to the bladder and rectum. The total dose received by the rectal mucosa from both radium applications usually ranges between 4000 and 6000 cGy. The nearest bladder mucosa may receive between 5000 and 7000 cGy. When whole-pelvis irradiation is used, the radium dose must be reduced to keep the total dose to the bladder and rectum within acceptable limits.

In conjunction with the development of a system of radium distribution, British workers have defined two anatomic areas of the parametria (see Fig. 3.34) where dose designation can be

Manchester technique   Paris technique   Stockholm technique

FIGURE 3.32 Three techniques of intracavitary brachytherapy.

FIGURE 3.33 Fletcher-Suit radium applicators: Ovoids and tandem with inserts.

FIGURE 3.34 Pear-shaped distribution of radiation delivered to tissues surrounding a typical radium application with the Manchester type of applicators. Points *A* and *B* are noted as reference points.

correlated with clinical effect. These are situated in the proximal parametria adjacent to the cervix at the level of the internal os and in the distal parametria in the area of the iliac lymph nodes and are designated point A and point B. **The description states that point A is located 2 cm from the midline of the** **cervical canal and 2 m superior to the lateral vaginal fornix.** The dose at point A is representative of the dose to the paracervical triangle, which correlates well with the incidence of sequelae and with the 5-year control rate in many studies. **Point B is 3 cm lateral to point A.** This point, together with the tissue superior to it, is significant when considering the dose to the node-bearing tissue. It is clear from what has been said relative to points A and B that they can represent important points on a curve describing the dose gradient from the radium sources to the lateral pelvic wall. This gradient is different for the various techniques. In a comparison of the physical characteristics of radio techniques, the ratio of the dose at point A to the dose at point B should help define physical differences. In addition, determining the dose at point A relative to the calculated dose at points identified as bladder trigone and rectal mucosa provides a means of assessing the relative safety of one application over another. The concepts of points A and B have been questioned by many authors, including Fletcher and Rutledge. They remain as imaginary points but seem to provide a framework in which therapy is planned. Again, the distribution of the disease must be the primary guide in planning therapy, and the total dose to either point A or point B is relative only to their position with regard to the disease distribution.

Whole-pelvis irradiation is usually administered in conjunction with brachytherapy (eg, intracavitary radium or cesium) in a dose range of 4000 to 5000 cGy. Megavoltage machines such as cobalt, linear accelerators, and the betatron have the distinct advantage of giving greater homogeneity of dose to the pelvis. In addition, the hard, short rays of megavoltage pass through the skin without much absorption and cause very little injury, allowing almost unlimited amounts of radiation to be delivered to pelvic depths with little if any skin irritation. Orthovoltage, because of its relatively long wavelength and low energy, has the disadvantage that doses to the skin are particularly high and, in delivering the required amount of radiation to the pelvis, may cause temporary and permanent skin changes. Thus, for pelvis irradiation, high-energy megavoltage equipment has definite advantages over orthovoltage and even low-energy megavoltage equipment.

Interstitial Therapy

In advanced carcinoma of the cervix, the associated obliteration of the fornices or contracture of the vagina may interfere with accurate placement of conventional intracavitary applicators. Poorly placed applicators fail to irradiate the lesion and the pelvis homogeneously. Syed and Feder have revived a solution to this problem by advocating transvaginal and transperineal implants. The technique uses a template to guide the insertion of a group of 18-gauge hollow steel needles into the parametria transperineally (Fig. 3.35). These hollow needles are subsequently "afterloaded" with iridium wires when the patient returns to her hospital room. Theoretically, this technique locates a pair of paravaginal interstitial colpostats in both parametria. This approach appears promising, but long-term studies illustrating an improved survival rate and reasonable morbidity are not available. Also, there is no report reflecting, prospectively, the effectiveness, in comparable groups of patients, of the interstitial technique versus the standard intracavitary approach.

Interstitial therapy may have particular value in the treatment of carcinoma of the cervical stump. Although carcinoma of the cervical stump has become a relatively rare disease, accounting for fewer than 1% of all gynecologic malignancies, it does create difficult problems in terms of optimal geometry for delivery of effective irradiation therapy. In some series of cervical cancer, the incidence of carcinoma of the cervical stump is approximately 10%. Prempree, Patanaphan, and Scott reported excellent results with absolute survival rates of 83.3% for stage I, 75% for stage IIa, and 62.5% for stage IIb using radiation therapy with an emphasis on parametrial interstitial implants in the more advanced diseases. Similar results have been obtained by Puthawala and associates.

Extended-Field Irradiation Therapy

Over the past 2 decades, attempts have been made to improve survival for more patients with advanced cervical cancer by identifying the presence of paraaortic lymph node metastases and applying extended-field irradiation to the area (Fig. 3.36). The en bloc pelvic and periaortic portals extend superiorly as far as the level of the dome of the diaphragm and inferiorly to the obturator foramen. **The width of the periaortic portion of the field is usually 8 to 10 cm, and the usual dose delivered is**

FIGURE 3.35 Diagram of the technique of interstitial therapy for advanced cervical cancer using a Syed-Noblett template.

FIGURE 3.36 Abdominal radiograph showing portals for extended-field irradiation in cervical cancer.

TABLE 3.21 Late Complications of Radiation Therapy With Approximate Incidence

Complication	Patients (%)
Sigmoiditis	3
Rectovaginal fistula	1
Rectal stricture	1
Small bowel obstruction	1
(with extended field)	20
Vesicovaginal fistula	1
Ureteral stricture	1

between 4000 and 5000 cGy in 4 to 6 weeks. A booster dose of 1000 cGy is often given to the pelvic field alone. Identification of paraaortic lymph node involvement was initially attempted by use of lymphangiography, but this technique did not find general acceptance because of varied accuracy from institution to institution and from radiologist to radiologist. Surgical localization of periaortic involvement has been more satisfactory.

Several reports have discussed survival and complications in patients with carcinoma of the cervix and periaortic metastases who received extended-field irradiation (Table 3.21). Piver and Barlow of Roswell Park Memorial Institute, Buffalo, reported on 20 women with previously untreated cervical cancer who received radical irradiation to the periaortic lymph nodes and pelvis after the diagnosis of periaortic lymph node metastases had been established by surgical staging. They noted that 90% of these patients received 6000 cGy to the periaortic nodes and pelvis in 8 weeks using a split-course technique. A later report shows that 30% died of complications of this therapy, and 45% died of recurrent disease. Only 25% of patients survived disease free for 16, 18, 24, and 36 months. The criticism may be that the dose is too high, yet a lesser dose might be ineffective, and four patients did survive. It is obvious that a safe yet effective dosage level for extended-field irradiation therapy has not yet been established.

Wharton and colleagues of the MD Anderson Hospital reported on 120 women treated with preirradiation celiotomy. Of these patients, 32 had severe bowel complications, and 20 (16.6%) eventually died as a result of the surgery or of the surgery and irradiation. Four of these patients died immediately as a result of the surgical procedure. Of 64 patients with positive nodes who were irradiated, 17% lived for 13 to 38 months after treatment. No patient had survived for 5 years. Wharton and associates further reported that in 36 women with positive nodes, it was possible to accurately determine the failure sites after completion of the full course of irradiation therapy. In 25 of these patients, distant metastases were the first evidence of treatment failure, 11 had disease or developed recurrence within the treatment fields, and disease of the pelvic wall was found in only two patients.

The role of surgical staging in removal of paraaortic or pelvic nodes in cervical cancer remains controversial. The results of the aforementioned experience would question significant benefit in view of the complications and survival. Retroperitoneal lymphadenectomy, compared with the intraperitoneal approach, has decreased complications mainly as a result of adhesions and possible bowel complications. More recently, patients with advanced disease have had the paraaortic nodes reevaluated so that extended fields could be added if necessary. The laparoscopic approach is currently being evaluated. Less invasive approaches such as lymphangiogram, CT, and MRI studies have also been evaluated. The sensitivity is less, and false-negative results may be as high as 24% in patients with stage IIIB disease. Many gynecologic oncologists will obtain a CT scan and, if the result is positive, do a fine-needle aspiration. If the result is negative, then surgical removal may be done. An alternative is to radiate the paraaortic areas prophylactically. This has been done with little or no survival benefit. All of the studies note that the severe complication rate essentially doubles (5%–10%) when radiation was given to the paraaortic area.

Experience has shown that doses of about 4500 cGy, particularly when administered in daily fractions of 150 to 180 cGy, are safely tolerated by the organs in the periaortic treatment volume, and a complication rate of 5% should be expected. Extraperitoneal surgery appears to be associated with less postradiation morbidity, probably because of reduced bowel adhesions. The issues of the utility of periaortic radiation and surgical staging in the management of cervical carcinoma are closely intertwined. Although many hypotheses have been raised to support or reject the use of surgical staging, it is clear that some patients with biopsy-proven periaortic node metastases can be cured with radiotherapy using extended fields. Approximately 20% of patients who receive extended-field radiotherapy survive cervical cancer metastatic to the periaortic lymph nodes. Rubin and colleagues had a 50% survival rate in a group of patients with stage Ib disease with documented periaortic lymph node involvement. In many reports, the true value of extended-field radiation is clouded because patients with periaortic node involvement often have advanced disease in which any node or regional therapy may have little effect on long-term survival.

The incidence of pelvic recurrence after irradiation alone for stages Ib, IIa, and IIb carcinomas of the cervix increases with the diameter of the tumor. Data from the MD Anderson Hospital showed an improved pelvic control rate, and a small increase in survival, when patients with the bulky, so-called barrel-shaped lesions were treated with preoperative irradiation followed by extrafascial hysterectomy. The subject continues to be controversial, with conflicting studies in the literature. Gallion and colleagues reported on 75 patients with "bulky, barrel-shaped" stage Ib cervical cancer; 32 patients received radiation alone, and 43 patients were treated with radiation followed by extrafascial hysterectomy. The incidence of pelvic recurrence was reduced from 19% to 2%, and extrapelvic recurrence was reduced from 16% to 7% in patients treated by combination therapy, which produced no increase in treatment-related complications. However, Weems and colleagues described 123 such patients treated from two different eras at his institution. Examination of pelvic control rates, and disease-free survival, showed no significant advantage in pelvic control, disease-free survival, or absolute survival for either treatment group when compared by stage and tumor size. Unfortunately, no large prospective randomized study has been done that could clarify this issue.

Radiation and Chemotherapy

Radiation therapy alone fails to control the progression of cervical cancer in 35% to 90% of women with locally advanced disease. Concurrent chemoirradiation has been used in the treatment of many cancers in an attempt to improve local control and eradicate distant metastases and has been successfully integrated into the therapeutic program of not only cervical carcinomas but also those of the head and neck and anal canal. The rationale for chemoradiation is based on the finding that tumor radiosensitivity can be enhanced through the formation of DNA-platinum adducts. There is a correlation of radiosensitivity with platinum sensitivity. Specifically, the therapeutic index may be improved by loading the tumor with platinum salts containing fast atomic ions. Mechanisms of drug–radiation interaction leading to enhanced radiation kill may include modification of the slope of the dose-response curve, inhibition of sublethal damage repair, inhibition of recovery from potentially lethal damage, alterations in cellular kinetics, decrements in tumor volume leading to improved blood supply and tissue oxygenation, and increased radiosensitivity.

Five phase III trials of concurrent chemoirradiation performed by the Gynecologic Oncology Group, the RTOG, and the Southwestern Oncology Group (SWOG) have demonstrated a reduction in the risk of recurrence by up to 50% in patients with locally confined bulky or advanced-stage cervical cancer, regional spread, or high-risk features after hysterectomy (Table 3.22). Three studies compared radiotherapy alone with radiotherapy plus cisplatin-based chemotherapy, one of which addressed the prescription of adjuvant therapy following radical surgery for early-stage tumors (Intergroup Trial, discussed previously). Excluding patients with nodal involvement by CT scan, GOG protocol 123 evaluated the benefit of preoperative chemoirradiation therapy (weekly cisplatin 40 mg/m^2; maximal weekly dose of 70 mg) compared with radiation therapy alone in patients with locally advanced disease confined to the cervix (ie, stage IB2). All patients underwent adjuvant hysterectomy. In this landmark study, the rates of both PFS ($P <0.001$) and OS ($P = 0.008$) were significantly higher in the combined therapy group at 4 years. Patients receiving radiosensitizing chemotherapy experienced higher frequencies of grade III and grade IV adverse hematologic effects and adverse GI effects. An update of GOG 123 was provided by Stehman and colleagues in which chemoradiation was found to significantly improve long-term PFS and OS without significantly increasing serious late effects.

TABLE 3.22 Five Pivotal Trials of Chemoradiation in Locally Advanced Cervical Cancer

Trial	Author	Year	Eligibility	Arms	Patients (n)	Complete Response		Median Survival	
GOG 85	Whitney et al.	1999	IIB-IVA§	Pelvic RT + cisplatin 50 mg/m^2 + 5-FU 4 g/m^2/96 hr (2 cycles)	177	60%	$P = 0.033$	65%	$P = 0.018$
				Pelvic RT + hydroxyurea 3 g/m^2 (2×/wk)	191	48%		50%	
						PFS at 4 yr		OS at 4 yr	
GOG 109*	Peters et al.	2000	IA2-IIA	Adjuvant pelvic RT + cisplatin 70 mg/m^2 + 5-FU adjuvant pelvic RT	127	80%	$P = 0.003$	81%	$P = 0.007$
					116	63%		71%	
						PFS at 4 yr		OS at 4 yr	
GOG 120	Rose et al.	1999	IIB-IVA§	Pelvic RT + cisplatin 40 mg/m^2/wk	176	60%	$P = <0.001$‖	60%	$P = 0.002–0.004$‖
				Pelvic RT + cisplatin 50 mg/m^2 + 5-FU 4 g/m^2/96 hr + hydroxyurea 2 g/m pelvic RT + hydroxyurea 3 g/m^2 (2×/wk)	173	60%		58%	
					177	45%		34%	
						PFS at 4 yr		OS at 4 yr	
GOG 123	Keys et al.	1999	IB2†	Preoperative pelvic RT + cisplatin 40 mg/m^2/wk	183	80%	$P <0.001$	86%	$P = 0.008$
				Preoperative pelvic RT	186	64%		72%	
						DFS at 5 yr		OS at 5 yr	
RTOG 90-01	Morris et al.	1999	IB‡–IIA tumor ≥5 cm IIB-IVA or positive pelvic nodes	Pelvic RT + cisplatin 75 mg/m^2 + 5-FU 4 g/m^2/96 hr (3 cycles Pelvic RT + extended-field RT	193	67%	$P <0.01$	73%	$P = 0.004$
					193	40%		58%	

*Intergroup: Gynecologic Oncology Group (GOG) 109/Southwestern Oncology Group (SWOG) 8797/ Radiation Therapy Oncology Group (RTOG) 91-12; no randomization.
†Negative nodes.
‡State IB lesions included bulky tumors and those with positive pelvic lymph nodes.
§Negative paraaortic nodes.
‖Platinum-based regimens compared with hydroxyurea.
5-FU, 5-Flurouracil; PFS, progression-free survival; OS, overall survival; RT, radiation therapy.

Morris and colleagues reported the results from RTOG protocol 90-01. In this study, the effects of pelvic radiation plus concurrent cisplatin and 5-FU were compared with pelvic radiation plus extended-field radiation therapy. This was the only trial to include chemotherapy during low-dose-rate brachytherapy. Eligibility requirements for this study differed from the previous GOG studies with the inclusion of patients with FIGO stage IB2 to IIA tumors. The estimated 5-year survival rates were 73% versus 58%, respectively, for patients treated with chemoirradiation therapy versus radiation therapy alone. A significant difference in disease-free survival was also seen in favor of the chemotherapy arm. The addition of chemotherapy to radiation therapy was effective in reducing both the frequency of local recurrences and distant metastases, with the latter observation refuting those detractors who claim that the benefit conferred by radiosensitizing chemotherapy is strictly a function of increasing the relative dose intensity of the radiation that can be delivered to the pelvis. These results have been sustained in an update of RTOG protocol 90-01 with 8 years of follow-up provided by Eifel and colleagues.

Two additional phase III trials have confirmed the superiority of cisplatin-based chemoirradiation for the treatment of locally advanced cervical cancer. Whitney and colleagues published the results of concurrent cisplatin plus 5-FU and pelvic radiation therapy versus hydroxyurea plus pelvic radiation therapy in women with FIGO stage IIB to IVA disease who had undergone surgical staging and were found to have negative common iliac and aortocaval lymph nodes (GOG protocol 85). Among 368 eligible patients, the median follow-up time among survivors was 8.7 years. Disease progression occurred in 43% of patients randomly assigned to cisplatin plus 5-FU versus 53% of patients randomized to hydroxyurea. PFS was significantly better among patients treated with the combined chemotherapy regimen ($P=0.033$), with 3-year survival rates of 67% (cisplatin–5-FU arm) versus 57% (hydroxyurea).

Rose and colleagues reported the results from the three-arm GOG trial of pelvic radiation therapy plus concurrent single-agent cisplatin versus cisplatin plus 5-FU plus hydroxyurea versus hydroxyurea alone (protocol 120). All patients had FIGO stage IIB to IVA cervical cancer with surgically confirmed negative common iliac and aortocaval lymph nodes. The median duration of follow-up was 35 months for 526 women included in the final analysis. Significant improvements in progression-free and OS were observed in patients randomly assigned to either cisplatin-containing arm. Effectively, the results from GOG protocol 85 and GOG protocol 120 were critical in supplanting hydroxyurea as the radiosensitizer of choice. In 2007, Rose and colleagues provided their own update of GOG 120 in which again it was found that the improvement in PFS and OS observed with cisplatin-based chemoradiation was sustained without significant increases in late toxicity (Table 3.23).

Because the combination of cisplatin plus 5-FU results in added toxicity, weekly single-agent cisplatin dosed at 40 mg/m^2 has emerged as the standard radiosensitizer in locally advanced cervical cancer. At present, radiosensitizing chemotherapy is recommended during that part of the treatment program when external-beam pelvic radiotherapy is administered.

TABLE 3.23   Updates and Ad Hoc Analysis of Pivotal Chemoradiation Trials in Cervical Cancer

Study	Description	Update
Intergroup trial	Adjuvant RT Adjuvant CRT	Absolute 5YS benefit for CRT: tumors >2 cm, ≥2 positive nodes
GOG 123	RT plus adjuvant hysterectomy CRT plus adjuvant hysterectomy	CRT significantly improves long-term PFS and OS; serious late effects not increased significantly
RTOG 9001	RT plus EFRTCRT	CRT: superior OS and DFS (IB–IIB); superior DFS (III–IVA); serious late effects not increased significantly
GOG 120	CDDP–RTCDDP/HU/5-FU–CDDP–HU	CDDP-based CRT improves long-term PFS and OS; no significant increase in late toxicity

CDDP, cisplatin; *CRT*, chemoradiation; *EFRTCRT*, extended field radiation therapy plus chemoradiation; *GOG*, Gynecologic Oncology Group; *HU*, hydroxyurea; *OS*, overall survival; *PFS*, progression-free survival; *RT*, radiation therapy; *RTCDDP*, radiation therapy plus cisplatin; *RTOG*, Radiation Therapy Oncology Group.

 Relative risk—with 90% CI

FIGURE 3.37 Relative risk estimate of survival from five phase-III, randomized controlled clinical trials of chemoradiation in women with cervical cancer. *GOG*, Gynecologic Oncology Group; *RTOG*, Radiation Therapy Oncology Group; *SWOG*, Southwestern Oncology Group.

These pivotal phase III trials not only identified a significant survival advantage associated with the addition of concurrent chemotherapy but also were noteworthy in that the degree of benefit achieved with chemotherapy was remarkably similar for each of the four trials that studied chemoirradiation for primary therapy (Fig. 3.37). The results changed the standard of care for the treatment of locally advanced cervical cancer and formed the basis for the 1999 National Cancer Institute (NCI) Clinical

Announcement (Practice Alert) in cervical cancer. At that time, NCI Director Richard D. Klausner, MD, stated the following: "The findings of these five trials are remarkably consistent. They are likely to change the standard of care for invasive cervical cancer."

A meta-analysis of 19 RCTs of chemoradiation versus radiation therapy alone containing a sample of 4580 patients treated from 1981 to 2000 was published in 2001 by Green and colleagues. In their report, the HRs for both PFS and OS favored chemoradiation (HR 0.61; P <0.0001 and HR 0.71; P <0.0001, respectively). The Cochrane review from 2005 analyzed 24 RCTs of 4921 patients. Chemoradiation was associated with a 10% absolute benefit in OS, a 13% absolute benefit in PFS, and a significant benefit was noted for local control. Acute hematologic and GI toxicity were reported more frequently with chemoradiation, but treatment-related deaths attributable to multimodality therapy were rare. Late effects were not able to be adequately determined in the Cochrane review. Most recently, a meta-analysis of 18 randomized trials containing 3517 patients again reported superiority of chemoradiation to radiation therapy alone in terms of relative risk (RR), 3-year survival, and 5-year survival. In this third meta-analysis, although GI toxicity, myelosuppression, and leukopenia occurred more frequently with the use of chemoradiation, there were no significant differences noted between the two modalities in terms of proctitis, cystitis, and nausea or vomiting.

A phase III experience from the Ion Chiricuta Cancer Institute in Romania involved 566 patients with FIGO IIB-IIIB lesions who were randomly assigned to pelvic radiation therapy (46 Gy [gray]) plus high-dose rate brachytherapy (10 Gy) with or without cisplatin (20 mg/m^2 × 5 days). The 5-year survival rate was significantly improved with the use of chemoradiation (74% vs. 64%; P <0.05), as was the local control rate (78% vs. 67%; P = 0.01).

In a 2007 study of practice patterns within the Gynecologic Cancer Intergroup, a global consortium of 14 cooperative groups, the mean external-beam radiation therapy dose was 47 Gy (3.5 Gy SD [standard dose]). The mean total dose to point A was 79.1 Gy (7.9 Gy SD), and the upper border for extended-field radiation therapy among 63% of respondents was T12 to L1. Approximately 85% used high-dose rate systems for vaginal brachytherapy. Of note, all groups reported using concurrent chemotherapy, with weekly cisplatin being the agent of choice for 83%.

The National Comprehensive Cancer Network (NCCN) Clinical Practice Guidelines in Oncology were updated in 2010 for cervical cancer. **For patients with selected bulky tumors, those with FIGO stage IB2 and IIA lesions (>4 cm), and those with FIGO stage IIB to IVA disease, Category 1 treatment constitutes pelvic radiotherapy plus concurrent cisplatin-containing chemotherapy plus brachytherapy.**

The latest phase III trial to study chemoradiation in the locally advanced cervical cancer population was conducted in Mexico by Duenas-Gonzalez et al. In their open-label, randomized phase III trial, the authors studied cisplatin-based chemoradiation followed by brachytherapy with and without concurrent gemcitabine (125 mg/m^2 weekly) and by adjuvant

cisplatin (50 mg/m^2 day 1) plus gemcitabine (1000 mg/m^2 days 1 and 8) every 21 days for two cycles. Grade 3 and 4 toxicities were more frequent in the investigational arm (86.5% vs. 46.3%; P <0.001), including two deaths possibly related to treatment toxicity. The PFS at 3 years for the 515 patients enrolled favored the investigational arm (74.4% vs. 65.0%; P = 0.029) and the overall hazard of progression was 0.68 (95% CI, 0.49-0.95; P = 0.0227), and the hazard of death was 0.68 (95% CI, 0.49–0.95; P = 0.0224). Despite these survival figures, the incorporation of gemcitabine into chemoradiation protocols has not been met with great enthusiasm worldwide. Currently, NRG Oncology (the former Gynecologic Oncology Group and Radiation Therapy Oncology Group) in collaboration with the Australian-New Zealand Gynecologic Oncology Group (ANZGOG) is studying the value of four cycles of adjuvant carboplatin plus paclitaxel in this population in the phase III randomized study known as the OUTBACK Trial.

Neoadjuvant Chemotherapy and Other Novel Treatment Approaches

Although multimodality therapy has emerged as the standard of care of patients with locally advanced disease, chemoradiation has some shortcomings related to access, efficacy, and tolerability in certain populations. Neoadjuvant chemotherapy is the most studied alternative treatment modality for FIGO stage IB2 to IVA and is discussed in detail later in this chapter. Other modalities under investigation include proton beam therapy, CyberKnife radiosurgery, IMRT, radiosurgery, radiohyperthermia, and the incorporation of antiangiogenesis and other targeted agents into chemoradiation protocols.

Kagei and colleagues treated 25 patients with FIGO stage IIB to IVA disease with external-beam radiation therapy plus proton beam irradiation. The median total tumor dose was 86 Gy. At a median follow-up period of 139 months (range, 11–184 months), the 10-year OS rates were 89% for stage IIB and 40% for stages IIIB/IVA. Grade IV GI and GU toxicities were reported in 4% of patients. Choi and colleagues treated 30 women with isolated paraaortic nodal metastases with the CyberKnife. Grade III to IV toxicity requiring hospitalization occurred in one patient. The 4-year OS and 4-year local control rates were 50.1% and 67.4%, respectively. A nonrandomized trial comparing 135 women with locally advanced disease treated with IMRT using FDG-PET/CT simulation to 317 non-IMRT patients was reported to have had no significant impact on recurrence-free survival, although the grade III to IV bowel and bladder toxicities were reportedly higher in the non-IMRT cohort (P = 0.0351). Although the radiobiologic rationale for these three investigational modalities is promising, there have been no randomized trials for the population under discussion.

As a result of limited access to sophisticated radiotherapy centers in resource-poor areas of the world, neoadjuvant chemotherapy has emerged as a viable alternative for treatment of women with locally advanced lesions. This approach was popularized by Sardi and colleagues in their "Buenos Aires protocol." In one of the first prospective randomized studies of neoadjuvant chemotherapy in early-stage cervical cancer, Sardi and colleagues reported their final results in 205 cases of stage

Ib carcinoma of the cervix. Patients were treated with radical hysterectomy followed by 50-Gy radiotherapy to the pelvis with or without neoadjuvant chemotherapy. In patients with stage Ib1, neoadjuvant chemotherapy did not improve overall resectability or survival compared with those not receiving chemotherapy. In patients with stage Ib2, there was 83.6% (51 of 61) partial or complete response to chemotherapy. OS after 9 years of follow-up was 61% for the control group (no chemotherapy) and 80% for the neoadjuvant group ($P < 0.01$). Resection was possible in 85% of the control group and 100% in the neoadjuvant group. Patients who responded to neoadjuvant therapy had an OS of 88% compared with 23% for nonresponders. Of interest, the stage Ib1, neoadjuvant groups had an 82% OS compared with 80% for stage Ib2. The control groups' survival rates were 77% and 61%, respectively. Neoadjuvant chemotherapy improved resectability and survival in the patients with stage Ib2. All patients received postoperative radiation.

The Cochrane Collaboration visited this subject originally in 2004 and returned to it recently. In their 2010 report, the authors identified 1072 patients from six trials (Table 3.24). Although PFS was significantly improved with neoadjuvant chemotherapy (HR, 0.76; 95% CI 0.62–0.94; $P = 0.01$), no OS benefit was observed (HR, 0.85; 95% CI 0.67–1.07; $P = 0.17$). Neoadjuvant chemotherapy was associated with a significant decrease in adverse pathologic findings, including lymph node status and parametrial infiltration. Total cisplatin dose and schedule did not influence the findings, nor did stage of disease. The authors concluded that it remains unclear whether neoadjuvant chemotherapy consistently offers a benefit over surgery alone for patients with early-stage or locally advanced cancer.

The latest Cochrane Collaboration review of six randomized trials of neoadjuvant chemotherapy with surgery for women with untreated early or locally advanced cervical cancer providing PFS data ($n = 1027$) and OS data ($n = 1071$) was reported by Rydzewska et al. in 2012. Both parameters were significantly improved among patients receiving neoadjuvant chemotherapy (hazard of progression, 0.75; 95% CI 0.61–0.93; $P = 0.008$) and hazard of death 0.77; 95% CI, 0.62–0.96; $P = 0.02$). The authors emphasized that despite the favorable results associated with neoadjuvant chemotherapy, their analysis was based on a small number of trials, and further research is clearly warranted.

TABLE 3.24   **Neoadjuvant Chemotherapy Plus Surgery Versus Surgery Alone: Hazard Ratios and Confidence Intervals for Overall Survival**

Study (Year)	Patients (n)	HR	95% CI
Sardi et al. (1997)	210	0.53	0.31, 0.92
Katsumata (2006)	134	1.12	0.56, 2.22
Cai (2006)	106	0.74	0.33, 1.65
Napolitano (2003)	288	0.84	0.51, 1.40
Total	**930**	**0.85**	**0.67, 1.07**

CI, Confidence interval; *HR,* hazards ratio.
Modified from Rydzewska L, Tierney J, Vale CL, Symonds PR. Neoadjuvant chemotherapy plus surgery versus surgery for cervical cancer. *Cochrane Database Syst Rev* 2010;1:CD007406.

A Cochrane Collaboration review identified six randomized controlled trials of radiotherapy versus radiohyperthermia for patients with locally advanced cervical carcinoma during the period from 1987 to 2009. Seventy-four percent of patients treated had FIGO stage IIIB tumors. The HRs for 3-year local recurrence and 3-year survival favored the 43°C hyperthermia arms (HR, 0.48; 95% CI 0.37–0.63; $P < 0.001$ and HR 0.6; 95% CI 0.45–0.99; $P = 0.05$, respectively). There were no significant differences in acute or late-grade III to IV toxicity. The review did indicate that these studies were limited by small numbers and important methodologic flaws.

Finally, a recent Cochrane Collaborative study focusing on the impact of hysterectomy for women with locally advanced disease treated with radiotherapy or chemotherapy or both was reported by Kokka et al. Seven randomized trials were identified involving 1217 patients. Although individual trials did not report a survival advantage among women undergoing hysterectomy after radiotherapy or concurrent chemoradiation, the meta-analysis of three trials ($n = 571$) of neoadjuvant chemotherapy and hysterectomy versus radiotherapy alone found that women who received neoadjuvant chemotherapy plus hysterectomy had a lower risk of death (HR, 0.71; 95% CI, 0.55–0.93).

Targeted therapy has been studied in two chemoradiation protocols. In 2012, the Gynecologic Oncology Group reported in the phase I protocol 9918 that the addition of anti-epithelial growth factor therapy using cetuximab (400 mg/m² loading dose followed by 250 mg/m²) to cisplatin-based chemoradiation was tolerable, but when added to extended-field radiation therapy for treatment of nodal metastases, there were eight dose-limiting toxicities, making the combination not feasible. In RTOG 0417, the antiangiogenesis agent bevacizumab (10 mg/kg IV every 2 weeks) was added to 49 patients treated with cisplatin-based chemoradiation for FIGO stage IB to IIIB disease. The 3-year OS, disease-free survival, and locoregional failure rates were 81.3%, 68.7%, and 23.2%, respectively. The paraaortic nodal failure rate at 3 years was 8.4%.

Suboptimal Treatment Situations

Several clinical situations pose unique challenges in the management of cervical cancer, causing some patients with invasive cancer of the cervix to receive suboptimal treatment:
1. Cancer in a cervical stump
2. Simple hysterectomy in the setting of invasive cervical cancer
3. Poor vaginal geometry for intracavitary radiation.

Cancer that occurs in a cervical stump is fortunately a diminishing problem because supracervical hysterectomies are performed less frequently. Carcinoma occurring in a cervical stump presents a special problem because often an optimal dose of intracavitary radium cannot be applied as a result of the insufficient place to insert the central tandem, which contributes significantly to the radiation dose to the central tumor and to the pelvic sidewall. Radical surgery is also more difficult; the bladder and rectum firmly adhere to the stump and may adhere to each other. Also, the ureters are more difficult to dissect cleanly from the parametrial tissue because of fibrosis from the previous surgery. The net result is an increase in the risk of significant surgical complications involving the ureters, bladder, and rectum. In modern gynecologic surgery, supracervical hysterectomy is rarely indicated, although in recent years, concerns regarding pelvic support and even sexual function have prompted some surgeons to consider the procedure.

In a report of the MD Anderson Hospital experience with 263 patients with carcinoma of the cervical stump, Miller and colleagues noted a 30% complication rate after full therapy with radiation. Urinary and bowel complications result from post-surgical adhesions; the absence of the uterus, which acts as a shield; and a tendency to emphasize external radiation therapy. We have had a similar experience, resulting in a preference for radical trachelectomy in patients with cancer of the cervical stump in whom stage and medical conditions allow. The increased technical difficulty of performing such a procedure seems to be outweighed by the low complication rate and comparable survival of patients.

A simple hysterectomy performed for invasive cervical cancer is not adequate therapy for most patients. This situation may occur because of poor preoperative evaluation or because the surgery was performed under emergency conditions without an adequate preoperative cervical evaluation. Such a situation may occur in a patient presenting with acute abdomen from ruptured tuboovarian abscesses. In any event, if an extensive cancer is found in the cervix, the prognosis is poor because optimal irradiation cannot be given with the cervix and uterus absent. An even more ominous situation occurs when a hysterectomy is performed with a "cut through" of the cancer—that is, the hysterectomy dissection passes through the cancer. The prognosis is uniformly poor in this event. In the examples just given, surgical cures are not obtained, and the probability of curative radiotherapy is greatly diminished.

In 1968, Durrance reported survival rates of 92% to 100% using postoperative radiation therapy in selected patients with presumed stage I or II disease after suboptimal surgery. Excellent survival rates were also reported by Andras and colleagues in 148 patients who had invasive cervical carcinoma found incidentally in the hysterectomy specimen. Of these patients, 126 were treated with postoperative radiation therapy. Patients with microscopic disease confined to the cervix had a 96% 5-year survival rate. Those with gross tumor confined to the cervix had an 84% 5-year survival. Patients with tumor cut through at the margins of surgical resection, but with no obvious residual cancer, had a 5-year survival rate of 87%. Patients with obvious residual pelvic tumor had a 47% 5-year survival rate. In 1986, Heller and colleagues reviewed the literature and reported equivalent survival rates in 35 patients who were also treated mainly with radiation.

Orr and colleagues have preferred radical parametrectomy, upper vaginectomy, and lymphadenectomy as the treatment of choice after a simple hysterectomy. We also prefer this approach, particularly because many of these patients are young and desirous of preserving optimal sexual function. We are also concerned about postoperative small bowel adhesions and the difficulty of delivering effective irradiation to the medial parametria in the absence of a uterus. Survival rates with either approach appear to be exceptionally good; undoubtedly, this clinical situation creates a bias for smaller lesions that may be easier to eradicate.

Adequate radiotherapy is also compromised in patients who have a vagina or cervix that cannot accommodate a complete intracavitary radiation application. This situation is encountered with atrophic stenotic pelvic structures. These patients are treated by inserting the tandem and ovoids in a compromised manner, such as insertion of the ovoids singly or independently of the central tandem. In any event, standard optimal doses are usually not obtained, and the possibility of sustaining a radiation injury is increased.

NEUROENDOCRINE AND OTHER UNCOMMON TUMORS OF THE CERVIX

Neuroendocrine (small cell) cervical cancer (Fig. 3.38) is a rare malignancy, representing fewer than 5% of all cases of cervical cancer. These tumors provide a therapeutic challenge for the clinician because they are characterized by frequent and early nodal and distant metastases. The pathologist's dilemma results from the large number of pathologic entities all described as "small cell cancers," including fully differentiated small cell nonkeratinizing SCC, reserved cell carcinoma, and neuroendocrine (oat cell) carcinoma. Neuroendocrine carcinomas, which can be identified by characteristic light and electron microscopic criteria, are indistinguishable from oat cell cancers of the lung. In addition, they appear to have the poorest prognosis of the various small cell cancers. Therefore, it is important to distinguish this particular subtype of cancer from the rest and to consider innovative approaches to treatment. **Neuroendocrine markers are commonly used to assist in classification, with up to 80% of tumors staining for synaptophysin, chromogranin, or CD56 (neural cell adhesion molecule).** At least in one series, Pap smear results were abnormal in only one of seven patients.

Abeler and colleagues reported on 26 cases of true neuroendocrine cervical carcinoma. The 5-year survival rate was 14% despite aggressive therapy, including surgery, radiation, and chemotherapy. Viswanathan and colleagues observed a 66%

FIGURE 3.38 Small cell carcinoma. (Courtesy of Ibrahim Ramzy, MD, University of California, Irvine (UCI), College of Medicine.)

relapse rate, with a course frequently characterized by the development of widespread hematogenous metastases. Locoregional recurrence outside irradiated fields was also frequently observed. In the group studied, the OS rate at 5 years was only 29%, with none of the patients who had disease more extensive than FIGO stage Ib1 or clinical evidence of lymph node metastases surviving their disease.

In our experience in the 1980s with 14 patients in stage Ib or IIa treated by radical hysterectomy with postoperative radiation therapy, all 14 have experienced recurrence, 12 before the 31st month after therapy. Innovative approaches to treating this subset of unfortunate patients are under study. Recently, Chan and colleagues updated our series and performed a multivariate analysis of different prognostic factors among 34 patients. His group documented that only those with early lesions amenable to extirpation were curable. The role of primary or postoperative radiation with or without chemotherapy is unclear and yields uniformly poor results, particularly in patients with advanced lesions.

Hoskins and colleagues treated 31 patients with small cell neuroendocrine carcinoma (SCNEC) using protocols containing etoposide, cisplatin, and radiation therapy with concurrent chemotherapy with and without the addition of carboplatin and paclitaxel. The reported 3-year failure-free rate for patients with early-stage disease (stage I and II) was 80%. Chang and colleagues have reported that regimens containing a combination of vincristine, doxorubicin, and cyclophosphamide or cisplatin and etoposide constitute active adjuvant therapies after radical hysterectomy. Zivanovic and colleagues examined the outcomes of 17 patients with SCNEC. The estimated 3-year PFS and OS rates were 22% and 30%, respectively. Median OS rates for early-stage disease (IA1–IB2) were 31.2 months and 6.4 months for those with advanced-stage disease (IIB-IV; $P = 0.034$). In the early-stage disease group, the 3-year distant recurrence-free survival rates were 83% for patients who received platinum-based combination chemotherapy and 0% for those who did not receive chemotherapy as part of their initial treatment ($P = 0.025$). These data support the role of chemotherapy for distant control as an addition to radiation therapy for local control. Of interest, combined modality treatment with definitive chemotherapy and radiotherapy are used in the current management of small cell lung cancer, with surgical resection playing a limited role in patients with stage I and stage II disease. It is unclear which patients, if any, should undergo radical hysterectomy for SCNEC of the cervix. Zivanovic and colleagues advise proceeding with combined modality therapy when the diagnosis is established by cervical biopsy, holding surgery in reserve to be used in the adjuvant setting if necessary. It should be recognized that there are advocates of primary radical hysterectomy for patients with early-stage tumors.

Finally, a recent case report by Lyons et al. describing the objective response when a neuroendocrine cervical cancer harboring a Kirsten rat sarcoma viral oncogene homolog (KRAS) mutation was treated with a mitogen-activated protein kinase kinase (MEK) inhibitor emphasizes a potential role for biomarker testing to further guide therapy. Provision of the molecular phenotype of these (and other) tumors is likely to provide the basis for future personalized therapy.

GLASSY CELL CARCINOMA, CARCINOSARCOMA, LYMPHOMA, AND MELANOMA

Glassy cell carcinoma of the cervix has also been classically regarded as a poorly differentiated adenosquamous carcinoma, which is infrequently diagnosed and associated with a poor outcome regardless of the modality of therapy. Many recurrences occur in the first year after therapy, and most have occurred by 24 months. Reported survival rates are more encouraging than are those associated with neuroendocrine carcinomas; rates have been seen to be as high as 50% for stage I disease in some series.

In the SEER report of 6549 cases of cervical carcinoma from 1973 to 1977, there were only 36 cases of cervical sarcoma, which is an incidence of 0.55%. Ninety-six cases of cervical sarcoma were reviewed by Rotmensch and colleagues, and no clear statement could be made regarding management, although surgery was consistently used for early-stage lesions. Laterza and colleagues reviewed the literature and described the outcomes of 33 patients with carcinosarcoma of the cervix, including two of their own (Fig. 3.39). Of 16 patients with stage I disease, eight were reported to be NED after a variety of treatment modalities, including surgery, radiation, or chemotherapy, alone or in combination. The impact of radiotherapy on survival is uncertain. Given the propensity for distinct histologic subtypes to respond to systemic regimens irrespective of organ site of origin (eg, small cell neuroendocrine carcinomas of the cervix and lung, malignant germ cell tumors of the ovary and testis), ifosfamide-based regimens, particularly ifosfamide plus paclitaxel, may be expected to exhibit some activity in this disease, similar to what has been reported in carcinosarcoma of the uterine corpus.

FIGURE 3.39 Carcinosarcoma. (From Laterza R, Seveso A, Zefiro F, et al. Carcinosarcoma of the uterine cervix: case report and discussion. *Gynecol Oncol* 2007;107(1 suppl):S98-100.)

FIGURE 3.40 Lymphoma. (From Szánthó A, Bálega J Já, Csapó Z, et al. Primary non-Hodgkin's lymphoma of the uterine cervix successfully treated by neoadjuvant chemotherapy: case report. *Gynecol Oncol* 2003;89:171-174.)

FIGURE 3.41 Melanoma. (From Kristiansen SB, Anderson R, Cohen DM. Primary malignant melanoma of the cervix and review of the literature. *Gynecol Oncol* 1992;47:398-403.)

Biomarker profiling may also be of value to understand the clinical behavior of these rare cancers. In a small series of three women with cervical carcinosarcoma, Gan et al. reported high levels of bcl-2 and surviving expression and decreased apoptosis using an apoptosis index. Dysregulation of apoptosis may facilitate the aggressive behavior of carcinosarcoma.

In contrast to systemic lymphomas, fever, night sweats, and weight loss rarely have been reported in cervical lymphoma (Fig. 3.40). Most present with abnormal vaginal bleeding or discharge, but pelvic pain and dyspareunia may also be present. The differential diagnosis of cervical lymphomas should include benign chronic inflammations, poorly differentiated and small cell cervical carcinomas, sarcomas, and lymphoma-like lesions. Immunophenotyping can be used to make the diagnosis.

The prognosis of extranodal lymphomas is usually poorer than that of nodal lymphomas as a result of inaccurate or delayed diagnosis. Early-stage diagnosis of cervical lymphoma has been associated with favorable outcomes. Some authors have suggested that surgical resection in localized lymphoma may improve survival, although this is unclear. The CHOP (cyclophosphamide, doxorubicin, vincristine, prednisone) regimen is the most commonly used regimen.

Malignant melanoma of the uterine cervix is a rare manifestation (Fig. 3.41). A careful survey should be done of the patient's skin and mucous membranes for a possible primary site. Almost 90% of the patients are asymptomatic, and vaginal bleeding is the main complaint among 10%. Most lesions present as an exophytic polypoid cervical mass with obvious coloring. **Immunohistochemistry can be used to identify melanin granules, and positive staining for S100, HMB 45, or Melan-A can help in establishing the diagnosis.** Although there is little consensus on the best approach for therapeutic management, the majority of patients have undergone radical hysterectomy with or without pelvic lymphadenectomy and upper vaginectomy. The efficacy of radiation therapy has not been established, although it has been used in the adjunctive and palliative settings. Likewise, the use of adjuvant chemotherapy

is under debate. To date, there have been no reports of immunotherapy, including the use of interferon, for this disease. The 5-year survival rate is very poor, not exceeding 40% of stage I and 14% of stage II.

The therapeutic landscape of cutaneous melanoma has been transformed with the introduction of checkpoint inhibitors (eg, anti-CTLA-4 ipilimumab and the antiprogrammed cell death 1 nivolumab and pembrolizumab). To date, there have been no reports of the efficacy of breaking immune tolerance in cervical melanoma but we may anticipate that they will be forthcoming.

SURVIVAL RESULTS AND PROGNOSTIC FACTORS FOR EARLY-STAGE AND LOCALLY ADVANCED DISEASE

For early-stage tumors, results may imply that one form of therapy (ie, radical surgery vs. radiotherapy) has advantages over the other, but considering the rather wide dispersion that, in fact, may be unrelated to treatment, we must maintain collective open-mindedness about the efficacy of individual therapeutic regimens. The best available figures for the two methods give results that are almost identical, and because the presence of other factors affect the samples being compared, large differences would be necessary to be significant. Individual physicians will probably continue to decide on the basis of personal preferences and comparison of complications and later disabilities.

The recovery rates of patients with operative SCC of the cervix depend on many factors, including the histologically documented extent of the carcinoma. Baltzer and associates studied 718 surgical specimens of patients with SCC of the cervix. Lymphatic and blood vessel invasion significantly influenced survival, blood vessel invasion being much more ominous. In their study, whereas 70% of the patients who demonstrated blood vessel invasion succumbed to the disease,

31% of the patients demonstrating only lymphatic invasion succumbed to the disease process. Other studies have not found prognostic significance for vascular invasion. A definite linkage was noted between the size of the carcinomas and the frequency of metastases. Fuller and colleagues drew similar conclusions. In their study of 431 patients who underwent radical hysterectomy for stages Ib or IIa carcinoma of the cervix at Memorial Sloan-Kettering Cancer Center, they found 71 patients who had nodal spread that correlated closely with increased primary tumor size, extracervical extension of tumor, and the presence of adenocarcinoma. Although these factors were recognized as having prognostic significance, the authors were unable to demonstrate that these detrimental effects could be overcome by postoperative pelvic radiation. Patients receiving postoperative irradiation therapy seemed to have some better local control, but the problem of systemic spread of disease resulted in little overall improvement in survival. In a similar study, Abdul-hayogu and associates reported on a series of patients with negative lymph nodes at the time of radical hysterectomy who subsequently developed recurrent disease. They too pointed out the histologic architecture of invasion as an important prognostic indicator. Recurrence was more likely in patients who had deep invasion of the cervical stroma, especially when it extended to the serosal surface (even when the parametria were not involved). Again, the volume of tumor correlated with the eventual prognosis for the patient. They suggested that these patients were in need of postoperative therapy, and radiation therapy for local control was recommended in the absence of any other demonstrated effective adjuvant modality for this set of circumstances. Gauthier and colleagues had similar results and, in a multifactorial analysis of clinical and pathologic factors, demonstrated that the depth of stromal invasion is the single most important determinant of survival.

The role of intraperitoneal tumor spread was evaluated by an Italian group. They evaluated 208 patients with advanced local disease who received neoadjuvant chemotherapy. There were 183 clinically responsive patients who underwent radical surgery; 7 (4%) and 13 (7%) showed macroscopic and microscopic peritoneal tumor, respectively. Multivariant analysis showed that the peritoneal tumor involvement, stage, pathologic parametrial involvement, and lymph node metastasis were independent factors associated with survival. About one-quarter of those with pelvic lymph node metastasis had intraperitoneal involvement compared with only 6% of node-negative patients. If intraperitoneal disease was present, survival was similar, irrespective of stage (Ib–IIb compared with III–IVa).

A study from Austria evaluated 166 patients with stage Ib cancers treated with radical hysterectomy. In a multivariant analysis, microvessel density, lymph node involvement, tumor size, and postoperative radiation remained independent prognostic factors for survival. LSI failed to be a prognostic factor. Of interest, patients with negative lymph nodes but increased microvessel density had similar survival to patients who were node positive but with low microvessel density. A study from Norway evaluated HPV DNA in 97 patients with squamous carcinoma (all stages). When corrected for stage and age, the prognosis was significantly poorer for HPV-18– and -33–positive tumors; however, overall, when all HPV-positive tumors were compared with HPV-negative tumors, no survival difference was noted.

When age was evaluated in the Annual Report, the OS rate in stage I decreased with age. Patients between 15 and 39 years of age in stage II had a worse survival rate compared with older patients. This was true for patients 30 to 49 years of age with stage IV cancers compared with patients of other ages. Mitchell and colleagues reviewed 398 patients with stages I to III cervical cancer of whom 338 patients were 35 to 69 years of age, and 60 patients were 70 years of age or older. Although elderly patients had a higher rate of comorbidity resulting in more frequent treatment breaks and less ability to receive definitive therapy with intracavity radiation, the 5-year actuarial disease-free and cause-specific survival rates were comparable between the two groups.

RECURRENT AND ADVANCED CARCINOMA OF THE CERVIX

It is estimated that approximately 35% of patients with invasive cervical cancer will have recurrent or persistent disease after therapy. The diagnosis of recurrent cervical cancer is often difficult to establish (Table 3.25). The optimal radiation therapy most patients receive makes cervical cytologic findings difficult to evaluate. This is especially true immediately after completion of radiation therapy. Suit, using mammary carcinomas in C3H mice, demonstrated that persistence of histologically intact cancer cells in irradiated tissue was not indicative of the regrowth of a tumor. Radiobiologically, a viable cell is one with the capacity for sustained proliferation. A cell would be classified as nonviable if it had lost its reproductive integrity, although it could carry out diverse metabolic activities. This reproductive integrity was demonstrated by the transplantation "take" rate when histologically viable tumor cells were transplanted into a suitable recipient. It was evident from these experiments in mice that relatively normal-appearing cancer cells can persist for several months after radiation therapy but that these cells are "biologically doomed." Thus, cytologic evaluation of a patient immediately after radiation therapy may erroneously lead to the supposition that persistent disease exists. In addition, subsequent evaluation of the irradiated cervix is difficult because of the distortion produced in the exfoliated cells, often called the *radiation effect*. Thus, histologic confirmation of recurrent cancer is essential. This can be accomplished by

TABLE 3.25 **MD Anderson Hospital Central Recurrence Rate for Carcinoma of the Cervix After Treatment With Radiation Therapy**	
Stage	**Patients (%)**
I	1.5
IIb	5
IIIa	7.5
IIIb	17

punch or needle biopsy of suspected areas of malignancy when they are accessible. An interval of at least 3 months should elapse after completion of radiation therapy. The clinical presentation of recurrent cervical cancer is varied and often insidious. Many patients develop a wasting syndrome with severe loss of appetite and gradual weight loss over a period of weeks to months. This is often preceded by a period of general good health after completion of radiation therapy. Because most recurrences of cancer occur within 2 years after therapy, the period of good health rarely lasts more than 1 year before the symptoms of cachexia become evident. Diagnostic evaluation at this time of suspected recurrence may include a chest radiograph and CT scan and complete blood count, blood urea nitrogen, creatinine clearance, and liver function tests.

Autopsy studies of the location of advanced recurrent and persistent disease have been reported (Figs. 3.42 and 3.43). After radical hysterectomy, about one-fourth of recurrences occur locally in the upper part of the vagina or the area previously occupied by the cervix. The location of recurrence after radiation therapy showed a 27% occurrence in the cervix, uterus, or upper vagina; 6% in the lower two-thirds of the vagina; 43% in the parametrial area, including the pelvic wall; 16% distant; and 8% unknown. Often one notes the development of ureteral obstruction in a patient who had a normal urinary tract before therapy. Although ureteral obstruction can be caused by radiation fibrosis, this is relatively rare, and 95% of the obstructions are caused by progressive tumor. Central disease may not be evident, and in the absence of other findings, a patient with ureteral obstruction and a negative evaluation for metastatic disease after therapy should undergo exploratory laparotomy and selected biopsies to confirm the diagnosis of recurrence. Patients with ureteral obstruction in the absence of recurrent malignancy should be considered for urinary diversion or internal antegrade ureteral stents.

The definition of primary healing after radiation therapy is a cervix covered with normal epithelium or an obliteration of the vaginal vault without evidence of ulceration or discharge. On rectovaginal examination, the residual induration is smooth

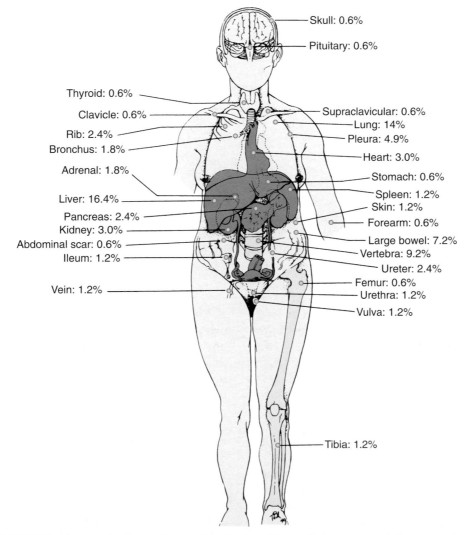

FIGURE 3.42 Metastatic sites of treated patients with cervical cancer and the percentage of involvement. (From Henriksen E. The lymphatic spread of carcinoma of the cervix and of the body of the uterus; a study of 420 necropsies. *Am J Obstet Gynecol* 1949;58:924-942.)

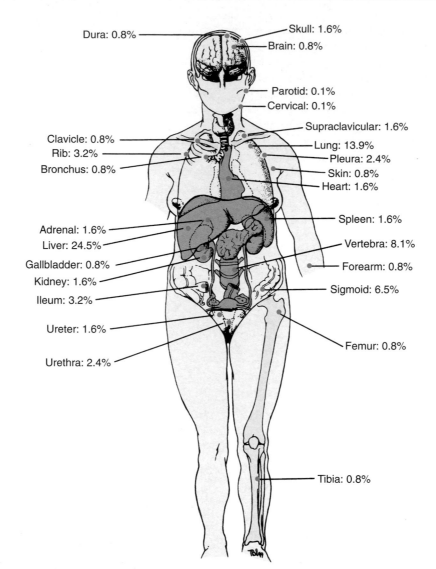

FIGURE 3.43 Metastatic sites of untreated patients with cervical cancer and the percentage of involvement. (From Henriksen E. The lymphatic spread of carcinoma of the cervix and of the body of the uterus; a study of 420 necropsies. *Am J Obstet Gynecol* 1949;58:924-942.)

with no nodularity. The cervix is greater than 2.5 cm in width, and there is no evidence of distant metastasis. The definition of persistent disease after radiation therapy is as follows:

1. Evidence of a portion of the tumor that was clinically present before treatment or
2. Development of a new demonstrable tumor in the pelvis within the treatment period.

The definition of recurrence after radiation therapy is a regrowth of tumor in the pelvis or distally, which is noted after complete healing of the cervix and vagina.

Recurrence after surgery is defined as evidence of a tumor mass after all gross tumor was removed and the margins of the specimen were free of disease. Persistent disease after surgery is defined as persistence of gross tumor in the operative field or local recurrence of tumor within 1 year of initial surgery. A new cancer of the cervix would be a lesion that occurs locally at least 10 years after primary therapy.

The triad of weight loss accompanied by leg edema and pelvic pain is ominous. Leg edema is usually the result of progressive lymphatic obstruction, occlusion of the iliofemoral vein system, or both. The clinician should consider the possibility of thrombophlebitis, but recurrent cancer is more likely. Patients characteristically describe pain that radiates into the upper thigh either to the anterior medial aspect of the thigh or posteriorly into the buttock. Other patients describe pain in the groin or deep-seated central pelvic pain. The appearance of vaginal bleeding or watery, foul vaginal discharge strongly suggests a central recurrence (Table 3.27). These lesions are among the more readily detectable recurrent cervical cancers, and histologic confirmation is easily obtained.

Fewer than 15% of patients with recurrent cervical cancer will develop pulmonary metastasis. When this does occur, patients will complain of cough, hemoptysis, and occasionally chest pain. In many cases, there will be enlargement of supraclavicular lymph nodes, especially on the left side. Needle aspiration of enlarged lymph nodes can be accomplished easily and avoids the necessity for an open biopsy of the area.

In almost every case, the diagnosis of recurrent cervical cancer must be confirmed histologically. CT-directed needle biopsies have provided us with a tool that avoids the necessity of more elaborate operative procedures. In addition to the standard radiographic evaluations, such as IVP and chest radiograph, the clinician may find more sophisticated studies such as lymphangiography and MRI helpful in localizing deep-seated areas of recurrent cervical cancer.

Bony metastases presenting clinically are particularly rare. In a study of 644 patients with invasive cervical carcinoma, Peeples and colleagues were able to find only 29 cases of remote metastases. Of these, 15 were to the lungs and only 12 were to the bone, which is an incidence of 1.8%. No bony metastases were found at initial staging and diagnosis. The earliest discovery of bone metastasis came 8 months after diagnosis. Therefore, a bone survey was not recommended as part of the staging examination for cervical cancer.

Blythe and associates reported on 55 patients who were treated for cervical carcinoma and who developed bony metastases. Radiographs were diagnostic in all except two of the patients. In 15 patients, a combination of radioactive scans and radiographs was used to establish the diagnosis. The most common mechanism of bony involvement from carcinoma of the cervix was extension of the neoplasia from periaortic nodes, with involvement of the adjacent vertebral bodies. The longest interval from the primary diagnosis until the discovery of bony metastases was 13 years. Of the patients, 69% were diagnosed within 30 months of initial therapy, and 96% died within 18 months. Of the 36 patients treated with radiation therapy, four received complete relief of symptoms, 24 gained some relief, and eight received no relief.

Van Herik and colleagues examined the records of 2107 cases of cervical cancer for recurrence after 10 years. Sixteen (0.7%) patients had a recurrence 10 to 26 years after the initial therapy. Of these patients, 25% had bony metastasis or extension of the recurrence into bone. The finding of metastasis after 10 years correlates with the findings of Paunier and associates, who indicated that 92.5% of deaths resulting from carcinoma of the cervix occur in the first 5 years after diagnosis. In addition, their cumulative death rate curve was flat after 10 years.

Deaths resulting from cancer of the cervix occur most frequently in the first year of observation and decrease thereafter. About half of all the deaths occur in the first year after therapy, 25% in the second year, and 15% in the third year, for a total of 85% by the end of the third year. Because more than three-fourths of the recurrences are clinically evident in the first 2 years after initial therapy, posttreatment evaluation done at frequent intervals during this critical period is mandatory. The patient should be examined every 3 to 4 months, and cervical cytologic testing should be done at these visits. In addition, particular attention should be paid to the parametria on rectovaginal examination to detect evidence of progressive disease. For several months after the completion of radiation therapy, the examiner may observe a progressive fibrosis in the parametria, creating the so-called horseshoe fibrosis. The amount of fibrosis may sometimes be alarming, but smoothness of the induration should be reassuring when compared with the nodular presentation of recurrent parametrial malignancy. Parametrial needle biopsies, with the patient under anesthesia, may be helpful when the palpatory findings are equivocal. Generous use of endocervical curettage at these follow-up visits is recommended, especially when central failure is suspected after radiation therapy. Every follow-up examination should include careful palpation of the abdomen for evidence of periaortic enlargement, hepatomegaly, and unexplained masses. Every follow-up examination should begin with a careful palpation of the supraclavicular areas for evidence of nodal enlargement. This frequently omitted portion of the examination will sometimes reveal the only evidence of recurrent disease.

The prognosis for patients with recurrent or advanced cervical cancer depends on the location of the disease. Of patients with recurrent cervical cancer, the most favorable for therapy after primary irradiation are those with a central recurrence. These patients are candidates for curative radical pelvic surgery, including pelvic exenteration. There will be further discussion of this group of patients later in this chapter. With the advent of sophisticated methods of radiation therapy, including improved methods of brachytherapy and supervoltage external irradiation therapy, patients with pure central recurrence have become a rarity.

Isolated lung metastases from pelvic malignancies have responded in very selected cases to lobectomy. Gallousis reported metastases to the lung from cervical cancer in 1.5% of 5614 cases reviewed, with solitary nodules present in 25% of the cases. A surgical attack for isolated pulmonary recurrence should be considered, especially if the latent period has been longer than 3 years.

Other patients who deserve serious consideration are those with radiation bowel injury. Over the past decade, the limits of human tolerance to radiation therapy have been reached, with treatment techniques for advanced disease that include large extended fields to the periaortic area. Many patients with advanced-stage primary lesions have been treated with large doses of pelvic radiation (6000–7000 cGy), often after intraabdominal surgery. With these techniques, standard radiation therapy can lead to a small but significant number of patients with chronic radiation injury to the large or small bowel. These patients often develop cachexia, which is indistinguishable from the clinical presentation of recurrent and progressive malignancy. These patients are often quickly and superficially diagnosed as having recurrent disease, and no further investigation is initiated. Careful investigation of these patients reveals a history of postprandial crampy abdominal pain causing anorexia and weight loss. The diagnostic evaluations discussed previously reveal no conclusive evidence of persistent malignancy. In most cases, these patients can be returned to health with appropriate bowel surgery, including internal bypass procedures. In every patient suspected of recurrent malignancy, an effort should be made to confirm this suspicion by biopsy (histologic confirmation), and patients who do not have a recurrence and who have radiation bowel injury should be identified.

Management and Prognosis

Persistent or recurrent carcinoma of the cervix is a discouraging clinical entity for the clinician, with a 1-year survival rate between 10% and 15%. Treatment failures are, as expected, much more common in patients with more advanced stages of the disease; therefore, most patients are unlikely candidates for a second curative approach with radical pelvic surgery. Cases of curative therapy applied to isolated lung metastases or lower vaginal recurrences are reported but occur rarely. Unfortunately, most recurrences are suitable for palliative management only.

Surgical Therapy: Radical Hysterectomy

Radical hysterectomy has been reported as therapy for patients with a small recurrent cervical carcinoma after radiation. Coleman's series of 50 patients from the MD Anderson Hospital were treated with radical hysterectomy (type II or III). Severe postoperative complications occurred in 42% of these patients. Of these patients, 28% developed urinary tract injury. The survival rate was 90% at 5 years for patients with lesions smaller than 2 cm as opposed to 64% in patients with larger lesions. Excessive morbidity can be limited if an omental pedicle is placed at the operative site at the end of the procedure, bringing in a new blood supply to the operative field that has undergone previous radiation therapy.

Pelvic Exenteration

In 1948, Brunschwig introduced the operation of pelvic exenteration for cancer of the cervix (Fig. 3.44). Since then, extensive experience with pelvic exenteration has been accumulated, and the techniques and patient selection have steadily improved so that now, 50 years later, this procedure has attained an important role in the treatment of gynecologic malignancies for a selected group of patients. It is now accepted as a respectable procedure that can offer life to selected patients when no other possibility of cure exists. The criticism of this procedure has been lessened by steadily improving mortality and morbidity and a gratifying 5-year survival record. Most important, however, is that patients who survive this procedure can be rehabilitated to a useful and healthful existence.

Although pelvic exenteration has been used for various pelvic malignancies, its greatest and most important role is in the treatment of advanced or recurrent carcinoma of the cervix. **Total exenteration** (Fig. 3.45) **with removal of the pelvic viscera, including the bladder and rectosigmoid, is the procedure of choice for carcinoma of the cervix recurrent or persistent within the pelvis after irradiation.** In select cases, the procedure may be limited to anterior exenteration (Fig. 3.46) with removal of the bladder and preservation of the rectosigmoid or posterior exenteration (Fig. 3.47) with removal of the rectosigmoid and preservation of the bladder. Cogent objections have been raised regarding these limited operations, especially in patients with carcinoma of the cervix recurrent after irradiation, because of the increased risk of an incomplete resection. In addition, patients in whom the bladder or rectum is preserved often have multiple complications and malfunctioning of the

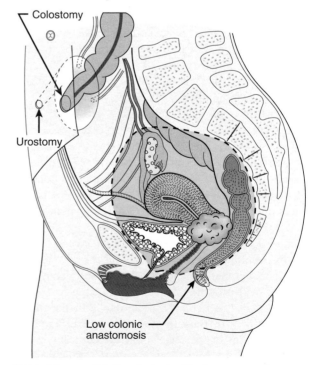

Shaded tissue within the *dashed outline* is permanently removed. Unshaded tissue within the *dashed outline* is first removed and then reconstructed.

FIGURE 3.45 Total exenteration with removal of all pelvic viscera. Fecal stream is diverted via a colostomy, and urinary diversion is via an ileal or sigmoid conduit or a continent pouch. (Modified from DiSaia PJ, Morrow CP, Townsend DE. Cancer of the vulva. *Calif Med* 1973;118:13-8.)

FIGURE 3.44 Specimen from an anterior exenteration done for recurrent cervical carcinoma; the specimen consists of the uterus, vagina, and bladder. (The anterior wall has been opened to expose bullous edema of the trigone.)

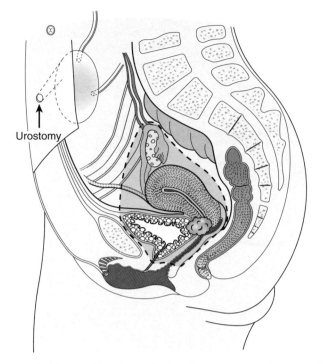

Shaded tissue within the *dashed outline* is permanently removed.

FIGURE 3.46 Anterior exenteration with removal of all pelvic viscera except the rectosigmoid. The urinary stream is diverted into an ileal or sigmoid conduit or a continent pouch. (Modified from DiSaia PJ, Morrow CP, Townsend DE. Cancer of the vulva. *Calif Med* 1973;118:13-8.)

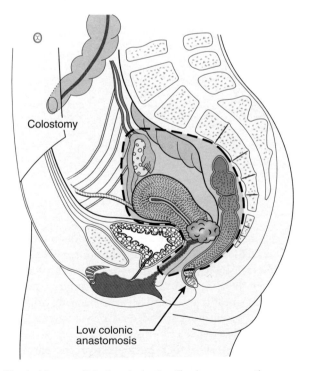

Shaded tissue within the *dashed outline* is permanently removed. Unshaded tissue within the *dashed outline* is first removed and then reconstructed.

FIGURE 3.47 Posterior exenteration with removal of all pelvic viscera except the bladder. The fecal stream is diverted via a colostomy. (Modified from DiSaia PJ, Morrow CP, Townsend DE. Cancer of the vulva. *Calif Med* 1973;118:13-8.)

preserved organ. Consequently, some surgeons have completely abandoned subtotal exenterations, and most oncologists use them very selectively.

One of the greatest technical advances in the evolution of pelvic exenteration is the intestinal conduit for diversion of the urinary stream. Originally, Brunschwig transplanted the ureters into the left colon just proximal to the colostomy, thus creating the so-called wet colostomy. The complication rate from this procedure, especially electrolyte imbalance and severe urinary tract infections, was unacceptable. Bricker popularized the use of an ileal segment conduit for urinary diversion. The incidence of both postoperative pyelonephritis and hypochloremic acidosis has been greatly reduced. Furthermore, the patients are dry and comfortable and therefore more easily rehabilitated. More recent developments have resulted in several techniques for creation of a continent reservoir, again using a segment of bowel (Fig. 3.48). Another significant advancement in surgical technique of these patients is the use of the intestinal stapling device. Whereas a permanent colostomy was a standard part of the exenterative procedure, today, it is rare. In many, if not most, cases, reanastomosis with the end-to-end anastomosis stapler can be performed, and the fecal stream continues through the anus.

Patient Selection

Only a few patients with recurrent cancer of the cervix are suitable for this operation (Table 3.26). **Metastases outside the pelvis, whether manifested preoperatively or discovered at laparotomy, are an absolute contraindication to pelvic exenteration. The triad of unilateral leg edema, sciatic pain, and ureteral obstruction is pathognomonic of recurrent and unresectable disease in the pelvis. The triad must be complete, however, to be entirely reliable. Weight loss, cough, anemia, and other aberrations suggestive of advanced disease are not sufficient justifications by themselves to discontinue efforts toward surgical management. Obesity, advanced age, and systemic disease may interdict extensive surgery in direct relation to the severity of these factors. Some patients are unsuitable because of psychological reasons, and a number of women who are otherwise candidates for pelvic exenteration elect to accept the fate of unresected recurrence. If the time from primary treatment to recurrence is short (<2 years), this usually indicates aggressive biologic activity of the tumor, and resectability is usually limited.**

Evaluation studies before surgery include chest radiography, CT scan of the abdomen and pelvis with intravenous contrast, creatinine clearance, liver function tests, and assessment of the patient's hemostatic mechanism. Any suspected disease outside the pelvis noted on any of the diagnostic studies should prompt an attempt at confirmation using a fine-needle biopsy technique. Bone survey and liver scan are not part of the "routine" evaluation.

Preparation for pelvic exenteration is often traumatic to patients with recurrent cervical cancer, especially when the procedure is aborted. The increased use of CT-directed fine-needle aspirants has contributed greatly to lowering the fraction of patients explored who are found to be unexenterable. At

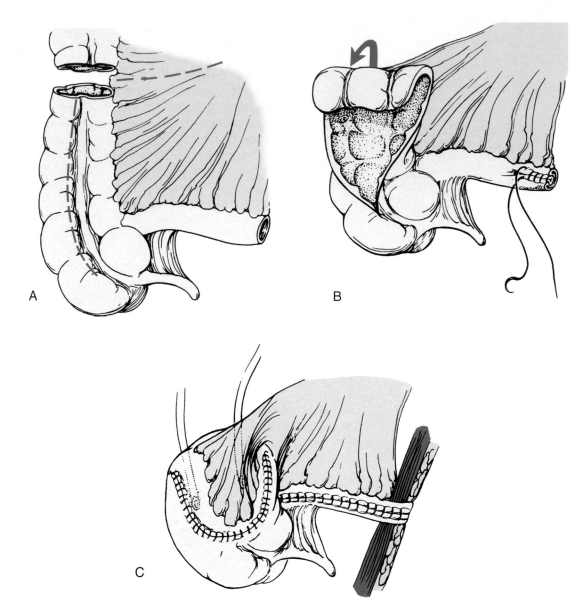

FIGURE 3.48 A–C, Construction of an Indiana pouch from the colon and the terminal ileum. (From Amis ES, Newhouse JH, Olsson CA. Continent urinary diversions: review of current surgical procedures and radiologic imaging. *Radiology* 1988;168:395-401.)

laparotomy, the entire abdomen and pelvis are explored for evidence of metastatic and intraperitoneal cancer (Fig. 3.49). The liver should be carefully inspected visually and by palpation. The lymph nodes surrounding the lower aorta are the first to be sampled if the exploration of the abdomen has revealed no evidence of disease. If the lower aortic area findings are negative, a bilateral pelvic lymphadenectomy is performed.

Morbidity and Mortality

Most of the morbidity and mortality directly related to exenteration occur within the first 18 months after the procedure. Many of the complications can be sequelae to any major surgery. These include cardiopulmonary catastrophes such as pulmonary embolism, pulmonary edema, myocardial infarction, and cerebrovascular accidents. The length of these surgical

procedures and the magnitude of blood loss definitely increase the incidence of cardiovascular complications. This category of complications usually occurs within the first week after the procedure. Then there is a period when sepsis is the greatest threat to the patient's health and life. This sepsis usually originates in the pelvic cavity with occurrence of a pelvic abscess or, more commonly, diffuse pelvic cellulitis.

One of the most serious postoperative complications of exenteration is small bowel obstruction related to the denuded pelvic floor. In the past decade, several techniques have been used in an effort to avoid the adherence of small bowel to this large raw surface, including mobilization of omentum (Fig. 3.50) or abdominal wall peritoneum to cover the pelvic floor (Fig. 3.51). When small bowel obstruction does occur, it is appropriately treated with conservative therapy. However, half

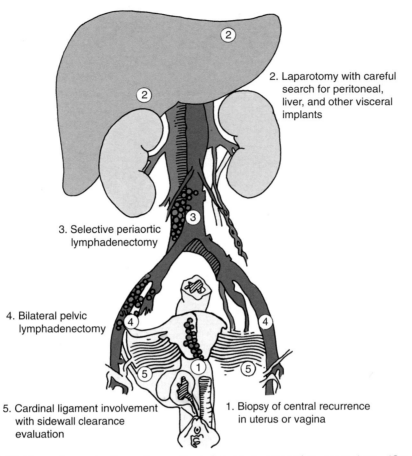

2. Laparotomy with careful search for peritoneal, liver, and other visceral implants

3. Selective periaortic lymphadenectomy

4. Bilateral pelvic lymphadenectomy

5. Cardinal ligament involvement with sidewall clearance evaluation

1. Biopsy of central recurrence in uterus or vagina

FIGURE 3.49 Steps in evaluation of a patient for an exenterative procedure. (Courtesy of A. Robert Kagan, MD, Los Angeles, CA.)

TABLE 3.26   Survival After Pelvic Exenteration

Author(s) (Year)	Institution	Patients Treated	Operative Deaths (%)	No. Surviving 5 Years* (%)
Douglas and Sweeney (1975)	New York Hospital	23	1 (4.3)	5 (22)
Parsons and Friedell (1964)	Harvard University	112	24 (21.4)	24 (21.4)
Brunschwig (1965)	Memorial Hospital	535	86 (16)	108 (20.1)
Bricker (1967)	Washington University	153	15 (10)	53 (34.6)
Krieger and Embree (1969)	Cleveland Clinics	35	4 (11)	13 (37)
Ketcham et al. (1970)	National Cancer Institute	162	12 (7.4)	62 (38.2)
Symmonds et al. (1975)	Mayo Clinic	198	16 (8)	64 (32.3)
Morley and Lindenauer (1976)	University of Michigan	34	1 (2.9)	21 (62)
Rutledge et al. (1977)	MD Anderson Hospital	296	40 (13.5)	99 (33.4)
Averette et al. (1984)	University of Miami			
	1966–1971	14	4 (28.5)	5 (36)
	1971–1976	45	15 (33.3)	10 (22)
	1976–1981	33	4 (12.1)	19 (58)
		65	6 (9.2)	15 (23)
Lawhead (1989)	Memorial Hospital	65	6 (9.2)	15 (23)
	1972–1981			
Soper et al (1989)	Duke University	69	5 (7.2)	28 (4.5)
Shingleton et al (1989)	University of Alabama	143	9 (6.3)	71 (50)
Sharma et al (2005)	Roswell Park Cancer Institute	48	2 (4.2)	16 (33)
Fotopoulou et al (2010)	Virchow University Hospital Berlin	47†	4 (8.5)	25 (53.2)‡
Total		**2012**	**248 (12.3)**	**663 (33.7)**

*In almost every series, the operative death rate and the 5-year survival rate improved dramatically in the later years of each series.

†Includes eight vaginal cancers.

‡Five-year survival not reached and therefore not included in the total.

TABLE 3.27   Signs and Symptoms of Recurrent Cervical Cancer

Weight loss (unexplained)
Leg edema (excessive and often unilateral)
Pelvic or thigh–buttock pain
Serosanguineous vaginal discharge
Progressive ureteral obstruction
Supraclavicular lymph node enlargement (usually on the left side)
Cough
Hemoptysis
Chest pain

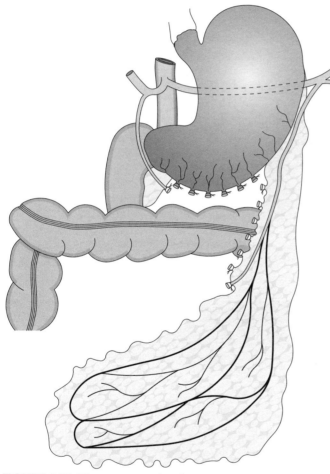

FIGURE 3.50 The omentum has been detached from the right transverse colon and the greater curvature of the stomach, keeping the left gastroepiploic vessels intact and creating a large "tongue of omentum" to cover the pelvic floor.

these patients come to reoperation, and the mortality rate of this group is approximately 50% in some series. The risk of bowel obstruction is increased by the presence of pelvic infection. Both conditions predispose to the development of small bowel fistulas, which always require reoperation and frequently are fatal. In general, complications are more common in patients who have recurrence after radiation therapy. Irradiated tissue is less likely to produce good wound healing, and the formation of granulation tissue is severely retarded.

The long-term morbidity from exenteration is predominantly related to urinary diversion. After the period of susceptibility to sepsis has passed, urinary obstruction and infection become the major nonneoplastic life-threatening complications. Pyelonephritis is common and should be treated promptly and vigorously. Periodic IVPs can be obtained to assess the collecting system for hydronephrosis. A mild degree of obstruction is frequently retained after construction of an ileal conduit, but progressive hydronephrosis will require correction to salvage renal function. The incidence of complications appeared to be less in patients in whom an unirradiated portion of bowel had been used for construction of the conduit.

Survival Results

The 5-year cumulative survival rate after pelvic exenteration varies in the literature from 20% to 62% (Table 3.26). Reported survival rates depend greatly on the circumstances of patient selection for exenteration. Cumulative survival rates are always improved when no patient is exenterated who has a positive pelvic node after pelvic irradiation. In general, however, both morbidity and mortality and the 5-year survival rate have improved steadily over the past 2 decades. The mortality rate in most centers is now well below 5%, and morbidity has been similarly lowered.

In 2009, 60 years after the first description of pelvic exenteration, Marnitz and colleagues surveyed and compared practice patterns in the United States and Germany. The number of exenterations performed in the 21st century was comparable in both countries, with centrally recurrent cervical cancer or persistent tumor after chemoradiation being the main indication. Whereas PET-CT is more commonly used in the United States, MRI is the preferred tool in Germany. Surgical staging is more commonly performed in the United States (61% vs. 32%). Exenteration for FIGO stage IVA disease was more commonly recommended in Germany (43% vs. 0%), as was the operation in the setting of fistulae involving the bladder or rectum (61% vs. 29%). In Germany, interdisciplinary treatment with general surgeons, urologists, plastic surgeons, and radiation oncologists is more common. Although there is a consensus to administer adjuvant therapy after exenteration for patients with positive margins or positive lymph nodes, adjuvant therapy is more frequently recommended in Germany (93%) than in the United States (74%).

In 2010, Spahn and colleagues reported the results of 37 anterior pelvic exenterations and six total pelvic exenterations performed at the University of Wurzburg in Germany. A continent urinary diversion was constructed in 16, and an ileal conduit was constructed in 27. Continent urinary diversion was not associated with higher complication rates than ileal conduit formation. The overall disease-specific 5-year survival rate was 36.5%. Survival correlated significantly with surgical margin status.

For vaginal reconstruction, vascularized muscle flaps are preferred to fill the empty pelvis, and developments in bioengineering tissue are likely to have applications in neovaginal creation. De la Garza and colleagues reported the successful performance of a total pelvic exenteration with a split-thickness

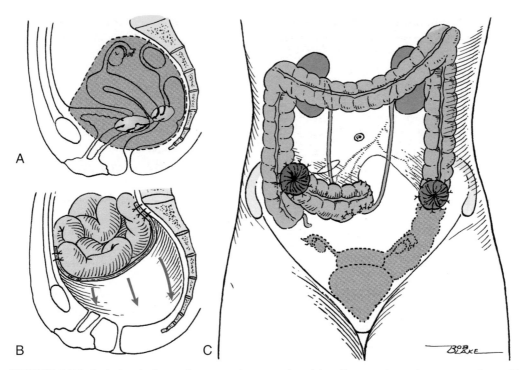

FIGURE 3.51 **A,** Lateral view of recurrent cancer involving the cervix and upper vagina with extension into the bladder and rectum. The *stippled area* indicates tissue to be removed by exenteration. **B,** A lateral view after pelvic viscera have been removed. The omental "carpet" is used to keep the intestines out of the pelvis during immediate postoperative period. With time, the omental "carpet" will descend into the pelvis, and the "carpet" will adhere to the pelvic floor. **C,** Urinary conduit and colostomy diversion after exenteration. *Dotted areas* of the sigmoid, bladder, and internal genitalia have been removed.

skin graft neovagina, continent orthotopic neobladder, and rectal anastomosis, resulting in no external ostomies and adequate sexual function.

Radiation

With recurrent disease outside the initial treatment field, irradiation is frequently successful in providing local control and symptomatic relief. External irradiation in moderate and easily delivered doses is usually effective in relieving pain from bone metastases. A dose of 3000 cGy delivered over 2 to 3 weeks is often sufficient to relieve pain from vertebral column or long-bone metastases.

Höckel and associates reported their experience with a combined operative and radiotherapy (CORT) for recurrent tumors infiltrating the pelvic wall. Although the combination therapy is not new, these authors surgically remove the recurrence more radically than previously reported. The bony pelvis and neurovascular support of the leg is preserved. Implantation of guide tubes, which exit from the skin for brachytherapy, is done after resection of the tumor. Considerable pelvic reconstruction is usually done. Although the indications and procedure are evolving, in the first 48 patients treated, survival probabilities are 50% and 44% after 3 and 5 years, respectively.

Reirradiation of pelvic recurrences of cervical cancer occurring within the previously treated field is a subject of some controversy. The results after reirradiation of patients with recurrent cervical malignancy have varied considerably.

Truelsen reported a 3-year cure rate of 1.7%. Murphy and Schmitz reported a 9% salvage rate in 1956, and Nolan and associates reported on the use of 60Co teleradiation with a 25% salvage rate. At the Roswell Park Memorial Institute, Murphy and Schmitz adopted the policy of reirradiating patients with recurrence, delivering a full or almost full course for a second time. Among the highly selected series of 46 patients, 9% to 10% were living and well at the end of 5 years. Only seven patients had biopsy-proven recurrences before treatment. Others have shown that the results of reirradiation depend on many factors, including the site of recurrence, initial clinical stage, and initial dose of radiation therapy.

Careful perusal of these reports suggests that most patients who benefited from reirradiation were those who received less than optimal radiation during initial therapy. This set of circumstances has become rare in recent times, when more sophisticated radiotherapy is being delivered in many areas of the United States. Therefore, reirradiation for recurrent disease is usually not a worthwhile consideration. The potential for necrosis and fistula formation with even moderate doses of reirradiation in the pelvis by external or interstitial sources can give very unfavorable results.

Recurrence after radical hysterectomy has been treated with radiation. In a study from Holland, 271 patients were treated with radical hysterectomy, and 27 recurred with 14 limited to the pelvis. Of note, adjuvant radiotherapy had been administered in 14 (52%) of the 27. In the four patients with isolated pelvic recurrence, only one died of disease, but all of the other patients with recurrences died of disease. The survivors were treated with radiation. In a study from the MD Anderson Cancer Center, 50 patients had recurrence after radical hysterectomy and were treated with radiation. OS rate was 33%. In the 16 patients with central disease, 12 (69%) remained disease free. The survival rate of 29 patients with squamous carcinoma was 51% compared with 14% for the 14 patients with adenocarcinoma ($P = 0.05$).

Chemotherapy

The management of disseminated cervical cancer has improved with the development of modern chemotherapy. Fig. 3.17 reviews the treatment of advanced or recurrent disease. Because concurrent platinum-based chemoradiation has become the standard of care for locally advanced disease, many recurrent tumors may therefore be platinum resistant. The GOG has completed eight multicenter, phase III randomized trials to study platinum-based therapies for recurrent and/or metastatic disease (Table 3.28). Drug discovery for the most part has fed into these phase III trial designs through the GOG's phase II series dedicated to exploring the activity and tolerability of cytotoxic compounds in cervical cancer.

The early trials of the GOG for recurrent and metastatic cervical carcinoma were designed to evaluate cisplatin dosing, schedules, and analogs. The next two trials evaluated the addition of ifosfamide, bleomycin, and mitolactol to cisplatin-based therapies. Among some of the lessons learned during the 1980s and 1990s governing chemotherapy for recurrent cervical cancer were that platinum-based therapies were most effective and that cisplatin was more active than carboplatin (19% vs. 15%, respectively). Two ways through which the RR could be increased without prolongation in survival included increasing

the platinum dose and/or adding ifosfamide to cisplatin. As a consequence of these first five phase III randomized clinical trials, single-agent cisplatin at 50 mg/m² emerged as the standard for recurrent disease, with a documented 19% RR on a 21-day schedule.

The combined regimen of cisplatin in combination with paclitaxel in GOG 169 yielded an impressive 36% RR, improvement in PFS, but no significant impact on OS compared with single-agent cisplatin. The next trial, GOG 179, compared single-agent cisplatin with cisplatin plus topotecan. The improvements observed in RR, PFS, and OS all favored the combined regimen, leading to FDA approval of the cisplatin 50 mg/m² plus topotecan 1.75 mg/m² days 1 to 3 in this population. In both GOG 169 and GOG 179, RRs were decreased in patients who had received prior platinum (Table 3.29). Because GOG 179 was conducted during the era of chemoradiation and GOG 169 was under way before the adoption of multimodality therapy, 57% of patients on GOG 179 received radiosensitizing platinum compared with 27% on GOG 169.

Gynecologic Oncology Group 204 compared four platinum-based doublets using paclitaxel, topotecan, gemcitabine, and vinorelbine. Because this study was activated before the data from GOG 179 were mature, cisplatin plus paclitaxel was selected as the control arm, primarily because of the 36% RR observed in GOG 169. None of the experimental arms outperformed the reference arm (Table 3.30 and Fig. 3.52). For this reason, cisplatin plus paclitaxel has been selected as the control arm for the succeeding trial, which was activated in April 2009 (GOG 240).

In GOG 240, the experimental arms were designed to answer two critical questions. The first is a chemotherapy question and concerns whether nonplatinum agents would have greater activity in the recurrent setting given the increased usage of

TABLE 3.28 Eight Phase III Randomized Trials in Recurrent Cervical Cancer Conducted by the Gynecologic Oncology Group

GOG Protocol	Study Chair	Year	Arms	Patients (n)	PR %	CR %	Overall %	Median Duration of Response (mo)	Median PFS (mo)
43	Bonomi et al.	1985	Cisplatin 50 mg/m² IV q21d	150	10.7	10	20.7	4.9	7.1
			Cisplatin 100 mg/m² IV q21d	166	18.7	12.7	31.4	4.1	7
			Cisplatin 20 mg/m² IV × 5d q21d	128	16.4	8.6	25	4.8	6.1
									Median Survival (mo)
64	Thigpen et al.	1989	Cisplatin 50 mg/m² 24 h continuous infusion	156	12	6	18	5.5	6.4
			Cisplatin 1 mg/min rapid infusion	164	11	6	17	4.5	6.2
								Median PFI (mo)	Median Survival (mo)
77	McGuire et al	1989	Carboplatin 340-400 mg/m² IV q28d	175	9.7	5.7	15.4	2.7	6.2
			Iproplatin 230–270 mg/m² IV q28d	177	6.8	4	10.8	3	5.5

TABLE 3.28 Eight Phase III Randomized Trials in Recurrent Cervical Cancer Conducted by the Gynecologic Oncology Group—cont'd

GOG Protocol	Study Chair	Year	Arms	Patients (n)	Objective Response			Median Duration of Response (mo)	Median PFS (mo)
					PR %	CR %	Overall %		
								Median PFS (mo)	Median Survival (mo)
110	Omura et al.	1997	Cisplatin 50 mg/m² IV q21d	140	11.4	6.4	17.8	3.2	8
			Cisplatin 50 mg/m² IV +	147	11.6	9.5	21.1	3.3	7.3
			mitolactol180 mg/m² PO days 2, 6 q21d	151	18.5	12.6	31.1	4.6	8.3
							P = 0.004	P = 0.003	
			Cisplatin 50 mg/m² IV + ifosfamide 5 g/m² 24-hr infusion + MESNA 6 g/m² q21d						
									Median Survival (mo)
149	Bloss et al.	2002	Cisplatin 50 mg/m² IV + ifosfamide 5 g/m² 24 hr infusion + MESNA 6 g/m² q21d	146	NS	NS	32.2	4.6	8.5
				141	NS	NS	32.1	5.1	8.4
			Bleomycin 30 units 24-hr infusion followed by cisplatin 50 mg/m² IV + ifosfamide 5 g/m² 24-hr infusion + MESNA 6 g/m² q21d						
									Median Survival (mo)
169	Moore et al.	2004	Cisplatin 50 mg/m² IV q21d	134	13	6	19	2.8	8.8
			Paclitaxel 135 mg/m² 24-hr infusion + cisplatin 50 mg/m² IV q21d	130	21	15	36	4.8	9.7
							P = 0.002	P <0.001	
									Median Survival (mo)
179	Long et al.	2005	Cisplatin 50 mg/m² IV q21d	145	10	13	13	2.9	6.5
			Topotecan 0.75 mg/m² days 1–3 + cisplatin 50 mg/m² IV q21d	148	16	10	26	4.6	9.4
							P = 0.004	P = 0.014	P = 0.017
			MVAC q4 wk	63	9	13	22	4.4	9.4
									Median OS (mo)
204	Monk et al.	2009	Paclitaxel 135 mg/m² 24-hr infusion + cisplatin 50 mg/m² q21d	103	26.2	2.9	29.1	5.82	12.87
			Vinorelbine 30 mg/m² days 1 and 8 + cisplatin 50 mg/m² q21d	108	18.5	7.4	25.9	3.98	9.99
			Gemcitabine 1000 mg/m² days 1 and 8 + cisplatin 50 mg/m² q21d	112	21.4	0.9	22.3	4.7	10.28
			Topotecan 0.75 mg/m² days 1–3 + cisplatin 50 mg/m² q21d	111	21.6	1.8	23.4	4.57	10.25

CR, complete response; *GOG*, Gynecologic Oncology Group; *IV*, intravenous; *MVAC*, methotrexate, vinblastine, doxorubicin, cisplatin; *NS*, not significant; *PFS*, progression-free survival; *PR*, partial response; *q*, every.

platinum-based chemoradiation initially for locally advanced cancers. Two phase II experiences using nonplatinum doublets have been described. In the United Kingdom, the Scotcerv trial piloted gemcitabine plus Taxotere, which, when presented at American Society of Clinical Oncology (ASCO), was not deemed to be suitable for further development. Tiersten and

colleagues reported on their experience with the nonplatinum doublet topotecan plus paclitaxel. It is important to note that the regimen was active in previously irradiated patients (RR, 26%) with acceptable toxicities. The laboratory work by Bahadori and colleagues demonstrating synergy between paclitaxel and microtubule-inhibiting agents (eg, topotecan or vinorelbine) underscored this regimen's potential.[12] This nonplatinum doublet is being studied by the Arbeitsgemeinschaft Gynakologische Onkologie (AGO).

The second question addressed by GOG 240 involves targeted therapy. Tumor angiogenesis as measured by microvessel quantification has been shown to be a prognostic factor in cervical cancer. A small case series by Wright and colleagues described the successful combination of bevacizumab with cytotoxic agents in the recurrent and metastatic setting among previously irradiated patients. Of note, the antiangiogenesis agent bevacizumab in combination with chemotherapy has been FDA approved first- and second-line therapy for metastatic colorectal cancer and untreated non–small cell lung cancer (NSCLC). The drug has also been studied by the GOG in primary advanced and platinum-sensitive recurrent ovarian

TABLE 3.29 **Association of Prior Platinum Exposure With Response Rates in Gynecologic Oncology Group (GOG) 169 and GOG 179**

GOG 179	No Prior Cisplatin (%)	Prior Cisplatin (57% of Patients) (%)
Cisplatin	20	8
Cisplatin + topotecan	39	15

GOG 169	No Prior Cisplatin	Prior Cisplatin (27% of Patients)
Cisplatin	26	5
Cisplatin + paclitaxel	37	32

TABLE 3.30 **Objective Response by Treatment Regimen in Gynecologic Oncology Group 204**

Tumor Response	Cis + Pac (%)	Cis + Vin (%)	Cis + Gem (%)	Cis + Topo (%)	Total
CR	3 (2.9)	8 (7.4)	1 (0.9)	2 (1.8)	14
PR	27 (26.2)	20 (18.5)	24 (21.4)	24 (21.6)	95
SD	50 (48.4)	46 (42.6)	54 (48.2)	53 (47.8)	203
PD	23 (22.3)	34 (31.5)	33 (29.5)	32 (28.8)	122
Odds ratio*	—	1.17	1.43	1.34	
95% CI	—	0.54, 2.58	0.65, 3.19	0.61, 2.98	

*Odds ratios for response are provided for the reference arm, Cis + Pac, to the experimental therapies.
CI, Confidence interval; *Cis*, cisplatin; *CR*, complete response; *Gem*, gemcitabine; *Pac*, paclitaxel, *PD*, progressive disease; *PR*, partial response; *SD*, stable disease; *Vin*, vinorelbine.
Modified from Monk BJ, Sill MW, McMeekin DS, et al. Phase III trial of four cisplatin-containing doublet combinations in stage IVB, recurrent, or persistent cervical carcinoma: a Gynecologic Oncology Group study. *J Clin Oncol* 2009;27:4649-4655.

FIGURE 3.52 Gynecologic Oncology Group 204 survival curve. (From Monk BJ, Sill MW, McMeekin DS, et al. Phase III trial of four cisplatin-containing doublet combinations in stage IVB, recurrent, or persistent cervical carcinoma: a Gynecologic Oncology Group study. *J Clin Oncol* 2009;27:4649-4655.)

FIGURE 3.53 Progression-free survival curves of bevacizumab from Gynecologic Oncology Group protocol 227C superimposed over progression-free survival curves of other agents studied by the Gynecologic Oncology Group in this patient population. (From Monk BJ, Sill MW, McMeekin DS, et al. Phase III trial of four cisplatin-containing doublet combinations in stage IVB, recurrent, or persistent cervical carcinoma: a Gynecologic Oncology Group study. *J Clin Oncol* 2009;27:4649-4655.)

carcinoma. A phase II evaluation of bevacizumab at 15 mg/kg q21 days was undertaken within the GOG (protocol 227C). The 26% RR of bevacizumab among previously irradiated patients was among the highest RRs noted within the GOG's phase II experience for recurrent cervical cancer (Fig. 3.53).

Given the potential shared tumor biology between NSCLC and cervical cancer, the activity of platinum plus paclitaxel with bevacizumab in NSCLC supported the inclusion of this regimen as one of the experimental arms in GOG 240. Assuming no interaction between the nonplatinum doublet and bevacizumab, a 2 × 2 factorial design was selected to answer both the chemotherapy question and the antiangiogenesis question. The schema for GOG 240 appears in Fig. 3.54. This study also prospectively evaluated important prognostic factors—including African American race, performance status greater than 0, pelvic disease, prior radiosensitizer, and time interval from diagnosis to first recurrence less than 1 year—that have been recently reported by Moore and colleagues in a multivariate pooled analysis of three prior phase III studies in this population (Table 3.31).

At 173 deaths in February 2012, the preplanned interim analysis occurred and was noteworthy for demonstrating that the substitution of topotecan for cisplatin did not significantly improve OS in the GOG 240 population, even among those who were platinum-naïve. However, at 276 deaths in December 2012, the database was locked again and a second analysis performed. **In February 2013, the NCI issued a press release indicating that the open-label, multinational, multi-center, phase III, randomized clinical trial, GOG protocol 240, had met its primary endpoint with the arms administering the fully humanized, antivascular endothelial growth factor (VEGF) monoclonal antibody bevacizumab being associated with a significant survival advantage when compared to chemotherapy alone.** The rationale to target tumor angiogenesis in cervical cancer was based on clinical, pathologic, and molecular phenomenon that characterize HPV-induced

cervical carcinogenesis along with therapeutic gains observed with antiangiogenesis drugs in phase I (eg, the fungal derived TNP-470 molecule) and phase II (bevacizumab; oral VEGF receptor tyrosine kinase inhibitor, pazopanib) trials in the recurrent cervical cancer population. In GOG 240, patients were treated every 21 days until progression. The American Society of Clinical Oncology accepted the abstract for the General Plenary 2013 but made a rare exception to their embargo policy and released the abstract into the public domain in March 2013, 3 months before the Annual Meeting. **Importantly, the incorporation of bevacizumab (15 mg/kg) with cisplatin–paclitaxel and with topotecan–paclitaxel led to a significant 3.7-month improvement in OS (17 vs. 13.3 months; HR, 0.71; 98% CI, 0.54–0.95; one-sided $P = 0.004$), a significant improvement in PFS (8.2 vs. 5.9 months; HR, 0.67; 95% CI, 0.54–0.82; two-sided $P = 0.002$), and superior ORR (48% vs. 36%; relative probability of response, 1.35; 95% CI, 1.08–1–1.68; two-sided $P = 0.008$)** (Fig. 3.55). Each of these gains was clinically meaningful and was not accompanied by a significant deterioration of QoL when measured by three QoL instruments that had undergone prior prospective validation in this population. **A vaginal fistula rate of 8.6% was observed among patients who received bevacizumab, all of whom had been previously irradiated.**

The results of GOG-240 led directly to US FDA approval on August 14, 2014 (without an Oncology Drugs Advisory Committee [ODAC]) for the population studied, as well as approval by regulatory agencies throughout the world, including the United Kingdom's Cancer Drug Fund; the European Union's European Medicines Agency; SwissMedic; and the Ministries of Health in Israel, Australia, Hong Kong, five Middle Eastern nations, Brazil, and 10 Latin American countries, including Mexico. The National Comprehensive Category Network (NCCN) Cervical Cancer Treatment Guidelines have listed both bevacizumab-containing triplets studied in GOG 240

GYNECOLOGIC ONCOLOGY GROUP PROTOCOL 240

A randomized phase III trial of cisplatin plus paclitaxel with and without bevacizumab versus the nonplatinum doublet, topotecan plus paclitaxel, with and without NCI-supplied bevacizumab, in stage IVb, recurrent, or persistent carcinoma of the cervix.

Activation Date – April 6, 2009   Target Accrual = 450

Study Chair: Krishnansu S. Tewari, MD (ktewari@uci.edu) Statistician: Michael Sill, PhD Pathologist: Helen Michael, MD
Co-Chairs: Harry J. Long, MD (Medical Oncology), Richard T. Penson, MD (Quality of Life), Michael J. Birrer, MD, PhD (Translational Research)
Scientific Collaborations: Steven Waggoner, MD. David H. Moore, MD. Kathleen M. Darcy, PhD, Bradley J. Monk, MD

PRIMARY OBJECTIVES
1. To determine whether the addition of bevacizumab to chemotherapy improves overall survival
2. To determine whether the non-platinum chemotherapy doublet consisting of topotecan plus paclitaxel improves overall survival compared with the regimen involving cisplatin plus paclitaxel
3. To determine the frequency and severity of adverse events as assessed by CTCAE version 3.0 for the regimens administered

SECONDARY OBJECTIVES
1. To estimate and compare the progression-free survival of patients treated by the regimens investigated on this study
2. To estimate and compare the proportion of patients with tumor responses by the regimens investigated on this study

HEALTH-RELATED QUALITY OF LIFE OBJECTIVES
To determine whether the addition of bevacizumab to chemotherapy or the substitution of cisplatin with topotecan improves the health-related QoL as measured by the FACT-Cx TOI and produces favorable toxicity profiles

ELIGIBILITY
Primary stage IVB or recurrent or persistent carcinoma of the cervix
Measureable disease
GOG PS 0-1

Cycles repeated q21 days to progression or toxicity

RANDOMIZE

REGIMEN I
Paclitaxel 135 mg/m^2 IV 24h d1
CDDP 50 mg/m^2 IV d2 OR
Paclitaxel 175 mg/m^2 IV 3h 1
CDDP 50 mg/m2 IV d^2 OR
Paclitaxel 175 mg/m^2 IV 3h d1
CDDP 50 mg/m^2 IV d1

REGIMEN II
Paclitaxel 135 mg/m^2 IV 24h d1
CDDP 50 mg/m^2 IV d2
Bevacizumab 15 mg/kg d2 OR
Paclitaxel 175 mg/m^2 IV 3h d1
CDDP 50 mg/m2 IV d^2
Bevacizumab 15 mg/kg d2 OR
Paclitaxel 175 mg/m^2 IV 3h d1
CDDP 50 mg/m^2 IV d1
Bevacizumab 15 mg/kg IV d1

REGIMEN III
Paclitaxel 175 mg/m^2 IV 3h d1
Topotecan 0.75 mg/m^2 30min d1–3

REGIMEN IV
Paclitaxel 175 mg/m^2 IV 3h d1
Topotecan 0.75 mg/m^2 30min d1–3
Bevacizumab 15 mg/kg IV d1

EXPLORATORY OBJECTIVE A: PROGNOSTIC MARKERS FOR PREDICTIVE MODELING
To evaluate the impact of age, race, performance status, stage, histology, grade, disease site, prior chemotherapy with primary radiation, and time to recurrence on RR, PFS, and OS

EXPLORATORY OBJECTIVE B: IMPACT ON SMOKING
To determine the prevalence of active smoking extent of nicotine dependence and to determine if smoking is an independent risk factor for PFS in this cohort

TRANSLATIONAL RESEARCH OBJECTIVES
1. To isolate circulating tumor cells recovered from blood and determine their association to measures of clinical outcome
2. To correlate angiogenesis markers in plasma, biomarkers of hypoxia, and single nucleotide polymorphisms with measures of clinical outcome
3. To develop an optimal prognostic model for PFS and OS using clinical covaniates, smoking status, and various biomarkers

Gynecologic Oncology Group

US NIH, 2010.

FIGURE 3.54 Gynecologic Oncology Group 240 schema.

	Chemotherapy (n = 225)	Chemotherapy + Bev (n = 227)
Events, n (%)	140 (62)	131 (58)
Median OS, mos	13.3	17.0
HR = 0.71 (97% CI; 0.54–0.94) P = 0.0035		
Median follow-up 20.8 mo		

FIGURE 3.55 Gynecologic Oncology Group 240 phase 3 randomized trial: progression=free survival for chemotherapy vs. chemotherapy plus bevacizumab.

TABLE 3.31 Multivariate Analysis of Prognostic Factors of Treatment Response in Recurrent, Persistent, and Metastatic Cervical Carcinoma*

	OR	95% CI	*P* Value
Race: black vs. nonblack	0.49	0.28–0.83	0.008
GOG performance 1 or 2 vs. 0	0.60	0.38–0.94	0.027
Site of disease: pelvic vs. nonpelvic	0.58	0.38–0.90	0.015
Radiosensitizer: yes vs. no	0.52	0.32–0.85	0.009
First recurrence within 1 year of diagnosis: yes vs. no	0.61	0.39–0.95	0.027

*Odds ratio (OR) in favor of treatment response estimated from logistic regression model, adjusted for covariates.
CI, Confidence interval; GOG, Gynecologic Oncology Group.
From Moore DH, Tian C, Monk BJ, et al. Prognostic factors for response to cisplatin-based chemotherapy in advanced cervical carcinoma: a Gynecologic Oncology Group Study. *Gynecol Oncol* 2010;116:44-49.

(cisplatin–paclitaxel–bevacizumab and topotecan–paclitaxel–bevacizumab) as Category 1.

We are seeing increasing evidence that therapy for metastatic cervical carcinoma does not need to be solely palliative. Qui and colleagues reported in 2007 on long-term survivors who presented with supraclavicular metastases. Additionally, in 2009, Takano and colleagues reported complete remissions in two patients with metastatic and recurrent cervical cancer. Before recurrence, one patient had received chemoradiation for locally advanced disease, and the other had been treated with adjuvant pelvic radiation after hysterectomy. Of note, both of these patients were treated with weekly paclitaxel (80 mg/m²) plus carboplatin (area under the concentration vs time curve [AUC] 2.0) (days 1, 8, and 15) and weekly bevacizumab (days 1, 8, 15, and 21). Notwithstanding significant unanticipated toxicities, the ongoing trials of the Arbeitsgemeinschaft Gynakologische Onkologie (AGO; ie, German Society of Gynaecologic Oncology), Japan Clinical Oncology Group (JCOG), and Gynecologic Oncology Group (GOG) have been positioned to further refine therapeutic options for this disease.

Targeted Therapies

Biologic therapy is attractive in cervical cancer because of the homogeneity of the disease brought on by virally driven carcinogenesis. Several translational studies indicate that in addition to the VEGF-dependent angiogenesis axis (discussed later), other important signal transduction pathways to consider targeting include the PI3KC/Akt/mTOR pathway, the Notch signaling pathway, and patients harboring homologous recombination deficiencies for whom poly-ADP-ribose polymerase (PARP) inhibitors may be active.

Angiogenesis Inhibitors

As discussed earlier, biologic therapy in the form of angiogenesis inhibitors may be useful in retarding tumor growth and progression and even eliminating small-volume residual disease. Evidence that angiogenesis plays an important role in locally advanced cervical cancer has accumulated in recent years. In one study of 111 patients, Cooper and colleagues identified tumor angiogenesis (as reflected by the tumor microvessel density [MVD]) as a significant prognostic factor within a Cox multivariate analysis, where it was associated with poor locoregional control and OS. Conversely, among 166 women who underwent radical hysterectomy for stage Ib tumors, Obermair and colleagues demonstrated enhanced 5-year survivorship when the MVD was less than 20 per high power field (HPF) (90% vs. 63% with MVD >20 HPF). The VEGF receptor expression has also been shown to correlate with MVD in cervical carcinomas.

Several small-molecule inhibitors are actively being studied in cervical cancer, although none of these agents is currently approved in cervical cancer. Pazopanib is an oral tyrosine kinase inhibitor with antiangiogenic activity. It targets VEGFR, PDGFR, and c-Kit. Another oral tyrosine kinase inhibitor, lapatinib, targets EGFR and HER2. Given existing evidence supporting a role for angiogenesis in cervical cancer and the observation that overexpression of EGFR correlates with poor outcome in this disease, Monk and colleagues studied these drugs in 230 patients with measurable stage IVB persistent or recurrent cervical carcinoma not amenable to curative therapy and at least one prior regimen. The randomization scheme included pazopanib 800 mg/day (*n* = 74) vs. lapatinib 1500 mg/day (*n* = 78) vs. pazopanib 400 mg/day plus lapatinib 1000 mg/day (*n* = 78). The futility boundary was crossed for the combined regimen at the planned interim analysis, and this arm was discontinued, leaving a total of 152 patients in the monotherapy arms. Pazopanib improved PFS (HR, 0.66; 90% CI 0.48, 0.91; *P* = 0.013) and OS (HR, 0.67; 90% CI 0.46, 0.99; *P* = 0.045; median OS for *P* is 50.7 weeks; L is 39.1 weeks) with RR for pazopanib of 9% and that of lapatinib of 5%. Pazopanib was generally well tolerated, with the most common grade III adverse effect reported being diarrhea.

One year after presentation of the GOG 240 results that demonstrated a survival advantage associated with the integration of bevacizumab with chemotherapy, Symonds et al. presented data on their randomized, blinded, phase II trial of Cediranib in Recurrent Cervical Cancer (CIRCCa). Cediranib is a tyrosine kinase inhibitor of VEGF receptors 1, 2, and 3. Patients received cediranib 20 mg orally daily or matched placebo in combination with carboplatin AUC5 and paclitaxel 175 mg/m² three times weekly. This was continued until documented disease progression or inability to tolerate adverse events. A total of 69 patients was randomized and 79% completed six cycles of chemotherapy. Median PFS for the cediranib and placebo arms were 35 weeks and 30 weeks, respectively (HR, 0.61; 80%CI, 0.41–0.89; *P* = 0.046). No significant difference in OS was demonstrated. The overall response rate with cediranib was 66% (80% CI, 53%–77%) compared with 42% with placebo (80% CI 30%–55%). Cediranib showed significantly more grade 3/4 neutropenia than placebo (31% vs. 9%, *P* = 0.019). Additionally, 50% experienced grade 2, 3, or 4 diarrhea, and 34% experienced grade 2, 3, 4 hypertension. Given its manageable toxicity but lack of demonstrated improvement in OS, further assessment of this agent may be warranted.

Immunotherapy

As discussed earlier, the therapeutic landscape of advanced melanoma has been effectively transformed through the introduction of checkpoint inhibitors. Clinical trials using the anti-programmed death cell 1 drugs pembrolizumab and nivolumab are currently being planned or are underway through the NRG Oncology cooperative group.

Therapeutic Human Papillomavirus Vaccine

Therapeutic vaccines target virus-infected cells using epitopes of major histocompatibility complex (MHC)–processed peptides. Through interaction with CD8+ lymphocytes and MHC I pathways, they engage the cellular machinery, resulting in production of cytotoxic T lymphocytes. The HPV oncoproteins E6 and E7 can be targeted for the development of antigen-specific vaccination. Molecular strategies to design a therapeutic vaccine can be based on bacterial or viral vectors, peptides, proteins, DNA, and even dendritic cells. They may be useful in inducing regression, halting progression of preinvasive disease, or eradicating subclinical residual neoplastic disease after therapy.

With respect to prophylactic HPV vaccines, in 2003, the World Health Organization convened a gathering of experts from both developing and developed countries to identify the appropriate endpoint measurements for HPV vaccine efficacy. The general consensus was that it would be desirable to have a globally agreed, measurable efficacy endpoint for considering deployment of HPV vaccines in public health settings. Because of the temporal lag between infection and the manifestation of invasive carcinoma, it was determined that a surrogate endpoint would be used to define the efficacy of HPV vaccines. Because persistent infection with the same high-risk HPV subtypes is considered a predictor for both moderate- or high-grade cervical dysplasias and invasive cervical cancer, it was determined that cervical intraepithelial neoplasia (CIN), rather than invasive cancer, would serve as the endpoint after HPV vaccine introduction.

Garcia and colleagues from the University of Arizona conducted a randomized, multicenter, double-blind, placebo-controlled trial in 161 women with biopsy-confirmed CIN II to III. Subjects received three intramuscular doses of placebo or ZYC101a, a vaccine containing plasmid DNA-encoding fragments derived from HPV-16 and -18 E6 and E7 oncoproteins. The vaccine was well tolerated and had demonstrable efficacy in promoting resolution of CIN II to III in women younger than age 25 years. Recently, Einstein and colleagues presented data from their phase II trial using the novel therapeutic vaccine HspE7. The fusion protein consists of a *Mycobacterium bovis* BCG heat shock protein (Hsp65) covalently linked at its C terminus to the entire sequence of HPV-16 E7. With an excellent safety profile on record, 32 HIV-negative women with CIN III were vaccinated. The investigators observed a 48% resolution of CIN III, 19% partial responses, and 33% of subjects with stable disease over a 4-month follow-up period.

A study by ADVAXIS conducted in India demonstrated no improvement in survival when cisplatin was added to their HPV-16 E7-based therapeutic vaccine. The immunotherapy platform being used by ADVAXIS is composed of an attenuated *Listeria monocytogenes* live vector that secretes an antigen-adjuvant fusion protein composed of truncated listeriolysin O and HPV-16 E7 oncoprotein. Through a shared evolution during which time *Listeria* has infected humans and humans in turn have acquired immunity to this bacterium, a profound, genetic ally-conserved, pathogen-associated immune mechanism has developed. Importantly, the first stage of GOG 265 (the open-label phase II trial of ADXS-HPV monotherapy in women with recurrent or persistent and metastatic cervical cancer) was notable for having a minimum of six patients alive (out of 26) at 12 months, allowing the trial to proceed to the second stage and is currently planning to enroll up to 38 additional patients. ADXS-HPV has also been greenlighted to be studied in HPV-induced head and neck carcinoma. At present, GOG Partners is developing a trial to study adjuvant ADXS-HPV in high-risk women treated with chemoradiation for locally advanced disease.

Human Papillomavirus–Targeted Tumor-Infiltrating T Cells

Stevanovic recently reported promising results from a small trial conducted at the NCI for women with metastatic cervical cancer who had been previously treated with platinum-based chemotherapy or chemoradiotherapy. Nine women were treated with a single infusion of tumor-infiltrating T cells selected when possible for HPV E6 and E7 reactivity (HPV-TILs). Cell infusion was preceded by lymphocyte-depleting chemotherapy and followed by administration of aldesleukin. Three of nine patients experienced objective tumor responses (two complete responses and one partial response). At the time of publication, the two complete responses were ongoing at 22 and 15 months after treatment. Importantly, HPV reactivity of T cells in the infusion product correlated positively with clinical response. Patients whose serum showed no reactivity did not respond to a single infusion of HPV-TILs. This approach using a novel autologous T-cell vaccine continues to be studied in this population.

For the bibliography list, log onto www.expertconsult.com ⟨http://www.expertconsult.com⟩

4

Endometrial Hyperplasia, Estrogen Therapy, and the Prevention of Endometrial Cancer

Lisa M. Landrum, MD, PhD, Rosemary E. Zuna, MD, Joan L. Walker, MD

OUTLINE

KEY POINTS

1. Atypia is the most worrisome feature in endometrial hyperplasia.
2. Complex hyperplasia with atypia has a concomitant risk of malignancy of more than 40%, many of which are high grade.
3. Estrogen therapy is the most effective treatment of postmenopausal vasomotor symptoms.
4. Estrogen is effective in the prevention and treatment of osteoporosis.

INTRODUCTION

The endometrium is a very dynamic tissue in reproductive age women. It is continuously changing in response to hormonal, stromal, and vascular influences, with the intended goal of implanting an embryo and supporting the nutritional needs of the developing pregnancy. Whereas estrogen stimulation is associated with the growth of proliferative endometrium (Fig. 4.1), progesterone produced by the corpus luteum after ovulation inhibits proliferation and stimulates formation of secretory endometrium (Fig. 4.2). Without conception and human chorionic gonadotropin (hCG) production, the corpus luteum fails to produce progesterone, and hormonal withdrawal allows endometrial breakdown and menses to occur. Continuous estrogen stimulation of the endometrium bypasses the normal recycling of the endometrium. Menarche and menopause represent transition times of varying lengths in women's lives when the absence of ovulation predisposes them to unopposed estrogen stimulation because no corpus luteum forms to secrete progesterone. Some women (≈5%) have polycystic ovarian disease, which is a prolonged anovulatory condition prone to estrogen excess. Obesity during menopause also produces a state of excess estrogen production. This is due to the peripheral

conversion, in the adipose tissues, of androgens secreted from the adrenal glands and ovaries into an estrogen, estrone, by the enzyme aromatase.

Unopposed estrogen stimulation yields a continuous spectrum of change from proliferative endometrium (Fig. 4.3) through many variations of endometrial hyperplasia until a malignant neoplasm develops. Endometrial cancer is defined by the ability to invade local tissue and metastasize (Fig. 4.4). Endometrial lesions show glandular and stromal variations in continuous change, presenting the challenge of classifying endometrial hyperplasia into distinct, reproducible categories that predict neoplastic risk, as well as response to progesterone therapy. Histopathologic classification of endometrial lesions provides a stratification of risk for progression to cancer by defined endometrial changes.

Understanding the pathophysiology of excess unopposed estrogen production helps the clinician better predict which women are at risk for endometrial cancer and provides windows of opportunity for implementation of prevention strategies. Selective estrogen receptor modulators (SERMs) such as tamoxifen and raloxifene and, more recently, aromatase inhibitors are widely used as both treatment and chemoprevention of breast cancer. These drugs have toxicities that the obstetrician/

FIGURE 4.1 Proliferative endometrium. Simple tubular endometrial glands are set in a prominent stroma. This pattern is associated with normal estrogen stimulation in a cycling woman (hematoxylin and eosin, 100× original magnification).

FIGURE 4.2 Secretory endometrium. Endometrial glands are present with a sawtooth pattern. Each gland is an individual unit set in endometrial stroma. The epithelium has intracytoplasmic glycogen secretion that is eventually extruded into the gland lumen (hematoxylin and eosin, 100× original magnification).

FIGURE 4.3 Benign endometrial hyperplasia (formerly simple hyperplasia without atypia). The endometrium shows an increase in the glandular epithelium usually caused by unopposed estrogen stimulation. This results in irregular and unpredictable gland outlines that are often cystic. There is abundant stroma, so that the gland-to-stromal ratio is little altered from normal (hematoxylin and eosin, 100× original magnification).

FIGURE 4.4 Endometrioid adenocarcinoma. Well-differentiated (International Federation of Gynecology and Obstetrics G1) endometrioid adenocarcinomas typically show a "back-to-back" glandular arrangement with little intervening stroma. The glands are lined by tall columnar cells (hematoxylin and eosin, 200× original magnification).

gynecologist will be required to manage. Although tamoxifen is an antiestrogen in breast tissue, it paradoxically has estrogen-like properties in the endometrium and increases the risk of endometrial cancer. It is also associated with thromboembolism and stroke. Although tamoxifen provides protection against bone loss, osteoporosis, and fractures, it does not appear to carry increased risk of myocardial infarction. There does appear to be an association with cataracts. Aromatase inhibitors block the cytochrome p450 CYP-19 enzyme responsible for the peripheral conversion of androgens to estrogens and result in estrogen deficiency. This accelerates menopausal bone loss, which could lead to osteoporosis and fractures; therefore, prevention of these toxicities is important when they are prescribed. Other side effects include hot flashes, sweats, edema, myalgias, and fatigue. Unfortunately, both tamoxifen and aromatase inhibitors accentuate menopausal symptoms.

Preventive health maintenance must balance all risks and benefits while maintaining quality of life and symptom control, and this is the central theme in this chapter. Many women want active control over these very important choices, balancing quality of life and their sexuality with factors such as cancer prevention and cardiovascular risk reduction.

CLINICAL PRESENTATION

The scientific explanation for the low incidence rates for endometrial hyperplasia is that it is a lesion that is usually unrecognized and asymptomatic until cancer develops. Until endometrial cancer screening becomes routine and cost effective, the true prevalence of the precursor lesions will remain unknown. Women with endometrial hyperplasias are identified by endometrial biopsy performed because of abnormal vaginal bleeding (menorrhagia or postmenopausal bleeding) or because a thickened endometrial stripe is found on transvaginal ultrasonography when ordered for another reason such as the identification of endometrial cells in the Pap test of a woman older than the age of 40 years.

There is evidence of exogenous or endogenous unopposed estrogen stimulation of the endometrium in most women with endometrial hyperplasia. The most common causes of excess estrogen are obesity, polycystic ovarian disease, or a prolonged perimenopause with anovulatory bleeding patterns. Some women have an ovarian neoplasm producing the estrogen stimulation, which is the classic presentation of a granulosa cell tumor. The development of hyperplasia secondary to anovulation at menarche is very uncommon and should be easily reversible, with normalization of cyclic menses with oral contraceptive pills. The age at presentation depends on the source of the excess estrogen. Endometrial hyperplasias and cancers that are associated with estrogen stimulation have a good prognosis. Endometrial cancers in women without evidence of excess estrogen are usually not associated with hyperplasia and can be associated with a tumor suppressor gene abnormality such as p53 associated uterine papillary serous carcinomas (Figs. 4.5 and 4.6). These are aggressive tumors, behaving similar to ovarian cancer with higher mortality rates.

Office endometrial biopsy has replaced the dilation and curettage (D&C) procedure for the diagnosis of endometrial hyperplasia or carcinoma. Historically, there was thought to be potential benefit of curettage as therapy, as well as providing more tissue for accurate histologic diagnosis. The use of "hormonal curettage" in which medical therapy with progesterone is followed by the withdrawal bleed provides the same benefit without the surgical cost or risk. Repeat office endometrial biopsy at 3-month intervals can reassure the patient and the clinician of the therapeutic effect of the hormonal therapy. An argument can be made that hysteroscopy and D&C for abnormal bleeding would potentially be more effective in identifying endometrial cancers, but there is no evidence that D&C reduces a woman's mortality risk. This outpatient office evaluation and management has become the usual and safest way to manage these patients until there is evidence that a hysterectomy is required. These management decisions are discussed further in later sections of this chapter.

FIGURE 4.5 Endometrial serous carcinoma in a polyp. There is an irregular, complex pattern of papillary epithelium arising in the tip of an endometrial polyp (hematoxylin and eosin, 20× original magnification).

FIGURE 4.6 Endometrial serous carcinoma. This tumor shows a complex pattern of highly atypical cells with large irregular nuclei and prominent nucleoli. Typically, the tumor shows a papillary configuration, with abnormal epithelium covering a thin connective tissue core (hematoxylin and eosin, 100× original magnification).

ENDOMETRIAL HYPERPLASIA: PATHOLOGIC DIAGNOSTIC CRITERIA

There are currently two systems of nomenclature for endometrial precursors, the 1994 World Health Organization (WHO94) schema and the endometrial intraepithelial neoplasia (EIN) system. Recently, the American College of Obstetrics and Gynecology and the Society of Gynecologic Oncology have published their "Committee Opinion" endorsing the EIN system but the community pathologists are not yet using this system. The International Society of Gynecological Pathologists (ISGYP),

TABLE 4.1   Classification of Endometrial Hyperplasia
Simple hyperplasia
Complex hyperplasia (adenomatous)
Simple atypical hyperplasia
Complex atypical hyperplasia (adenomatous with atypia)

From World Health Organization, Kurman RJ, ed. *Blaustein's Pathology of the Female Genital Tract*, ed 4, Springer, New York, 1994.

FIGURE 4.7 Endometrial intraepithelial neoplasia (formerly atypical complex hyperplasia). The tissue shows a marked increase in the gland-to-stromal ratio with complex glandular outlines and nuclear atypia in the lining epithelium (hematoxylin and eosin, 100× original magnification).

International Federation of Gynecology and Obstetrics (FIGO), a schema is commonly used to classify endometrial hyperplasia into four categories based on architectural structure and cytologic features. The architecture is either simple or complex, and the cytologic features are described as with or without atypia. This yields four separate diagnoses (Table 4.1): simple hyperplasia without atypia (see Fig. 4.3), complex hyperplasia without atypia, simple hyperplasia with atypia, and complex hyperplasia with atypia (AEH) (Fig. 4.7). The terms *adenomatous* and *cystic-glandular hyperplasia* have been discarded, and when the abbreviation AEH is used, it refers to atypical endometrial hyperplasia (AEH), which reflects the two categories of hyperplasia with cytologic atypia (simple hyperplasia or complex hyperplasia with atypia). The presence of atypia appears to be the most important criteria for progression to adenocarcinoma or the coexistence of endometrioid adenocarcinoma. The rates of coexisting endometrioid adenocarcinoma with AEH are reported to be as low as 13% and as high as 43%.

The pathologic diagnosis of these lesions is usually made with a small sampling of the endometrium in the office using an endometrial biopsy device. This small tissue sample then has to be categorized by the pathologist. A prospective study of the reproducibility of the diagnosis of AEH (both simple and complex) was undertaken by the Gynecologic Oncology Group (GOG). Women with the diagnosis of AEH who agreed to have a hysterectomy within 12 weeks of diagnosis of AEH were enrolled. The study population included 302 eligible cases with a median age of 57 years; 31% were 50 years of age or younger. The endometrial biopsy specimens were re-reviewed by three gynecologic pathologists independently (study panel diagnosis) in a blinded protocol. They agreed to categorize the endometrium as normal (cycling, menstrual, or atrophic), nonatypical hyperplasia (disordered proliferative, simple or complex hyperplasia), atypical hyperplasia (simple or complex), adenocarcinoma, or inadequate for evaluation. Two of three study pathologists had to agree on one of the above five diagnoses for a study panel diagnosis to be established. Correct diagnosis was determined by consensus agreement on the hysterectomy specimen during a simultaneous panel review with a multiheaded microscope. The results found only 40% of the cases had all three pathologists in agreement. The reproducibility was lowest for the diagnosis of AEH (kappa 0.28), and better for adenocarcinoma (kappa 0.51). Reproducibility was best for D&C (kappa 0.47; confidence interval [CI] 0.41:0.53) compared with small sampling devices (kappa 0.26–0.36). Two of three study panel members agreed with the referring institution diagnosis of AEH in 38% of cases. The study panel diagnosis was less severe in 25% of cases and adenocarcinoma in 29% of cases. The most important outcome for this study was the finding that 43% of the enrolled participants were found to have adenocarcinoma in their uteruses at the time of hysterectomy. The second most important finding was the rate of adenocarcinoma in each study panel majority diagnosis category: normal or nonatypical hyperplasia, 14 of 74 (18.9%); AEH, 45 of 115 (39.1%); and adenocarcinoma, 54 of 84 (64.3%). The uterine examination revealed the presence of some risk factors for metastatic disease present in 43 cases, including myometrial invasion or grade 2 or 3 lesions.

The natural history of simple hyperplasia without atypia is likely to follow a benign course. It is often seen in women near menopause when anovulatory cycles are common. The removal of the estrogenic stimulation or treatment with progestogens favorably influences the outcome. The majority of lesions will regress (60%) without treatment, and 84% will regress with progestin therapy. Only 3% are believed to progress to cancer. In the absence of atypia, the goal of treatment is to prevent progression to cancer in a small population of patients and to control abnormal uterine bleeding. The duration of treatment and best agent for progestin therapy have not yet been identified; however, medroxyprogesterone acetate (MPA) is typically used because there is the most clinical experience with it. Other progestin preparations that have been effectively used in hyperplasia without atypia include levonorgestrel-releasing intrauterine device and estrogen-progestin contraceptives in patients who desire to retain fertility. Complex hyperplasia is also expected to regress (56%) when atypia is not present. Atypical hyperplasia has a 36% progression rate, and even with progestins, 27% have been reported to progress, but it is uncertain if this is coexistent cancer that is eventually identified. Fifty-five percent of atypical hyperplasia is expected to regress with progestin therapy. A study among Finnish women notes that a treatment regimen including continuous progestin rather than cyclical (10–14 days/month) progestin appears to reduce risk of endometrial cancer in a postmenopausal population. It is assumed that unless the estrogen stimulation ceases, the progestin therapy may need to be lifelong. Alternatively, a hysterectomy is necessary to prevent the development of endometrioid adenocarcinoma (Fig. 4.4) or type I cancer (estrogen dependent). This estrogen-induced cancer is the most common histologic type and the least aggressive form of uterine malignancy and should be preventable, as well as successfully treated when detected.

The EIN system developed by International Endometrial Collaborative Group classifies endometrial precursors based on their clonal origin, noninvasive growth patterns, and risk of concurrent carcinoma. For a diagnosis of EIN to be made, the following criteria must be met: area of glands exceeds the stroma, cytology differs between the crowded focus and the normal background endometrium, the size of the lesion exceeds 1 mm and benign pathology with overlapping features such as polyps or effects of exogenous estrogen can be eliminated. This system is not universally adopted at this time, but there is some evidence that the clinical outcome prediction and the interobserver reproducibility using EIN may be improved over the 1994 WHO schema.

Endometrial carcinomas of the serous papillary variety arise in a background of atrophic endometrium. These cancers are not associated with excess estrogen and have been classified as type II (estrogen independent) endometrial cancers. Serous papillary adenocarcinoma is less likely to be identified at an early stage compared with endometrioid histologic types. These lesions are typically associated with mutations in the p53 tumor suppressor gene that results in accumulation of inactive p53 protein in the cell (Fig. 4.8). Unlike normal cells or most endometrioid cancers, immunostaining with antibodies to p53 will be positive in the majority of serous cancers. Endometrial hyperplasia is not a precursor to serous carcinoma. Rather, the precursor has been identified as endometrial intraepithelial carcinoma (EIC). Serous EIC (Fig. 4.9) can even be multifocal with disease found in the ovaries, fallopian tubes, and peritoneal cavity when no invasive component is found in the uterus. Comprehensive surgical staging is recommended because of the difficulty in establishing the diagnosis of invasive cancer intraoperatively. Postoperative therapy can be recommended after adequate histologic evaluation.

MANAGEMENT DECISIONS FOR ATYPICAL ENDOMETRIAL HYPERPLASIA (ENDOMETRIAL INTRAEPITHELIAL NEOPLASIA)

The patient's age, fertility plans and need for contraception, comorbidities, and personal preferences play a role in the management of these lesions. Hysterectomy is indicated when fertility is not desired and AEH is identified. AEH is commonly found with coexisting undiagnosed cancer already present in the uterus or progressing to endometrial cancer in untreated

FIGURE 4.8 p53 immunostain of endometrial intraepithelial neoplasia. Endometrial serous carcinoma is typically accompanied by p53 mutations that allow accumulation of p53 protein in the cells that can be identified by immunostaining. Normal cells do not stain positively for p53 because the amount of normal protein is below the threshold of the staining test (immunoperoxidase stain for p53 with DAB chromogen, 200× original magnification).

FIGURE 4.9 Endometrial intraepithelial carcinoma. This is the precursor lesion for serous carcinoma of the endometrium with markedly atypical, crowded epithelium with little architectural abnormality. This lesion is often observed on the surface of otherwise benign endometrial polyps (hematoxylin and eosin, 100× original magnification).

women. As previously discussed, the GOG reported that 43% of 306 women who had a community-based diagnosis of AEH on endometrial biopsy and proceeded without medical treatment to hysterectomy had endometrial cancer on final pathology. Although 63% (77 of 123) of the cancers identified were grade I lesions confined to the endometrium, 31% were myoinvasive, and 11% had deep myometrial invasion into the outer 50% of the myometrium. It is possible that future validation of a new EIN scoring system or another molecular marker will allow more precise predictability for the neoplastic potential and the coexistence of cancer before hysterectomy.

The complexity of the surgical management of AEH is underappreciated. Intraoperative decision making, using frozen section to determine the operative interventions, is never ideal, considering difficulty of the diagnosis and the variety of skill and expertise of the pathologist and gynecologists. It is to be expected that the postoperative diagnosis of cancer will be obtained in a substantial number of these cases. The recommendation is that the patient should be informed of the 20% to 45% risk of underlying malignancy, and hysterectomy is required for the final diagnosis. The patient should be counseled about the desire to keep her ovaries or have them removed based on her age, family history, and other medical conditions or comorbidities. Genetic counseling and testing for Lynch syndrome may also be reasonable as a factor to consider in this decision-making process. Vaginal hysterectomy may be all that is required, or laparoscopically assisted hysterectomy with bilateral salpingo-oophorectomy can be considered. For the vast majority of patients with AEH, lymphadenectomy and complete surgical staging results in overtreatment and increased surgical risk. Endometrial cancers associated with AEH are usually low-grade, early stage lesions with a low risk of lymphatic metastasis. The risk of a high-risk uterine cancer in women with a biopsy of AEH ranges from 5% to 7%. In the event that high-grade cancer or deep myometrial invasion is found, reoperation may be offered for comprehensive surgical staging and removal of retained ovaries. Staging can usually be accomplished laparoscopically. This should be necessary in approximately 15% of the cases when cancer is identified and depends on the entire health history of the individual. Staging based on intraoperative assessment of myometrial invasion and grade of tumor is an appropriate strategy for institutions experienced in this approach. Supracervical hysterectomy, morcellation, and endometrial ablation are unacceptable for treatment of AEH because of the high prevalence of occult endometrial cancer in these patients. Women who desire childbearing, refuse hysterectomy, or have medical conditions that make hysterectomy an undesirable first choice can be treated hormonally. Megestrol 160 mg/day, in divided doses, has been the drug of choice with acceptable results even in the face of complex endometrial hyperplasia with atypia. It is unclear whether the treatment should be continuous or cyclic, but there are theoretical advantages to the endometrial shedding provided by the progesterone withdrawal bleed. The endometrium needs to be reevaluated histologically, by office biopsy or D&C, at approximately 3-month intervals for at least 1 year. Lifelong prevention strategies must be emphasized with the patient. The pathologist finds the evaluation of the endometrial sampling more straightforward if it is not complicated by exogenous hormonal influences. For this reason, it is best to withdraw the patient from the progestogen for 7 to 14 days to allow withdrawal bleeding before endometrial biopsies. The biopsy or D&C should be scheduled for after the withdrawal bleeding ceases.

In 2012, a systematic review identified 391 subjects from 45 studies with hyperplasia or grade 1 endometrial cancer who desired fertility and were treated with progestins. Seventy-eight percent of patients demonstrated a response to therapy with 53% of patients demonstrating a durable, complete response. The complete response rate was significantly higher for those with hyperplasia at 65% than for those women with carcinoma (48%). The American Congress of Obstetricians and Gynecologists (ACOG) Practice Bulletin on endometrial cancer includes this general guideline: The new Endometrial Intraepithelial Neoplasia ACOG Practice Bulletin (May 2015) offers multiple options for women with contraindications for hysterectomy, including medroxyprogesterone acetate, depot medroxyprogesterone, micronized vaginal progesterone, megestrol acetate, or levonorgestrel intrauterine system.

Women with AEH and endometrial cancer who desire to maintain their fertility may be treated with progestin therapy. After therapy, they should undergo serial complete intrauterine evaluation approximately every 3 months to document response. Hysterectomy should be recommended for women who do not desire fertility.

Local therapy of the endometrium with a progestin-containing intrauterine device (Mirena) is encouraging. In a recent multicenter randomized trial in Norway, 170 women with endometrial hyperplasia were randomized to one of three treatment arms: levonorgestrel intrauterine system (LNG-IUS), oral MPA 10 mg administered 10 days per cycle, or continuous oral MPA 10 mg/day for 6 months. At the end of 6 months, women in all treatment regimens showed significant therapeutic response, but the highest numbers of responders were noted in the LNG-IUS group (100%) and the continuous MPA group (96%) compared with the cyclical MPA group (69%). Gallos et al. reported a 12-year comparative cohort study of 344 patients with endometrial hyperplasia who received conservative management with progestins for complex or AEH because of desire for fertility or who were medically unsuitable for surgery. For the group of women treated with LNG-IUS ($n = 250$), 94.8% achieved regression of hyperplasia compared with 84% of women treated with oral progestins. Of note, the patients with a body mass index of 35 or greater were most likely to have a relapse of hyperplasia or fail to regress to a normal endometrium. In conclusion, management decisions in women with AEH are complex and require an understanding of the risk of invasive endometrial adenocarcinoma, the reproductive desires of the patient and her comorbidities, and the risks for surgical management. Ideally, minimally invasive techniques can be used to complete hysterectomy with bilateral salpingo-oophorectomy. The finding of adenocarcinoma in the uterus requires consultation with a gynecologic oncologist to determine whether observation, reoperation for surgical staging, or adjuvant therapy based on uterine factors should be considered.

MANAGEMENT OF ENDOMETRIAL HYPERPLASIA WITHOUT ATYPIA

The diagnosis of simple or complex hyperplasia without atypia requires hormonal management and is not an indication for

TABLE 4.2 Hormonal Treatment for Endometrial Intraepithelial Neoplasia*

Hormonal Agent	Dosage and Length
Medroxyprogesterone acetate	10–20 mg/day or cyclic 12–14 days per month
Depot medroxyprogesterone	150 mg intramuscularly every 3 months
Micronized vaginal progesterone	100–200 mg/d or cyclic 12–14 days per month
Megestrol acetate	40–200 mg/day
Levonorgestrel intrauterine system	52 mg in steroid reservoir over 5 years

*Previously known as atypical endometrial hyperplasia.
Modified from Committee on Gynecologic Practice, Society of Gynecologic Oncology. Endometrial intraepithelial neoplasia. ACOG Committee Opinion No. 631. American College of Obstetricians and Gynecologists. *Obstet Gynecol* 2015;125(5):1272-1278 and Trimble CL, Method M, Leitao M, Lu K, et al. Management of endometrial precancers. Society of Gynecologic Oncology Practice Committee. *Obstet Gynecol* 2012;120:1160-1175.

hysterectomy. These lesions are generally reversible with progestogen (synthetic progestin or progesterone). The classification of progestogens is seen in Table 4.2. The initial approach is generally to treat in a cyclic fashion with the progestin given for 14 days of the month to deliver predictable cyclic withdrawal menses. Women, including teenagers who are premenopausal and sexually active, are usually best treated with a regimen that provides contraception such as Depo-Provera or oral contraceptives. Women who want to conceive are likely to be anovulatory and require ovulation induction agents after withdrawal bleeding is produced with a progestogen. Reassurance can be obtained from a reduction of menstrual flow and a bleeding pattern that is appropriately timed with the cyclic therapy. It is extremely important to counsel anovulatory women about the lifelong risk of endometrial cancer and methods for surveillance and prevention. Twenty-five percent of endometrial cancers occur in the premenopausal age range, and 5% are in women 40 years of age and younger. These cancers may be part of the polycystic ovarian syndrome or the anovulatory transition before menopause, and are all theoretically preventable with proper counseling and active management. Premenopausal endometrial cancer patients should also be counseled about the possibility of Lynch syndrome. A family history should be taken, and if endometrial and colon cancers are frequent in the family, the patient should be referred to genetic counseling. Colonoscopy is often recommended to endometrial cancer patients because of the association with colon cancer. There is a dramatic rise in the incidence rate of endometrial hyperplasia and endometrial cancer at 45 years of age and peaking at 65 years of age. This is likely because of the combined effects of estrone (estrogen) production in the peripheral adipose tissue, particularly in obese women, and to the absence of progesterone that is caused by the loss of ovulatory function in menopause.

PREVENTION OF ENDOMETRIAL CANCER

Endometrial stimulation by estrogens unopposed by progestins leads to endometrial hyperplastic conditions in a dose- and time-dependent manner. Experimental evidence has been obtained from prospective clinical trials conducted to identify the appropriate doses and schedules of hormone replacement therapies. Kurman reported a randomized trial of 1176 postmenopausal women receiving 1 mg of estradiol orally and either placebo or various doses of norethindrone acetate. Women treated with estradiol alone (247 evaluable participants) for 12 months had a 12.2% rate of simple hyperplasia without atypia, 1.6% had complex hyperplasia without atypia, and 0.8% had complex atypical hyperplasia. Norethindrone acetate at all doses used in this trial nearly eliminated that risk. The North American Menopause Society support the addition of a progestogen whenever estrogen is prescribed for menopausal symptoms in women with an intact uterus for the prevention of estrogen-induced hyperplasia and adenocarcinoma. Unfortunately, progestogen has undesirable side effects, and women have been known to discontinue this component of their prescribed hormone replacement (see Table 4.2).

The prevention of endometrial cancer has been complicated by the publication and early closure of the estrogen plus progestin (E + P) component of the Women's Health Initiative (WHI). This randomized placebo-controlled clinical trial evaluated conjugated equine estrogens (CEEs), 0.625 mg, plus MPA, 2.5 mg orally per day (hormone replacement therapy [HRT]). This trial enrolled 16,608 women with a range of 50 to 79 years of age for an average of 5.2 years to determine the primary outcomes of coronary heart disease (CHD), invasive breast cancer, and a global index (including stroke, pulmonary embolism [PE], endometrial cancer, colorectal cancer, hip fracture, and death from other causes). In May 2002, the data safety monitoring committee recommended premature closure of the trial because of the adverse outcomes of breast cancer and cardiovascular complications, including CHD, stroke, and PE. Of note, the overall mortality rate was not affected. The absolute excess risk per 10,000 person-years attributable to HRT was seven CHD events, eight strokes, eight PE, eight invasive breast cancers, and a reduction of five hip fractures. These risks need to be reviewed with women choosing HRT.

The WHI trial with CEE alone versus placebo had a very different outcome. There was a nonsignificant reduction in breast cancer risk ($P = 0.06$), and the CHD risk was unaffected (hazards ratio [HR], 0.91; CI 0.75–1.12), strokes were increased (HR, 1.39; CI 1.10–1.77), and hip fractures were reduced (HR, 0.61; CI 0.41–0.91). This places women with intact uteruses and their physicians in a difficult situation of balancing the risks. Women with uteruses can decide to accept the potential risks of the addition of a progestin or may choose to take unopposed estrogen and follow the endometrium yearly with transvaginal ultrasonography or endometrial biopsy. Unopposed estrogen use gives a woman a relative risk (RR) of endometrial cancer of three times the general population for less than 5 years of use and RR of 10 after 10 years of use. The risk decreases but remains elevated after discontinuing the drug. Alternatively, other progestins and progesterone formulations are available that may carry a different but as yet unknown risk of breast cancer. Micronized progesterone is available as oral 100- or 200-mg capsules (Prometrium) and has been approved by the Food and Drug Administration (FDA) for use in combination with estrogen for relief of menopausal symptoms. The dosage of 200 mg for 12 days per month in a cyclic fashion causes withdrawal bleeding in a predictable manner. The regimen of CEE 0.625 mg/day with oral micronized progesterone at a dose of 200 mg/day for 12 days per month failed to see any increase in endometrial hyperplasia with 3 years of follow-up. A vaginal progesterone gel is available that is only FDA approved for infertility use but has been studied in small numbers of menopausal women. An additional provocative alternative is to use the progestin-containing intrauterine system (Mirena is FDA approved for contraceptive use only) and unopposed estrogen, which has been studied prospectively in menopausal women. These women were only followed for 1 year, and they were able to convert proliferative endometrium to atrophic endometrium while using continuous estradiol 50 mcg/day via the transdermal route.

The official position statement of the North American Menopause Society is that a progestogen should be added to estrogen therapy for all postmenopausal women with intact uteruses. The type, route, or regimen can be individualized to minimize side effects while providing adequate endometrial protection.

BENEFITS AND RISKS OF ESTROGEN REPLACEMENT THERAPY

Quality of Life, Vasomotor Symptoms, and Sexual Function

The WHO and the Stages of Reproductive Aging Workshop (STRAW) working group define menopause as the permanent cessation of menstrual periods that occurs naturally or is induced by surgery, chemotherapy, or radiation. Menopausal transition is the time of an increase in follicle-stimulating hormone and increased variability in cycle length. Postmenopause begins at the time of the final menstrual period but is not recognized until 12 months of amenorrhea has occurred. The National Institutes of Health in the "State of the Science Conference Statement: Management of Menopause-Related Symptoms" defines menopausal symptoms as vasomotor symptoms, vaginal dryness and painful intercourse, and sleep disturbance. Estrogen is the most consistently effective therapy for vasomotor symptoms, vaginal dryness, sleep disturbances, and improved quality of life, and a subset of women may find an improved mood with estrogen therapy. Testosterone has been demonstrated to improve libido, especially in women who have undergone oophorectomy; however, the long-term risks have not been studied. Antidepressants, clonidine, and gabapentin have been studied in treatment of hot flashes with some efficacy.

Symptom control is the most common reason for initiating estrogen therapy and remains undisputed as the most appropriate indication for prescribing estrogen at the time of natural or surgical menopause. The epidemiology community recommendations are that the patient should be told that hormone replacement should be for symptom control only, prescribed at the lowest effective dose, and for the shortest duration of use possible. Women should consider tapering off after 5 years of use to avoid the adverse events of thromboembolic disorders, breast cancer, stroke, and cardiovascular events (myocardial infarction, death). Women must be active participants in the decision-making process regarding estrogen use or estrogen plus progestogen use. They must experience the symptoms, recognize the reasons they are choosing to use these agents, and actively make the decision that the benefit is worth the small risk. Their own social situation or individual risk profile may influence their personal decisions.

The WHI reported the symptoms manifested by 8405 women between 8 to 12 months from the date the HRT participants were asked to discontinue CEE plus medroxyprogesterone acetate. These women were mailed a survey, and 21.2% responded that they had moderate-to-severe vasomotor symptoms, which was significantly different (CI 4.92–6.89) compared with placebo. They also reported pain and stiffness (Adjusted odds ratio [AOR] 2.16), and these symptoms were reported by more than 10% of respondents. Other withdrawal effects were feeling tired, difficulty sleeping, and a feeling of bloating or gas. Depression was also significantly increased after withdrawal of hormone replacement ($P <0.001$).

The WHI documented the beneficial effects experienced from HRT in women with uteruses. Relief of hot flashes (85.7%), night sweats (77.6%), vaginal or genital dryness (74.1%), and joint pain or stiffness (49.1%) compared with placebo effects ranged from 57.7% to 38.4%, respectively. Women taking HRT were more likely to complain of breast tenderness (9.3%) and vaginal bleeding (51%) than those on placebo (2.4% vs. 5%, respectively).

In conclusion, the data summarized in the WHI are not generalizable to 45- to 55-year-old women with menopausal symptoms. These women must prioritize their own situations and health risks and quality of life benefits. Most will find the best symptom relief from estrogen use. Alternatives to estrogen include progestogens, antidepressants (venlafaxine, paroxetine, fluoxetine), clonidine, and the anticonvulsant gabapentin. Over-the-counter remedies frequently used include isoflavones, black cohosh, and vitamin E. None of the alternatives resolve the entire menopausal syndrome, including sexual dysfunction.

Estradiol may also be delivered by a silicone ring placed in the vagina (Estring, Femring). The Estring (Pfizer US Pharmaceuticals) contains 2 mg of estradiol and on average 0.02 mg/day is released over a 90-day period. Studies have demonstrated a median plasma estradiol increase from 4.5 pmol/L before insertion to 12.5 pmol/L at steady state. The comparison with a 0.05 mg Estraderm patch was 10-fold greater serum concentrations of estradiol in users of the patch. A study of endometrial thickness in 60 postmenopausal women over a 12-month period showed a thickness of 2.8 mm before Estring and 2.6 mm thickness after 12 months of use. This is reassuring to women unable to tolerate progestins. Another randomized controlled study (RCT) demonstrated a decrease in urinary tract infections with the use of Estring. The use of Estring may be preferred for women wanting local therapy for vaginal dryness symptoms and an inability to take progestins or a history of breast cancer. Femring is available when an increase in vaginal dose is desired.

Estrogen alone does not always resolve the sexual dysfunction complaints after bilateral salpingo-oophorectomy. Testosterone has been demonstrated in clinical trials to help with decreased sexual desire, arousal, and orgasmic response, but at present, there is no FDA approval for libido in women. A recent study evaluated the efficacy and safety of testosterone treatment in 814 postmenopausal women with hypoactive sexual desire not receiving estrogen therapy. Patients were randomized to receive testosterone by patch (150 or 300 mcg/day) or placebo. At 24 weeks, efficacy was measured, and the group of women receiving 300 mcg/day of testosterone reported significantly greater sexual satisfaction compared with the placebo group and the group treated with 150 mcg/day of testosterone. The rate of adverse events related to androgens, specifically unwanted hair growth, was also highest in this group. Furthermore, breast cancer was diagnosed in four women treated with testosterone compared with none of the women who received placebo. The long-term effects of testosterone, including effects on the breasts, remain unclear. The FDA has recently approved flibanserin to treat acquired, generalized hyposexual desire disorder in premenopausal but not postmenopausal women.

Osteoporosis

Osteoporosis is a disease characterized by low bone mass and microarchitectural deterioration of bone tissue, which leads to increased bone fragility and increased fracture risk. Low bone mass is related to a low peak bone mass (mainly under genetic influence) and to decrease in bone mass, which occurs after menopause and with aging. Menopause induces an accelerated bone loss within 5 to 8 years followed by a linear rate of bone loss. Bone density readings are standardized to healthy women of similar age. Osteopenia is defined as bone loss of greater than 1 standard deviation (SD) from the mean, and osteoporosis is bone loss greater than 2 SDs from the mean.

Osteoporosis prevention strategies should begin before 40 years of age because of a decline from peak bone mass. An even more dramatic loss of bone occurs at menopause with the loss of estrogen support of osteoblastic activity. Women should take active measures to protect their bones by regular weight-bearing exercise (at least 30 minutes three times a week), calcium supplementation (1500 mg elemental calcium for postmenopausal women), and adequate vitamin D supplementation (800–1200 IU/day). At menopause, a baseline bone density is recommended and then repeated every other year unless osteopenia or osteoporosis is detected. Estrogen replacement therapy (ERT) has been the traditional main strategy to prevent this deterioration in bone strength. A number of medications are approved by the FDA for the prevention or treatment of osteoporosis. Bisphosphonates such as alendronate (Fosamax), risedronate (Actonel), and ibandronate (Boniva) act by preventing bone resorption by blocking the action of osteoclasts.

Gastrointestinal side effects (reflex, esophagitis, esophageal ulcers) have been a primary concern for patients taking oral bisphosphonates. These drugs should be taken first thing in the morning on an empty stomach with a full 8-oz glass of water. The patient should then wait a full hour before eating or taking any other medications. Lying down or eating before the recommended time increases risk for gastrointestinal distress. There are also theoretical concerns that prolonged therapy with bisphosphonates leads to oversuppression of bone remodeling, which allows microdamage to accumulate and increase skeletal fragility. Microscopic crack frequency is increased in animals treated with high doses of bisphosphonates, although this has yet to be demonstrated in biopsies taken from postmenopausal women treated with long-term use. SERMs such as raloxifene (Evista) bind with high affinity to estrogen receptors and promote estrogen-like activity on bone. Unfortunately, raloxifene has the same thromboembolic risk of estrogen without the benefit of menopausal symptom relief. Drugs approved for treatment only include calcitonin (Miacalcin), which is administered by nasal spray, and teriparatide (Forteo), which is administered through daily subcutaneous injections. Both of these pharmacologic agents serve to increase bone formation.

Two anatomic areas are of interest in the bone remodeling process. The first is the axial skeleton, which is composed primarily of trabecular bone. The second is the appendicular skeleton, which is composed primarily of cortical bone. The remodeling cycle is the same in both types of bone. However, because of the greater surface area, approximately 40% of trabecular bone, as opposed to 10% of the cortical bone, is in "turnover" each year. The osteoclast is responsible for the resorption of old bone, which results in the formation of a resorption cavity. Osteoblasts are then attracted to the cavity, where they secrete osteoid, which is primarily type I collagen. The collagen is mineralized mainly with calcium, thus producing new bone with an appropriate mechanical strength. Under normal circumstances, the amount of bone removed is replaced with fresh bone; however, this process can become uncoupled if osteoclasts remove more bone than can normally be replaced by osteoblasts, resulting in net loss of bone mass. In menopausal women, accelerated bone loss is associated with high bone turnover rate and increased osteoclast activity. Estrogen may inhibit osteoclast activity and increase proliferation of osteoblasts as well as collagen production.

The beneficial effects of estrogen in preventing or treating postmenopausal osteoporosis are well recognized. At the same time, there is growing recognition that osteoporosis is a major public health problem in the United States. It is estimated that approximately 8 million women in the United States have osteoporosis and another 14 million are at risk because they have low bone mass. Osteoporosis causes more than 1.5 million fractures each year, including 300,000 hip, 700,000 vertebral, and 200,000 wrist fractures. These fractures are seen mainly in women. For a 50-year-old woman, the lifetime risk of fracture of any of the three is 40%. Traditional risk factors for osteoporosis include estrogen deficiency; fair complexion; high caffeine intake; low calcium intake; small, thin build; smoking; inadequate physical activities; and multiple disease processes and drugs. The acute and long-term medical care expenses associated with these fractures cost the nation an estimated $17 billion in 2005. The cumulative cost over the next 2 decades is estimated to be $474 billion. An excess mortality rate associated with hip fracture is 12% to 20% during the first year after the injury. Fewer than half of patients with hip fractures ever return to their prefracture activity level. Many require assistance and have lost their independence and require long-term domiciliary care. Vertebral fractures may be asymptomatic in 50%, but successive fractures can lead to loss of height, kyphotic distortion of posture, and chronic back pain. Approximately 10% of patients with hip fractures die of surgical complications within 6 months of fracture. Approximately 25% of all white women older than 60 years of age have spinal compression fractures resulting from osteoporosis. The risk of hip fracture is 20% by the age of 90 years, and hip fractures are about 2.5 times more common in women than in men. An increased rate of loss of both cortical and cancellous bone is associated with menopause. In a follow-up study of 82 postmenopausal women 5 to 10 years after their first examination, Meema and coworkers concluded that (1) as a group, menopausal women lost bone, and the beginning of this loss is less related to age than to loss of ovarian function; (2) the rate of loss was not significantly correlated with age; and (3) the bone loss was prevented by estrogen administration (ie, 0.625 mg of conjugated estrogens).

Nachtigall and associates conducted a 10-year double-blind prospective study to evaluate the effects of ERT. They took a sample population of 84 pairs of randomly chosen postmenopausal patients who were matched for age and diagnosis. Half of the patients received conjugated estrogens and cyclic progesterone, and the other half received a placebo. The estrogen-treated patients whose therapy was started within 3 years of menopause showed improvement or no increase in osteoporosis. The patients in the control group demonstrated an increase in osteoporosis. A subsequent report by the same authors showed that there was no statistically significant difference in the incidence of thrombophlebitis, myocardial infarction, or uterine cancer in the two groups. Indeed, there was a lower incidence of breast cancer in the treated group. Estrogen-treated patients did show a higher incidence of cholelithiasis. The low number of cases precludes drawing any real conclusions from the data on diseases of low frequency. The study excludes a high incidence of complications from estrogens.

In another crossover study comparing the effects of estrogen-progestin therapy with those of placebo, bone mineral content increased during the 3 years of combination hormone therapy but continued to decrease in the placebo-treated group (Fig. 4.10). When the placebo was given to some of the estrogen-progestin group, bone density decreased, but the placebo-treated women had an increase in bone mineral content after being given estrogen-progestin therapy. Other factors are also important in preventing osteoporosis, such as adequate dietary calcium, exercise, and vitamin D. Many case control studies have noted considerable protection from hip fracture with HRT (Table 4.3).

FIGURE 4.10 Estrogen–progestin versus placebo crossover study. Bone mass in postmenopausal women in response to randomization to estrogen plus progestin supplementation versus placebo at time zero and again at 24 months. Women were 49 to 51 years of age and were taking 500 mg of calcium daily. (From Christiansen C, Christensen MS, Transbøl I. Bone mass in postmenopausal women after withdrawal of oestrogen/gestagen replacement therapy. *Lancet* 1981;1(8218):459-461.)

TABLE 4.3 Case-Control Studies of Hormone Replacement Therapy in the Prevention of Hip Fracture

Authors	Relative Risk
Hutchinson et al.	0.70
Weiss et al.	0.43–0.77
Paganini-Hill et al.	0.42
Kreiger et al.	0.50
Kiel et al.	0.34–0.65
Naesser et al.	0.79
Kanis et al.	0.55

Colorectal Cancer

Colorectal cancer is the third most common cancer and the third leading cause of cancer deaths in US women. Several epidemiologic studies have noted that HRT may reduce the risk of colorectal cancers. The WHI demonstrated an HR of 0.63, demonstrating slight protection from colorectal cancer in their E + P arm but not in the estrogen alone study (HR, 1.08). There appear to be some biologic reasons why estrogen may be protective. Bile acids are thought to initiate or promote malignant changes in the epithelium of the colon. Exogenous estrogen decreases secondary bile acid production. Estrogen also decreases serum levels of insulin-like growth factor-1, which is an important mitogen associated with colorectal cancer. Both case-control and prospective studies have been reported. Kampman and associates reported the largest case-controlled study with 815 colon cancer and 1019 population base controls in postmenopausal women. After adjusting for multiple risk factors, they noted an 18% decrease in risk of colon cancer in HRT users compared with the nonusers (RR, 0.82; CI 0.67–0.99). In the large study of the American Cancer Society, 897 deaths from colon cancer were identified during 7 years of follow-up of 422,373 postmenopausal women. The authors reported a 29% decrease in risk of colon cancer deaths in hormone users compared with nonusers (R, 0.71; CI 0.61–0.83). In the review and meta-analysis by Grodstein and colleagues, 18 studies were evaluated. They found a 20% decrease of colon cancer in ERT users compared with the nonusers (RR, 0.8; CI 0.72–0.92) and a 19% decrease in rectal cancer (RR, 0.79; CI 0.72–0.92). Ten studies provided data on timing of hormone use. Current users had an RR of 0.66 (CI 0.59–0.74) compared with that of the nonusers. In the Nurses' Health Study, current users noted an RR of 0.65; in past users, the RR was 0.84 (nonsignificant). Among past users, the decreased risk continued during the first 4 years after quitting ERT; however, 5 years or more after stopping ERT, the risk was similar to that of nonusers (RR, 0.92; CI 0.70–1.21). The effect of ERT on colon cancer risk was evaluated in the California Teachers Study among 56,864 postmenopausal women. There was noted to be significantly lower risk for colon cancer in women who had used ERT within the past 15 years than women that had never used hormones (RR, 0.64; CI 0.51–0.80). Five studies evaluated the duration of current use and found similar apparent protection for all women currently on ERT, regardless of duration. Four studies evaluated ERT and colorectal adenoma. Most studies noted a significantly decreased risk of development of adenomas in women on ERT. This decrease did not appear to be caused by increased surveillance (sigmoidoscopy) in the ERT users. In several, but not all, studies, there was a suggestion that colorectal cancers increased in women who were taking tamoxifen.

Most recently, extended follow-up data from the WHI was published that reviewed both incidence and mortality of colorectal cancer in women treated with E + P. This analysis revealed that, although fewer colorectal cancers were diagnosed in the E + P group, the patients more commonly had positive lymph nodes and advanced stage at diagnosis, translating into more deaths. So, although the incidence of colorectal cancers was lower, the mortality rate was greater. These data address the importance of not only identifying the incidence of colorectal cancer but also the influence of tumor characteristics, stage, and mortality rate. Overall, the findings do not suggest a clinically meaningful benefit in reducing mortality from colorectal cancer.

Cardiovascular Disease

Cardiovascular morbidity (ie, heart disease and stroke) constitutes the most frequent cause of death among women in the United States. It is estimated to account for approximately 292,188 deaths in the United States in 2009—that is, one in every four female deaths. Cardiovascular risks factors can be found, and potentially modulated, in women. High cholesterol levels are present in 50% of women, and high blood pressure is observed in 32% of all women, with 45% of black women having high blood pressure. The prevalence of cardiovascular

TABLE 4.4 Effect of Estrogen Treatment on Cardiovascular Morbidity in Menopausal Women

Authors	Year	Relative Risk
Bush et al.	1983	0.4
Bush et al.	1987	0.3
Wilson et al.	1985	1.3–32*
Stampfer et al.	1985	0.3
Colditz et al.	1987	0.42

*Smokers.

diseases increases dramatically with age, starting at a low level of 17.6% for women 35 to 44 years of age, 36.6% for women 45 to 55 years of age, 56.5% for women 55 to 64 years of age, and 75% for women 65 to 74 years of age. The possible effects of estrogen and progestin on the incidence of cardiovascular disease in women is the subject of ongoing research. Most of the cohort studies suggest that ERT effectively diminishes the risk of cardiovascular disease in women who are 50 to 60 years of age, but protection decreases with age (Table 4.4). Unfortunately, the studies (WHI, Heart and Estrogen/Progestin Replacement Study [HERS]) reveal that initiating estrogen therapy in women with established vascular disease (mean ages of 63–67 years) will not prevent cardiovascular events or deaths. These studies are unable to be generalized to estrogen use in the younger perimenopausal age groups, and the cohort and epidemiologic studies reveal some benefit, but use of progestin consistently decreases benefit.

Prevention of cardiovascular disease includes smoking cessation, blood pressure control, weight control, exercise, and blood sugar and cholesterol control. Blood cholesterol level is the main risk factor for cardiovascular disease in postmenopausal women. A high positive correlation has been found between levels of low-density lipoprotein (LDL) and coronary morbidity. Conversely, the level of high-density lipoprotein (HDL) shows a high negative correlation with the probability of coronary disease and with the extent of damage to the coronary vessels. Matthews has shown the beneficial effects of ERT on LDL and HDL levels. In a prospective study, he showed clearly a corresponding rise in HDLs and a decrease in LDLs in postmenopausal patients treated with ERT. The association of increased HDL and decreased LDL levels with reduced risk of cardiovascular disease is well documented for both men and women.

Lobo reported on the impact of different dosages of MPA on metabolism and hemostasis in postmenopausal women treated with conjugated estrogens. In this prospective, double-blind study, 525 women were randomized to five treatment regimens at 26 sites in the United States and Europe. All participants received 0.625 mg of conjugated estrogens daily for up to 13 cycles; four groups also received MPA, either 2.5 or 5 mg/day continuously or 5 or 10 mg/day for the last 14 days of each cycle. Effects on lipid and carbohydrate metabolism and coagulation were evaluated.

All of the treatment groups experienced increases in HDL cholesterol (HDL-C), the HDL2-C subfraction, and apolipoprotein A-1 compared with baseline; however, at each time point, the increases from baseline in the conjugated estrogens–only group were significantly greater than were those for the conjugated estrogens–MPA groups. Additionally, all treatment groups had significant decreases in LDL cholesterol (LDL-C) and apolipoprotein B. Decreases from baseline in total cholesterol (TC) levels were significantly greater than were those in the conjugated estrogens–only group. HDL3-C levels increased significantly from baseline in the conjugated estrogens–only group but not in the other treatment groups. Triglyceride levels increased significantly in all groups. The mean increase in the MPA-treated groups was less than that in the conjugated estrogens–only treatment group. Although MPA modified some of the effects of conjugated estrogens on lipid metabolism, the direction of changes in lipid parameters was unaltered.

Additional data on the conjugated estrogens regimen were reported in the results of the Postmenopausal Estrogen/Progestin Intervention (PEPI) trial. In this 3-year, randomized, double-blind, placebo-controlled trial, the investigators evaluated differences in selected heart disease risk factors among 875 postmenopausal women who received placebo, conjugated estrogens, or one of three conjugated estrogens–progestin regimens. One of the regimens used in this study was identical to that present in conjugated estrogens.

The investigators reported that after 3 years of therapy, women taking the conjugated estrogens regimen experienced significant increases in HDL-C levels compared with those taking the placebo. However, the increases were significantly less than those experienced by women taking conjugated estrogens alone. Compared with the placebo, LDL-C values were significantly decreased in women taking the conjugated estrogens, with no significant difference between groups. TC levels decreased significantly among women taking the conjugated estrogens regimen compared with those taking the placebo. Significant increases in serum triglyceride levels occurred in all treatment groups compared with the placebo group. There were no significant changes in blood pressure, fasting insulin levels, or 2-hour insulin levels between treatment groups. Treatment groups had significant increases in 2-hour glucose levels and significant decreases in fasting glucose levels compared with the placebo group. In paired comparisons, women in the placebo group had greater increases in fibrinogen than did women in the active treatment groups; no significant differences were present among the active treatment groups. Among their findings, the investigators concluded that "… oral estrogen taken alone or with MPA … is associated with improved lipoprotein and lower fibrinogen levels compared with placebo and the magnitude of these differences is likely to be clinically significant."

Multiple studies have evaluated HRT and CHD. In 1998, an overview by Barrett-Connor and Grady included 25 studies. Overall, the RR of CHD for women who took ERT compared with those who never took ERT was 0.70 (CI 0.65–0.75). When HRT was evaluated, the RR was 0.66 (0.53–0.84) compared with the nonusers. This analysis evaluated cohort case control and angiographic studies. The apparent benefit is limited mainly to current or recent use. These findings are consistent across diverse populations and various study designs.

The US National Health and Nutritional Examination Survey (NHANES-1) evaluated HRT and death from all cardiovascular disease in 1944 white women 55 years of age or older who were monitored for up to 16 years. After adjusting for risk factors of CHD, the risk of death from CHD was 0.66 (0.48–0.90) in the HRT users. The study by Ettinger and associates noted similar findings. In their patient population followed for 25 years, the death from any cause in HRT users compared with nonusers was 0.54, which was mainly due to a reduction in CHD (RR, 0.40) and other cardiovascular diseases (RR, 0.27).

Many studies, including the PEPI RCT, have noted that estrogen therapy in postmenopausal women decreased serum TC, LDL, and Lp(a) lipoproteins. HDL and triglyceride concentrations increase. The route of administration does affect serum lipids. Transdermal application has less effect on the serum lipid concentrations than the oral route. The type of progestins can also affect the serum lipids. Synthetic progestins tend to blunt the beneficial effects on the HDL but not decrease it below the baseline. Micronized progesterone does not decrease HDL compared with estrogen alone. Estrogen tends to decrease plasma fibrinogen concentrations as it does anticoagulant proteins, antithrombin III, and protein S. There also appears to be a decrease in the antifibronolytic protein plasminogen B activator inhibitor type I with an overall increased potential for fibrinolysis. In some reports, factor VII was also lowered with estrogen. The net effect on coagulation depends on the type of estrogen, dose, and duration of treatment.

The Global Consensus Statement on menopausal hormone therapy released a statement in 2013 recommending the use of estrogen therapy as the most effective treatment for vasomotor symptoms associated with menopause, and the benefits are more likely to outweigh the risks before age 60 years. Estrogen is effective and appropriate for the prevention of osteoporosis-related fractures in at risk women before age 60 years. They recommend the lowest dose and shortest treatment duration to achieve goals. This statement is based on the results of a round table meeting between representatives of the major international menopausal societies to reach consensus on core recommendations regarding HRT.

Two large trials (WHI and HERS) have now demonstrated that estrogen cannot protect against myocardial infarction or death in women with preexisting heart or vascular disease. In fact, the thromboembolic properties of estrogen likely increase risk when preexisting vascular lesions are present, predisposing women to stroke, myocardial infarction, and death. The WHI demonstrated in a trial of 16,608 women randomized to combined estrogen plus progestin (HRT) versus placebo at a mean age of 63.6 years. The absolute excess risk per 10,000 person-years attributable to HRT was seven CHD events, eight strokes, eight PEs, eight invasive breast cancers, and a reduction of five hip fractures. The WHI trial also had women without uterus treated with CEE alone versus placebo (n= 10,739), and they had a very different outcome. There was a nonsignificant reduction in breast cancer risk (P = 0.06), and CHD risk was unaffected (HR, 0.91; CI 0.75–1.12), strokes were increased (HR, 1.39; CI 1.10–1.77), and hip fractures were reduced (HR, 0.61; CI 0.41–0.91).

The HERS was designed to determine if HRT could reduce cardiovascular events in women with known coronary artery disease (CAD). A total of 2763 women with preexisting CAD and an average age of 67 years were enrolled and randomized to conjugated estrogen 0.625 mg plus MPA 2.5 mg/day versus placebo. After 4.1 years of follow-up, there was no significant difference in the primary outcomes of CHD events or in any secondary outcome. There was a time trend of higher risk of events in the first year of use and a decrease in events in years 3 through 5. HERS II was a longer term follow-up study of the same participants that could not substantiate any benefit of HRT with longer use. It has been speculated that the initial increase in risk of cardiovascular events with HRT might be due to prothrombotic effects of the hormonal therapy. There may be a beneficial effect on the inhibition of progression of atherosclerosis because of the effects on lipoprotein cholesterol; therefore, those who were doing well on the medication were not asked to discontinue it. The conclusion of HERS and HERS II was that postmenopausal hormone therapy should not be used to reduce the risk for CHD events in women with CHD.

Manson et al., for the WHI investigators, published the summary of CHD outcomes. This report also emphasized the increased risk of CHD events during the first year of use and recommended against prescribing HRT for the prevention of cardiovascular disease. The problems with these trials are that the participants were older than the usual women prescribed HRT, and they were recruited because of their increased risk of CAD events. This makes the results of HERS and WHI applicable to a similar population of high-risk women, and the conclusions may not be generalizable to younger women initiating HRT at the onset of menopausal symptoms. Prevention of CAD may have a different pathophysiology than the progression from CAD to death. The epidemiologic and cohort data are criticized for the likely enrollment of healthier and more active women and may also not represent all women of a similar age.

Cardiovascular risk reduction recommendations are smoking cessation, exercise, and weight control along with blood pressure and cholesterol management. Aspirin has recently been shown to lower the risk of stroke without affecting the risk of myocardial infarction or death from cardiovascular causes in most women. In this randomized trial of 39,876 healthy women 45 years of age or older, participants received 100 mg or aspirin or placebo on alternate days for 10 years and were monitored for cardiovascular events. There was a 17% reduction of strokes for the entire study population randomized to aspirin (RR, 0.83; CI 0.69–0.99; $P = 0.04$). There was benefit for prevention of myocardial infarction only in women 65 years of age and older at enrollment (RR, 0.66; CI 0.44; 0.97; $P = 0.04$). The conclusion of this study is that physicians should perform a careful risk assessment to determine who is likely to benefit from aspirin versus likely to be harmed by the increase of gastrointestinal hemorrhage requiring transfusion ($P = 0.05$)

The 2013 ACOG committee recommended that HRT should not be used for the primary or secondary prevention of CHD, but rather women should be prescribed estrogen or estrogen plus a progestogen (when a uterus is present) at the onset of moderate or severe menopausal symptoms. The dose should be the lowest necessary to achieve the symptom control desired, and the duration of therapy should be 5 years or less. Discontinuation of this medication is not without side effects, and withdrawal symptoms may be minimized by a tapering schedule over a long period of time. It is accepted, however, that when a woman is on therapy, the risk of continuing such treatment is low, and the risk is greatest during the first year or two after initiating treatment, especially when preexisting vascular disease may already be present.

ESTROGEN REPLACEMENT THERAPY FOR ENDOMETRIAL AND BREAST CANCER SURVIVORS

Estrogen Replacement Therapy for Endometrial Cancer Survivors

Historically, HRT has been contraindicated for patients who have been treated for cancer of the uterus. Although estrogen administration has not been shown to have adverse effects on patients who have been treated for endometrial cancer, many physicians continue to be reluctant to administer this medication to these women. No data in the literature substantiate the detrimental effects of estrogen in these patients. It is not unusual for women with endometrial cancer to have severe symptoms because of withdrawal of estrogen at the time of their diagnosis and surgical treatment.

The GOG conducted a prospective trial to evaluate the potential risk of estrogen replacement in women after treatment of endometrial adenocarcinoma. This randomized clinical trial of ERT (CEE 0.625 mg orally per day, Premarin) compared with placebo in women treated for stage I and II endometrial cancer closed after the WHI was halted prematurely in 2002 because of decrease in accrual and lack of feasibility. Before study closure, 1236 eligible women were randomized, and the median follow-up was 35.7 months. The median age at endometrial cancer diagnosis was 57 years (range, 26–91 years). Compliance with medication for the entire treatment period was 41%, and for those on the ERT arm, 71% knew to which arm they had been randomized. A summary of the results on the ERT arm demonstrated endometrial cancer recurrence in 14 patients (2.3%); eight patients (1.3%) developed a new malignancy, one of which was breast cancer. There were 26 deaths (4.2%) on the estrogen arm; five were due to endometrial cancer. An important finding is that women with stage I and II endometrial cancer are more likely to die of causes unrelated to the cancer diagnosis; therefore, other health issues must take priority when planning for preventive health maintenance (Table 4.5). Women on the placebo arm of this study suffered 19 deaths (3.1% not statistically different), and four were due to endometrial cancer. Ten placebo patients developed a new malignancy (1.6%), three of which were breast cancer. Although there were no significant

TABLE 4.5 Gynecologic Oncology Group Randomized Trial of Estrogen in Endometrial Cancer Recurrence and Survival

	Treatment Group			
	Placebo*	%	ERT*	%
Alive, NED	591	(95.6)	583	(94.3)
Alive with disease recurrence	8	(1.3)	9	(1.5)
Total deaths	19	(3.1)	26	(4.2)
Endometrial cancer	4	(0.6)	5	(0.8)
MI or CHD	4	(0.6)	3	(0.5)
Pulmonary embolism	0	(0.0)	2	(0.3)
Other	6	(1.0)	9	(1.5)
Unknown	5	(0.8)	7	(1.1)

*618 evaluable patients in each treatment group
CHD, Coronary heart disease; *ERT,* estrogen replacement therapy; *MI,* myocardial infarction; *NED,* no evidence of disease.
From Barakat RR, Bundy BN, et al; Gynecologic Oncology Group Study. Randomized double-blind trial of estrogen replacement therapy verses placebo in stage I or II endometrial cancer: a gynecologic oncology group study. *J Clin Oncol* 2006;24(4):587.

differences in recurrence between the ERT and placebo arms for all comers, further investigation suggested that racial disparities in outcome may exist. With a median follow-up of 3 years, recurrent disease was noted in 5 of 56 black patients on the ERT arm compared with only 8 of 521 white patients. The RR of recurrence among blacks in the ERT group was 11.2 (95% CI, 2.86–43.59; $P = 0.0005$) after adjustment for age, body mass index, and tumor grade.

This study was admittedly underpowered for the endpoints of new breast cancer or endometrial cancer recurrence, but at least women can be informed that the rate of recurrence of endometrial cancer was equally low on each arm of this study. The exception to this may lie with ERT for specific subgroups. Although the number of outcome events was limited in this study, these findings suggest that the use of ERT in black women should be judicious and given only after appropriate patient education. The decision to prescribe estrogen must be individualized based on symptom control and quality of life concerns that only the patient can assess.

Many physicians do not hesitate to give ERT in patients with well-differentiated or superficially invasive cancers because recurrences are generally very low in these patients. There is greater hesitancy to treat poorly differentiated or deeply invasive cancers with ERT. This is also true for patients with extrauterine disease. The belief is that because recurrence is more frequent, ERT may increase the risk. The data suggest the opposite. Patients with high-risk factors and taking ERT had a lower recurrence rate than did those who were not taking ERT. Although theoretically a possible advantage, it does not appear that the addition of a progestin to estrogen is beneficial. We initially followed this routine of a combination of E + P; however, for several years now, we have not done so, and we have noticed no difference in outcomes.

The optimal time to begin ERT after treatment has not been determined. Some suggest waiting for at least 2 years because most patients who will develop recurrences will have done so. The data currently suggest no benefit in waiting. Within a few days of surgical treatment, many patients will develop disturbing vasomotor symptoms. These symptoms can be prolonged with subsequent adverse symptomatology, such as vaginal thinness and dryness, which can lead to unpleasant intercourse. As a result, symptoms can be treated as soon as they become troublesome.

In 1993, the ACOG released the following statement: "In women with a history of endometrial cancer, estrogens could be used for the same indications as for any other woman, except that the selection of appropriate candidates should be based on prognostic indicators and the risk the patient is willing to assume." In the absence of good prospective studies, this statement appropriately leaves the issue with the patient and the physician.

Fear of medicolegal liability because of the contraindication of estrogen in breast and endometrial cancer in the package insert requires that physicians document a lengthy discussion of the risks and benefits and have the patient actively participate in the decision and understand the process of informed consent needed for this therapy.

Hormonal Therapy for Breast Cancer Survivors

Women diagnosed with breast cancer are faced with many challenging decisions, especially if they are premenopausal. They are asked to review their family history to determine if they may have developed breast cancer because of a genetic predisposition (*BRCA1* or *BRCA2* gene) transmitting risk of familial breast and ovarian cancer. Genetic counseling and testing may then be recommended to properly counsel the patient and her family members about the benefits and risks of prophylactic mastectomy and bilateral salpingo-oophorectomy. This places premenopausal breast cancer patients in the unique position of being asked to undergo surgery to remove their ovaries to prevent ovarian cancer, when they may be told they cannot take estrogen replacement for the menopausal symptoms that will occur postoperatively. Appropriate estrogen or testosterone replacement (or both) after premenopausal oophorectomy is not condoned in this population by oncologists. The challenges to the patient's emotional well-being while facing a life-threatening illness with new menopausal symptoms, sexual dysfunction, and potential problems with her marriage all at the same time, are overwhelming. The benefits to bilateral salpingo-oophorectomy in a *BRCA1* or *BRCA2* carrier are the potential reduction in risk of breast cancer recurrence, as well as the 90% risk reduction from ovarian cancer. If symptom control from the surgery was feasible, this would be a great benefit. The risks of estrogen and androgen withdrawal can be decreased libido, lubrication, hot flashes, insomnia, and depression, and some women conclude that the benefit is not worth the risk. For this reason, the age at which prophylactic oophorectomy should be planned is not known in genetic carriers and must be individualized. Some allow patients a reversible trial period of Depo-Lupron to simulate menopause to help them with this decision-making process.

The treatment of breast cancer may consist of tamoxifen, aromatase inhibitors, local radiation, and chemotherapy. Some argue that the purpose of the chemotherapy is to destroy ovarian function. Oophorectomy may be able to replace the benefit of chemotherapy, but this has not yet been adequately scientifically compared. Women are also eligible for treatment with aromatase inhibitors if they are menopausal, which has demonstrated a 43% reduction in breast cancer recurrence after completion of 5 years of tamoxifen.

There is increasing concern for the long-term morbidity of the standard breast cancer therapies, which are poorly captured in research trials. Women report cognitive function impairment from chemotherapy, as well as fatigue, weight gain, osteoporosis, and sexual dysfunction. Further study is required in this area to determine prevention strategies, including bone density testing frequency, calcium and vitamin supplementations, benefits of bisphosphonates, bone density monitoring, and prevention of cognitive dysfunction and sexual dysfunction.

The use of tamoxifen for the treatment or prevention of breast cancer has many known consequences, including thromboembolic disease, strokes, and endometrial cancer. The expected annual rate of endometrial cancer in breast cancer patients is 1 per 1000. Patients taking tamoxifen have an excess risk of 2 per 1000 or a total risk of 3 per 1000 per year. Studies on the appropriate monitoring of women on tamoxifen have demonstrated that transvaginal ultrasonography and routine annual endometrial biopsies increase a woman's risk. The current recommendation is to "do no harm" by conducting a routine annual gynecologic examination with cervical cytology and inquire about symptoms such as bleeding or discharge.

For many years, it has been stated that ERT in patients who have had breast cancer is absolutely contraindicated, yet the data are inconsistent in substantiating this admonition. During the past couple of decades, there has been increasing evidence that ERT can protect against osteoporosis and colon cancer, and recent data suggest benefits in the prevention of Alzheimer disease, macular degeneration, and tooth loss. Because the benefits of ERT are substantial and no data are available to note detrimental effect in patients with breast disease, these authors firmly believe that a reappraisal of the admonition against ERT in patients with breast cancer is needed. Historically, it has been the dictum that women who have had breast cancer should not, under any circumstances, receive ERT. When one looks in the literature for data to support this recommendation, there is a huge void. In 1989, Wile and DiSaia suggested that in the absence of prospective study of ERT in breast cancer survivors, one could analyze situations when these patients were exposed to high levels of estrogens at a time when they may have been harboring breast cancer cells. These situations were defined as pregnancy coexistent with breast cancer, pregnancy subsequent to breast cancer, breast cancer in previous and current users of oral contraceptives, and breast cancer in women receiving ERT. After extensive evaluation of these situations, there appears to be very little, if any, relationship. A total of 234,190 new cases of breast cancer were projected to be diagnosed in the United States in 2015. More and more of these individuals fortunately are surviving their cancer; in many, long-term survival of more

than 90% of these patients can be expected. Because many will survive their cancer, they will experience old age. We must address the advisability of HRT in this setting.

In fact, some data suggest that ERT in breast cancer patients is not deleterious. Historically, we must remember that before cytotoxic agents, postmenopausal women with metastatic or recurrent cancer received estrogen as a first line of therapy. We now understand that its effectiveness depended to a certain extent on the receptor status of the cancer. At least seven prospective, randomized double-blind studies have compared estrogen with tamoxifen in patients with recurrent or metastatic breast cancer. The response rate of estrogen and tamoxifen is essentially the same. In prospective randomized studies comparing estrogen and tamoxifen as adjuvant therapy, the recurrence rate was essentially the same. It appears that we have a very short medical history memory.

At least six retrospective studies have evaluated HRT in women with breast cancer. These patients were recurrence free at the time, and they were given estrogen to combat vasomotor symptoms or to prevent the chronic illness of cardiovascular disease, osteoporosis, and colon cancer. In this selected group of more than 500 patients, there have been 30 (6%) recurrences and only seven (1%) deaths. In the authors' study of 145 patients in which patients with in situ, stage I to IV cancer were treated, there have been 13 (9%) recurrences. Patients with both node-positive and node-negative disease were treated. Of the 96 node-negative patients, 11 recurred, but only one of 34 node-positive patients to date has had a recurrence. Recurrence was noted in 1 of 15 patients in whom the lymph nodes were not pathologically evaluated. It appears that evaluation of the receptor status in patients who had this performed did not have an impact one way or the other with regard to recurrences (Table 4.6).

In addition, there have been three case-controlled studies and three cohort-type studies (Table 4.7) in which recurrences and deaths were similar in both the patients in the ERT and control groups. A cohort study of 125 patients with breast cancer who received HRT after cancer therapy were compared with 362 patients with breast cancer who did not receive HRT. Patients were matched for stage, age, and year of diagnosis. All stages were included, although 78% had carcinoma in situ (CIS) (14%) or stage I and II cancers. There was a survival advantage for HRT users compared with non-HRT users with

TABLE 4.6 Hormone Replacement Therapy in Women With Breast Cancer

Author	Recurrence (%)	Deaths (%)
Stoll	0/65 (0)	0
Powles	2/35 (8)	0
Sellin	1/49 (2)	0
Bluming	12/189 (6)	1 (1)
Brewster et al.	13/145 (9)	3 (2)
Natrajan	2/50 (4)	3 (6)
Totals number from the 6 noted studies	30/533 (6)	7 (1)

TABLE 4.7 Hormone Replacement Therapy Following Breast Cancer

	Recurrence		Deaths	
	ERT (%)	Controls (%)	ERT (%)	Controls (%)
CASE CONTROLLED				
Wile and DiSaia	1/25 (4)	2/50 (4)	1 (4)	2 (4)
DiSaia et al.	6/41 (14)	7/82 (8)	2 (5)	6 (7)
Eden et al.	6/90 (7)	30/108 (17)	0	11
COHORT				
Dew et al.	?/167	/1472	2 (1)	167 (13)
Espie et al.	5/120	/240	*	*

*No difference in disease-free survival.
ERT, Estrogen replacement therapy.

an odds ratio of 0.28 (CI 0.11–0.71). Six endometrial cancers were subsequently diagnosed in the patients who took HRT.

In 1997, two randomized clinical trials were started in Sweden to assess the risks of HRT after a diagnosis of breast cancer. Interestingly, these similarly designed trials in a homogenous population of Swedish women arrived at different conclusions. The HABITS (Hormonal Replacement Therapy After Breast Cancer—Is It Safe?) trial was designed as a randomized, non-placebo noninferiority study to compare combined estrogen–progesterone treatment for menopausal symptoms with best management without HRT in women previously treated for stage 0 to 2 breast cancer. Patients were treated for 2 years and then asked to stop treatment. After a median follow-up of 4 years, there was an increased risk of a new breast cancer event in the HRT group compared with the group without HRT with a relative hazard of 3.5 (CI 1.5–8.1). Of 219 patients in the HRT group, 26 new breast cancer events were noted. In the no HRT group, there were eight new breast cancer events in 215 women. This corresponds to an absolute difference of 14% in the cumulative incidence of a new breast cancer event at 5 years. Based on these findings at the interim analysis, the decision was made that HRT represented an unacceptable risk for women with a history of breast cancer, and the trial was terminated in 2003.

The Stockholm trial was a randomized open study in postmenopausal women with a history of breast cancer randomized to receive HRT with a cyclic estrogen–progesterone regimen for 5 years (n = 188) or no HRT (n = 190). In contrast to the HABITS trial, the Stockholm trial found that the risk of breast cancer recurrence was not associated with the use of HRT in patients with early stage breast cancer with a risk hazard of 0.82

(CI 0.35–1.9). Despite these findings, the Stockholm steering committee prematurely closed this trial based on considerations related to patient safety and difficulty recruiting patients in light of the HABITS results. It is unclear why these two similarly designed studies arrived at different conclusions, but with significant heterogeneity between the two studies (P = 0.02), it is unlikely that this can be explained by chance alone. It should be noted that the proportion of lymph-node positive patients was higher in the HABITS trial compared with the Stockholm trial (26% vs. 16%, respectively). Furthermore, only 21% of patients in the HABITS trial received adjuvant tamoxifen therapy compared with 52% of patients in the Stockholm trial. The distinctions in these clinical characteristics may have contributed to the differences in results of the two studies.

In conclusion, the risk of recurrent breast cancer in postmenopausal women receiving ERT is unclear. In postmenopausal women with previously treated breast cancer, consideration of ERT is an option but must be reviewed with caution. In other words, there must be informed consent. Women are interested in information for which they can make informed decisions. To not even discuss replacement therapy with these individuals is not in their best interest. In the United States today, more than 36,000 women who are younger than 50 years of age will develop breast cancer. Most, if not all, will go on cytotoxic chemotherapy, and a significant number will become amenorrheic even though they are younger than 35 years of age. Unfortunately, if amenorrhea occurs while they are on chemotherapy, permanent ovarian failure occurs in the vast majority. Even in the very young (younger than 40 years of age), 86% will have ovarian failure. We therefore are seeing an increasing number of young women who are going through chemotherapeutic-induced premature menopause. A significant number of these women will be cured of their breast cancer; however, because of the premature menopause, they may have significant vasomotor symptoms that are much greater than those expected with natural menopause. Long-term benefits of replacement therapy may even be greater because of the premature menopause. These patients should be made aware of the rationale for replacement (ie, the benefits and risks) so that intelligent decisions can be made. Breast cancer patients may be the ideal candidates for the vaginal slow-release forms of estradiol rings. Estring contains a very low dose of estradiol, which can successfully treat vaginal atrophy symptoms and only increase plasma estradiol levels to one tenth the amount of a 0.05 Estraderm patch. If menopausal symptoms remain intolerable, Femring has a higher estradiol dose of 0.05 mg/day and may provide some relief of symptoms as well.

For the bibliography list, log onto www.expertconsult.com ⟨http://www.expertconsult.com⟩

5

Adenocarcinoma of the Uterine Corpus

William T. Creasman, MD, David Scott Miller, MD, FACOG, FACS

KEY POINTS

1. Adenocarcinoma of the endometrium is the most common gynecologic malignancy and is increasing in incidence. The mortality rate form this disease is also increasing.
2. Classically, endometrial cancer is divided into two histologic types: type I is endometrioid, and type II is consists of uterine papillary serous carcinoma (UPSC), clear cell (CC), and other more aggressive histologic types.
3. The mainstay of treatment is surgery with removal of the uterus tubes and ovaries with staging.
4. Adjuvant therapy is often given. Radiation or chemotherapy is used depending on the clinical scenario.
5. Endometrial cancer is commonly inherited through a DNA mismatch repair defect, which is known as Lynch syndrome. All patients with endometrial cancer should be evaluated for this possibility.

INCIDENCE

In the United States, cancer of the uterine corpus is the most common malignancy unique to women. It was estimated by the American Cancer Society that uterine cancer will develop in approximately 60,050 women in 2016 in the United States, making it the fourth most common cancer in women. The increased incidence of carcinoma of the endometrium has been apparent only during the past 3 decades. In reviewing the predicted incidence for the 1970s, the American Cancer Society noted a 1.5-fold increase in the number of patients with endometrial cancer; however, there was a decline in incidence during the late 1980s. In the past several years, the incidence has remained constant. During the period of increased incidence, predicted deaths from this malignant neoplasm actually decreased slightly. More recently, deaths from uterine cancer have increased. In 1990, the American Cancer Society estimated 4000 deaths from this cancer, increasing to 10,470 in 2016. An estimation of the most common new cancers and the percentage of female deaths for 2009 in the United States is shown in Fig. 5.1. The increased use of estrogen has been implicated in the apparent increased incidence during the 1970s and early 1980s; however, Norway and Czechoslovakia report a 50% to 60% increase, respectively, in endometrial cancer even though estrogens are rarely prescribed or are not generally available there. However, the increasing prevalence of overweight and obesity in women, especially in developed countries, may account for this apparent increase. Regardless of the reason for the increased number of women with corpus cancer, this malignant neoplasm has become an important factor in the care of the female patient.

EPIDEMIOLOGY

Endometrial adenocarcinoma occurs during the reproductive and menopausal years. The mean age for patients with adenocarcinoma of the uterine corpus is 63 years; most patients are between the ages of 50 and 59 years (Fig. 5.2). Approximately 5% of women will have adenocarcinoma before the age of 40 years, and **20% to 25% will be diagnosed before menopause.** Bokhman suggested that there are two pathogenic types of endometrial cancer. **The first type arises in women with obesity, hyperlipidemia, and signs of hyperestrogenism, such as anovulatory uterine bleeding, infertility, late onset of menopause, and hyperplasia of the stroma of the ovaries and endometrium. The second pathogenic type of disease arises in women who have none of these disease states or in whom**

FIGURE 5.1 Common new cancer cases and deaths in women for 2010 in the United States. (Modified from American Cancer Society. *Cancer Facts and Figs. 2010.* Atlanta, 2010, American Cancer Society.)

FIGURE 5.2 Carcinoma of the corpus uteri; patients treated in 1999 to 2001. Age distribution by mode of staging. (Modified from Creasman WT, Odicino F, Maisonneuve P, et al. Carcinoma of the corpus uteri. FIGO 26th Annual Report on the Results of Treatment in Gynecological Cancer. *Int J Gynecol Obstet* 95(1):S105-S143, 2006.)

TABLE 5.1	Endometrial Cancer Risk Factors
Risk Factors	**Risk**
Obesity	2.5–4.5×
Nulliparity	
Compared with one child	2×
Compared with five or more children	3×
Late menopause	2.4×

TABLE 5.2	Multiple Risk Factors	
Risk		
Nulliparous		Parous
Top 15% in weight	5× more than	Lower two thirds in weight
Menopause at 52 years		Menopause before 49 years

the disease states are not clearly defined. Bokhman's data suggest that patients with the first pathogenic type mainly have well-differentiated or moderately differentiated tumors, superficial invasion of the myometrium, high sensitivity to progestins, and a favorable prognosis (85% 5-year survival rate in his material). The patients who fall into the second pathogenic group tend to have poorly differentiated tumors, deep myometrial invasion, a high frequency of metastatic disease in the lymph nodes, decreased sensitivity to progestin, and poor prognosis (58% 5-year survival rate).

Multiple risk factors for endometrial cancer have been identified, and MacMahon divides them into three categories:

- Variants of normal anatomy or physiology
- Frank abnormality or disease
- Exposure to external carcinogens

Obesity, nulliparity, and late menopause are variants of normal anatomy or physiology classically associated with endometrial carcinoma. These three factors are evaluated in regard to the possible risk of developing endometrial cancer in Table 5.1. If a patient is nulliparous and obese and reaches menopause at age 52 years or older, she appears to have a fivefold increase in the risk of endometrial cancer above that of a patient who does not satisfy these criteria (Table 5.2).

The type of obesity in patients with endometrial cancer has been evaluated. In a study from the University of South Florida, **it was noted that women with endometrial cancer had greater waist-to-hip circumference ratios, abdomen-to-thigh skin ratios, and suprailiac-to-thigh skin ratios than those of** matched control women. As these ratios increased, the relative risk (RR) of endometrial cancer increased. The researchers concluded that upper-body fat localization is a significant risk factor for endometrial cancer. In a large multicenter case-control study of 403 endometrial cancer cases and 297 control cases, Swanson and associates confirmed and amplified these findings. Women whose weight exceeded 78 kg had a risk 2.3 times that of women weighing less than 58 kg. For women weighing more than 96 kg, the RR increased to 4.3. Upper-body obesity (waist-to-height ratio) was a risk factor independent of body weight. Patients in the highest quartile of both weight and waist-to-thigh circumference had a risk of 5.8 times. The amount of body fat has been associated with decreased circulating levels of both progesterone and sex hormone–binding proteins. There was a strong inverse association between sitting height and risk of endometrial cancer. This may be related to sex hormone–bound globulin (SHBG), which appears to be depressed in women with endometrial cancer. The level of SHBG is progressively depressed with increasing upper-body fat localization. With lower SHBG, there is a higher endogenous production of non–protein-bound estradiol. Because endometrial cancer is related to obesity, dietary habits appear to be important. Data suggest that the levels of estriol, total estrogens, and prolactin were lower and those of SHBG were higher in postmenopausal women who were vegetarians. In a case-control study, Levi and colleagues evaluated dietary factors in 274 patients with endometrial cancer and 572 control subjects from two areas in Switzerland and northern Italy. Extensive dietary history was obtained. Their data confirmed the relationship between obesity and endometrial cancer. In relation to diet, they noted an increased association with total energy intake. After correction for total energy intake, a risk was present with the frequency of consumption of most types of meats, eggs, beans, added fats, and sugar. **Conversely, significant protection was noted with an elevated intake of most vegetables, fresh fruits, whole grain bread, and pasta.** This reflected a low risk with increased intake of ascorbic acid and beta-carotene. Of dietary interest is that the intake of olive oil seemed beneficial in Switzerland but resembled other added fats in the Italian women. It has been previously noted that the amount and type of dietary fat influence estrogen metabolism because estrogen reabsorption from the bowel seems to be increased by diets rich in beef or fats.

Diabetes mellitus and hypertension are frequently associated with endometrial cancer. Elwood and colleagues reported an RR of 2.8 associated with a history of diabetes after controlling for age, body weight, and socioeconomic status. High levels of insulin-like growth factor I, coupled with elevated estrogen levels, are thought to have neoplastic potential that accounts for the observed increased risk of endometrial cancer. High blood pressure is prevalent in older obese patients but does not appear to be a significant factor by itself, even though 25% of patients with endometrial cancer have hypertension or arteriosclerotic heart disease.

As extensively detailed in Chapter 4, **the relationship of unopposed estrogen and endometrial cancer is well documented. Fortunately, the addition of a progestin appears to be protective. The adequacy of progesterone is important in prevention of endometrial cancer.** In a study from Sweden, at the end of 5 years, excess risk of endometrial cancer was 6.6, but with combined estrogen progestin (E + P), the RR was 1.6 for 11 to 15 days of progestin, 2.9 for 10 days of use, and 0.2 if continuous E + P was given. The Million Women study from the United Kingdom reported its findings of endometrial cancer and hormone replacement therapy (HRT). This study, which first reported on HRT and breast cancer, has been severely criticized mainly on methodology factors. The study had an average follow-up of 3.4 years, during which 1320 incident endometrial cancers were diagnosed. At time of recruitment, 22% of HRT users (total number was 320,953 women) last used continuous combined therapy, 45% last used cyclic combined therapy with progestogen usually added for 10 to 14 days per month, 19% last used tibolone, and 4% used estrogen alone. **Compared with nonusers, the RRs of endometrial cancer were 0.71, confidence interval (CI) 0.56 to 0.90, $P = 0.005$; 1.05, CI 0.91 to 1.22; 1.79, CI 1.43 to 2.25, $P <0.001$; and 1.45, CI 1.02 to 2.06, $P = 0.04$, respectively.** Of note, the adverse effects of tibolone and estrogen only were greatest in the nonobese women, and the beneficial effects of combined HRT were greatest in obese women. Although the risk of unopposed estrogen is present, women taking estrogen who develop endometrial cancer appear to have favorable prognostic factors. Several but not all studies suggest that risk factors such as multiparity and obesity are lower in the estrogen users. **Stage of disease and histologic grade appear to be lower in estrogen users.** With correction for stage and grade, estrogen users still have less myometrial invasion than nonestrogen users do. The poor prognostic subtypes, such as clear cell carcinoma and adenosquamous cancer, appear less frequently in estrogen users. As a result, **survival rates with estrogen-related endometrial cancer are much better than those of non–estrogen-related cancers.** In fact, some studies note just as good if not better survival in estrogen users than in women with nonestrogen, nonendometrial cancers.

Data indicate that the use of combination oral contraceptives decreases the risk for development of endometrial cancer. The Centers for Disease Control and Prevention evaluated endometrial cancer cases of all women aged 20 to 54 years from eight population-based cancer registries and compared them with control patients selected at random from the same centers. A comparison of the first 187 cases with 1320 control cases showed that **women who used oral contraceptives at some time had a 0.5 RR of developing endometrial cancer compared with women who had never used oral contraceptives.** This protection occurred in women who used oral contraceptives for at least 12 months, and **protection continued for at least 10 years after oral contraceptive use.** Protection was most notable for nulliparous women. **These investigators estimated that about 2000 cases of endometrial cancer are prevented each year in the United States by past or current use of oral contraceptives.** Of interest, cigarette smoking appears to decrease the risk for developing endometrial cancer. In a population-based case-control study of women aged 40 to 60 years, Lawrence and associates found a significant decline in RR of endometrial carcinoma with increased smoking ($P >0.05$).

The RR decreased by about 30% when one pack of cigarettes was smoked per day and by another 30% when more than one pack was smoked per day. The effects of smoking did not appear to vary with menstrual status or exogenous estrogen. There was a fourfold increase in smoking-related odds ratio with body weight; the greatest reduction in risk by smoking was in the heaviest women. However, the estimated risk increased 12-fold in overweight women who were nonsmokers and whose primary source of estrogen was peripheral conversion of androgen to estrogen. Although smoking apparently reduces the risk for development of early-stage endometrial cancer, this advantage is strongly outweighed by the increased risk of lung cancer and other major health hazards associated with cigarette smoking.

Incidence and survival are higher in white women compared with black women. Reasons for these differences are unexplained. An analysis of the Gynecologic Oncology Group (GOG) database evaluated this factor in 600 white and 91 black women with clinical stage I or stage II endometrial cancer. A larger number of the African American women were diagnosed after age 70 years, and they had a higher proportion of UPSC and clear cell histologic types; the black women also had more advanced disease, grade, vascular space involvement, depth of invasion, and lymph node metastases than the white women did. The survival rate (5-year) was 77% for white women and 60% for black women. Survival difference remained even in high-risk groups such as grade III tumors (59% vs. 37%, respectively). The unadjusted hazard rate was 2.0, which was statistically significant. With adjustment for age, cell type, and extent of disease, the RR dropped to 1.2. **The adjusted risk rate suggests that race is not a significant factor; nevertheless, race does denote an increased risk for poor prognostic factors, which clinically may be important.**

Tamoxifen is used to prevent or treat breast cancer. Tamoxifen was first introduced in clinical trials in the early 1970s and was approved in 1978 by the US Food and Drug Administration (FDA) for treatment of advanced breast carcinoma in postmenopausal woman. Tamoxifen, although labeled an antiestrogen, is known to have estrogenic properties and truly is a weak estrogen. Women receiving tamoxifen also appear to have some protection from osteoporosis and heart disease (decreased lactate dehydrogenase and cholesterol), similar to women receiving estrogen replacement therapy. Extensive experience with this drug has been reported. It is estimated that more than 4 million women in the United States have taken tamoxifen for almost 8 million women-years of use. One of its major benefits is that in women taking tamoxifen, there has been a substantial decrease in the incidence of a second cancer in the opposite breast compared with similar women who were taking a placebo.

The Early Breast Cancer Trialists Collaborative Group (EBCTCG) has produced an important meta-analysis of 194 randomized trials of adjuvant chemotherapy or endocrine therapy with at least 15 years of follow-up. The analysis evaluated the effects of adjuvant tamoxifen on breast cancer recurrence and survival. It was shown that 5 years of tamoxifen therapy, compared with no adjuvant therapy, reduced the 15-year probability of breast cancer recurrence (from 45% to

33%) and breast cancer mortality (from 35% to 26%). In addition, tamoxifen has been shown to provide a preventive benefit in women at risk for developing breast cancer.

There has been a considerable amount of discussion in the literature concerning the association of tamoxifen with endometrial cancer. At least three studies (Fisher and colleagues, Powels and colleagues, and Veronesi and colleagues) evaluating the prophylactic use of tamoxifen in women without breast cancer have reported an association between tamoxifen use and endometrial cancer. In addition, several cases of endometrial cancer have been described in women receiving tamoxifen. In a prospective, randomized study of the National Surgical Adjuvant Breast and Bowel Project (NSABP), 2843 patients with node-negative estrogen receptor–positive invasive breast cancer were randomly assigned to receive a placebo or 20 mg/day of tamoxifen. An additional 1220 tamoxifen-treated patients were registered and given the drug. The average time in the study was 8 years for the randomly assigned patients and 5 years for the registered patients. Of the 1419 patients randomly assigned to tamoxifen, 15 developed uterine cancer, of which two were sarcomas. One patient randomly assigned to receive tamoxifen did not take the drug and developed endometrial cancer 78 months after randomization. In the placebo group, two developed endometrial cancer; however, both were receiving tamoxifen at the time of their uterine malignant disease. One patient had a breast recurrence and was prescribed tamoxifen, and the other was given tamoxifen after colon cancer. Two of the patients with endometrial cancer had been taking tamoxifen for only 5 and 8 months before their diagnosis of uterine disease was made. Five patients in the tamoxifen group developed endometrial cancer after the drug had been discontinued for 7 to 73 months. In the registered patients who received tamoxifen, eight uterine tumors (seven endometrial) were subsequently diagnosed. Three of these patients had been taking tamoxifen for less than 1 year (2 months, 2 months, and 9 months). The authors determined the average annual hazards ratio (HR) of endometrial cancer per 1000 women in their population of patients. This was 0.2 per 1000 in the placebo group and 1.6 per 1000 for the randomized tamoxifen-treated patients. In the registered patients receiving tamoxifen, the average annual hazard rate was 1.4 per 1000, similar to that of the randomized tamoxifen-treated group. The hazard rate of endometrial cancer in the placebo group was low compared with the Surveillance, Epidemiology, and End Results (SEER) data and with previous NSABP randomized tamoxifen–placebo studies; these data suggest that the average annual hazard rate is 0.7 per 1000.

These data, based on a limited number of patients with endometrial cancer while receiving tamoxifen, suggest that there may be an RR of 2.3 for development of endometrial cancer while receiving tamoxifen. This does not take into account the well-known fact that women who develop breast cancer are at an increased risk for development of endometrial cancer irrespective of subsequent treatment. The RR of 1.72 to more than 3 has been reported. The risks and benefits of the prevention of recurrences and new breast cancer in comparison to new endometrial cancers were evaluated in the NSABP study. **The benefits suggest that 121 fewer breast-related events** per 1000 women treated with tamoxifen were seen compared with 6.3 endometrial cancers per 1000 women. Therefore, the benefit from tamoxifen is apparent.

It was initially suggested that the rate of endometrial cancers associated with tamoxifen use might be equal to that associated with unopposed estrogen replacement therapy. Because tamoxifen is a weak estrogen, similar characteristics of endometrial cancer were also implied (ie, well-differentiated superficially invasive cancers). Barakat and associates reviewed five studies, including the study by Magriples, the NSABP, their own data from Memorial Sloan-Kettering Hospital, and two studies from overseas. A total of 103 patients were evaluated in regard to histologic features, grade of tumor, International Federation of Gynecology and Obstetrics (FIGO) staging, and deaths from uterine cancer; an increase was not found in poor prognostic histologic findings, tumor differentiation, or stage compared with what would be expected in a similar group of non–tamoxifen-treated patients with uterine cancer. Jordan, in an evaluation of the SEER data and of tamoxifen-associated endometrial cancer in the literature, reported similar findings.

It is suggested that all women, irrespective of whether they are taking tamoxifen, should have yearly gynecologic examinations. The endometrium should be evaluated if the patient is symptomatic. We concur with the American College of Obstetricians and Gynecologists (ACOG) committee opinion that does not recommend endometrial sampling or ultrasound evaluation of the endometrium just because an individual is taking tamoxifen. This possible concern of tamoxifen and endometrial cancer may lessen in the near future because the aromatase inhibitors (AIs) may appear to be better than tamoxifen in the prevention of recurrent or contralateral breast cancer. Several clinical trials have demonstrated the comparable if not greater efficacy of AIs compared with tamoxifen. Although tamoxifen remains an option for adjuvant therapy for postmenopausal women, AIs are thought to be more effective in preventing breast cancer recurrence in the first 2 years after surgery. AIs reduce estrogen levels in postmenopausal women by inhibiting or inactivating aromatase, the enzyme that synthesizes estrogens from circulating androgens. AIs should be avoided in premenopausal women, including those who have experienced chemotherapy-induced amenorrhea. Whereas tamoxifen is a partial agonist, AIs are not agonists and are not associated with estrogenic-related thromboembolic events and uterine cancers. The activity of third-generation agents anastrozole, letrozole, and exemestane is generally considered comparable. Although AIs are associated with a significant risk of osteoporosis, they do not increase the risk of gynecologic problems. In one large adjuvant therapy trial (the Anastrozole, Tamoxifen Alone or in Combination Trial [ATAC]), anastrozole was associated with fewer cerebrovascular events (2.0% vs. 2.8%), endometrial cancers (0.2% vs. 0.8%), thromboembolism (3% vs. 4%), hot flashes (41% vs. 36%), and vaginal bleeding (5% vs. 10%) compared with tamoxifen. The role of AIs as prophylaxis is being investigated, but data are lacking at the present time.

Although most cases of endometrial cancer are sporadic, hereditary endometrial cancer has been identified in association with hereditary nonpolyposis colon cancer (HNPCC), also known as Lynch II syndrome. This is an autosomal-dominant inherited cancer that involves a germline mutation in one of the genes in the DNA mismatch repair gene family, which includes *MSH2, MLM1*, and *MSH6*. Fortunately, HNPCC accounts for only 1% to 5% of all colorectal cancers but it is associated with a 39% to 54% lifetime risk of developing colon cancer. There is a lifetime risk of 30% to 61% of developing endometrial cancer in those with HNPCC. There is also an increased risk of ovarian cancers and other nongynecologic cancers. In a study by Lu and associates, they noted that about half the time, the endometrial or ovarian cancer appeared before the colon cancer. In both instances, the age at diagnosis was in the early 40s. There was a median of 11 years between the gynecologic cancer and the colon cancer. About 14% of the time, the gynecologic and colon cancers were diagnosed simultaneously. Several "red flags" should prompt an evaluation for HNPCC. These include any individual with a personal or family history of colon cancer at an early age of onset (usually before age 50 years) or endometrial cancer at an early age of onset (premenopausal or before age 50 years) and two or more HNPCC-related cancers in an individual or family. Assessing a patient's risk for hereditary cancer is an important process, beginning with screening for the "red flags" of hereditary colon (and endometrial) cancer. Individuals with any of the "red flags" should enter into a discussion about genetic testing to determine if this is appropriate for them. Medical management strategies can be tailored depending on the genetic testing results and may include increased surveillance, chemoprevention, and prophylactic surgery. The Cancer Study Consortium suggests colonoscopy every 1 to 3 years beginning at age 25 years in individuals with this hereditary disorder. The data suggest that if surveillance is done, survival rates are improved. Women should be offered surveillance with ultrasound and endometrial sampling from age 25 to 35 years, although there are no data to suggest this will improve survival if endometrial cancer is diagnosed by these means. As reported by Schmeler and colleagues, risk-reducing surgery consisting of removal of the uterus and bilateral ovaries has been shown to decrease the risk of uterine and ovarian cancer in these high-risk patients.

DIAGNOSIS

Routine screening for uterine adenocarcinoma and its precursors is not recommended. Women receiving HRT (estrogen and progesterone) do not need endometrial biopsy before institution of therapy or during replacement therapy unless abnormal bleeding occurs. Monthly withdrawal bleeding after progestin is not considered abnormal bleeding. However, break through bleeding should be evaluated. The use of continuous estrogen alone increases the risk of adenocarcinoma. Estrogen plus progesterone appears to decrease the risk of adenocarcinoma and therefore is the preferred treatment. In asymptomatic high-risk patients, periodic screening may be advisable. All postmenopausal women with uterine bleeding must be evaluated for endometrial cancer, although only 20% of these patients will have a malignant genital neoplasm. As the patient's age increases after menopause, there is a progressively increasing

probability that her uterine bleeding is caused by endometrial cancer. Feldman and associates found that age was the greatest independent risk factor associated with endometrial cancer or complex hyperplasia. In women aged 70 years or older, the odds ratio was 9.1. If complex hyperplasia was present, the odds ratio increased to 16. When a woman was older than 70 years, her chance of having cancer when vaginal bleeding was present was about 50%. If she was also nulliparous and had diabetes, the risk was 87%. A perimenopausal patient who may have abnormal uterine bleeding indicative of endometrial cancer is frequently not evaluated because the patient or her physician interprets her new bleeding pattern as resulting from menopause. **During this time in a woman's life, the menstrual periods should become lighter and lighter and farther and farther apart.** Any other bleeding pattern should be evaluated with carcinoma of the endometrium in mind. A high index of suspicion must be maintained if the diagnosis of endometrial cancer is to be made in a young patient. Prolonged and heavy menstrual periods and intermenstrual spotting may indicate cancer, and endometrial sampling is advised. Most young patients who develop endometrial cancer are obese, in many instances massively overweight, often with anovulatory menstrual cycles.

Historically, fractional dilation and curettage (D&C) has been the definitive diagnostic procedure used in ruling out endometrial cancer. **Today, most advocate the routine use of the endometrial biopsy as an office procedure to make a definitive diagnosis and spare the patient hospitalization and an anesthetic.** Several studies have indicated that the accuracy of the endometrial biopsy in detecting endometrial cancer is approximately 90%. Cytologic detection of endometrial cancer by routine cervical Papanicolaou (Pap) smear has generally been poor in comparison with the efficacy of the Pap smear in diagnosing early cervical neoplasia. Several studies in the literature indicate that only one-third to half of the patients with adenocarcinoma of the endometrium have abnormal Pap smear results on routine cervical screening. The main reason for the poor detection with the cervical Pap smear is that cells are not removed directly from the lesion. When a cytologic preparation is obtained directly from the endometrial cavity, malignant cells are present in higher numbers than those found if routine cervical or vaginal smears are obtained. Techniques that obtain only a cytologic preparation are generally inadequate if they are used alone.

Several commercial apparatuses are available for sampling the endometrial cavity on an outpatient basis. If diagnosis of endometrial cancer can be made on an outpatient basis, the patient can avoid hospitalization and a minor surgical procedure. Devices that remove tissue for histologic evaluation have generally been good if tissue is obtained from the endometrial cavity. Stovall and colleagues used the Pipelle instrument to evaluate 40 patients known to have endometrial cancer. Ninety percent of the women were postmenopausal. Only in one patient was cancer not identified with the Pipelle. This patient had a prior D&C that revealed a grade I lesion. The Pipelle diagnosis was atypical adenomatous hyperplasia, and the hysterectomy specimen revealed a focus of adenocarcinoma in situ.

The pathologist noted that the obtainable tissue was acceptable for analysis in 100% of patients. Discomfort was recorded as mild in 80%, and only two patients (5%) reported severe pain. Goldchmit and coworkers reported similar accuracy with the Pipelle in 176 consecutive patients undergoing D&C. Whereas endometrial biopsy and D&C appear to be equivalent in terms of diagnosing cancer, the accuracy of endometrial biopsy appears to be inferior to D&C in predicting final posthysterectomy tumor grade. In a recent study by Leitao and colleagues, 18% of endometrial biopsy specimens were upgraded on final hysterectomy specimen, but only 9% of D&C specimens were upgraded. In symptomatic patients in whom inadequate tissue (or no tissue at all) is obtained for pathologic evaluation, a D&C must be considered.

Hysteroscopy has been suggested as adjuvant in making the diagnosis of endometrial cancer and in establishing the extent of disease. Hysteroscopy has been used frequently in the evaluation of patients with abnormal uterine bleeding and has the advantages of allowing the physician to see the pathologic lesion and direct biopsy, identify other competing diagnoses (fibroids, polyps), and perform the procedure on an outpatient basis. Clark and colleagues analyzed data from 65 primary studies on the use of hysteroscopy to diagnose endometrial cancer and endometrial disease (cancer, hyperplasia, or both), including more than 26,000 women. All of the patients had abnormal premenopausal or postmenopausal uterine bleeding. Using endometrial histologic findings as a reference, a positive hysteroscopy result was associated with a 72% probability of endometrial cancer, but a negative result reduced this probability to 0.6%. The corresponding probabilities for endometrial disease were 55% with a positive result and 3% with a negative result. The accuracy of hysteroscopy tended to be higher among postmenopausal women and in an outpatient setting. They concluded that hysteroscopy is highly accurate and thereby clinically useful in diagnosing endometrial cancer in women with abnormal uterine bleeding and is moderately useful in diagnosing endometrial disease. Because many patients with endometrial cancer can be diagnosed with office biopsy, that is our preferred first diagnostic step. If the biopsy result is negative and further evaluation is needed, we proceed to hysteroscopy. With its use, surgeons can direct biopsies of focal lesions that might be missed by D&C. Hysteroscopy can also be used to evaluate the endocervical canal.

Ultrasonography has been suggested as a diagnostic tool in evaluating women with irregular bleeding, particularly postmenopausal patients (Fig. 5.3). The endometrial stripe as seen with transvaginal ultrasonography appears to be indicative of endometrial thickness. Several studies suggest that if a thin endometrial stripe is present, a histologic diagnosis is not necessary because atrophic endometrium would be present. Granberg and associates evaluated 205 women with postmenopausal bleeding, 30 postmenopausal asymptomatic women, and 30 postmenopausal patients with known endometrial cancer. In the two groups of 60 patients, the endometrial thickness was 3.2 (mean) versus 17.7, respectively. In the group of 205 women, 18 were found to have endometrial cancer. No cancers were present in the endometrium that had an endometrial thickness

FIGURE 5.3 A, Ultrasound image of the uterus showing the "triple line" indicating the thickness of the endometrium. B, Ultrasound of the uterus showing a "thickened endometrium" of more than 10 mm. C, Saline instillation of the endometrial cavity notes a well-defined submucous fibroid and not thickened endometrium.

of 8 mm or less. There was considerable overlap of endometrial thickness by all histologic groups. The authors noted that if a cutoff of 5 mm was used, no false-negative findings were present. With this measurement, the positive predictive value was 87%, with specificity of 96% and sensitivity of 100% for identifying endometrial abnormalities. It has been suggested that if ultrasonography could save a large number of

endometrial biopsies, there would be a large cost savings with less discomfort to the patient. As previously noted, significant pain with the newer disposable endometrial biopsy techniques affects only a small number of patients, and a certain number of patients, because of considerable endometrial thickness, will require endometrial sampling anyway. Clark and colleagues investigated the cost-effectiveness of initial diagnostic strategies for postmenopausal bleeding. A decision analytic model was constructed to reflect current service provision, which evaluated 12 diagnostic strategies using endometrial biopsy, ultrasonography (4- and 5-mm endometrial thickness cutoff), and hysteroscopy. Diagnostic probability estimates were derived from systematic quantitative reviews, clinical outcomes from published literature, and cost estimates from local and National Health Service sources. The main outcome measure was the cost per additional life year gained (£/LYG). Compared with carrying out no initial investigation, a strategy based on initial diagnosis with ultrasonography using a 5-mm cutoff was the least expensive (£11 470/LYG). Initial investigation with endometrial biopsy or ultrasonography using a 4-mm cutoff was comparably cost-effective (<£30,000/LYG vs. ultrasonography with a 5-mm cutoff). The strategies involving initial evaluation with test combinations or hysteroscopy alone were not cost-effective. They concluded that women presenting for the first time with postmenopausal bleeding should undergo initial evaluation with ultrasonography or endometrial biopsy.

Unfortunately, endometrial cancer has been identified when the endometrial thickness is less than 5 mm. Although studies may evaluate several hundred patients, most do not have many cancer patients included. Wang and associates reviewed the ultrasounds of 52 women who were diagnosed with UPSC, clear cell and other high-grade carcinomas. Of the 52, 34 (65%) had a thickened endometrium measuring 5 mm or more; in nine (17%) the endometrium was less than 5 mm, and in an additional nine women (17%) the endometrium was indistinct. In the women with a nonthickened endometrium, other ultrasound abnormalities were noted: intracavitary fluid or lesion, myometrial mass, enlarged uterus, or adnexal mass. **Multiple factors can affect endometrial thickness. These include estrogen use, E + P use, body mass index (BMI), diabetes, poor histotype, race, and postmenopausal status.** The Committee on Gynecologic Practice of the ACOG issued an opinion on the role of transvaginal ultrasonography in the evaluation of postmenopausal bleeding. They concluded that women with postmenopausal bleeding may be assessed initially with either endometrial biopsy or transvaginal ultrasonography. This initial evaluation does not require performance of both tests. Transvaginal ultrasonography can be useful in the triage of patients in whom endometrial sampling was performed but tissue was insufficient for diagnosis. When transvaginal ultrasonography is performed for patients with postmenopausal bleeding and an endometrial thickness of less than or equal to 4 mm is found, endometrial sampling is not required. Meaningful assessment of the endometrium by ultrasonography is not possible in all patients. In such cases, alternative assessment should be completed. When bleeding persists despite negative initial evaluations, additional assessment is indicated.

The reliability determining endometrial thickness in postmenopausal patients does not appear to be applicable to women taking tamoxifen. **In all studies, the endometrium in a tamoxifen-treated patient is considerably thicker than in a non–tamoxifen-treated patient.** Histologic evaluation revealed an atrophic endometrium in a large number of these tamoxifen-treated patients. Lahti and colleagues evaluated 103

asymptomatic postmenopausal patients (51 receiving tamoxifen and 52 control participants) with ultrasonography, hysteroscopy, and endometrial histologic examination. In the tamoxifen group, 84% had an endometrial thickness on ultrasonography of 5 mm or more versus 19% in the non-tamoxifen group (51% vs. 8% >10 mm, respectively). Hysteroscopy findings noted that 28% of uterine mucosa was atrophic versus 87% in the non-tamoxifen control group. Histopathologic examination noted atrophic endometrium in 60% of tamoxifen-treated patients versus 79% of control subjects. **The biggest difference between the two groups was the finding of polyps in 18% of the tamoxifen group versus 0% of the control group; this appears to be a frequent finding in the tamoxifen-treated patient.** So-called megapolyps measuring up to 12 cm have been described. Other uterine diseases have been attributed to tamoxifen, including increased uterine volume, lower impedance to blood flow in uterine arteries, endometriosis, focal periglandular condensation of stromal cells, and epithelial metaplasia. Data now suggest that the markedly thickened endometrium (≤40 mm) in patients receiving tamoxifen is not thickened endometrium but proximal myometrium.

Ultrasonography has also been evaluated as a means for determining depth of myometrial invasion. Gordon and associates studied 15 known patients with endometrial cancer by ultrasonography and magnetic resonance imaging (MRI). By use of criteria of greater than 50% myometrial wall involvement as deep invasion and less than 50% as superficial invasion, ultrasonography was judged to be more accurate than MRI in five studies; MRI was better in three, both were equally accurate in four, and neither was accurate in three. It has been suggested by some that ultrasonography can accurately predict myometrial invasion in about 75% of cases. Although knowing the depth of invasion preoperatively would be important information to the clinician, the data from studies as noted before would currently appear to be too premature or too costly to use routinely. **We prefer to evaluate depth of myometrial invasion intraoperatively with gross examination or frozen section.**

Pathology

Careful evaluation of the uterus by the pathologist is essential for proper diagnosis and treatment of corpus cancer (Fig. 5.4). Gross inspection of a bivalved uterus at the time of hysterectomy can offer an impression of the size of the lesion, its location (involvement of fundus, lower uterine segment, or cervix), and the depth of tumor penetration into the myometrium (depth of invasion). A clinically enlarged uterus may be caused by increasing tumor volume, but this should not be the only gauge for significant local disease. Obviously, many patients can have enlarged uteri because of factors other than adenocarcinoma. Carcinoma of the endometrium may start as a focal discrete lesion, as in an endometrial polyp. It may also be diffuse in several different areas, in some situations involving the entire endometrial surface. As the tumor grows, it can become larger or spread within the endometrium or myometrium. Endometrial cancer may disseminate to regional lymph nodes, by embolization or direct extension into the pelvis or vagina, or hematogenously to distant organs (Fig. 5.5). The risk of spread

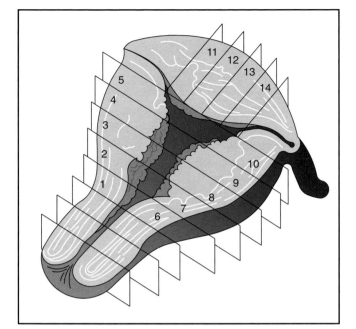

FIGURE 5.4 Pathologic evaluation of endometrial cancer. (Courtesy of Paul Underwood, MD.)

is related to several factors, including depth of invasion into the myometrium, tumor grade, and histologic type.

Adenocarcinoma, the most common histologic type, is usually preceded by a predisposing lesion, atypical endometrial hyperplasia (Table 5.3). Only hyperplasias with cellular atypia are considered precursors of adenocarcinoma of the endometrium. For most patients with endometrioid-type tumors, particularly grade I or II lesions, and hyperplasia, hyperestrogenism is the etiologic basis. Pathologically, endometrial cancer is characterized by the presence of glands in an abnormal relationship to each other, with the hallmark of little,

TABLE 5.3 Endometrial Carcinoma Subtypes	
Type	**Number (%)**
Endometrioid	6231 (84)
Adenosquamous	317 (4.2)
Mucinous	74 (0.9)
Uterine papillary serous	335 (4.5)
Clear cell	185 (2.5)
Squamous cell	28 (0.04)
Other	285 (3.8)

From Creasman WT, Odicino F, Maisonneuve P, et al. Carcinoma of the corpus uteri. *Int J Gynecol Obstet.* 2003 Oct;83 Suppl 1:79-118. No abstract available.

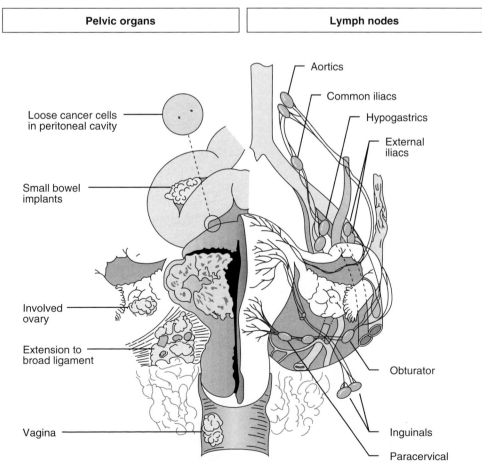

FIGURE 5.5 Spread pattern of endometrial cancer with particular emphasis on potential lymph node spread. Pelvic and periaortic nodes are at risk, even in stage I disease.

if any, intervening stroma between the glands. There can be variations in the size of the glands, and infolding is common. The cells are usually enlarged, as are the nuclei, along with nuclear chromatin clumping and nucleolar enlargement. Mitosis may be frequent. Differentiation of adenocarcinoma (mild, moderate, and severe, or grades I–III) is important prognostically and is incorporated into FIGO surgical staging (Fig. 5.6). Most studies suggest that 60% to 65% of all endometrial cancers are of this subtype.

FIGURE 5.6 Histologic patterns of differentiation in endometrial carcinoma. **A,** Well-differentiated (G1). **B,** Moderately differentiated (G2). **C,** Poorly differentiated (G3). (Courtesy of Gregory Spiegel, MD.)

For almost a century, it has been recognized that a squamous component may be associated with an adenocarcinoma of the endometrium. This occurs in about 25% of patients. Historically, patients with a squamous component were further stratified according to whether the squamous component appeared benign (designated adenoacanthoma [AA]) or malignant (designated adenosquamous carcinoma [AS]). It was suggested that AA indicated a good prognosis and those with AS had a poor survival. Today, this distinction has been questioned concerning its prognostic importance. **Zaino and coworkers, in reporting data from the GOG, suggest that the notation of squamous component irrespective of differentiation does not affect survival.** Patients with clinical stage I and stage II cancers were evaluated, and 456 with typical adenocarcinoma (AC) and 175 with squamous differentiation (AC + SQ) were identified. The latter were subdivided into 99 with AA and 69 with AS. Multiple known prognostic factors were compared with differentiation of glandular and squamous component of the tumor. Age, depth of myometrial invasion, architecture, nuclear grade, and combined grade were similar for AC and AC + SQ, although patients with AA were better differentiated than those with AS and had less myometrial invasion. Both glandular and squamous differentiation correlated with frequency of pelvic and paraaortic node metastasis. Nodal metastasis, when it was stratified for grade and depth of invasion, was similar in AC and AC + SQ patients. **The differentiation of squamous component is closely correlated with the differentiation of the glandular element, and the glandular element is a better predictor of outcome.** It would therefore appear that the previous designation of AA and AS has no added predictive property than differentiation of glandular component and probably should be dropped as a diagnostic term. **The authors suggest the term** *squamous differentiation* **instead, with differentiation of the glandular component noted as the important prognostic factor.** Subsequently, Abeler and Kjorstad reviewed 255 cases and made the same recommendations.

Secretory adenocarcinoma (Fig. 5.7) is an uncommon type of endometrial cancer. It usually represents well-differentiated carcinoma with progestational changes. It is difficult to differentiate it from secretory endometrium. Survival is good and comparable to that associated with the pure adenocarcinoma. Although it is an interesting histologic variant, the separation of the entity as it relates to treatment and survival is probably not warranted.

Increasing emphasis has been placed on the importance of the **histologic subtype serous adenocarcinoma of the uterus, known as uterine papillary serous carcinoma (UPSC). This subtype represents fewer than 10% of all adenocarcinomas but is a highly aggressive carcinoma of the uterus.** Unlike the more common variants, UPSC is not associated with hyperestrogenism and frequently develops in the setting of atrophic endometrium. **It is more commonly seen in older and nonwhite patients. Hendrickson, in the early 1980s, noted that in more than 250 endometrial cancers, only 10% had histologic features of UPSC, but these accounted for 50% of all treatment failures.** The histopathologic appearance resembles a high-grade serous carcinoma of the ovary that has a

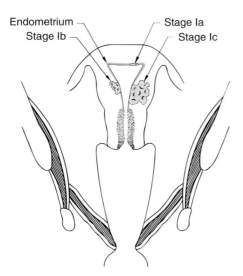

Stage Ia: Tumor limited to endometrium
Stage Ib: Invasion to less than half the myometrium
Stage Ic: Invasion to more than half the myometrium

Stage I

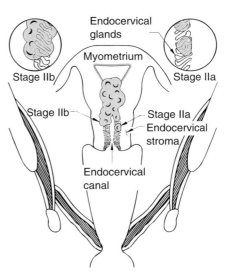

Stage IIa: Endocervical glandular involvement only
Stage IIb: Cervical stroma invasion

Stage II

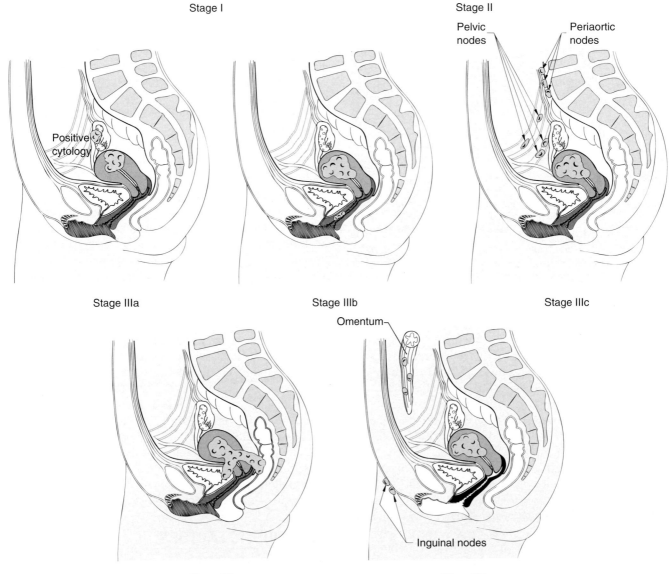

Stage IIIa

Stage IIIb

Stage IIIc

Stage IVa

Stage IVb

FIGURE 5.7 High-power view of well-differentiated secretory carcinoma invading the inner third of the myometrium. (Courtesy of William M. Christopherson, MD, Louisville, KY.)

FIGURE 5.9 Clear cell carcinoma of the endometrium. Clear cell component is quite evident. (Courtesy of Gregory Spiegel, MD.)

FIGURE 5.8 Serous adenocarcinoma. The similarity to ovarian carcinoma is apparent. (Courtesy of Gregory Spiegel, MD.)

propensity for vascular or lymphatic vascular space involvement (LVSI). Well-formed papillae are lined by neoplastic cells with grade III cytologic features (Fig. 5.8). Differentiation between papillary architecture and syncytial metaplasia with benign endometrial alterations must be made because **the papillary architecture alone does not designate UPSC.** The uterus may appear grossly normal but can have extensive myometrial invasion. Most UPSC tumors are aneuploid and have a high S-phase, and can be pure or admixed with other histologic types (endometrioid, clear cell, carcinosarcoma).

Clear cell carcinomas (Fig. 5.9) are also infrequent in number but have distinct histologic criteria. Clear cell tumors are characterized by large polyhedral epithelial cells that may be admixed with typical non–clear cell adenocarcinomas. Some authorities accept the mesonephritic-type hobnail cells as part of this pattern, but others believe that this histologic type should be excluded from the clear cell category. Silverberg and DeGiorgi and Kurman and Scully suggested a worse prognosis for clear cell adenocarcinoma than for pure adenocarcinoma. This was

confirmed in studies by Christopherson and coworkers. Even in stage I disease, only 44% of patients with clear cell carcinomas survive 5 years. Neither the FIGO classification nor nuclear grade correlates with survival. Photopulos and associates, in a review of their material, noted that their patients with this entity were older and tended to have a worse prognosis. They did note that patients with stage I clear cell carcinomas had a 5-year survival rate similar to that of patients with stage I pure adenocarcinoma of the endometrium.

Tumor Grade

In addition to histologic type, pathologists assign a measure of tumor differentiation, known as grade, to endometrial cancers. Grade I lesions are well differentiated, are frequently associated with estrogen excess, closely resemble hyperplastic endometrium, and are generally associated with a favorable prognosis. Grade III lesions are poorly differentiated, do not resemble normal endometrium, and frequently have a poorer prognosis. Grade II tumors are moderately well differentiated and have an intermediate prognosis. Both architectural criteria and nuclear grade are used to classify. Architectural grade is related to the proportion of solid tumor growth, with grade I having an adenocarcinoma in which less than 5% of the tumor growth is in solid sheets, grade II having 6% to 50% of the neoplasm arranged in solid sheets of neoplastic cells, and grade III having greater than 50% of the neoplastic cells in solid masses. Regions of squamous differentiation are excluded from this assessment. The FIGO rules for grading state that notable nuclear atypia, inappropriate for architectural grade, raises the grade of a grade I or grade II tumor by one. By convention, serous and clear tumors are considered grade III or high-grade tumors.

PROGNOSTIC FACTORS

After hysterectomy and lymph node dissection, clinical-pathologic characteristics are commonly used to predict risk of recurrence and to optimize therapy. Multiple factors have been

TABLE 5.4 Prognostic Factors in Endometrial Adenocarcinoma

Histologic type (pathology)
Histologic differentiation
Stage of disease
Myometrial invasion
Peritoneal cytology
Lymph node metastasis
Adnexal metastasis

TABLE 5.5 2009 International Federation of Gynecology and Obstetrics Staging System for Carcinoma of the Endometrium

Stage I*		Tumor Contained to the Corpus Uteri
	Ia	No or less than half myometrial invasion
	Ib	Invasion equal to or more than half of the myometrium
Stage II		Tumor invades the cervical stroma but does not extend beyond the uterus[†]
Stage III*		Local and/or regional spread of tumor[‡]
	IIIa	Tumor invades the serosa of the corpus uteri and/or adnexa
	IIIb	Vaginal and/or parametrial involvement
	IIIc	Metastases to pelvis and/or paraaortic lymph nodes
	IIICI	Positive pelvic nodes
	IIIC2	Positive paraaortic lymph nodes with or without positive pelvic lymph nodes
Stage IV*		Tumor invades bladder and/or bowel mucosa and/or distant metastases
	IVa	Tumor invasion of bladder and/or bowel mucosa
	IVb	Distant metastases, including intraabdominal metastases and/or inguinal lymph nodes

*Includes grades 1, 2, or 3.
†Endocervical glandular involvement only should be considered as stage I and no longer as stage II.
‡Positive cytology has to be reported separately without changing the stage.

TABLE 5.6 5-Year Survival in Endometrial Cancer: Surgical Stage

Stage	Patients (n)	5-Year Survival (%)
Ia	1063	91
Ib	2735	90
Ic	1219	81
IIa	364	79
IIb	426	71
IIIa	484	60
IIIb	73	30
IIIc	293	52
IVa	47	15
IVb	160	17

From Pecorelli S, ed. FIGO Annual Report, years 1996–98. *Int J Gynecol Obstet* 2003;83:95.

TABLE 5.7 Distribution of Endometrial Carcinoma by Stage (Surgical)

Stage	Patients (%)
I	3839 (73)
II	574 (11)
III	694 (13)
IV	166 (3)

From Pecorelli S, ed. *J Epidemiol Biostat* 2001;6:47.

identified for endometrial carcinoma that has prognostic value (Table 5.4). Essentially all reports in the literature agree stage (extent of disease spread), grade of tumor, and depth of invasion are important prognostic considerations. Before 1988, endometrial cancer was clinically staged with stage assignments based on uterine size and clinical extent of disease. Because of the considerable discrepancy between the clinical extent of disease spread and pathologic spread noted after surgical staging, FIGO adopted a surgical-pathologic staging classification in 1988. In 2009, FIGO updated the staging system (Table 5.5). FIGO staging classification attempts to categorize patients into prognostic groups based on extent of disease and tumor grade.

Stage of Disease: Depth of Invasion, Cervical Involvement, Adnexal Involvement, and Nodal Metastasis

Staging of patients with malignancies is designed to have prognostic value by classifying the size and extent of tumor. The survival rate in regard to stage of disease has been consistent,

and Table 5.6 and Fig. 5.10 show the 5-year survival rate reported by FIGO (FIGO 1988 staging). The patterns of disease spread in endometrial cancer was evaluated in a prospective study performed by the GOG (GOG protocol 33) and reported by Creasman. This study is required reading for physicians who care for patients with endometrial cancer. GOG protocol 33 was a surgical-pathologic study of 621 patients with clinical stage I endometrial cancer who were uniformly treated with total abdominal hysterectomy (TAH), bilateral salpingo-oophorectomy (BSO), peritoneal cytologic evaluation, and selective pelvic and paraaortic selected lymphadenectomy. Before this study, it was presumed most patients with endometrial cancer were at risk for nodal metastases, and nearly all patients required some form of pelvic radiation therapy (either preoperatively or postoperatively). The study demonstrated important relationships between pathologic factors and risk of nodal disease. For example, factors associated with nodal disease included higher tumor grade, deeper myometrial invasion, cervical involvement, (+) cytology, and LVSI. Because of this study, FIGO accepted a surgical-based staging system, including lymphadenectomy, of endometrial cancer in 1988.

For endometrial cancer, FIGO staging reflects the progression of disease within the uterus and at extrauterine sites. Approximately 75% of patients with endometrial cancer present with disease limited to the uterus (Table 5.7). For stage I disease, depth of tumor invasion into the myometrium is an important prognostic factor. **The degree of myometrial invasion is a consistent indicator of tumor virulence** (Fig. 5.11). DiSaia and

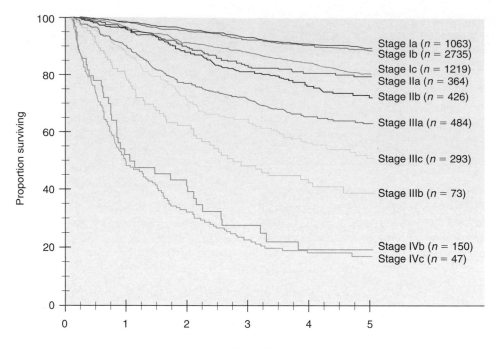

FIGURE 5.10 Carcinoma of the corpus uteri for patients treated in 1990 to 1992 (International Federation of Gynecology and Obstetrics). Survival by surgical stage (*n* = 5694). (From Pecorelli S, ed. FIGO Annual Report, years 1996–98. *Int J Gynecol Obstet* 2003;83:95. © International Federation of Gynecology and Obstetrics.)

Myometrial invasion

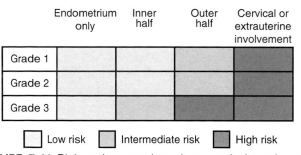

FIGURE 5.11 Risk assignment based on surgical staging and extent of disease in patients with endometrial cancer.

TABLE 5.8 Relationship Between Depth of Myometrial Invasion and Recurrence in Patients With Stage I Endometrial Carcinoma

Endometrial only	7/92 (8%)
Superficial myometrium	10/80 (13%)
Medium myometrium	2/17 (12%)
Deep myometrium	15/33 (46%)

Modified from DiSaia PJ, Creasman WT, Boronow RC, Blessing JA. Risk factors in recurrent patterns in stage I endometrial carcinoma. *Am J Obstet Gynecol* 1985;151:1009.

TABLE 5.9 Relationship Between Depth of Myometrial Invasion and 5-Year Survival Rate (Stage I)

Stage	Patients	5-Year Survival (%)
IaG1	698	93
IbG1	1030	88
IcG1	442	87
IaG2	229	91
IbG2	1307	93
IcG2	485	84
IaG3	66	75
IbG3	280	82
IcG3	247	66

From Pecorelli S, ed. FIGO Annual Report, years 1996–98. *Int J Gynecol Obstet* 2003;83:95.

associates noted that recurrences were directly related to depth of myometrial invasion in patients with stage I cancer treated primarily with surgery (Table 5.8). The Annual Report of FIGO demonstrated a decrease in the survival rate as myometrial penetration increased (Table 5.9). Lutz and coworkers determined that the depth of myometrial penetration was not as important as the proximity of the invading tumor to the uterine serosa. Patients whose tumors invaded to within 5 mm of the serosa had a 65% 5-year survival rate, but patients whose tumors were more than 10 mm from the serosa had a 97% survival rate. The depth of myometrial invasion is associated with the other prognostic factors, such as the grade of the tumor. As noted by DiSaia and associates, the survival rate of patients with poorly differentiated lesions and deep myometrial invasion is poor in contrast to that of patients who have well-differentiated lesions but no myometrial invasion. This suggests that virulence of the tumor may vary considerably, and as a result, therapy should depend on the combination of prognostic factors.

Location of the tumor within the endometrial cavity is important because tumors low in the cavity may involve the cervix earlier than fundal lesions. The prognosis for women with cervical involvement (stage II) is worse than with stage I disease. Cervical involvement is often a surrogate marker for extrauterine disease spread or for risk of local recurrence. Data from GOG 33 showed that those with disease of the lower uterine segment had a higher incidence of pelvic lymph node metastases (16%) than do those with only fundal disease (8%). There is a similar frequency of paraaortic nodal metastases: a 16% incidence from disease of the lower uterine segment and a 4% incidence when only fundal disease is present. Previously, endocervical curettage (ECC) was commonly used to determine whether the patient had cervical involvement. Many false-positive results occur with this technique, however. In addition, the prognostic significance of endocervical glandular spread (formerly stage IIa) has been challenged. The new surgical staging adopted by FIGO in 2009 includes only patients with cervical stromal invasion in the stage II category. In some cases, cervical biopsy or ECC is required in the pretreatment planning of a patient with suspected cervical involvement.

Patients with stage III or IV disease may have a heterogeneous mix of disease characteristics. It is well recognized that endometrial cancer can and frequently does metastasize to the adnexa. Patients with adnexal or serosal involvement are categorized as having stage IIIA disease and are considered to have a higher risk of peritoneal recurrence. In GOG 33, 5% of patients had adnexal involvement. Adnexal metastasis was significantly associated with involved pelvic (32%) and paraaortic (20%) lymph nodes. In a large surgical trial comparing laparoscopy with open staging (GOG Lap 2 trial), 5% of 2616 patients enrolled were found to have stage IIIA disease (FIGO 1988 staging). In an analysis of 222 patients with clinical stage I carcinoma of the endometrium reported by DiSaia and colleagues, 16 (7%) were found to have metastasis in the adnexa. This finding correlated with many but not all of the other prognostic factors. Spread to the adnexa did not seem to be related to the size of the uterus. The grade of the disease did not appear prognostically important in regard to this in that 6% of patients with grade I tumors had adnexal disease compared with only 10% if poorly differentiated carcinoma was present. The depth of invasion did appear to be significant, however, in that only 4% of patients with only the endometrium involved had adnexal spread compared with 24% who had adnexal metastases if deep muscle was involved. If tumor was limited to the fundus of the uterus, only 5% of patients had disease in the adnexa; however, if the lower uterine segment or the endocervix was involved, one-third had spread to the adnexa. When metastasis was present in the adnexa, 60% of patients had malignant cells in the peritoneal cytologic fluid compared with only 11% if the adnexa were not involved. Recurrences appeared in only 14% of these individuals who did not have metastasis to the adnexa compared with recurrences in 38% of patients with adnexal metastasis.

Metastatic spread to lymph nodes (stage IIIC) has prognostic and therapeutic implications. It is clear that lymphadenectomy, to date, is the most sensitive way to identify nodal disease. The

TABLE 5.10 Grade vs. Positive Pelvic and Aortic Nodes

Grade (n)	Pelvic Nodes (%)	Aortic Nodes (%)
G1 (180)	5 (3)	3 (2)
G2 (288)	25 (9)	14 (5)
G3 (153)	28 (18)	17 (11)

Modified from Creasman WT, Morrow CP, Bundy BN, et al. Surgical pathologic spread patterns of endometrial cancer: a Gynecologic Oncology Group study. *Cancer* 1987;60:2035.

TABLE 5.11 Maximal Invasion and Node Metastasis

Maximal Invasion (n)	Pelvic Nodes (%)	Aortic Nodes (%)
Endometrium only (87)	1 (1)	1 (1)
Superficial muscle (279)	15 (5)	8 (3)
Intermediate muscle (116)	7 (6)	1 (1)
Deep muscle (139)	35 (25)	24 (17)

Modified from Creasman WT, Morrow CP, Bundy BN, et al. Surgical pathologic spread patterns of endometrial cancer: a Gynecologic Oncology Group study. *Cancer* 1987;60:2035.

GOG 33 study demonstrated that as the depth of tumor invasion or tumor grade increased, the frequency of pelvic and paraaortic nodal metastases also increased (Tables 5.10 and 5.11). For all 621 patients, 58 (9%) had positive pelvic nodes, and 34 (6%) had positive paraaortic nodes. Patients with grade 1, 2, and 3 tumors had pelvic nodal metastases of 3%, 9%, and 18% respectively. Similarly, patients with no myometrial invasion, inner one-third, middle one-third, and outer one-third invasion had 1%, 5%, 6%, and 25% pelvic nodal disease, respectively. The highest risk group included patients with grade III tumors and outer one-third invasion who had pelvic nodal involvement in 34% of cases (Table 5.12). Without a lymphadenectomy, one may grossly estimate the probability of nodal involvement based on these data to select for or against the use of adjuvant therapy. This strategy potentially results in undertreatment or overtreatment of patients, however. In two large prospective randomized trials, routine lymphadenectomy resulted in the identification of more patients with nodal disease (9%–13%) compared with when only clinically suspicious nodes were removed (1%–3%). It is clear that patients with nodal disease have a poorer prognosis (3- to 5-year survival rate of 50%–75%) and different patterns of failure (nodal, distant) than patients with negative nodes (3- to 5-year survival rate of 80%–95%, vaginal cuff failures predominate). Patients with nodal involvement include those with pelvic nodal disease (IIIC1) or any paraaortic involvement (IIIC2). The substaging was created in 2009 given the belief of different outcomes associated with different levels of nodal involvement. The number of involved nodes and the extent of resection of grossly involved nodes also affect outcome. In addition, Mariani and McMeekin have suggested that patients with positive nodal

TABLE 5.12 Frequency of Pelvic and Paraaortic Nodal Disease*

Depth of Invasion	Grade		
	Grade I (n = 180)	Grade II (n = 288)	Grade III (n = 153)
Endometrium only (n = 86)	0%/0%	3%/3%	0%/0%
Inner third (n = 281)	3%/1%	5%/4%	9%/4%
Middle third (n = 115)	0%/5%	9%/0%	4%/0%
Outer third (n = 139)	11%/6%	19%/14%	34%/23%

*Pelvic nodal positivity/paraaortic nodal positivity.
Modified from Creasman WT, Morrow CP, Bundy BN, et al. Surgical pathologic spread patterns of endometrial cancer: a Gynecologic Oncology Group study. *Cancer* 1987;60:2035.

TABLE 5.13 Relationship Between Tumor Differentiation and 5-Year Survival Rate, Stage I (Surgical)

Grade	Survival (n = 5017) (%)
1	91
2	90
3	81

From Pecorelli S, ed. FIGO Annual Report, years 1996–98. *Int J Gynecol Obstet* 2003;83:95.

TABLE 5.14 Correlation of Differentiation and Myometrial Invasion in Stage I Cancer

Myometrial Invasion	Grade		
	1 (%)	2 (%)	3 (%)
None	24	11	11
Superficial	53	45	35
Mid	12	24	16
Deep	10	20	42

Modified from Creasman WT, Morrow CP, Bundy BN, et al. Surgical pathologic spread patterns of endometrial cancer: a Gynecologic Oncology Group study. *Cancer* 1987;60:2035.

disease plus other stage III defining features (positive cytology, adnexal or serosal involvement) have a much poorer prognosis than those with nodal disease only. Patients with stage IV or distant disease spread (intraperitoneal, lung, liver) have a particularly poor prognosis, with 5-year survival rate of less than 20%. The extent of surgical resection has been suggested to alter the prognosis in patients with advanced-stage disease. As with ovarian cancer, the extent of resection of disease reflects the biology of the tumor, aggressiveness of the surgery, and response to postoperative therapies.

Tumor Grade

The degree of histologic differentiation (tumor grade) of endometrial cancer is a sensitive indicator of prognosis and is included in FIGO stage assignment. The Annual Report on the Results of Treatment in Gynecological Cancer has evaluated survival in regard to grade in patients with clinical stage I adenocarcinoma of the endometrium (Table 5.13). Tumor grade is inversely related to survival decreases; as grade increases, survival is poorer. In their review of 244 patients with stage I disease, Genest and colleagues noted that patients with grade I disease had a 5-year survival rate of 96%. This dropped to 79% and 70% for grade II and grade III, respectively. Data presented by Morrow for outcomes in patients enrolled on GOG 33 show that recurrence-free survival markedly diminishes with increasing grade, with progression-free survival (PFS) at 48 months being approximately 95%, 85%, and 68% for grade I, II, and III tumors, respectively. Grade of tumor also correlates with other factors of prognosis. Table 5.14 shows the relationship between differentiation of the tumor and depth of myometrial invasion as reported by Creasman from the GOG 33 study. As the tumor

becomes less differentiated, the chances of deep myometrial involvement increase. However, exceptions can occur: Patients with a well-differentiated lesion can have deep myometrial invasion, but patients with a poorly differentiated malignant neoplasm might have only endometrial or superficial myometrial involvement.

Lymphovascular Space Involvement

Hanson and colleagues described 111 patients with stage I endometrial cancer and found capillary-like space (CLS) involvement in 16. This was most frequently found in patients with poorly differentiated tumors with deep invasion. These patients had a 44% recurrence rate compared with 2% if the CLS was not involved. This was an independently significant prognostic factor. In the GOG study of 621 patients, it was shown that 93 (15%) had CLS involvement. **The incidences of pelvic and paraaortic node metastases were 27% and 19%, respectively.** This compares with a 7% occurrence of pelvic node metastasis and a 3% occurrence of paraaortic node metastasis when there is no CLS involvement. In risk models predicting risk of recurrence in node-negative, early-stage endometrial cancer, the GOG has suggested that LVSI is an important risk factor. In the Post-Operative Radiation Therapy in Endometrial Cancer (PORTEC) trial, LVSI was considered a factor associated with distant site of failure.

Tumor Size

Schink and coworkers evaluated tumor size in 91 patients with stage I disease. The incidence of lymph node metastases in patients with tumor size less than 2 cm was only 6%. If the tumor was larger than 2 cm in diameter, there were nodal metastases of 21% and up to 40% if the entire endometrium was involved. Patients with lesions greater than 2 cm in size and less than half myometrial invasion had no nodal metastasis. Using multivariate analysis, the authors showed that tumor size was an independently significant prognostic factor. Watanabe and associates did not find cancer size was predictive of lymph node metastasis. Gynecologic oncologists from the Mayo Clinic have developed a risk model predicting nodal metastases and have suggested that grade I and II tumors that are smaller than 2 cm are particularly low risk for nodal disease.

Peritoneal Cytology

The importance of peritoneal cytology in endometrial cancer is controversial. In GOG 33, 76 (12%) had malignant cells identified by cytologic examination of peritoneal washings. Of these patients, 25% had positive pelvic nodes compared with 7% of patients in whom no malignant cells were found in peritoneal cytologic specimens ($P > 0.0001$). It is true that peritoneal cytology, to a certain degree, mimics other known prognostic factors—that is, if peritoneal cytologic specimens are positive, other known poor prognostic factors may also be identified. In addition, data from GOG 33 also suggested that the RR for recurrence with positive cytology was 2.4 ($P = 0.02$).

Given the relationship of positive cytology with other known risk factors, it is important to evaluate data sets coming from patients who undergo complete surgical staging. Saga and colleagues reported on a series of 307 (32 with positive cytology, 275 with negative cytology) patients with endometrioid-type cancer, all who underwent complete staging and had negative lymph nodes. The authors reported that 5-year survival rate was 87% with positive cytology compared with 97% with negative cytology. Most patients with positive cytology received chemotherapy postoperatively. Havrilesky et al. reported on experience from Duke University. Patients with positive cytology alone ($n = 37$) were compared with patients with adnexal or serosal involvement ($n = 20$). The 5-year survival rate was similar between the groups (62% positive cytology, 68% adnexal or serosal disease), but in a multivariable analysis, cytology was an independent predictor of recurrence and poorer survival. This study included patients with nonendometrioid histologies, and lymphadenectomy was not routinely performed. In another review of the literature, Wethington demonstrated that in endometrioid-type tumors with low risk factors (superficial invasion, grade I or II); the recurrence rate was only 4%. By comparison, 32% of patients with higher grade tumors or deeper invasion and positive cytology had a recurrence. These results suggest that for at least a subset of cytology patients, the risk of recurrence approximates that driven by other uterine factors (depth of invasion, tumor grade). In 2009, FIGO dropped cytology as a stage IIIA defining characteristic.

Milosevic and colleagues reviewed 17 studies. In 3820 patients, the prevalence of positive cytologic findings was 11%. **The three largest studies totaling more than 1700 patients (Haroung and associates, Turner and colleagues, Morrow and coworkers) using multivariate analysis noted that the finding of malignant cells on cytologic examination was independently significantly associated with either recurrence or reduced survival.** Pooled odds ratio for the entire series was 4.7 (CI, 3.5–6.3) for disease recurrence. All studies note the highest correlation of malignant cytologic specimens with extrauterine disease. **It does appear that with multivariate analysis, the presence of malignant cells is an important prognostic factor even when disease is limited to the uterus.**

Optimal therapy has not been determined to date. Historically, intraperitoneal ^{32}P or oral progestins have been used to manage disease in patients with positive cytology. Today, uterine risk factors are largely used to define postoperative adjuvant therapy independent of cytology status and, increasingly, in otherwise low-risk patients (endometrioid-type tumors, negative nodes), observation is often considered. Chemotherapy has also been used in the adjuvant setting for patients with positive cytology.

Molecular Indices

Hormone receptors. Historically, estrogen and progesterone receptors were the first "targets" describing the molecular biology of endometrial cancer. Using multivariate analysis to analyze hormone receptor status, Creasman and associates noted that in stage I and stage II cancers, progesterone receptor–positive status was a highly significant, independently prognostic factor in endometrial cancer. Without progesterone receptor status in the model and with the evaluation of estrogen receptor status in its stead, estrogen receptor–positive status was an independent prognostic factor but not to the degree of progesterone receptor–positive status. Hormone receptor status may closely mirror grade, however.

Today there is an explosion of research into the molecular makeup of endometrial cancer. Cytogenetic studies have described gross chromosomal alterations, including changes in the number of copies of specific chromosome. The extent of abnormalities in a given tumor is relatively low. About 80% have normal diploid DNA content. Aneuploidy in 20% is usually associated with high-grade, extrauterine disease, high-risk histotypes, and poor prognosis. So-called loss of heterozygosity occurs at a relatively low frequency compared with other solid tumors. When chromosomal loss of heterozygosity does occur, underlying molecular genetic defects have been observed on 17p and 10q that correlate with mutational inactivation of *TP53* and *PTEN*, respectively. **Individual tumors with a greater number of gains and losses are associated with a poorer prognosis, and some changes seen in cancer are also present in atypical hyperplasia but not simple hyperplasia lesions.**

Mutational activation or aberrant expression of some oncogenes has been described but to a lesser degree than tumor suppressor genes. The *RAS* gene family is the most commonly identified oncogene aberration in human cancers and is present in 10% to 30% of endometrial cancers. This mutation appears to occur early in the neoplastic process, and the incidence is the same in endometrial hyperplasia. Correlation of *RAS* mutation to survival has produced conflicting results. About 10% to 15% of endometrial cancer has overexpression of ERBB-2

(HER2/neu) protein. **Overexpression appears to be confined to high-grade or advanced-stage tumors.**

The *FMS* oncogene encodes a tyrosine kinase, which serves as a receptor for macrophage colony-stimulating factor (m-CSF). Expression of *FMS* correlates with advanced-stage, high-grade, and deep myometrial invasion. Expression of *C-MTC,* which has been observed in normal endometrium and endometriosis, has a higher expression in secretory endometrium. Several studies suggest amplification is present in a fraction of endometrial cancers.

Mutation of TP53 tumor suppressor gene, the most common genetic abnormality currently recognized in human cancers, is present in 10% to 30% of endometrial cancers. Overexpression or mutation (or both) is associated with prognostic factors. In a study of more than 100 endometrial hyperplasia specimens, TP53 mutation was not present. PTEN mutation analysis in endometrial cancer indicates that this gene is somatically inactivated in 30% to 50% of all tumors, the most frequent molecular genetic alteration defined in endometrial cancer. There does appear to be a correlation between microsatellite instability and PTEN mutation. PTEN mutation is observed in 20% of endometrial hyperplasias, suggesting that this is an early event in the development of some type I endometrial cancers.

Inherited mutations in gene encoding DNA mismatched repair proteins, primarily MSH2 and MLM1, are responsible for HNPCC, for which endometrial cancer is the second most common cancer in women with these mutations. Cancers in these individuals are characterized by frame shift mutations in multiple microsatellite repeat sequences throughout the genome. This instability is also seen in 20% of sporadic endometrial cancers. In these sporadic cancers, acquired mutation in mismatched repair genes is rare. Endometrial cancers that exhibit microsatellite instability tend to be type I, which has a more favorable prognosis. This microsatellite instability is present in some cases of complex hyperplasia associated with endometrial cancer but is not seen in UPSC cancers.

Type I endometrial cancers are commonly described to include tumors seen in obese and nulliparous women, are well differentiated, are superficially invasive, and frequently carry a good prognosis. These tumors also share several common molecular changes and tend to have the following genetic features: diploid, low allelic imbalance, K-RAS, MLH1 methylation, and PTEN. In contrast, type II with poor prognostic pathologic features have aneuploid, high allelic imbalance, K-RAS, TP53, and HER2/neu changes.

Recently, array-based technology has allowed a more comprehensive characterization of endometrial cancers. It should be noted that these new technologies are in their infancy, although multiple papers using these techniques have been reported, many with DNA microassay. The effects of exogenous PTEN expression in endometrial carcinoma cell lines lacking PTEN function has been studied by Matsushima-Nishiu and associates. They observed increased expression in 99 genes and repression of 72 genes, many of which are known to be involved in cell proliferation, differentiation, and apoptosis, suggesting the potential power of expression profiling identifying molecular pathways affected by critical cancer-related genes. Proteomic profiling, which is the study of intact and fragmented proteins and their function, is being evaluated. Newer technologies allow the creating of proteomic fingerprints that reflect in serum what is happening in the end organs. The biochip is playing a major role in this evaluation. As little as 1 μL of serum can be evaluated, and this technology is very sensitive to low molecular weight protein regions. The results of The Cancer Genome Atlas (TCGA) Research Network has further improved our understanding of the molecular characteristics of endometrial cancer. They described four molecular subtypes, including (1) POLE (ultra-mutated) tumors, (2) microsatellite unstable tumors, (3) copy-number high tumors with mostly TP53 mutations, and (4) a remaining group without these alterations. For protocol 210, the GOG has collected material (tissue, serum, urine) on a large number of endometrial cancer patients stored in its tumor bank for in-depth research using these newer technologies, which will hopefully allow us to understand the malignant process.

Correlation of Multiple Prognostic Factors

The GOG 33 protocol identified the extent of disease spread identified at surgery correlated with outcomes. Although single factors were associated with recurrence, the combination of factors could also establish risk. For example, Morrow showed that patients with no risk factors (LVSI, cervical involvement, adnexal involvement, nodal disease) had a very low risk of recurrence, but 20% with one, 43% with two, and 63% with three or more factors recurred. In multivariate analysis, patients with disease limited to the uterus were at increased risk for recurrence if there were deep myometrial invasion, vascular space involvement, or positive washings. Fig. 5.11 is the author's attempt to compartmentalize these risk factors into risk categories for predicting prognosis and guiding decisions for adjuvant therapy. The lines between categories are somewhat porous, consistent with most clinical situations.

Data from three randomized trials evaluating the use of postoperative pelvic radiation therapy have been useful in shaping models predicting risk of recurrence after surgery. Aalders identified a subset of the 95 of 540 (18%) patients enrolled in a randomized trial of vaginal cuff brachytherapy with or without pelvic radiation therapy with grade III tumors and greater than 0% myometrial invasion to be particularly notable for risk of recurrence. Patients with these factors had a pelvic recurrence rate of 20% with vaginal brachytherapy alone compared with 5% with the combination of pelvic and vaginal radiation. It is interesting that approximately 15% of patients with these tumor characteristics failed at a distant site, regardless of radiation technique. The PORTEC trial compared pelvic radiation therapy with observation after hysterectomy without lymph node dissection in patients with endometrial cancer. In this trial of 714 patients, a subset of patients with grade III tumors (10%), age older than 60 years (72%), or greater than 50% depth of invasion (59%) was identified in which having two of three factors defined a high-risk group. The locoregional failure rate was 23% in this group who underwent surgery followed by observation compared with 5% after pelvic radiation therapy. There was no difference in distant sites of recurrence

TABLE 5.15 High-Intermediate Risk Model: Early-Stage Endometrial Cancer

Age	Risk Factor
Any age + 3 factors	LVSI
≥50 years + 2 factors	Grade II or III tumor
≥70 years + 1 factor	Outer one-third invasion

LVSI, Lymphovascular space invasion.
Modified from Keys HM, Roberts JA, Brunetto VL, et al. A phase III trial of surgery with or without adjunctive external pelvic radiation therapy in intermediate risk endometrial adenocarcinoma: a Gynecologic Oncology Group study. *Gynecol Oncol* 2004;92:744-751.

FIGURE 5.12 Total abdominal hysterectomy and bilateral salpingo-oophorectomy showing large polypoid adenocarcinoma of the endometrium with deep myometrial invasion.

(~5% each group) or in cancer-related deaths (8% observation, 11% radiation). The GOG conducted a randomized trial (GOG 99) of observation versus pelvic radiation in a group of patients with surgically documented negative nodes and any amount of myometrial invasion. Depending on patient age and number of risk factors (LVSI, grade I or II tumor, outer one-third myometrial invasion) (Table 5.15), a high-intermediate (H-IR) risk group could be identified. The H-IR group accounted for one-third of all patients enrolled but two-thirds of recurrences. Perhaps equally important was the identification that two-thirds of the patients enrolled who did not have H-IR features had an incredibly low risk of recurrence (2%–3%), suggesting that in addition to defining high-risk groups, low-risk groups that may avoid postoperative adjuvant therapy may also be identified.

The value of risk models is that they can be applied to an individual patient incorporating all of the information (age, uterine characteristics) to provide a reasonable estimate of risk of recurrence and probability of benefit of selected adjuvant therapy. Research is under way to identify molecular markers that may augment clinical-pathologic information in establishing risk. Other cancer types (breast, prostate, bladder) have well-validated disease-specific nomograms predicting risk and benefit to adjuvant therapy. Similarly, developed and validated models for endometrial cancer are needed.

TREATMENT

Surgical Management of Endometrial Cancer

We prefer to sample the endometrium in symptomatic postmenopausal patients as the first diagnostic technique. **If histologic findings are "negative," the patient is observed. A D&C is done only if the patient continues to be symptomatic after the negative biopsy result.** After a tissue diagnosis of endometrial cancer is established, the patient should be assessed for surgical options of therapy. Most patients require routine blood counts (CBC), metabolic profile, and a metastatic evaluation with chest radiography. Routine use of computed tomography (CT) or MRI scans has not shown to be useful and should be reserved for unusual situations (high-risk tumor types, evidence of intraperitoneal disease, positive chest radiograph). Most patients with endometrial cancer are candidates for definitive surgery, including surgical staging (lymphadenectomy). Routes

of hysterectomy include vaginal, abdominal, laparoscopic (total or assisted), and robotic and have broadened the surgical options for patients.

The surgical evaluation of most patients with endometrial cancer requires a thorough inspection of the peritoneal cavity, collection of cytologic washings, and pelvic and paraaortic lymphadenectomy (PALA) in addition to hysterectomy. Cytologic evaluation of peritoneal fluids, or washings, has been a common surgical step in staging endometrial cancer because of associations with extrauterine disease and prognosis. After the peritoneal cavity is opened, an assessment of the amount of peritoneal fluid in the pelvis is made. If none is present, 100 to 125 mL of normal saline solution is injected into the pelvis. This can be done easily with a bulb syringe. The saline solution is admixed in the pelvis, withdrawn with the syringe, and sent for cytologic evaluation. We continue to recommend that peritoneal cytologic evaluation be performed in all patients undergoing surgery for endometrial cancer, although FIGO no longer uses cytology as a stage-defining characteristic. Omental biopsy may be considered in patients with gross spread to the omentum or adnexa or in cases with high-risk histologies such as serous or clear cell tumors. Approximately 10% of all patients will be found with nodal metastasis when surgically staged, but only 1% to 3% will be found to have nodal disease if nodes are evaluated only when clinically suspicious. In a large GOG study of 621 staged patients, 6% of patients with clinical stage I disease were noted to have intraperitoneal disease.

The definitive treatment for patients with endometrial cancer is hysterectomy. The hysterectomy should be extrafascial, and removal of the upper vagina does not appear to decrease vault recurrences (Fig. 5.12). Extirpation of the uterus removes the primary tumor and can provide important information that can be used to estimate risk of spread to lymph nodes or risk of recurrence. Removal of the adnexa is thought to be important given that approximately 5% of endometrial cancers have metastatic disease to the ovaries, fallopian tubes, or both.

In addition, synchronous ovarian and endometrial cancers are not infrequent, particularly in younger patients. Historically, total abdominal hysterectomy (TAH) and bilateral salpingo-oophorectomy (BSO) have been the hallmarks of therapy for endometrial cancer. There are no data to suggest that the route of hysterectomy influences recurrence-free or overall survival (OS) outcomes for patients; as such, the hysterectomy (abdominal, laparoscopic, and robotic) is the safest and facilitates rapid recovery and thus is suggested.

Several studies note the role of vaginal hysterectomy in highly selected patients with endometrial cancer for whom surgical staging cannot be performed safely (morbid obesity, significant cardiopulmonary medical comorbidities, advanced age). Because factors associated with the choice of vaginal hysterectomy (morbid obesity, medical comorbidities) are often associated with favorable uterine characteristics (low-grade lesions, smaller uterus), it is not surprising that survival rates are comparable to those of the abdominal approach. Chan and coworkers reviewed 51 medically compromised patients treated with vaginal hysterectomy and reported 3- and 5-year disease-specific survival rates of 91% and 88%, respectively. Of note, approximately 50% of women could not have the ovaries removed at the time of vaginal hysterectomy. Smith evaluated 63 patients with obesity or medical comorbidities and found that vaginal hysterectomy was safe and well tolerated in this patient population. Vaginal hysterectomy may represent a reasonable tradeoff for patients who may not tolerate other approaches or for whom surgical staging is not being considered (atypical hyperplasia, some patients with grade I cancers).

Over time, there has been a more widespread use of lymphadenectomy in the management of patients with endometrial cancer. Lymph node dissection provides the best estimate of spread of disease (vs. palpation or use of imaging studies), the lymph node status is prognostically important (as evident from the different survival rates seen with different stages of disease), and patients who are found to have positive or negative nodes receive different postoperative therapy vs. patients with unknown status of lymph nodes. In a joint statement by ACOG and the Society of Gynecologic Oncologists (SGO) in 2005, both organizations suggested that most women with endometrial cancer should undergo systematic surgical staging, including bilateral pelvic and PALA. Today, debate continues as to which patients (all, none, or some) benefit most from lymphadenectomy and the technique (pelvic, pelvic and paraaortic, level of paraaortic dissection) that should be performed.

The extent of the lymph node dissection is thought to be important. Early studies were conducted with selective lymphadenopathy or lymph node sampling (only visibly enlarged lymph nodes are selectively removed). Some data suggest that a true lymphadenectomy (complete skeletonization of vessels) should be performed. It seems intuitive that a sufficient number or distribution of nodes needs to be removed to represent an adequate sampling. When lymphadenectomy is done, the retroperitoneal spaces in the pelvis are opened in routine fashion. The vessels are outlined, and the lymph node–bearing tissue along the external iliacs from the bifurcation to the inguinal ligament is removed. The obturator fossa anterior to the

obturator nerve is cleaned of lymphoid tissue. Lymph nodes along the common iliacs are also removed. The left and right paraaortic nodes are approached by retracting the small intestine into the upper abdomen and incising the peritoneum over the upper common iliac artery and lower aorta. The main vessels are outlined, and the ureter is retracted laterally. On the right, the tissue overlying the vena cava and the aorta are removed en bloc, beginning at the bifurcation of the aorta and extending caudad. On the left, the left common nodes are frequently quite lateral. Using this technique, one should have a total of 20 to 30 pelvic and paraaortic lymph nodes available for histologic evaluation. The upper limit of the dissection (unless enlarged nodes are noted above this area) is usually the inferior mesenteric artery (IMA), but some surgeons suggest that the dissection should extend to the level of the renal vessels.

The extent of nodal dissection to include paraaortic nodes is also thought to be important in endometrial cancer. There appear to be two nodal drainage basins—pelvic and paraaortic. Studies indicate that when lymph nodes are positive, approximately 50% to 60% of the time paraaortic nodes are involved. In a retrospective study from the Mayo Clinic, 137 patients at high risk for nodal involvement who underwent PALA (PAL+) were compared with those who did not undergo surgical evaluation of the paraaortic nodes (PAL–). **The 5-year survival rate was 85% for PAL+ patients compared with 77% for PAL– patients. In 51 patients with pelvic or paraaortic node metastasis, survival was 77% for PAL+ patients compared with 42% in the PAL– group. It is generally thought that the rate of isolated paraaortic lymph node metastasis is less than 5%; metastasis isolated to the paraaortic lymph node and metastasis above the IMA are seen.** Mariani and colleagues reported on a study of 482 patients with endometrial cancer at the Mayo Clinic. A total of 281 underwent lymphadenectomy to the renal vessels, and 22% had positive lymph nodes; of these, 51% had both positive pelvic and paraaortic nodes, 33% had positive pelvic nodes only, and 16% had isolated involvement of the paraaortic nodes. Of note, 46% of those with isolated paraaortic lymph nodes were only positive above the IMA, and 77% had at least one metastatic node located above the level of the IMA. However, the authors do report that there were no positive lymph nodes detected in those with grade I or II tumors with a tumor size of smaller than 2 cm with less than 50% invasion, raising the question of the benefit of lymphadenectomy in the truly low-risk group. Abu-Rustum and colleagues demonstrated a 1% risk of isolated paraaortic lymph node metastasis in both the low- and high-grade tumors. Based on these and other reports, PALA does have an important role in comprehensive staging. For high-risk patients, the data suggest even a therapeutic role for paraaortic lymph node dissection. However, prospective trials are needed to confirm this concept for patients with early-stage endometrial cancer with high-risk features.

Since 1988 when FIGO changed endometrial staging from clinical to surgical, there have been questions raised as to whether the lymphadenectomy is only diagnostic, which is an important determinate, or whether it also could be therapeutic. **Kilgore and associates, in evaluating 649 patients, noted that those who underwent multiple-site lymph node removal had**

FIGURE 5.13 Survival by nodes sampled and risk groups: multiple-site pelvic node sampling versus no nodes. Low-risk group, $P = 0.026$; high-risk group, $P = 0.0006$. (From Kilgore LC, Partridge EE, Alvarez RD, et al. Adenocarcinoma of the endometrium: survival comparisons of patients with and without pelvic node sampling. *Gynecol Oncol* 1995;56:29.)

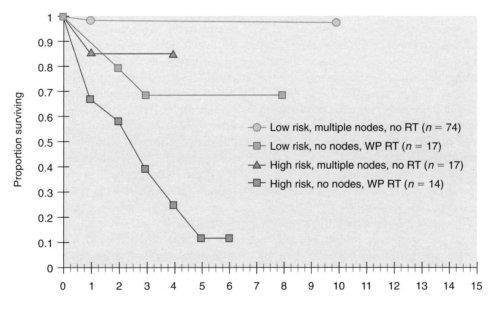

FIGURE 5.14 Survival comparisons of multiple-site pelvic node sampling with whole-pelvic (WP) radiation therapy (RT): multiple nodes without RT versus no nodes plus WP RT. Low-risk group, $P = 0.003$; high-risk group, $P = 0.041$. (From Kilgore LC, Partridge EE, Alvarez RD, et al. Adenocarcinoma of the endometrium: survival comparisons of patients with and without pelvic node sampling. *Gynecol Oncol* 1995;56:29.)

significantly better survival rates than those patients who had no lymph nodes removed (Figs. 5.13 **and** 5.14). **Lymph node removal resulted in a better survival rate than for those without lymph node removal plus postoperative radiation.** Cragun and colleagues reported that patients with grade III or poorly differentiated cancers with more than 11 lymph nodes removed had an improved survival (hazard ratio [HR], 0.25) and PFS (HR, 0.26) compared with those with fewer than 11 lymph nodes removed. However, the number of lymph nodes removed was not predictive of survival outcome in those with grade I and II tumors. This association between lymphadenectomy and improved survival remained when controlling for adjuvant radiation treatment, emphasizing the impact of extensive lymph node dissection. A retrospective review by

Chan and colleagues of more than 12,000 patients showed an increased 5-year survival rate for the intermediate- and high-risk group that underwent an extensive lymph node dissection. However, there was no benefit of nodal dissection seen in the low-risk group.

Removal of nodes involved by tumor has been supported as a therapeutic option. In a study reported by Havrilesky et al., 91 patients were identified with stage IIIc disease. There were 39 with microscopic involvement of the lymph nodes and 52 with grossly enlarged nodes. After surgery, 92% received some type of adjuvant therapy with 85% receiving radiation therapy. **The survival rate (5 years) was 58% in the 39 with microscopic lymph nodes, 48% in 41 patients with grossly positive lymph nodes completely resected, and only 22% in the 11 with unresected lymph nodes. The authors believed that these data suggested a therapeutic benefit for lymphadenectomy. Similarly, in a small study of 41 patients, Bristow and coworkers noted disease-free survival was improved if patients with bulky adenopathy underwent complete resection of involved nodes compared with patients who had gross residual disease in lymph nodes remaining after surgery (37.5 vs. 8.8 months; $P = 0.006$).** Onda and colleagues carried out thorough pelvic and paraaortic lymphadenectomies on 173 patients with stage I to III endometrial cancer. The average numbers of lymph nodes removed were 38 pelvic and 29 paraaortic. There were 30 patients (17%) with positive nodes: 10 to pelvis only, two paraaortic only, and 18 with metastasis to both pelvic and paraaortic nodes. Selected patients received radiation therapy with extended fields, combination chemotherapy, or both. In the 10 patients with only pelvic metastasis, the 5-year survival rate was 100%; it was 75% in those with paraaortic involvement. **The authors suggest that, although postoperative treatment may contribute to these excellent results, systematic pelvic and PALA was a contributing factor.**

One of the important effects of lymph node dissection is that it identifies that most patients with negative lymph nodes are at very low risk for recurrence. As such, lymph node dissection has allowed for modifications of postoperative therapy away from pelvic radiation therapy. In one study, Mohan and associates evaluated 159 stage I patients who had full pelvic lymphadenectomy (PLA) and received vaginal brachytherapy rather than the more traditional pelvic radiation. In general, vaginal brachytherapy is a quicker therapy (1–3 days vs. 5–6 weeks for pelvic radiation) and is associated with fewer side effects. In the Mohan study, the 15-year OS was 92%, and the recurrence rate was 4%, all at distant sites. **Podratz and associates reviewed four studies that used thorough lymphadenectomies in moderate- and high-risk patients who did not receive postoperative radiation therapy. There were 20 recurrences (7%) in 305 patients; only five recurrences were local or regional, with four being in the vagina. Those four did not receive postoperative brachytherapy but were salvaged with subsequent radiation.**

The disadvantages of a lymph node dissection include that the performance of lymph node dissection requires a specially trained surgeon, has the potential to increase complications (postoperative ileus, lymphedema), and has not been prospectively validated to improve outcomes. Two recent phase III trials compared the use of lymph node dissection or not in patients with endometrial cancer. In a large multicentric study (ASTEC study), 1408 patients were randomly assigned to abdominal hysterectomy or bilateral salpingo-oophorectomy with or without PLA. A median follow-up period of 37 months was obtained. There was no difference in survival between the two groups. This was an intent-to-treat study and has been criticized as having a relatively large noncompliance in regard to lymphadenectomy and subsequent therapy. In the lymphadenectomy arm, almost a half had no nodes or a small number (≤9) removed. This study was further complicated by the fact that many of these patients were secondarily randomly assigned into a postoperative radiation study, not taking into consideration surgical findings. PALA was not the standard management, although some patients had these nodes removed.

The second study was published by Pierluigi Benedetti Panici. The Italian study randomly assigned 514 stage I patients to systematic PLA or no lymphadenectomy. Although 13% of patients in the lymphadenectomy arm had known metastasis versus 3% in the no-lymphadenectomy arm, there was no difference in recurrence or OS. The protocol required a minimum of 20 lymph nodes to be removed; however, the lymphadenectomy was limited to the pelvis, although PALA could be removed at the discretion of the surgeon. Postoperative radiation was left to the discretion of the treating physician. Adjuvant therapy was similar in the two groups. Whether or not this had an effect on survival is unknown because this was not standardized.

A study from Japan (SEPAL study) was published in early 2010. This was a study of PLA ($n = 325$ patients) versus PALA ($n = 346$ patients) in endometrial cancer. It was not a randomized study; however, one hospital did only pelvic nodes and the other pelvic and paraaortic. Lymphadenectomy was certainly adequate for using the number of lymph nodes removed as a parameter. The survival rate was significantly better ($P >0.001$) in women receiving the PLA and PALA. This was seen in intermediate- and high-risk patients but not in low-risk patients. In a multivariant analysis, the PLA plus PALA reduced the risk of death compared with PLA only. In the high-risk group, patients receiving chemotherapy plus PLA plus PALA had a better survival than patients receiving chemotherapy plus PLA only. PLA plus PALA and adjuvant chemotherapy were independently associated with improved survival.

The Cochrane Database subsequently concluded that there was no overall statistical difference between PFS and OS in patients who had a lymphadenectomy versus those who did not but did report more morbidity for those patients who had a lymphadenectomy. Cochrane only considered the ASTEC and the Italian study in reaching this conclusion. The extent of the lymphadenectomy appears to be critical in evaluating studies in determining an appropriate surgical procedure for patients with endometrial cancer. Multiple studies confirm that both pelvic and paraaortic lymph nodes are at risk for metastasis.

Patients with stage II carcinoma of the endometrium, because of extension of disease into the endocervix, will have a greater propensity for lymph node metastasis. For example, in the GOG 33 protocol, 16% of patients with cervical involvement had positive pelvic lymph nodes versus 8% with a fundal location of tumor. Even in patients with occult cervical involvement, 19% of patients had lymph node metastases. In addition, parametrial and vaginal involvement are thought to be more common when the cervix is involved. As such, surgery in the form of radical hysterectomy and lymphadenectomy has been advocated when there is gross cervical involvement with tumor. Because many cases of cervical involvement are occult and only recognized after surgery, simple hysterectomy with lymphadenectomy appears to be adequate surgery in most cases. Postoperative radiation therapy can be planned, depending on surgical-pathologic findings, including use of pelvic radiation or vaginal cuff brachytherapy, both, or neither.

In 1993, Childers and others pioneered laparoscopic lymph node removal in conjunction with vaginal hysterectomy and bilateral salpingo-oophorectomy. In the hands of those who acquired those surgical skills, the outcomes appeared comparable, and some advantages were gained, such as short hospitalization and rapid postoperative recovery. A large GOG study comparing the laparoscopic approach versus laparotomy has been completed. Walker and colleagues published the results of GOGLAP2, which randomly assigned patients between laparoscopic versus open laparotomy surgical staging. Laparoscopy was initiated and completed without conversion in 74%. Conversion from laparoscopy to laparotomy was secondary to poor visibility in 15%, metastatic cancer in 4%, and bleeding in 3%. Patients randomly assigned to undergo laparoscopy had significantly fewer moderate to severe postoperative (14% vs. 21%) complications and similar rates of intraoperative complications. Length of hospital stay was significantly shorter for those randomized to undergo laparoscopy (median 3 days vs. 4 days), but operative time was significantly longer (median, 204 minutes vs. 130 minutes). Pelvic and paraaortic nodes were removed in 92% of patients undergoing laparoscopy and 96% of patients undergoing laparotomy, and cytology was performed in 96% vs. 98%. Neither treatment arm demonstrated an improved ability to detect metastatic disease. Quality-of-life evaluation found a better body image and return to normal activities for the patients undergoing laparoscopy. Laparoscopic surgical staging is feasible and safe for patients with uterine cancer and results in fewer complications and shorter hospital stays. A reduction in paraaortic node evaluation is a potential risk of laparoscopic staging. Recurrence rates were lower than anticipated; the estimated 3-year recurrence rate was 11% with laparoscopy and 10% with laparotomy, and the estimated 5-year OS rate was almost identical in both arms (90%). Today, advancements of laparoscopic surgery, including use of a robotic surgical platform, have been suggested as the next step. Robotic surgery offers three-dimensional graphics, improved ergonomics, and greater dexterity of surgical instruments. Robotic surgery may extend the applications of laparoscopy, especially in obese patients or patients in whom a vaginal component is more difficult. However, no randomized trials have confirmed equivalence or superiority of robotic assistance.

Surgical staging has now been accepted as standard therapy in patients with endometrial cancer unless clinical conditions suggest otherwise. Of the 6260 patients with endometrial cancer reported to the last Annual Report of FIGO, 94% were surgically staged. It is appreciated that institutions reporting to the Annual Report are academic ones and that most patients with endometrial cancers, at least in the United States, have their primary surgery at academic hospitals. Because endometrial cancer staging has been determined by surgical staging, it has been suggested by some that these are patients who are at low risk (ie, grade I) for lymph node metastasis and that lymphadenectomy is not worthwhile. Increasing data suggest that even in grade I disease, as noted on endometrial biopsy, a significant number of patients have full surgical staging findings that would have an impact on further therapy. **Ben-Shachar and colleagues, in evaluating 181 grade I endometrial cancers, found that 19% had grade change on hysterectomy specimen, 11% had extrauterine disease, 4% had lymph node metastasis, and 26% on final evaluation had high-risk intrauterine factors. Of note, the authors believed because of full surgical staging that 12% needed and received adjuvant therapy, and 17% who may have received postoperative treatment did not based on full surgical findings.** Geisler and associates found in 349 patients that of those with grade I lesions, 16% had positive nodes and 3% had positive paraaortic nodes only. Of all positive nodes, **31% occurred in grade I lesions. As a result of these and other studies, many believe that all patients with endometrial cancer should have the benefit of full surgical staging, which includes peritoneal cytology, bilateral pelvic lymphadenectomy and PALA, and total abdominal hysterectomy and bilateral salpingo-oophorectomy.** Obviously, complete evaluation of the entire peritoneal cavity and its contents should be performed, and any suspicious areas should be pathologically evaluated.

Straight and associates reported on a large number of patients who were surgically staged. Low-risk factors, stage IaG1 and 2, were present in 103 patients. None received postoperative therapy, and none had recurred. **Intermediate risk was defined as stage IaG3 and all stage I and Ic cancers. There were 440 patients of whom 93% received no further therapy. Twenty-eight patients received postoperative therapy, and one (4%) had a recurrence compared with 5% of those not radiated.** The latter patients received therapy at the time of recurrence, and 62% were successful. **The Annual Report (2003) noted 5-year survival rates with surgery only of 93%, 91%, 73%, 79%, and 73%, respectively, for stages Ia, Ib, Ic, and IIa, and IIb. This compares with 89%, 91%, 83%, 83%, and 75%, respectively, if surgery plus postoperative radiation is used.** There is a suggestion that in stage Ic, the survival rate is somewhat better when postoperative radiation is added than surgery alone. What factors went into decision making regarding postoperative therapy is unknown. In a multi-institutional study, 220 surgically staged Ic patients were identified. High-risk histotypes were excluded. Adjuvant radiation was used in 99 (45%), 56 brachytherapy only, and 19 whole-pelvis radiation, and 24 received both. **OS rates between those treated with surgery and surgery plus radiation was similar (92% vs. 90%).**

Radiation Therapy

Radiation therapy has been the mainstay of adjuvant therapy for endometrial cancer. Historically, nearly all patients received

TABLE 5.16　Radiation in Early-Stage Carcinoma of the Endometrium

	Local Recurrence (%)	Survival (%)
Aalder		
Surgery + VCB (n = 277)	7*	91
Surgery VCB + RT (n = 263)	2†	89
Creutzberg (PORTEC)		
Surgery (n = 300)	14†	85
Surgery + RT (n = 354)	4†	81
Keyes (GOG 99)		
Surgery (n = 202)	4	86
Surgery + RT (n = 190)	2	92
ASTEC/NCIC CTG EN.5		
Surgery ‡(n = 454)	6§	84
Surgery + RT (n = 452)	3§	84

*P <0.01.
†P <0.001.
‡50% received vaginal brachytherapy.
§P = 0.038.

GOG, Gynecologic Oncology Group; PORTEC, Post-Operative Radiation Therapy in Endometrial Cancer; RT, pelvic radiation therapy; VCB, vaginal cuff brachytherapy.

some form of preoperative or postoperative radiation therapy given the perception of risk for recurrence was high. Whereas GOG 33 defined relationships between depth of invasion and tumor grade and extrauterine spread after surgical staging, it also showed that most patients were not at risk for extrauterine disease spread. As such, the routine use of pelvic radiation therapy became increasing questioned. To date, four large prospective randomized studies have compared external pelvic radiation with observation or vaginal brachytherapy in women with endometrial cancer (Table 5.16). Aalders and colleagues compared vaginal cuff brachytherapy with or without pelvic radiation in 540 patients with early-stage endometrial cancer. Patients did not undergo lymph node dissection. The addition of pelvic radiation therapy reduced local failures (2% vs. 7%), but there was no difference in 5-year survival rate between the groups (89% pelvic, 91% brachytherapy). Onsrud et al. updated the long-term follow-up for these patients. After a median 20.5 years of follow-up, no statistically significant difference was revealed in OS rate between treatment groups. However, women younger than age 60 years had significantly higher mortality rates after external-beam radiotherapy (EBRT) (HR, 1.36; 95% CI, 1.06–1.76) than the control group. The risk of secondary cancer increased after EBRT, especially in women younger than age 60 years (HR, 2.02; 95% CI, 1.30–3.15). The authors concluded that there was no survival benefit of external pelvic radiation in early-stage endometrial carcinoma. In women younger than age 60 years, pelvic radiation decreased survival and increased the risk of secondary cancer. Thus, adjuvant EBRT should be used with caution, especially in women with long life expectancies.

In the Dutch PORTEC trial, Creutzberg et al. enrolled 714 patients with grade I lesions with greater than 50% myometrial

invasion, grade II lesions with any amount of invasion, or grade III with less than 50% invasion. Patients were randomly assigned postoperatively to receive either external radiation or observation. None of the patients were surgically staged, and all histologies were eligible. In the 654 eligible for follow-up, **local and regional recurrences were less frequent in the radiation therapy group (4% vs. 14%) than in the observational group, but the 5-year survival rates were similar, 81% versus 85%, respectively.** Long-term follow-up is also available for this trial. As published by Creutzberg et al., after 15 years, there remained no survival advantage and a trend for long-term risk of second cancers. EBRT should be avoided in patients with low- and intermediate-risk EC.

The GOG performed a phase III trial, #99, of surgery with or without adjunctive external pelvic radiation in intermediate-risk endometrial adenocarcinomas. These included all women with any degree of myometrial invasion, any grade, and no evidence of lymph node metastasis (stage Ib, IC, IIA occult, and IIB occult). All patients were required to have surgical staging with histologic evaluation of the lymph nodes. A total of 202 received no radiation (NAT), and 190 received pelvic radiation. The median follow-up period was 69 months. There were 15% total recurrences in the NAT group compared with 6% to 8% in the radiation group (P = 0.007). Local recurrences were 9% versus 2%, respectively. The OS at 48 months was 86% for NAT and 92% for radiation, with intercurrent diseases accounting for half or more of the deaths in both groups. **Deaths from disease were 8% in both the NAT versus radiation group.** Grade III and IV toxicity by treatment was 5% versus 14% in the NAT and radiation, groups, respectively. In 12 of the 13 women who had isolated vaginal recurrences, the NAT arm were treated with radiation, and five have died of disease. An high intermediate (H-IR) subgroup appeared to derive the best benefit from pelvic radiation, with 27% of H-IR patients followed with observation compared to 13% after pelvic radiation, recurring. All other eligible patients were considered low–intermediate risk and had recurrence rates less than 1% to 3% regardless of the use of radiation therapy. The most recent data from a pooled trial of the MRC ASTEC and NCIC CTG EN.5 randomized trials also showed no survival advantage for adjuvant EBRT in the treatment of endometrial cancer (5-year survival rate ~84% both groups). In this study including 906 patients randomly assigned to pelvic radiation or observation, 30% of patients underwent lymphadenectomy, and 50% received vaginal brachytherapy. Pelvic radiation reduced local failures (6% with observation vs. 3% after pelvic radiation). In a subsequent Cochrane review on the use of adjuvant radiation therapy for stage I endometrial cancer, the authors concluded that there is no survival advantage with routine use of pelvic radiation therapy and that benefits must be balanced against the toxicity and morbidity of therapy. In addition, risk factors within stage I groups (grade III, outer 50% invasion) should be considered in an effort to better select populations who may get the best benefit.

Essentially all studies evaluating pelvic radiation therapy show improved local control rates compared to observation. The local control, however, is largely a result of reduction in

TABLE 5.17   Survival Rate in Stage I Carcinoma of the Endometrium With Regard to Grade and Treatment

Grade	Survival	
	Surgery Only (%)	Combined Therapy (%)
1	1295/1375 (94)	2284/2389 (96)
2	488/510 (96)	1490/1721 (87)
3	100/135 (74)	398/498 (80)

From Pettersson F, ed. *Annual report on the results of treatment in gynecological cancer, vol 21.* Stockholm, 1991, International Federation of Gynecology and Obstetrics.

TABLE 5.18   Recurrences in Stage I Carcinoma of the Endometrium With Regard to Depth of Invasion and Treatment

Recurrence	Surgery and Radium	Surgery and External Radiation
Endometrium only	6/88 (7%)	0/4 (0%)
Inner and mid thirds	3/68 (4%)	9/29 (31%)
Outer third	3/9 (33%)	11/24 (46%)

Modified from DiSaia PJ, Creasman WT, Boronow RC, Blessing JA. Risk factors in recurrent patterns in stage I endometrial carcinoma *Am J Obstet Gynecol* 1985;151:1009.

vaginal cuff recurrences. A considerable amount of data has been collected to evaluate vaginal recurrence and survival rate with surgery alone or combined therapy when mainly preoperative application of brachytherapy and surgery were used. Data have also been evaluated concerning the grade of the tumor (Table 5.17) and, in some instances, the depth of myometrial involvement (Table 5.18). In patients who had postoperative irradiation, there appeared to be a lower incidence of vaginal vault recurrences, although there does not appear to be much difference in the grade I and grade II lesions. Vaginal vault recurrence did not appear to affect survival. Recently, results of a randomized prospective trial comparing adjuvant EBRT versus vaginal brachytherapy in 427 patients with intermediate-risk early-stage endometrial cancer have been reported (PORTEC-2). No differences in recurrence rate (vaginal failure 2% with pelvic radiation, 0.9% with vaginal brachytherapy) or OS (3-year survival rate ~90% both groups) were observed between the two treatment arms, suggesting that patients with intermediate-risk early-stage endometrial cancer can be treated with adjuvant vaginal brachytherapy alone. Although these findings have led many clinicians in the United States to move away from the routine use of EBRT in early-stage endometrial cancer, it is important to note that in the patients who did not undergo a lymph node dissection, pelvic failure rates were higher in vaginal brachytherapy group (3.5% vs. 0.7%), and the study excluded higher risk patients such as those with grade III or deeper invasion tumors. The most recently reported study comparing pelvic radiation followed by vaginal cuff brachytherapy to vaginal cuff brachytherapy alone for "medium-risk"

endometrial cancer by Sorbe et al. showed results similar to PORTEC-2, demonstrating that pelvic radiation reduced locoregional relapse rates (1% vs. 5%, P = 0.013) with no difference in OS. Sorbe et al. also reported a randomized trial of vaginal brachytherapy versus no further treatment in patients with low-risk endometrial cancer (grade I or II endometrioid cancer with <50% invasion). There was no significant reduction in vaginal recurrence in the group receiving brachytherapy (3% vs. 1%).

Chemotherapy

The role of chemotherapy in endometrial cancer is evolving. Traditionally reserved for patients with recurrent or disseminated cancer, chemotherapy has become increasingly used in the first-line management of patients with advanced-stage and high-risk early-stage disease. Historically, radiation therapy has been the adjuvant of choice for patients at risk of recurrence. Although the overall prognosis of patients in adjuvant radiation trials has been favorable, 3% to 23% of patients have a recurrence at distant sites, demonstrating the need for effective systemic therapy.

Drug Development

Progestins have been an important systemic therapy given response rates in up to one-third of patients and low toxicity. The identification of active cytotoxic chemotherapy regimens has led to a reevaluation of chemotherapy. Phase II studies have identified several single agents with activity in advanced or recurrent endometrial cancer. In a report of the GOG experience, Thigpen and colleagues noted that 37% with advanced or recurrent cancer experienced an objective response with use of doxorubicin alone. Unfortunately, response lasted only 7 months. The Eastern Cooperative Oncology Group achieved only a 19% response rate in its doxorubicin trial; however, a dosage lower than the GOG dosage was used. When one evaluates the doxorubicin data, one notes that only about 10% of patients who received this drug had a complete response rate. Patients designated as giving a partial response had survival rates no greater than those of patients who had no response to this cytotoxic agent. Likewise, phase II studies have identified platinum agents (cisplatin, carboplatin) and taxanes (paclitaxel) to have significant activity.

Combining two or more active agents has been an important strategy. Phase III studies have shown better response rates when the agents were combined compared with used alone. Several chemotherapy combinations have been used in recurrent or advanced endometrial cancer. The GOG, in a randomized trial, #107, compared doxorubicin with or without cisplatin. The combination produced tumor response in 66% versus 35% for the single agent, with median progression-free intervals of 6.2 and 3.9 months, respectively. **The GOG reported a 45% response rate (22% complete response) for the combination of doxorubicin and cisplatin in advanced or recurrent endometrial cancer compared to 17% response for doxorubicin alone.** The European Organization for Research and Treatment of Cancer Gynecological Cancer Cooperative Group (EORTC-GCCG) compared doxorubicin alone with doxorubicin and cisplatin. Response rate was 17% and 57%, respectively. The GOG (GOG 163) has compared doxorubicin and cisplatin with doxorubicin and paclitaxel (24-hour infusion) with filgrastim in advanced or recurrent endometrial cancer. A total of 317 patients randomly assigned to the two regimens. Response rates were similar (40% vs. 43%). PFS was median 7.2 versus 6 months, and OS was median 12.6 versus 13.6 months. Toxicities were also similar. **A phase III study by the GOG (177) compared doxorubicin plus cisplatin with or without paclitaxel plus filgrastim (TAP) in advanced endometrial cancer. There were 273 women registered, and objective responses were 57% versus 34% ($P < 0.01$); PFS (median, 8.3 vs. 5.3 months, $P < 0.01$) and OS (median, 15.3 vs. 12.3 months, $P = 0.037$) were improved with the triple combination TAP regimen.** This study marked for the first time a statistically significant improvement in response rate, PFS, and survival with a combination regimen in endometrial cancer. However, the three-drug regimen required a 2-day treatment and the use of growth factors on day 3 and was associated with moderate peripheral neuropathy. The GOG has presented a randomized trial, #209, comparing the three-drug TAP regimen with carboplatin plus paclitaxel (TC). PFS (median TC vs. TAP, 14 vs. 14 months; HR, 1.03) and OS (median TC vs. TAP, 32 vs. 38 months; HR, 1.01) results for TC were not inferior to TAP. Health-related quality of life differences, when they were present, favored TC over TAP by a small margin.

Advanced Disease

Drug development trials are largely designed to assess the efficacy of new drugs or combinations in patients with incurable disease (recurrent, disseminated). The concept of using chemotherapy in patients with advanced but potentially curable disease was once considered controversial. Treatment of patients with stage III or IV disease depends largely on the extent of surgical resection. Patients with stage III or IV disease and resection to less than 1 to 2 cm residual may be treated with curative intent with chemotherapy, radiation, or a combination of the two. The GOG studied patients (GOG 122) with stage III or IV endometrial cancer with 2 cm or less residual disease (distant metastases were excluded). After surgery, patients were randomly assigned to receive doxorubicin and cisplatin every 3 weeks for eight courses or whole-abdominal radiation with 3000 cGy to the whole abdomen. A boost to the pelvic and paraaortic lymph node region (1500 cGy) could be given for positive nodes. As reported by Randall et al., 2 years after therapy, the OS rate was improved by 11%, and the cancer-free survival rate was improved by 13% with chemotherapy compared with those treated with radiation therapy. Side effects were more common in the chemotherapy-treated patients.

In an effort to build on improvements noted with the first-line chemotherapy into the management of patients with advanced endometrial cancer, the GOG performed a randomized trial (GOG 184) comparing volume-directed radiation (pelvic radiation with or without extended field to cover paraaortic lymph nodes) followed by six cycles of doxorubicin–cisplatin with or without paclitaxel chemotherapy. The results showed no improvement in PFS with the addition of paclitaxel

to pelvic radiation plus cisplatin and doxorubicin except in patients with gross residual disease. Although the results of GOG 184 may seem to conflict with the results of GOG 177, several important observations can be made. First, the addition of pelvic radiation therapy may supplant the benefit of adding paclitaxel the two-drug regimen seen in GOG 177. Second, this trial demonstrates the feasibility of combining multiagent cytotoxic chemotherapy with adjuvant radiation. The role of radiation therapy in advanced disease is addressed in GOG0258, which randomized carboplatin and paclitaxel with or without radiation therapy. This study has finished the accrual phase, and results are awaited.

Factors associated with response to chemotherapy have been studied. Behbakht and colleagues evaluated prognostic factors in 137 patients with advanced disease (stage III and stage IV). Multivariate analysis noted age, parametrial involvement, and abdominal metastasis as significant prognostic indicators. An increased frequency of advanced stage was also noted with UPSC histology. Unfortunately, multiple therapies were used, and conclusions concerning treatment cannot be made. Kadar and associates evaluated 58 patients with surgical stage III and stage IV disease. Extrapelvic peritoneal metastasis and positive peritoneal cytologic findings affected survival. If either of these factors was present, the 2-year survival rate was only 25% compared with 83% if they were not present. Postoperative therapy varied, but it did not appear to have any effect on survival.

Adjuvant Therapy: High-Risk Disease

Given the results of GOG 122, new considerations for chemotherapy in a variety of settings have been considered. Today, the role of adjuvant chemotherapy in intermediate- and high-risk early-stage endometrial cancers is increasingly considered. Several trials have assessed the role of chemotherapy in high-risk endometrial cancer. The Japanese GOG group performed a randomized trial of chemotherapy (at least three cycles of cyclophosphamide, doxorubicin, cisplatin [CAP regimen]) versus pelvic radiation in patients with endometrial cancer. Most patients had stage Ic or II disease (75%), but patients with IIIa and IIIc disease were included. For all patients, there was no difference in PFS or OS between the regimens. The study did identify a group of patients with higher risk features (Ic or grade III, stage II or III with depth of invasion >50%) for whom PFS and OS were significantly improved in the chemotherapy arm. Maggi and colleagues performed a similar study comparing five cycles of CAP chemotherapy with pelvic radiation in 340 patients with endometrial cancer. In this trial, 62% of patients had stage IIIa to IIIc disease. The 5-year PFS and OS were not statistically different between the groups. Neither of these studies used paclitaxel, an agent that in phase II and III studies appears to offer improved efficacy.

The role of adjunctive chemotherapy in addition to surgery and radiation therapy has been addressed by the GOG in patients with high-risk stage I and occult stage II endometrial cancers. Morrow et al. reported on 181 patients treated with TAH and BSO, peritoneal cytologic evaluation, and selective pelvic and PALA followed by external irradiation (pelvic with or without extended field) and were then randomly assigned to receive doxorubicin 60 mg/m^2 every 3 weeks for eight doses. Patients participating in the doxorubicin arm of the protocol had a higher incidence of metastases to pelvic nodes (20% vs. 10%) than did those in the no doxorubicin arm; otherwise, the risk factors were equal between the two groups. There were recurrences in 22 of 92 (23%) in the doxorubicin arm versus recurrences in 23 of 89 (26%) in the nondoxorubicin arm. Of patients with recurrences, those who received doxorubicin had a greater chance of metastasis to the abdomen than did those not receiving it (40% vs. 17%). However, distant metastases occurred more frequently without the use of doxorubicin than with it (56% vs. 18%). The small sample size (and reduced power), the heterogeneous population, and the use of single-agent doxorubicin (as opposed to combination therapy) are weaknesses of the study. The Radiation Oncology Group (RTOG) and the EORTC have both published data on patients with high-risk early-stage endometrial cancers treated with adjuvant radiation therapy with or without adjuvant platinum-based chemotherapy. Both trials suggest that adjuvant radiation combined with adjuvant chemotherapy in high-risk early-stage endometrial cancers is feasible and may result in better OS.

Based on the experience with current studies, two important trials assessing the role of chemotherapy have been developed. The PORTEC-3 trial is an ongoing randomized phase III trial comparing concurrent chemoradiation followed by adjuvant paclitaxel–carboplatin chemotherapy versus pelvic radiation alone. The GOG completed a randomized phase III trial (GOG 249) comparing vaginal brachytherapy plus adjuvant carboplatin and paclitaxel versus pelvic radiation. Neither the PORTEC-3 trial nor GOG 249 required lymph node dissection as part of the inclusion criteria. However, full surgical staging was encouraged in the GOG trial. The results of these trials will elucidate the role of adjuvant chemotherapy combined with adjuvant radiation in high-risk early-stage endometrial cancer.

Hormones

Progestins have been used for more than 30 years, and the objective responsiveness of recurrent carcinoma of the endometrium to these hormones has been substantiated (Fig. 5.15). Historically, approximately one-third of all patients with recurrent carcinoma of the endometrium are said to respond to the hormone, although patients with well-differentiated tumors have a response rate much higher than that of patients with moderately or poorly differentiated lesions. The GOG described 420 patients with advanced or recurrent endometrial carcinoma treated with medroxyprogesterone acetate (MPA) 50 mg three times a day. Of the 219 patients with objective measurable disease, there were only 17 complete responders (8%) and 13 partial responders (6%). More than half of the patients remained stable, and one-third progressed. The median survival time was 10.5 months. Grade I lesions responded more frequently than poorly differentiated carcinomas did. The GOG evaluated, in a randomized phase III trial (#81), MPA at 1000 mg/day compared with 200 mg/day. In almost 300 patients, there was no difference in response rate or survival between the two groups. Lentz reported another GOG trial, #121, of high-dose megestrol

FIGURE 5.15 Patient with right hilar metastases that resolved completely on progestin therapy.

TABLE 5.19   Correlation of Tumor Differentiation With Receptor Content

Differentiation	ER and PR Positive (%)
Well	28/40 (70)
Moderate	21/38 (55)
Poor	11/27 (41)

ER, Estrogen receptor; *PR*, progesterone receptor.
From Creasman WT, Soper JT, McCarty KS Jr, et al. Influence of cytoplasmic steroid receptor content on prognosis of early stage endometrial carcinoma *Am J Obstet Gynecol* 1985;151:922.

acetate (800 mg/day) in patients with advanced or recurrent endometrial carcinoma. Of 58 patients, 13 (24%) responded; six (11%) had a partial response. Four of the responses lasted more than 18 months and were primarily between the grade I and grade II lesions.

More recently, considerable interest has been shown in the presence of specific estrogen and progesterone receptors in neoplastic human uterine tissue. These receptors are definitely present and vary from tumor to tumor. It has been shown that there is a greater number of both estrogen and progesterone receptors in well-differentiated lesions than in poorly differentiated ones (Table 5.19). In a small group of patients, it was noted that about one-third of those with recurrent cancer had a positive receptor site analysis to both estrogen and progesterone. The receptor data may therefore correlate with clinical findings of responsiveness to progesterones in patients with recurrent cancer. Preliminary data suggest an excellent correlation (Table 5.20). Obviously, considerable additional data are needed to verify these findings; however, the prospects are excellent. If

TABLE 5.20 Response to Progestin Therapy in Regard to Receptor Content	
Receptor Content	Progestin Response (%)
Positive	44/55 (80)
Negative	4/76 (5)

Based on papers by Ehrlich et al., Benraad et al., Creasman et al., Kauppila, Pollow et al., and Quinn et al.

direct correlation can be substantiated, the receptor site analysis can guide the type of progestin therapy or chemotherapy given for recurrent endometrial cancer. If receptor site analysis is positive for both estrogen and progesterone, a patient's chances of responding to progestins are extremely good, even if she has a poorly differentiated lesion. However, if the receptor site analysis is negative, the data suggest that the patient's response to progestins may be extremely low, making it more advisable to go directly to cytotoxic agents without wasting time on progestin therapy. Kauppila noted from five studies in the literature that 89% of progesterone receptor–positive tumors were hormonally responsive compared with only 17% of progesterone receptor–negative tumors. The GOG noted that 4 of 10 (40%) estrogen receptor–positive, progesterone receptor–positive tumors responded to progestins compared with 5 of 41 (12%) progesterone receptor–negative tumors.

Progestin therapy may be administered in several different ways; MPA (Depo-Provera), 400 mg intramuscularly at weekly intervals, oral MPA (Provera) in the range of 150 mg/day, and megestrol acetate (Megace) 160 mg/day are recommended progestins. Progestins are continued indefinitely if an objective response is obtained. If progression of disease is noted, progestins should be discontinued, and chemotherapy should be considered.

Progestins have been evaluated as adjunctive therapy in the hope of preventing recurrences. Lewis and coworkers, in a randomized study, treated endometrial cancer patients postoperatively with MPA or placebo. The 4-year survival rate was similar in the two groups. Kauppila, in describing more than 1100 patients who received adjunctive progestin therapy for 2 years after surgery and radiation therapy, found that even in stage I low-grade tumors, recurrences did appear; it was their belief that prophylactic progestins were not of benefit to these patients. In a prospective study of 363 patients with stage I disease who received adjuvant MPA for 12 months, DePalo and colleagues compared survival with that of 383 patients with stage I disease who did not receive MPA postoperatively; there was no difference in survival between the two groups. In a British study in which 429 patients with stage I or stage II cancers were randomized between postoperative MPA and observation, no difference in survival was seen after 5 years. A Cochrane Database review concluded that current evidence did not support the use of adjuvant progestin therapy in the primary treatment of endometrial cancer.

With only modest response to progestins, other hormonal agents have been evaluated. Tamoxifen has been shown to bind estrogen receptors and thereby block access of the estrogen into the nucleus. It has also been suggested that tamoxifen can increase the number of progesterone receptors in vivo. Combined results of several small studies noted a response rate of 22% (complete response rate of 8%) in 257 patients. These studies suggest that grade I lesions are more responsive than other grades of tumors. Progestins plus tamoxifen have been evaluated in combination in recurrent carcinoma of the endometrium. Tamoxifen, 40 mg/day, with intermittent Provera, 200 mg/day on alternate weeks, had a 33% response rate with a median PFS of 3 months and median survival of 13 months (GOG 0119). A phase II trial of megestrol acetate, 160 mg orally for 3 weeks, alternating with tamoxifen, 40 mg/day for 3 weeks, until disease progression showed an overall response rate of 27% with a median PFS of 2.7 months and median OS of 14 months (GOG 0153). The response rate was 38% in patients with histologic grade I tumors, 24% in those with grade II, and 22% among patients with grade III. Although tamoxifen is theoretically attractive (it causes an increase in progesterone receptors for better progestin effect), studies of small groups of patients have not produced favorable results. The use of tamoxifen is interesting in view of the reports of endometrial cancer in patients taking tamoxifen. This is in contrast to in vitro data suggesting that tamoxifen does not stimulate and in fact may inhibit established endometrial cell line growth.

Gonadotropin-releasing hormone (GnRH) analogues have been evaluated in the treatment of endometrial cancer in a small number of patients. These analogues suppress gonadotropins with a reduction in estrogen but not cortisol levels. Gallagher and associates treated 17 patients with recurrent endometrial cancer who had received previous progesterone therapy; six (35%) had a response that continued for a median of 20 months. Further study is needed, but it appears that GnRH analogues may have a direct inhibitory effect on cancer cells.

Special Circumstances
Multiple Malignant Neoplasms
Simultaneous or subsequent primary cancers involving the breast, ovary, and large intestines occur more frequently in patients with endometrial cancer than might be expected. The reverse also appears to be true, in that women with breast or ovarian cancer have a higher than expected risk for development of subsequent primary cancers of the endometrium. As a result, the recommendation in a patient with one of these malignant neoplasms is to evaluate the other organ sites at the time of diagnosis or during follow-up visits. Appropriate screening, such as mammography, should be emphasized.

Simultaneous malignant neoplasms of the ovary and endometrium are noted in about 8% of patients with carcinoma of the uterus, and twice that rate is noted in patients with ovarian carcinoma. Ovarian involvement in cases in which endometrial cancer is present has been reported to be as high as 40% of autopsy specimens and 15% of specimens obtained at the time of hysterectomy and bilateral salpingo-oophorectomy. In approximately one-third of cases of endometrioid carcinoma of the ovary, endometrial carcinoma has also been noted. When the occurrence is simultaneous, the question arises whether these are simultaneous multiple malignant neoplasms or one is metastatic from the other. It appears that if metastasis is present, it is more common for it to go from the endometrium to the ovary than from the ovary to the endometrium. Metastasis to the ovary is suspected if the endometrial carcinoma involves significant myometrium, particularly with lymphatic or vascular channel invasion, or if the tumor is on the ovarian surface. If, however, the corpus carcinoma is small and limited to the endometrium or superficial myometrium, with associated atypical hyperplasia, and the ovarian tumor is centrally located, the tumors are probably independent of each other. Most common tumors are the endometrioid type, but they can occasionally be of different histologic types in the two organs. Most studies suggest that most of the synchronous ovarian and corpus carcinomas are independent primary tumors. The survival of patients with what is believed to be multiple primaries mimics the excellent prognosis of the individual cancer, suggesting that the two tumors are probably each stage I and not stage III. This has certainly been true when the simultaneous endometrial and ovarian carcinomas are of the endometrioid type. In one study, the survival was 100% of the 16 patients described. It appears that when such a situation is encountered (ie, when there is no evidence of direct extension of either tumor), myometrial invasion is usually absent or superficial, there is no lymphatic or blood vessel invasion, there is atypical hyperplasia of the endometrium frequently associated with the cancer, both tumors are usually confined to the primary sites and have minimal spread, and tumor is predominantly within the ovary or the endometrium. Whether the histologic type is uniform or dissimilar, therapy should be appropriate for stage I disease, which in many instances may be treated adequately with surgery only (hysterectomy and bilateral salpingo-oophorectomy with appropriate surgical staging).

Uterine Papillary Serous Carcinoma

Much debate has surrounded the biology and clinical behavior of UPSC tumors. There is a common perception that UPSC tumors behave differently than similarly staged patients with endometrioid tumors. Given the relative rarity of UPSC tumors, most series reported in the literature have been small, retrospective series covering a long time period using variable levels of surgical staging and a variety of postoperative therapies. Older studies that did not include comprehensive surgical staging suggest that nearly 50% of "early staged" cases of UPSC recurred. One explanation for this finding is that for UPSC tumors, extrauterine disease spread is common at diagnosis, even in clinically stage I disease. One of the larger series by Goff and associates identified 50 patients with UPSC, 33 pure UPSC and 17 admixed with other histologic types. Unlike endometrioid tumors, UPSC tumors have a greater frequency of disease spread at presentation. In the Goff series, 72% had extrauterine disease; lymph node metastasis was found in 36% with no myometrial invasion, 50% with less than half invasion, and 40% with outer half invasion. **Of particular significance was the fact that 14 patients (28%) had disease limited to the endometrium, yet 36% had lymph node metastasis, 43% had intraperitoneal disease, and 50% had positive peritoneal**

TABLE 5.21	Upstaging of Serous Carcinoma of the Uterus	
Author	Patients (*n*)	Patients Upstaged (%)
Mallipeddi	9	8
Lee	10	10
Carcangiu	64	32
Cirisano	53	26
Gehrig	16	10
Kato	28	19
Sutton	10	4
Gallion	13	6
Chen	13	5
Goff	50	36
Sherman	41	19
Frank	9	7
Ward	20	8
Total	339	190 = 56%

cytologic findings, essentially equal to the findings in patients with outer-half myometrial invasion. In this study, the only significant predictor of extrauterine disease was LVSI. The propensity for extrauterine spread even in the absence of invasion is not an unusual feature in UPSC tumors. Chan evaluated 100 patients with UPSC tumors and identified 12 without myometrial invasion who had complete staging. Of these patients, six were found to have extrauterine disease spread. A pooled analysis of several studies (Table 5.21) showed that **approximately 50% of cases will be upstaged with comprehensive staging.** It is not surprising that if patients with UPSC tumors do not undergo surgical staging, unrecognized disease spread will be a common occurrence, and survival for "early-stage" patients will be poorer.

Some suggest that in appropriately staged patients, outcomes of UPSC/CC tumors are comparable to patients with high-risk endometrioid tumors. Creasman and colleagues using the FIGO Annual Report database compared patients with surgically staged I UPSC and CC carcinomas with those with endometrioid G3 cancers. Of 3996 surgically stage I cancers, there were 148 UPSC, 59 CC (5% of all stage I), and 325 G3 (8%) cancers. These were more IA cancers (no myometrial invasion) with UPSC and CC than G3. **Five-year survival rates for UPSC and CC were 72% and 81% respectively, compared with 76% for G3 lesions.** Postoperative radiation therapy improved survival somewhat (6%–8%), but the difference was not significant. The role of chemotherapy was not defined in this study because few patients had this treatment. Huh et al. reported on 60 patients with comprehensively staged stage I UPSC cases and showed that 5-year OS for patients treated by surgery alone was 66%, and it was 59% by radiation alone. Of interest, there was no recurrences in a small group (*n* = 7) treated with chemotherapy. Nickels Fader evaluated data from a pooled multi-institutional dataset of 206 surgically staged, stage I to II UPSC patients. A variety of postoperative therapies were used, including observation after surgery, chemotherapy, radiation, and combinations of chemotherapy and radiation.

Of all patients 21% recurred, including 11% of patients with no myometrial invasion.

The peritoneal cavity and distant sites (lung, liver) are common sites of failure in UPSC tumors. In an effort to improve peritoneal coverage whole-abdominal radiation has been studied extensively in this disease. In a small phase II study of whole-abdominal radiation, Sutton reported 5-year PFS of only 38% in stage I or II disease. In GOG 122 (whole-abdominal radiation vs. chemotherapy), chemotherapy was superior for all patients, including the subset with UPSC/CC tumors. Given the histologic similarity and propensity for intraperitoneal disease spread like ovarian cancer, several investigators have advocated use of systemic chemotherapies active in ovarian cancer for UPSC tumors. Levenback and colleagues from MD Anderson treated 20 patients with UPSC using cisplatin, doxorubicin, and cyclophosphamide. This included patients with measurable disease (advanced and recurrent disease) and adjuvant therapy. Only two of 11 patients with measurable disease had an objective response. The 5-year survival rate for all patients was 23%. Paclitaxel and carboplatin have been increasingly used, and several series suggest improvements in outcomes with this regimen. For example, Huh et al. demonstrated no recurrences in 12 patients with stage I disease treated with platinum-based therapy, and Kelly showed that 0 of 15 patients had a recurrence with IB UPSC tumors treated with platinum chemotherapy compared with 10 of 13 who did not receive chemotherapy. In a review of the GOG phase III experience of advanced or recurrent endometrial cancers by McMeekin et al., there was no difference noted in response rate to chemotherapy based on histologic type (endometrioid vs. UPSC/CC).

The optimal therapy for UPSC/CC tumors remains to be determined. Chemotherapy alone or in combination with radiation is being investigated. Given unique molecular findings in UPSC and CC tumors, it is also hoped that targeted therapies may offer a unique option in this disease.

Carcinosarcoma

Clinical profile. Most patients with uterine carcinosarcoma present with postmenopausal bleeding. As in other cases of postmenopausal bleeding, histologic evaluation by endometrial biopsy or curettage is mandatory and will establish the diagnosis. Not infrequently, a large polypoid mass may extend from the endometrial cavity protruding through the cervical os, which can be easily biopsied (Fig. 5.16). Carcinosarcomas have both malignant epithelial and mesenchymal elements, but on small biopsies, the epithelial component may be the only one recognized preoperatively (Figs. 5.17 and 5.18). Some patients may present without bleeding but with an enlarging pelvic mass as a result of tumor and hematometrium. Patients with advanced-stage disease may present similarly to patients with ovarian cancer with pleural effusions, ascites, adnexal masses, and evidence of intraperitoneal disease spread.

Preoperative assessment with imaging studies is controversial. At a minimum, chest radiography is recommended given the potential for distant disease spread. For common endometrial cancers, routine preoperative CT scans have not been shown to alter clinical management, but data are limited for

patients with carcinosarcoma. Consultation with a gynecologic oncologist should strongly be considered in cases with a preoperative diagnosis of carcinosarcoma.

Surgical management. The surgical management for patients with uterine carcinosarcoma should include collection of cytologic washings, hysterectomy with bilateral salpingo-oophorectomy, and pelvic and paraaortic lymph node dissection. Patients with carcinosarcoma of the uterus should be staged according to the 2009 FIGO staging system for endometrial cancer. Extrauterine disease spread in carcinosarcoma is not uncommon. In one analysis of the SEER data from 1988 to 2004, 40% of cases were classified as having stage III or IV disease. When gross extrauterine disease is encountered, many advocate a debulking surgery akin to what is used to manage ovarian cancer.

The GOG prospectively evaluated disease distribution in 530 patients with clinical stage I or II uterine sarcomas. All patients underwent collection of pelvic washings, hysterectomy, and pelvic and paraaortic lymph node dissection. In the subgroup of 301 patients with carcinosarcoma, extrauterine disease was found commonly; 21% were identified with positive cytologic washing, 37% had myometrial invasion into the outer half of the myometrium, 12% had adnexal metastases, and 17% had

FIGURE 5.16 Uterine carcinosarcoma with a polypoid mass filling the uterine cavity and with deep myometrial invasion. (Courtesy of Dr. Pablo Souza, University of Oklahoma.)

FIGURE 5.17 Close-up view of specimen in Fig. 5.16 showing carcinosarcoma with tumor filling the endometrial cavity. (Courtesy of Dr. Pablo Souza, University of Oklahoma.)

nodal involvement. Compared with a similar surgical staging study conducted by the GOG evaluating endometrial cancer patients, positive cytology was found in only 12%, deep myometrial invasion in 22%, adnexal involvement in 5%, and nodal metastases in 9% of cases (Table 5.22). For carcinosarcoma,

FIGURE 5.18 Photomicrograph of carcinosarcoma of the uterus. Within the tumor are two discrete malignant populations: a high-grade epithelial component (**A**) and a stromal component (**B**). (Courtesy of Dr. Pablo Souza, University of Oklahoma.)

after surgical staging, 59% were stage I, 21% were stage II, 9% were stage III, and 11% were stage IV. In almost every case, when extrauterine metastases are encountered, only the epithelial component of the tumor was present.

Carcinosarcomas frequently carry a poor prognosis. In some cases managed without complete surgical staging, unrecognized disease spread may account for poorer outcomes. For example, in the 1988 to 2004 SEER database, of 3962 cases of carcinosarcoma, only 53% underwent lymph node dissection. For patients with apparent uterine confined disease, 5-year cancer-specific survival was 59% for stage Ia (no myometrial invasion), 54% for stage IB, and 38% for stage Ic. Even in series with uniform use of staging recurrences are common, indicating that unrecognized disease spread occurs frequently. In the GOG series, 53% of all patients with carcinosarcoma and 40% with stage I disease had a recurrence within 3 years of diagnosis. As in endometrial cancer, survival was related to the presence of nodal metastases, to the depth of myometrial invasion, and to whether the lower uterine segment or cervix was involved. Patients with adnexal involvement also had a poor prognosis. Ferguson reported a series of 42 patients in stage I who all underwent pelvic nodal dissection and found 3-year disease-free survival and OS were 42% and 62%, respectively, even though nearly all patients received some form of postoperative adjuvant therapy.

Although many believe carcinosarcoma to actually represent a metaplastic high-grade or undifferentiated endometrial cancer (and not a true sarcoma), some data indicate a different clinical behavior between uterine carcinosarcoma and high-grade (grade III, serous, or clear cell) endometrial cancers. Amant and colleagues compared 104 patients with grade III, UPSC, or clear cell endometrial cancers with 33 patients with carcinosarcoma. Among patients with stage I or II disease, patients with carcinosarcoma had a poorer survival rate and a higher incidence of pulmonary metastases. Carcinosarcoma was also an independent predictor of survival with an HR of 3.2 for recurrence compared with the other histologies. In a population-based comparison between carcinosarcoma and grade III endometrioid cancers, patients with carcinosarcoma had poorer survival compared with endometrioid cancers when compared stage by stage. For example, the 5-year survival rate was 38% versus 68% for patients with stage IC disease. Some have argued that based on the differences in clinical behavior, carcinosarcoma should be studied separately from high-risk endometrial cancers.

TABLE 5.22 Frequency and Distribution of Disease Spread in Patients With Uterine Malignancies

	Carcinosarcoma (%) (n = 301)	Leiomyosarcoma (%) (n = 59)	Endometrial Adenocarcinoma (%) (n = 621)
Deep myometrial invasion	37	—	22
Positive peritoneal cytology	21	5	12
Adnexal involvement	12	3	5
Nodal metastases	17	3.5	9

From Major FJ, Blessing JA, Silverberg SG, et al. Prognostic factors in early-stage uterine sarcoma: a Gynecologic Oncology Group study. *Cancer* 1993;71:1702; Creasman WT, Morrow CP, Bundy BN, et al. Surgical pathologic spread patterns of endometrial cancer: a Gynecologic Oncology Group study. *Cancer* 1987;60:2035.

Patterns of failure after surgery alone or after adjuvant therapies can help to inform how to best direct therapies for patients with cancers. For example, local therapies such as pelvic radiation may reduce local (vaginal or pelvic) failures but have no or minimal effect on the frequency that cancers recur at distant sites (lung, liver, abdominal cavity). In the GOG study (#20), 40% of patients received postoperative pelvic radiation therapy, with 17% of these patients having a recurrence in the pelvis, 16% at an extrapelvic location, and 19% in the lung (Table 5.23). In the 60% of patients who received no radiation, 24% had a pelvic recurrence, 24% had an extrapelvic recurrence, and 10% recurred in the lung. In the GOG trial, therapy was not randomized but was selected by the physician. Pelvic recurrences usually develop within the first 12 to 18 months after diagnosis and surgery. In a series of 23 carcinosarcoma patients with surgically staged, stage I disease who received no postoperative therapy, 11 patients were noted to have recurrence. The median time to recurrence in these patients was 13 months, and patterns of failure showed that three patients had an isolated pelvic recurrence, three had an isolated distant recurrence, and five had both local and distant failures.

Adjuvant Therapy

Postoperative radiation therapy or chemotherapy has been used to reduce the risk of recurrence in patients with uterine sarcoma. In older studies, all types of uterine sarcomas were commonly grouped together so that the effect of therapy on a particular histologic type of sarcoma was largely unknown. Historically, radiation therapy has been most commonly used in an effort to reduce pelvic failures. When radiation therapy is given, 4500 to 6000 cGy to the pelvis has been advocated, with some also recommending intravaginal brachytherapy to deliver a boost to the vaginal cuff or entire vagina. Preoperative radiation is infrequently used and typically reserved for cases with bulky cervical involvement or parametrial extension.

Several series have shown improved rates of local control with the use of radiation without necessarily improving survival rates compared with patients managed without radiation. In a prospective GOG study (#20) that included patients with stage I or II uterine sarcomas of all types, 156 patients were randomly assigned to postoperative treatment with doxorubicin or not. Pelvic radiation was permitted at the physician's discretion. In this study, which included 93 patients with carcinosarcoma, 47% of patients' disease recurred with or without the use of pelvic radiation therapy (Table 5.24). Pelvic radiation did appear to reduce local recurrences. Similarly, there was not a statistically significant difference in recurrence rates, PFS, or survival in patients who did or did not receive doxorubicin. More recently, EORTC enrolled 224 patients with stage I or II uterine sarcomas (including 91 with carcinosarcoma) and randomly assigned patients to observation vs. pelvic radiation therapy after surgery. For the group as a whole, there was no difference in disease-free survival or OS between the two treatment groups. For patients with carcinosarcoma, improved local control was noted with pelvic radiation therapy. The study found that after observation, 47% of patients with carcinosarcoma developed a local recurrence versus 24% after pelvic radiation. Distant sites of failure remained a significant problem regardless of treatment (35% after radiation; 29% with observation).

TABLE 5.23   Patterns of Failure in Uterine Sarcomas

Site of First Failure	Carcinosarcoma (n = 301)		Leiomyosarcoma (n = 59)	
	No Radiation (n = 182)	Radiation (n = 119)	No Radiation (n = 46)	Radiation (n = 13)
Pelvis	24%	17%	17%	0
Extrapelvic	24%	16%	29%	8%
Lung	10%	19%	37%	54%
Other	11%	7%	4%	15%

Adapted from Major FJ, Blessing JA, Silverberg SG, et al. Prognostic factors in early-stage uterine sarcoma: a Gynecologic Oncology Group study. *Cancer* 1993;71:1702.

TABLE 5.24   Gynecologic Oncology Group Randomized Trial of Doxorubicin Versus No Further Therapy in Completely Resected Stage I and Stage II Uterine Sarcoma: Rates of Recurrence

	Adjuvant Doxorubicin (n = 75)		No Chemotherapy (n = 53)	
CS (n = 90)	39%		51%	
LMS (n = 52)	44%		61%	
	Adjuvant Doxorubicin (n = 75)		No Chemotherapy (n = 53)	
	Radiation (n = 31)	No Radiation (n = 44)	Radiation (n = 28)	No Radiation (n = 53)
All sarcoma types (n = 156)	39%	43%	57%	51%
	Radiation ± Chemotherapy (n = 59)		No Radiation ± Chemotherapy (n = 97)	
All sarcoma types (n = 156)	47%		47%	

CS, Carcinosarcoma; *LMS*, leiomyosarcoma.
Modified from Omura GA, Blessing JA, Majors F, et al. A randomized clinical trial of adjuvant Adriamycin in uterine sarcoma: a Gynecologic Oncology Group study. *J Clin Oncol* 1985;3:1240.

Because a common site of failure is at a distant site from the pelvis, the use of adjuvant local irradiation, although improving local control, may ultimately have no effect in increasing the OS rate. Systemic therapy using chemotherapy with or without radiation has been evaluated in adjuvant settings. The selection of drugs or regimens likely to be beneficial is based on information from studies performed with patient populations with advanced or recurrent disease. To date, ifosfamide, cisplatin, and paclitaxel have shown the most promise for development for carcinosarcomas. Kanjeekal and colleagues reviewed the literature on the chemotherapy for uterine sarcomas and noted that for carcinosarcoma, the most promising regimens would likely include platinum-based combinations. Drawing on experience from patients with advanced and recurrent carcinosarcoma, which found that the combination regimen of ifosfamide and cisplatin produced nearly a doubling in response rate and a modestly prolonged PFS compared with ifosfamide alone (GOG0107), the GOG initiated a randomized trial comparing three cycles of ifosfamide and cisplatin with whole-abdominal radiation therapy (WART) (GOG0150). Eligible patients could have had stage I to IV disease provided no residual disease greater than 1 cm remained after surgery. For the group as a whole, stage was one of the most important prognostic factors, with 37% of patients with stage I disease versus 80% with stage IV disease having a recurrence by 5 years. The crude 5-year rate of recurrence rate was 58% for patients treated by WART versus 52% for chemotherapy. After adjusting for stage and age, the recurrence rate was 29% lower for chemotherapy; however, the results did not achieve statistical significance (relative hazard, 0.789; CI 0.48–1.04; $P = 0.245$). Despite this, the authors concluded the results supported further evaluation of combination chemotherapy in future research trials. A retrospective review by Makker and colleagues of 49 patients with stage I to IV disease treated by radiation alone versus chemotherapy ± radiation suggested that the inclusion of chemotherapy into an adjuvant regimen improved PFS and OS compared with chemotherapy alone.

Management of Recurrent Disease

Not unlike with surgical development, the development of chemotherapy in uterine sarcomas began with studies combining all uterine sarcoma types. This strategy appeared justified because, regardless of tumor type, about half the patients with early-stage uterine sarcoma developed a recurrence. Given its importance in patients with soft tissue sarcomas, doxorubicin has been used extensively in patients with uterine sarcomas. The GOG performed a randomized trial comparing doxorubicin with or without DTIC (dimethyl triazenoimidazole carboxamide) in 226 patients with stage III, stage IV, and recurrent sarcomas of the uterus. There was no difference in response rate, PFS, or survival between doxorubicin and doxorubicin plus DTIC-treated groups. Response rate for leiomyosarcoma was 25% versus 15% for carcinosarcoma, and survival time of patients with leiomyosarcoma was significantly longer than that of patients with other cell types. This study was important because it suggested that there was a difference between

sarcomas types and response to different agents. With the recognition that there are differences in prognosis and response between the histologic types, carcinosarcoma and leiomyosarcoma are now studied in separate chemotherapy trials.

The first GOG trial to evaluate carcinosarcomas as a separate group was reported by Thigpen and coworkers (#26-C). This phase II study evaluated cisplatin in 28 patients with advanced or recurrent disease who had received prior chemotherapy and had measurable disease. The response rate was 18%, with two patients obtaining a complete response. A subsequent phase II study used cisplatin in a similar group of 63 patients who had not received prior chemotherapy and noted a response rate of 19% (8% complete response).

As a result of activity seen in soft tissue sarcomas, ifosfamide was selected for evaluation in uterine sarcomas. Using ifosfamide with the uroprotective agent mesna (2-mercaptoethane sodium sulfate), Sutton reported for the GOG on 28 patients with advanced or recurrent carcinosarcoma who had not received prior chemotherapy (#87-B). He described a 32% response rate, including 18% of patients with a complete response. Given these promising results, interest in studying combination regimens in this disease resurfaced. The GOG evaluated ifosfamide and mesna with and without cisplatin in patients with advanced, persistent, or recurrent carcinosarcomas in a phase III study (#108). The study evaluated 194 patients and found that response rate for ifosfamide alone was 36% compared to 54% for the combination. Patients treated with cisplatin had a modest improvement in median PFS (6 months vs. 4 months), but there was no statistically significant improvement in survival (ifosfamide, 9 months vs. ifosfamide plus cisplatin, 10 months, median survival). The combination regimen produced greater incidences of neutropenia, anemia, and peripheral neuropathy.

Paclitaxel has been evaluated in 44 patients with advanced or recurrent disease who all had received one prior chemotherapy regimen. Curtin et al. for the GOG reported an 18% response rate with acceptable toxicity. The GOG has subsequently conducted a phase III trial comparing ifosfamide with and without paclitaxel (#161). This trial enrolled 179 eligible patients with stage III, IV, or recurrent carcinosarcoma who had not received prior chemotherapy. The combination regimen produced higher response rates (45% vs. 29%), longer PFS (median, 5.8 months vs. 3.6 months), and longer survival times (median, 13.5 months vs. 8.4 months). There was a 31% decrease in the HR of death (0.69; 95% CI 0.49–0.97; $P = 0.03$). The combination regimen produced more neuropathy and thrombocytopenia and required 3 days for infusion. Because there is interest in improving convenience and cost and reducing toxicity, other regimens have been evaluated in patients with carcinosarcoma. Powell reported on a phase II study, GOG0232-B, evaluating the combination of paclitaxel with carboplatin in 46 patients with advanced or recurrent carcinosarcoma. The response rate was 54% (13% complete response), and 59% of patients completed six or more cycles of therapy. The GOG has completed but not yet reported a phase III trial (#261) comparing ifosfamide–paclitaxel with paclitaxel–carboplatin in untreated patients.

Follow-Up

After surgery, with or without adjuvant therapy, patients with endometrial cancer should enter a routine surveillance program. We advocate for patients to be seen every 3 to 4 months for the first 2 years and then yearly. Most recurrences manifest within 2 years, making closer surveillance during this time reasonable. Surveillance visits should include a focused review of systems (questions related to pelvic, leg, or back pain; vaginal bleeding urinary changes; changes in bowel habits) and physical examination, including pelvic examination. Routine Pap smear collection of the vaginal cuff is controversial. We tend to perform Pap smears as a sampling of the vaginal cuff in an effort to afford early detection of vaginal cuff recurrences. Some have suggested that routine Pap smears are not cost-effective and that most recurrences are clinically palpable or associated with patient symptoms. In addition, after radiation (vaginal or pelvic), vaginal cuff recurrences are uncommon, and radiation may produce cytologic changes occasionally difficult to classify. Most low- and intermediate-risk patients do not require routine, scheduled imaging studies to evaluate for recurrence. Patients with new complaints or worsening of abdominal and pelvic complaints may be considered for additional studies (CT scans, colonoscopy). It has been suggested by some that CA-125 can be used to monitor therapy in patients with advanced or recurrent adenocarcinoma of the endometrium, much as is done in ovarian cancer. Niloff and colleagues and others have noted that CA-125 is elevated in as many as three-fourths of these patients.

Data are limited in regard to monitoring. Fanning and Piver did note in 21 women that clinical response, in addition to subsequent relapse, correlated with CA-125 levels of patients with advanced or recurrent disease. Monitoring with CA-125 is helpful, primarily in patients with high risk for recurrent disease, as in patients with recurrent disease receiving therapy who have a proven elevation of their serum value.

Even though the most patients with endometrial carcinoma do not experience recurrence or die of disease, the number of endometrial cancer deaths has risen over the past several years. Patients identified with recurrence are assessed for treatment options. Long-term disease control of recurrent disease is a function of site of recurrence. Patients with recurrence at a distant site or with multiple sites of recurrence are best treated with hormonal or chemotherapy, as discussed earlier, in a palliative setting. Isolated vaginal cuff recurrences may occur, particularly in patients in whom postoperative radiation was not used. Provided no other disease spread is noted, 60% to 80% of patients with vaginal cuff recurrences can achieve long-term disease control with the use of surgery, radiation therapy, or both. Patients with pelvic sidewall or isolated paraaortic recurrences may have long-term disease control, but overall prognosis is poorer than with vaginal recurrence. Rarely, patients with vaginal or pelvic recurrence after radiation therapy may be offered pelvic exenteration with the hopes of cure.

For the bibliography list, log onto www.expertconsult.com ⟨http://www.expertconsult.com⟩.

6

Sarcoma of the Uterus

D. Scott McMeekin, MD, William T. Creasman, MD

OUTLINE

KEY POINTS

1. Uterine sarcomas are uncommon tumors. The most common tumors are leiomyosarcomas (LMSs) (59%) and endometrial stromal sarcomas (ESSs) (33%). Other sarcomas comprise less than 8% of the remaining.

2. The standard treatment for any sarcoma is removal of the uterus tubes and ovaries if possible.

3. The prognosis of LMSs is poor; even at an early stage, adjuvant therapy has not been shown to affect survival.

4. ESSs are often hormonally responsive.

CLASSIFICATION

Sarcomas are uncommon tumors arising from mesenchymal elements and are distinguished from carcinomas that arise from epithelial elements. Uterine sarcomas are thought to arise primarily from two tissues: endometrial stroma and the uterine muscle itself. When endometrial mesenchymal tissue undergoes malignant transformation, it may be accompanied by a malignant epithelial component (carcinosarcoma [CS], formerly referred to as malignant mixed Müllerian tumor), it may be associated with a benign-appearing epithelial component (adenosarcoma), or it may have no recognizable epithelial component (endometrial stromal sarcoma [ESS]). Tumors arising from malignant transformation of uterine smooth muscle are known as uterine leiomyosarcomas (LMSs). Other sarcomas, such as angiosarcoma and fibrosarcoma, arise in supporting tissues and are rare.

INCIDENCE AND EPIDEMIOLOGY

The Surveillance, Epidemiology, and End Results (SEER) database notes that LMSs account for 59% of 8365 cases reported. ESSs are represented by 33%, and other sarcomas account for 8%. The peak age for all sarcomas was 45 to 54 years with the peak age for LMS being slightly older than 55 years.

In previous editions, classification of sarcomas included CS, LMS, and ESS as the three most common uterine sarcomas with CS being the most common. **Convincing evidence now suggest that CSs are not true sarcomas but are derived from epithelial cells and therefore are now included as a type 2 endometrial cancer category. Although there are minor other types of uterine sarcoma, their occurrence is such that they will not be included in this chapter.**

Sarcomas arising within the uterus are relatively rare and account for 3% to 8% of uterine cancers. According to the SEER, the age-adjusted incidences for all sarcomas (per 100,000 women age 35 years and older) in US women were 2.68 for Native American, Asian, and Hispanic; 3.58 for white; and 7.02 for black women. By comparison, the incidence for epithelial uterine cancers, per 100,000 women, is roughly nine for black women and 20 for white women. Uterine sarcomas represented 8% of primary uterine malignancies in the most recent analysis of the SEER database. Harlow and coworkers had previously reported from SEER databases covering 1973 to 1981 that suggested an annual incidence of only 1.7 cases per 100,000 women. Sarcomas have been traditionally thought to represent only 3% to 5% of all uterine tumors. The increasing incidence of uterine sarcomas noted in the SEER studies may reflect better diagnosis and perhaps a true increase in an aging population.

The type and frequency of uterine sarcomas are related to both age and race. LMS can occur at an early age, has an incidence plateau in middle age, and declines thereafter. In a large prospective surgical-pathologic study conducted by the Gynecologic Oncology Group (GOG) evaluating patients with all types of sarcomas, the median age of patients with LMS was 55 years compared with 65 years for those with CS. Brooks and coworkers suggested that white women were older at the time of diagnosis of their sarcomas compared with black women.

Using SEER data (1992–1998), Sherman and Devesa reported on racial differences in uterine malignancies. They found that for all histopathologic categories, the age-adjusted incidence of uterine cancers (per 100,000 women) was 23 for non-Hispanic white, 14 for white Hispanic, and 15 for black women. In contrast, LMSs are more common in black women. For LMSs, ESSs, and adenosarcomas combined, the incidence was 1.24 for black versus 0.79 for non-Hispanic white women. Harlow and associates found the same trend reporting on an earlier SEER data set. It has also been suggested that blacks present with stage I disease less commonly than whites. Given that uterine sarcomas are rare and form a heterogeneous group, little is known about other risk factors favoring development of these tumors.

LEIOMYOSARCOMA

Clinical Profile

Many of these patients experience perimenopausal bleeding, are found to have a pelvic mass on examination, and will be thought to have uterine leiomyomas. Giuntoli and coworkers, reporting on the Mayo Clinic experience of 208 patients with uterine LMS collected over a 23-year period, found that vaginal bleeding was the most common symptom (56%) followed by a palpable pelvic mass (54%) and pelvic pain (22%). **A commonly described "clinical pearl" has been the relationship of a rapidly enlarging uterus to LMS. The data to support such an observation are mixed, however.** Parker and associates evaluated 1332 patients who underwent surgery for presumed leiomyoma. In the group of 371 patients who had rapid uterine growth, only one case (0.2%) of LMS was identified. Similarly, in a subgroup of 198 patients who had carefully documented rapid uterine growth, no cases of LMS were found. Leibsohn and coworkers reported on 1432 patients undergoing hysterectomy for bleeding related to uterine leiomyomas and identified 7 (0.49%) patients with LMS.

Because LMS arises within the uterine smooth muscle, biopsy of the malignant tissue is difficult, and many lesions are found only at final pathology. In Leibsohn et al.'s series none of the seven patients with LMS were identified on preoperative biopsy and in only three cases was there an intraoperative suspicion of sarcoma. Various authors have reported that LMS may be present in the submucosa of the uterus in 30% to 50% of patients, but even at that, biopsy diagnosis is not easily accomplished. Schwartz and coworkers described the tumors to be both broad based and pedunculated and that in 19 of 20 cases, the LMS was confined to one mass.

Because of the difficulty in establishing a preoperative diagnosis and the high frequency of uterine leiomyoma in the population, it is not unexpected that several case reports have detailed the finding of LMSs in patients who have undergone conservative management of symptomatic leiomyomas by myomectomy, after Lupron treatment before myomectomy, and after vascular embolization of presumed leiomyomas. These cases speak to the importance of pretreatment counseling of patients who undergo such therapies.

There is considerable discussion about the histologic criteria necessary for the diagnosis of LMS (Fig. 6.1). LMSs must be

FIGURE 6.1 Photomicrograph of uterine leiomyosarcoma demonstrating the malignant lesion at the top right, normal endometrium at the bottom left, and normal myometrium between them.

TABLE 6.1   **Metastatic Potential of Smooth Muscle Tumors of the Uterus**

Mitotic Figures/10 hpf	Atypia*	Diagnosis	Metastatic Potential
1–4	Any degree	Leiomyoma	Very low
5–9	None	Leiomyoma with high mitotic activity	Very low
5–9	Grade 1	Smooth muscle tumor of uncertain malignant potential	Low
5–9	Grade 2 or 3	Leiomyosarcoma	Moderate
≥10	Grade 1	Leiomyosarcoma	High
≥10	Grade 2 or 3	Leiomyosarcoma	Very high

*Grade based on a scale of 1 to 3.
From O'Connor DM, Norris HJ. Mitotically active leiomyomas of the uterus. *Hum Pathol* 1990;21:223.

distinguished from a variety of benign smooth muscle tumors (Table 6.1). The predominant differentiating features between benign and malignant tumors include mitotic activity (as gauged by the number of mitotic figures per 10 high-power fields [hpf]), cellular atypia, and necrosis. Leiomyoma, cellular leiomyoma, and bizarre leiomyoma (also called atypical or symplastic leiomyoma) are considered to be benign. These entities are distinguished from LMS mainly by the mitotic count of the tumor. Although cellular leiomyomas and bizarre leiomyomas may appear at first sight to be malignant, they contain fewer than 5 mitoses/10 hpf on histologic evaluation, and the prognosis is excellent with surgery only. Smooth muscle tumors of uncertain malignant potential (STUMP) include a group of smooth muscle tumors with 5 to 9 mitoses/10 hpf that can exhibit a variable behavior.

Intravenous leiomyomatosis is a rare smooth muscle tumor characterized by nodular masses of histologically benign smooth muscle cells growing within venous channels that are lined by epithelium; arteries are not involved. Treatment involves surgical removal, and the prognosis is good.

Recurrences are unusual and are usually managed successfully with further surgical excision.

Benign metastasizing leiomyoma is another rare condition in which smooth muscle tumor deposits are found in the lung, lymph nodes, or abdomen and appear histologically like a benign leiomyoma. Most women have a history of pelvic surgery for benign leiomyomas years before these metastatic sites are recognized. Surgical excision has been the primary treatment.

Norris and Taylor believed that mitotic count was extremely important in that if fewer than 10 mitoses/10 hpf were identified, the lesion was benign regardless of the degree of cellular atypia; if more than 10 mitoses/10 hpf were present, the prognosis was grave. More recently, Norris and Taylor stated that tumors with fewer than 5 mitoses/10 hpf can rarely metastasize. In a follow-up study from the Armed Forces Institute of Pathology, O'Connor and Norris evaluated 73 smooth muscle tumors of the uterus with 5 to 9 mitotic figures/10 hpf but lacking cytologic atypia. They concluded that the metastatic rate was too low to consider these as being sarcoma. Several of their patients were treated only with myomectomies with excellent results. Lissoni and colleagues have suggested extending this philosophy to additional patients.

Kempson and Bari believe that the mitotic count is important but state that prognosis is poor if more than 5 mitoses/10 hpf are identified. Their experience with tumors containing 5 to 9 mitoses/10 hpf indicates that the tumors usually behave aggressively and will metastasize. These authors believe that the degree of cellular atypia is of limited value by itself in determining the malignancy of smooth muscle tumors. In tumors with higher mitotic counts, there were usually a greater number of very atypical cells. This atypia was also seen in tumors with 5 to 9 mitoses/10 hpf. Tumors with fewer than 5 mitoses/10 hpf were thought to be benign regardless of the atypia of the cells. None of Kempson and Bari's patients with fewer than 5 mitoses/10 hpf had disease outside the uterus, but distant disease was a common finding if more than 5 mitoses/10 hpf were noted. The presence of coagulative necrosis, especially with diffuse significant atypia, suggests strongly that the lesion is a LMS regardless of the mitotic count.

However, Silverberg believes that the mitotic count alone cannot be used as a strict histologic criterion because he had patients with fewer than 10 mitoses/10 hpf who succumbed to their disease. He emphasized that the grade of the tumor, which reflects the cytologic atypia, is a better criterion than mitotic count alone. Toledo and Oliva point out that mitotic rate alone is not sufficient to predict prognosis. Although mitotic rate and nuclear atypia are important features, tumor cell necrosis is a unique feature of LMS. Most uterine LMS with necrosis will show high mitotic rate and atypia. Essentially all investigators note the gravity of the situation if intravascular invasion or disease outside the uterus is found. Silverberg believes that the single most important prognostic indicator is the menopausal status of the patient. Women who are premenopausal when the diagnosis is made tend to have a much better prognosis than that of women who are postmenopausal, even when criteria such as blood vessel invasion, growth pattern, grade, and mitotic counts are considered. LMSs occur in young patients and tend to be more localized when they are first diagnosed, and they probably exhibit a slower growth pattern than CSs or ESSs do.

Surgical Management

Planning the surgical management of LMS is difficult because many cases go unrecognized preoperatively. Patients commonly undergo myomectomy or hysterectomy for presumptive leiomyomas, which are subsequently identified as a sarcoma. When a preoperative diagnosis is known, hysterectomy should be performed. Retention of the ovaries in premenopausal patients has not shown to worsen outcome in several retrospective series and may be considered. Surgical staging with lymph node dissection is controversial, but most authorities tend to recommend biopsy of suspicious nodes only. When LMS is recognized postoperatively, reexploration for the purposes of completing surgical staging is not recommended. After diagnosis, evaluation of the chest with chest radiography or computed tomography is reasonable given the propensity of spread to the lungs. Goff and colleagues found that 10% of patients with LMS had lung metastases at presentation.

Data on patterns of spread for LMS are limited by the rarity of the tumor. Goff and coworkers found that 16 of 21 patients had stage I disease at surgery, and only patients with disseminated intraabdominal disease had nodal involvement. Giuntoli and coworkers reported that only 34 of 208 patients in the Mayo Clinic series had pelvic nodal dissections performed, and of the four with positive nodes, extrauterine disease was reported in three. The GOG sarcoma study on patterns of spread found that in 59 surgically staged patients, 5% had positive extrauterine spread to peritoneal cytology, 3% had adnexal involvement, and 3.5% had nodal metastases (Table 6.2). After surgical staging, 83% were stage I, and only 13% of patients were upstaged based on biopsies. In 2009, the Federation of International Gynecologists and Obstetricians (FIGO) introduced a new staging system for LMS, ESS, and adenosarcoma. For LMS, stage reflects tumor size and extrauterine spread (see Table 6.2).

Leiomyosarcomas most commonly spread hematogenously. Corscaden and Singh reported the results of autopsies of 15 patients who died of LMS of the uterus. Of these patients, 100% had intraabdominal visceral involvement, 80% had lung or pleural metastases, 40% had paraaortic nodal involvement, 33% had renal metastases, and 20% had liver metastases. In the GOG study, the most common first site of recurrence was the lung (41%), and only 13% had a pelvic failure (Table 6.3).

The prognosis for LMS is poor, even for early-stage disease. Vardi found that of the total group of 32 patients, 44% died of disease within the first 3 years after diagnosis. There was a 63.6% 5-year survival rate in women in whom diagnosis was made while they were premenopausal compared with a 5.5% 5-year survival in postmenopausal women. The GOG found that only 31% of patients remained disease free at 3 years. Gadducci and coworkers found that 39% of patients with stage I or II disease had a recurrence, with a median time to recurrence of 18 months. Berchuck and coworkers reported that only 29% of patients with stage I or II disease remained free of disease, with a median follow-up period of 7.5 years. Although almost all deaths and recurrences are during the 4 years after diagnosis, Gallup and coworkers reported a recurrence 25 years after initial therapy. Contrary to an older perception, these data indicate that LMSs have a poorer prognosis than CSs.

Predictors of outcome have been assessed by several groups. The GOG found that patients with greater numbers of mitoses were associated with an increased risk of recurrence such that 79% of patients with more than 20 mitoses/hpf recurred compared with 61% with 10 to 20 mitoses/hpf. Patients who present with extrauterine disease also have a very poor prognosis. Berchuck and coworkers found no survivors beyond 2 years in this group of patients. Gadducci and coworkers assessed 126 patients collected from a multi-institutional study and identified stage, mitotic count, and age as independent prognostic factors predicting recurrence. Giuntoli and coworkers found that high grade, advanced stage, and having had ovaries removed at surgery were independent predictors of poorer survival.

Adjuvant Therapy

For patients with LMS, no adjuvant therapy has been shown to be effective in prolonging survival. As with other high-risk uterine cancers, LMSs have been managed postoperatively by radiation therapy or chemotherapy. Berchuck and coworkers found that among patients receiving any form of adjuvant therapy, 83% recurred compared with 68% who underwent surgery alone. Given the propensity for hematogenous spread, radiation does not adequately address the high frequency of distant sites of failure (lung, liver, abdominal cavity). Supporters of radiation note that pelvic control may be obtained, which can prevent bulky pelvic recurrences and improve patient comfort and quality of life. The GOG reported that only three of 13 patients who received radiation remained without recurrence, but no pelvic failures were seen. Giuntoli and coworkers performed a subset analysis within their large series of patients, identifying 31 patients who received adjuvant radiation therapy. In a comparison with 31 well-matched patients who did not receive radiation, there was not a statistically significant difference in survival between the groups, although the 5-year survival rate for those receiving radiation was 60% compared with 40% without radiation therapy. In the only prospective randomized trial, the European Organization for Research and Treatment of Cancer (EORTC) showed in the subgroup of 103 patients with LMS, there was no improvement of local control with radiation (local recurrence; 20% after radiation vs. 24% after surgery alone). Of note, most patients developed distant sites of failure.

Given the importance of distant failures in this disease, chemotherapy has been used to manage early-stage LMSs. In the GOG adjuvant trial evaluating the role of doxorubicin with or without radiation, 61% of patients with LMS treated without doxorubicin compared with 44% who received chemotherapy had a recurrence. This study **was too small to specifically evaluate the importance that histology played in response to therapy. With the identification of an active combination regimen of docetaxel plus gemcitabine for patients with advanced or recurrent disease, early data suggest that this regimen may hold promise in an adjuvant setting.** In one series of 18 patients with stage I or II LMS, 59% remain progression free at 3 years.

Hensley et al. reported results of a phase II study of 23 patients completely resected LMS treated with four cycles of gemcitabine and docetaxel. In patients with uterus-limited disease, the 2-year progression-free survival (PFS) rate was

---

TABLE 6.2   Federation of International Gynecologists and Obstetricians 2009 Staging Classification for Uterine Sarcomas

Stage I (tumor limited to uterus)*
  IA: <5 cm tumor size
  IB: ≥5 cm tumor size

For Leiomyosarcoma
  IA: tumor limited to endometrium or endocervix without myometrial invasion
  IB: tumor invades <50% myometrium
  IC: tumor invades ≥50% myometrium

For Endometrial Stromal Sarcoma and Adenosarcoma
Stage II (tumor extension into the pelvis)
  IIA: adnexal involvement
  IIB: other extrauterine pelvic disease
Stage III (tumor invades abdominal tissues)
  IIIA: one site of involvement
  IIIB: >1 site of involvement
  IIIC: metastasis to pelvic and/or paraaortic lymph nodes
Stage IV (tumor invades bladder and/or rectum, and/or distant metastasis)
  IVA: involvement of bladder and/or rectum
  IVB: distant metastasis

*For stage I disease, two substages are used based on tumor type. Modified from Mutch DG. Meeting Report—the new FIGO staging system for cancers of the vulva, cervix, endometrium and sarcomas. *Gynecol Oncol* 2009;115:325-328 and FIGO Committee. FIGO staging for uterine sarcomas. *Int J Gynecol Obstet* 2009;104:179.

TABLE 6.3   Frequency and Distribution of Disease Spread in Patients With Uterine Malignancies

	Carcinosarcoma (%) (n = 301)	Leiomyosarcoma (%) (n = 59)	Endometrial Adenocarcinoma (%) (n = 621)
Deep myometrial invasion	37	—	22
Positive peritoneal cytology	21	5	12
Adnexal involvement	12	3	5
Nodal metastases	17	3.5	9

59%. GOG 277 evaluated 47 women with uterine-limited disease with four cycles of doxorubicin followed by four courses of gemcitabine and docetaxel. At a median follow-up period of 27.4 months, a 78% 2 year PFS was noted with a median PFS of 39.3 months.

Hensley and coworkers more recently enrolled 46 with resected uterus-limited high-grade uterine LMS who received four cycles of gemcitabine and docetaxel. If confirmed disease free after four cycles, they then received four cycles of doxorubicin. At 2 years, PFS was 78% of patients; it was 57% at 3 years. Bevacizumab was added to the gemcitabine–docetaxel regimen in 25 women with combined complete and partial response of 44%. GOG 250 enrolled patients with LMS in a phase III placcbo-controlled study to evaluate the addition of bevacizumab to gemcitabine and docetaxel. The addition of bevacizumab failed to improve PFS, overall survival, or OR. Currently, there is a randomized trial of adjuvant chemotherapy versus observation in women with LMS limited to the uterus (GOG 277).

Multiple single agents have been tried and have been unsuccessful. Recently, there has been an increased interest in the study of biologic targets, including mTOR (mammalian target of rapamycin) inhibitors, with modest results. Multikinase inhibitors that affect the vascular endothelial growth factor pathway to date have been unsuccessful.

Management of Recurrent Disease

Data from randomized phase III trials conducted by the GOG, which included advanced and recurrent uterine sarcomas of all types, helped to identify the differential sensitivity of LMSs compared with CSs to different agents. In the trial comparing doxorubicin with and without dacarbazine (DTIC), patients with LMSs were found to have longer survival times compared with patients with other types when treated with a doxorubicin-containing regimen. In a subsequent study using doxorubicin with or without cyclophosphamide, histologic type was not found to be a prognostic indicator. Given that 80% of all patients died of disease within 2 years, the GOG adopted a strategy of performing phase II trials with the hope of identifying active agents that could later be tested in randomized studies. The rarity of LMSs, however, has made randomized study of this tumor more difficult.

Historically, doxorubicin and ifosfamide have demonstrated the most activity in patients with recurrent disease with responses ranging from 25% to 33% for doxorubicin and 18% for ifosfamide when used as single agents. Sutton et al. and the GOG published the results of a phase II study combining ifosfamide and mesna and doxorubicin, showing an overall response rate of 30%. The duration response was 4 months, and the regimen produced substantial toxicity. Paclitaxel has been studied in LMSs, with an 8% response seen in patients who had received prior chemotherapy and a 9% response in those who were chemotherapy naïve. A novel combination of gemcitabine with docetaxel has shown a 53% response rate in a small phase II trial of patients that included 29 patients with uterine LMS. This regimen was subsequently evaluated in two phase II trials. In one trial of 39 patients with advanced or recurrent LMS who

had received no prior chemotherapy, the regimen produced a 36% response rate and a median PFS of 4.4 months. In a similar population of 48 patients who had received one prior chemotherapy regimen, a 27% response rate was noted. In both studies, myelosuppression was the most common toxicity.

Targeted biologic agents are also being explored, although no agent has yet to demonstrate activity in this tumor type. A randomized trial comparing the docetaxel plus gemcitabine regimen with or without the antivascular endothelial growth factor antibody bevacizumab is currently ongoing. Patients with late recurrences of LMS in the form of isolated pulmonary metastases are candidates for thoracotomy and sequential resection of the lesions. Five-year survival rates of 30% to 50% have been reported after such therapy.

Recently, several reports have appeared in the medical as well as lay literature in which women with a preoperative diagnosis of leiomyoma were treated with minimally invasive surgery including morcellation, and the final pathology noted a uterine malignancy. Most of these cancers were LMS. Because preoperative diagnosis of LMS is very imprecise compared with other uterine malignancies and occur in peri- or early menopause, a benign preoperative diagnosis could be easily made. These cases have resulted in disseminated disease with poor prognosis. As a result, several studies have evaluated the incidence of malignancy associated with a hysterectomy or myomectomy done for presumed benign disease. In reported studies of women undergoing hysterectomy or myomectomy for a myometrial mass, the prevalence of sarcoma is about 1 in 500 (0.2%) in most studies and reviews. Most sarcomas were LMS. The largest study of unexplained malignancy in women undergoing morcellation was from the US insurance database including 232,882 women undergoing minimally invasive hysterectomy noted morcellation was performed in 36,470 (15.7%). Among those in which morcellation was performed, 99 cases (0.34%) of uterine cancer were found. The prevalence of cancer in this series for women younger than the age of 40 years was 1 in 1500 and 1 in 1100 for women 40 to 44 years of age. Unfortunately, histology of uterine cancer cases was not reported. Data from a national US hospital database of 41,777 women undergoing myomectomy included 3220 who underwent power morcellation, and 0.09% had uterine cancer. Occult uterine cancer was 1 in 2337 in women younger than 40 years, 1 in 702 in those age 40 to 49 years, 1 in 154 in those age 50 to 59 years, and 1 in 31 in women age 60 years or older. Studies have noted morcellation is associated with the worst prognosis with uterine sarcoma. A meta-analysis of four observational studies in women with uterine sarcoma found morcellation compared with no morcellation was associated with higher recurrence rate (61% vs. 39%) and mortality rate (48% vs. 29%). **These data support the US Food and Drug Administration guideline that power morcellation should not be used in peri- and postmenopausal women (November 2014).**

More recent data by Wright et al. using a Markov model suggest that morcellation may be beneficial in women younger than the age of 40 years and not beneficial in older women. Contained morcellation in a containment bag is a potential emerging technique that may put this controversy to rest.

ENDOMETRIAL STROMAL SARCOMA

Clinical Profile

Endometrial stromal tumors are rare mesenchymal tumors composed of cells that resemble endometrial stromal cells of the proliferative endometrium. The most common symptom of ESS is irregular vaginal bleeding. Asymptomatic uterine enlargement, pelvic pain, or a palpable mass are also common symptoms. The tumors are generally soft, fleshy, smooth, polypoid masses that may protrude into the endometrial cavity. The multiple-polyp form of the neoplasm has also been described, as has the characteristic yellow color of many of these lesions. On occasion, the uterine wall is diffusely enlarged by tumor without the presence of an obvious tumor mass. Preoperative diagnosis remains challenging because endometrial biopsy may not identify the lesion in many cases.

In the past, endometrial stromal tumors were largely grouped as either endolymphatic stromal myosis or ESS. Endolymphatic stromal myosis was distinguished from stromal sarcomas by the minimal extent of tumor infiltration into the myometrium, the lack of metastases, and an indolent clinical behavior. There was significant histologic overlap between the two entities that made diagnosis difficult, however. Currently, endometrial stromal tumors are classified into two groups based on their metastatic potential. Stromal nodules are benign proliferations with the appearance indistinguishable from endometrial stroma of proliferative endometrium. They tend to be well-circumscribed lesions smaller than 15 cm and do not demonstrate infiltrating margins or vascular space invasion. They behave like benign lesions without reported recurrences or metastases. Stromal sarcomas represent the second type of stromal neoplasm. Stromal sarcomas demonstrate local invasiveness or vascular and lymphatic space involvement and infiltrate and separate the muscle fibers of the uterus. Stromal sarcomas have traditionally been divided into low- and high-grade ESSs, largely based on the mitotic activity. Today there is a greater recognition that most high-grade tumors should be classified as undifferentiated endometrial sarcomas.

Low-grade endometrial stromal sarcoma (LGESS), previously described as endolymphatic stromal myosis, can have an infiltrating growth pattern that on gross examination can project out in a wormlike fashion into the myometrium or into pelvic blood vessels. On microscopic examination, there is little or no cellular atypia, and there are few if any mitoses (Figs. 6.2 and 6.3). Although metastasis can occur, the clinical course is usually indolent, and surgery only is usually adequate treatment. Low-grade sarcomas may recur, but their clinical course is marked by late recurrences, typically more than 5 years from diagnosis, with recurrences up to 25 years having been reported. In a review of 72 cases of LGESS, 88% of patients remained alive at 80 months.

High-grade ESS traditionally has been distinguished from LGESS by having 10 or greater mitoses per 10 hpf based on work by Norris and Taylor. From a review of 17 stromal sarcomas, Kempson and Bari noted that 10 tumors contained more than 20 mitoses/10 hpf, and 9 of 10 patients died of disease. Seven patients had tumors that contained 5 mitoses or fewer/10

FIGURE 6.2 Low-power photomicrograph of a low-grade endometrial stromal sarcoma with invasion into the myometrium.

FIGURE 6.3 High-power view of low-grade endometrial stromal sarcoma shown in Fig. 6.2.

hpf, and none have developed a recurrence. Kempson and colleagues subsequently reviewed 109 cases of ESS and found that stage was the predominant predictor of behavior, even more so than the number of mitoses. For example, disease in 45% of stage I patients with rare mitosis and minimal atypia recurred. In this series, as long as the stromal cells appeared bland (similar to normal proliferative endometrial stromal cells), the 10 mitoses/10 hpf cutoff was not predictive of recurrence or survival. Leath and colleagues demonstrated that the clinical behavior of high-grade endometrial stromal sarcoma (HGESS) is frequently aggressive, with more patients presenting with advanced stage (extrauterine disease, 61% vs. 32%) and poorer survival compared with LGESS. Today there is a belief that many HGESS tumors are in fact undifferentiated endometrial sarcomas. These tumors show myometrial invasion and nuclear pleomorphism and have a high mitotic rate and extensive necrosis but lack smooth muscle or endometrial stromal differentiation.

Surgical Management

The standard management for patients with stromal sarcoma is hysterectomy and bilateral salpingo-oophorectomy. The role of nodal dissections is unresolved, largely because there are a scarcity of data when complete surgical staging has been performed. Goff and associates found no nodal disease, but only seven patients were evaluated. In the GOG surgical staging series, 52 stromal sarcomas were included, but the frequency of nodal disease was not reported. Data suggest that bilateral salpingo-oophorectomy should be performed. Several investigators have suggested that recurrences were higher in patients who had ovaries preserved. In 2009, the FIGO introduced a new staging classification for ESSs (see Table 6.3).

Patients with LGESS tend to present with disease confined to the uterus, with stage I or II disease being reported in approximately 70% of series. In contrast, patients with HGESS had stage I or II disease in 40% to 50% of cases. In a retrospective review of 52 cases of LGESS by Piver and colleagues, 47% of stage I patients developed recurrence after surgery. Despite this, the 5-year survival rates were 88% for stage I and 100% for stage II patients. Gadducci and coworkers evaluated 66 patients with stromal sarcomas, including 26 with LGESS and 40 with HGESS. For 20 patients with stage I or II low-grade tumors, 25% recurred (median follow-up period, 86 months), all in the pelvis. The median time to recurrence was 36 months, with a range of 4 to 108 months. For LGESS, 5-year survival rates have ranged from 80% to 100 even though 20% to 40% of patients eventually have a recurrence. Piver and coworkers reported on patterns of failure in stage I patients whose disease recurred, with 12 of 19 recurrences being in the pelvis, 3 of 19 being at distant sites, and 4 of 19 with combined pelvic and distant failures.

The prognosis for HGESS is comparable to LMSs. Gadducci and coworkers reported 5-year disease-free survival (DFS) rate of only about 20% for this group of patients. The median time to recurrence is shorter than with LGESS, with a median time of 7 months. Mitotic count was an independent predictor of survival with patients with 10 to 20 mitoses/10 hpf having a 2-year DFS of approximately 60% compared with approximately 10% if there were 20 mitoses or more/10 hpf. Other investigators have suggested 5-year survival rate between 20% and 55% for HGESS. Recurrences in the pelvis, abdomen, and lung are commonly seen, with the majority including at least some distant site of failure. A study of 24 patients with HGESS from the Mayo Clinic found that prognosis was related to the extent of disease, size of primary tumor, and grade. Mitotic count was not a prognostic factor, nor was DNA pattern.

Adjuvant Therapy

As with other uterine sarcomas, adjuvant therapy has been evaluated to reduce recurrences. Gadducci and coworkers had no recurrences in five patients with low-grade disease who received adjuvant therapy versus 5 of 15 (33%) who did not. In the Piver et al. study, five patients with low-grade disease received postoperative pelvic radiation, and no recurrences were seen. Piver et al., noting the sensitivity of advanced or recurrent disease to progestins, suggested that adjuvant progestin therapy may be an effective strategy. In the large multi-institutional series by Leath and coworkers, 30 of 72 patients received adjuvant hormonal therapy and survival curves suggested a possible benefit associated with its use.

Berchuck and coworkers reported recurrence rates of 57% with adjuvant chemotherapy or radiation therapy versus 56% who did not receive adjuvant therapy in 25 patients with stage I ESS (high and low grade). Gadducci and coworkers noted no benefit to adjuvant therapy in stage I or II high-grade tumors. Given the rarity of ESS, no prospective study has been performed to identify active agents to be used in adjuvant treatment. As with other sarcoma types, radiation therapy may have a role in reducing pelvic recurrences but with an unknown effect on survival.

Management of Recurrent Disease

Although initial studies did allow for patients with ESS, the small numbers of such patients included does not allow for interpretation of results. Low-grade endometrial sarcomas have a high frequency of progestin receptors, making progestational agents reasonable. Piver and associates found that progestins produced a 46% response rate in a small number of patients with LGESS treated at recurrence. Responses lasted from 2 to 104 months. Recurrences of LGESS should be considered for local resection when they develop in the pelvis. For HGESS, limited success has been reported with drugs commonly used for uterine sarcomas including ifosfamide and doxorubicin.

OTHER SARCOMAS

Clement and Scully described 100 cases of adenosarcoma of the uterus. This is an unusual tumor with low malignant potential. Similar to other endometrial lesions, adenosarcoma usually presents with abnormal vaginal bleeding. On gross evaluation, the tumor is usually a polypoid mass that can fill the endometrial cavity. Involvement of the cervix and myometrium is less commonly seen. In 2009, the FIGO introduced a new staging classification for adenosarcomas (see Table 6.3). Histologic evaluation notes benign or atypical neoplastic glands with a sarcomatous stroma. In 78% of patients, the sarcomatous stroma was homologous. The stromal mitotic rate was 1 to 40/10 hpf. Extensive stromal fibrosis was common. Myometrial invasion was present in only 15, and it was deeply invasive in only four. Recurrence became apparent in 23 patients and in one-third appeared 5 years after diagnosis. Recurrence was confined to the vagina, pelvis, or abdomen, with two exceptions. Of those with recurrence, only 11 died with tumor. Only the presence of myometrial invasion was associated with an increased risk of recurrence. A variant of adenocarcinoma is a pattern that has been called adenosarcoma with sarcomatous overgrowth. This is characterized by overgrowth of the neoplasm by a pure sarcomatous component occupying at least 25% of the lesion. It is an ominous feature with reported recurrence rates exceeding 50% compared with the usual adenosarcoma.

Pure heterologous uterine sarcomas are rare. Of these, rhabdomyosarcoma is the most common followed by chondrosarcoma and osteosarcoma. Rhabdomyosarcoma is derived from primitive myogenic precursors and is the most common soft tissue tumor in children and adolescents; 21% occur in genitourinary sites, and 20% of these in the uterus. Therapy has evolved from radical surgery and radiation therapy to more reliance on chemotherapy. Some authors have reported successful preservation of reproductive functions.

For the bibliography list, log onto www.expertconsult.com ⟨http://www.expertconsult.com⟩.

7

Gestational Trophoblastic Disease

Emma L. Barber, MD, John T. Soper, MD

OUTLINE

KEY POINTS

1. Gestational trophoblastic disease (GTD) describes a spectrum of neoplastic conditions derived from the placenta, including hydatidiform moles, postmolar gestational trophoblastic neoplasia (GTN), gestational choriocarcinoma, placental site trophoblastic tumor (PSTT), and epithelioid trophoblastic tumor (ETT).

2. GTN is the most curable gynecologic malignancy.

3. Complete hydatidiform moles are completely derived from the paternal genome and most frequently have a diploid 46XX karyotype.

4. Partial moles are composed of both paternal and maternal genomes, resulting in triploidy, and most frequently have the 69XXX karyotype. Partial moles have evidence of fetal development, which differentiates them from complete moles.

5. Malignant GTN is more common after a complete molar pregnancy than a partial molar pregnancy.

6. Human chorionic gonadotropin (hCG) values should be followed for 6 months after molar pregnancy evacuation to detect postmolar GTN.

7. GTN is defined by a plateaued, rising, or prolonged persistence of elevated hCG values after molar evacuation; histologic diagnosis of choriocarcinoma, invasive mole, PSTT, or ETT; or identification of metastatic disease after molar evacuation.

8. GTN is staged based on the World Health Organization prognostic score as either low risk (≤6) or high risk (≥7).

9. Low-risk GTN is treated with actinomycin D or methotrexate. Cure rates approach 100%.

10. High risk GTN is treated with EMA/CO (etoposide, methotrexate, actinomycin D, cyclophosphamide, and vincristine) chemotherapy. Cure rates are greater than 90%.

Gestational trophoblastic disease (GTD) comprises a spectrum of neoplastic conditions derived from the placenta. Whereas hydatidiform moles, gestational choriocarcinoma, and placental site trophoblastic tumor (PSTT) are histologic diagnoses, postmolar GTN is defined by clinical and laboratory criteria. The disease entities included in GTD have a wide variation in behavior, but GTN specifically refers to those with the potential for tissue invasion and metastases.

Gestational trophoblastic disease has been recognized since antiquity. Individual hydropic molar villi (Fig. 7.1) were sometimes identified as separate fetuses. In the early 19th century, Velpeau and Boivin recognized hydatidiform mole as a

FIGURE 7.1 Complete hydatidiform mole, gross specimen. Note the diffuse hydropic placental villi, which make up almost the entire specimen. (Courtesy of David Mutch, MD.)

TABLE 7.1   Features of Partial and Complete Hydatidiform Moles

Feature	Partial Mole	Complete Mole
Karyotype	Most commonly 69,XXX or −,XXY	Most commonly 46,XX or −,XY
Pathology		
Fetus	Often present	Absent
Amnion, fetal RBC	Usually present	Absent
Villous edema	Variable, focal	Diffuse
Trophoblastic proliferation	Focal, slight to moderate	Diffuse, slight to severe
CLINICAL PRESENTATION		
Diagnosis	Missed abortion	Molar gestation
Uterine size	Small for dates	50% large for dates
Theca-lutein cysts	Rare	25%–30%
Medical complications	Rare	10%–25%
Postmolar GTN	2.5%–7.5%	6.8%–20%

GTN, Gestational trophoblastic neoplasia; *RBC,* red blood cell.

cystic dilation of the chorionic villi. In 1895, Marchand demonstrated that hydatidiform mole and less frequently normal pregnancy preceded the development of choriocarcinoma. In the early 20th century, Fels identified elevated chorionic gonadotropic hormones in the urine of women with hydatidiform moles.

Before the mid-1950s, the prognosis for women with GTN was dismal, and there were no effective treatments. In the 1940s, Hertz demonstrated that fetal tissues required large amounts of folic acid and that their growth could be inhibited by methotrexate. However, it was not until 1956 that Li reported the first sustained remission in a patient with choriocarcinoma treated with methotrexate.

Since that report, GTN has been recognized as the most curable gynecologic malignancy. Reasons for this include (1) identification and development of quantitative assays for human chorionic gonadotropin (hCG) in serum and urine allowed hCG to become the prototype for tumor markers; (2) sensitivity of GTN to various chemotherapeutic agents; and (3) identification of risk factors allowing individualization of treatment, often using multimodality treatment with chemotherapy combined with surgery or radiation therapy (or both) in selected cases.

In general, GTD represents a derangement in the development of the conceptus, associated with unregulated trophoblastic proliferation and invasion, with the propensity for hematogenous metastasis in GTN. The diseases are characterized by paraneoplastic disorders from secretion of gestational hormones, most notably hCG. GTD is the only group of female reproductive neoplasms derived from paternal genetic material (androgenic origin).

Although largely unclear, the etiology of GTD likely involves genetic abnormalities involved in fertilization. Abnormalities in differentiation and pronuclear cleavage, decidual implantation, myometrial invasion, and host immunologic tolerance are also involved. Several candidate tumor suppressor genes (eg, DOC-2/hDab2), chromosomal loci (e.g., 7qp12-7q11,23 and

9q13,3-13,4), and oncogenes (eg, CD9) have been implicated in the pathogenesis of GTD.

HYDATIDIFORM MOLE

Two distinct forms of molar pregnancies, complete (CM) and partial (PM) moles, are currently recognized (Table 7.1). Cytogenetic studies have conclusively demonstrated that they are completely separate but related entities. Despite the cytogenetic, pathologic, and clinical differences outlined in Table 7.1, the clinical management of patients with CMs and PMs is similar.

Epidemiology

The incidence of molar pregnancies in the United States is approximately 1 in 1500 pregnancies. Race or ethnicity, age, socioeconomic status, diet, and prior reproductive history all influence the risk. The most reliable studies suggest that the incidence of hydatidiform mole is slightly less than 1 in 1000 pregnancies in most of the world, 1.2 in 1000 in South Africa, as high as 2 in 1000 in Japan, 7 in 1000 deliveries in Malaysia and the Philippines, and possibly higher in Saudi Arabia. The reported incidence of molar pregnancies among various ethnicities and races may be biased as a result of dependence on hospital records, particularly from tertiary referral centers, rather than population-based studies. Historically, GTD was thought to occur more frequently in the Asian population; however, recent population-based studies in Japan have shown a decreasing incidence of GTD in Japan, even with a relatively homogeneous population.

Extremes of reproductive age are associated with increased risk of molar pregnancy. Based on an analysis of 2202 patients with hydatidiform moles compared with a contemporary control group including all types of pregnancy events, a Duke study found a significantly higher incidence of molar pregnancy in women younger than 15 years and older than 40 years of age.

Other studies have confirmed the peak incidence of molar pregnancies at the extremes of maternal reproductive age. Some of these studies noted an increased risk associated with increasing paternal reproductive age for CM but not for PM.

Dietary factors associated with an increased risk of hydatidiform mole may include a low-protein diet and vitamin A deficiency, although these factors are difficult to separate from effects of lower socioeconomic class alone. Berkowitz and colleagues have suggested that a deficiency of animal fat and fat-soluble vitamin carotene is associated with increased risk of molar pregnancies. Populations with a high prevalence of vitamin A deficiency have been noted to have higher incidences of hydatidiform mole. Although carotene-rich vegetables are available in these countries, the lack of dietary fat needed for carotene absorption may result in an overall carotene-deficient condition.

Prior molar pregnancy also increases the risk of recurrent molar pregnancy. Women with a single previous molar pregnancy have more than 10 times the risk of having another molar pregnancy compared with those who have never had one. Based on data by Bagshawe and colleagues, after having had one molar pregnancy, the risk for a second was 1 in 76; after two molar pregnancies, the risk for a third was 1 in 6.5. Sand reported that the risk of a third molar pregnancy was 28%. Goldstein and colleagues noted that 9 of 1339 patients (1 in 150) had at least two consecutive molar pregnancies. Other centers have reported that the incidence of a second molar pregnancy is as high as 1 in 50 women with one prior molar pregnancy.

With recurrent molar pregnancies, there is also an increased risk of developing malignant GTN, although patients with consecutive molar pregnancies may have subsequent normal pregnancies. Berkowitz and colleagues noted that four of their patients with consecutive molar pregnancies later had full-term pregnancies. Lurain noted that five of eight patients with consecutive molar pregnancies later had normal full-term pregnancies.

In a case-controlled study from Baltimore, factors found to be associated with GTN included professional occupation, history of prior spontaneous abortions, and the mean number of months from antecedent pregnancy to the index pregnancy. Contraceptive history, irradiation, ABO blood groups, and smoking factors of the male partner were not associated with development of GTN. Among PMs, no clinical factor such as gravidity, parity, age, uterine size, gestational age at diagnosis, or hCG levels at presentation were associated with development of GTN.

Cytogenetics and Pathology

Molar pregnancies consist of CMs and PMs. In most series, CM and PM comprise approximately 70% and 30% of molar pregnancies, respectively.

Complete hydatidiform moles are completely derived from the paternal genome (see Table 7.1). Most frequently, CMs have a diploid 46, XX genome with exclusively androgenetic markers on the chromosomes, implying duplication of a

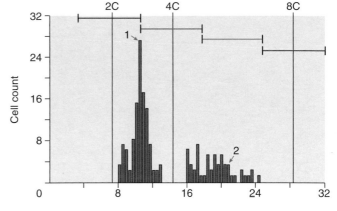

FIGURE 7.2 Flow cytometry of a partial mole. Note the peak at 3C, indicating triploidy. (Courtesy of Dr. Rex Bentley, Duke University Medical Center.)

haploid sperm chromosomal complement in the fertilized ovum. Approximately 5% of CMs have a 46,XY androgenetic genome, indicating that dispermic fertilization occurs in some. The mechanism for exclusion of the maternal polar body from the nucleus of the fertilized ovum is unknown. No 46,YY moles have been reported, but aneuploid karyotypes, such as tetraploidy, have been associated with CM. Fetal red blood cells (RBCs) are not observed in microscopic sections of CM, because the fetus never develops a cardiovascular system.

In contrast, PMs are composed of both paternal and maternal genomes (see Table 7.1). Usually, two paternal haploid sets of chromosomes are combined with one maternal set, resulting in **complete triploidy** (Fig. 7.2). The 69,XXX karyotype is most common, but some PM, have a 69,XXY karyotype, implying dispermic fertilization. Sometimes other aneuploid karyotypes are observed in PM but none with duplication of the Y chromosome. All karyotypes reported for PM feature a maternal haploid set and multiples of the paternal chromosomal complement. Gross or histologic evidence of fetal development such as fetal RBCs is a feature of PM that differentiates it from CM.

Other histopathologic features of CM and PM differ. CMs have diffuse villous edema, often with central cisterna formation (Fig. 7.3). Trophoblastic proliferation is usually diffuse (Fig. 7.4) but may vary in extent. Histologic evidence of a fetus is lacking. Histologic features of PM can be subtle, and many PMs are probably underdiagnosed erroneously as spontaneous abortions. A PM exhibits focal, varying degrees of hydropic villi with scalloping and trophoblastic inclusions within the villi (Fig. 7.5). Focal trophoblastic proliferation is usually subtle compared with CM. Fetal RBCs are observed within vessels of the villi (Fig. 7.6), and sometimes a fetus can be grossly identified. The fetus is usually nonviable and rarely survives beyond 20 weeks of gestation. The difference in the amount of trophoblastic proliferation between CM and PM is related to their different clinical presentations. Malignant GTN occurs in 2.5% to 7.5% of patients with PM compared with approximately

FIGURE 7.3 Low-power photomicrograph of a complete mole illustrating diffuse hydropic change of the villi, which have marked paucity of stroma in the central zone of each villus (cisternae formation). Sheets of trophoblast cell are adjacent to the villi. (Courtesy of Dr. Rex Bentley, Duke University Medical Center.)

FIGURE 7.5 This low-power photomicrograph of a partial hydatidiform mole contains enlarged placental villi with stromal edema, scalloping at the edge of the villi, and trophoblastic inclusions within the stroma of the villi. Minimal trophoblastic proliferation is present. (Courtesy of Dr. Rex Bentley, Duke University Medical Center.)

FIGURE 7.4 High-power photomicrograph of a complete mole. The villus (upper left) is associated with sheets of trophoblast cells, containing the multinucleated syncytiotrophoblasts and the small, polygonal cytotrophoblast cells. Production of human chorionic gonadotropin occurs mainly in the syncytiotrophoblast cells. (Courtesy of Dr. Rex Bentley, Duke University Medical Center.)

FIGURE 7.6 In this high-power photomicrograph of a villus from a partial mole, small vessels within the stroma are seen containing nucleated fetal red blood cells. (Courtesy of Dr. Rex Bentley, Duke University Medical Center.)

6.8% to more than 20% after evacuation of a CM mole (see Table 7.1).

Other techniques have been developed to differentiate CM from PM. These include karyotyping, flow cytometry, fluorescence in situ hybridization, and amplification of short tandem repeat loci. Additionally, p57 immunohistochemistry is absent in CM but present in PM because it is paternally imprinted but maternally expressed. Although most cases of molar pregnancy can be classified as CM or PM using histopathology alone, histologic differences may not be apparent if the diagnosis is made early in gestation. In this scenario, molecular genetic techniques may be critical for accurate diagnosis.

Presentation and Symptoms

Irregular bleeding is the hallmark symptom of hydatidiform moles. Nearly all patients with moles have delayed or irregular menses for varying time periods. Vaginal bleeding usually occurs during the first trimester. The bleeding may vary from spotting to hemorrhage requiring blood transfusion. In earlier series, bleeding occurred in 73% to 100% of molar pregnancies including CM and PM. Expulsion of recognizable molar vesicles may accompany vaginal bleeding when the gestation approaches the second trimester.

There is increasing information that the presentation of moles may be changing as a result of earlier and improved diagnostic tests, including early ultrasound and hCG serum assays. The New England Trophoblastic Disease Center (NETDC) group compared symptoms in CM treated at their institution from 1994 to 2013 to those treated from 1988 to 1993. Patients in the more recent cohort were less likely to present with vaginal bleeding, 46% versus 84% in the earlier cohort. Patients in the recent cohort were also more likely to be diagnosed with a molar pregnancy at less than 11 weeks (56% vs. 41%). However, earlier diagnosis did not result in decreased rates of GTN.

Other symptoms include nausea and vomiting caused by the high levels of hCG. Nausea and vomiting were reported in almost one-third of patients with hydatidiform mole in older studies. However, in the most recent series from the NETDC, 14% of 180 patients presented with hyperemesis from 1994 to 2013. Curry and colleagues also reported hyperemesis in 14% of patients.

Preeclampsia-like symptoms in the first trimester of pregnancy are nearly pathognomonic of a hydatidiform mole. Symptoms of headache with hypertension, hyperreflexia, and proteinuria define preeclampsia. Preeclampsia was present in 1% of patients in the NETDC cohort and in 12% of the patients in the study by Curry and colleagues. Fortunately, eclampsia in the setting of hydatidiform mole is rare.

Molar pregnancy is also associated with other medical comorbidities such as tachycardia and hypertension from hyperthyroidism or shortness of breath and chest pain from acute respiratory distress syndrome. Hyperthyroidism occurs rarely but can be very severe. Laboratory evidence of hyperthyroidism can occur in as many as 10% of patients; however, clinical manifestations are less frequent. Hyperthyroidism is caused by the production of elevated levels of normal hCG by molar tissue. hCG has structural homology with the thyroid-stimulating hormone (TSH) molecule and binds to TSH receptors, which results in thyroid hyperfunction. Furthermore, Yoshimura and colleagues demonstrated that the isoforms of hCG produced by molar pregnancies have higher thyrotrophic activity compared with the hCG produced by normal pregnancies. Clinical manifestations of hyperthyroidism disappear after the molar pregnancy is evacuated. Antithyroid therapy may be indicated for a short period to control hyperthyroidism during molar evacuation. Specifically, the use of beta-blockers to prevent tachycardia may be indicated.

Acute respiratory distress caused by trophoblastic pulmonary embolization can also occur. It is very rare, occurring in only 2% of patients in the NETDC cohort. These patients often have coexisting pathology that may alter cardiac or pulmonary function such as preeclampsia, hyperthyroidism, and anemia, and this combination can contribute to acute cardiopulmonary decompensation. Respiratory distress is most often associated with a large volume of molar tissue and uterine enlargement greater than 16 weeks' gestational size.

Theca-lutein cysts are caused by hyperstimulation of the ovaries by excessive hCG production. Traditionally, approximately 15% to 25% of patients with unevacuated molar pregnancies present with theca-lutein cysts larger than 6 cm. More recent series have shown rates of theca-lutein cysts at presentation of 6% to 9%. Although theca-lutein cysts will resolve after molar evacuation, there may be considerable lag behind the decline of hCG levels. Surgical intervention is rarely required for acute torsion or bleeding. Patients who develop theca-lutein cysts have a higher incidence of postmolar GTN. Furthermore, patients with the combination of enlarged ovaries with a large for gestational age uterus results are at a high risk for malignant GTN. Up to 57% of patients with this combination require subsequent therapy for postmolar GTN.

Classically, a patient with a hydatidiform mole was said to have a uterine size excessive for gestational age. Historically, this was found in more than 50% of patients with CM; however, approximately one-third of patients have uteri smaller than expected for gestational age. In the NETDC cohort from 1994 to 2013, uterine size was excessive for dates in only 24%.

Similar to the comparative study performed by NETDC, Mangili and colleagues from Italy compared clinical features of molar pregnancies between two historical cohorts, 1970 to 1982 versus 1992 to 2004. The later cohort had significantly less vaginal bleeding on presentation (51% vs. 74%, P <0.0001), fewer with increased uterine volume (29% vs. 51%, P <0.0001), and fewer with theca-lutein cysts (13% vs. 21%, P = 0.03). There was no difference in rates of hyperemesis or preeclampsia. Because molar pregnancies are diagnosed at an increasingly early gestational age, clinical symptoms are less frequent. As a result, there is increasing reliance on histopathologic analysis to identify cases of molar pregnancies.

The previously outlined conditions are seen mainly in patients with CM. Patients with PM usually do not exhibit excessive uterine size, theca-lutein cysts, preeclampsia, hyperthyroidism, or respiratory problems. In most patients with PM, the clinical and ultrasound diagnosis is usually a missed or incomplete abortion. PMs are often underdiagnosed because of the lack of clinical suspicion and the often subtle or focal nature of the pathologic changes in the placental tissues. Therefore, products of conception from missed or incomplete abortions should be thoroughly examined by pathologists to prevent a missed diagnosis of PM. Cytogenetic testing may be required to accurately diagnose GTD.

Diagnosis

Patients with CM are often clinically diagnosed by characteristic ultrasound features and a markedly elevated hCG. In contrast, the majority of patients with PM and an increasing proportion of patients with CM are clinically misdiagnosed as missed abortion. A quantitative hCG of greater than 100,000 IU/L, an enlarged uterus with absent fetal heart sounds, and vaginal bleeding suggest a diagnosis of hydatidiform mole. However, a single hCG determination is not diagnostic. A single high hCG value may be seen with a normal single or multiple pregnancy, especially if there has been bleeding or disruption of the placenta. Therefore, an isolated hCG value alone should not be

FIGURE 7.7 Transabdominal ultrasound image of an unevacuated complete mole, illustrating the characteristic mixed echogenic pattern in the uterus. (Courtesy of John Soper, MD.)

FIGURE 7.8 Gross specimen in a patient treated for complete hydatidiform mole with primary hysterectomy. (Courtesy of John Soper, MD.)

used as the sole determining factor in diagnosing hydatidiform mole. Conversely, a "normal" hCG level for an anticipated gestational age does not exclude the possibility of a molar pregnancy.

Ultrasonography has replaced all other radiographic means (eg, amniography or uterine angiography) for diagnosis of hydatidiform mole. Molar tissue typically is identified as a diffuse mixed echogenic and vesicular pattern replacing the placenta (Fig. 7.7), traditionally labeled a "snowstorm appearance." Recently, with increasing use of early ultrasonography, classic features may be subtle or lacking in cases of early CM or PM. In a recent series based on histopathologic identification of molar pregnancies, 52% of patients were diagnosed based on ultrasound examination before evacuation of the uterus. In another series, the abundant vesicular pattern and "snowstorm appearance" were absent in 10% of CM pregnancies and only subtly present in 63% of CM based on ultrasonography performed at mean gestational age of 7 weeks and 6 days.

The largest study to date, from Charing Cross Hospital in the United Kingdom, assessed more than 1000 cases of GTD from 2002 to 2005 and found an overall 44% detection rate by ultrasonography of molar pregnancies before evacuation. The overall detection rate was 35% to 40% before 14 weeks of gestation and 60% after 14 weeks. The sensitivity was 44%, and the specificity was 74%. The positive predictive value was 88%, and the negative predictive value was 23% for detecting molar pregnancy of any type. Detection rates were higher for CM versus PM and for later gestations. Nonetheless, fewer than 50% of molar pregnancies were diagnosed by ultrasonography in first-trimester scans.

In a smaller series from St. George's in London, the sensitivity of ultrasonography for the diagnosis of a CM was 95% and 20% for PM. Another series evaluated the use of both ultrasound and hCG values to diagnose hydatidiform mole. When ultrasonography was used alone, 42% of patients with molar pregnancies did not have a definite diagnosis on first

examination. When the hCG value was above a threshold of 82,350 mIU/mL and was used with the initial ultrasound findings, 89% of hydatidiform moles were correctly identified (Fig. 7.8). A combined algorithm using hCG, clinical history, examination, and imaging is required to make the diagnosis of hydatidiform mole.

Several reports have been made of a hydatidiform mole arising in ectopic sites, such as the fallopian tube. These patients present with classic symptoms and signs of ectopic pregnancy, including occasionally with tubal rupture and hemorrhagic shock. Tubal GTD was diagnosed in 16 (0.8%) of 2100 women with GTD who were managed at the NETDC. Various authors have warned that the current trend of treating ectopic pregnancies with conservative surgery or single-dose methotrexate necessitates close monitoring of serum hCG levels to avoid missing the diagnosis of ectopic GTD.

Evacuation

Given the subtle presentation of GTD in the modern era, the diagnosis of molar pregnancy will increasingly be made only after histologic evaluation of uterine curettings. Curettage is

TABLE 7.2   Management of Hydatidiform Mole

Evacuation: suction D&E (or hysterectomy in selected patients)

Postevacuation quantitative hCG level and chest radiography

Monitor quantitative hCG levels every 1–2 weeks until three normal values or criteria for GTN

After hCG level is normal for three values, then monitor hCG levels every 1–3 months for 6 months

Initiate chemotherapy for GTN using indications listed in Table 7.4:

1. Plateaued or rising hCG values
2. Histologic diagnosis of choriocarcinoma, invasive mole, or placental site trophoblastic tumor
3. Persistent hCG >6 months after evacuation
4. Metastatic disease

D&E, Suction dilation and evacuation; *GTN,* gestational trophoblastic neoplasia; *hCG,* human chorionic gonadotropin.

FIGURE 7.9 Ultrasound image demonstrating a large theca-lutein ovarian cyst associated with a complete hydatidiform mole. These usually contain multiple thin septations and have an appearance similar to iatrogenic ovarian hyperstimulation during ovulation induction. Theca-lutein cysts regress spontaneously after evacuation of the molar pregnancy, but regression often lags behind human chorionic gonadotropin level decline. (Courtesy of John Soper, MD.)

often performed for a suspected incomplete spontaneous abortion. When GTD is diagnosed, patients should be monitored with serial hCG measurements. Baseline postevacuation chest radiography should be considered. For patients in whom hydatidiform mole is suspected before evacuation, the following laboratory evaluation is recommended (Table 7.2): complete blood count with platelet determination, clotting function studies, renal and liver function studies, blood type with antibody screen, and hCG level. A pre-evacuation chest radiograph should also be obtained.

Evacuation of molar pregnancies should be performed expeditiously. Medical complications are observed in approximately 25% of patients with molar pregnancy and uterine enlargement of greater than 14 to 16 weeks' gestational size. The molar pregnancy should be evacuated as soon as possible after stabilization of any medical complications. The choice of facilities for molar evacuation should be based on the expertise of the physician, uterine size, and ability of the facility to manage existing medical complications. In most patients, the preferred method of evacuation is suction dilation and evacuation (D&E) (see Table 7.2).

Medical induction of labor with oxytocin or prostaglandin and hysterotomy are not recommended for evacuation because they increase blood loss and may increase the risk for malignant sequelae compared with suction D&E. The Charing Cross group reported a significant trend toward more frequent evacuation by suction curettage compared with sharp curettage or medical induction for molar evacuation over their study interval. Postmolar GTN developed in 5.9%, 3.8%, and 9.1% of their patients evacuated with suction curettage, sharp curettage, and medical induction, respectively (*P* <0.05 for increased postmolar GTN in the medical induction group). Furthermore, many patients require D&E to complete the evacuation of the mole after medical induction of labor.

Evacuation is usually performed under general anesthesia, but local or regional anesthesia may be used for a cooperative patient with a small uterus. After serial dilatation of the cervix, uterine evacuation is accomplished with the largest cannula that can be introduced through the cervix. Most providers begin

curettage in the lower uterine segment, allowing the uterus to contract progressively as the pregnancy is evacuated. Evacuation may be accompanied by significant blood loss during evacuation of tissue, particularly with increasing gestational age. Intravenous (IV) oxytocin is begun after the cervix is dilated and continued for serval hours postoperatively to assist with uterine contractility. Other uterotonics such as methylergonovine or misoprostol may be used if needed. After completion of suction D&E, gentle sharp curettage may be performed. Repeat uterine evacuation by D&E has been performed for persistent GTD, defined in the United Kingdom as failure of hCG to normalize within 4 to 6 weeks or an increase in hCG any time after primary D&C. The utility of repeat second D&C is controversial. It may subject patients to surgical complications, when hCG may normalize given more time. Additionally, it does not comply with current International Federation of Gynecology and Obstetrics (FIGO) guidelines for treatment of GTN.

Hysterectomy is an alternative to suction D&E for molar evacuation in selected patients who do not wish to preserve childbearing (Fig. 7.9). The adnexa are routinely preserved, and theca-lutein cysts should be left in situ unless they are torsed or ruptured and actively bleeding. Hysterectomy reduces, but does not eliminate, the risk of malignant postmolar sequelae. The risk of postmolar GTN after hysterectomy remains approximately 3% to 5%; therefore, these patients should be monitored postoperatively with serial hCG levels.

Risk Factors for Postmolar Gestational Trophoblastic Neoplasia

Many of the risk factors for development of postmolar GTN indirectly reflect the amount of trophoblastic proliferation at the time of evacuation. High pre-evacuation hCG levels, uterine size larger than expected by dates, and theca-lutein cysts (see Fig. 7.9) increase the risk. Many of these factors interact. The combination of theca-lutein cysts and uterus larger than expected for dates increases the risk of postmolar GTN to 57%. Other series have used multivariate analysis to identify other risk factors for postmolar GTN and have found that age, parity, initial uterine size, presence of theca-lutein cysts, and initial hCG concentration were not independent prognostic factors.

Multiple risk factors have been incorporated into scoring systems that seek to categorize patients and predict which patients will develop postmolar GTN. However, many of these efforts have not been successful. Parazzini and colleagues found that, although 15% of their patients had risk factors that classified them as "high risk," these patients accounted for a minority of the cases of postmolar GTN. Of note, despite the earlier diagnosis and decreasing symptom burden among patients in the modern era with molar pregnancies, there has not been a decrease in the incidence of postmolar GTN. This implies that other molecular biologic mechanisms may be responsible for the development of postmolar GTN rather than the amount of trophoblastic proliferation at the time of evacuation. Most centers do not treat "high-risk" molar pregnancies with postevacuation chemotherapy to prevent the development of postmolar GTN; rather, they rely on surveillance with serial hCG levels to diagnose postmolar GTN and then treat it when encountered.

Postmolar Surveillance

After molar evacuation, it is important to monitor all patients to diagnose and treat postmolar GTN promptly. Serial quantitative serum hCG measurements should be performed using one of several commercially available assays capable of detecting hCG to baseline values (<5 mIU/mL). Ideally, serum hCG levels should be obtained every 1 to 2 weeks until three consecutive values are normal. hCG can then be measured at 1- to 3-month intervals until 6 months after the initial normal value (see Table 7.2). Reliable contraception is highly recommended during monitoring of hCG values. Chest radiography is indicated if the hCG level rises. Patients with a histologic diagnosis of malignant GTN (choriocarcinoma, invasive mole, or PSTT), the development of metastatic disease, a rising hCG value, or a plateauing of the hCG values over several weeks' time are diagnosed with postmolar GTN, as discussed later. Whereas approximately 15% to 20% of patients develop postmolar GTN after evacuation of a CM, 1% to 5% of patients develop postmolar GTN after a PM.

Postmolar surveillance by serial hCG monitoring after achieving normal values allows identification of patients who develop late GTN. Although rare instances of long latent periods between molar evacuation and postmolar GTN have been

reported, the vast majority of episodes of GTN after hydatidiform moles occur within approximately 6 months of evacuation. The NETDC analyzed 1029 patients followed with hCG assays after CM evacuation at their institution. Postmolar GTN occurred in 153 (15%) patients. Only two women developed postmolar GTN after normalization of hCG levels, and both were followed by an older assay with a sensitivity of 10 mIU/mL.

None of their 82 (95% confidence interval [CI], 0%–4.5%) patients who were followed with an hCG assay with a sensitivity of 5 mIU/mL developed postmolar GTN after their hCG values normalized. However, a substantial number of their patients were excluded from analysis because of incomplete follow-up, including 817 patients lost to follow-up after normalization of hCG and 60 patients lost to follow-up before hCG values normalized. The same group of investigators reported that patients with PM had spontaneous normalization of hCG, with a median time of 46 days, and suggested that surveillance in this group may also be abbreviated.

Kerkmeijer and colleagues from the Netherlands reported that 74.6% patients with molar pregnancies attained spontaneous normalization of hCG after evacuation. Only one case of GTN occurred out of 265 patients who obtained two normal hCG levels. They conclude that hCG surveillance can also be curtailed after normalization of values. Within the same database, they found that no GTN occurred in patients with CM who obtained spontaneous normalization of weekly hCG levels within 2 months after evacuation. Because this total experience is relatively small and plagued by incomplete follow-up, it is prudent to recommend continued surveillance after molar evacuation with hCG monitoring for 6 months after normalization of hCG values. However, it should be noted that the risk of postmolar GTN is quite low after normalization.

Although early pregnancies after molar evacuation are usually normal gestations, an early pregnancy obscures detection of an elevated hCG caused by GTN. Oral contraceptives do not increase the incidence of postmolar GTN or alter the pattern of regression of hCG values. Special consideration should be given to oral contraceptive pills as the contraceptive of choice because they suppress the luteinizing hormone (LH) surge by preventing ovulation. LH shares an alpha subunit with hCG, and thus an LH surge may lead to a false-positive hCG value. In a randomized study conducted by the Gynecologic Oncology Group (GOG), patients treated with oral contraceptives had half as many intercurrent pregnancies during hCG surveillance as those using barrier methods. Furthermore, the incidence of postmolar GTN was lower in patients using oral contraceptives.

After completion of surveillance documenting remission for 6 months, pregnancy can be encouraged and hCG monitoring discontinued. Patients with a history of molar pregnancy remain at an elevated risk of GTN after all future pregnancies. Thus, pathologic examination of all future pregnancies is recommended, including placental examination and examination of the products of conception. Patients should also obtain a serum hCG value at 6 weeks after any pregnancy event (delivery or spontaneous or therapeutic abortion).

Prophylactic Chemotherapy After Molar Evacuation

Two randomized studies have evaluated prophylactic chemotherapy after molar evacuation. Kim and colleagues reported that a single course of methotrexate–folinic acid reduced the incidence of postmolar GTN from 47.4% to 14.3% (P <0.05) in patients with high-risk molar pregnancies, but the incidence was not reduced in patients with low-risk molar pregnancies. Patients who received prophylactic chemotherapy but developed GTN required more chemotherapy than those who had not been exposed to prophylactic chemotherapy. In the study by Limpongsanurak, a single course of actinomycin D was compared with observation in patients after evacuation of high-risk molar pregnancies. Postmolar GTN was 50% in the control group compared with 13.8% in the treatment group (P <0.05). In both studies there were no deaths in the treatment or control groups caused by GTN or treatment toxicity.

However, there are anecdotal cases of fatalities caused by prophylactic chemotherapy, and prophylactic chemotherapy does not eliminate the need for postevacuation follow-up. Furthermore, patients are exposed to drugs most frequently used to treat postmolar GTN, which could lead to relative chemoresistance. Receipt of chemotherapy is also associated with decreased quality of life, cost, and morbidity. In compliant patients, the low morbidity and mortality achieved by monitoring patients and instituting chemotherapy only in patients with postmolar GTN appears to outweigh the potential risk and small benefit of routine prophylactic chemotherapy. Exceptions to this are scenarios in which hCG follow-up is not possible because of patient or system factors; prophylactic chemotherapy may be considered in these cases.

Coexistent Molar Pregnancy With a Normal Fetus

Coexistence of a genetically normal fetus with molar change of the placenta is relatively rare (Fig. 7.10), occurring in 1 in 22,000 to 1 in 100,000 pregnancies. The majority of the literature covering this relatively rare entity consists of case reports and case series. Both CM and PM with a coexistent normal fetus have been reported. A variety of criteria have been used to evaluate these pregnancies. Many of the reports that antedated the histologic and cytogenetic distinction between CM and PM likely included twin gestations with coexistent fetus and molar gestation in addition to singleton PM. Although there might be an increased incidence of coexisting molar pregnancy and fetus related to an increase in multifetal pregnancies caused by ovulation induction for infertility, this may only reflect reporting bias.

Most of these are diagnosed antepartum by ultrasound findings of a complex, cystic placental component distinct from the fetoplacental unit. However, in a few cases, the diagnosis is not suspected until examination of the placenta after delivery. Medical complications of hydatidiform mole appear to be increased, including hyperthyroidism, hemorrhage, and pregnancy-induced hypertension.

Compared with singleton hydatidiform moles, twin pregnancy with a fetus and mole has an increased risk for postmolar

FIGURE 7.10 Gross photo of a fetus and mole.

GTN and a higher proportion of patients develop high-risk GTN requiring multiagent chemotherapy. In patients with a coexistent mole and fetus who continue pregnancy beyond 12 weeks, the subset that develop early complications leading to termination of the pregnancy before fetal viability has a markedly increased risk of postmolar GTN compared with patients whose pregnancy continues into the third trimester.

Among 72 patients collected by a national survey of physicians in Japan, 24 patients underwent first-trimester evacuation with 20.8% subsequently developing postmolar GTN. In comparison, 45.2% of 31 patients who required evacuation during the second trimester and 17.6% of the 17 who delivered in the third trimester developed postmolar GTN (P <0.05). Nine (50%) of the 18 patients with proven androgenic mole in association with a fetus subsequently were treated for postmolar GTN, but this increased risk may have been a result of selection bias. Major congenital abnormalities have not been reported in surviving infants.

For patients with coexistent hydatidiform mole and fetus suspected by ultrasonography, there are no clear guidelines for management. Ultrasonography should be repeated to exclude retroplacental hematoma, other placental abnormalities, and degenerating myoma and to fully evaluate the fetoplacental unit for evidence of a PM or gross fetal malformations. If the diagnosis is still suspected and continuation of pregnancy is desired, fetal karyotype should be obtained, chest radiography should be performed to screen for metastases, and serial serum hCG values should be followed.

Patients are at an increased risk for medical complications of pregnancy requiring evacuation, including bleeding, premature labor, and pregnancy-induced hypertension. They should be counseled about these risks and the increased risk of postmolar GTN after evacuation or second-trimester delivery. If fetal karyotype is normal, major fetal malformations are excluded by ultrasonography, and there is no evidence of metastatic disease, it is reasonable to allow the pregnancy to continue unless pregnancy-related complications force delivery. After delivery, the placenta should be histologically evaluated, and the patient should be followed closely with serial hCG values, as one would with a singleton hydatidiform mole.

GESTATIONAL TROPHOBLASTIC NEOPLASIA

GTN is defined by a plateaued, rising, or prolonged persistence of elevated hCG values after molar evacuation; histologic diagnosis of choriocarcinoma, invasive mole, PSTT, epithelioid trophoblastic tumor (ETT); or identification of metastatic disease after molar evacuation. Prompt diagnosis of malignant GTN is important because a delay in diagnosis may increase the patient's risk and decrease response to treatment. All patients with malignant GTN should undergo a complete evaluation aimed at identifying metastatic sites (Table 7.3) and other clinically important prognostic factors. Several classification systems have been used to determine prognostic groups and assist in the triage of management for individual patients. The FIGO revised its staging system for patients with malignant GTN in 2000 to reflect prognostic factors other than simple anatomic distribution of disease.

Diagnosis

Between half and two-thirds of cases of GTN that require treatment follow evacuation of CM or PM. Because these patients are treated on the basis of hCG levels rather than hysterectomy, the distribution of histologic lesions is not known.

TABLE 7.3   Distribution of Metastatic Sites From Gestational Trophoblastic Neoplasia

Metastatic Site	Number	(%)	(% Metastatic)
Nonmetastatic	195	54	
Metastatic	136	46	
Lung only	110		81
Vagina only	7		5
Central nervous system*	9		7
Gastrointestinal*	5	—	4
Liver*	2	—	1.5
Kidney*	1	—	0.7
Unknown†	4	—	3

*Concurrent lung metastases, highest risk site recorded.
†Rising human chorionic gonadotropin after hysterectomy for hydatidiform mole, no identifiable metastases.
Modified from Soper JT, Clarke-Pearson DL, Hammond CB. Metastatic gestational trophoblastic disease: prognostic factors in previously untreated patients *Obstet Gynecol* 1988;71:338.

Whereas approximately 50% to 70% of patients with postmolar GTN have persistent or invasive moles, 30% to 50% have postmolar gestational choriocarcinoma.

Gestational choriocarcinoma (Fig. 7.11) derived from term pregnancies, spontaneous abortions, and ectopic pregnancies accounts for the vast majority of the other cases of malignant GTN. PSTT (Fig. 7.12) and ETT are rare forms of GTN that can follow any pregnancy event.

Invasive moles are characterized by the presence of edematous chorionic villi with trophoblastic proliferation that invades directly into the myometrium. Metastasis of molar vesicles may occur. Usually invasive moles undergo spontaneous resolution after many months, but they are treated with chemotherapy to prevent morbidity and mortality caused by uterine perforation, hemorrhage, or infection. Gestational choriocarcinoma is a pure epithelial malignancy, comprising both neoplastic syncytiotrophoblast and cytotrophoblast elements without chorionic villi (see Fig. 7.11). Gestational choriocarcinomas are highly malignant, and chemotherapy is indicated.

Placental site trophoblastic tumors are rare. These tumors are characterized by absence of villi with proliferation of intermediate trophoblast cells (see Fig. 7.12). The syncytiotrophoblast population observed in choriocarcinoma is lacking in PSTT, with relatively lower levels of intact hCG secreted by these tumors. In general, PSTTs are not as sensitive to chemotherapy. Fortunately, most patients present with disease confined to the uterus and can be treated with hysterectomy.

Women with postmolar GTN are usually diagnosed early in the course of disease by serial hCG monitoring. In contrast, patients with malignant GTN after nonmolar gestations traditionally presented with predominantly nongynecologic symptoms, including hemoptysis or pulmonary embolism, cerebral hemorrhage, gastrointestinal (GI) or urologic hemorrhage, or metastatic malignancy of an unknown primary site. The index

FIGURE 7.11 High-power photomicrograph of gestational choriocarcinoma, illustrating the dimorphic population of the polygonal cytotrophoblast and the multinucleated syncytiotrophoblast cells. (Courtesy of Dr. Rex Bentley, Duke University Medical Center.)

FIGURE 7.12 High-power photomicrograph of placental site trophoblastic tumor treated with hysterectomy. Sheets of anaplastic polygonal cells with frequent mitoses infiltrate the smooth muscle of the uterine wall. (Courtesy of Dr. Rex Bentley, Duke University Medical Center.)

pregnancy event may have occurred years before presentation or may have been a subclinical spontaneous abortion. In a series from the NETDC, the presentation of choriocarcinoma after term gestation in the modern era (1996–2011) was compared with an earlier period (1964–1996). They found 30% of women in the modern era were asymptomatic and diagnosed by an incidental positive pregnancy test result or placental pathology compared with 2% in the previous time period ($P = 0.001$). The possibility of malignant GTN should be suspected in any woman of reproductive age who presents with metastatic disease from an unknown primary site or cerebral hemorrhage. Under these circumstances, the diagnosis is facilitated by a high index of suspicion that, coupled with serum hCG testing and exclusion of a concurrent pregnancy, confirms the diagnosis without need for tissue biopsy.

Before the development of effective chemotherapy, 10% of patients required hysterectomy after molar evacuation for the treatment of invasive molar pregnancy or choriocarcinoma. Other prechemotherapy reports indicated a mortality rate of more than 20% among patients with invasive mole. Since the development of chemotherapy, between 15% and 36% of patients in the United States are treated after molar evacuation based on inclusive hCG level criteria for initiating chemotherapy in an attempt to limit the morbidity and mortality caused by postmolar GTN. In contrast, Bagshawe and colleagues used very conservative hCG criteria to initiate chemotherapy and reported treating only approximately 8% of their patients after molar evacuation.

The pattern of hCG regression after evacuation of hydatidiform mole is most often used to make a diagnosis of postmolar GTN. After evacuation, most patients have an initial decrease in hCG levels and should be followed with serial hCG values every 1 to 2 weeks. Almost every series has treated patients on the basis of a confirmed hCG rise. In many studies, however,

chemotherapy was initiated on the basis of an hCG level plateau of relatively short (<3 weeks) duration. Kohorn noted that 15% of his patients had hCG plateaus after molar evacuation that lasted at least 2 weeks followed by spontaneous regression without intervention. In a trial of actinomycin D, Schlaerth and colleagues observed that 25% of their patients had a substantial spontaneous decrease in hCG levels on the day that chemotherapy was initiated. Based on the correlation between hCG level and tumor burden, Kohorn has suggested an approach using shorter observation periods for patients with high hCG level plateaus but allowing longer periods of observation for those who have hCG plateaus at levels under 1000 mIU/mL.

In some studies, an additional criterion for initiating chemotherapy after molar evacuation has been persistence of hCG for an arbitrary length of time, ranging between 6 weeks and 6 months after evacuation. The initial reports of chemotherapy from the National Institutes of Health (NIH) used persistence of hCG for more than 60 days after molar evacuation as an indication for chemotherapy treatment. Many series have documented that persistence of hCG for more than 60 days after evacuation increases the risk for developing postmolar GTN. However, 60% to 64% of patients with delayed regression of hCG beyond 60 days will ultimately undergo spontaneous hCG regression, with no deaths in those who began therapy more than 60 days from molar evacuation. Furthermore, groups reporting from the United Kingdom, where care for GTD patients is centralized, follow patients with elevated hCG levels for up to 6 months without an increase in morbidity or mortality among those treated after this prolonged follow-up.

Lurain and colleagues from the John I. Brewer Trophoblastic Disease Center reported their experience with 738 patients with complete hydatidiform moles. In their study, 80.7% of patients had spontaneous regression of hCG values to normal, although only 65% had done so by 60 days. An additional 27.9% reached normal values during the next 110 days. Overall, 142 (19%) were treated with chemotherapy because of rising or plateauing hCG levels. Of these, 125 had invasive moles, and 17 had choriocarcinomas. Only 15% of the 142 treated patients, or 3% of the total, developed metastases outside of the uterus. Morrow and Kohorn treated a higher proportion of their patients (36% and 27%, respectively) using hCG criteria derived from regression curves compared with studies that use the individual patient's hCG regression pattern. It appears that use of hCG regression curves may result in treatment of more patients than necessary, and it did not prevent metastatic disease.

In an effort to provide uniformity to the diagnosis of postmolar GTN, the FIGO conducted workshops among members of the Society of Gynecologic Oncologists, International Society for the Study of Trophoblastic Disease, and International Gynecologic Cancer Society to formulate its current recommendations for evaluation and staging this disease. The current FIGO requirements for making a diagnosis of postmolar GTN are as follows (Table 7.4):

1. Four values or more of plateaued hCG (±10%) over at least 3 weeks: days 1, 7, 14, and 21
2. A rise of hCG of 10% or greater for 3 values or more over at least 2 weeks: days 1, 7, and 14

TABLE 7.4   Diagnosis and Evaluation of Gestational Trophoblastic Neoplasia

Diagnosis of GTN

After molar evacuation: four values or more of plateaued hCG (±10%) over at least 3 weeks: days 1, 7, 14, and 21

After molar evacuation: a rise of hCG of 10% or greater for three values or more over at least 2 weeks: days 1, 7, and 14

After molar evacuation: persistence of hCG beyond 6 months

The histologic diagnosis of choriocarcinoma, invasive mole, or PSTT

Metastatic disease without established primary site with elevated hCG (pregnancy has been excluded)

Evaluation of GTN

Complete physical and pelvic examination; baseline hematologic, renal, and hepatic functions

Baseline quantitative hCG level

Chest radiograph or CT scan of chest

Brain MRI

CT or MRI scan of abdomen and pelvis

CT, Computed tomography; *GTN,* gestational trophoblastic neoplasia; *hCG,* human chorionic gonadotropin; *MRI,* magnetic resonance imaging; *PSTT,* placental site trophoblastic tumor.

3. Histologic diagnosis of choriocarcinoma
4. Persistence of hCG beyond 6 months after mole evacuation

The level and duration for observation of the hCG plateau beyond 3 weeks would be determined at the discretion of the treating physician. Observation of hCG level plateau for longer than 3 weeks was permitted because this does not appear to have an adverse effect on survival.

Recently, laboratory assays for hyperglycosylated hCG have been found to be highly sensitive for differentiating active GTN or choriocarcinoma from inactive or "quiescent" GTD in patients with hCG level plateaus. These newer assays, developed by Cole and associates at the US hCG Reference Service at the University of New Mexico, may allow earlier diagnosis of postmolar GTN in the future.

The majority of centers in the United States treat patients if metastases are identified. In contrast, Bagshawe and colleagues in the United Kingdom followed patients with pulmonary nodules conservatively and based treatment decisions on hCG regression patterns. Although the overall results from this policy were excellent, outcome for patients with pulmonary metastases was not detailed. In the United States, where care is decentralized, identification of metastases is included as an indication for initiation of therapy.

"Phantom" Human Chorionic Gonadotropin

Rarely, women present with persistently elevated hCG levels but are subsequently found to have a false-positive hCG assay result, sometimes after receiving chemotherapy or surgery for presumed malignant GTN. Most patients with "phantom" hCG present with low-level hCG elevations, but occasionally values as high as 200 to 300 mIU/mL have been recorded. The false-positive hCG values result from nonspecific heterophile antibodies that interfere with the hCG immunometric sandwich

assays. Many of these patients have an undefined previous pregnancy event and do not have radiographic evidence of metastatic disease. Serial hCG values usually do not substantially vary, despite prolonged observation, and do not substantially change with therapeutic interventions such as surgery or chemotherapy.

"Phantom" hCG may also present after evacuation of a hydatidiform mole or after a clearly defined pregnancy event, such as an ectopic pregnancy. It should be suspected if hCG values plateau at low levels and do not respond to therapeutic maneuvers such as methotrexate. Evaluation should include study of serum hCG using a variety of assay techniques at different dilutions of patient serum combined with a urinary hCG level if the serum level is above threshold for the urinary assay. Heterophile antibodies are not excreted in the urine. Therefore, if they are the cause of serum hCG level elevation, urinary hCG values will not be detectable. False-positive hCG assays are also not affected by serial dilution of patient sera and have markedly different values using different assay techniques, with the majority of assays reflecting undetectable hCG. Other techniques are available to inactivate or strip the patient's serum of heterophile antibodies, and many current assays now incorporate these techniques to reduce the incidence of false-positive results. It is important to exclude the possibility of "phantom" hCG before subjecting these patients to hysterectomy or chemotherapy for GTN.

The "Hook Effect"

Instead of being a false-positive test result such as a phantom hCG due to heterophile antibodies, the "hook effect" causes a false-negative hCG value. hCG immunoassays rely on a sandwich assay approach. A sandwich assay approach means that the hCG molecule binds to antibodies attached to a matrix and then additional free-floating "reporter" antibodies bind to the hCG attached to the matrix, and this sandwich of both antibodies on the same molecule is how the hCG level is measured. In the "hook effect," the assay is overwhelmed by very high levels of hCG, generally greater than 1,000,000 mIU/mL. The large number of hCG molecules bind not only to the antibodies on the matrix but to the reporter antibodies as well. Many fewer or no "sandwiches" are created, and the hCG result will either be falsely low or falsely negative. The "hook effect" can be overcome by serial dilution of the serum before using an hCG immunoassay, and this is standard practice in many laboratories; however, if a false-negative hCG is suspected, serial dilution of the patient's serum should be performed.

Pretherapy Evaluation

In contrast to epithelial endometrial cancer, GTN usually spreads by hematogenous dissemination. Venous metastasis can occur in the subvaginal venous plexus, resulting in vaginal metastases (Fig. 7.13), or in the main uterine venous system with metastases to the parametrium and lungs. Although direct shunting into the systemic circulation may occur, the majority of disseminated metastases develop only after pulmonary metastases have become established. The brain, liver, GI tract, and kidneys are the distant organs most often affected, but

FIGURE 7.13 Vaginal metastasis of malignant gestational trophoblastic neoplasia (GTN), presenting as vaginal bleeding with a discolored submucosal mass underlying the urethra. Vaginal metastases of GTN are highly vascular and should not be biopsied. (Courtesy of John Soper, MD.)

metastases to virtually every organ have been reported. Although lymphatic spread can occur, it is relatively uncommon. The hematogenous pattern of metastatic involvement is important when considering the radiographic evaluation of patients with GTN (see Table 7.3).

Pretherapy evaluation of the patient with GTN (see Table 7.4) includes assessment of history for clinical risk factors, examination, laboratory evaluation, and radiographic survey for potential sites of metastatic disease and number of lesions. Clinical risk factors important for assigning staging and treatment include duration of disease interval from antecedent pregnancy, type of antecedent pregnancy, and previous treatment. Because of different clinical characteristics, patients with histologically proven ETT and PSTT are classified separately from patients with gestational choriocarcinoma or postmolar GTN.

The laboratory evaluation should include a pretherapy hCG value. It should be emphasized that the hCG level obtained immediately before instituting treatment for malignant GTN is the one used for staging—not the hCG level obtained at the time of molar evacuation.

Vaginal metastases of GTN are diagnosed by physical examination. These lesions usually involve the mucosa of the anterior vagina and present as dark, often blue, soft nodules (see Fig. 7.13). Ulceration or active bleeding may be present. Because of the highly vascular nature of these lesions, biopsy is not recommended. If the vagina is the only site of metastasis, the majority of these lesions respond to chemotherapy. A few patients require vaginal packing or selective embolization using interventional radiology to control active hemorrhage.

The recommended radiographic staging evaluation for patients with GTN includes evaluation of the abdomen and pelvis with computed tomography (CT) or magnetic resonance imaging (MRI) and contrasted MRI of the brain. Ultrasonography of the pelvis should also be obtained to exclude the possibility of intrauterine pregnancy before instituting chemotherapy. Both ultrasound and MRI studies of the uterus can be used to identify intrauterine tumors and foci of myometrial invasion by GTN, but they are not sensitive or specific enough to replace serum hCG level monitoring for establishing the diagnosis of GTN or for following patients during treatment.

Approximately 45% of patients have metastatic disease when GTN is diagnosed. As indicated by the anatomic sites of metastatic disease encountered among patients initially treated for malignant GTN (see Table 7.3), the lungs are the most frequent site of extrauterine metastasis (Fig. 7.14). Although the majority of patients with high-risk metastatic sites have pulmonary metastases on chest radiograph or symptoms of metastatic involvement, a full metastatic evaluation is recommended for all patients rather than relying on a negative chest radiograph alone to make a determination of nonmetastatic GTN.

Between 29% and 41% of patients treated for nonmetastatic GTN have pulmonary metastases identified on chest CT that are not detected by chest radiography. The prognostic importance of occult pulmonary metastases is debated when they are the only sites of extrauterine metastases. However, many series of patients treated for high-risk metastases include patients who initially presented with normal chest radiographs. It would be a tragedy to miss the diagnosis of a high-risk metastasis in a patient and delay appropriate aggressive initial therapy.

Although operative procedures may be integrated into the treatment of patients with malignant GTN, they are rarely indicated for establishing the diagnosis or staging. Performing a secondary D&C before beginning chemotherapy in a patient with postmolar GTN is controversial. The experience at the University of Southern California indicated that it had an effect on the treatment in only 20% of patients and was complicated by uterine perforation requiring hysterectomy in 8% of patients. In contrast, Pezeshki and associates analyzed 544 women undergoing a second uterine evacuation for presumed postmolar GTN. After a second evacuation, 368 (68%) entered spontaneous remission. Of 251 patients with a histologic diagnosis of persistent GTD, 96 (38%) required chemotherapy compared with 39 (18%) of 219 with negative histology at the second D&C. A GOG study attempted to answer this question definitively. They prospectively enrolled 64 low-risk nonmetastatic GTN patients and performed a second curettage as initial management of GTN. Only preliminary results are currently available. The authors found that 38% underwent a surgical cure and did not need additional treatment, but 55% underwent progression. They observed one uterine perforation and one grade 3 hemorrhage. Four patients underwent transformation to a PSTT, which would have not been discovered without repeat curettage. The results of this study indicate that a surgical cure is possible but less likely than progression of disease and thus will likely not alter current practice patterns regarding repeat curettage. Many clinicians in the United States treat

FIGURE 7.14 Pulmonary metastases of gestational trophoblastic neoplasia can present as solitary (A) or diffuse (B) pulmonary nodules. (Courtesy of John Soper, MD.)

TABLE 7.5 Clinical Classification System for Patients With Malignant Gestational Trophoblastic Neoplasia

Category	Criteria
Nonmetastatic GTN	No evidence of metastases; not assigned to prognostic category
Metastatic GTN	Any extrauterine metastases
Good-prognosis metastatic GTN	Short duration (<4 months)
	No brain or liver metastases
	Pretherapy hCG <40,000 mIU/mL
	No antecedent term pregnancy
	No prior chemotherapy
Poor-prognosis metastatic GTN	Any one risk factor:
	Long duration (>4 months)
	Pretherapy hCG >40,000 mIU/mL
	Brain or liver metastases
	Antecedent term pregnancy
	Prior chemotherapy

GTN, Gestational trophoblastic neoplasia; hCG, human chorionic gonadotropin.

patients with postmolar GTN without performing a second D&C because of the concern for preservation of fertility. Other operative procedures such as laparoscopy, thoracotomy, or craniotomy are rarely justifiable to establish the primary diagnosis of GTN.

Classification and Staging

The classification and staging of malignant GTN has evolved over the past 50 years. The Clinical Classification System, based on risk factors, was frequently used in the United States (Table 7.5). In this system, patients with nonmetastatic disease are not assigned into a prognostic group because of uniformly good outcome using simple single-agent chemotherapy. The risk factors used in this system were derived by retrospective analysis of resistance to single-agent methotrexate and actinomycin D regimens among women treated for metastatic GTN at the NIH. Hammond and colleagues subsequently reported essentially 100% survival among women who presented with good-prognosis metastatic GTN treated with single-agent therapy. He noted a survival rate of 70% among patients with metastatic poor prognosis disease initially treated with multiagent chemotherapy compared with only 14% survival for patients in this category who initially received single-agent therapy. Poor tolerance of multiagent therapy was noted in the group of poor-prognosis patients receiving initial single-agent regimens, with toxicity causing death in half of these patients.

A staging system was adopted by the World Health Organization (WHO) in the early 1980s based on the experience at the Charing Cross Hospital in London between 1957 and 1973. Bivariate analysis was used to identify prognostic factors among patients treated with predominantly single-agent chemotherapy regimens. In the original study, patient age, antecedent pregnancy, interval from antecedent pregnancy, hCG level, ABO blood type, size of the largest tumor, sites and number of metastases, and type of prior chemotherapy were each found to

TABLE 7.6 Prognostic Index Score Compared With Clinical Classification System*

Clinical Classification	Low Risk (<5)	Medium Risk (5–7)	High Risk (>8)	Total Clinical Classification
Nonmetastatic GTN	99.5% (217)	100% (10)	—	99.7% (227)
Metastatic GTN				
Good prognosis	100% (86)	100% (5)	—	100% (91)
Poor prognosis	100% (8)	90.5% (21)	68.4% (38)	79.1% (67)
Total WHO	99.8% (311)	94.4% (36)	68.4% (38)	

*Data presented as life table survival percentage (number of patients).
GTN, Gestational trophoblastic neoplasia; WHO, World Health Organization.
Modified from Soper JT, Evans AC, Conaway MR, et al. Evaluation of prognostic factors and staging in gestational trophoblastic tumor. *Obstet Gynecol* 1994;84:969.

correlate with prognosis. The prognostic index applied a weighted score to each of these factors, which were assumed to act independently. The sum of component scores was then used to determine the individual patient's risk category.

Multivariate analyses have not confirmed that the factors have independent effects on prognosis. Paternal blood-type information is not uniformly available and was omitted in generating WHO score values by many investigators. Others modified the weighted scoring system using a highest risk score of 6 for each prognostic factor while not changing the total score for assigning patients into risk categories. Furthermore, the WHO prognostic index score provided for reassignment of a score among patients who have previously received treatment for GTN, which might obscure the prognostic effects of some of the other clinical factors on primary treatment. Finally, there was no uniformity in assessing size of the largest tumor or assigning number of metastases. Despite these limitations, modifications of the WHO prognostic index score were useful for predicting risk groups of patients with malignant GTN.

In Table 7.6, the Clinical Classification System and WHO prognostic index score are compared among patients who presented for initial treatment of GTN at Duke University Medical Center before 1990. The Clinical Classification System had a greater sensitivity for identifying patients at risk for treatment failure and death (see Table 7.6). Although the WHO prognostic index score was able to provide slightly better discrimination of patients with poor prognosis metastatic disease in low-, intermediate-, and high-risk populations, stratification into three categories was considered less important than identifying patients at risk of failure for initial therapy. Using multivariate analysis, both systems were roughly equivalent for stratifying patients into risk groups.

In the early 1980s, the FIGO proposed an anatomic staging system for malignant GTN (Table 7.7). Although this system recognized the stepwise development of metastatic disease, it did not incorporate any of the other prognostic factors into the FIGO stage. Although stage I patients uniformly had low-risk disease and stage IV patients had uniformly high-risk disease, there was considerable overlap of outcome within stages II and III. Revision of the FIGO staging in 1992 recognized hCG level and time from antecedent pregnancy as risk factors. These factors generated substages within each stage. Although this revised system did correlate with outcome, it resulted in a

TABLE 7.7 Anatomic International Federation of Gynecology and Obstetrics Staging System for Gestational Trophoblastic Neoplasia

Stage	Criteria
I	Disease confined to the uterus
II	Disease outside of uterus but is limited to the genital structures
III	Disease extends to the lungs with or without known genital tract involvement
IV	All other metastatic sites

Modified from Kohorn EI. The new FIGO 2000 staging and risk factor scoring system for gestational trophoblastic disease: description and critical assessment. *Int J Gynecol Cancer* 2000;11:73.

proliferation of substages, was confusing for clinicians, and is therefore of questionable importance.

In 2000, the FIGO revised its staging system for GTN again. The original anatomic stages were retained, but the 1992 risk factors were replaced by a risk factor score that used a modification of the WHO prognostic index score (Table 7.8). Patients with histologically diagnosed PSTT and ETT were reported separately, reflecting the distinct tumor biology of these lesions. Changes to the WHO classification included elimination of ABO blood group risk factors and a change in the risk score for liver metastasis from 2 to 4, reflecting the worse prognosis for patients with liver metastasis. Radiographic staging studies were standardized. Finally, the three risk groups of the WHO prognostic index score were consolidated into two groups: low risk with a score of 6 or less and high risk with a score of 7 or greater. Hancock and colleagues retrospectively compared the outcomes of patients according to the risk score categories generated by the modified WHO prognostic index score and the proposed FIGO score. The consolidated risk categories generated by the FIGO score correlated better with outcome than did the modified WHO prognostic index score.

The current FIGO system counts and measures pulmonary metastases only if they are visible on chest radiograph. Other recommended studies include CT scan of the abdomen and pelvis, ultrasonography of the uterus, and MRI or contrasted CT scan of the brain. It is important to realize that the hCG level used to generate the risk score refers to the level recorded at the time GTN is diagnosed *rather than hCG at the time of*

TABLE 7.8 The Revised International Federation of Gynecology and Obstetrics 2000 Scoring System for Gestational Trophoblastic Neoplasia*

FIGO Score	0	1	2	4
Age (years)	<40	≥40		
Antecedent pregnancy	Hydatidiform mole	Abortion	Term pregnancy	
Interval from index pregnancy (months)	<4	4–6	7–12	≥13
Pretreatment hCG (mIU/mL)	<1000	1000–<10,000	10,000–100,000	≥100,000
Largest tumor size including uterus (cm)		3–5	≥5	
Site of metastases	<3	Spleen, kidney	Gastrointestinal	Brain, liver
Number of metastases identified	0	1–4	5–8	>8
Previous failed chemotherapy			Single drug	≥2 drugs

*The total score for a patient is obtained by adding the individual scores for each prognostic factor. Total score 0–6 = low risk; >7 = high risk. From Kohorn EI. The new FIGO 2000 staging and risk factor scoring system for gestational trophoblastic disease: description and critical assessment. *Int J Gynecol Cancer* 2000;11:73.

molar evacuation. Under the new FIGO system, reporting of patients includes both anatomic stage and FIGO risk score. For example, a 30-year-old patient with nonmetastatic GTN diagnosed 5 months after molar evacuation with an hCG level of 8000 mIU/mL would be recorded as a FIGO stage I: 2. Likewise, a 40-year-old patient with index term pregnancy 7 months previously, hCG of 200,000 mIU/mL, 2 brain metastases, 10 lung lesions, and uterine tumor measuring 6 cm would be FIGO stage IV: 17.

Adoption of the current revision of FIGO staging for GTN will allow uniformity for evaluation and reporting of outcomes. With accumulation of data through FIGO, it is hoped that multivariate analysis can confirm or refute the prognostic importance of individual factors used to generate the risk scores. Although these changes are important on an international scale and are the standard for reporting results of treatment, they are of lesser importance for the practicing general obstetrician/gynecologist initially encountering patients with malignant GTN. For these clinicians, the most important decisions revolve around identification of patients who should be referred out of the community to a specialist for treatment of high-risk disease. Because the clinical classification system (see Table 7.5) is relatively simple, it may be the best system for use by the generalist for the purpose of appropriate referral.

Treatment of Nonmetastatic and Low-Risk Metastatic Gestational Trophoblastic Neoplasia

Primary remission rates of patients treated for nonmetastatic or low-risk GTN are similar using a variety of chemotherapy regimens (Table 7.9). Essentially all patients with low-risk GTN can be cured, usually without the need for hysterectomy. Randomized comparisons of all the regimens detailed in Table 7.9 have not been completed, and comparison of the results may not be valid because of slightly different criteria used to make the diagnosis of nonmetastatic GTN by different investigators. Patients with metastatic GTN who lack any of the clinical high-risk factors or have a total FIGO risk score of 6 or lower have low-risk disease and can be treated successfully with initial single-agent chemotherapy regimens.

Methotrexate 0.4 mg/kg/day given by intramuscular (IM) injection for 5 days, with cycles repeated every 12 to 14 days,

TABLE 7.9 Chemotherapy Regimens for Nonmetastatic and Low-Risk Metastatic Gestational Trophoblastic Neoplasia

Agent and Schedule	Dosage
Methotrexate*	
Weekly	30–50 mg/m² IM
5 day/every 2 weeks	0.4 mg/kg IM (maximum, 25 mg/day total dose)
Methotrexate–folinic acid rescue	Methotrexate 1 mg/kg IM, days 1, 3, 5, 7; and Folinic acid 0.1 mg/kg IM, days 2, 4, 6, 8
Every 2 weeks	
Methotrexate infusion–folinic acid	Methotrexate 100 mg/m² IV bolus; and Methotrexate 200 mg/m² 12 hour infusion with 15 mg PO every 6 hours for four doses
Every 2 weeks	
Dactinomycin†	
5 day/every 2 weeks	9–13 mcg/kg/day IV (maximum dose, 500 mcg/day)
Bolus, every 2 weeks	1.25 mg/m² IV bolus
Etoposide‡	
5 day/every 2 weeks	200 mg/m²/day PO

*Dose based on ideal body weight, maximum 2 m².
†Potential extravasation injury, gastrointestinal toxicity common.
‡Alopecia, small leukemogenic risk.
IM, Intramuscular; *IV,* intravenous; *PO,* oral.

was the regimen originally used to treat GTN at the NIH. Hammond and colleagues reported the NIH experience treating 58 patients with nonmetastatic GTN. Only four (7%) patients had disease resistant to this regimen, and three of these were salvaged with single-agent actinomycin D. In Lurain's series from the Brewer Trophoblastic Disease Center, all 337 patients with nonmetastatic GTN were cured using this regimen. Only 10.7% of 253 patients initially treated with 5-day IM methotrexate therapy required a second agent, only 1.2% needed multiagent chemotherapy, and only 0.8% required hysterectomy to achieve a complete remission. Factors significantly associated with the development of methotrexate resistance included pretreatment serum hCG in excess of 50,000 mIU/mL, nonmolar antecedent pregnancy, and histopathologic diagnosis of choriocarcinoma. Others have used 5-day IM methotrexate, reporting similar results. If patients have abnormal liver function, methotrexate should not be used because it is metabolized in the liver. Significant hematologic suppression, cutaneous toxicity, mucositis, alopecia, GI toxicity, and serositis are frequently seen in patients receiving the 5-day methotrexate regimen.

Patients with low-risk GTN and metastasis have higher failure rates. DuBeshter and colleagues used single-agent methotrexate or actinomycin D to treat 48 patients with low-risk metastatic GTN at the NETDC. All patients achieved sustained remission, but 51% required a second drug, 14% needed combination chemotherapy, and 12% required surgery to remove drug-resistant disease. Among 52 patients with low-risk metastatic GTN treated initially with the 5-day methotrexate regimen at Duke University Medical Center, 60% achieved primary remission within a median three cycles of methotrexate chemotherapy. Patients were treated with actinomycin D for documented methotrexate resistance or toxicity with equal frequency. All patients achieved remission, with only 4% requiring multiagent regimens. Likewise, Roberts and Lurain treated 92 patients for low-risk metastatic GTN at the Brewer Trophoblastic Disease Center. Among their 70 patients who were initially treated with chemotherapy alone, 24.6% developed chemoresistant disease, and 9.8% had therapy changed because of toxicity. Overall, 78% achieved remission using the primary regimen with or without hysterectomy. However, all eventually achieved remission, and only one (1.1%) required multiagent chemotherapy.

Bagshawe and Wilde first reported the use of alternating daily doses of IM methotrexate (1 mg/kg) and leucovorin factor or folinic acid (0.1 mg/kg) for four doses of each agent in an attempt to reduce the toxicity of daily methotrexate regimens. Whereas toxicity sparing may be true for high doses of methotrexate, Rotmensch and colleagues evaluated methotrexate levels in patients after daily methotrexate therapy compared with levels in patients receiving alternating daily doses of methotrexate and folinic acid, with a higher daily dose of methotrexate given in the methotrexate–folinic acid regimen. They noted that whereas patients on the methotrexate–folinic acid regimen had higher peak methotrexate levels after treatment with the higher methotrexate dose, trough levels were both subtoxic and subtherapeutic 24 hours after methotrexate administration. This finding alone might explain the therapeutic and toxicity benefit described for the low-dose methotrexate–folinic acid regimen used for treatment in GTN.

At Charing Cross Hospital in London, 347 of 348 (99.7%) low-risk patients treated with methotrexate and folinic acid survived; however, 69 (20%) had to change treatment because of drug resistance, and 23 (6%) patients needed to change because of drug-induced toxicity. An analysis of the data from the Southeastern Trophoblastic Disease Center at Duke University indicated that 8 (27.5%) of 29 patients developed resistance to methotrexate with folinic acid given at 14-day intervals compared with 3 (7.7%) of 39 treated with standard 5-day

methotrexate for nonmetastatic disease. Although this difference was statistically significant, a similar proportion of patients was changed to a second agent in each group because a larger number of patients receiving 5-day methotrexate changed therapy because of toxicity. Wong and colleagues also compared 5-day methotrexate with methotrexate with folinic acid, resulting in comparable sustained remission rates. In their series, however, patients who received methotrexate–folinic acid achieved remission earlier but experienced a higher incidence of hepatic toxicity compared with patients receiving the 5-day regimen.

McNeish and associates, reporting from the Charing Cross system, reviewed the results of 485 patients with low-risk GTN (prognostic index score <8, using their modification) treated with cyclical IM methotrexate–folinic acid, and the overall survival rate was 100%. Whereas two-thirds achieved remission with primary chemotherapy, 150 patients were changed to an alternative agent because of chemoresistance. In patients with chemoresistant disease and hCG levels less than 100 mIU/mL, therapy was changed to single-agent actinomycin D, with 89% responding to actinomycin D, and the remaining patients were salvaged with multiagent regimens. If hCG levels were greater than 100 mIU/mL, patients were treated with a multiagent regimen containing etoposide, with 98.9% responding to the first salvage regimen and all patients entering sustained remission.

Berkowitz and colleagues, at the NETDC, used IM methotrexate with folinic acid rescue in 185 patients with GTN. Ninety percent of 163 patients with nonmetastatic disease and 68% of 22 patients with low-risk metastatic disease were placed into complete remission with this regimen. Rather than recycling treatment at fixed intervals, they treated patients based on hCG level response. More than 80% were placed into remission with only one course of chemotherapy. All patients with methotrexate resistance achieved remission with other agents. Other investigators have used higher doses of IV methotrexate (300–500 mg/m^2) followed by oral or IV folinic acid every 6 hours for 24 hours, resulting in primary remission rates of 45% to 86% in patients with nonmetastatic or low-risk metastatic GTN. Overall cure rates in these series were excellent, and toxicity was minimal. A major disadvantage with these regimens is the need for a prolonged (up to 12-hour) IV infusion.

Oral methotrexate is readily absorbed via the GI tract. Barter reported a retrospective analysis of 15 patients treated solely with oral methotrexate 0.4 mg/kg for 5-day cycles that were repeated every 14 days. The primary remission rate was 87% with minimal toxicity. Concerns about patient compliance and the possibility of unpredictable absorption in individual patients have led to infrequent use for this mode of treatment in GTN.

In a prospective phase II trial, the GOG reported an 82% primary remission rate for patients treated with weekly IM methotrexate given at a dose of 30 to 50 mg/m^2. Remission was achieved within a median seven cycles of therapy. There was no apparent benefit for increasing the dose up to 50 mg/m^2. It was concluded that the weekly methotrexate regimen was most cost effective among several alternative methotrexate or actinomycin D schedules when taking efficacy, toxicity, and cost into consideration. Hoffman and colleagues confirmed the low toxicity and overall remission rates for patients treated with this regimen. In the experience reported by Hoffman and colleagues, weekly methotrexate was compared with methotrexate–folinic acid, producing equivalent primary remission rates. Total doses of methotrexate required to induce remission were lower in the weekly methotrexate group. They also concluded that weekly methotrexate was minimally toxic and equally effective and is their preferred regimen for nonmetastatic GTN.

In contrast to IM methotrexate regimens used for treating ectopic pregnancies, chemotherapy for GTN is given every week until hCG values have achieved normal levels, and then an additional course is administered after the first normal hCG value has been recorded. Hematologic indices must be monitored carefully during chemotherapy, but significant hematologic toxicity is infrequent among patients treated with the weekly methotrexate regimen.

Other investigators have used 5-day courses of IV actinomycin D (9–13 mcg/kg/day) as primary therapy for nonmetastatic or low-risk GTN with equally good results. They believe that toxicity from 5-day actinomycin D is less than that from 5-day methotrexate regimens. However, alopecia, nausea, and significant myelotoxicity can result. Furthermore, extravasation of actinomycin D during administration can result in severe local soft tissue damage.

Treatment of nonmetastatic and low-risk metastatic GTN with actinomycin D (1.25 mg/m^2) given as a single IV bolus dose every 2 weeks, generally referred to as pulse or bolus actinomycin D, had equal remission rates in retrospective series to 5-day courses of IV actinomycin D. The GOG reported a phase II study of this regimen. Of 31 patients who were treated, 29 (94%) achieved remission after an average of 4.4 (range, 2–15) courses of therapy. The two patients who failed to respond to pulse therapy were subsequently cured by alternative treatment. The frequency of toxicity was quite low. The advantages of pulse actinomycin D over other treatment schedules include ease of administration, greater patient convenience, and improved cost effectiveness. Moreover, the single bolus administration appears to reduce the risk of extravasation injuries compared with 5-day IV administration.

Other investigators have alternated courses of 5-day IM methotrexate with 5-day IV actinomycin D in an attempt to limit toxicity and improve primary remission rates. Rose and Piver combined their experience using this approach in nine patients with a literature review of 40 patients treated in this manner. All patients were cured with primary therapy when the two regimens were alternated. However, given the relatively small numbers of patients and selectivity of reporting small series of patients in the literature, one cannot conclude that this strategy is superior to beginning therapy in patients with GTN using a single agent and changing to the alternative only if chemoresistance or toxicity is encountered.

Oral etoposide and 5-fluorouracil (5-FU) are frequently used in Asia for primary treatment of patients with nonmetastatic and low-risk metastatic GTN, but they are not often used in the United States. Among patients treated with a 10-day continuous IV infusion of 5-FU, Sung and colleagues reported

a 93% primary remission rate. Acute toxicity included diarrhea, nausea and vomiting, hepatotoxicity, and stomatitis. Wong and colleagues reported a 98% primary remission rate among patients treated with 5-day courses of oral etoposide 100 mg/m^2, recycled at 14-day intervals. Toxicity included frequent alopecia, myelosuppression, and GI toxicity. Furthermore, patients exposed to etoposide have a low but significant risk of developing acute myelogenous leukemia. Based on considerations of convenience, cost, and toxicity, these agents are not usually used as initial therapy for low-risk GTN in the United States.

Few randomized trials have been conducted in patients with low-risk GTN. Lerkhachonsuk and colleagues randomly assigned 49 stage I low-risk patients to the 5-day IV actinomycin D or IM alternating methotrexate–folinic acid. Six women in the methotrexate arm required cross-over to actinomycin D because of rising liver function test (LFT) results. All 20 women in the actinomycin D arm achieved remission versus 14 (73.6%) in the methotrexate–folinic acid arm ($P = 0.02$). Whereas mucositis and alopecia were more frequent in the actinomycin D group, elevations of LFT results were more frequent in the methotrexate–folinic acid group.

Yarand and colleagues randomly assigned 131 women with FIGO low-risk GTN to pulsed weekly IM methotrexate (30 mg/m^2) versus biweekly IV bolus actinomycin D (1.25 mg/m^2). Primary remission rates were 48% versus 90% ($P <0.01$), respectively. The mean number of treatment cycles needed to achieve remission was lower in the actinomycin D group (4.8 vs. 6.8). Toxicity was reported as low in each of the treatment arms.

A larger GOG phase three trial of weekly methotrexate versus pulsed actinomycin D in 240 women confirmed these results. Biweekly actinomycin bolus was superior to methotrexate in producing a complete response of 70% for the actinomycin arm and 53% for weekly methotrexate ($P = 0.01$). An increased FIGO risk score, increased hCG, and metastatic disease were associated with a higher primary failure rate.

The performance of 5-day methotrexate has also been compared with actinomycin D. A retrospective series by Mousavi reported on 75 women with low-risk GTN who received either actinomycin D or 5-day methotrexate. Complete response rates were 90% for actinomycin D and 68% for methotrexate ($P = 0.018$). However, the mean numbers of chemotherapy courses were 3.1 in the methotrexate group and 5.3 in the actinomycin group ($P = 0.01$). An ongoing GOG trial is examining pulse actinomycin D versus multiday methotrexate regimens to answer this question in a randomized fashion.

Among patients with nonmetastatic and low-risk GTN, early hysterectomy will shorten the duration and amount of chemotherapy required to produce remission. Therefore, each patient's desire for further childbearing should be evaluated at the onset of treatment. Hysterectomy may be performed during the first cycle of chemotherapy (Fig. 7.15). However, further chemotherapy after hysterectomy is mandatory until hCG values are normal.

Treatment for nonmetastatic and low-risk metastatic GTN is outlined in Table 7.10. Most centers in the United States begin

FIGURE 7.15 Hysterectomy specimen in a 39-year-old woman with nonmetastatic gestational trophoblastic neoplasia who underwent surgery during her first course of methotrexate. She entered complete remission 4 weeks after initial therapy. (Courtesy of John Soper, MD.)

TABLE 7.10 Management of Low-Risk Gestational Trophoblastic Neoplasia

Initiate single-agent methotrexate or dactinomycin regimen (see Table 7.9).
Consider hysterectomy if fertility is not desired.
Monitor hematologic, renal, and hepatic indices before each cycle of chemotherapy.
Monitor serum hCG levels weekly during therapy.
Change to alternative single-agent if resistance or severe toxicity to first agent.
If resistance to alternative agent:
1. Repeat metastatic evaluation
2. Consider hysterectomy if no extrauterine metastases
3. Multiagent therapy (MAC or EMA/CO; see text)
Remission: three consecutive weekly hCG values in the normal range
1 or 2 cycles of maintenance or consolidation chemotherapy

EMA/CO, Etoposide, methotrexate, actinomycin D, cyclophosphamide and vincristine; *hCG,* human chorionic gonadotropin; *MAC,* methotrexate, actinomycin D, and cyclophosphamide.

therapy with the bolus actinomycin D regimen or methotrexate. Weekly hCG values should be monitored during treatment, along with hematologic and metabolic studies to monitor for toxicity. Chemotherapy is repeated until hCG levels normalize, and at least one cycle of chemotherapy is given as maintenance chemotherapy to prevent recurrence. Reliable contraception should be used to prevent a new pregnancy during chemotherapy and hCG monitoring after remission. Again, consideration should be given to oral contraceptives given the effect of the LH surge on hCG assay measurement.

Patients for whom hCG levels have plateaued or are rising during therapy should be switched to an alternative single-agent regimen after radiographic restaging. If there are new metastases or failure of the alternative single-agent chemotherapy, the patient should be treated with a multiagent regimen. Hysterectomy should be considered for the treatment of disease that is refractory to chemotherapy and confined to the uterus.

The overall cure rate for patients with nonmetastatic and low-risk GTN approaches 100%. The majority of women who wish to preserve fertility can be cured without hysterectomy. When chemotherapy is given for an additional one to two cycles after the first normal hCG value, recurrence rates are less than 5%.

High-Risk Metastatic Gestational Trophoblastic Neoplasia

Patients with metastatic disease and one or more of the clinical classification system risk factors or a FIGO risk score of 7 or greater have high-risk disease. They require multiagent chemotherapy. It should be emphasized that patients with high-risk metastatic GTN should have their treatment directed by individuals who have experience in treating this relatively rare disease, preferably in a trophoblastic disease center. Survival in modern series is greater than 94%. In contrast to patients with nonmetastatic or low-risk metastatic GTN, early hysterectomy does not appear to improve the outcome in women with high-risk metastatic disease.

Aggressive treatment with multiagent chemotherapy is standard of care for high risk GTN. Triple therapy (Table 7.11) with methotrexate, actinomycin D, and either chlorambucil or cyclophosphamide (MAC) was the standard regimen for many years in the United States, producing sustained remission rates of 63% to 73%. Studies from the Southeastern Regional and the Brewer Trophoblastic Disease Centers in the 1970s documented the importance of initial combination chemotherapy for these patients; whereas single-agent regimens followed by multiagent chemotherapy produced only 14% to 39% remissions, patients with high-risk GTN treated initially with MAC chemotherapy had remission rates of 65% to 70%.

In the late 1970s, the Charing Cross group developed a complex, alternating regimen using cyclophosphamide, hydroxyurea, actinomycin D, methotrexate–folinic acid, vincristine, and doxorubicin (CHAMOCA). Sustained remissions were reported in 56% to 83% of patients with high-risk GTN using modifications of this regimen with an overall impression of reduced toxicity compared to MAC. However, when the GOG performed a randomized trial of MAC versus CHAMOCA, the

TABLE 7.11 Triple-Agent (MAC) Chemotherapy for High-Risk Gestational Trophoblastic Neoplasia

Day	Drug	Dose
1–5	Methotrexate	15 mg IM
	Actinomycin D	500 mcg IV
	Chlorambucil	8–10 mg PO
	OR	
	Cyclophosphamide	3 mg/kg IV
15–22	Begin next cycle	

IM, Intramuscular; *IV,* intravenous; *MAC,* methotrexate, actinomycin D, and cyclophosphamide; *PO,* oral.

TABLE 7.12 Alternating Weekly EMA/CO Chemotherapy for High-Risk Gestational Trophoblastic Neoplasia

Day	Drug	Dose
1	Etoposide	100 mg/m² IV
	Methotrexate*	100 mg/m² IV bolus
	Methotrexate	200 mg/m² IV infusion over 12 hours
	Actinomycin D	350 mcg/m² IV
2	Etoposide	100 mg/m² IV
	Actinomycin D	350 mcg/m² IV
	Folinic acid	15 mg PO, IM or IV every 12 hours × 4 doses; begin 24 hours after methotrexate bolus
8	Cyclophosphamide	600 mg/m² IV
	Vincristine	1 mg/m² IV
15	Begin next cycle	

EMA/CO, Etoposide, methotrexate, actinomycin D, cyclophosphamide and vincristine; *IM,* intramuscular; *IV,* intravenous; *PO,* oral.
*Methotrexate is sometimes given as a 12-hour IV infusion at a dose of 500–1000 mg/m² for treatment of brain metastases, with folinic acid rescue increased to 15 mg every 6 hours × 48 hours or 30 mg every 12 hours × 48 hours.

TABLE 7.13 Management of High-Risk Gestational Trophoblastic Neoplasia

Evaluate for high-risk metastases: brain, liver, kidney.
Stabilize medical status of patient.
Multiagent therapy with EMA/CO (see Table 7.12) or MAC
- Aggressive recycling may require cytokine support.
Management of brain metastases (see text)
- Consider gamma knife radiation if isolated brain lesion.
- CNS-dosed methotrexate
Management of liver metastases (see text)
- Consider selective angiographic embolization.
Monitor hCG weekly during therapy.
- At least three cycles of maintenance chemotherapy after hCG values normalize

CNS, central nervous system; *EMA/CO,* etoposide, methotrexate, actinomycin D, cyclophosphamide and vincristine; *hCG,* human chorionic gonadotropin; *MAC,* methotrexate, actinomycin D, and cyclophosphamide.

primary remission rates were comparable at 73% and 65%, respectively. Of note, five of six patients who failed MAC were salvaged compared with only one of seven patients failing CHAMOCA. Perhaps initial exposure to marginally effective additional agents in CHAMOCA adversely affected the efficacy or tolerance of savage regimens. Furthermore, the CHAMOCA regimen had significantly more acute life-threatening toxicity, with a 45% incidence of grade 4 toxicity compared to only 9% with MAC (P <0.05).

More recent regimens have incorporated etoposide into primary combination chemotherapy for GTN. Alternating weekly chemotherapy (Table 7.12) with etoposide, methotrexate–folinic acid rescue, actinomycin D–cyclophosphamide, and vincristine (EMA/CO) was first developed by the Charing Cross group. Their initial report documented 86% survival rate for patients with high-risk GTN after primary treatment with EMA/CO. In their most recent series published in 2014, Agarwal and colleagues included 196 patients with high-risk

GTN treated with EMA/CO between 1995 and 2010. The overall survival rate was 94% with a median follow-up of 4.7 years. Other smaller retrospective series have reported complete response rates of 65% to 94% among patients with high-risk GTN treated initially with EMA/CO. As a result of these reports, EMA/CO has become the most widely used regimen for treatment of patients with high-risk GTN.

Toxicity from EMA/CO includes universal alopecia and rare stomatitis and nausea and vomiting. Myelosuppression is often the acute dose-limiting acute toxicity. Several investigators have used stem cell support with granulocyte colony-stimulating factor to avoid dose reductions or treatment delays during EMA/CO therapy.

Platinum-containing regimens have also been found to be active in treating GTN. Cisplatin combined with etoposide and actinomycin D (PEA) demonstrated complete responses in 57% to 100% of patients with high-risk GTN. A 1-day course of cisplatin and etoposide (EP) was originally substituted for CO and combined with EMA to treat patients with refractory GTN. Surwit and Childers successfully treated four high-risk patients initially with EMA/EP, but concerns about acute toxicity have kept it from becoming widely accepted as primary therapy. It should be emphasized that MAC and EMA/CO are the two regimens that have been most extensively evaluated for the treatment of high-risk GTN (Table 7.13), but these have never been compared in a randomized trial. The majority of the literature for other regimens has been in the form of retrospective analyses of relatively small numbers of patients using slightly different definitions of "high-risk" GTN. Regardless of the regimen selected, aggressive recycling of multiagent therapy is the cornerstone for management of patients with high-risk disease (see Table 7.13).

Management of cerebral metastases is controversial. Radiation therapy has been used concurrently with chemotherapy in an attempt to limit acute hemorrhagic complications from these metastases. Brain irradiation combined with systemic chemotherapy is successful in controlling brain metastases, with cure rates up to 75% in patients who initially present with brain metastases. However, a similar primary remission rate has also been reported among patients treated with combination regimens that incorporated high-dose systemic methotrexate combined with intrathecal methotrexate infusions without brain irradiation. It should be noted that at Charing Cross Hospital, whole-brain irradiation is not used, and a recent series reports an 85% prolonged remission rate using central nervous system (CNS) dosing of chemotherapy alone. They note that the cognitive complications from whole-brain radiation should be considered, especially in young patients, and recommend against whole-brain radiation given the similar rate of cure compared with whole-brain radiation series that they report in their study. Targeted gamma knife radiation is another tool that clinicians can use to treat brain metastases, although this is a relatively new technology and is not as well studied.

The best treatment for liver or other high-risk sites of metastases has not been established. Even with intense chemotherapy, additional surgery may be necessary to control hemorrhage from metastases, remove chemoresistant disease, or treat other complications to stabilize high-risk patients during therapy.

The Charing Cross group reviewed the role of induction low-dose etoposide-cisplatin in combination with EMA/CO chemotherapy. Patients with high-risk metastatic GTN have a high disease burden, and early deaths (<4 weeks from diagnosis) have been observed in response to initial multiagent chemotherapy. Therefore, Charing Cross instituted a policy of using low-dose induction chemotherapy with cisplatin (20 mg/m²) and etoposide (100 mg/m²) to minimize the overwhelming amount of cell death that patients experience upon chemotherapy initiation. They successfully significantly reduced the rates of early death when patients received induction EP to 0.7% versus 7.6% when patients were treated initially with EMA/CO alone.

Treatment of patients with high-risk GTN who have developed chemoresistant disease is extremely challenging and is largely determined by prior chemotherapy exposure and cumulative toxicity from prior treatment. Patients who have not been exposed to etoposide-containing regimens are usually treated with EMA/CO, with remission rates of 71% to 82% reported for this group in several studies. The Charing Cross group used EMA/EP to treat 34 high-risk patients previously exposed to EMA/CO, reporting remission rates of 95% in patients with hCG level plateau during EMA/CO compared to 75% for those with rising hCG levels. Myelosuppression is more severe in patients receiving regimens for salvage than when they are used as primary therapy.

Variations of combination regimens used in the treatment of testicular and ovarian germ cell tumors have been used as salvage therapy in patients with GTN. Etoposide–platinum (± bleomycin ± doxorubicin) and vinblastine–bleomycin–cisplatin have remission rates reported between 50% and 86% in a small series of patients treated with these regimens, but they have long-term survival rates of usually less than 50% and considerable myelosuppression when used in a salvage setting. Ifosfamide-containing chemotherapy produced responses in four of five patients reported by Sutton and colleagues, but

TABLE 7.14 Surveillance During and After Therapy of Gestational Trophoblastic Neoplasia

Monitor serum quantitative hCG levels every week during chemotherapy:
1. Response: >10% decline in hCG during 1 cycle
2. Plateau: ±10% change in hCG during 1 cycle
3. Resistance: >10% rise in hCG during 1 cycle or plateau for 2 cycles of chemotherapy
   - Evaluate for new metastases.
   - Consider alternative chemotherapy (see text).
   - Consider extirpation of drug-resistant sites of disease.

Remission: three consecutive normal weekly hCG values
1. Maintenance chemotherapy (see text)

Surveillance of remission:
1. hCG values every 2 weeks × 3 months
2. hCG values every month to complete 1 year of follow-up
3. Physical examination every 6–12 months for at least 3–5 years

hCG, Human chorionic gonadotropin.

only one patient had a sustained remission. Anecdotal case reports and small series of patients also indicate activity of paclitaxel regimens, high-dose chemotherapy with autologous bone marrow or colony-stimulating factor support, and 5-FU/actinomycin D in treating drug-resistant disease.

Chemotherapy is continued until hCG values have normalized, and this is followed by at least three courses of maintenance chemotherapy in the hope of eradicating all viable tumor (Table 7.14). Despite using sensitive hCG assays and maintenance chemotherapy, up to 13% of patients with high-risk disease will develop recurrence after achieving an initial remission.

Surgery

Brewer and associates reported that the survival rates of patients treated with hysterectomy were 40% for women with nonmetastatic choriocarcinoma and only 19% for those with metastatic choriocarcinoma before effective chemotherapy was developed. The majority of their patients died of progressive disease within 2 years of surgery. The emergence of effective chemotherapy has lessened the importance of surgical procedures for primary management of malignant GTN. However, many procedures remain useful adjuncts when integrated into the management of these patients.

Primary or delayed hysterectomy can be integrated into management to remove central disease, and surgical extirpation of metastases may cure highly selected patients with drug-resistant disease. Surgical procedures are often required during therapy of patients with high-risk disease to treat complications of the disease, such as hemorrhage or abscess, and allow stabilization during chemotherapy. Percutaneous angiographic embolization can allow relatively noninvasive control of hemorrhagic complications of pelvic tumors or metastatic lesions.

Most patients with malignant GTN are in their peak reproductive years and do not wish sterilization. Furthermore, the majority can be cured with chemotherapy alone. Hammond and colleagues reported an overall 100% sustained remission rate among 194 patients treated at Duke University Medical Center for nonmetastatic or low-risk metastatic GTN. Of these, 162 wished to retain fertility, and 89% were able to avoid hysterectomy. All 32 women treated with primary hysterectomy combined with methotrexate or actinomycin D single-agent chemotherapy regimens entered sustained remission.

Compared with similar patients who had low-risk disease and were treated with chemotherapy alone, patients receiving primary hysterectomy had shorter durations of chemotherapy and lower total dosage of chemotherapy, roughly equivalent to one cycle of chemotherapy. Suzuka and associates also analyzed the total dosage of chemotherapy in women treated with etoposide for low-risk GTN. They found that the total dosage of etoposide was decreased in women with nonmetastatic disease treated with adjuvant hysterectomy compared with those who were treated with chemotherapy alone, again roughly equivalent to a single cycle of chemotherapy. In other series, hysterectomy was incorporated into the primary therapy of approximately 25% of patients with low-risk GTN.

Primary adjuvant hysterectomy was not effective in reducing chemotherapy requirements or improving cure rates for women with high-risk GTN. These patients usually present with disseminated disease, and hysterectomy would be expected to contribute much less to reduction of tumor burden compared with patients with low-risk GTN. Therefore, the major role of primary hysterectomy should be as part of primary treatment for women with low-risk nonmetastatic GTN and no desire for future fertility.

Delayed hysterectomy is often considered for patients who fail to respond to primary chemotherapy. In the Duke experience reported by Hammond and colleagues, almost all of the patients with low-risk GTN who were treated with a delayed hysterectomy because of resistance to primary chemotherapy achieved remission without requiring multiagent chemotherapy. Others have reported that salvage hysterectomy is effective in producing remissions in most patients with nonmetastatic or low-risk metastatic disease. Control of extrauterine disease is central in the success of salvage hysterectomy for these patients.

Placental site trophoblastic tumor and ETT are much more rare than invasive mole or gestational choriocarcinoma. In contrast to other forms of GTN, production of hCG is lower, and these tumors are usually resistant to conventional chemotherapy regimens. Papadopoulos and colleagues noted that two-thirds of their patients were cured after surgery alone if PSTT was confined to the uterus. Hysterectomy should be integrated into the primary management of PSTT unless there are widespread metastases.

The majority of women undergoing hysterectomy for malignant GTN have been treated with abdominal hysterectomy, with or without preservation of the adnexa. Ovarian removal is not required because GTN rarely metastasizes to the ovaries, and these tumors are not hormonally influenced. Vaginal hysterectomy may be considered in women with nonmetastatic GTN who have a small uterus and low hCG levels, but it does not allow assessment of the upper abdomen for occult metastases. Laparoscopic-assisted vaginal hysterectomy or total laparoscopic hysterectomy allows surveillance of the upper abdomen and have a shorter acute convalescence than abdominal hysterectomy.

More conservative myometrial resections combined with uterine reconstruction can be considered in highly selected patients with nonmetastatic chemoresistant GTN who wish to avoid hysterectomy. Previous anecdotal reports of local myometrial resections of invasive moles have documented the use of resection and uterine repair for primary therapy of nonmetastatic GTN and PSTT. Because of the high cure rates reported after chemotherapy alone in low-risk GTN patients, it is more rational to consider these as salvage procedures in women with localized chemoresistant disease. Each patient considered for this procedure should be carefully evaluated for systemic metastases, and the uterine lesion should be localized using a combination of color-flow ultrasonography, MRI, and hysteroscopy. Intraoperative frozen sections should be used to assess surgical margins. Small lesions associated with low hCG levels are more likely to be completely excised with a conservative myometrial resection than lesions larger than 2 to 3 cm in diameter.

The most frequently used surgical procedure for removal of extrauterine metastases is thoracotomy with pulmonary wedge resection. Although this can safely be performed in conjunction with chemotherapy, it is not necessary to resect lung metastases in the majority of patients. Radiographic evidence of tumor regression often lags behind hCG response to treatment, and some patients have persistent pulmonary nodules months after completion of therapy. In women with low-risk GTN, the overall risk of recurrence is less than 5%. Even though women with persistent pulmonary nodules may be at an increased risk for recurrence, these patients can be safely followed with serial hCG levels without surgical resection.

Many series of patients with GTN treated with thoracotomy include patients whose disease was not suspected until after resection of a pulmonary nodule. As in the case of brain, liver, or renal metastases, any woman of reproductive age who presents with an apparent metastatic malignancy of unknown primary site should be screened for the possibility of GTN with a serum hCG level. Excisional biopsy is not indicated to histologically confirm the diagnosis of malignant GTN if the patient is not pregnant and has a high hCG value. Given the vascular nature of these lesions, biopsy can have significant morbidity.

Resection of pulmonary nodules in highly selected patients with drug-resistant disease may successfully induce remission. Immediately before performing pulmonary resection, it is important to exclude the possibility of active disease elsewhere by performing a comprehensive metastatic survey. Patients with isolated, unilateral nodules associated with low hCG values are much more likely to benefit from thoracotomy with pulmonary resection than patients with bilateral or multiple unilateral lesions or those with disease in other locations. Tomoda and colleagues reported that 14 (93%) of their 15 patients with isolated nodules and low hCG values survived after pulmonary resection compared with none of four patients with either hCG values greater than 1000 mIU/mL or evidence of active disease elsewhere. Others have reported that hCG level remission within 1 to 2 weeks of surgery portends a favorable outcome.

FIGURE 7.17 Nephrectomy specimen with a large hemorrhagic metastasis of choriocarcinoma involving the superior pole. (Courtesy of John Soper, MD.)

FIGURE 7.16 Brain magnetic resonance image of a patient presenting with high-risk metastatic gestational trophoblastic neoplasia, pulmonary metastases, and seizures associated with a solitary brain metastasis. She is in remission after surgical resection of this brain lesion during her first cycle of chemotherapy followed by multiple cycles of chemotherapy with high-dose methotrexate combinations, platinum–taxane, and hysterectomy. (Courtesy of John Soper, MD.)

Brain metastases (Fig. 7.16) occur in 8% to 15% of patients with metastatic GTN and are associated with a worse prognosis than vaginal or pulmonary metastases. Metastases from GTN tend to be highly vascular and have a tendency for central necrosis and hemorrhage. A significant portion of early deaths is caused by CNS metastases of GTN with acute neurologic deterioration before effective therapy is initiated or very early in the course of treatment. The major goals of treatment include early detection of brain metastases through complete radiologic metastatic survey, stabilization of the patient's neurologic status, and initiation of therapy. Craniotomy solely for the purpose of tissue confirmation is not justified if GTN is clinically diagnosed on the basis of metastatic disease associated with an elevated hCG level.

In series of patients with brain metastases of GTN reported from the United States, brain irradiation has usually been integrated into treatment in an attempt to prevent hemorrhage and neurologic deterioration. However, Rustin and colleagues recommended an approach using early craniotomy with excision of isolated lesions combined with high-dose systemic and intrathecal chemotherapy to treat patients with brain metastases. In their experience, brain irradiation was not used routinely. Both primary radiation therapy combined with chemotherapy and the approach emphasizing early surgical intervention appear to have similar efficacy in previously untreated patients. More recently, a series from Charing Cross reported on their results using high dose methotrexate chemotherapy within

EMA/CO and EMA/EP regimens and no brain radiation or initial surgical resection. They reported an 85% overall survival rate for these patients and caution against the long-term cognitive complications from whole-brain radiation and intrathecal methotrexate. In sharp contrast to the outlook for women with brain metastases from other solid tumors, up to 85% of women with brain metastases presenting for primary therapy from malignant GTN will be cured. Craniotomy for resection of drug-resistant brain lesions is only rarely performed. In these patients, it is important to exclude active disease elsewhere before attempting surgical resection. Sometimes craniotomy is required for women who require acute decompression of CNS hemorrhagic lesions to allow stabilization and institution of therapy.

Surgical removal of metastatic disease at other sites is occasionally beneficial for primary or salvage therapy of malignant GTN. Because PSTT and ETT are more often resistant to conventional chemotherapeutic agents, multiple surgical resections of metastatic sites may be required in highly selected patients to produce a cure. In general, resection of distant metastases is unlikely to be successful if there is evidence of disseminated disease resistant to chemotherapy.

Vaginal metastases of malignant GTN are highly vascular, originating via metastasis through the submucosal venous plexus of the vagina. These should not be biopsied or resected unless they represent the only site of drug-resistant disease. Biopsy of a metastatic vaginal lesion often results in massive hemorrhage. Packing or angiographic localization with selective embolization is usually used in an attempt to control bleeding from vaginal metastases during initial therapy.

Renal metastases occur in 1% to 20% of patients treated for metastatic GTN. They are usually associated with other high-risk factors and disseminated disease. All three survivors with renal metastases treated at Duke University Medical Center had nephrectomy incorporated into initial therapy (Fig. 7.17);

however, three of the five fatalities also underwent nephrectomy. Survivors had limited metastatic involvement elsewhere compared with patients with renal metastases who died. The role for nephrectomy appears limited because others have reported patients with high-risk metastatic GTN involving the kidneys who entered remission after treatment with etoposide-containing chemotherapy regimens alone.

Fewer than 5% of patients with metastatic GTN have initial involvement of other intraabdominal organs or the GI tract. Liver metastases are the most common intraabdominal metastases. The overall survival rate for these patients is as high as 55% when they receive EMA/CO chemotherapy. Occasional patients will develop intraabdominal bleeding from metastatic disease that requires resection for stabilization. Selective angiographic embolization techniques should be considered as an option if possible. Only rarely will resection of isolated liver metastases be feasible for treatment of drug-resistant disease because most patients will have other sites of active disease or diffuse involvement of the liver.

With the development of advanced interventional radiology techniques, selective angiographic localization and embolization techniques have been used to conservatively manage hemorrhage from active sites of metastatic GTN and to treat intrauterine arteriovenous malformations (AVMs) that rarely develop after treatment of GTN. Vaginal metastases are the site of active disease most often treated with selective angiographic embolization, when simple packing or suturing techniques have failed to control hemorrhage. Grumbine and colleagues managed a patient with liver metastases with the prophylactic placement of a catheter in the hepatic artery for balloon occlusion or embolization in the event of rupture, and others have successfully used selective embolization to treat hemorrhage from hepatic metastases. Lang used selective catheter placement for chemoembolization in three patients with liver metastases and two with pelvic tumors from GTN. All had chemoresistant GTN and relatively localized persistent tumors. Two of the patients with liver metastases achieved long-term remissions, with minimal hematologic toxicity recorded during treatment.

Angiographic abnormalities in the uterus caused by GTD can persist for many months after evacuation of hydatidiform mole or treatment of malignant GTN. The occurrence of intractable bleeding from intrauterine AVM after successful treatment for GTD is a relatively rare complication. Lim and colleagues reported 14 patients treated over a 20-year interval with selective angiographic embolization for this indication. Hemorrhage was initially controlled with the first procedure in 11 (78%), and six (45%) patients required a second embolization for treatment of recurrent bleeding, but only two (15%) patients required hysterectomy. Successful term pregnancies have been reported after this procedure.

Radiation Therapy

Radiation therapy has a limited role in the management of patients with malignant GTD. Radiation is used most frequently to treat patients with brain or liver metastases in an effort to minimize hemorrhagic complications from disease at these sites.

Brace first reported control of brain metastases using 2000-cGy whole-brain irradiation for patients with GTN treated at the NIH with single-agent regimens. He reported five (24%) survivors among 21 patients treated for brain metastases; three required retreatment for recurrent symptoms of intracranial disease. Whole-brain irradiation has been used in the majority of series of patients with brain metastases reported from the United States. Most series report administration of between 2000 and 4000 cGy in 10 to 20 equal fractions that are given concurrently with combination chemotherapy, with reduced field boosts given in selected patients. Total doses correlate with control of CNS metastases. Schecter and colleagues reported that the 5-year actuarial local control rate for patients given doses less than 2200 cGy was only 24%, significantly worse than 91% local control among patients given 2200 to 6000 cGy.

Survival rates of 50% to 75% are reported in series of patients who initially presented with brain metastases and received combined chemoradiation. Survival of these patients is influenced in part by the extent and subsequent control of extracranial disease in addition to the extent of CNS involvement. Small and colleagues reported that women who were asymptomatic at presentation had a 100% survival rate compared with only 38% survival rate in those who presented with symptoms from brain metastases, a significant difference. Evans and associates reported that patients with new brain metastases diagnosed at the time of recurrence or who developed brain metastases during chemotherapy had survival rates of only 38% and 0%, respectively. These groups had significantly worse survival than the 75% survival rates of their patients who presented with brain metastases for primary therapy.

Chronic central nervous system toxicity such as mental retardation has been reported among long-term survivors of leukemia and other tumors treated with a combination of whole-brain irradiation and concurrent moderate-dose methotrexate regimens. These reports have diminished the enthusiasm for combining whole-brain radiation with chemotherapy regimens that incorporate infusions of 300 to 1000 mg/m^2 of methotrexate used to treat GTN, such as EMA/CO. Stereotactic treatment of individual brain metastases could be considered in these circumstances. A 6- to 12-hour infusions of methotrexate greater than 500 mg/m^2 result in therapeutic cerebrospinal fluid levels of methotrexate, suggesting that doses of methotrexate in these ranges should be used when whole-brain radiation is not used. The group at Charing Cross Hospital reported 85% survival for patients who received primary therapy with this approach.

Hepatic metastases are identified in 2% to 8% of patients presenting for primary therapy of malignant GTN (Fig. 7.18). Involvement of the liver constitutes a poor prognostic factor, as evidenced by survival rates of 40% to 55% for women with primary liver involvement and dismal survival rates for those who develop new liver metastases during therapy. These are highly vascular and tend to produce catastrophic intraabdominal hemorrhage. In an attempt to minimize this risk, patients treated at Duke University Medical Center for liver metastases received approximately 2000-cGy whole-liver irradiation concurrently with MAC chemotherapy. Administration of

FIGURE 7.18 Multiple liver metastases in a woman presenting less than 4 weeks after term delivery with lung, brain, and liver metastases of gestational trophoblastic neoplasia. Selective hepatic arterial embolization was required to control bleeding from the hepatic metastases; note the fluid density around liver from intraabdominal blood. This patient was treated aggressively with multimodality therapy and placed into remission. (Courtesy of John Soper, MD.)

chemotherapy was limited in only one of 15 patients because of hepatitis, but the survival rate was very poor among these patients, with only two (13%) survivors overall and no survivors among patients who developed liver metastases during therapy. Bakri and colleagues reported survival in none of their patients who were treated with MAC combined with whole-liver radiation compared with survival in five of eight patients who were treated with etoposide-based combination regimens. Modern series have reported survival of approximately 55% among patients treated with etoposide-based regimens without hepatic irradiation. Thus, liver radiation is not used in management of GTN.

Radiation therapy is occasionally administered to other sites of disease in an attempt to treat drug-resistant foci, with anecdotal responses to multimodality therapy. However, the overall efficacy of radiation therapy to sites other than the brain is unclear. Most of the successes probably reflect the summation of an aggressive multimodality approach to individual patients with high-risk metastatic GTN.

It must be emphasized that cure rates of greater than 90% for patients with high-risk metastatic GTN are reported from centers that specialize in the treatment of women with this relatively rare malignancy. Patients with high-risk disease present multiple challenges for management. They often require a highly individualized approach to address the extent of their disease and treatment toxicity. All women with high-risk disease should be treated by physicians experienced in the management of patients with GTN who can coordinate all aspects of therapy.

Placental Site Trophoblastic Tumor

This rare tumor has the potential to metastasize and cause death. Approximately 100 cases have been reported in the literature. It may be diagnosed after abortion, mole, or normal pregnancy. Bleeding, the most common symptom, can appear shortly after termination of pregnancy or years later. Bleeding is often accompanied by uterine enlargement, and the diagnosis of pregnancy is often entertained. The result of a pregnancy test may be positive, but these tumors characteristically produce lower levels of intact hCG than other forms of GTD. Gross uterine findings may vary from a diffuse nodular enlargement of the myometrium, which is usually well circumscribed, to a large polypoid projection into the uterine cavity with involvement of the myometrium. Invasion may extend to the serosa or even with direct extension to the adnexa. Microscopically, it is difficult to differentiate from benign trophoblastic infiltration. PSTT is characterized by mononuclear infiltration of the uterus and its blood vessels with occasional multinucleated giant cells. The predominant cell is an intermediate trophoblast with large polyhedral cells and pleomorphic nuclei. Occasionally, syncytial trophoblast giant cells are present. Mitotic counts have not been a reliable prognostic factor.

Placental site trophoblastic tumors must be distinguished from choriocarcinoma and can occasionally be interpreted as sarcomas. Histochemical stains for human placental lactogen are usually diffusely positive but only focally positive for hCG. The serum hCG, although elevated enough to give a positive pregnancy test result, is often low, even with metastasis; therefore, it is a poor predictor of prognosis. Free beta-chain hCG may have elevated levels, but these are not routinely measured with current hCG assays. Most of these tumors behave in a locally aggressive fashion, although they may metastasize, with at least 20 deaths reported, indicating approximately a 15% to 20% mortality rate. Metastases have been reported at various sites. Some patients may be cured with a D&C only, but a hysterectomy is considered optimal therapy and is usually adequate in most situations. Swisher and Drescher reported a complete response to EMA/CO in a patient with metastasis to lung and vagina. In their review, two of seven patients treated with EMA/CO had a complete response.

In a review by Chang and associates of 88 patients with placental site tumor, 58 of 62 patients with FIGO stage I and II survived and were treated mainly with a hysterectomy with or without chemotherapy. Apparently, 9 of 10 patients survived after a D&C alone. Only 7 of 21 patients with stage III or IV disease survived. All received chemotherapy, and only six received a hysterectomy. Leiserowitz and Webb reported a patient whose tumor was localized with ultrasonography and MRI and treated with local excision and uterine reconstruction. Surgical-free margins were present, and the patient has had three subsequent pregnancies, including two spontaneous abortions and one term delivery.

Epithelioid Trophoblastic Tumor

Epithelioid trophoblastic tumor is a very rare form of GTN. The first report describing this tumor was published in 1998. The tumor is characterized histologically by a nested, corded, and nodular growth pattern that is normally not deeply invasive and differentiates it from PSTT. ETT is similar to PSTT in that it grows slowly, is resistant to chemotherapy, and produces low levels of hCG. The tumors often present in the lower uterine segment and often have positive staining for p63 and cytokeratin, causing them to be confused with squamous cell carcinoma of the cervix. Surgery in the form of hysterectomy is the mainstay of treatment for ETT, and most patients who present with disease confined to the uterus alone will be cured with hysterectomy alone. The mortality rate from ETT is low with one series reporting a 13% mortality rate with a range of 1 to 39 months of follow-up.

OTHER CONSIDERATIONS

Future Childbearing

After effective treatment for malignant GTN, molar pregnancies occur in only about 1% to 2% of subsequent pregnancies, and many patients have subsequently had normal gestations without difficulty (Table 7.15). Because of the increased risk for the development of a mole in subsequent pregnancies, it is reasonable to evaluate these pregnancies with first-trimester ultrasonography. A particular dilemma has been noted in women undergoing ovulation induction after previous molar gestations. In such cases, patients have occasionally developed repeated hydatidiform moles or malignant GTN subsequent to the implementation of assisted reproductive technologies. In one such patient, in vitro fertilization (IVF) of oocytes retrieved showed a significantly high incidence of abnormal fertilization, resulting in the development of triploid embryos. The authors suggested the possible association of an oocyte defect predisposing to abnormal fertilization resulting in the high incidence of triploid embryos. Investigators have proposed the use of intracytoplasmic sperm injection (ICSI) with preimplantation genetic diagnosis or donor oocyte IVF as therapeutic alternatives in these cases.

It appears that the pregnancy outcomes in women with a history of molar gestations are no different from the outcomes in women who have no such history with respect to term live births, first- and second-trimester abortions, anomalies, stillbirths, prematurity, and primary cesarean section rate (Table 7.15). For women with prior molar gestations, subsequent pregnancy outcome appears similar irrespective of whether the mole is complete or partial.

Treatment of malignant GTN with chemotherapy is compatible with the preservation of fertility and is not associated with an increased risk of congenital malformations. Ayhan and colleagues from Turkey reported on 49 women who had received chemotherapy for GTN and subsequently became pregnant a total of 65 times with 42 (64.7%) term births and three (4.6%) molar pregnancies. No congenital malformations or obstetric complications were observed. Of the 63 patients in the Southeastern Trophoblastic Center study of poor prognosis metastatic GTN, only 19 were able to preserve their reproductive capacity. Only four of these patients had subsequent pregnancies that resulted in one spontaneous abortion and four normal deliveries. In a recent study from the NETDC, an increased risk of still birth in future pregnancies was noted for patients who received chemotherapy for treatment of GTN; however, the overall risk remained low for this group at 1.3%.

In the Charing Cross experience of women treated with EMA/CO, 56% of women who were in remission for at least 2 years and had fertility-conserving therapy achieved pregnancy after completing EMA/CO. At the time of the report, there were 112 live births, including three babies with congenital abnormalities. Woolas and colleagues updated the outcome data of posttreatment reproductive intent and outcome from 1121 GTN survivors. Of 728 women who had tried to become pregnant, 607 reported at least one live birth, 73 conceived but had not registered a live birth, and 48 did not conceive. No differences were apparent among the 392 women who received methotrexate as single-agent chemotherapy and the 336 treated with multiple-agent chemotherapy. Women who had registered a live birth were significantly younger. They concluded that standard chemotherapy protocols in the treatment of malignant GTN have minimal impact on the subsequent ability to reproduce.

Coexistence of Normal Pregnancy and Gestational Trophoblastic Neoplasia

Rare cases of metastatic GTN coexisting with normal gestations have been reported; some have been treated successfully with delivery and subsequent chemotherapy. In one case, a patient with a normal intrauterine pregnancy of 27 weeks' gestation had a coexisting pulmonary metastatic choriocarcinoma. Treatment with single-agent methotrexate during pregnancy resulted in favorable outcomes for both the mother and the child.

Transplacental Fetal Metastases

Rare cases (only 15 to 20 cases have been reported and only five since 1990) of maternal GTN metastatic to the fetus have been described. The diagnosis of widely metastatic disease in the delivered neonate may occur in the absence of metastatic GTN in the mother (found only in retrospective examination of the term placenta) or precede diagnosis of metastatic GTN in the mother.

TABLE 7.15 Fertility After Treatment for Gestational Trophoblastic Neoplasia		
Desired fertility	109/122 (89%) patients	
Reproductive Outcome		
Infertility	62/109 (57%) patients	
Pregnancies	47/109 (43%) patients	57 pregnancies
Normal infants		45*/57 (79%)
Spontaneous abortion		7/57 (12%)
Therapeutic abortion		3/57 (5%)
Mole		2/57 (4%)

*Two sets of twins.
Modified from Hammond CB, Weed JC Jr, Currie JL. The role of operation in the current therapy of gestational trophoblastic disease. *Am J Obstet Gynecol* 1980;136:844-858.

Survivorship Issues After Successful Treatment of Gestational Trophoblastic Neoplasia

Survivors of nonmalignant and malignant GTN may be at risk for unique physical and psychosocial problems. This generally relates to the increased risk of developing secondary malignancies after treatment with agents such as etoposide and to issues related to reproductive capacity.

Rustin conducted a population-based study in the United Kingdom analyzing the incidence of secondary malignancies after successful treatment of malignant GTN. Using a sophisticated epidemiologic design, an overall 50% excess of risk (relative risk [RR], 1.5; 95% CI, 1.1–2.1; $P <0.011$) was observed. The risk was significantly increased for myeloid leukemia (RR, 16.6; 95% CI, 5.4–38.9), colon (RR, 4.6; 95% CI, 1.5–10.7), and breast cancer (RR, 5.8; 95% CI, 1.2–16.9) when the survival exceeded 25 years. The risk was not significantly increased among the 554 women who received single-agent therapy (RR, 1.3; 95% CI, 0.6–2.1). Leukemias only developed in patients who received etoposide plus other cytotoxic drugs.

Savage and coworkers conducted a survey of all patients treated at Charing Cross Hospital between 1958 and 2000 and obtained data for 1903 patients. They found significantly increased risks of leukemia, melanoma, meningioma, and oral cancer among survivors who received EMA/CO but no increased risk of malignancy among patients who received single-agent methotrexate and folinic acid. They also found no difference in rates of early menopause for patients receiving methotrexate but increased rates of early menopause among patients receiving EMA/CO reaching 13% at 40 years old and 36% at 45 years old.

Wenzel and colleagues reported on 76 women with GTN from the New England Trophoblastic Disease Center in regard to chronic psychosocial effects. Across all levels of disease, they found that patients with GTN experience clinically significant levels of anxiety, anger, fatigue, confusion, and sexual problems and are significantly affected by pregnancy concerns for protracted periods.

For the bibliography list, log onto www.expertconsult.com ⟨http://www.expertconsult.com⟩.

Invasive Cancer of the Vulva

Thomas J. Herzog, MD

KEY POINTS

1. Invasive vulvar cancer is a relatively rare tumor, accounting for 4% of all female genital malignant neoplasms.
2. Squamous cell carcinoma of the vulva develops by human papillomavirus- (HPV-) dependent and HPV-independent pathways.
3. Sentinel lymph node biopsy represents the largest innovation in the care of vulvar cancer patients in the past decade.
4. The standard of care is pelvic lymph node irradiation for patients with positive inguinal nodes.
5. Recurrence may be local or distant, and more than 80% will occur in the first 2 years after therapy, demanding initial close follow-up.

Invasive vulvar cancer is a relatively rare tumor, accounting for 4% of all female genital malignant neoplasms with the American Cancer Society reporting just over 5100 cases resulting in 1080 deaths in 2015 in the United States. With the exception of the rare sarcomas, the peak incidence is in women between 65 and 75 years old (Fig. 8.1); in some series, almost half are 70 years of age or older. Although classically a disease of elderly women, the trend in recent years is an increasing prevalence among younger women, which cannot be accounted for by immune suppression alone. Human papillomavirus (HPV) is a key age-dependent risk factor that causes preinvasive disease in the form of vulvar intraepithelial neoplasia (VIN) that is often associated with a history of tobacco use. HPV-related VIN lesions are rarer in older women, and these malignancies may be associated with chronic vulvar dystrophies, such as lichen sclerosis, although a direct association remains unproven. No race or culture is spared, and gravidity and parity appear unrelated in the pathogenesis of this neoplasm. Vulvar cancer is common in poor and elderly women in most parts of the world, and this has led to the hypothesis that inadequate personal hygiene and medical care are contributing factors in disease development.

Younger patients frequently have early stromal invasion associated with diffuse VIN. Choo found 17 patients younger than age 35 years with invasive carcinoma of the vulva. Of these, eight had microinvasion. Al-Ghamdi and coworkers evaluated 21 patients younger than age 40 years with invasive vulvar cancer and found that most, but not all, had associated HPV. Outcomes in these populations were excellent. Lanneau and colleagues have corroborated these results in 56 women younger than age 45 years with squamous cell carcinoma (SCC) of the vulva. They concluded that vulvar cancer in this population is associated with early-stage disease, HPV, VIN, and smoking.

SCC of the vulva develops by HPV-dependent and HPV-independent pathways. The association between HPV and both preinvasive and invasive urogenital lesions has been well described. Susceptibility of the cervical, vaginal, and vulvar epithelium is referred to as the "field effect," which is more pronounced in tobacco users and in patients who are immunocompromised, such as those with HIV/AIDS, or organ transplant recipients. The association of condyloma acuminatum with vulvar carcinoma is well known, but no cause and effect relationship has been confirmed as yet. HPV is suspected in the etiology of squamous neoplasia of the vulva, as it is in lesions

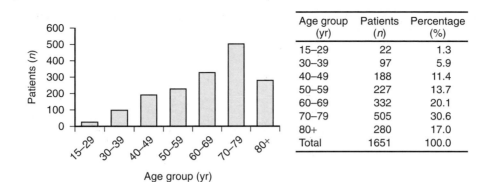

Age group (yr)	Patients (n)	Percentage (%)
15–29	22	1.3
30–39	97	5.9
40–49	188	11.4
50–59	227	13.7
60–69	332	20.1
70–79	505	30.6
80+	280	17.0
Total	1651	100.0

FIGURE 8.1 Carcinoma of the vulva: patients treated from 1999 to 2001. (Adapted from Beller U, Quinn MA, Benedet JL, et al. Carcinoma of the vulva. FIGO 26th Annual Report on the Results of Treatment in Gynecological Cancer, *Int J Gynaecol Obstet* 95(Suppl 1):S7–S27, 2006.)

of the cervix. Bloss and colleagues looked at the clinical and histologic features of vulvar carcinomas analyzed for HPV status. Of 21 invasive carcinomas of the vulva analyzed, 10 were found to contain HPV-16 DNA. Others have confirmed this observation, suggesting that HPV DNA associations with malignant changes of the vulva are similar to those observed elsewhere in the genital tract. Although the incidence of vulvar cancer has remained relatively stable over the past several decades, the incidence of VIN has increased, especially that associated with HPV. Hoang and coworkers contrast these multicentric HPV related precursors with VIN of the differentiated type that occurs in postmenopausal women, often in a background of lichen sclerosis or chronic inflammatory dermatoses associated with a high number of somatic mutations, particularly in TP53. In a recent review, Sznurkowski pointed out the need to better understand the relationship between vulvar cancer and HPV for not only causation but also for developing potential therapeutics.

Many previously reported associated features seen in patients with vulvar cancer, such as diabetes, obesity, hypertension, and arteriosclerosis, may just reflect the increased incidence of these diseases associated with aging.

INVASIVE SQUAMOUS CELL CARCINOMA

Histology

The overwhelming majority of all vulvar cancer is squamous in origin. The vulva is covered with skin, and any malignant change that appears elsewhere on the skin can occur in this region. Table 8.1 depicts the incidence of vulvar neoplasia from several collected studies in the literature. The following discussion focuses mainly on SCC because of its preponderance, but as a generalization, the other lesions can be treated similarly, except as noted.

Clinical Presentation and Diagnosis

Squamous cell vulvar cancer usually arises from an area of intraepithelial neoplasia that subsequently develops into a small nodule that may break down and ulcerate (Figs. 8.2 and 8.3). On other occasions, small, warty, or cauliflower-like growths evolve, and these may be confused with condyloma

TABLE 8.1   Incidence of Vulvar Neoplasms by Histologic Type*

Tumor Type	Incidence (%)
Squamous	86.2
Melanoma	4.8
Sarcoma	2.2
Basal cell	1.4
Bartholin gland	
Squamous	0.4
Adenocarcinoma	0.6 ⎫ 1.2
Adenocarcinoma	0.6 ⎭
Undifferentiated	3.9

*Based on 1378 reported cases.
Modified from Plentl AA, Friedman EA. *Lymphatic System of the Female Genitalia.* Philadelphia, 1971, WB Saunders.

TABLE 8.2   Signs and Symptoms of Vulvar Cancer

Sign or Symptom	Incidence (%)
Pruritus	45.0
Mass	45.0
Pain	23.0
Bleeding	14.0
Ulceration	14.0
Dysuria	10.0
Discharge	8.0
Groin mass	2.5

acuminatum. **Long-term pruritus or a lump or mass on the vulva is present in more than 50% of patients with invasive vulvar cancer** (Table 8.2). Biopsy must be done of all suspicious lesions of the vulva, including lumps, ulcers, and pigmented areas, even in the patient not complaining of burning or itching (Table 8.3).

A significant delay in diagnosis and appropriate treatment is common. **Several series of carcinoma of the vulva report delays of 2 to 16 months after onset of symptoms** before

FIGURE 8.2 Squamous cell carcinoma arising in a bed of lichen sclerosis.

FIGURE 8.3 Small, well-localized lesion of the vulva.

TABLE 8.3 Indications for Excisional Biopsy of Vulvar Lesions
1. Change in surface area of nevus
2. Change in elevation of a lesion: raised, thickened, or nodular
3. Change in color: especially brown to black
4. Change in surface: smooth to scaly or ulcerated
5. Change in sensation: itching or tingling

FIGURE 8.4 A, Large ulcerating squamous cell malignancy of the vulva with destruction of the clitoris and the urethra. **B,** Large exophytic squamous cell carcinoma of the vulva.

medical attention is sought. Further delay can occur when medical treatment of vulvar lesions continues without biopsy for definitive diagnosis.

Fortunately, vulvar cancer is commonly indolent, extends slowly, and metastasizes fairly late. Hence, there is an opportunity for preventing the development of advanced stages of this disease through patient and physician education.

Location and Spread Pattern

Primary disease can appear anywhere on the vulva. Approximately 70% arise primarily on the labia. Disease more commonly occurs on the labia majora; however, it may appear on the labia minora, clitoris, or perineum. The disease is usually localized and well demarcated, although it can occasionally be so extensive that the primary location cannot be determined (Fig. 8.4). Multifocal growth pattern in invasive SCC of the vulva is uncommon, except for the so-called "kissing lesions" that can occur.

FIGURE 8.5 Verrucous carcinoma of the vulva.

FIGURE 8.6 Photomicrograph of a tumor nodule invading a vulvar lymphatic.

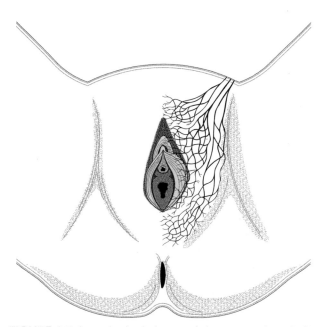

FIGURE 8.7 Lymphatic drainage of the external genitalia.

Verrucous carcinoma of the vulva (Fig. 8.5) is a special and unusual variant of SCC that is locally invasive but nonmetastasizing. The lesion, which may involve the cervix, vagina, and the vulva, presents as a warty, fungating, ulcerated mass with a bulky, elevated appearance reminiscent of a benign HPV lesion. Identification of this variant is important because the biologic behavior of the disease influences therapy. Condyloma may initially be diagnosed on microscopic examination, but distinction from ordinary condylomata is aided by the absence of fibrovascular cores within the proliferating papillary masses of tumor. There is usually a uniform lack of malignant features histologically. Adequate material, including underlying stroma for pathologic evaluation, is necessary to differentiate verrucous carcinoma from condyloma. Tumor may invade deeply into the underlying tissue, often requiring extensive surgery, and has a propensity to recur locally. Woodruff noted a lack of lymph node metastases in 27 patients, including a literature review, who were treated with radical vulvectomy and inguinal lymphadenectomy. As a result, a more conservative approach is advocated with wide local excision and tumor-free margins as the therapeutic aim. Lymphadenectomy is of questionable value except when nodes are obviously involved. Historically, it has been thought that radiotherapy is contraindicated because of its ineffectiveness, and reports have indicated that it can incite more aggressive behavior by this tumor.

Fundamental to the understanding of therapy for invasive cancer of the vulva is thorough knowledge of the lymphatic drainage of this region. **In general, the four histologic types of invasive cancer primarily metastasize via the lymphatic route** (Fig. 8.6). Lymphatic drainage of the external genitalia begins with minute papillae that connect to a multilayered meshwork of fine vessels that extend over the entire labium minus, the prepuce of the clitoris, the fourchette, and the vaginal mucosa up to the level of the hymenal ring (Fig. 8.7). Drainage of these lymphatics extends toward the anterior portion of the labium minus, where they emerge into three or four collecting trunks whose course is toward the mons veneris, bypassing the clitoris. Vessels from the prepuce anastomose with these lymphatics. Similarly, vessels from the labium majus proceed anteriorly to the upper part of the vulva and mons veneris, there joining the vessels of the prepuce and labium minus. These lymphatic vessels abruptly change direction, turning laterally, and terminate in ipsilateral or contralateral femoral nodes. Drainage is usually limited initially to the medial upper quadrant of the femoral node group. The nodes are medial to the great saphenous vein above the cribriform fascia and in turn may drain secondarily to the deep femoral group. The next echelon of nodes is the pelvic/iliac nodes.

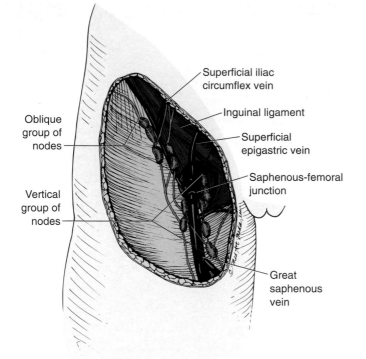

FIGURE 8.8 The superficial inguinal lymph nodes can be divided into the horizontal group and the perpendicular group.

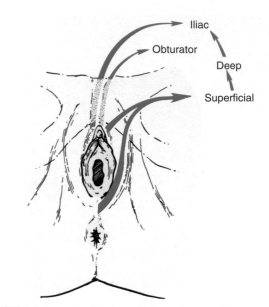

FIGURE 8.9 Lymphatic spread of a vulvar malignancy. See the text for details.

The superficial inguinal lymph nodes are located immediately beneath the integument and Camper fascia, with an average of 8 to 10 in number. Most authors agree that these nodes are the primary drainage for the vulva, thereby containing the sentinel lymph node (SLN) (Fig. 8.8). The deep femoral nodes, which are by classic teaching located beneath the cribriform fascia, are the secondary node recipients and are involved before drainage into the deep pelvic nodes. The **Cloquet node**, the last node of the deep femoral group, is located just beneath the Poupart ligament. The multilayered meshwork of lymphatics on the vulva itself is always limited to an area medial to the genitocrural fold (Fig. 8.9). Lymphatic drainage of the vulva occurs via a progressive systematic mechanism, and therapy can be planned according to where in the lymphatic chain tumor is present.

Borgno and colleagues examined 100 inguinal lymphadenectomy specimens at autopsy and demonstrated that the deep femoral nodes are always situated within the openings in the fascia at the fossa ovalis, and no lymph nodes are distal to the lower margin of the fossa ovalis, under the fascia cribrosa. The clinical implication is that a carefully performed deep femoral lymphadenectomy does not require removal of the fascia lata (cribriform fascia) because no lymph nodes are to be found between the femoral vein and artery lateral to the artery or distal to the lower margin of the fossa ovalis beneath the cribriform fascia. They also found that the node of Cloquet or Rosenmüller, which is the uppermost node among the deep femoral lymph nodes, was absent in 54% of dissections. Borgno and colleagues also demonstrated that during surgery, when

TABLE 8.4	Incidence of Positive Nodes		
Series	Cases (*n*)	Positive Groin or Pelvic Nodes (%)	Positive Pelvic Nodes (%)
Morley (1976)	374	37.0	—
Curry et al. (1980)	191	30.0	4.7
Simonsen (1984)	122	50.0	10.0
Sutton et al. (1991)	150	24.0	—
Homesley (1994)	277	29.2	—
Creasman et al. (1997)	1553	31.0	—

traction is persistently applied to the lymphovascular fat tissue above the cribriform fascia, all inguinal nodes can be removed. No nodal tissue was found when the cribriform fascia and the fat beneath were submitted separately for pathologic review. Hudson and colleagues confirmed this finding in cadaveric dissections, and Micheletti and coworkers found supporting evidence with embryologic studies.

Although lymphatics draining from the clitoris directly to the deep pelvic lymph nodes are described, their clinical significance appears to be minimal. It is unusual to find a case in which metastasis is present in the pelvic lymph nodes without metastatic disease in the inguinal lymph nodes even when the clitoris is involved. Curry and associates noted clitoral involvement in 58 patients of 191 studied; none had positive deep pelvic nodes without concomitant inguinal node involvement. Similar results were observed in a study of 38 patients, with carcinomas of the clitoris by Ericksson and coworkers, who found also that the deep inguinal or femoral nodes were never positive in the absence of positive superficial inguinal nodes.

The incidence of positive inguinal and pelvic nodes varies considerably, as noted in Table 8.4. Unfortunately, most of

TABLE 8.5 Groin Node Versus Tumor Diameter			
Feature	N	Positive Groin Nodes	%
TUMOR DIAMETER			
≤2.0 cm	190	36	19
>2.0 cm	390	163	43
INVASION			
≤5 mm	272	57	21
>5 mm	286	137	48
CLINICAL EXAMINATION			
N0-1	477	114	23
N2-3	111	89	80

From Homesley HD, Bundy BN, Sedlis A, et al. Prognostic factors for groin node metastasis in squamous cell carcinoma of the vulva (a Gynecologic Oncology Group study). Gynecol Oncol 1993;49:279,.

TABLE 8.6 Federation of International Gynecologists and Obstetricians Staging of Invasive Cancer of the Vulva	
Stage	Description
I	Tumor confined to the vulva
IA	Lesions ≤2 cm in size confined to the vulva or perineum and with stromal invasion ≤1.0 mm*; no nodal metastasis
IB	Lesions >2 cm in size confined to the vulva or perineum with stromal invasion greater than 1.0 mm*; no nodal metastasis
II	Tumor of any size with extension to adjacent perineal structures (1/3 lower urethra, 1/3 lower vagina, anus); no nodal metastasis
III	Tumor of any size with or without extension to adjacent perineal structures (1/3 lower urethra, 1/3 lower vagina, anus) with positive inguinofemoral lymph nodes
IIIA	(i) With 1 lymph node metastasis (≥5 mm), or (ii) With 1–2 lymph node metastasis(es) (<5 mm)
IIIB	(i) With ≥2 lymph node metastases (≥5 mm), or (ii) With ≥3 lymph node metastases (<5 mm)
IIIC	With positive nodes with extracapsular spread
IV	Tumor invades other regional (2/3 upper urethra, 2/3 upper vagina) or distant structures
IVA	Tumor invades any of the following: (i) Upper urethra or vaginal mucosa, bladder mucosa, rectal mucosa, or fixed to pelvic bone, or (ii) Fixed or ulcerated inguinofemoral lymph nodes
IVB	Any distant metastasis, including pelvic lymph nodes

*The depth of invasion is defined as the measurement of the tumor from the epithelial–stromal junction of the adjacent most superficial dermal papilla to the deepest point of invasion.

these studies were unstaged, although, in general, the larger the tumor, the greater the propensity for inguinal and pelvic node metastases. Morley noted a 21% incidence of lymph node involvement if there was a T1 lesion (<2 cm in diameter) versus 45% with a T2 lesion (>2 cm but limited to the vulva). Malfetano and colleagues reported the incidence of inguinal node metastases in patients with stage III and stage IV lesions to be 53% and 90%, respectively. Clinical evaluation of the groin is somewhat more accurate than tumor size. **Homesley found that approximately 24% of patients with clinically nonsuspicious nodes had positive nodes when dissected, and approximately 75% of patients with suspicious (palpable, fixed, or ulcerated) groins had positive nodes.** Table 8.5 demonstrates the association between inguinal lymph node involvement and tumor size, depth of invasion, and clinical examination. Of note, these data did not evaluate laterality or unifocal versus multifocal lesions.

Staging

Many staging systems have been applied to invasive cancer of the vulva. Significant discrepancy exists between clinical and surgical-pathologic evaluation of lymph node status. Iversen demonstrated that overdiagnosis (clinically suspicious but pathologically negative nodes) occurred in 40 of 258 patients (15%). Of the 100 patients with metastasis to the inguinal lymph nodes, lymph node involvement was clinically unsuspected in 36 patients. Patients with "micrometastasis" (lymph node involvement not suspected clinically but positive microscopically) had a significantly better survival rate than did those with gross metastasis. As a result of these repeated findings, it was suggested that staging be based on surgical-pathologic evaluation instead of clinical evaluation alone. Federation of International Gynecologists and Obstetricians (FIGO) staging of vulvar cancer dates back to 1969. In 1988, FIGO replaced the clinical staging system with a surgical-pathologic, or tumor–node–metastasis (TNM), classification system. The most recent 2009 FIGO staging for carcinoma of the vulva (Table 8.6)

further characterizes the number and type of lymph node metastases. Previous studies noted decreased survival among individuals with bilateral lymph node metastasis; thus, laterality was incorporated into the staging system. However, recent studies have demonstrated that the number of lymph node metastases and extracapsular spread are predictive of survival regardless of laterality. It is important to consider that many reports in the literature use older staging systems, and thus data must be evaluated within the context of the staging system used.

Donaldson and colleagues demonstrated that lesion size predicted incidence of lymph node metastasis (19% metastasis for lesion <3 cm and 72% for lesion >3 cm). Likewise, tumor grade correlated with node metastasis (one-third of well-differentiated tumors had metastasis compared with 75% for poorly differentiated lesions). Of 38 patients, 11 (29%) had node involvement if invasion of the primary lesion was 5 mm or smaller compared with 17 of 28 (61%) if invasion was larger than 5 mm. If the tumor did not involve lymphatic or vascular spaces, only 2 of 33 (6%) had positive nodes, but 26 of 33 patients (79%) with lymphatic or vascular space involvement had metastasis to the regional lymph nodes. None of 25 patients with lesions invading less than 5 mm and without lymphatic or vascular space involvement had lymph node metastasis.

Tabbaa and associates reported the largest cohort study to evaluate the effect and prognostic performance of the 2009

FIGO staging. They reported FIGO stage I, II, III, and IV 5-year overall survival (OS) rates of 84%, 75%, 48%, and 9%, respectively. The 5-year OS rate was 85% for patients without LN metastasis, and for patients with three or more lymph node metastases, the 5-year OS rate was 30%. They surmised that bilateral nodal disease does not appear to impact cause-specific survival, justifying its omission from the 2009 staging system, and that separating node-positive stage III from node-negative stage II cases appears justified.

Sentinel Lymph Node Biopsy

Sentinel lymph node biopsy (SLNB) represents the largest innovation in the care of patients with vulvar cancer in the past decade. The use of the SLN technique in the evaluation of vulvar cancer was first described in the late 1970s based initially on the experience in penile cancers followed by the successes reported in breast cancer and melanoma. The past 20 years have witnessed a myriad of reports featuring SLN techniques in the management of gynecologic cancers, including vulvar cancer, that have provided experienced clinicians with a standard of care option for surgical lymph node management in appropriately selected patients. The concept of SLNs depends on reliable prediction of a tracer substance identifying the primary nodal drainage of the tumor. The assumption is that if the SLN is negative for malignancy then the other nodes will be negative thus precluding the need for full nodal dissection and thereby significantly reducing the procedural related short-term infection and wound breakdown and long-term edema associated with inguinal femoral lymph node dissection (IFLND).

Only approximately 30% of early stage vulvar cancers have positive nodes with IFLND, which thus exposes a large number of women to ostensibly an unnecessary morbid procedure wherein up to two-thirds of patients experience lymphedema. Therefore, reducing the radicality of groin lymphadenectomy by SLNB merits investigation, validation, and implementation as a reliable alternative to full nodal dissection that requires balancing the slightly higher groin recurrence rates of SLNB versus the significantly greater morbidity of IFLND.

Concerns raised in adopting SLNB as the standard of care include first, the reliability of SLN detection. How feasible is this technique in terms of how often does one detect an SLN, and which technique should be used in terms of injection site and tracer selection? Second, what is the reliability of a negative SLN to predict that all the other inguinal nodes are likewise negative for malignancy? In other words, what is the potential for a false-negative result, whereby a SLNB does not demonstrate metastases but additional groin dissection discovers lymphatic spread? Finally, what is the groin recurrence rate? This question is critical because untreated groin metastases will result in groin recurrences that are most often fatal. It is important to recall that the gold standard for the rate of groin relapse in a node-negative groin is 0.3% based on Homesley et al.'s Gynecologic Oncology Group (GOG) experience. The data for detection rate, sensitivity, or false-negative results can be considered from the perspective of each groin, viewed as a separate entity, or from the patient's perspective whereby the outcomes of SLNB are considered for both groins as a unit.

Another concept to consider is the role of nodal ultrastaging with very fine sectioning and use of immunohistochemistry (IHC) as an adjunct to conventional staining, in which the SLN is subjected to far greater scrutiny in terms of pathologic sectioning than nodes removed via traditional IFLND. Nodal yield from traditional IFLND is much greater in number, and these nodes are not usually subjected to these labor-intensive techniques because of time and resource constraints. Also, a statistical concept known as the false-negative predictive value (FNPV), defined as (1- Negative predictive value), needs to be understood to properly consider the burgeoning SLNB literature in the management of vulvar cancer.

Several small studies were instrumental in validating the feasibility of SLNB, with the original lymphatic mapping data being published by Levenbach and colleagues in 1994. Recent studies have continued to demonstrate improved outcomes for SLNB over time. Initial mapping studies of SLNB in vulvar cancer evaluated 21 patients with isosulfan blue dye only, and an SLN was identified in only 86% of patients and 66% of groins. Addition of lymphoscintigraphy (LSG) with radiolabeled technetium significantly improved the SLN detection rate. A collective review of the literature in 2002 noted a detection rate of 92% with the combined technique. Frumovitz and colleagues reported on 52 women who underwent SLNB 1993 and 1999; 14 had a recurrence. Eight of the recurrences (15.4%) were on the vulva, three (5.8%) in the groin, and three (5.8%) distant. The pattern of recurrence is similar to that seen with standard approaches, although the rate of relapse in the groin appears high.

One of the first large prospective multicenter observational trials to assess SLNB was the GROINSS-V I study reported by Van der Zee and associates that included 403 assessable patients using the combined technique. Eligible patients had T1 or T2 lesions smaller than 4 cm, invasion greater than 1 mm, and clinically nonsuspicious inguinofemoral lymph nodes. SLNB was performed, and if the SLN result was negative, then an IFLN was not performed; only when SLN metastases were identified was an IFLND performed either at time of surgery based on frozen section or subsequently based on final pathologic analysis of the SLN. A total of 623 groins in 403 patients were evaluated. The authors selected 276 selected patients with unifocal vulvar disease and a negative SLN to describe in detail, and the 3-year survival rate was 97%, with a mean follow-up of 35 months. Adjuvant radiotherapy was administered to the groin and pelvis when more than one lymph node demonstrated metastasis or extracapsular nodal tumor growth was identified. Those who underwent SLNB had a FNPV of 2.9% with a false-negative rate of 6%. **The groin recurrence rate for those with negative SLNs was 2.3%.** Patients with unifocal lesions had only a 2% recurrence rate compared with 12% for those with multifocal lesions on the vulva. Lymphedema was noted in 2% for SLNB versus 25% in those with positive SLN who underwent full IFLND. Wound breakdown and recurrent cellulitis occurred in 12% and 0.4% versus 34% and 16% for SLNB versus completion IFLND procedures respectively. Ultrastaging with three sections per mm was performed only on SLNs that were negative on routine histopathologic examination. Ultrastaging significantly increased detection of nodal metastases. Routine pathologic examination detected 95 (58%) of the 163 groins with metastatic SLNs, and ultrastaging detected the remaining 68 (42%) groins demonstrating metastatic SLNs.

A subset analysis of the GROINSS-V I study conducted by Oonk and colleagues demonstrated that the risk of non-SLN metastases increased with increasing size of SLN metastasis. Also, the risk of non-SLN metastases was higher when the SLN was found to be positive with routine pathology than with ultrastaging. The 5-year disease-specific survival rates were 97% for women with isolated tumor cells in the SLN, 88% for those with SLN metastases smaller than 2 mm, 70% for those with metastases measuring 2 to 5 mm, and 69% for those with metastases larger than 5 mm. No cutoff provided complete assurance that the non-SLNs would be free of metastases thus given the high risk of mortality if such nodes are missed; **additional groin treatment remains the current recommendation for all patients with SLN involvement.**

GOG 173 reported by Levenback and associates included 452 women who underwent SLNB followed by IFLND irrespective of SLNB findings. Eligibility criteria included SCC confined clinically to the vulva with at least 1 mm of invasion and tumor size up to 6 cm in greatest diameter. Patients with groin nodes that were clinically suggestive of cancer were excluded. Every woman underwent intraoperative lymphatic mapping using isosulfan blue dye; however, 2 years into the study, the protocol was amended to require preoperative LSG and intraoperative radiolocalization, which previously had been optional. Nodes were subjected to ultrastaging by serially sectioning them into 3-mm blocks with at least two sections 40 microns apart per block. The use of frozen section was discouraged. If routine hematoxylin and eosin staining was negative for metastatic disease on the first slide, IHC cytokeratin staining was performed on the second slide. A total of 772 groin dissections were performed (320 = bilateral and 132 = unilateral) in 452 women of whom 418 exhibited at least one SLN. Incidence of node positivity among women with at least one SLN identified was 32%. Of the 132 women with positive nodes, 11 had false-negative findings on SLNB (8.3%; 90% confidence interval [CI], 4.7%–13.4%); thus, the sensitivity was 92%. Importantly, this study showed that the false-negative rate for SLNB increased significantly when tumor size was 4 cm or larger (7.4% vs. 2% for tumors <4 cm). They also demonstrated a favorable FNPV of 3.7%, which was the primary statistical endpoint of this trial. This FNPV is comparable to that observed in breast cancer, but salvage rates for that disease are more favorable. This study highlighted the role of pathologic analysis as 23% of the positive nodes were missed on conventional staining and required IHC for detection of cancer. SLN ultrastaging is also important via step sectioning, which significantly increases the chance of finding metastases, according to Puig-Tintore et al.

Coleman et al. published a subset analysis of patients from GOG 173 that examined the importance of the location of the primary tumor relative to the midline and the role of LSG, which was optional in this study. A total of 234 patients were eligible with 64 having lateral lesions (>2 cm from midline) and thereby undergoing only unilateral IFLND after SLNB; the 105

women with midline and 65 with near-midline lesions (<2 cm distance from midline) underwent bilateral completion IFLND. Bilateral groin drainage using LSG was discovered in 22% of lateral, 58% of near-midline, and 70% of midline tumors. At mapping, no SLNs were found in contralateral groins among patients with near-midline and midline tumors who had unilateral-only LSGs, yet groin metastases were found in four of 32 patients with midline tumors undergoing contralateral dissection; none were found in 27 patients with near-midline tumors. They concluded that the likelihood of detectable bilateral drainage using preoperative LSG decreases as a function of distance from midline. Patients with near-midline primary tumors exhibiting unilateral drainage on LSG may safely undergo unilateral SLN. Further validation of this concept is indicated.

A Cochrane review of SLNB in vulvar cancer management was reported by Lawrie et al. that assessed the diagnostic test accuracy of various techniques using traceable agents for SLNB to diagnose groin lymph node metastasis in women with FIGO stage IB or higher vulvar cancer. A total of 34 studies evaluating 1614 women and approximately 2396 groins were included in the analysis. Use of blue dye only provided a sensitivity of 0.94 (68 women; 95% CI 0.69–0.99); for mixed tracers, sensitivity was 0.91 (679 women; 95% CI 0.71–0.98); and for technetium only, it was 0.93 (149 women; 95% CI 0.89–0.96). Sensitivity for combined tests was 0.95 (390 women; 95% CI 0.89–0.97). Negative predictive values (NPVs) for all index tests exceeded 95%. Mean detection rate for blue dye alone was 82%, compared with 95%, 96%, and 98% for mixed tests, technetium only, and combined tests, respectively. It was estimated that for 100 women hypothetically undergoing SLNB assuming groin metastases prevalence of 30% for the combined or technetium only tests, one and two women with groin metastases might be "missed," and for mixed tests, three women with groin metastases would occur as false-negative results. This review concluded that there are only minor differences in diagnostic test accuracy between the technetium and combined tests. Combined testing may reduce the number of false-negative results compared with technetium alone. It must be recognized that there is a learning curve to successful SLNB, and combined tests may further increase detection for less experienced surgeons. Blue dye alone may be associated with more FNs compared with tests that include technetium. They further concluded that SLNB would reduce the need for full IFLND by 70% in patients with early vulvar cancer, but long-term survival data are needed.

A systematic review was presented by Meads et al. to assess the accuracy of SLNB with technetium 99 and/or blue dye–enhanced LSG. A total of 29 studies that included 1779 women were analyzed. Most studies used technetium-99 combined with blue dye. Pooling when appropriate revealed mean SLN detection rates of 94% for technetium, 69% for blue dye alone, and 98% for both. SLNB revealed a pooled sensitivity of 95% (95% CI 92%–98%) with an NPV of 97.9% in studies using technetium with blue dye, ultrastaging, and IHC with inguinal lymphadenectomy as reference. Less morbidity was reported for those undergoing SLNB. The authors concluded that SLNB should be done in carefully selected patients with technetium and blue dye with ultrastaging and IHC. They further concluded that patients must make an informed choice between the slightly higher groin recurrence rates of SLNB versus the higher morbidity with full lymphadenectomy.

Another systematic review by Hussanzade et al. included 49 studies and reported a false-negative rate by patient and groin perspectives of 8%. Pooled NPVs were 97% for patient- and groin-based analyses. They pointed out that those with palpable groin nodes had lower detection rates and sensitivity with SLNB. They concluded that SLNB with radioactive tracer plus blue dye was accurate in appropriately selected patients with exclusion of those with clinically suspicious inguinal nodes. They also raised the concern of an increased FN rate for midline tumors.

Slomovitz and colleagues performed a review recently that declared SLNB as the standard of care for early stage vulvar cancer secondary to lymphedema rates of 30% to 70% after traditional IFLND combined with the robust prospective data from GOG 173 and the GROINSS-V I studies that confirmed the feasibility and utility of SLNB with similar false-negative rates of 6% for tumors smaller than 4 cm. Important differences between these studies include the fact that GROINSS-V had smaller tumors (T1 or T2 <4 cm) versus GOG 173 in which T1 and T2 tumors measuring 2 to 6 cm were included. Mapping techniques also differed because GROINSS-V required both dye and tracer as well as a minimum threshold of 10 cases for skill verification versus blue dye only was required initially with no skill verification in GOG 173. The authors concluded that the groin relapse rate attributable to a false-negative SLNB for primary vulvar tumors smaller than 4 cm was less than 3%.

Covens and associates convened a working group panel that performed an additional systematic review with meta-analysis whereby they reported a per groin detection rate for SLNB using radiocolloid tracer and blue dye of 87% and a false-negative rate of 6.4%. They recommended SLNB for women with unifocal tumors smaller than 4 cm with clinically nonsuspicious groin nodes, provided that conditions of specific infrastructure and SLN experience and volume are met. The groin recurrence rates are 6.6% for superficial IFLND and 1.4% for complete IFLD versus 3.4% for SLNB. Expert panel recommendations from this paper included using radiocolloid with blue dye and not using blue dye alone secondary to low detection rates. Four quadrant intradermal injections into normal tissue at the margins of the tumor were recommended. Near-infrared tracers (eg, indocyanine green [ICG]) as well as the role of frozen sections require further study. Radiocolloids can be injected 30 min to 24 hours before surgery, depending on the size of the radiocolloid, and manufacturer directions, and blue dye should be injected in the same location as the radiocolloid after induction of anesthesia. A node that has more than five times the background radioactivity should be used to identify an SLN. Pathologically, the panel advocated for SLN ultrastaging by serially sectioning into 3-mm blocks and at least two sections 40 µm apart from each block. If routine hematoxylin and eosin staining is negative for metastatic disease on the first slide, IHC cytokeratin staining should be performed subsequently. Finally, the panel endorsed omission of IFLND in the contralateral side to a positive node when the SLN has been negative in that contralateral side, although they acknowledged that data are limited.

Some issues with SLNB remain less clear, but data are emerging. What is the risk of contralateral non-SLN metastasis in patients with unilaterally positive SLNs? Woelber and colleagues addressed this question in 140 patients, 124 with bilateral and 16 with unilateral SLN dissection. A median number of two SLNs with a range of one to seven per groin were dissected. Of 33 patients with unilaterally positive SLNs, 28 (85%) underwent complete bilateral IFLND despite a contralateral negative SLN, and none demonstrated contralateral non-SLN metastasis. Of the remaining five patients, three received postoperative radiotherapy to the groins. One woman (3.6 %), however, did develop groin recurrence in the initially SLN-negative, fully dissected groin after 19 months. These data support the omission of contralateral IFLND if negative contralateral SLN is found, but clearly further study is needed before altering current guidelines that mostly advocate for bilateral IFLND in these circumstances because these numbers are small and possibly confounded by groin irradiation.

Another unanswered question with SLNB heretofore has been the effect on long-term survival. This issue was recently addressed by te Grootenhuis and associates, who reported the long-term follow-up from the GROINSS-V I study with a median follow-up period of 105 months. The overall local vulvar recurrence rates were 27% at 5 years and 40% at 10 years after primary treatment. These recurrence rates are high considering that these were patients with unifocal tumors smaller than 4 cm. Notably, 89% of patients underwent wide excision versus only 10% who underwent radical vulvectomy for the primary tumor. For SLNB-negative patients, recurrence rates were 25% and 36% at 5 and 10 years, respectively, but SLNB positive patients demonstrated 33% and 46% recurrence rates at 5 and 10 years, respectively. A total of 39 (15%) SLNB-negative patients underwent IFLND secondary to a local recurrence. The isolated groin recurrence rates were 2.5% for SLNB-negative patients and 8% for SLNB-positive patients at 5 years of follow-up. The overall 10-year disease-specific-survival rates were 91% for SLNB-negative patients versus 65% for SLNB-positive patients. For all patients, 10-year disease-specific survival rate decreased from 90% for patients without a local recurrence to 69% for those with a local recurrence.

Additional questions with SLNB remain including optimal imaging techniques such as ultrasonography, computed tomography (CT), magnetic resonance imaging, positron emission tomography/CT, and most recently, single-photon emission computed tomography (SPECT) preoperatively, that would best exclude clinically suspicious nodes that are thought to considerably increase the FN rate for SLNB. Nodes that are totally replaced by tumor may not be identified by mapping because of blockage of lymphatic channels by tumor, thereby resulting in a false-negative result. The role of prior local recurrences as well as prior SLNB also are poorly understood in terms of the accuracy of repeating SLNB. Furthermore, the clinical consequences of micrometastases are unclear. As SLN metastasis size increases, the probability of non-SLN metastases increases, which correlates with decreasing survival. SNLB appears to be cost effective in separate reports (McCann et al. and Erickson et al.); nonetheless, Sutton and associates performed a model-based economic analysis that clearly showed that IFLND was most cost effective and dominated all other strategies considering 2-year OS, but when morbidity-free outcomes were considered, then SLNB using a combined identification technique with ultrastaging and IHC was superior.

Future directions in optimizing SLNB will include development of novel tracers and dyes such as fluorescent dyes (eg, ICG) for enhanced SNL identification. Additionally, ongoing trials GROINSS-V-II and GOG270 will address the potential role of adjuvant groin irradiation as a substitute for completion IFLND in those with positive SLNB. It is noteworthy that this trial suspended accrual in 2010 because of higher than allowable groin recurrences in the cohort of patients with positive SLNB who received adjuvant radiotherapy. At the time of suspension, 10 groin recurrences were identified in 82 such patients. Extensive analysis of these cases revealed that tumor metastases size (≥2 mm) and extranodal extension were associated with a statistically higher rate of groin recurrence. The trial was reopened for accrual after amending the eligibility criteria. Only those with micrometastases remain eligible for radiation; those with macrometastases are to undergo IFLND.

In summarizing, if an SLN is not identified and in any case in which the mapping procedure appears inadequate, SNLB should be abandoned in favor of complete IFLND. Patient selection is crucial to success. Patients should have a negative metastatic workup. Table 8.7 summarizes factors that affect the success of SNLNB. Ideal candidates have unifocal T_1 or T_2 primary tumors smaller than 4 cm in diameter and clinically nonsuspicious groin nodes. SNLB performance characteristics from select studies are summarized in Table 8.8. The standard has been that if a positive SLN is found on one side, then a complete groin dissection should be done bilaterally; however, emerging evidence supports omission of full contralateral IFLND if the contralateral SLN is negative. Fig. 8.10 proposes a potential management algorithm for SLNB. Clearly, these management schemes require individualization as well as constant vigilance of emerging literature that may alter recommendations.

SENTINEL NODES

Management

Overall, management of invasive vulvar cancer has witnessed an evolution from large en bloc resection associated with high morbidity to more conservative approaches, such as radical local resection, separate groin incisions, and now SLNB to minimize complications such as wound breakdown and infection, lymphocele formation, and chronic lymphedema. Way originally reported improved survival in carcinoma of the vulva by use of the en bloc dissection of radical vulvectomy plus inguinal and pelvic lymphadenectomy, which subsequently became the mainstay of treatment in vulvar cancer. The corrected 5-year survival rate for stage I and stage II disease has been reported by many authors to be approximately 90%. This so-called "longhorn" or "butterfly" en bloc resection has evolved into a significantly more tailored approach depending on size and laterality of the lesion, resulting in similar cure rates with lower morbidity. Modified radical vulvectomy is the current approach to resect the primary lesion with a 2-cm margin, sparing a significant amount of normal tissue, especially with smaller lesions. Lymph nodes are resected via separate incisions. Well-lateralized lesions, defined as more than 1 cm from the midline, can be managed with local radical excision or modified radical vulvectomy and ipsilateral inguinofemoral lymph node dissection (LND). Homesley and coworkers presented the GOG experience with such lesions (Table 8.9) and confirmed the low incidence of contralateral node involvement, making ipsilateral inguinal lymphadenectomy a rational approach. However, central lesions must be evaluated with bilateral LND. This is

TABLE 8.7 Factors Influencing Sentinel Lymph Node Biopsy Success

Vulvar tumor size
Unifocal vs. multifocal vulvar tumor
Previous primary resection
Previous groin dissection
Palpable groin nodes
Tracer: dye vs. radiocolloid vs. ICG
Radiopharmaceutical dose
Lateral vs. midline lesion
Ultrastaging
Cytokeratin IHC
Subcutaneous injection
Operator experience

ICG, Indocyanine green; *IHC*, immunohistochemistry.

TABLE 8.8 Select Studies of Sentinel Lymph Nodes

Author, Study, Year	Patients (n)	SLN Detection Rate (%)	Sensitivity (%)	NPV (%)
Van der Zee et al., GROINSS-V I, 2008	403	NR*	98	97
Levenback et al., GOG 173, 2012	452	93%	92	96[†] 98[‡]
Lawrie, review, 2014	1614 (aggregated)	98	95	98
Meads, review, 2014	1779 (aggregated)	97.7	95	97.9
Hussanzade, review, 2013	981 (aggregated)	94.4	92	98
Covens, review, 2015	1087 (aggregated)	87	94	NR

*Combined Tc and blue dye.
[†]Overall.
[‡]Tumors <4 cm.
GOG, Gynecologic Oncology Group; *GROINSS-V I*, GROningen INternational Study on Sentinel nodes in Vulvar cancer I; *NR*, not reported; *NPV*, negative predictive value; *SLN*, sentinel lymph node.

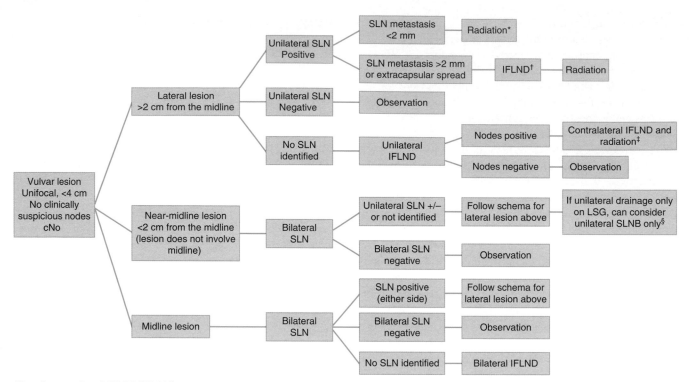

*Pending results of GROINSS-V II.
†Most recommend bilateral IFLND until final results of GROINSS-V II.
‡Depending on number and location of nodes.
§This concept requires further validation.

FIGURE 8.10 A potential management algorithm for sentinel lymph node (SLN) biopsy. *cNo,* no clinically suspicious nodes; *GROINSS-V II,* GROningen INternational Study on Sentinel nodes in Vulvar cancer II; *IFLND,* inguinal femoral lymph node dissection; *LSG,* lymphoscintigraphy.

TABLE 8.9 **Unilateral Lesions: Percentage of Positive Groin Nodes by Tumor Thickness**

Tumor Thickness (mm)	Ipsilateral Positive Only	Contralateral Positive Only	Bilateral Positive	Total	Patients (*n*)
<2	6.8	0.0	0.0	6.8	59
3–5	20.4	1.9	2.8	25.0	108
6-10	28.8	3.8	11.3	43.8	80
>11	36.7	6.7	6.7	50.0	30
Total	**21.7**	**2.5**	**5.1**	**29.2**	**277**

From Homesley HD, Bundy BN, Sedlis A, et al. Prognostic factors for groin node metastasis in squamous cell carcinoma of the vulva (a Gynecologic Oncology Group study). *Gynecol Oncol* 1993;49:279.

based on the lymphatic drainage of the vulva confirmed by anatomic studies demonstrating contralateral lymphatic drainage of lesions near the anus and clitoris, thus warranting the evaluation of both groins in central lesions.

Adjuvant therapy is based on surgicopathologic findings after radical vulvectomy and evaluation of appropriate lymph nodes. Historically, if metastasis was noted in the groin nodes, pelvic LND was performed. This practice has been largely abandoned in favor of pelvic radiation therapy to treat the next nodal chain when groin nodes are involved. The pelvic nodes are essentially never involved with metastatic disease when the inguinal nodes are uninvolved. A study by Curry et al. showed that of 191 patients, only nine (5%) had positive pelvic nodes, and all nine patients also had metastatic disease in the groin nodes. The

GOG (Homesley et al.) performed a prospective randomized study in patients with vulvar carcinoma who had positive groin nodes; 114 patients with positive inguinal nodes were randomly assigned to receive radiotherapy versus ipsilateral pelvic node dissection. The group treated with radiotherapy had a 68% relative 2-year survival rate, and the group undergoing pelvic node dissection had a 54% relative 2-year survival rate. **Thus the standard of care became pelvic lymph node irradiation** (Fig. 8.11) **for patients with positive inguinal nodes.**

A randomized GOG trial by Stehman and colleagues attempted to evaluate groin irradiation versus groin dissection for patients with N0/N1 nodes. This study was closed prematurely when interim monitoring demonstrated an excess groin failure rate in the radiation arm. Although this study's radiation

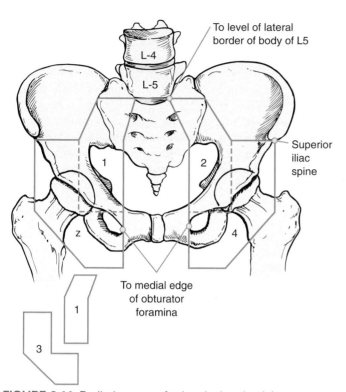

FIGURE 8.11 Radiation ports for inguinal and pelvic treatment. *1, 2,* anteroposterior pelvic and inguinal port; *3, 4,* anterior boost, or "wing." (From Prolog. *Gynecologic Oncology and Surgery,* 2nd ed. 1991, The American College of Obstetricians and Gynecologists, p 51.)

prescription has been criticized, a Cochrane Database Systematic Review (van der Velden and Ansink, 2005) concluded that follow-up studies do not support better disease control with radiation of the intact groin and that LND continues to be the cornerstone of therapy. There may still be some role for radiation therapy, especially in patients who are not surgical candidates, although the risks of groin failure and hip fracture must be considered (Katz et al., 2003).

Boronow also emphasized the possible role of primary radiation therapy in vulvar and vaginal cancers. His report dealt mostly with advanced disease involving vaginal tissues, necessitating an exenterative procedure if a primary surgical approach was used. As an alternative, he recommended surgical extirpation of the lymph nodes with a combination of external and interstitial irradiation for control of the central lesion. In a small, highly individualized series, this approach appeared promising. Similar reports by Fairey and associates and Hacker and colleagues substantiated this. Although neoadjuvant radiation has gained acceptance in this setting, significant challenges remain. Low anterior and posterior fields must be used, resulting in intense exposure of the vulvar skin because the axis of the x-ray beam runs parallel to (and often within) the skin and mucous membrane. Vulvitis may result, and interruption of therapy is often necessary because of the patient's discomfort. Similarly, radiating enlarged, grossly positive inguinal nodes becomes technically difficult. Surgical removal of enlarged nodes with subsequent radiation therapy to the area has been

our preference. **Requisite preoperative doses of 45 to 50 Gy to either the groin or vulvar areas significantly complicates any subsequent surgery because wound healing is impaired. Delaying surgical intervention for 4 to 6 weeks after radiation may reduce these risks.**

Neoadjuvant concurrent chemoradiation therapy to provide optimal reduction in the size of the central lesion has also been evaluated. Russell and coworkers described 25 women with locoregionally advanced squamous cancer of the vulva. All patients received external-beam radiation and synchronous radiopotentiating chemotherapy. Complete clinical response was obtained in 16 of 18 previously untreated patients and in four of seven patients with recurrent disease. Concurrent chemoradiation with cisplatin and 5-fluorouracil (5-FU) has been prospectively evaluated by the GOG and found to be highly effective. Moore and colleagues reported on 73 patients with T3 or T4 tumors who would have required ultraradical surgery to clear disease. Resection was accomplished after chemoradiation in 69 of 71, and only three patients required urinary or fecal diversion. Montana and colleagues reported the companion trial for patients with unresectable groin nodes. Many of these poor-prognosis patients experienced progression or intercurrent death during chemoradiation. Still, 38 of 40 who completed treatment had resectable disease, and 15 of 37 had negative lymph nodes.

It has been suggested that in selected stage IV carcinomas of the vulva, ultra-radical surgery may be applicable. Cavanagh and Shepherd, in a review of their data and the literature, identified 53 patients since 1973 who were treated with exenteration and radical vulvectomy. Most of the patients were young, and 47% were alive without recurrence at 5 years. In their series, Cavanagh and Shepherd found all survivors to have negative pelvic lymph nodes.

Technique of Radical Vulvectomy

The goal of radical vulvectomy is to remove the primary lesion to the depth of the perineal fascia with a 2-cm circumferential margin. Ipsilateral or bilateral inguinofemoral lymph nodes are harvested based on the size and laterality of the lesion, as discussed previously. The single-incision technique is described in Fig. 8.12 and can be modified to incorporate one or both groins. Today, most limit the skin incision to the inguinal area, thereby preserving the bridge of skin between the inguinal and vulvar incisions (three-incision technique, Fig. 8.13). All tissue is removed from the inguinal lymph node bundles. An 8-cm incision is made parallel to the inguinal ligament two fingerbreadths (4 cm) beneath the inguinal ligament and two fingerbreadths (4 cm) lateral to the pubic tubercle (Fig. 8.14). The incision is carried down through the Camper fascia, and at this point, skin flaps are bluntly and sharply dissected superiorly and inferiorly, allowing access to the fat pad containing the superficial nodes. The SLNs are located in the fatty layer of tissue beneath the Camper fascia, in part anterior to the cribriform plate and protruding from beneath the fascia lata (Fig. 8.15). The dissection should be carried superiorly to the inguinal ligament and inferiorly to a point approximately 2 cm proximal to the opening of the Hunter canal. The dissection should be carried laterally to the sartorius muscle and medially to the adductor longus muscle fascia (Fig. 8.16). Blunt dissection facilitates identification of the cribriform fascia, which is most easily identified just below the inguinal ligament or in the area of the saphenous opening. The cribriform fascia unites with the fascia lata, and thus is contiguous with the fascia on the surface of the adductor longus and sartorius muscles; this may facilitate its identification. The portion of the fascia covering the femoral triangle is perforated by the saphenous vein, by lymph nodes of the vertical set, and by numerous blood and lymphatic vessels, hence the name *cribriform fascia*. If the

dissection is carried out properly, the adventitia of the femoral vessels should not be clearly seen except through the vessel openings mentioned earlier.

Bell showed that a complete inguinal dissection could be achieved while leaving the fascia intact. He and his co-investigators retrieved a mean of 10 nodes per groin without removing the cribriform fascia. Borgno and colleagues demonstrated that the deep inguinal or femoral nodes are exposed in the fossa ovalis and other openings of the cribriform fascia, allowing access to all inguinal nodes with this technique. The result is that a dissection that uses the boundaries of the femoral triangle and is

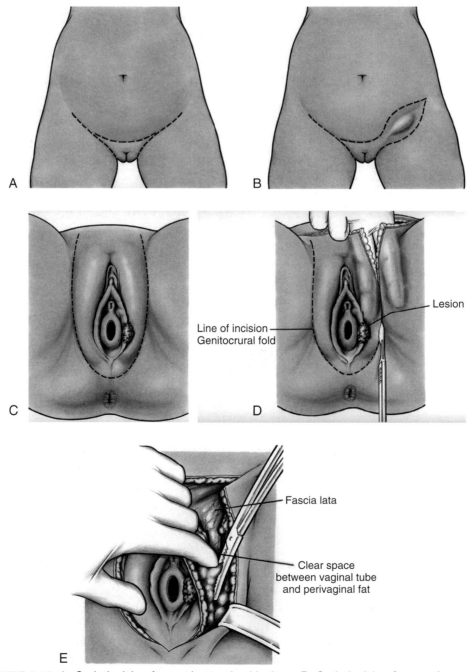

FIGURE 8.12 A, Groin incision for moderate-sized lesions. **B,** Groin incision for a patient with a matted left inguinal node. **C** and **D,** Vulvar incision along the genitocrural fold. **E,** Clamping the perivaginal tissue.

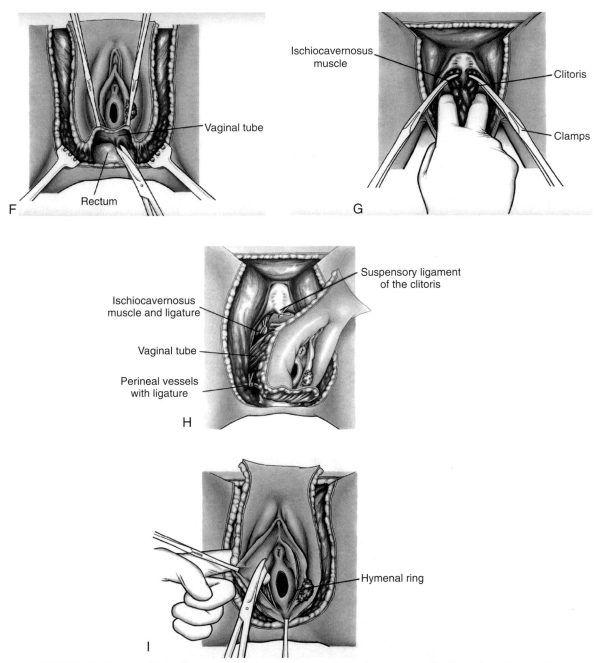

FIGURE 8.12, cont'd F, The vagina being separated from the rectum. G, Clamping the ischio-cavernosus muscle and the crura of the clitoris. H, The mobilized specimen is prepared for excision. I, Excision along the inner margin of the specimen.

FIGURE 8.13 Three-incision technique for vulvar cancer.

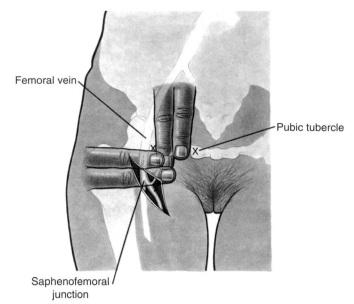

FIGURE 8.14 Incision can be made as noted so that superficial inguinal nodes can be removed easily. (Modified from Cabanas RM. An approach to the treatment of penile carcinoma. *Cancer* 1977;39:456. Copyright © 1977 American Cancer Society. Reprinted by permission of Wiley-Liss, Inc., a subsidiary of John Wiley & Sons, Inc.)

carried out to the level of the cribriform fascia with optimal traction on the lymphovascular fat bundle of the inguinal area **will produce a specimen that contains all of the inguinal and femoral nodes.**

Frozen-section analysis can be obtained if the initial plan is to perform an ipsilateral LND and suspicious nodes are encountered during the dissection. If metastatic disease is confirmed, a contralateral LND is performed. Closed-suction drains are then placed in the groin dissection, and the skin incision is closed by means of a running delayed absorbable suture. The LND is typically performed first, and attention is then turned to the vulvectomy.

A complete radical vulvectomy is accomplished by defining the margin of dissection. The mons is incised anteriorly, extending medially to the genitocrural fold and posteriorly midway between the anus and posterior fourchette. A bloodless space can be dissected between vulvar fat and the subcutaneous tissue of the thigh using a finger dissection (see Figs. 8.12, *C* and *D*). The tissue is transected and ligated with 0 or 2-0 delayed absorbable suture at the level of the fascia of the thigh (see Fig. 8.12, *E*). The posterior dissection is performed sharply (see Fig. 8.12, *F*). Special attention is directed to the location of the anus and rectum. It is sometimes helpful for the operator to place a double-gloved finger in the rectum to ascertain its

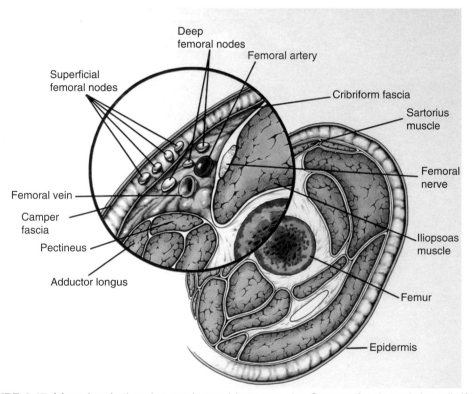

FIGURE 8.15 Many inguinal nodes are located between the Camper fascia and the cribriform fascia, as noted on cross-section through the femoral triangle. Additional nodes are clustered in the foramen ovalis in the part protruding from beneath the plane of the cribriform fascia. (Modified from Cabanas RM. An approach to the treatment of penile carcinoma. *Cancer* 1977;39:456. Copyright © 1977 American Cancer Society. Reprinted by permission of Wiley-Liss, Inc., a subsidiary of John Wiley & Sons, Inc.)

FIGURE 8.16 The *right side* demonstrates the two groups of lymph nodes making up the "sentinel" nodes. The *left side* notes the limits of the dissection with the cribriform fascia removed. The triangle that is dissected in a full inguinal lymphadenectomy is clearly identified on the patient's left side. The inguinal ligament forms the base of the triangle, and the opening of the Hunter canal becomes the apex. The triangle is bound laterally by the sartorius muscle and medially by the adductor muscles and fascia.

location and avoid damage during this part of the procedure. The clitoris is then isolated, and its suspensory ligament is clamped, divided, and suture ligated at its inferior attachment to the pubic bone. It is often helpful at this point to attempt to isolate the ischiocavernosus muscle and divide this structure as laterally as possible (see Fig. 8.12, *G*). The pudendal artery and vein are ligated bilaterally. At this point in the procedure, only the vagina remains attached to the vulva (see Fig. 8.12, *H*). A decision about the amount of vagina to be removed should be made relative to the location and size of cancer and based on knowledge of the lymphatic drainage of the vulva. Every effort should be made to avoid resection of the urethra unless it is close to the cancer. If it is indicated, the distal 1 to 2 cm of this organ can be removed without damage to the functional sphincter. The perineal defect is closed primarily with mattress sutures of 0 or 2-0 delayed absorbable suture. Tension on this closure can be prevented, if necessary, by sharp and blunt mobilization of the vaginal barrel or subcutaneous tissue of the thigh. The most anterior extent of the dissection may be allowed to granulate secondarily for large defects if closure would result in significant tension. This prevents distortion of the urethra and alteration of the urinary stream. If the defect is too large for primary closure, intraposition of a split-thickness skin graft or rhomboid or rotational flaps can be used.

Multiple studies have demonstrated that the classical radical vulvectomy can be safely modified depending on the laterality and extent of the lesion without compromising outcomes if a 1 to 2-cm circumferential margin is maintained. If a unilateral lesion is present, radical local excision or modified radical vulvectomy can be performed. If presurgical clinical examination reveals tumor less than 1.0 cm from structures that will not

be surgically removed, then the potential of an inadequate surgical margin is high, and preoperative radiation or concomitant chemotherapy and radiation should be considered.

Morbidity Associated With Treatment of Vulvar Carcinoma

In the early series of Way, the operative mortality rate approached 20%. In the past 2 decades, this has been reduced to 1% to 2%. This procedure is commonly carried out in the ninth and tenth decades of life with surprising safety. However, morbidity remains high and most commonly includes wound breakdown, lower extremity lymphedema, lymphocyst formation, decreased pelvic support, and decreased sexual function.

Wound breakdown occurs in more than 50% of patients in most series. This aspect of morbidity is usually limited to skin loss at the margin of the groin incision. Podratz and colleagues at the Mayo Clinic noted impaired primary wound healing in 148 of 175 patients (85%) who were treated with radical vulvectomy and inguinal lymphadenectomy. Removing lesser amounts of skin and decreasing the undermining of the skin flaps have reduced the incidence of wound breakdown. Routine prophylactic antibiotics and the use of closed-suction drainage aid in wound healing and decrease the incidence of wound cellulitis and wound breakdown. Careful débridement and vigorous care to keep the wounds clean and dry optimize healing. Bed rest for 1 to 3 days after extensive resections may be considered but must be balanced against the increased risks of thromboembolism and pulmonary complications.

Lymphedema of the lower extremities is another potential major problem (see Fig. 8.17). Historically, lymphedema was much more common in patients who underwent inguinal and

FIGURE 8.17 Marked lymphedema of the left leg after inguinal and pelvic lymphadenectomy.

FIGURE 8.18 Severe edema of the vulva after radiation therapy with necrosis at the site of the primary lesion.

pelvic lymphadenectomy. Podratz and colleagues reported that varying degrees of lymphedema of the lower extremities occurred in 69% of their patients. This debilitating long-term complication can be reduced by routine use of custom-made elastic support hose during the first postoperative year while collateral pathways of lymph drainage develop. Streptococcal lymphangitis in the lower extremities is associated with lymphedema; thus, Rutledge and colleagues recommended low-dose prophylactic antibiotic therapy after lymphadenectomy. Zhang and colleagues confirmed Plaxe's observation that sparing of the saphenous vein reduces the incidence of chronic lymphedema and does not compromise the outcome, with similar recurrence rates in patients undergoing complete resection versus preservation of the saphenous vein during inguinal lymphadenectomy.

Boccardo and associates reported performing multiple lymphatic-venous anastomoses after IFLND in 25 patients with vulvar cancer and melanoma of the trunk with blue dye injection into the thigh preoperatively. Afferent lymphatic channels to the blue nodes were anastomosed to a collateral branch of the great saphenous vein. They reported no lymphocele or infectious complications, and only one patient had long-term lower limb lymphedema. Further study is needed of this technique.

Lymphocysts in the groin are infrequent and usually resolve spontaneously. The incidence can be reduced by careful ligation of all the lymph-bearing tissue during the groin dissection and by maintaining closed-suction drains in these spaces postopera-

tively until drainage is less than 30 cc/day. On occasion, intermittent aseptic aspiration of the fluid facilitates resolution.

Complication rates have been reduced significantly with the use of modified radical excisions and smaller groin incisions as well as use of SLN techniques. Multiple series (Rouzier et al., 2003; Gaarenstroom et al., 2003; Gould et al., 2001) have shown that wound cellulitis occurs in 25% to 39% of patients, wound breakdown in 17% to 31% of patients, and lymphedema in 28% to 39% of patients. SLN techniques have further reduced morbidity significantly.

Morbidity is also associated with radiation therapy. The use of radiation therapy as a priori treatment, especially in patients with fixed inguinal nodes, can result in significant vulvar edema. This is especially true when low fields are used to include vulvar disease. Fig. 8.18 illustrates severe edema in a patient treated primarily with radiation therapy. Necrosis (at 5 o'clock) is a residual from the large lesion-occupying that area before irradiation. Pelvic radiation therapy also increases risk of pelvic fracture, especially in older women. Baxter et al. reported more fractures occurred in patients treated for anal cancer followed by rectal cancer and cervical cancer. Although the risk in vulvar cancer was not specifically evaluated because of small numbers, all women undergoing pelvic radiation had a higher rate of pelvic fracture than women with pelvic malignancies who did not undergo irradiation, and nearly 90% of fractures involved the hip.

Symptoms related to stress incontinence and the development of cystocele or rectocele are sometimes reported by patients undergoing surgery or radiation for the treatment of vulvar cancer. These conditions are secondary to the loss of the support of the lower end of the vagina and subsequent enlargement of the introitus. The findings may also simply reflect the increased frequency of pelvic visceral prolapse among older women.

Removal of significant vulvar tissue, particularly the clitoris, can result in decreased sexual satisfaction. With small lesions in which the clitoris is not involved, resection with preservation of the clitoris should be performed.

Survival Results

Survival in cancer of the vulva is directly related to the extent of disease. In addition, because this malignant neoplasm is initially diagnosed in elderly women, many patients succumb to intercurrent disease while tumor free. In stage I and stage II disease, the corrected 5-year survival rate should approach 90%. A 75% corrected 5-year survival rate for all stages of vulvar cancer is commonly reported.

Regardless of stage, nodal status is of particular prognostic significance. In many series, if the lymph nodes are negative irrespective of stage, more than 90% of these patients will survive 5 years (corrected survival), but only 40% to 50% will survive if the lymph nodes are positive (Table 8.10). The large National Cancer Data Base (NCDB) study reported a stage I 5-year survival rate of 93% and 87% for stage II. In patients with negative nodes, irrespective of size or primary lesion, the 5-year survival rate was 90%. The survival rate was 55% with one positive node, 59% with two or three positive nodes, and 33% with four positive nodes. In patients with positive nodes, the survival rate was 62% if the primary lesion was 2 cm or smaller and 43% if the primary lesion was larger than 2 cm. OS results by stage are found in Fig. 8.19.

Curry and associates noted that patients with three or fewer involved unilateral groin nodes had a 5-year survival rate of 68% (17 of 25) versus 0% (0 of 5) if more than three nodes had metastases. None of the patients with three or fewer involved nodes had pelvic node metastases. Boyce and associates and Shimm and coworkers reported similar results, with prognosis worsening not only with an increase in the number of positive nodes but also to a lesser extent with bilateral inguinal node involvement. Of the patients with more than four unilateral nodes, 50% had pelvic node metastasis, and if bilateral groin nodes were involved, 26% had positive pelvic nodes. In patients with positive pelvic nodes, the survival rate is poor. Collected series indicate that only one-fifth of patients with pelvic node metastasis survived 5 years (Table 8.11).

Features of nodal metastasis have been noted by some investigators to carry prognostic significance. Raspagliesi and associates evaluated features that included FIGO stage, depth of invasion, grade, lymph node status, lymphovascular space involvement (LVSI), DNA ploidy, and patient age and found that lymph node status and LVSI were both significant independent prognostic factors. Pathologic analysis of metastatic lymph nodes determined that the percentage of nodal replacement and extracapsular spread were both statistically significant also, but the number of positive nodes and laterality were not significant. Similarly, Fons and colleagues confirmed that extracapsular spread was an important prognostic factor. In addition, the significance of bilateral lymph node involvement was lost when the total number of metastatic nodes was taken into account. In other words, the number of metastatic nodes is more important than their location—either unilateral or bilateral. FIGO staging modifications for vulvar cancer included degree of tumor burden within metastatic lymph nodes, number of involved nodes, and presence of extracapsular lymph node spread (Table 8.6). Tumor size is now included in stage I substaging, rather than stage I and stage II, and laterality of lymph node metastasis is no longer included.

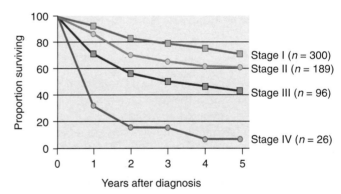

FIGURE 8.19 Carcinoma of the vulva: patients treated from 1990 to 1992. (From the Annual Report of Gynecological Cancer. FIGO, Vol 23, 1998.)

TABLE 8.10 Survival Rates for Carcinoma of the Vulva

Series	Status of Nodes	Patients (n)	Percentage Surviving Positive	Percentage Surviving Negative
Boyce et al. (1985)	Positive	30	50	
	Negative	49		82
Shimm et al. (1986)	Positive	33	52	
	Negative	65		77
Cavanagh et al. (1990)	Positive	77	39	
	Negative	126		85
Creasman et al. (1997)	Positive	444	49	
	Negative	983		90

TABLE 8.11 Survival Rates for Patients With Positive Pelvic Nodes

Series	5-Year Survival Rate (%)
Way (1957)	2/9 (22.2)
Green et al. (1958)	2/16 (12.5)
Way (1960)	3/8 (37.5)
Merrill and Ross (1961)	1/3 (33.3)
Collins et al. (1963)	1/6 (16.7)
Franklin and Rutledge (1971)	3/12 (25.0)
Morley (1976)	1/6 (16.7)
Curry et al. (1980)	2/9 (22.2)
Boyce et al. (1985)	0/6 (0)
Shimm et al. (1986)	0/7 (0)
Total	**15/82 (18.3)**

Mahner and associates recently presented a large series examining the impact of nodes on outcome that detailed a 10-year experience from the AGO composed of 1249 women who had lymph node assessments. Of the node-positive patients, 39% had one, and 23% had two positive nodes. Three-year progression-free survival (PFS) rate of node-positive patients was 35%, and OS was 56% compared with 75% and 90% in node-negative patients. Those with positive nodes who received postoperative radiation to the groin and other fields demonstrated improved survival (3-year PFS, 40% vs. 26%), but improved treatments such as adding chemotherapy are needed to overcome these poor outcomes.

Tolerance of the Elderly Patients to Therapy

The rate of SCC of the vulva increases with age, often affecting patients in the eighth through tenth decades of life. As the average lifespan of women increases, gynecologic malignant neoplasms in geriatric patients have become more common. The reason for the increase in incidence of cancer in this population has not been clearly established, although multiple factors may be involved, including decreased immunosurveillance, longer duration of environmental carcinogenic exposures, and an accumulation of tumorigenic mutations.

Elderly patients should not be categorically excluded from appropriate aggressive therapies; nonetheless, treatment may require modifications to accommodate comorbidities and functional status. Surgical therapy such as radical vulvectomy and inguinal lymphadenectomy is generally well tolerated by elderly patients.

Recurrence

Recurrence may be local or distant, and more than 80% occur in the first 2 years after therapy, demanding initial close follow-up. Oonk et al. noted that 65% of recurrences were found during scheduled follow-up visits and that half of those patients were asymptomatic. Recurrences found during scheduled follow-ups tended to be smaller. Local recurrence is more common with larger tumors and positive capillary-lymphatic space involvement (Table 8.12). More than half of the recurrences are local and near the site of the primary lesion. Recurrence is more common in patients with large primary tumors or metastatic disease in the lymph nodes at initial surgery. The margin of resection has also long been recognized to be a significant prognostic factor. The goal is to achieve a tumor-free margin of 1 cm or more to minimize local recurrence risk. One needs to account for approximately 20% specimen shrinkage with tissue fixation and slide preparation; thus, an 8-mm margin with fixed tissue will correspond to the desired surgical margin of 1 cm. Data from Heaps and colleagues as well as de Hullu et al. and Rouzier et al. established this relationship. The high incidence of local recurrence demands careful attention to adequate margins in the removal of the primary lesion. Some recurrences on the vulva occur at a site remote from the primary excision. Rouzier and colleagues (2001) noted that these patients, who may actually have new primary lesions, had a better prognosis than those who recurred earlier and near the site of the prior excision.

TABLE 8.12 Sites of Recurrence After Modified Radical Operation

Author	Patients (n)	Local (%)	Bridge (%)	Groin (%)	Distant (%)
de Hullu et al. (2002)	238	18 (8)	1 (0.4)	2 (0.8)	12 (5)
Gonzalez-Bosquet et al. (2005)	330	64 (19)	—	8 (2.4)	37 (11)
Maggino et al. (2000)	502	100 (20)	—	35 (6.9)	25 (5)
Oonk et al. (2003)	238	49 (20)	2 (0.8)	6 (2.5)	8 (3)
Rouzier et al. (2002)	215	26 (17)	7 (3.3)		

Radical wide local excision and the triple-incision technique may lead to a slightly increased risk for local recurrence (van der Velden et al., 2004). Care must be given to excising the entire lesion with at least a 1- to 2-cm margin. In many instances, local recurrences can be successfully treated by local excision or interstitial irradiation. Patients with recurrent local disease in the lymph node area or distant disease are difficult to treat, and the salvage rate is poor. Simonsen reported a 40% salvage rate with local recurrence and an 8% survival rate at 5 years with regional metastases. Both groups were treated with a combination of surgery and radiation therapy. Prempree and Amornmarn demonstrated similar results using radiation alone. Disease limited to the introitus resulted in the best prognosis: six of six patients survived. As expected, extensive recurrences have the poorest prognosis, especially when bone involvement occurs. Patients with distant recurrences have been treated with platinum-based chemotherapy, and a 30% overall response rate has been achieved. Responses are more likely outside the radiation field.

EARLY VULVAR CARCINOMA

Andreasson and Nyboe constructed three different models of groups at low risk for metastasis in SCC of the vulva region. They concluded that a distinct profile of low-risk patients would require data from large accruals of patients and international collaboration. Based on such studies, the International Society for the Study of Vulvovaginal Disease (ISSVD) proposed the following pathologic definition of microinvasive carcinoma of the vulva: "a squamous carcinoma having a diameter of less than 2 cm, as measured in the fresh state, with a depth of invasion of less than 1 mm, measured from the epithelial-stromal junction of the most superficial adjacent dermal papilla to the deepest point of invasion." LVSI by tumor excludes the lesion from this definition, and groin nodes should be clinically nonsuspicious. The current staging system classifies these lesions as stage Ia. Microinvasive, or stage Ia, lesions are managed with wide local excision and do not require inguinal lymphadenectomy because lymph node metastasis is extremely rare.

Assessing the depth of invasion is obviously critical in assuring microinvasion and, unfortunately, there remains considerable inconsistency regarding pathologists' measurement methodology. The preferred method measures from the most superficial dermal–epidermal junction of the most superficial adjacent dermal papilla as required in the FIGO staging system. Others have used a method that measures from the surface of the lesion; although this method is simpler, it appears not to be as reflective of true invasion. The importance of LVSI adjacent to the vulvar carcinoma in predicting lymph node metastasis, or prognosis, remains controversial. However, data support the hypothesis that LVSI by tumor at the site of the primary is associated with an increased frequency of lymph node metastasis. There does not appear to be a definitive correlation between tumor differentiation and lymph node metastasis and survival. There may be an association between depth of tumor invasion and tumor differentiation, with deeply invasive tumors being more undifferentiated. More study of this issue is needed.

Podratz and colleagues reported a 5-year survival rate of 90% if the primary lesion was smaller than 1 cm, 89% if the lesion was 1 to 2 cm, and 83% if the lesion was 2 to 3 cm. They found that the 5- and 10-year survival rates of patients with stage I disease were independent of the extent of the surgical procedure, **suggesting that local radical resection with adequate margins is feasible without sacrifice of curability.**

Stehman and colleagues reported the GOG experience with 121 patients with stage I disease and invasion less than 5 mm treated with a modified radical vulvectomy and superficial inguinal lymphadenectomy. There were 19 recurrences, including five groin-only recurrences and seven deaths. Gordiner reported nine groin recurrences in 104 patients treated with superficial dissection. In these nine patients, the median number of nodes removed per groin was seven, but there were four groins with zero to two nodes. In contrast, in Kirby and coworkers' report, only an average of 2.7 nodes was retrieved per groin. The difference among all these reports is likely to be in the extent of the inguinal lymphadenectomy. Our suggestions for management are presented in Figs. 8.20 to 8.22.

PAGET DISEASE

Paget disease was first described by Sir James Phillips in 1874. Involvement of the vulva is rare. It most often occurs in women in the seventh decade of life but can be seen in young patients. **Pruritus and tenderness are the most common presenting symptoms.** These symptoms may be present for years before the patient seeks medical attention. The vulvar lesion may be localized to one labium or involve the entire vulvar epithelium. It is not unusual for the disease process to extend to the perirectal area, buttocks, inguinal area, or mons. Extension into the vagina has been reported.

Clinical and Histologic Features

On examination, the vulvar lesions are usually hyperemic, sharply demarcated, and thickened, with foci of excoriation and induration. The vulvar skin is often thick and smooth, leading to the impression of leukoplakia. It is not unusual for the hyperemic areas associated with a superficial white coating to give the impression of "cake-icing effect." This finding

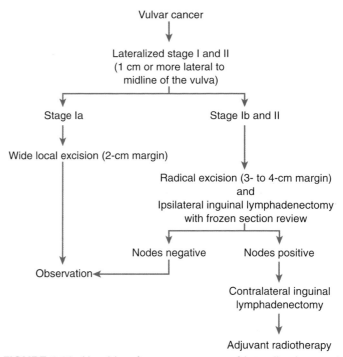

FIGURE 8.20 Algorithm for management of lateralized stage I or II vulvar cancer.

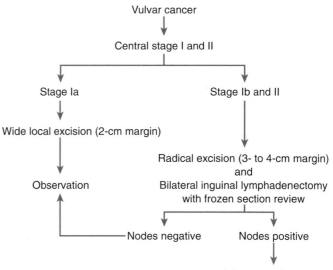

FIGURE 8.21 Algorithm for management of central stage I or II vulvar cancer.

is classic and, if present, is almost pathognomonic for Paget disease (Fig. 8.23). **Typically, areas of leukoplakia are mixed with patches of redness where excoriation has occurred secondary to intense pruritus.** Vulvar changes are usually superficial, but palpation may indicate thickness or a mass-like effect under the epithelial changes, raising concern of an underlying adenocarcinoma. If clinical findings are suspicious, adequate biopsy of the lesion relative to width and depth of tissue must be obtained to enable adequate histologic evaluation. One

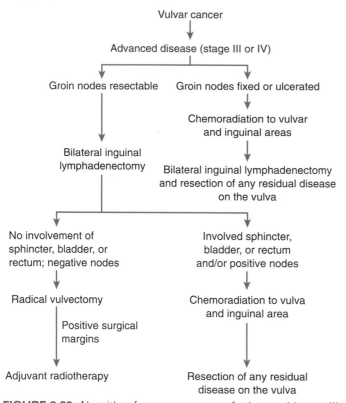

FIGURE 8.22 Algorithm for management of advanced (stage III or IV) vulvar cancer.

FIGURE 8.23 Paget disease of the vulva involving the lower half of the left labium major and labium minor. The white medial portion is characteristic of "cake-icing effect." The red medial aspect is also commonly seen and called "violaceous coloring."

should perform a needle aspiration of any thickness or mass that is palpated beneath the skin involved with Paget disease.

Historically, it appears that there are two separate lesions: intraepithelial extramammary Paget disease and pagetoid changes within the skin associated with an underlying adenocarcinoma. Lopes Filho et al. reported that of all extramammary Paget disease, approximately 65% is observed in the vulva. More recently, invasive Paget disease has been described based on the depth of invasion. Minimally invasive Paget disease is defined by Paget cells that have invaded the basement membrane into the underlying dermis to less than 1 mm. Invasive vulvar Paget disease is a lesion in which the Paget cells invade the basement membrane into the underlying dermis greater than 1 mm. Therapy for these two lesions is considerably different, and a definitive diagnosis is therefore imperative.

A thickened, often acanthotic, epidermis is the typical histologic finding. **Characteristic large cells with clear granular cytoplasm are found within the epidermis** (Fig. 8.24). A single layer of squamous cells often separates the Paget cells from the epidermis, but neoplastic cells may be in immediate contact with the dermis. Intraepidermal formation of glands with true lumens may also be present. The hair follicles may also be involved with Paget cells. These cells contain intracytoplasmic mucin demonstrated by Mayer's mucicarmine or Alcian blue. A mixed inflammatory infiltrate of variable intensity composed usually of lymphocytes and plasma cells is present in the upper dermis. IHC is helpful in distinguishing Paget from Bowen disease and amelanotic superficial spreading melanoma.

FIGURE 8.24 Histologic picture of Paget disease of the vulva. Large cells with clear cytoplasm are apparent in the epidermis. Note the heavy lymphocytic infiltration in the dermis.

Clinical Course and Management

If only intraepithelial Paget disease is present, the clinical course may be prolonged and indolent, often associated with recurrence of intraepithelial disease. Rarely, the disease can have an invasive component or be associated with an underlying adenocarcinoma of underlying apocrine glands. The latter is not actually Paget disease but rather a secondary infiltration of the vulvar skin with pagetoid cells from the primary adenocarcinoma. Paget disease with an underlying adenocarcinoma can be aggressive, with metastasis to the regional lymph nodes and distant spread.

The literature has been confusing with regard to the association of invasive carcinoma and concomitant intraepithelial Paget disease. Early reports suggested invasive underlying adenocarcinomas in up to 20% of patients with histologically confirmed pagetoid cells in the vulvar skin. Recent literature suggests a much lower incidence. Similarly, older studies suggest that up to 25% of patients have a concomitant carcinoma at another site, such as the breast, colon, anus, or cervix. Here, too, recent studies have not confirmed such strong associations, with only a rare patient having a simultaneous lesion. In a review of 100 cases from eight institutions, Fanning and colleagues noted 12% of patients with invasive vulvar Paget disease and 4% with an underlying primary vulvar adenocarcinoma. A review of the literature noted an underlying adenocarcinoma in 8% and 10% with invasive Paget disease of the vulva; 20 patients had a total of 26 nonvulvar malignant neoplasms. The authors postulated that the nonvulvar cancers were probably more related to advanced age of the patients and not necessarily to Paget disease. Note that this infrequent association with an underlying cancer is in contradistinction to the more than 90% association observed between mammary Paget and underlying breast cancer.

Because Paget disease without an underlying adenocarcinoma appears to be a true intraepithelial neoplasia, it can be treated as such. Wide local excision to include the entire lesion is usually sufficient. **Even with apparently wide margins, it is not unusual to find Paget disease extending to the edge of the surgical margin, and recurrences are common.** In the Fanning et al. study, 31 of 84 patients with intraepithelial disease developed a recurrence. Radical vulvectomy, hemivulvectomy, and wide local excision were used as treatment. Recurrence rates were similar with all three treatments. Because of the high recurrence rate and challenges in evaluating the margin grossly, intraoperative frozen section of the margins has been recommended in the past (Fig. 8.25). Unfortunately, this approach is time and labor intensive without leading to an improved outcome. Fishman and colleagues evaluated 14 patients with Paget disease who underwent a total of 25 operations. Margin status was determined by frozen section in eight, with an average of 5.5 biopsies per patient to achieve a negative margin. Visual inspection was used to determine the margin in the remaining 17 patients. Frozen section was incorrect in three of eight (37.5%), and visual inspection was wrong in six of 17 (35%). Furthermore, outcome was not significantly different with respect to the margin status. A total of two of five (40%) with a positive margin and three of nine (33%) with a negative margin experienced recurrences.

New lesions can be handled in the same manner as the primary disease—that is, by wide local excision. Studies show that removal of full-thickness skin plus a microscopic amount of subcutaneous fat routinely results in an operative specimen that is 6 mm thick (Fig. 8.26). Because the base of the hair follicles in vulvar skin is at a depth of 4 mm, full-thickness resection should remove cells that may have involved hair shafts.

FIGURE 8.25 Diagram of the vulva with an area of Paget disease involving the right labium majus. The two parallel lines lateral to the lesion represent the surgical margin sent intraoperatively for frozen section analysis. The margin is serially cut in a clockwise fashion, labeled, and analyzed. If any segment of the margin reveals Paget disease, the resection is extended in that direction. (From Bergen S, DiSaia PJ, Liao SY, et al. Conservative management of extramammary Paget's disease of the vulva. *Gynecol Oncol* 1989;33:151.)

Lesions can be extensive in both primary and recurrent settings, and treatment should be determined accordingly. A skin graft to cover the removed tissue may be necessary. DiSaia and coworkers described two patients who developed recurrent Paget disease in the middle of a split-thickness skin graft. Retrodissemination of pagetoid cells from peripheral persistent disease was proposed as the likely mechanism of recurrence.

Besa and coworkers reported good results when radiotherapy was used in conjunction with surgery or for patients for whom surgery was not possible. A dose of 50 to 55 Gy appeared adequate. Voigt and colleagues reported a dramatic response of extramammary Paget carcinoma in a man with chemotherapy using carboplatin and 5-FU with folinic acid.

Patients in whom an underlying adenocarcinoma is identified in association with Paget disease of the vulva should be treated in the same manner as patients with other invasive malignant neoplasms of the vulva. This usually includes radical vulvectomy and inguinal lymphadenectomy. If the lymph nodes have no evidence of metastatic disease, the prognosis is good; however, if metastases are present in the lymph nodes, the prognosis is guarded.

FIGURE 8.26 Schematic of vulvar skin anatomy showing the extension of skin appendages into the subdermal adipose tissue. (From Bergen S, DiSaia PJ, Liao SY, et al. Conservative management of extramammary Paget's disease of the vulva. *Gynecol Oncol* 1989;33:151.)

TABLE 8.13 High-Risk Group for Development of Melanoma

Increased risk with one or more of the following:
- Family history of melanoma
- Poor or no tanning ability, often with a history of sunburn in adolescence

Unusual moles with any of the following characteristics:
- Dark (blue-black) look
- Speckled or splotchy color pattern
- Jagged or fuzzy border
- Recent change in size, shape, or color of a mole
- Any mole larger than a dime

TABLE 8.14 Clark's Staging Classification of Melanoma by Levels

Level	Definition
I	In situ melanoma: All demonstrable tumor is above the basement membrane in the epidermis.
II	Melanoma extends through the basement membrane into the papillary dermis.
III	The tumor fills the papillary dermis and extends to the reticular dermis but does not invade it.
IV	The tumor extends into the reticular dermis.
V	The tumor extends into the subcutaneous fat.

MELANOMA

Melanoma of the vulva is rare but represents the second most common malignant neoplasm of the vulva. This malignant neoplasm probably arises from a lesion containing junctional or compound nevi. Tables 8.13 to 8.15 define the high-risk group and describe the characteristics of pigmented lesions of the vulva or any skin that determine the need for excisional biopsy.

Characteristically, vulvar melanomas are usually pigmented and raised, and they may be ulcerated (Fig. 8.27). In a nationwide study of 198 women from Sweden, vulvar

---

TABLE 8.15 Lymph Node Metastasis and Clark's Level of Vulvar Melanoma

Clark's Level (*n*)	Nodes Examined (%)	Positive Nodes (%)
I (38)	3 (8)	0 (44)
II (80)	30 (60)	3 (10)
III (70)	38 (54)	6 (16)
IV (90)	55 (61)	13 (23)
V (45)	31 (69)	9 (29)

Modified from Creasman WT, Phillips JL, Mench HR. A survey of hospital management practice for vulvar melanoma. *J Am Coll Surg* 1999;188:670.

melanoma was overrepresented by 2.5 times compared with cutaneous melanoma. **Most vulvar melanomas are on the labia majora or clitoris.** Of all melanomas, 46% of lesions were in glabrous (nonhairy) skin, 12% in hairy skin, and 35% in both areas. The median age of patients with these lesions is 65 years in a series reported by Tasseron and coworkers. In a large NCDB study of melanoma of the vulva, age ranged from 7 to 97 years with a median of 66 years; in this study, 50% were 70 years old

or older, and macroscopic amelanotic tumors were present in 27% of patients. Patients may experience pruritus, bleeding, or enlargement of a pigmented area. Melanomas are often misdiagnosed as undifferentiated SCCs, especially when they are histologically amelanotic. The histologic diversity of melanoma can make the diagnosis challenging. In difficult cases, ultrastructural analysis with electron microscopy and immunohistochemistry (especially with S-100 protein and HMB antibody) in conjunction with histologic evaluation can establish the diagnosis.

Prognosis is related to the size of the lesion, depth of invasion, and margin status. A 50-year experience with vulvar and vaginal melanomas was reported by Seifried and associates in which they found that disease-free survival was dependent on tumor thickness, mitotic rate, ulceration status, and pathologic clearance margin. The Clark classification, which uses histologic levels, is commonly used for melanomas elsewhere on the skin and is of prognostic benefit for the vulva also (Table 8.16). In 1970, Breslow recognized that survival was relative to the greatest thickness of the invasive portion of the melanoma by micrometer measure (Fig. 8.28). The Breslow technique appeals to many because of its simplicity. In 1975, Chung and associates

FIGURE 8.27 Melanoma of the vulva. A typical pigmented neoplasm is present.

TABLE 8.16 Correlation of Melanoma Thickness With Survival

Thickness (mm)	8-Year Survival Rate (%)
<0.85	100
0.85–1.5	99
1.5-4	66
>4	25–35

From Jaramillo BA, Ganjei P, Averette HE, et al. Malignant melanoma of the vulva. *Obstet Gynecol* 1985;66:398; Day CL, Lew RA, Mihm MC Jr, et al. The natural break points for primary tumor thickness in clinical stage I melanoma. *N Engl J Med* 1981;305:1155.

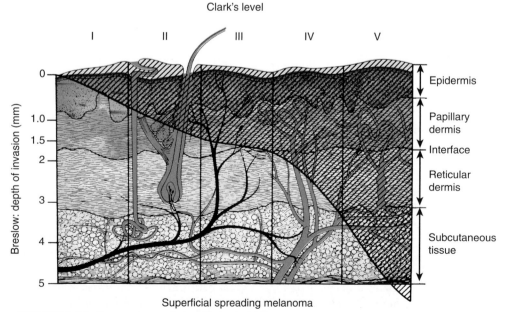

FIGURE 8.28 Comparison of the Clark and Breslow classifications for skin melanomas.

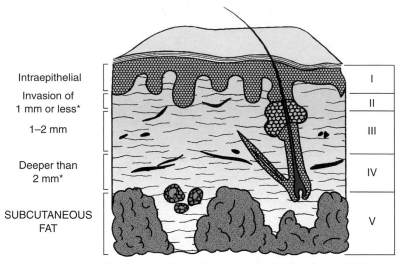

Intraepithelial

Invasion of
1 mm or less*

1–2 mm

Deeper than
2 mm*

SUBCUTANEOUS
FAT

I

II

III

IV

V

*As measured from the granular layer of surface epithelium.

FIGURE 8.29 Chung system of reporting melanoma involvement.

described a third system of reporting level of involvement of vulvar melanoma (Fig. 8.29). Survival rates are influenced by histology as well. Five-year survival rates for superficial spreading and nodular melanomas were 71% and 38%, respectively; 10-year survival rates were 66% and 25%, respectively.

Historically, it had been suggested that all patients with melanoma of the vulva be treated with radical vulvectomy and inguinal and pelvic lymphadenectomy. More conservative approaches are now advocated. In the 596 patients described by the NCDB, surgery was used in more than 90% of patients with stage 0 to stage III disease. Local excision was performed mainly in early stage (stage 0 and stage I) disease. Lymph node evaluation was performed in more than 50% of the patients, with greater frequency for patients with advanced disease. Radical local excision with a margin of 2 cm for thin lesions (≤7 mm) and 3 to 4 cm for thicker lesions appears to be adequate for most well-circumscribed melanomas. Because prognosis is directly related to depth of invasion, therapy can be tailored accordingly. If the disease is intraepithelial, the cure rate should approximate 100%. Clark level I or II melanomas may be adequately treated with wide local excision. As the melanoma extends deeper, the chance of lymph node metastasis increases, and the prognosis worsens considerably. Podratz and colleagues reported that 10-year survival rates associated with Clark's level II, III, IV, and V tumors were 100%, 83%, 65%, and 23%, respectively. In the 323 patients described by the NCDB who had a Clark level determination, 157 had lymph nodes evaluated. Most were in level II to level V, and as expected, **metastasis increased as level of invasion increased** (Table 8.17). In the patients with negative nodes, survival of level I to level IV was 88%, 77%, 88%, and 85%, respectively. Interestingly, four of seven patients with positive nodes survived. Using the Breslow method, Jaramillo and coworkers and Day and coworkers reported nearly 100% survival rate in patients with lesions smaller than 1.5 mm in thickness, 65% to 70% survival rate in patients with lesions 1.5 to 4 mm, and 25% to 35% survival rate

TABLE 8.17	Lymph Node Metastasis and Clark's Level of Vulvar Melanoma	
Clark's Level	**Nodes Examined**	**Positive Nodes**
I (n = 38)	3 (8%)	0 (44%)
II (n = 80)	30 (60%)	3 (10%)
III (n = 70)	38 (54%)	6 (16%)
IV (n = 90)	55 (61%)	13 (23%)
V (n = 45)	31 (69%)	9 (29%)

Modified from Creasman WT, Phillips JL, Mench HR. A survey of hospital management practice for vulvar melanoma. *J Am Coll Surg* 1999;188:670.

TABLE 8.18	Correlation of Melanoma Thickness With Survival of Patients
Thickness (mm)	**8-Year Survival Rate (%)**
<0.85	100
0.85–1.5	99
1.5-4	66
>4	25–35

From Jaramillo BA, Ganjei P, Averette HE, et al. Malignant melanoma of the vulva. *Obstet Gynecol* 1985;66:398; Day CL, Lew RA, Mihm MC Jr, et al. The natural break points for primary tumor thickness in clinical stage I melanoma. *N Engl J Med* 1981;305:1155.

in patients with lesions larger than 4 mm (Table 8.18). Trimble and colleagues described 80 patients with a median follow-up time of 193 months. The 10-year survival rates for Chung level I to V were 100%, 81%, 87%, 11%, and 33%, respectively.

Verschraegen and colleagues reported that 32 of 51 patients ultimately had a recurrence of their melanoma. Both Clark's and Breslow's assessments were predictive. The type of operation performed did not impact the recurrence rate. The role of lymphadenectomy in this disease is probably more prognostic than therapeutic, and strong consideration can be given for SLN dissection as used for melanoma arising from other parts of the body. If disease is limited to the vulva, regardless of its extent, and the lymph nodes are negative, the survival rate is good. Most patients with positive inguinal or pelvic nodes eventually succumb to the disease.

Standard management of primary disease includes surgical resection, but there is a lack of consensus in the published literature regarding additional treatment options. Radiation, chemotherapy, biologic agents and, most recently, an array of immunologic therapies have been implemented in high-risk and recurrent settings. Recommendations can be extrapolated from the experience in nongenital cutaneous melanomas. Therapy should be tailored to the individual patient.

Rouzbahman and colleagues characterized the molecular features of 33 vulvar and 11 vaginal melanomas and found BRAF mutations in 8%, C-KIT mutations in 28%, NRAS mutations in 28%, and TP53 mutation in only 7.6% of the vulvar cases. Thus, the mutational analysis differed in distribution from other primary melanomas, and such analyses may lead to novel molecularly based therapeutics.

SARCOMA

Sarcoma of the vulva is rare, and the experience is limited even in large referral institutions. The source of these tumors can be any of the supporting mesenchymal structures of the vulva. Symptoms and findings can be similar to those noted with SCC, or patients can present with a well-circumscribed mass. In a review of 12 patients, DiSaia and colleagues noted that vulvar sarcoma occurred more often in younger patients (mean age, 38 years) than other vulvar malignant neoplasms. A variety of histologic subtypes have been reported, all exceedingly rare, including leiomyosarcoma; rhabdomyosarcoma; malignant fibrous histiocytoma; epithelioid sarcoma; dermatofibrosarcoma protuberans; and, even more rare, Kaposi sarcoma. The clinical course of these tumors tends to be similar to sarcomas occurring in other anatomic locations. The histologic grade appears to be the most important factor in prognosis. Whereas undifferentiated tumors often grow rapidly and metastasize early, well-differentiated tumors may be cured with local resection or follow an indolent course. Primary therapy consists of radical excision with adequate margins and bilateral inguinal lymphadenectomy except in the low-grade lesions, in which node involvement is rare. Patients undergoing wide local excision are at risk for local recurrence and should be observed closely. Recurrences can be managed with re-resection, chemotherapy, radiation, or combined modalities tailored to the individual patient.

BARTHOLIN GLAND CARCINOMA

Adenocarcinoma of the Bartholin gland is a rare lesion occurring in only about 1% of all vulvar malignant neoplasms (Fig. 8.30). Peak incidence is in women in their mid-60s, although it has been reported in a teenager. Because of its location, the tumor can be of considerable size before the patient is aware of symptoms. Dyspareunia may be one of the first symptoms,

FIGURE 8.30 Adenocarcinoma of the Bartholin gland with local skin metastasis.

although the finding of a mass or ulcerative lesion may be the first indication. **An enlargement in the Bartholin gland area in a postmenopausal woman should be considered a malignant neoplasm until proved otherwise.** The lesion can spread into the ischiorectal fossa and to the inguinal nodes by the usual lymphatic spread pattern for vulvar cancer and via posterior spread to the pelvic nodes directly. Almost half of all carcinomas of Bartholin gland origin are SCCs. Every attempt should be made to differentiate between a true Bartholin gland cancer and a primary SCC of the vulva arising in proximity to the Bartholin gland. The prognosis is good if lymph node metastasis is not present.

Therapy includes radical resection with a large, wide, extensive dissection around the gland and inguinal lymphadenectomy. To have adequate margins, there may be a need to remove a considerable amount of vagina and, on occasion, part of the rectum. Pelvic lymphadenectomy is not indicated. A more conservative approach in selected patients with early disease may be appropriate. The largest series reported by Copeland and associates included 36 patients of whom 27 had squamous histology whose 5-year survival rate was 84%. Of 30 patients with LNDs, 14 (47%) had nodal metastasis, and 11 remain free of disease. Disease recurred in nine patients (six local recurrences, two distant, one local and distant), and four were treated successfully. Less impressive results were reported by Wheelock et al. in a series of 10 patients of whom nine underwent radical vulvectomy with bilateral inguinal lymphadenectomy. A total of five of the nine patients had positive lymph nodes of whom four died of disease. Recently, Bhalwal and colleagues reported on 33 women accessioned over 18 years with Bartholin gland carcinoma of whom 88% had squamous histology and 12% exhibited adenocarcinomas. Compared with those with primary vulvar cancers, those with Bartholin gland carcinoma were younger, had later stages of disease at diagnosis, and were more likely to receive radiation. Nonetheless, despite diagnoses at more advanced stages, patients with Bartholin gland cancers seem to have similar oncologic outcomes and survival rates to patients with vulvar carcinomas not related to the Bartholin gland.

Adenoid cystic carcinoma of the Bartholin gland is rare and manifested by frequent local painful recurrences and slowly progressive disease, including pulmonary metastasis, sometimes many years after initial therapy. The characteristic perineural and lymphatic invasion seen in these tumors are likely responsible for the pain and high recurrence rate. Recommended primary treatment ranges from wide local excision to radical vulvectomy and inguinal lymphadenectomy followed by careful monitoring. Local recurrences are best treated by surgery. As with some other rare tumors, radiation and chemotherapy can be considered individually, especially in refractory cases and in those with distant metastasis.

BASAL CELL CARCINOMA

Basal cell carcinoma usually presents in the eighth decade of life, comprising approximately 1.4% of all vulvar cancers. Clinical presentation often includes itching, irritation, or soreness and a lesion that bleeds and then seems to heal. The process repeats itself as the lesion slowly increases in size. No specific etiology or risk factors have been identified. Most lesions are small, and the most common location is the anterior hair-bearing aspect of the labia majora. A typical lesion has a rolled, pearly border showing fine telangiectatic vessels on the surface with central ulceration (Fig. 8.31). These lesions typically behave like they do elsewhere on the body, with local invasion being the rule. Stromal infiltration is usually circumscribed and orderly with a slow and indolent growth rate. Lymphatics are rarely involved, and metastases are rare.

FIGURE 8.31 Basal cell carcinoma.

Primary treatment consists of wide local excision and primary closure without the need to surgically evaluate regional lymph nodes. Close follow-up is important. In resecting large lesions, skin grafting may be required. In the rare cases of very large lesions or clinically involved lymph nodes, successful response to preoperative radiation has been reported. Basal cell carcinoma must be differentiated pathologically from baso-squamous cell carcinoma, which must be treated as one would treat a SCC of the vulva.

For the bibliography list, log onto www.expertconsult.com ⟨http://www.expertconsult.com⟩.

9

Invasive Cancer of the Vagina

Marilyn Huang, MD, Brian M. Slomovitz, MD, MS, FACOG, Robert L. Coleman, MD

OUTLINE

KEY POINTS

1. Primary carcinoma of the vagina comprises 3% of gynecologic malignancies.
2. Metastatic disease to the vagina develops more commonly than primary disease.
3. Most disease is treated with radiation therapy and in a similar fashion to cervical cancer.

The vagina, in sharp contrast to the uterine cervix and other gynecologic organs, rarely undergoes malignant transformation. **Primary cancer of the vagina is uncommon, accounting for only 3% of gynecologic malignancies** (Table 9-1). Vaginal cancers in the United States occur in about 4000 women and account for 900 deaths each year.

When primary vaginal cancer occurs, it is usually in the upper third of the vagina (Table 9-2) and is most commonly an epithelial carcinoma. The mean age of diagnosis is approximately 65 years old with an incidence **between 35 and 90 years and more than 50% of the cases occurring between the seventh and ninth decades of life** (Fig. 9.1). By convention, any primary malignant neoplasm involving both the cervix and vagina is classified as cervical cancer.

Squamous cell carcinoma (SCC) is the most frequent histologic subtype (78%). Adenocarcinoma (6%), melanoma (3%), and sarcoma (3%) have all been described as primary vaginal cancers (Table 9-3). The relationship of diethylstilbestrol (DES) intrauterine exposure to clear cell adenocarcinoma of the vagina has resulted in the reporting of significant numbers of cases of vaginal adenocarcinoma in both exposed and unexposed individuals. A personal history of radiation therapy contributes to the development of vaginal sarcomas.

The principal focus of this chapter is squamous cancers. Rare histologies are discussed later in the chapter. However, the clinical evaluation and staging for vaginal tumors are the same for all types of vaginal cancers.

SQUAMOUS CELL CARCINOMA OF THE VAGINA

Epidemiology

Similar to cervical cancer, epidemiologic evidence suggests that vaginal cancer has a strong relationship with human papilloma virus (HPV) infection. **HPV subtype 16 presence has been associated with up to two-thirds of all new cases of vaginal cancer.** Approximately one-third of women who develop vaginal cancer will have a history of cervical dysplasia or cervical cancer more than 5 years earlier. A study from the University of South Carolina found that the median interval between cervical disease and development of vaginal cancer was 14 years, and 16% of patients had a history of prior radiation. Proposed mechanisms for developing vaginal cancer with a remote history of cervical cancer include occult residual disease, radiation-induced tumorigenesis, and a new primary cancer in a high-risk individual. A large retrospective cohort of more than 130,000 women with cervical intraepithelial neoplasia 3 (CIN3) demonstrated a significantly increased risk of vaginal cancer compared with women within the same population and time period (incidence ratio, 6.8). Similarly, of the 153 women treated for vaginal cancer, 34 had a prior history of cervical cancer. In general, a new vaginal lesion 5 years or more after treatment of cervical cancer constitutes a new primary vaginal cancer.

The natural course of vaginal intraepithelial neoplasia (VAIN) is not well understood because most patients are treated

TABLE 9.1 Incidence of Vaginal Cancer

Series	Malignant Genital Neoplasms (*n*)	Vaginal Cancer (%)
Smith (1955)	8199	1.5
Ries and Ludwig (1962)	14,785	2.1
Smith (1964)	6050	1.8
Wolff and Douyon (1964)	4665	1.8
Rutledge (1967)	5715	1.2
Palumbo et al. (1969)	2305	1.9
Daw (1971)	564	1.9
Gallup et al. (1987)	Not given	3.1
Manetta (1988)	2149	1.3
Eddy (1991)	2929	3.1

TABLE 9.2 Involvement of Vagina

Series	Upper Third	Middle Third	Lower Third
Livingstone (1950)	34	4	42
Bivens (1953)	22	3	14
Mobius (1956)	89	0	29
Arronet et al. (1960)	14	8	3
Whelton and Kottmeier (1962)	20	13	19
Blunt (1965)	13	15	10
Daw (1971)	24	14	13
Benedet (1984)	46	3	19
Manetta et al. (1990)	22	8	16
Eddy et al. (1991)	33	5	8
Total	**317 (56%)**	**73 (13%)**	**173 (31%)**

TABLE 9.3 Histologic Distribution of Primary Vaginal Cancer

Cell Type	Percentage
Squamous	85
Adenocarcinoma	6
Melanoma	3
Sarcoma	3
Miscellaneous	3

after they are diagnosed. Up to 99% of VAIN 1 and 93% of VAIN 2/3 result from HPV, with HPV-16 subtype being the most common. Thus, risk factors for vaginal cancer are similar to those for cervical neoplasia: multiple lifetime sexual partners, early age at first intercourse, and smoking. Between 3% and 7% of cases of VAIN progress to invasive carcinoma despite treatment. Chronic vaginal irritation has been suggested to contribute to the etiology of vaginal cancer; however, the mechanism by which this promotes carcinogenesis is not well understood and has not been extensively studied.

Screening

The diagnosis of vaginal cancer may often be missed in women who have had a prior hysterectomy. It is particularly important that the lateral "horns" of the upper vaginal vault be thoroughly examined. For some patients, this may require use of an endocervical speculum to ensure a complete evaluation of the vaginal apices.

The Papanicolaou (Pap) test is effective in detecting vaginal cancer in asymptomatic women. The American Cancer Society recommends that Pap screening for cervical cancer may be discontinued in women who have had a hysterectomy for conditions other than cervical dysplasia or cancer. However, women with a history of cervical dysplasia or cervical cancer are at increased risk, and Pap testing should be continued whether or not they may have had a hysterectomy.

For a screening test to be effective, the incidence of the disease must be sufficient to justify the cost. Because the incidence of vaginal cancer is so low, routine screening is not cost effective. **However, development of vaginal cancer is possible even in women with a history of hysterectomy for benign disease.** Bell and colleagues described 87 patients with primary cancer of the vagina, 31 of whom had undergone total hysterectomy for benign disease. Benedet and colleagues found that 19 of their 97 patients (20%) with vaginal cancer had surgery for benign diseases. Peters et al. reported that 38% (25 of 68) of the patients in their series had undergone prior hysterectomies for benign disease. Guidelines aside, these observations underscore the need to individualize vaginal cancer cytologic screening by careful consideration of estimated risks and benefits of such clinical activity.

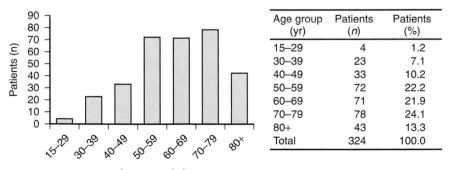

Age group (yr)	Patients (*n*)	Patients (%)
15–29	4	1.2
30–39	23	7.1
40–49	33	10.2
50–59	72	22.2
60–69	71	21.9
70–79	78	24.1
80+	43	13.3
Total	324	100.0

FIGURE 9.1 Carcinoma of the vagina: patients treated from 1999 to 2001. Number of cases by age group. (From IJGO (International Journal of Gynecology and Obstetrics): vol 95, suppl 1, Nov 2006, pages S29–S42.)

Signs and Symptoms

The signs and symptoms of invasive vaginal cancer (Fig. 9.2) are similar to those of cervical cancer. Many women may be asymptomatic. **Painless vaginal discharge, often bloody, is the most frequent symptom in most series.** Postcoital or postmenopausal vaginal bleeding is the initial symptom in many patients with invasive lesions, and a gross lesion is obvious on speculum examination. Patients may also present with watery, blood-tinged, or malodorous vaginal discharge. Urinary symptoms (pain and frequency) are more common than with cervical cancer because neoplasms that are lower in the vagina are close to the vesicle neck, with resulting compression of the bladder at an earlier stage of the disease. Tenesmus is commonly associated with posterior vaginal lesions. Approximately 5% to 10% of women are asymptomatic, with disease diagnosed on suspected physical examination and confirmed by biopsy.

Diagnostic Considerations

All patients presenting with a vaginal cancer need a full workup to rule out metastatic disease. Medical history should emphasize history of cancer, radiotherapy, and surgery. Physical examination, including an adequate pelvic examination (under anesthesia if necessary), should be performed. The diagnosis is often missed on first examination, especially if the lesion is small and covered by the blades of the speculum. Definitive diagnosis is made by histologic confirmation on biopsy.

In patients with an abnormal Pap test result and no gross abnormality, careful vaginal colposcopy is necessary. To differentiate between an early vaginal cancer and VAIN III, it is often necessary to perform a partial upper vaginectomy as reapproximated vaginal tissue at the time of hysterectomy may bury the lesion.

Hoffman and associates reported on 32 patients with VAIN III who underwent an upper vaginectomy; 28% had invasive carcinoma.

FIGURE 9.2 Lesion of the posterior fornix in squamous cell carcinoma.

Metastatic carcinoma to the vagina occurs more often than primary disease because more than 80% of malignant vaginal lesions are metastasis from other sites. In 269 patients with metastatic vaginal cancer, Mazur et al. found that 84% were from genital sites, and the remaining 16% were most commonly metastatic from the gastrointestinal tract or breast. The cervix (32%) and endometrium (18%) are the most common primary sites of cancer. Whereas endometrial carcinomas and choriocarcinomas often metastasize to the vagina, rectal and bladder cancers directly invade the vagina.

When the primary site of growth is in the vagina and does not involve surrounding organs (eg, vulva or cervix), the tumor is considered a primary vaginal cancer. Special consideration needs to be made for patients with a remote (>5 years) or questionable history of a gynecologic malignancy (especially cervical cancer) who present with a vaginal lesion. Patients with a history of endometrial cancer and a vaginal lesion with a histologic diagnosis of adenocarcinoma consistent with recurrence are diagnosed with recurrent endometrial cancer.

After being diagnosed with vagina cancer, patients should be examined for evidence of local or distant spread in a manner analogous to that of cervical cancer. All patients should have at least the following diagnostic studies in addition to a thorough history and physical examination: chest radiography, intravenous pyelography, cystoscopy, and proctosigmoidoscopy, the last two depending on the location of disease. A computed tomography (CT) scan or magnetic resonance imaging (MRI) can replace the pyelography, cystoscopy, and proctosigmoidoscopy. If bone pain is present, further radiographs are warranted. Although staging is clinical, not surgical, an imaging evaluation should be performed to evaluate lymph node metastasis, distant metastasis, and the genitourinary system.

Staging

Most vaginal cancers are staged using the International Federation of Gynecology and Obstetrics (FIGO) combined with the American Joint Committee on Cancer (AJCC) TNM system (Fig. 9.3); a summary of the staging classification last updated January 2010 follows:

Stage 0   Carcinoma in situ, intraepithelial carcinoma
Stage I   Carcinoma is limited to the vaginal wall
Stage II   Carcinoma has involved the subvaginal tissue but has not extended onto the pelvic wall
Stage III Carcinoma has extended onto the pelvic wall
Stage IV   Carcinoma has extended beyond the true pelvis or has involved the mucosa of the bladder or rectum; bullous edema or tumor bulge into the bladder or rectum is not acceptable evidence of invasion of these organs
Stage IVa Spread of the growth to adjacent organs or direct extension beyond the true pelvis
Stage IVb Spread to distant organs

Vaginal cancer is staged clinically. By the FIGO system, tumors that involve the cervix or vulva are not considered

Stage 0

Stage I

Stage II

Stage III

Stage IV

FIGURE 9.3 Staging diagrams for vaginal cancer.

primary vaginal cancers and are classified as either cervical or vulvar primaries. Although FIGO does not specify the stage of patients with inguinal lymph node involvement, the AJCC assigns patients with T1 to T3 tumors with positive inguinal lymph nodes to stage III. Involvement of the pubic symphysis is also classified as stage III. Similar to cervical cancer staging, FIGO does encourage the use of advanced imaging modalities to guide therapy.

Patterns of Spread

Vaginal cancer metastasizes by direct extension, lymphatic dissemination, and hematogenous spread. The pelvic soft tissues, pelvic bones, bladder, and rectum are commonly involved via direct extension in patients with locally advanced disease. The lymphatic vasculature of the vagina begins as an extremely fine capillary meshwork in the mucosa and submucosa (Fig. 9.4). In the deep layers of the submucosa and muscularis, there is a similar parallel but coarser network. Irregular anastomoses have been demonstrated between the two. Both systems drain into small trunks that coalesce at the lateral aspect of the vagina and form a number of collecting trunks. It is at this point that the efferent lymph drainage channels of the organ originate. The lymphatic trunks of the upper vagina drain into the iliac and eventually the paraaortic lymph nodes. A lymphatic network that anastomoses with the regional lymph nodes of the femoral triangle principally drains the lower vagina. All lymph nodes in the pelvis may at one time or another serve as primary sites or regional drainage nodes for vaginal lymph and its contents.

Because most patients with vaginal cancer are treated with radiation, the incidence of lymph node involvement is not well recorded. However, retrospective studies demonstrate that 30% to 35% of patients with vaginal cancer have lymph node metastasis. Paraaortic spread is almost exclusively seen in patients with concomitant pelvic node metastases.

Imaging and Vaginal Cancer

Imaging such as CT, MRI, and positron emission tomography (PET) are often used to guide therapy. MRI is particularly useful in delineating tumor size and extent of spread to the paravaginal or parametrial involvement given its superior soft tissue resolution. PET imaging has become a standard diagnostic tool in the initial staging of cervical cancer and for posttreatment surveillance and has similar applicability for vaginal cancer. Metabolic imaging with PET has been shown to be more sensitive than CT and MRI, specifically for cancer of the head and neck, lung, esophagus, and cervix. In a study from Washington University, Lamoreaux and associates found that PET imaging detected primary and metastatic lesions more often than CT scans. In vaginal cancers, PET is more sensitive for detecting primary vaginal tumors and involved inguinal or pelvic lymph nodes. We recommend that all patients with vaginal cancer have imaging, and PET/CT with or without pelvic MRI is a reasonable option for these patients.

Sentinel Lymph Node Dissection

Patients with vaginal cancer rarely undergo lymph node dissection. Sentinel lymph node evaluation is a technique to determine

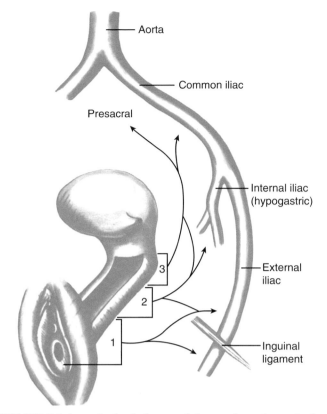

FIGURE 9.4 Lymphatic drainage of the vagina: channels from the lower third drain into the femoral and external iliac nodes (*1*); the channels from the middle third drain into the hypogastric nodes (*2*); channels from the upper third drain into the common iliac, presacral, and hypogastric nodes (*3*). (Modified from Plentl AA, Friedman EA. *Lymphatic System of the Female Genitalia.* Philadelphia, 1971, WB Saunders.)

if there is microscopic nodal metastasis. Frumovitz and colleagues evaluated the utility of radiocolloid and blue dye injection in 14 women with newly diagnosed vaginal cancer. The authors found that lymphatic drainage from the primary tumor does not always follow the predicted lymphatic channels. Pretreatment lymphoscintigraphy did improve treatment planning in this small study. However, because of the lack of data, incorporation of sentinel lymph node dissection into the treatment plan should be limited to research protocols.

Prognostic Features

Our understanding of vaginal cancer and improved radiation techniques have increased survival rates (Fig. 9.5 and Table 9-4). **Several investigators believe that age at time of diagnosis is one of the most important prognostic factors.** Reflecting intolerance of aggressive multimodality therapy and attendant comorbidities, age acts as a surrogate of clinical outcome. Although not well described, performance status likely reflects a factor with greater precision in determining the impact of chronologic age. Tumor histology may also have prognostic relevance. Vaginal melanomas and sarcomas have the poorest

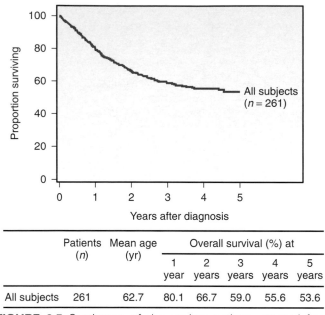

Patients (*n*)	Mean age (yr)	Overall survival (%) at				
		1 year	2 years	3 years	4 years	5 years
All subjects 261	62.7	80.1	66.7	59.0	55.6	53.6

FIGURE 9.5 Carcinoma of the vagina: patients treated from 1990 to 1992. Five-year survival rates. (From IJGO (International Journal of Gynecology and Obstetrics): vol 95, suppl 1, Nov 2006, pages S29-S42.)

TABLE 9.4   Vaginal Cancer: Comparison of Survival Rates

		STAGE AND SURVIVAL (%)				
Authors	Cases (*n*)	I	II	III	IV	All Stages
Krepart (1978)	14*	65	60	35	39	51.8
Nori et al. (1981)	36*	71	66	33	0	42.8
Perez and Camel (1982)	105*	81	42	30	9	50.8
Prempree (1982)	80*	78	57	39	0	8.8
Puthawala et al. (1983)	27*	100	75	22	0	56.8
Benedet et al. (1983)	75*	71	50	15	0	45.8
Reuben et al. (1985)	68*	79	52	54	0	49.8
Gallup et al. (1987)	28*	100	50	0	25	42.8
Eddy (1991)	84*	70	45	35	28	50.8
Stock et al. (1995)	100*	67	53	0	15	46.8
Creasman et al. (1998)	792*	73	58	58	58	

*5-year survival rate.

prognosis compared with SCC and adenocarcinomas. However, survival differences among the different histologies have not been well documented due to rarity of cases.

Stage, tumor location, and tumor size also appear to affect prognosis. In a review of 843 patients with vaginal cancer, patients with stage I disease had a 64% to 90% 5-year survival rate; rates were 31% to 80% for stage II, 0% to 79% for stage III, and 0% to 62% for stage IV. In this study, lesions of the distal vagina had a poorer prognosis than those originating in the proximal vagina. In a review of 104 patients, Smith (1964) found 6.8% survivors among 29 patients with cancer of the

lower third of the vagina, 25% of 48 patients with tumors of the middle third, and 37% of 27 patients with lesions of the upper third. In 1958, Merrill and Bender reported a 29% survival rate in 14 patients with upper third lesions and an 11% rate in nine patients with distal third involvement. More recently, Tewari and colleagues (2001) reported better survival for patients with lesions smaller than 3 cm compared with those larger than 3 cm. Chyle et al. found that tumor size larger than 5 cm was associated with a higher local recurrence rate compared with smaller tumors.

In 2005, Frank and colleagues at MD Anderson Cancer Center reported their 30-year experience treating patients with vaginal cancer. In this series of 193 patients, disease-specific survival and pelvic disease control rates were correlated with stage (I, II, or III/IV) and tumor size (<4 cm or >4 cm).

Intuitively, lymph node status at the time of diagnosis would portend a worse prognosis; however, this has not been well evaluated. In one study by Pingley et al., the 5-year survival rate for patients without lymph node involvement was 56% compared with 33% for patients with lymph node involvement. Furthermore, as in radiation therapy trials of cervical cancer patients, time to treatment initiation and total treatment time also affect vaginal cancer survival. Lee and associates found that the pelvic control rate was 97% if the treatment was completed within 63 days compared with 54% if treatment lasted longer than this time.

In a review of the Surveillance, Epidemiology, and End Result (SEER) population-based cancer registry, 2149 women with vaginal cancer between 1990 and 2004 were identified. Advanced stage, tumor size larger than 4 cm, aggressive histologies (eg, melanoma), and combined treatment modality (vs. surgery alone) were associated with a worse prognosis.

Management

Until the 1930s, vaginal cancers were considered incurable. With advances in radiation therapy, cure rates for even advanced cancers approach those for cervical cancer. Early stage vaginal cancers (stages I and II) treatment approaches include surgical resection or definitive radiotherapy. Bilateral pelvic lymphadenectomy is required given the high risk of occult nodal spread. Surgical series have reported rates of pathologic nodal involvement for stage I of 6% to 14% with stage II of 26% to 32%. Advanced-stage vaginal cancers are mainly managed with definitive radiation therapy. The use of neoadjuvant chemotherapy for locally advanced vaginal cancers has only been reported as case reports and small series with most patients relapsing and dying of disease. Consideration for up front exenteration may also be considered in carefully selected patients with resectable advanced-stage disease.

Prevention

Although the potential effect of HPV vaccines may not be as high for vaginal cancer as it may be for cervical cancer, vaccinating young women against HPV, specifically types 16 and 18, should help to reduce the incidence of HPV-related vaginal disease.

Stage 0 and I

Vaginal intraepithelial neoplasia usually occurs at the vaginal apex, is multifocal, and is common in patients with a history of cervical dysplasia. Treatment options for patients with VAIN include surgery (wide local excision or vaginectomy), 5% fluorouracil cream, local ablation (eg, laser, cryotherapy, electrodiathermy), and intracavitary radiation (Table 9-5).

Creasman and associates reported the results of the National Cancer Data Base (NCDB), a large central registry of hospital data, for 10 years (1984–1994). There were 4885 cases, with 1242 carcinomas in situ (CIS) representing 26% of all vaginal lesions. CIS was almost exclusively treated with surgery; only 5% were treated with radiotherapy. Brown and colleagues reported no new cases of in situ or invasive carcinoma of the vagina developing after radiation therapy for CIS or early invasive carcinoma. Their report discouraged overly aggressive therapy for early-stage tumors because of the good prognosis for these lesions and the adverse effects of high-dose irradiation on the pliability of the vagina and on sexual function. Lee and Symmonds reported the results of 66 patients treated previously with wide local excision or partial vaginectomy and seven patients with multicentric disease treated with total vaginectomy. Only one patient developed recurrence; recurrence was vaginal carcinoma, which resulted in the patient dying of disease. In young, sexually active patients with diffuse involvement of the vaginal epithelium, total or subtotal vaginectomy with split-thickness skin graft reconstruction of the vagina often allows for excellent long-term results. When radiation therapy is chosen, patients who have CIS and superficial stage I tumors can be treated with intracavitary insertion alone.

Surgical management is an option for lesions 0.5 cm or less in patients with invasive carcinoma. For early lesions, particularly in the upper vagina (see Fig. 9.2), surgery may be preferred in many patients. Peters et al. have described superficially invasive SCC of the vagina as a lesion that invades less than 2.5 mm from the surface, lacking involvement of lymphovascular spaces, and occurring in a background of CIS. Their experience with six patients suggests that local therapy was sufficient, and no attempt was made to treat pelvic nodes either surgically or with irradiation. This conservative approach might allow preservation of optimal sexual function in young patients who have these early invasive SCC and adenocarcinoma lesions.

There are no randomized trials defining treatment exclusively for vaginal cancer because of its rarity. Treatment approaches have been largely extrapolated from cervical and anal cancers. For invasive carcinoma thicker than 0.5 cm, total vaginectomy and lymphadenectomy have been performed in the past. If the patient did not have a prior hysterectomy, a radical hysterectomy and upper vaginectomy would need to be performed. However, pelvic external-beam radiotherapy and interstitial implants may be appropriate for some patients, especially those with tumors larger than 2 cm and those involving the mid to lower portion of the vagina. Patients with small stage I cancers (<2 cm) who are not good surgical candidates can adequately be treated with brachytherapy alone. For large vaginal tumors (>2 cm), options for radiating the primary lesion are tailored by physician preference and extent of disease. **Bulky stage I cancers (>2 cm) of the upper portion of the vagina in patients with intact uteri are treated with techniques similar to those used for carcinoma of the cervix.** External irradiation in a dose of 4500 to 5000 cGy is generally recommended with another 2500 cGy given as intracavitary or interstitial brachytherapy in bulky stage I and stage II cancers (see Table 9-5). For young patients who require radiation therapy, pretreatment laparotomy or laparoscopy with ovarian transposition and surgical staging is a rational approach.

Stage II to IVa

For patients who have stage II to IV vaginal cancer, treatment is tailored to the extent of the disease, and the radiation therapy plan should reflect consideration of the depth of invasion of the lesion. Proper planning of radiation therapy and individualization of treatment plans are essential to minimize the more serious complications of acute and long-term radiation sequelae in these organs. The difficulty in applying radiation systems to vaginal cancer led some, such as Wertheim and Brunschwig, to advocate for radical exenteration surgery as primary therapy. However, the complications associated with this radical procedure, especially in older patients, have become a serious limiting factor to surgical approach. **Patients with advanced-stage disease should be treated with external irradiation and brachytherapy.** External irradiation to the pelvis is usually sufficient, and paraaortic extension is not routinely administered. Groin radiation is often considered if the tumor involves the lower third of the vagina or in the presence of metastatic groin disease. Perez and associates evaluated 149 patients with vaginal carcinoma and clinically negative lymph nodes who were not treated with groin radiation. In the group of patients with tumors confined to the upper

TABLE 9.5	Radiotherapy for Vaginal Cancer	
Stage	External Irradiation	Vaginal Therapy
0	Surgical excision preferred for localized disease	7000-cGy surface dose
I		
1- to 2-cm lesion		Brachytherapy irradiation, 6000–7000 cGy*
Larger lesions	4000–5000 cGy of the whole pelvis	Brachytherapy delivering 3000–4000 cGy
II	4000–5000 cGy of the whole pelvis	Same as for stage I
III	5000 cGy of the whole pelvis (optional 1000–2000 cGy through reduced fields)	Brachytherapy implant, 2000–3000 cGy (if tumor regression is satisfactory)
IV (pelvis only)	Same as for stage III	Same as for stage III

*Surgical excision for selected sites on 1- to 2-cm lesions may be used instead of brachytherapy.

vagina, there were no recurrences compared with an 8% recurrence rate in those patients whose tumor involved the lower third of the vagina.

If the uterus is intact and the lesion is in the upper vagina, an intrauterine tandem and ovoids would be appropriate. If the patient has had a hysterectomy, interstitial radiation alone or in combination with intracavitary therapy optimizes dose distribution.

For patients who can be treated with brachytherapy only, a minimum of 6000 to 7000 cGy is delivered to the neoplasm in 5 to 7 days. Pelvic and groin radiation consists of a total of 45 to 50.4 Gy given in 1.8-Gy fractions daily. Use of concomitant sensitizing chemotherapy is discussed in the following section.

If there is metastatic lymph node involvement to the pelvic or groin lymph nodes, external radiation is given to a dose of 60 to 66 Gy. In addition, adenopathy greater than 2 cm may be best controlled with excision. The deep nodes must be included in the treatment fields because large tumors have a high incidence of regional lymphatic metastasis. After receiving 5000 cGy, the patient with a large lesion should be reevaluated for an additional 1000 to 2000 cGy of external radiation to reduced field. Higher radiation doses, however, are associated with greater vaginal toxicity. **Newer treatment planning protocols using intensity-modulated radiation therapy may yield higher tumor control with less local normal tissue effects.** Long-term morbidity outcomes with this technology are awaited.

Radiation therapy alone for locally advanced vaginal cancers generate relatively poor outcomes because of predominantly local failures. Chemoradiation is standard of care for patients with locally advanced carcinoma of the cervix. Because the natural history, histology, and risk factors are similar for vaginal cancer, chemosensitization with weekly cisplatin has been recommended in patients receiving radiation for advanced-stage disease. Prospective studies will likely not be performed given the rarity of this disease. There are several small retrospective series that demonstrated high locoregional control rates after chemoradiation therapy with no increase in radiation-related long-term side effects compared to radiation alone. A single institution series of 71 patients treated with definitive radiation therapy with ($n = 20$) or without ($n = 51$) concurrent chemotherapy, the addition of chemosensitization resulted in improvement in 3-year disease-free survival (43 vs. 73%) and 3-year overall survival (56 vs. 79%). However, given the lack of high-quality data, radiation therapy alone is reasonable if the patient is not a candidate for cisplatin-based chemotherapy. A phase III clinical trial of ribonucleotide reductase inhibitor triapine is currently being conducted by the NRG-GOG (Gynecologic Oncology Group) in women with stage IB2, II, or IIIB-IVA or stage II-IVA vaginal cancer (NCT02466971). Women with advanced-stage vaginal cancer are eligible.

Chemotherapy

Studies are limited regarding the experience with chemotherapy for patients with vaginal cancer. In a phase II GOG study, 26 patients with progressive or recurrent vaginal carcinoma were treated with cisplatin (50 mg/m^2 every 3 weeks). There was minimal, insignificant activity, particularly in the patients with

SCC. Other agents that have been used for the treatment of vaginal cancer include 5-fluorouracil (5-FU), mitomycin-C, epirubicin, or combinations of two of these agents.

A small series of patients with stage II vaginal carcinoma treated with neoadjuvant chemotherapy followed by radical surgery has been reported by Panici and colleagues. Eleven patients were treated with paclitaxel 175 mg/m^2 and cisplatin 75 mg/m^2 for three courses followed by surgery. There were a 27% complete response rate and a 64% partial response rate. At a median follow-up of 75 months, two (18%) patients had a recurrence, and one died of disease.

Special Considerations

Although one is often dealing with a radiosensitive neoplasm in a relatively radioresistant bed (the vagina), serious limitations exist. The proximity of relatively radiosensitive normal tissues, such as the bladder and rectum, provides a challenge to the therapist, especially in the treatment of tumors in the lower third of the vagina. Therapy must be individualized, and radical surgery should be reserved for treatment failures (Fig. 9.6).

The incidence of complications after radiation therapy or surgery for vaginal cancer can be substantial. Serious complications consist primarily of rectal stenosis, rectovaginal fistulas, and severe rectal bleeding often requiring diversion. As many as 35% of patients experience cystitis or proctitis during or shortly after therapy, but symptoms usually resolve spontaneously. A few patients have extensive vaginal necrosis that usually resolves with prolonged conservative management.

Frank and associates found that the incidence of major complications associated with radiation were associated with FIGO stage. Four percent of stage I patients, 9% of stage II patients, and 21% of stage III/IVa patients had major complications. Patients who are sexually active should be encouraged to continue regular intercourse. For others, vaginal dilators should be used to maintain vaginal patency during and after therapy.

Survival and Recurrence

A study by Rutledge in 1967 reported 3- and 5-year survival rates of 42% and 44%, respectively, for patients treated primarily with radiotherapy. Comparable survival results at 5 years were reported by Prempree and colleagues, who used radiotherapy for stage I (83%), stage II (63%), stage III (40%), and stage IV (0%) lesions; their absolute 5-year cure rate for all stages was 55.5%.

In 1982, Perez and Camel reported their long-term follow-up of patients treated with radiation therapy for invasive carcinoma of the vagina. The actuarial disease-free 5-year survival rates for stage I (39 patients) were 90%; stage IIa (39 patients), 58%; stage IIb (21 patients), 32%; stage III (12 patients), 40%; and stage IV (8 patients), 0%. Of 39 patients with stage I carcinoma, 37 (95%) showed no evidence of vaginal or pelvic recurrence. Most of them received interstitial or intracavitary therapy or both; the addition of external-beam irradiation did not significantly increase survival or tumor control. In stage IIa (paravaginal extension), tumor was controlled in 22 of 34 patients (64.7%) with a combination of brachytherapy and external-beam irradiation; only two of five (40%) treated with

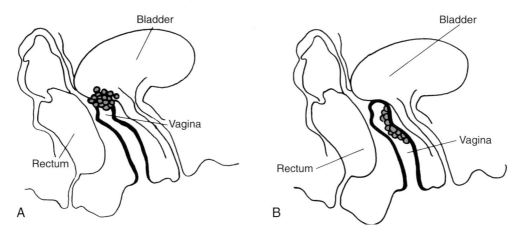

FIGURE 9.6 Diagrammatic representation of typical locations of vaginal cancer in a previously hysterectomized patient illustrating the proximity of the bladder and urethra. **A,** Lesion at the vaginal apex. **B,** Lesion at the upper anterior vaginal wall. (Courtesy of A. Robert Kagan, MD, Los Angeles, CA.)

TABLE 9.6 Primary Vaginal Carcinoma: Local Control and Disease-Free Survival by Stage

FIGO Stage	Local Control (%)	5 YEARS Disease-Free Survival Rate (%)	Patients (n)
I	23	72	67
II	58	62	53
III	9	0	0
IV	10	21	15

FIGO, International Federation of Gynecology and Obstetrics.
From Stock RG, Chen AS, Seski J. A 30-year experience in the management of primary carcinoma of the vagina: analysis of prognostic factors and treatment modalities *Gynecol Oncol* 1995;56:45.

brachytherapy alone exhibited tumor control in the pelvis. The incidence of complications was 9.7% for all stages.

In 1991, Eddy and coworkers published similar results for stage I and stage II lesions of the vagina treated with curative radiotherapy and reported 5-year survival rates of 78% for patients assigned to stage I and 71% for patients assigned to stage II. In addition, Stock and colleagues (1995) reported local control rates of 72% for stage I and 62% for stage II disease (Table 9-6). In the large database (NCDB) reported in 1998, the 5-year relative survival rates were 96% for stage 0, 73% for stage I, 58% for stage II, and 36% for stage III and IV. Women with stage I disease who were treated with surgery had a 5-year survival rate of 90% compared with 63% for patients treated with radiotherapy and 79% for patients treated with surgery and radiotherapy.

In the study from MD Anderson, the 5-year disease-specific survival rate was 85% for patients with stage I disease, 78% for stage II, and 58% for stage III/IVa. In this study, external-beam radiation fields and dose were determined by evaluating

distribution of gross disease and possible sites of microscopic paravaginal and nodal disease.

Sinha and colleagues from Indiana University reviewed their experience with treating vaginal cancers. Overall survival rates were similar to the MD Anderson study (stage I, 92%; stage II, 82%; and stages III and IVA, 20%; $P = 0.0005$). Because of the poor prognosis associated with advanced stage disease, these investigators suggested routine use of combined chemotherapy and radiation as a treatment strategy for these patients.

Vaginal cancers appear to behave similar to cervical or vulvar cancer by first recurring locally. More than 80% of patients with recurrent disease have pelvic recurrence noted clinically, and most recurrences appear within 2 years of primary therapy. Distant sites of involvement occur later and much less frequently. Effective treatment for previously irradiated but locally recurrent or persistent vaginal cancer patients requires radical surgery (ie, pelvic exenteration). However, for those with extrapelvic recurrence, the long-term prognosis is poor. Chyle and colleagues reported a 12% 5-year survival rate after first recurrence. Rubin and associates reported on 33 patients with recurrent vaginal cancer. Eighteen had recurrent disease in the pelvis; 15 were extrapelvic recurrences. At the time of the report, 30 patients had died of disease. The average length of survival from recurrence was 8 months. In the past, chemotherapy for recurrent SCC of the vagina has been relatively ineffective. In the only GOG study of recurrent vaginal cancer, Thigpen and coworkers described 16 patients with SCC of the vagina treated in a phase II study of cisplatin 50 mg/m^2 intravenously every 3 weeks. The results were disappointing. There was only one responder, and this was a complete responder who had extrapelvic disease and who had received no prior therapy. Most of the patients with recurrence in previously irradiated fields showed no response; five of the remaining 15 patients had stable disease.

In the SEER study, an apparent survival advantage was seen with the incorporation of chemoradiation (patients treated since 2000) compared with radiation alone (patients treated between 1990 and 1994).

RARE HISTOLOGIES

Adenocarcinoma and Clear Cell Adenocarcinoma

Approximately 6% of vaginal cancers are adenocarcinomas. Before 1965, clear cell adenocarcinoma of the cervix in women younger than age 30 years was reported only rarely, and vaginal clear cell adenocarcinoma was unknown. In April 1970, Herbst and Scully reported seven cases of primary vaginal adenocarcinoma in patients between the ages of 15 and 22 years. These seven cases exceeded the number of cases in the world literature in adolescent girls born before 1945. Because of this case clustering, an epidemiologic study of the patients and their families was initiated to identify associative factors. With the addition of another patient to the study, it was discovered that the mothers of seven of the eight patients with vaginal adenocarcinoma had been treated with DES, a nonsteroidal synthetic estrogen, in the first trimester of the relevant pregnancy. Since that time, additional cases of vaginal and cervical adenocarcinoma have been reported in patients whose mothers ingested nonsteroidal estrogen during pregnancy. DES and related drugs were used to support high-risk pregnancies and reduce fetal wastage in the mid-1940s and 1950s, but their use then declined. The incidence of DES-induced clear cell carcinoma peaked in the mid-1970s.

As of 1992, 594 cases of vaginal and cervical (≈40% involve the cervix) adenocarcinoma have been accessioned by the registry established by Herbst and colleagues. Among the cases in which a maternal history was obtainable, the proportion that was positive for medication with DES or chemically related estrogens was approximately two-thirds. Progestins had been administered in six of the cases, and a steroidal estrogen had been administered in another three cases. The risk for development of these carcinomas in DES-exposed female patients through the age of 24 years has been estimated to be 0.14 to 1.4 per 1000. Of the cases, 90% have occurred in patients 14 years of age or older. About 68% of the individuals with clear cell adenocarcinoma of the cervix and 86% of those with primary vaginal tumors had a history of hormone exposure. In addition, there was a lower risk for cancer among women whose mothers began DES after the 12th week of pregnancy. It is not known how many exposed women are in the United States, but estimates place this population at 0.5 million to 2 million.

Patients 15 years of age and younger appeared to have more aggressive carcinomas than those of patients 19 years of age and older. Abnormal bleeding was the initial symptom in most of the patients, but 20% were asymptomatic, and carcinomas were discovered on routine pelvic examinations. Cytologic testing has proved useful, but a false-negative rate of up to 20% has been reported, probably because of the heavy polymorphonuclear infiltration seen with these lesions. The carcinomas may occur anywhere on the vagina or cervix, but most have been in the upper part of the vagina, particularly on the anterior wall (Fig. 9.7). **Adenosis (the presence of glandular epithelium or its mucinous products in the vagina) has been found accompanying vaginal clear cell adenocarcinoma in virtually all cases.** Adenosis is benign tissue, but it may be the nonneoplastic precursor of the clear cell adenocarcinoma in some cases,

FIGURE 9.7 Clear cell adenocarcinoma (radical hysterectomy and upper vaginectomy specimen). Note the involvement of the cervix and the anterior wall of the upper vagina.

although direct transitions from adenosis to cancer have not been identified. The same observations apply to cervical eversion (ectropion, "congenital erosion") and clear cell adenocarcinoma of the cervix.

Both surgery and radiation have been effective in treating these tumors (Table 9-7), although follow-up for many of these patients is limited. Incidence of lymph node metastases is fairly high, with approximately 16% in stage I and 30% or more in stage II. The clear cell adenocarcinomas tend to remain superficial, suggesting the possibility that this disease can be treated locally, especially if the lesion is small.

The Registry for Research on Hormonal Transplacental Carcinogenesis has reported a study examining the effectiveness of various forms of therapy for early-stage vaginal clear cell adenocarcinomas. Of 219 patients with stage I vaginal clear cell adenocarcinomas, 20% received local therapy, and 80% underwent conventional therapy. Actuarial survival rates at 5 and 10 years for patients treated with local therapy and conventional therapy were equivalent (92% and 88%, respectively). This study indicated that for certain early cancers, local therapy, which can conserve reproductive function, is an effective mode. Another study showed that pregnancy does not appear to affect the prognosis or behavior of clear cell adenocarcinoma. However, one instance of pelvic node metastasis has been reported in a patient with invasion of less than 3 mm.

If the cancer is confined to the cervix, upper vagina, or both, radical hysterectomy with upper vaginectomy and pelvic lymphadenectomy with retention of the ovaries is the recommended therapy. In young patients, avoidance of pelvic irradiation is desirable in view of the increased risks of long-term morbidity (radiation-induced carcinogenesis and progressive vasculitis) in patients surviving many decades after full-dose pelvic irradiation and the possible decrease of optimal vaginal function.

More extensive tumors and lesions involving the lower two-thirds of the vagina, including the pelvic nodes and parametrial tissues, are more suitable for radiation. Although some

TABLE 9.7 Suggested Management of Clear Cell Adenocarcinoma of the Cervix and Vagina

Stage	Surgery	Radiation
CERVIX		
Ib	Radical hysterectomy with clear vaginal margins and bilateral pelvic lymphadenectomy	5000 cGy of the whole pelvis in patients with positive pelvic nodes
IIa	Radical hysterectomy with bilateral pelvic lymphadenectomy and upper vaginectomy	5000 cGy of the whole pelvis in patients with positive pelvic nodes
IIb	Consider exenteration for radiation failures	5000 cGy of the whole pelvis, tandem, and ovoids
IIIa and IIIb	Consider exenteration for radiation failures	6000 cGy of the whole pelvis, tandem, and ovoids
IV	Individualize	
VAGINA		
I (upper third of vagina)	Radical hysterectomy with bilateral pelvic lymphadenectomy and upper vaginectomy	5000 cGy of the whole pelvis in patients with positive nodes
I (lower two-thirds of vagina)	Radical hysterectomy with bilateral pelvic lymphadenectomy and total vaginectomy with vaginal reconstruction	5000 cGy of the whole pelvis, vaginal application, or interstitial implant
II	Consider exenteration for radiation failures	5000 cGy of the whole pelvis, interstitial implant
III	Consider exenteration for radiation failures	6000 cGy of the whole pelvis, interstitial implant
IV	Individualize	

TABLE 9.8 5- and 10-Year Survival Rates for 588 Patients With Clear Cell Adenocarcinoma of the Vagina and Cervix by Stage

Stage	5-Year Survival Rate (%)	10-Year Survival Rate (%)
I	91	85
IIa	80	67
IIb	56	47
II (vagina)	82	67
III	37	25
IV	0	0

From Herbst AL. Neoplastic diseases of the vagina. In Mishell DR Jr, Stenchever MA, Droegemuller W, et al. eds. *Comprehensive Gynecology*, 3rd ed. St. Louis, 1997, Mosby Year Book.

Survival percentages are highly correlated with tumor stage. The following percentages were found for patients at these stages:

Stage I	91%
Stage II vaginal	82%
Stage IIa cervical	80%
Stage IIb cervical	56%
Stage III	37%

The overall survival rate of 80% is somewhat better than the 65% crude survival rate reported for SCC of the cervix and much higher than the 35% to 45% overall survival rate reported for SCC of the vagina. The better prognosis might be the result of early detection because it occurs mainly in young patients exposed to DES (Table 9-8).

Recurrent Adenocarcinoma

A higher proportion of clear cell adenocarcinomas metastasize to the lungs and supraclavicular area compared with squamous cancers. In the study by Herbst and colleagues, 346 patients were analyzed for frequency, site, and treatment of recurrent disease. Of the 346 patients, 20 were never free of disease after initial therapy, and 19 had died at the time of the report. Recurrence developed in 58 patients, and diagnosis was made in most of these within 3 years after primary tumor treatment: 60% had recurrence in the pelvis, almost half of these being in the vagina; 36% (21 patients) had recurrence in the lungs; and 20% (12 patients) had recurrence in the supraclavicular lymph nodes. Surgery and radiation have been effective in the control of pelvic recurrences in some cases.

The results of chemotherapy are disappointing. Objective responses (>50% reduction of tumor size for longer than 3 months) were observed in 8 of 34 cases in which chemotherapy regimens were analyzed. Two patients who received doxorubicin (Adriamycin) had objective remissions, but an alkylating agent was also given in one of these. Two patients who received combination chemotherapy (5-FU, methotrexate, vincristine, cyclophosphamide, and prednisolone; and 5-FU, dactinomycin, and cyclophosphamide) also had objective remissions. No total

experienced surgeons have used radical hysterectomy with total vaginectomy and split-thickness skin graft vaginal reconstruction in this group of patients, it is difficult to get negative surgical margins (especially on the bladder). Herbst and coworkers reported a discouraging 37% recurrence rate among 22 patients treated by conventional irradiation, but 21 of these 22 patients had large vaginal adenocarcinomas and probably would not have been good surgical candidates for vaginectomy. Pelvic exenterations are reserved for radiation failures in patients with central persistence of the neoplasm and involvement of the lower two-thirds of the vagina.

Transvaginal local excision of stage I vaginal adenocarcinoma, which is associated with higher recurrence rates than transabdominal approaches, appears to be an inferior treatment. Some institutions have attempted radiation treatment with transvaginal cone or implant, especially for small vaginal tumors after local excision. The identification of the risk for pelvic lymph node spread, even in cases of small stage I tumors, led to the recommendation that retroperitoneal node dissection be carried out before the local treatment. Follow-up of many of the cases is limited. Therefore, comparing the efficacy of various modes of therapy is difficult.

remissions were observed. There were no responses in nine cases in which a progestational agent alone was used.

In a 1981 report by Herbst, follow-up data of 409 patients for periods up to 15 years were published. In this study, 55 patients had an initial recurrence in the pelvis (60% of the total group with recurrence) up to 7 years after initial therapy. This emphasizes the importance of prolonged follow-up. Of the 58 patients with recurrences, 12 survived 3 years or longer after treatment of their first recurrence. A second recurrence was observed in 17 of the patients, and 12 of them died within 1 year of the diagnosis. However, three patients had survived longer than 2 years after treatment of their second recurrence.

Primary adenocarcinoma of the vagina can occur unrelated to intrauterine DES exposure. Some cases that were thought to have arisen in association with vaginal adenosis or from foci of endometriosis generally resembled endocervical or endometrial carcinomas. Because of their content of clear cells, others were considered to be of mesonephric origin. A few exceptional cases may have arisen from Gartner duct remnants and thus may have truly been mesonephric in origin. Therapy for these adenocarcinomas is presently analogous to that for their squamous counterpart.

Vaginal metastases from adenocarcinoma of other pelvic and abdominal organs are more common than primary vaginal cancers. Lesions of cervical and endometrial origin are most common. Ovary, tube, colon, rectum, and renal cell neoplasms can also be present with vaginal metastasis.

Malignant Melanoma

Malignant melanoma of the vagina is rare and represents fewer than 0.5% of all vaginal malignant neoplasms and 0.4% to 0.8% of all malignant melanomas in women. The main presenting symptoms is vaginal bleeding, but vaginal discharge, and a blue-black or black-brown mass, plaque, or ulceration may also occur. The tumors are predominantly located in the lower third of the vagina, commonly on the anterior wall. These malignancies typically occur at a mean age of 60 years (range, 22–84 years), and almost all reported cases have been in white women. Lesions may be single or multiple, pigmented or nonpigmented, and arising from melanocytes present in the epithelium of the vagina (Fig. 9.8).

Multiple therapies have been attempted during the past several decades, and surgery remains the treatment of choice. The surgical approach must be tailored to the location of the lesions. The NCDB report noted 192 patients with vaginal melanoma; 95 (49%) were 70 years of age or older. Surgery was used as the first course of treatment in 66%, and 40% received radiotherapy. External radiation was more frequently used to treat advanced melanoma cases. Neoplasms that involve the lower third of the vagina are usually treated similarly to vulvar melanoma, with radical vulvectomy, partial vaginectomy, and inguinal and deep node dissection. Neoplasms that involve the upper two-thirds of the vagina require some form of exenteration for optimal results. Radiation therapy in general has not proved effective, and the results of chemotherapy have been equally disappointing; thus, the radical surgical approach remains the primary therapy when it is applicable.

FIGURE 9.8 An exenteration specimen showing an open uterus, tubes, and ovaries with multifocal melanotic lesions of the vagina in a patient who underwent vaginectomy with her exenteration.

Survival figures for this group of lesions are difficult to determine because of the infrequent occurrence of this disease. Patients with negative nodes who have disease involving the upper two-thirds of the vagina and who are treated by exenteration have about a 50% probability of surviving 5 years or longer. The overall survival rate for vaginal melanoma is about 15%. Lymph node metastases portend a poorer prognosis. Many patients have advanced disease at the time of diagnosis.

Treatment must be based on the extent of the disease, location, tolerance of the patient, and depth of invasion. Increasing emphasis is placed on the depth of invasion. Superficial lesions (Clark's level I and level II) can be managed with less than exenterative-type surgery, but more deeply invasive tumors must be managed with extended radical surgery with some expectation of a favorable outcome, as reported by Van Nostrand and associates. Survival appears to be more favorable with depths of invasion of less than 2 mm. In the NCDB report, the 5-year survival rate for 76 patients whose diagnosis was made between 1985 and 1989 was 14%. The number of diagnoses with Clark's level information was small (51 patients). The 3-year relative survival rate by Clark's level without regard to node status or presence of metastasis was as follows:

Level II	45% (11 patients)
Level III	36% (5 patients)
Level IV	27% (4 patients)
Level V	14% (9 patients)

No level I was reported.

The dissection of lymph nodes that are clinically negative for melanoma of the vagina, urethra, and vulva continues to

be controversial. For level I and level II lesions, there appears to be little value in lymphadenectomy if nodes are clinically negative. Whether or not there is a role for selective sampling via lymphatic mapping and sentinel node localization is not known. However, in the few vulvovaginal primary lesions mapped, groin sentinel nodes have been isolated. Such dissections may provide prognostic information without extensive morbidity seen with inguinofemoral lymphadenectomy. Patients with level IV and level V lesions with positive nodes rarely survive, but local control may be achieved with lymphadenectomy. Recurrences develop primarily in the pelvis and lung. The interval to recurrence varies, but it is usually less than 1 year. Survival from point of recurrence averages 8 months. Recent advances in immunotherapy for the treatment of melanoma may lead to improved prognosis and survival in this cohort.

Sarcoma

Spindle cell sarcomas of the vagina, such as leiomyosarcoma and fibrosarcoma, occur rarely. Tavassoli and Norris reported 60 smooth muscle tumors of the vagina. Only five neoplasms recurred, and these were all larger than 3 cm, with more than five mitotic figures per 10 high-power fields (hpf). Local excision was the treatment of choice when the tumor was well differentiated and well circumscribed and the margins were not infiltrated. In general, these lesions behave like their corresponding cell types on the vulva in that the well-differentiated lesions have a much better prognosis than the pleomorphic types, which tend to have a poor prognosis regardless of therapy. The vagina, similar to the vulva, has a rich lymphatic and vascular network, possibly contributing to the early dissemination of these neoplasms (especially the pleomorphic types). In general, hematogenous dissemination occurs surprisingly late in the course of the disease, so that the importance of local therapy is underlined. However, after local excision of a circumscribed lesion and postoperative local radiation therapy, the value of pelvic radiation therapy is unclear. In most instances when it has been successfully applied, the lesions were well differentiated and well circumscribed, suggesting that surgery itself was curative.

An unusual and tragic lesion that predominantly affects children is sarcoma botryoides (Fig. 9.9). These lesions are usually multicentric and tend to arise in the anterior wall at the apex of the vagina. There is a tendency for this tumor to originate higher in the genital tract in older patients. In all patients, the tumor may be multifocal, but this is rare and should not be taken as a basis for extensive surgery.

Whereas these lesions were formerly treated by exenterative procedures, equal success has been obtained in recent years with less radical surgery and adjuvant chemotherapy, with or without radiotherapy. There were 30 sarcomas reported in children from the NCDB, 32 patients were between the ages of 20 and 49 years, 36 patients were between 50 and 69 years, and 37 patients were 70 years or older. The diagnosis was embryonal rhabdomyosarcoma in 70% of the children ($n = 21$), infantile embryonal carcinoma in 20% ($n = 4$), and rhabdomyosarcoma in 10% ($n = 3$). More than three-quarters of the children received

FIGURE 9.9 Sarcoma botryoides (rhabdomyosarcoma) in a 3-year-old child.

chemotherapy, including four-fifths who were treated surgically. The 12 children whose diagnosis was made between 1985 and 1989 were younger than 5 years, and their 5-year survival rate was 90%.

A combination of vincristine, dactinomycin, and cyclophosphamide appears to be effective in this disease and results in a marked reduction in tumor size when the drug combination is used as initial therapy, permitting more conservative surgery. Although there is continued use of external radiation therapy in many centers, its role in managing sarcoma botryoides of the female genital tract remains unclear. Small lesions appear to be adequately treated with chemotherapy and surgery. A combination of chemotherapy and radiation therapy without surgery has been reported by Flamant and colleagues to be curative of localized vaginal lesions.

The tendency for genitourinary rhabdomyosarcoma to spread to regional lymph nodes is well established. The Intergroup Rhabdomyosarcoma Study reported a 26% incidence of known lymph node metastasis. The pelvis is the most common site for primary recurrences.

Leiomyosarcoma was the most frequent type of sarcoma for adults, accounting for 50% of the cases in patients aged 20 to 49 years and for 35% in those aged 70 years or older. Adjuvant chemotherapy was used less with increasing age, but radiotherapy was used most frequently for older patients. Survival rates decreased with increasing age. The relative 5-year survival rates were 84% for those aged 20 to 49 years and 48% for those 50 to 69 years. Those older than 70 years had a 2-year relative survival rate of only 30%.

Endodermal Sinus Tumor

This rare carcinoma occurring in the vaginas of infants is most likely of germ cell origin. Norris and coworkers use the term *mesonephroma* or *mesonephric carcinoma* because of an alternative theory of the origin of this carcinoma. The disease usually occurs in infants younger than 2 years, and survival rates have been poor, with fewer than 25% of patients alive at 2 years. Lesions most often occur on the posterior vaginal wall or fornices. Combination therapy (surgery and chemotherapy) appears appropriate. **Patients who have vaginal endodermal sinus tumors are usually seen because of vaginal bleeding or discharge and have polypoid or sessile tumors.** In the majority of cases, the differential diagnosis of endodermal sinus tumor is that of embryonal rhabdomyosarcoma (sarcoma botryoides). This is the most common vaginal tumor of children and almost always develops in patients younger than 5 years; the average age at the time of diagnosis is 3 years. The characteristic grape-like appearance of sarcoma botryoides differs from the usual endodermal sinus tumor. In addition, the edematous and cellular areas that are composed of immature skeletal muscle cells characteristic of embryonal rhabdomyosarcoma bear no resemblance to the histologic appearance of endodermal sinus tumor.

Young and Scully described 32 patients with endodermal sinus tumors. At the time of the report, 18 had died of their disease despite radical surgical therapy. Six patients were treated by surgery and then received vincristine, dactinomycin, and cyclophosphamide. Of these six patients, two also received radiation therapy. All were alive and free of disease 2 to 9 years after surgery. Copeland and associates have reported similar results with the same combination. Thus, chemotherapy after conservative surgical excision can be effective in controlling this neoplasm.

Special Considerations

Pride and Buchler suggested that **vaginal carcinoma might occur more frequently in patients who received pelvic irradiation 10 years or longer before the appearance of the new lesion.** Of patients previously treated for cervical cancer, those who had received radiation therapy (>5 years previously) were more likely to develop vaginal cancer than were those whose cervical cancers had been treated surgically, according to Murad and colleagues. Abnormal vaginal cytologic findings are common after radiation, and many have ignored these dysplastic lesions as if they were routine results of irradiation therapy. However, a study from MD Anderson suggested that 30% of these "dysplastic" or "intraepithelial" lesions will progress to invasive cancer if they are left untreated. In this report, 28 patients with dysplasia or carcinoma in situ of the vagina after previous pelvic radiation therapy were observed for progression, and nine developed invasive carcinoma. The median length of time from diagnosis of the intraepithelial lesion to invasion was 34 months. Therefore, treatment of these intraepithelial lesions by local excision is warranted. Laser vaporization or topical chemotherapy with 5-FU should be seriously considered.

For the bibliography list, log onto www.expertconsult.com ⟨http://www.expertconsult.com⟩.

10

Adnexal Masses

Camille C. Gunderson, MD, Robert S. Mannel, MD, Philip J. Di Saia, MD

OUTLINE

KEY POINTS

1. Adnexal masses are common, and careful evaluation is required before a therapeutic intervention is planned.
2. Masses are classified based on the workup for risk of malignant potential. Of all the variables, age is probably the most predictive of cancer.
3. There are many markers that help in determining how likely the mass represents a cancer, and these should be considered preoperatively.
4. It is important to be prepared for the possibility that any mass is malignant.
5. Arrangements should always be made for this possibility if the patient goes to the operating room.

ADNEXAL MASSES

The adnexae consist of the fallopian tubes, broad ligament, ovaries, and structures within the broad ligament that are formed from embryologic rests. Detection of pelvic abnormalities is more frequent in women of reproductive age because these patients have serial examinations as part of periodic screening for cancer (ie, Pap testing) and contraceptive counseling. Management of an adnexal mass is complex because of the scope of the disorders it encompasses and the numerous therapies that may be appropriate (Table 10.1). The risk of malignancy and the fundamental concept that early diagnosis and treatment in cancer are related to reduced mortality and morbidity propel the system. An adnexal mass often involves ovarian substance because of the propensity of the ovary for neoplasia. Fewer neoplasms occur in the fallopian tube, although that structure may commonly be involved in an inflammatory process that manifests as an adnexal mass. It is estimated that

5% to 10% of women in the United States will undergo a surgical procedure for a suspected ovarian neoplasm during their lifetime, and 13% to 21% of these women will be found to have an ovarian malignant neoplasm. The overwhelming majority of adnexal masses are benign, and it is important to determine preoperatively whether a patient is at high risk for ovarian malignant disease to minimize the number of operative procedures performed for self-limited processes.

Evaluative Approach

Patients may present with an adnexal mass in a variety of clinical settings. Some may be symptomatic (pelvic pain or pressure) as a result of the mass, others may have a mass identified as part of a workup for another condition (computed tomography [CT] scan performed for back pain), and some have a mass incidentally identified as part of a normal well-woman examination. In addition, masses are occasionally identified during pregnancy as a result of the number of prenatal ultrasounds

TABLE 10.1   Differential Diagnosis of Adnexal Mass

Organ	Cystic	Solid
Ovary	Functional cyst	Neoplasm
	Neoplastic cyst	Benign
	Benign	Malignant
	Malignant	
	Endometriosis	
Fallopian tube	Tubo-ovarian abscess	Tubo-ovarian abscess
	Hydrosalpinx	Ectopic pregnancy
	Paraovarian cyst	Neoplasm
Uterus	Intrauterine pregnancy in a bicornuate uterus	Pedunculated or interligamentous myoma
Bowel	Sigmoid or cecum distended with gas or feces	Diverticulitis
		Ileitis
		Appendicitis
		Colonic cancer
Miscellaneous	Distended bladder	Abdominal wall hematoma or abscess
	Pelvic kidney	Retroperitoneal neoplasm
	Urachal cyst	

TABLE 10.2   Pelvic Findings in Benign and Malignant Ovarian Tumors

Clinical Findings	Benign	Malignant
Unilateral	+++	+++
Bilateral	+++	+++
Cystic	+++	+++
Solid	+++	+++
Mobile	+++	+++
Fixed	+++	+++
Irregular	+++	+++
Smooth	+++	+++
Ascites	+++	+++
Cul-de-sac nodules	—++	+++
Rapid growth rate	—++	+++

that are performed. A patient with a mass is approached differently depending on the clinical scenario. The approach of what to do in the setting of adnexal mass can be broken down into two fundamental questions: (1) What is the suspicion that the mass is malignant? and (2) Is the patient symptomatic? Understanding these two issues helps focus treatment planning into a decision for surgery versus observation.

To determine the appropriate intervention for an adnexal mass, a thorough evaluation, including a complete history and physical examination, liberal use of transvaginal ultrasonography, and judicious use of serum tumor markers, should be performed. Pelvic examination should always be performed under optimal circumstances. The patient's bladder should be empty. It is not unheard of for a patient with 10-cm midline mass to have the mass disappear with catheterization of the bladder. The rare pelvic kidney should always be kept in mind as a possible cause of a pelvic mass. Tragic reports of excision of such a mass in a patient with one kidney are found in the literature. Whenever possible, the rectum and rectosigmoid should also be empty when a pelvic examination is done. This avoids the misdiagnosis of fecal material as an adnexal mass. Detection of an adnexal mass is greatly facilitated by a rectovaginal examination (see Fig. 3.13), which allows more complete access to the cul-de-sac and to the more superficial areas of the pelvic basin. Knowledge of the size, shape, contour, and general location of the mass within the pelvis helps the physician arrive at the most likely diagnosis. Benign tumors are commonly smooth walled, cystic, mobile, unilateral, and smaller than 8 cm (7 cm is the exact diameter of a new tennis ball). Malignant tumors are usually solid or semisolid, bilateral, irregular, fixed, and associated with nodules in the cul-de-sac. Ascites usually is found with malignant neoplasms (Table 10.2). Koonings and

coworkers showed that the risk of malignant disease was 2.6-fold greater for women with bilateral neoplasms than for women with unilateral neoplasms.

The patient's symptoms may derive from the physical nature of the mass by producing pressure against the bladder or rectum and increasing abdominal distention. Pain may be acute or chronic in nature. It may be a result of rapid size change and can be caused by torsion, hemorrhage into the mass, or rupture. Pain may also be a result of associated inflammatory processes from tubo-ovarian abscess or diverticular abscess. The nature and severity of the pain and other associated symptoms frequently lead to operative intervention, irrespective of the risk for malignancy.

Classifying the Mass

The complete evaluation of a patient with an adnexal mass requires that the physician assemble and analyze all of the available information from the history, examination, imaging studies, and tumor markers. One goal is to characterize the mass based on its malignant potential. Management then depends on a combination of many factors, including age and menopausal status of the patient, morphologic characteristics of the mass by ultrasonography, clinical findings, and patient desires. Classically, features associated most commonly with benign masses include young age, absence of symptoms (nausea, vomiting, weight loss, changes in urinary frequency, pain), unilateral and unilocular cystic masses, and normal cancer antigen 125 (CA-125) level. Despite these factors, it is clear that no single characteristic guarantees that a mass will be benign. Increasingly, models taking into account all available information have shown the best ability to predict benign versus malignant masses.

Of all variables, however, age is probably the most important factor for predicting the potential for malignancy. For example, Moore and colleagues showed in one large prospective series of 531 patients with adnexal masses for whom surgery was to be performed that 7% of premenopausal versus 39% of postmenopausal patients had a diagnosis of an epithelial ovarian malignancy on final pathology. The differential diagnosis of an adnexal mass varies with the age of the patient. In premenarchal girls and postmenopausal women, an adnexal mass should be considered highly abnormal and must be immediately investigated. In premenarchal patients, most neoplasms are germ cell in origin and require immediate surgical exploration. Stromal, germ cell, and epithelial tumors are seen in postmenopausal women. It was once dogma that a postmenopausal patient with any enlargement of the ovary be considered to have "cancer until proven otherwise." In an era before pelvic ultrasonography, examining a patient with a "palpable postmenopausal ovary" was thought pathognomonic for ovarian cancer. Today, with common use of imaging studies, it has been shown that adnexal masses in postmenopausal women are more frequent than previously recognized, and many of these are benign. Greenlee and colleagues demonstrated in a prevalence study of more than 15,000 women older than 55 years of age who underwent pelvic ultrasonography that 14% had an adnexal cyst at initial screening. As with patients in all age groups, a complete evaluation can better characterize the risk of malignancy. (See section on postmenopausal ovary.)

One of the most common modalities used for characterizing an adnexal mass is pelvic ultrasonography. Pelvic ultrasonography may be performed transabdominally (better for larger masses extending out of the pelvis) or transvaginally (best for masses in the cul-de-sac or pelvis) to characterize masses. Many adnexal masses have characteristic appearances that define them as benign or suspicious for malignancy. The ultrasonography shows size, mass morphology, unilateral or bilateral involvement, and associated findings such as ascites. Ultrasonography is the most valuable initial tool and should be considered the first choice in assessing an adnexal mass by imaging. In some cases, CT or magnetic resonance imaging (MRI) may augment information on the mass and provide additional relevant anatomic information (eg, description of upper abdominal findings and information on adenopathy and ureteral patency). Masses may be described as purely cystic (so-called simple cyst), solid, or mixed solid–cystic (so-called complex cyst). The risk of malignancy increases with increasing complexity. Large series have shown that simple cysts have a very low risk of malignancy. Cysts with septations and no solid component also have been shown to have a low risk of malignancy. Malignancy is more commonly associated when a cyst wall or septation is thickened or has nodularity or the cyst contains solid components.

Much research has been devoted to developing accurate biomarkers that can detect malignancy and better characterize adnexal masses. To date, no single marker has been shown to be accurate in distinguishing a mass as benign or malignant. Information from tumor markers may be useful in characterizing the potential risk of malignancy so appropriate therapy may be offered (eg, surgery vs. observation), and patients may be appropriately triaged to specialists who are trained to perform complete surgical staging and debulking as needed.

One of the most widely used serum biomarkers for ovarian cancer is CA-125. CA-125 is used to monitor response of therapy and to assess for possible recurrence in patients with a known diagnosis of ovarian cancer. It is elevated in approximately 80% of patients with nonmucinous, epithelial ovarian cancers. It is elevated in only approximately 50% of stage I ovarian cancers, however. In combination with examination and serial pelvic ultrasonography, CA-125 has been evaluated in several large screening studies including asymptomatic women at risk for ovarian cancer to identify those with unrecognized disease. These studies show that CA-125 may augment the information from ultrasonography alone. CA-125 testing has limited sensitivity and specificity, making routine CA-125 testing problematic. Conditions associated with peritoneal or serosal inflammation or irritation of any etiology may be associated with CA-125 level elevations. In addition to ovarian cancer, CA-125 levels may be elevated by a number of other malignancies and benign conditions, including endometriosis, uterine leiomyomata, benign adnexal masses, tubal inflammation or infection, liver disease or hepatitis, congestive heart failure, menses, and pregnancy. Because most of these conditions are seen in younger women, CA-125 testing in premenopausal women is particularly difficult to interpret. A higher sensitivity has been reported in postmenopausal women, in whom CA-125 levels greater than 50 mL have been associated with a high risk of ovarian malignancy. In a prospective study comparing ultrasonography with CA-125 levels to characterize patients with persistent adnexal masses ($n = 1066$), Van Calster reported ultrasound pattern classification correctly classified 93% of tumors as benign or malignant compared with 83% by CA-125 testing. Histologic diagnoses most commonly misclassified by CA-125 testing were fibromas, endometriosis, abscess, and borderline tumors. CA-125 information in the setting of an adnexal mass may provide information in conjunction with patient symptoms, examination, and imaging studies as to whether to offer observation or perform surgery, make referral to specialists, or perform additional testing.

The CA-125 to carcinoembryonic antigen (CEA) ratio is now being considered helpful in deciphering the site of neoplastic origin. CEA is generally a marker for gastrointestinal (GI) malignancy but is also a marker for the rare entity of mucinous ovarian cancer. A ratio greater than 25 is generally consistent with ovarian origin.

OVA1 Test

The OVA1 test is a biomarker panel that measures five proteins (CA-125, β_2-microglobulin, apolipoprotein A1, prealbumin, and transferrin); it was approved by the Food and Drug Administration in 2009 to better classify adnexal masses to assist physicians with making referral to gynecologic cancer specialists. The concept is that an abnormal test result should prompt referral to specialists trained in staging and debulking of ovarian cancer. The OVA1 test produces a score from 0 to 10, with a cutoff of 5 for premenopausal and 4.4 for postmenopausal women. In a pivotal trial of 516 patients, OVA1 testing augmented information from radiologic imaging and laboratory testing. The Society of Gynecologic Oncologists (SGO) in September 2009 noted support for testing that resulted in appropriate referral of patients but also noted that OVA1 testing has not been validated as a screening tool and should not be used in this manner.

HE4

Human epididymis protein 4 (HE4) is a novel tumor marker for recurrence that is indicated for women with known ovarian cancer who have been treated. HE4 is a glycoprotein produced in normal glandular epithelium of the reproductive tract, renal tubules, and respiratory epithelium. HE4 levels appear to be less susceptible to peritoneal irritation, perhaps reducing false-positive findings. For example, in one study, HE4 levels were not increased in patients with endometriosis. HE4 testing has been investigated in combination with CA-125 levels to increase sensitivity and specificity of biomarker testing. In combination with patient menopausal status and CA-125 and HE4 testing, Moore and coworkers reported a sensitivity of 94% for all patients.

Multimodality Approach

Because no single test or finding in a vacuum is accurately predictive of a benign or malignant status of an adnexal mass, combining all information is our best option. Jacobs and associates introduced the concept of the Risk of Malignancy Index (ROMI) in 1990 combining demographic, sonographic, and tumor marker data into the assessment of a patient with an adnexal mass. It was a simple, reproducible system that has been modified and studied in several large trials. In a systematic review of the literature of ROMI, Geomini et al. suggested that all models have acceptable sensitivity and specificity, but the best predictors accounted for data from ultrasound findings, menopausal status, and CA-125 level. One modification proposed by Tingulstad and coworkers created a formula of U × M × CA-125 level, where U = ultrasound score (higher-risk morphology = 3, low-risk morphology = 1), M = menopausal status (postmenopausal = 3, premenopausal = 1), and CA-125 level is the actual testing value. van den Akker and coworkers reported a prospective observational study of 548 women with adnexal masses using this modified ROMI with a threshold value of 200 and achieved a sensitivity of 81% and specificity of 85%. They found that using the ROMI, they could accurately refer 80% of ovarian cancers to specialists using a threshold value of 200. In 2015, the United Kingdom Collaborative Trial published its risk of ovarian cancer algorithm (ROCA), in which they evaluated CA-125 velocity for ovarian cancer detection in contrast to a single-threshold rule. They found that emphasis of biomarker velocity within the algorithm led to 85.8% sensitivity and 99.8% specificity, leading to a doubling in the number of screen-detected cancers in comparison to use of a fixed CA-125 cutoff value.

Differential Diagnosis

The differentiation between benign (Table 10.3) and malignant ovarian enlargements is often the exclusive decision of the pathologist, but a short discussion of these lesions is pertinent even in a textbook of oncology. Although functional ovarian cysts are usually asymptomatic, they can on occasion be accompanied by a minor degree of lower abdominal discomfort, pelvic pain, or dyspareunia. In addition, rupture of one of these fluid-filled structures can result in additional peritoneal irritation and possibly an accompanying hemoperitoneum; however,

TABLE 10.3 Benign Ovarian Tumors
• Nonneoplastic tumors
• Germinal inclusion cyst
• Pregnancy luteoma
• Endometrioma
• Neoplastic tumors derived from coelomic epithelium
• Cystic tumors
• Serous cystoma
• Mucinous cystoma
• Mixed forms
• Fibroma, adenofibroma
• Brenner tumor
• Tumors derived from germ cells
• Dermoid (benign cystic teratoma)

this is rarely serious. More intense lower abdominal discomfort results when these ovarian tumors undergo torsion or infarction. Similar to functional cysts of the ovary, benign ovarian neoplasms do not produce any symptoms that readily differentiate them from malignant tumors or from various other pelvic diseases. Although these tumors are more likely to twist, resulting in infarction, malignant neoplasms may have the same fate. Indeed, one of the most unfortunate features of benign ovarian neoplasms is that they are indistinguishable clinically from their malignant counterparts. Although it is not known whether malignant ovarian tumors arise de novo or develop from benign tumors, there is strong inferential evidence that at least some benign tumors will become malignant. All too often, the first symptom of cancer in an ovarian tumor is increasing abdominal distention, although benign ovarian neoplasms may become apparent because of increasing abdominal girth, and indeed the "giant tumors" of the ovary are often benign mucinous cystadenomas. Benign mucinous cystadenomas weighing up to 300 lb have been reported.

EXTRAOVARIAN ADNEXAL MASSES

Given the proximity in the pelvis, a variety of nonovarian structures may be responsible for the appearance of an "adnexal mass." This category includes disorders of the uterus, fallopian tubes, intestines, and adjacent structures. The process that creates the mass can be congenital, functional, neoplastic, or inflammatory. It is important to keep a broad differential diagnosis of the adnexal mass and to use all of the information available based on the history, physical examination, and imaging studies. On occasion, extragenital lesions, which are often large and cystic, are found on pelvic examination; exploratory laparotomy is indicated because of the size alone. These extragenital lesions include peritoneal cysts, omental cysts, retroperitoneal lesions, and diseases of the GI tract (cecum, appendix, sigmoid, and even small bowel, any of which can fall into the pelvis and become adherent). Retroperitoneal disorders may also be palpated on pelvic examination. Retroperitoneal sarcomas, lymphomas, and teratomas of the sacrococcygeal areas are commonly noted on rectovaginal examination and misdiagnosed as an adnexal mass.

Uterine Masses

Pregnancy should always be kept in mind as a cause of uterine enlargement. Most physicians are familiar with the unreliability of a menstrual history, and any patient of reproductive age with a pelvic mass should first have pregnancy ruled out by any of a variety of pregnancy tests or by detection of a fetus with ultrasound examination.

Myomas of the uterus are the most common uterine neoplasms (Fig. 10.1). They are usually discrete, relatively round tumors that are firm to palpation and may be single or multiple. Myomas may be located within the myometrium (intramural), just beneath the endometrial lining (submucosal), or on the surface of the uterus (serosal). A myoma may frequently be found in the broad ligament attached to the lower uterine segment by a thin pedicle. This will often confuse the examiner and suggest that the mass originates in the ovary or tube. In the United States, myomas are found in at least 10% of white women and 30% to 40% of black women older than age 35 years. In the postmenopausal group, it is said that the incidence increases to 30% in white women and 50% in black women. Fortunately, these neoplasms usually shrink after menopause, especially in patients not receiving high doses of exogenous estrogen stimulation. It appears that most of these benign neoplasms are somewhat estrogen dependent. Growth is commonly seen during pregnancy, probably secondary to elevated hormone levels. Degeneration, infarction, and infection can occur in these lesions, and these complications are associated with considerable lower abdominal pain. Sarcomatous elements, associated with myomas less than 0.1% of the time, are most often recognized postoperatively. Symptoms of associated sarcomatous elements may include a rapidly enlarging pelvic mass, often accompanied by pain and tenderness. The mean age at diagnosis of these lesions is 50 to 55 years, with a range of 25 to 85 years.

A recent enlargement of the uterus in a postmenopausal patient is rarely caused by fibroids, particularly if the enlargement develops in a short time ("rapid" growth). The use of hormone replacement therapy in and of itself is not an explanation for such an enlargement. The most probable diagnosis is a malignant neoplasm, and physicians must prepare to do an appropriate surgical procedure even if the result of dilatation and curettage (D&C) is negative.

Other conditions that can cause enlargement of the uterus are adenomyosis and endometrial carcinoma or sarcoma. Endometrial carcinoma can enlarge the uterus to as much as four times normal size. Most patients with endometrial cancer describe abnormal vaginal bleeding, and the diagnosis can be made appropriate endometrial sampling (office biopsy or D&C).

Tubal Masses

Neoplasms arising from the fallopian tube are rare. More commonly, adnexal masses secondary to tubal disease are inflammatory or represent an ectopic pregnancy. Distinction between tubal and ovarian masses on the basis of examination alone is often difficult. In the acute phase of salpingitis, the fallopian tube is distended by grossly purulent material. This infection may be secondary to gonorrhea or other organisms, including anaerobes. As the salpingitis process progresses, the adjacent ovary may become involved, creating a so-called tubo-ovarian abscess. Although this acute process may resolve, the patient is often subject to reinfection. As a result of repeated chronic infectious processes, the tubal ostia may close or firmly adhere to the adjacent ovary, and the fallopian tube fills with a clear fluid. As the structure distends, it creates a mass that can easily be mistaken for an ovarian cyst. Although the symptoms of acute pelvic inflammatory disease are distinct (pelvic pain, fever, increased vaginal discharge, and abnormal uterine bleeding), the symptoms of chronic pelvic infection may be subtle. Even the traditional elevation of the erythrocyte sedimentation rate or leukocyte count may be absent in as many as 30% of patients with chronic pelvic inflammatory disease and adnexal masses.

A cystic mass in the adnexal region may be neither ovarian nor tubal in origin but caused instead by remnants of embryologic structures. The parovarium, located within the portion of the broad ligament containing the fallopian tube, consists of vestigial remnants of the Wolffian duct. Paraovarian cysts are found as distal remnants of the Wolffian duct system. They are characteristically located between the fallopian tube and the ovary; when large, they are often found with the fallopian tube

Pedunculated

Intramural

Submucous

Pedunculated submucous

Subserous

Adenomyoma

Cervical

Intraligamentary

Necrotic

Malignant degeneration

Cystic

Red degeneration

FIGURE 10.1 Myomas can be seen initially in multiple sizes and states of growth, disease, and degeneration. (Courtesy of Erle Henriksen, MD, Los Angeles, CA.)

stretched over the top of the cyst. These paraovarian cysts are most commonly unilocular and filled with clear yellow fluid. They often persist into the postmenopausal period and can appear as cystic structures in the adnexa on imaging studies done for other complaints.

Approximately 98% of ectopic pregnancies are tubal. Unfortunately, a pelvic mass can be found on examination in fewer than half the cases of tubal pregnancy. Rupture usually occurs when the distended fallopian tube reaches a diameter of 4 cm. Tubal pregnancy must be distinguished from pelvic inflammatory disease, torsion of the adnexa, and bleeding corpus luteum cysts because all produce pain or abnormal bleeding.

Carcinoma limited to the fallopian tube is rare and accounts for fewer than 0.5% of all female genital tract malignant neoplasms. Historically, most of these neoplasms were discovered by serendipity, with a preoperative diagnosis of ovarian neoplasm being most common. On gross evaluation, the fallopian tube is usually enlarged, smooth walled, and sausage shaped. On occasion, patients present with the symptom of several weeks of profuse watery vaginal discharge, the so-called hydrops tubae profluens. However, it is now known that the fallopian tube and, more specifically, the fimbriae is the origin of most high-grade serous carcinomas of the ovary. This has become apparent over recent years as women with hereditary risk underwent risk-reducing surgery and represents a shift away from incessant ovulation as the leading hypothesis of epithelial ovarian carcinogenesis.

Adnexal Masses of Nongynecologic Origin
Bowel

By far the most common entity of the GI tract that initially appears to be an adnexal mass is fecal material in the sigmoid colon or cecum, which may on initial pelvic examination be palpated as a soft, mobile, tubular mass. Patients should be reexamined after appropriate cleansing enemas to confirm or rule out this possibility.

Inflammatory disorders of the large and small intestine can also be detected on pelvic examination. Diarrhea, nausea and vomiting, anorexia, or passage of blood or mucus per rectum should suggest these GI tract disorders. Patients with diverticulitis, even with abscess formation, sometimes exhibit remarkably minor symptoms initially. Careful questioning to detect subtle changes in GI symptoms is often rewarding. Periappendiceal abscesses may be formed as a result of rupture of the appendix and present as pelvic masses. Unfortunately, they vary in location, although they are generally found on the right side of the pelvis and are usually fixed, firm, and tender to palpation. Diverticulitis is a more common disorder with increasing age. Although it is usually located in the sigmoid colon, the mass may be midline or right sided. Inflammation of the ileum (regional ileitis) may occasionally present as a right-sided adnexal mass as the loops of thickened and inflamed ileum become fixed in the pelvis.

Gastrointestinal malignant disease is suggested by the presence of blood in the stool, anemia, and alterations in bowel habits. Neoplasms of the large intestine are particularly common with increasing age, and 60% to 70% occur on the left side

within the reach of a palpating finger or flexible sigmoidoscope. However, carcinoma of the cecum often presents as a right-sided adnexal mass, and on examination, induration and irregularity may be found in the involved area. An elevated serum CEA level should raise suspicion for GI malignancy, particularly when the CA-125 to CEA ratio is less than 25. If one suspects GI origin of the mass, appropriate endoscopic or radiographic studies usually help in the definitive diagnosis.

OVARIAN MASSES
Functional Cysts

The cyclic ovarian function of a reproductive-age women continually produces follicular growth and resorption. Among the most frequently found "masses" involving the adnexa are the nonneoplastic cysts related to the process of ovulation that are sometimes referred to as functional cysts. They are by far the most common clinically detectable enlargements of the ovary occurring during the reproductive years. If ovulation does not occur, a clear fluid-filled follicular cyst (Fig. 10.2) lined by granulosa cells may result that can reach a size as large as 10 cm in diameter. These cysts usually resolve spontaneously within a few days to 2 weeks but can persist longer. When ovulation occurs, a corpus luteum is formed that may become abnormally enlarged through internal hemorrhage or cyst formation. The masses are of great significance because young women will have cysts on their ovaries at essentially all times (in varying sizes, numbers) during the reproductive years, and occasionally the cysts can produce pain and discomfort, and a mass will be noted on examination or ultrasonography. Clinical sequelae of these benign physiologic processes can also bring patients to the physician's attention because the masses may undergo torsion; acutely hemorrhage into the mass; or grow to sufficient size to produce pain, pressure, or bloating symptoms. The clinical challenge is that these functional cysts cannot be readily distinguished from true neoplasms on clinical grounds alone. Ultrasound evaluation typically shows a thin-walled, simple-appearing, anechoic cyst without solid component or septations. A hemorrhagic cyst may also show more complexity on ultrasonography given the presence of blood and fibrin stranding.

In addition, such cysts are often associated with variable delays in the onset of menses and confusion regarding the possibility of pregnancy. Theca-lutein cysts result from overstimulation of the ovary by hCG and on histologic examination are characterized by extensive luteinization of the stroma surrounding the follicle. Although theca-lutein cysts do not commonly occur in a normal pregnancy, they are often associated with hydatidiform moles and choriocarcinoma. Gross examination of the ovary containing theca-lutein cysts shows a structure almost completely replaced by lobulated thin-walled cysts that vary in size and are smooth and yellow.

Corpus luteum, follicular, and theca-lutein cysts are benign and represent an exaggerated physiologic response of the ovary. In most instances, they involute over time, but they do need to be included in the differential diagnosis. Luteomas of pregnancy are often large and solid but are not neoplastic

FIGURE 10.2 A, Follicular cyst (8 cm) with fimbria. B, Microscopic view of a follicular cyst as seen in A. (Courtesy of Ibrahim Ramzy, MD, University of California, Irvine, CA.)

masses originating in the ovary during pregnancy. Most cases are discovered at cesarean section in the last 2 months of pregnancy. The exact origin of luteomas have not been established. It is probably a hCG-dependent nonneoplastic hyperplasia and usually regresses after delivery. Therefore, surgical excision of these lesions at the time of cesarean section is not necessary.

Polycystic (sclerocystic) ovaries contain multiple follicle cysts with hyperplasia and luteinization of theca interna surrounding the cysts and atretic follicles. The ovaries are two to five times normal size with a thickened capsule. The condition is found most frequently in association with the Stein–Leventhal or polycystic ovarian syndrome.

Endometriotic Cysts

Endometriosis is a condition in which implants of normal-appearing endometrial glands and stroma are found outside their normal location in the uterine cavity. Presumptive evidence of endometriosis is also supported by significant

scarring in the pelvis and the presence of hemosiderin-laden macrophages in the cyst wall or peritoneum. The most common sites for endometriosis are the ovaries, the supporting ligaments of the uterus, and the peritoneum of the cul-de-sac and bladder. Endometriosis is most common in women 35 to 45 years of age and is more common in white and nulliparous women. Endometriotic cysts sometimes may be distinguished from ovarian neoplasms by patient history (history of endometriosis or symptoms suggestive of endometriosis, including dysmenorrhea, pelvic pain, or infertility) and examination findings (nodularity of the uterosacral ligaments). Pelvic pain is by far the most usual symptom of endometriosis. Although physical activity and sexual intercourse usually increase the discomfort, the amount of endometriosis present does not seem to correlate with the intensity of the symptoms. For some, pain produced from small peritoneal implants appears to be incapacitating. Ultrasonography may show a homogenous echo, sometimes referred to as having a "ground-glass appearance," and on occasion may be misinterpreted as a solid mass. Septations and wall nodularity are also seen commonly. Of note, CA-125 levels are frequently elevated in patients with endometriosis. The morphologic complexity on ultrasonography coupled with CA-125 level elevations make endometriotic cysts among the most common masses incorrectly thought to be suspicious for malignancy on workup. During surgery, the ovary may be enlarged and cystic. The lumen contains blood of varying color, depending on the amount and age of the hemorrhage. In most instances, it is dark brown (chocolate cyst). In at least 50% of cases, both ovaries are involved. These cysts rarely exceed a diameter of 12 cm. They are frequently adherent to surrounding structures.

Benign Ovarian Neoplasms

The ovary is composed of tissue derived from coelomic epithelium, germ cells, and mesenchyme, and any one of these components may undergo neoplastic change (benign or malignant). Morphologically, neoplasms can be divided into solid and cystic types based on ultrasonography and gross appearances. The most common benign cystic neoplasms of the ovary are serous and mucinous cystadenomas and cystic teratomas (dermoids). Benign cystadenomas may vary in size from 5 to 50 cm and are thin walled, ovoid, and frequently unilocular. Benign neoplasms do not spontaneously regress, nor do they have the potential to disseminate or metastasize. Whether some begin neoplasms are premalignant is a source of controversy. Intraepithelial neoplasia has been reported in otherwise benign serous cystadenomas; in early stage invasive epithelial cancer, several authors have described the presence of transitional changes from normal epithelium to intraepithelial neoplasia to invasive cancer.

Serous Cystadenoma

Serous cystadenomas are more common than the mucinous type of tumor, but as a rule, they do not attain the large size characteristic of their mucinous counterparts. On gross evaluation, the cyst fluid is usually thin, watery, and yellow tinged. The surface of the cyst is usually smooth and frequently

FIGURE 10.3 A, Gross photograph of an opened serous cyst adenoma that contained 500 mL of clear straw-colored fluid. Note the papillary projections on the inner surface, especially on the right. **B,** Microscopic view of a serous cystadenoma with a few papillary projections from the surface.

FIGURE 10.4 Barium enema film of a patient with a large mucinous cystadenoma of the right ovary filling the pelvis and lower abdomen.

unilocular (Fig. 10.3). Septations dividing the cyst can be seen, however. Some serous tumors may have small papillary projections on the surface of the cyst wall, which at times are so numerous that a cauliflower pattern is produced. Large, frond-like solid projections or nodules or areas of necrosis should raise the concern for malignancy. On microscopic examination, the epithelium is usually of the low columnar type with cilia. Particularly characteristic of this type of cyst are small calcific granules, the so-called psammoma bodies, which are an end product of degeneration of the papillary implants. Associated fibrosis may lead to the so-called cystadenofibroma.

Many serous cystadenomas of the ovary are asymptomatic and are discovered as an incidental finding during routine pelvic examination or through imaging studies performed for another reason. Symptoms may develop because of the size of the mass (pain, pressure on the bladder or rectum) or as a result of rupture or torsion. Ultrasound appearance is frequently similar to a large functional cyst, unilocular and simple.

Mucinous Cystadenoma

Mucinous cystadenomas (Fig. 10.4) may become huge, with some (Fig. 10.5) reported to weigh more than 300 lb. On gross evaluation, the masses are round or ovoid with smooth capsules that are usually translucent or bluish to whitish gray. The interior is divided by a number of discrete septa into loculi containing in general a clear, viscid fluid. Papillae are rarely noted. However, on microscopic examination, the lining of the epithelium is of a tall, pale-staining secretory type with nuclei at the basal pole; the presence of goblet cells is common. The cells are found to be rich in mucin if suitable stains are obtained. It is believed that this type of cyst usually arises from simple metaplasia of the germinal epithelium. It may occasionally arise from a teratoma in which all the other elements have been lost. It rarely occurs from a Brenner tumor in which there has been mucinous transformation of the epithelium.

Bilaterality may be found in as many as 10% of patients with serous cystadenomas, in contrast with mucinous cystadenomas, for which there is essentially no significant incidence of bilaterality. This information is helpful when the surgeon needs to make a judgment about surgical inspection of the opposite ovary in a young woman desirous of further childbearing. If the other ovary is of normal size, shape, and configuration, surgical evaluation is not needed.

FIGURE 10.5 Mucinous cystadenoma. **A,** Gross appearance. **B,** Histologic section showing tall epithelial lining with pale-staining nuclei at basal pole. (A, Courtesy of Ibrahim Ramzy, MD, University of California, Irvine, CA.)

Dermoid Cyst (Benign Cystic Teratoma)

Dermoid cysts are rarely large (typically <10 cm), are often bilateral (15%–25%), and occur with disproportionate frequency in younger patients. On gross evaluation, there is a thick, opaque, whitish wall; on opening of the cyst, one frequently finds hair, bone, cartilage, and a large amount of greasy fluid, which rapidly becomes sebaceous on cooling. On microscopic examination, various amounts of mature ectoderm, mesoderm, and endoderm may be present. Stratified squamous epithelium, hair follicles, sebaceous and sudoriferous glands, cartilage, neural and respiratory elements, and indeed all elements normally seen in fetal life may be present. Sequelae include growth of the mass, rupture (Fig. 10.6), and malignant degeneration. Malignant degeneration occurs in benign cystic teratomas in 1% to 3% of these tumors, and it is usually of a squamous type. These neoplasms are thought to arise from early ova that have been triggered by some type of

FIGURE 10.6 **A,** Ruptured dermoid cyst with sebaceous material seen. **B,** Photomicrograph of a mature teratoma (dermoid) of the ovary.

parthenogenetic process. Imaging evaluation of teratomas can be useful. For example, abdominal radiographs may demonstrate calcifications (teeth, bone), and CT imaging is excellent at showing fat densities commonly seen with dermoids. Ultrasound appearance is variable, and complex morphology with hyperechoic areas is common.

Removal of the ovary or cyst is recommended, and given the young age of many patients with mature teratoma, cystectomy (open or laparoscopically) in a patient desirous of further childbearing is standard. In most instances, a significant portion of normal ovary can be preserved and reconstituted. Care must be taken to remove the entire capsule of the neoplasm to avoid recurrence. In our experience, bilaterality is relatively rare when the opposite ovary is normal in appearance and is usually identified by preoperative ultrasonography. We do not recommend bivalving or opening a normal-appearing contralateral ovary in these circumstances. Care should be taken to prevent spillage of the contents of the dermoid cyst because this material can cause a chemical peritonitis. Because many of the masses are found in pregnant patients undergoing routine prenatal ultrasonography, conservative management until delivery is reasonable. Caspi reported on 49 women with ultrasonographically diagnosed ovarian cystic teratoma smaller than 6 cm in pregnancy who were followed for change in size. A total of 68 pregnancies resulted. None of the classic complications of dermoid cysts such as torsion, dystocia, or rupture occurred. The authors concluded that such small lesions are safe to just follow, especially in pregnancy.

Fibroma

Benign solid tumors of the ovary are usually of connective tissue origin (fibromas, thecomas, or Brenner tumors). They vary in size from small nodules found on the surface of the ovary to large neoplasms weighing several thousand grams. On physical examination, these neoplasms are usually firm, slightly irregular in contour, and mobile. The occurrence of fibromas (Fig. 10.7) is not at all infrequent. Sometimes they are first noted as small nodules on the ovarian cortex. In other instances, they can be extremely large, filling the entire pelvis and lower abdomen. The tumors are characterized by their firmness and resemblance to myomas, and they are frequently misdiagnosed as such. The cut surface has a homogeneous grayish-white and firm appearance, although areas of cystic degeneration are common in larger tumors. On microscopic examination,

one finds stellate or spindle-shaped cells arranged in fusiform fashion. The cells are uniformly well differentiated with nothing to suggest malignancy. Hyalinization is frequent, particularly in the larger tumors, and if fat stains are done, admixtures of theca cells may be seen. Meigs syndrome is characterized by ascites, hydrothorax, and an ovarian tumor that was originally believed to be specifically a fibroma; however, many other types of ovarian tumors are now known to be associated with this syndrome, such as Brenner tumors and Krukenberg tumors. The cause of Meigs syndrome is not completely understood, but it seems that the hydrothorax occurs by certain lymphatics through the diaphragm. After removal of the ovarian neoplasm, there is a prompt resolution of both abdominal and pleural fluid.

Brenner Tumor

Brenner tumor (Fig. 10.8), an uncommon type of ovarian neoplasm, is grossly identical to a fibroma. Frequently, the tumor is an incidental finding in an otherwise unremarkable ovary. On microscopic examination, one finds a markedly

FIGURE 10.7 Ovarian fibroma. **A,** Gross appearance: solid white lesion with a firm cut surface and fallopian tube. **B,** Histologic section: whorls of fibromatous matrix. (Courtesy of Ibrahim Ramzy, MD, University of California, Irvine, CA.)

FIGURE 10.8 Brenner tumor. **A,** Gross appearance: solid, firm, white cut surface. **B,** Histologic section: hyperplastic fibromatous matrix interspersed with nests of epithelioid cells. (Courtesy of Ibrahim Ramzy, MD, University of California, Irvine, CA.)

hyperplastic fibromatous matrix interspersed with nests of epithelioid cells. The epithelioid cells under high magnification show a "coffee bean" pattern caused by the longitudinal grooving of the nuclei. The cell nests show a frequent tendency toward central cystic degeneration, producing a superficial resemblance to a follicle. Although it was originally believed that Brenner tumors arise from simple Walthard cell rests, it has been conclusively demonstrated that Brenner tumors can arise from diverse sources, including the surface epithelium, rete ovarii, and ovarian stroma itself. It was originally stressed that Brenner tumors were uniformly benign, but there have been scattered reports in the past several decades of a number of malignant Brenner tumors. Brenner tumors are generally thought to be hormonally inert, but several cases in recent years have been associated with postmenopausal endometrial hyperplasia, and a frequent estrogen effect has been attributed to this neoplasm. These lesions are managed by simple excision.

MANAGEMENT OF ADNEXAL MASSES

Observation versus Surgery

Optimal management for patients with adnexal masses can be achieved by combining all available information from the history, examination, and diagnostic studies to create an accurate differential diagnosis. The presence and severity of symptoms are other important considerations. For example, a patient with a 6-cm unilocular cyst may be initially observed expectantly, but a similar patient with severe pain may need urgent surgery. In addition, consultation with additional specialists (gynecologic oncologist, urologist, general surgeon) may be required based on suspicion of malignancy or the differential diagnosis being considered.

Decisions that must be considered are as follows:

1. Does the patient require surgical evaluation (vs. observation)?
2. After a decision for surgery has been made, is a specialist referral or consultation required, and what type of surgical procedure is planned (open vs. minimally invasive)?
3. If observation has been elected, at what intervals and with what thresholds for changing course would be considered?

Deciding which patients need surgical exploration can best be done by considering the characteristics of the adnexal mass. In reproductive-age women, 95% of ovarian cysts smaller than 5 cm in diameter are nonneoplastic. In addition, functional cysts are seldom larger than 7 cm in diameter and are usually unilateral and freely mobile. A physician can presume that during the reproductive years, an adnexal mass as described earlier is a functional or hyperplastic change of the ovary rather than a true neoplasm. The transitory existence of functional cysts is of prime importance in distinguishing them from true neoplasms. Tradition and clinical experience have shown that functional cysts usually persist for only a few days to a few weeks, and reexamination during a later phase of the menstrual cycle has been a reliable procedure in confirming this diagnosis. Many gynecologists prescribe oral contraceptives to accelerate the involution of the functional cyst on the presumption that these cysts are gonadotropin dependent. The unconfirmed theory is that the inhibitory effect of the contraceptive steroids

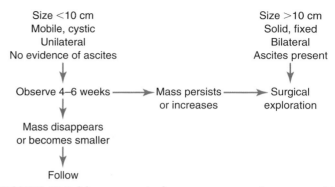

FIGURE 10.9 Management of a premenopausal woman with an adnexal mass.

on the release of pituitary gonadotropins shortens the lifespan of these cysts, hastening their identification as functional or nonneoplastic lesions. In an era before the use of ultrasonography, Spanos conducted a careful study of 286 patients who had adnexal cysts. Combination oral contraceptives were prescribed, and the women were reexamined in 6 weeks. In 72% of the women, the masses disappeared during the observation period. Of the 81 patients whose masses persisted, none were found to have a functional cyst at laparotomy. The fact that five of the removed tumors were malignant underscores the importance of avoiding an unnecessary delay in the operative investigation of these patients. In general, masses larger than 10 cm in diameter should be surgically explored regardless of concerns for malignancy because these masses are not likely to be functional and seldom resolve spontaneously. Our practice is to reassess young women with suspected functional cysts with a repeat examination and ultrasonography in 6 to 8 weeks. If the cyst resolves, no further therapy is indicated. If the cyst persists, the patient is counseled regarding surgical evaluation (Fig. 10.9).

Data also have accumulated showing that some patients with nonfunctional cyst adnexal masses may be conservatively followed with serial observation and not undergo surgery. For example, postmenopausal women with unilocular cysts smaller than 5 cm and normal CA-125 levels may be considered for observation because the risk for malignancy is very low. In addition, many of the masses will resolve spontaneously. In some older patients with concurrent medical comorbidities, avoiding surgery may be a safer strategy. Patients undergo serial repeat pelvic ultrasonography every 3 to 6 months with CA-125 testing. Surgical intervention is recommended if the morphology becomes complex, the size increases, or the CA-125 level increases outside of normal range. Saunders and colleagues at the University of Kentucky evaluated a series of 1319 patients (25% premenopausal, 75% postmenopausal) with 2870 septated ovarian cysts without solid or papillary projections. On serial follow-up, 39% of cysts resolved (mean duration to resolution, 12 months). Of 1756 cysts that persisted, 128 surgeries were performed, and no case of ovarian cancer was identified. The most common histopathologies were serous cystadenoma, mucinous cystadenoma, and endometrioma. The authors suggested that patients with septated cysts without solid components are at low risk for ovarian cancer and may be followed.

TABLE 10.4 Adnexal Mass: Indications for Surgery
• Ovarian cystic structure >5 cm that has been observed 6–8 weeks without regression
• Any solid ovarian lesion
• Any ovarian lesion with papillary vegetation on the cyst wall
• Any adnexal mass >10 cm in diameter
• Ascites
• Palpable adnexal mass in a premenarchal or postmenopausal patient
• Torsion or rupture suspected

TABLE 10.5 Society of Gynecologic Oncologists and American College of Obstetricians and Gynecologists Referral Guidelines for Women With a Newly Diagnosed Pelvic Mass
Premenopausal Patients (<50 Years Old)
CA-125 >200 units/mL
Presence of ascites
Evidence of intraperitoneal or distant metastasis (based on examination or imaging studies)
Family history (first-degree relative) of breast or ovarian cancer
Postmenopausal Patients (>50 Years)
1. Elevated CA-125 level
2. Ascites
3. Evidence of intraperitoneal or distant metastasis (based on examination or imaging studies)
4. Family history (first degree relative) of breast or ovarian cancer

Adapted from ACOG Practice Bulletin. Management of adnexal mass. *Obstet Gynecol* 2007;110:207.

Masses that raise a suspicion for malignancy require surgical intervention (Table 10.4). In addition, consultation with a specialist trained in the management of ovarian cancer should be considered. Patients with associated hallmarks of ovarian cancer, including peritoneal or omental implants, ovarian caking, and markedly elevated CA-125 levels, frequently have advanced ovarian cancer and require care from physicians specialized in surgical debulking techniques. In other tumors with the potential for malignancy, surgical evaluation should be considered, and consultation is advised. Conditions raising the concern of possible malignancy include the following:

1. Bilateral adnexal masses
2. Complex masses, especially including solid components, thick septations, or mural nodules
3. Premenopausal patients with complex masses that persist or grow after period of observation
4. Postmenopausal patients with simple masses larger than 5 cm or complex masses of any size
5. Masses associated with elevated tumor markers
6. Symptomatic masses

In a joint publication, the American College of Obstetrics and Gynecology (ACOG) and the SGO suggested referral guidelines to triage patients with adnexal masses to specialists in the care of ovarian cancer. The guidelines are shown in Table 10.5. The SGO performed a multisite, retrospective validation trial assessing the guidelines in 1035 women undergoing surgery for an adnexal mass. The prevalence of ovarian cancer was 31%. When using the referral guidelines, the positive predictive values were 34% for premenopausal and 60% for postmenopausal women. The negative predictive value was approximately 92% for each group. Others have criticized the guidelines for largely detecting cases of advanced cancers and missing many cases of early stage cancers (when appropriate staging would be desired).

Minimally Invasive Surgery for Adnexal Masses

Minimally invasive surgery (MIS), either laparoscopic or robotic, is the preferred approach for a presumptively benign adnexal mass. With the use of specific ultrasound criteria, benign masses can be predicted with a high degree of certainty, especially in premenopausal women. Careful selection of patients is critical for the appropriate use of MIS for removal of adnexal masses. The patient's age, the clinical examination, tumor markers, and the ultrasound findings provide important information that helps determine the appropriate operative approach. MIS should be used cautiously in the presence of any mass with clinical or ultrasonographic characteristics suggestive of malignancy, especially an adnexal mass in a postmenopausal woman associated with an elevated serum CA-125 value.

All patients scheduled for MIS with an adnexal mass should also consent to possible laparotomy. If the preoperative risk for finding malignancy is high enough, referral to a surgeon prepared to proceed with staging or surgical debulking if malignant disease is uncovered is warranted. Cell washings are obtained from the pelvis and upper abdomen and saved for proper staging if a malignant neoplasm is found. Any lesions or suspicious areas are sampled and sent for frozen section analysis. If an unexpected malignancy is found, appropriate biopsies and photo documentation can be taken, and referral can be made to a cancer specialist. The main reasons for conversion from laparoscopy to laparotomy are extensive adhesions or intraoperative complications.

Nezhat and colleagues reported their experience with 1209 patients with adnexal masses who were managed laparoscopically. Of 1011 cases with surgical management, ovarian cancer was discovered intraoperatively in four. The management of a cystic mass included aspiration of fluid, which was sent for cytologic examination, followed by opening of the cyst and inspection of the wall for any irregular thickening. Frozen section biopsy specimens were obtained if the surgeon thought any surfaces were suspicious. An ovarian cystectomy–oophorectomy was then performed, and tissue was sent for permanent histologic examination. The Nezhat et al. study suggests that experienced surgeons using intraoperative histologic sampling may safely evaluate adnexal masses laparoscopically.

Hasson reported another series of 102 women with ovarian cysts who were managed laparoscopically. In 83 of the women, laparoscopic fenestration and biopsy were done, with or without coagulation or removal of the cyst lining. Only 1 of 56 functional, simple, or paraovarian cysts recurred during the study. Two of the 18 ovarian endometriomas treated with fenestration and coagulation or removal of the lining recurred, and eight of nine such lesions recurred with treatment by fenestration alone. There were no surgical complications.

Canis et al. reported on their group's experience with 247 adnexal masses suspicious at ultrasound examination; 17 patients were evaluated by laparotomy and 230 by laparoscopy. Of the 230 women triaged to laparoscopy, the procedure was completed laparoscopically in 204 women. Women who were treated by laparoscopy included 7 of 37 malignant tumors and 191 of 210 benign masses. One case of tumor dissemination occurred after a laparoscopic adnexectomy and morcellation of a grade 1 immature teratoma. This study demonstrated the feasibility of laparoscopy for management of a suspicious adnexal mass, thus sparing the patient the known morbidity of a laparotomy. Some surgeons prefer to manage cystic ovarian masses with a mini laparotomy. A small incision (3–5 cm) is made over the mass, and the cyst fluid is aspirated with a long needle, trocar, or suction cannula after draping the field with dry laparotomy pads (Fig. 10.10, A). The collapsed mass can then be removed through the small incision (Fig. 10.10, B) and

A

B

FIGURE 10.10 A, Aspiration of a large 40-cm simple cyst at laparotomy. The area around the puncture site is surrounded with dry laparotomy sponges. **B,** Collapsed cyst extracted through an 8-cm incision.

submitted to pathology. Spill is minimal with this approach, but thorough irrigation of the surgical field is recommended before closure. Our preferred approach is to place the mass into a bag inserted laparoscopically to enable aspiration and extraction of the mass without intraperitoneal spill and with use of a truly minimally invasive approach.

SPECIAL CIRCUMSTANCES

Adnexal Masses in Childhood

The differential diagnosis of an adnexal mass in children and adolescents also includes benign and malignant processes. Table 10.6 outlines the frequencies of adnexal masses in young women and children. Fig. 10.11 outlines the process of differentiating between benign and malignant masses in childhood. Whenever possible, conservative or MIS is preferred to preserve endocrine and reproductive functions. Dermoid cysts are among the most common ovarian masses in both pediatric and adolescent patients. These tumors are bilateral in 15% to 25% of cases. Two percent of dermoids (teratomas) have malignant components; these are usually found in adolescent patients but can also be found in childhood. A complete workup of a pelvic mass in this age group should include imaging and determination of serum levels of tumor markers such as CA-125, α-fetoprotein, lactate dehydrogenase, and β-hCG. The differential diagnosis should consider acute appendicitis, intussusception, gastroenteritis, chronic constipation, genitourinary problems, and pelvic infection.

In a study by Ehren and colleagues, 63 children and adolescents with benign or malignant ovarian tumors were described. Abdominal pain was the most common complaint; 22% had torsion. The most common sign on initial examination was a palpable abdominal mass (45 of 54 patients). Benign teratoma was the final diagnosis in 41 of the patients (65%), and 29 had

TABLE 10.6 Frequency Distribution of Adnexal Masses in Childhood

Mass	Age of Patient at Diagnosis (0–20 yr)	%
Nonneoplastic	335	64
Simple or follicular cyst	117	23
Corpus luteum cyst	143	28
Other*	75	14
Neoplastic	186	36
Benign	144	28
Malignant	42	8
Germ cell	17	3
Stromal	9	2
Epithelial	14	3
Gonadoblastoma	2	1
Total	**521**	

*Endometrioma, polycystic ovary syndrome, pelvic inflammatory disease, or ectopic pregnancy.
Modified from Van Winter JT, Simmons PS, Podratz KC. Surgically treated adnexal masses in infancy, childhood, and adolescence. *Am J Obstet Gynecol* 1994;170:1780.

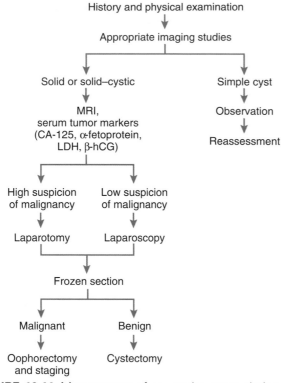

FIGURE 10.11 Management of an ovarian mass during childhood. *β-hCG,* β human chorionic gonadotropin; *CA-125,* cancer antigen 125; *LDH,* lactate dehydrogenase; *MRI,* magnetic resonance imaging.

FIGURE 10.12 Comparison of the size of the ovary during progressive periods of a woman's life. (From Barber HRK, Graber EA. Gynecological tumors in childhood and adolescence. *Obstet Gynecol Surv* 1973;28:357. Copyright © 1973 The Williams & Wilkins Co, Baltimore.)

TABLE 10.7 **Symptoms at Initial Presentation of 521 Adnexal Masses in Children**	
Symptom	No. of Patients
Pain*	271
Mass†	151
Menstrual irregularity‡	71
Dysmenorrhea	50
Amenorrhea, primary	12
Amenorrhea, secondary	35
Increased abdominal girth	34
Urinary complaints§	16
Hirsutism	13
Premature sexual development	6

*Mass was secondarily discovered in 150 of these patients.
†Without accompanying pain.
‡Metrorrhagia, menorrhagia, oligomenorrhea.
§Frequency, dysuria, suprapubic pressure.
Modified from Van Winter JT, Simmons PS, Podratz KC. Surgically treated adnexal masses in infancy, childhood, and adolescence. *Am J Obstet Gynecol* 1994;170:1780.

calcification apparent on abdominal radiography. All patients younger than 12 years with ovarian neoplasms had germ cell lesions, although an epithelial tumor has been reported in a 4-year-old patient. Two patients experienced precocious puberty, and of note, both had embryonal carcinoma. In this 63-patient study, appendicitis was the most usual misdiagnosis. Twenty-one percent had malignant tumors. Breen and Maxson noted that 35% of ovarian tumors in children were malignant.

Van Winter and associates reported on 521 adnexal masses in infancy, childhood, and adolescence; 92% were benign, including 335 nonneoplastic and 144 of 186 (77%) neoplastic lesions. The frequency of ovarian malignant neoplasms correlated inversely with the patient's age. Germ cell, stromal, and epithelial malignant neoplasms accounted for 40%, 21%, and 33%, respectively, of the 42 cancers. Nonconformance between preoperative and postoperative diagnoses was noted in 94 cases. The most common preoperative diagnosis necessitating reassignment was acute appendicitis. During the last decade of this study, ultrasonography and CT did not miss a single malignant neoplasm. The majority of these patients presented with a pain or a mass (Table 10.7).

It is important to note that when adnexal torsion is identified in a pediatric patient, the first step should be untwisting of the adnexa rather than immediate resection. The surgeon should then carefully inspect the adnexa for 10 to 15 minutes to assess viability. Often, the adnexa will revascularize and immediately demonstrate improved perfusion, and thus the standard of care is now considered to be ovarian preservation. Celik et al. prospectively followed 14 girls who underwent conservative management of torsion; they found that 13 of 14 girls had resumption of normal ovarian size and folliculogenesis. No recurrence of torsion was noted.

Postmenopausal Ovary

During the postmenopausal years, when the ovaries become smaller and quiescent after cessation of menses, the presence of a palpable ovary must alert the physician to the possibility of an underlying malignant neoplasm. Physiologic enlargement and functional cysts should not be present in late postmenopausal ovaries. The postmenopausal gonad atrophies to a size of 1.5 × 1 × 0.5 cm on average (Fig. 10.12), and at that size, it should not be palpable on pelvic examination. The possibility of malignant disease must therefore be carefully assessed when

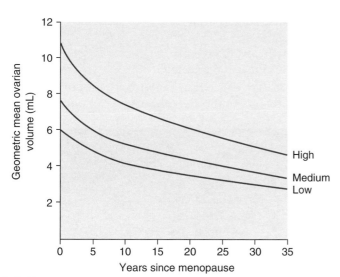

FIGURE 10.13 The 95th centiles for high, medium, and low expected ovarian volumes (geometric means) based on data from 2221 postmenopausal women. (From Goswamy RK, Campbell S, Royston JP, et al. Ovarian size in postmenopausal women. *Br J Obstet Gynaecol* 1988;95:795. Reproduced by permission of the Royal College of Obstetrics and Gynaecologists.)

TABLE 10.8 **Frequency of Simple Ovarian Cysts in Asymptomatic Postmenopausal Women**			
Author	Women (*n*)	Cysts (*n*)	Women With Cysts (%)
Wolf et al.	149	22	14.8
Conway et al.	1769	116	6.6
Andolf and Jorgensen	534	30	5.6
Aubert et al.	622	36	5.7
Bailey et al.	7705	256	3.3

From Oyelese Y, Kueck AS, Barter JF, Zalud I. Asymptomatic postmenopausal simple ovarian cyst. *Obstet Gynecol Surv* 2002;57:803. © 2002 by Lippincott Williams & Wilkins, Inc.

FIGURE 10.14 A 5-cm adenofibroma found in surgery in a postmenopausal woman and detected preoperatively and diagnosed by ultrasonography as a solid mass. (Courtesy of Ibrahim Ramzy, MD, University of California, Irvine, CA.)

an ovary is palpable in a postmenopausal woman. Goswamy and colleagues studied ovaries from 2221 postmenopausal women with regard to ovarian volumes (Fig. 10.13). They noted that there were three ranges of volume and that volume appeared to be increased in obese and multiparous women.

Adnexal masses are usually evaluated by ultrasonography, and suspicious masses should be surgically evaluated (Fig. 10.14). When surgery is performed, the approach should be made with the assumption that the patient may have an early ovarian carcinoma. Cytologic washings should be obtained, and careful exploration of the abdomen should be done, as in any patient being staged for ovarian cancer. If laparotomy is chosen, a vertical abdominal incision is recommended, which allows

for careful assessment of the upper abdomen. Small simple cysts are not uncommon in the adnexae of postmenopausal asymptomatic women who undergo pelvic imaging. Wolf and colleagues identified unilocular cysts ranging in size up to 5 cm in 22 of 149 (14.8%) asymptomatic postmenopausal women. Conway and colleagues performed transvaginal sonography on 1769 similar asymptomatic women and found 116 (6.6%) simple cysts up to 5 cm in diameter. Others have had a similar outcome (Table 10.8).

Castillo et al. evaluated 8794 asymptomatic postmenopausal women with ultrasonography and identified 215 women with simple adnexal cysts (2.5%). Of 104 women who underwent conservative observation, 44% had spontaneous resolution of the cysts during follow-up, and of women with cysts that did not resolve, 70% of the cysts remained the same size, 17% increased, and 17% decreased. Of 45 women who underwent surgery, one was identified with an ovarian cancer. The authors suggested that the risk of malignancy in simple cysts is low and that conservative management is reasonable.

Lerner and colleagues accurately predicted a benign outcome in 247 of 248 patients studied. They used color-flow Doppler analysis to improve the accuracy of ultrasonic characterization of ovarian masses. However, this technique has not been as accurate when used by others. Shalev and coworkers described 55 postmenopausal women who underwent operative laparoscopy for an adnexal cyst that was not complex and when the serum CA-125 level was normal. All of the 55 cysts were benign. During the same period, 75 women underwent exploratory laparotomy for complex cysts or an elevated serum CA-125 level. Of the 75 women, 23 had malignant lesions. Size is an important determinant of malignant potential. Cysts smaller than 5 cm in diameter are rarely malignant, but cysts larger than 5 cm in diameter have a high probability of malignancy in postmenopausal patients.

A diagnosis of ovarian cancer should be considered when a postmenopausal woman presents with a pelvic mass. The presence of ascites, which can be detected clinically or by ultrasound examination, markedly increases the probability of a diagnosis of malignancy. In addition, CA-125, although nonspecific in the population of premenopausal patients, is sensitive in postmenopausal patients when it is used in combination with a clinical impression and an abnormal ultrasound finding. Early surgical intervention is a key component in the treatment of these patients, and extensive diagnostic testing should be discouraged.

Borderline Malignant Epithelial Ovarian Neoplasms

In the past 4 decades, clear evidence has been presented that there is a group of epithelial ovarian tumors with histologic and biologic features intermediate between those of clearly benign and those of frankly malignant ovarian neoplasms. These borderline malignant neoplasms account for approximately 15% of all epithelial ovarian cancers. In the younger population, these lesions tend to occur more frequently than the obviously malignant epithelial ovarian carcinomas, which are seen more frequently in older patients (Fig. 10.15). There is a 10-year survival rate of more than 95% for stage I lesions in these borderline neoplasms. However, symptomatic recurrence and death may occur as many as 20 years after therapy in a few patients.

Borderline serous epithelial tumors (Fig. 10.16) occupy an intermediate position between the benign serous cystadenomas and the frankly malignant serous cystadenocarcinomas in their histologic features and prognostic aspects. On gross evaluation, the borderline serous tumors are similar to the previously described benign serous cystadenomas, which have papillary projections, but the borderline tumors possibly show an increased incidence of bilaterality. In addition, the papillary component is usually more abundant in the borderline lesions than in the perfectly benign serous cystadenoma. Survival in these lesions differs significantly from that in their obviously malignant counterpart (Fig. 10.17).

The histologic criteria characterizing the borderline tumors can be summarized as follows:

1. Stratification of the epithelial lining of the papillae
2. Formation of microscopic papillary projections or tufts arising from the epithelial lining of the papillae
3. Epithelial pleomorphism
4. Atypicality
5. Mitotic activity
6. No stromal invasion present.

In 1973, Hart and Norris reported a series of borderline mucinous tumors confined to either ovary or both ovaries at

FIGURE 10.16 Borderline serous carcinoma. **A,** Gross appearance. **B,** Histologic section showing stratification of the epithelial lining in papillary projections.

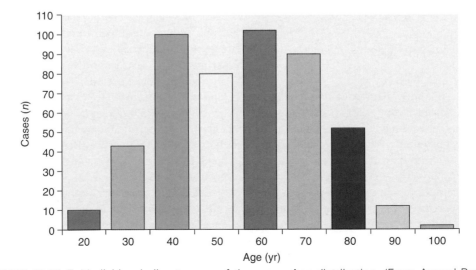

FIGURE 10.15 Epithelial borderline tumors of the ovary. Age distribution. (From Annual Report Gynecological Cancer. FIGO, Vol 22, 1994.)

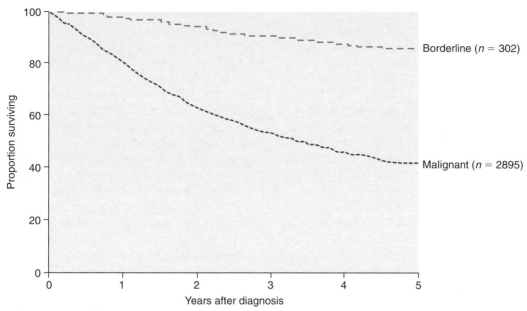

FIGURE 10.17 Carcinoma of the ovary: patients treated from 1900 to 1992. Survival by histology (n = 3197). (From FIGO Report. J Epidemiol Biostat Vol 3, 1998. Reprinted with permission of the publisher, Taylor & Francis Ltd., http://www.tandf.co.uk/journals.)

the time of diagnosis, with a corrected 10-year actuarial survival rate of 96%. These neoplasms do not differ significantly from their benign counterparts in gross appearance. They are multilocular, cystic, frequently voluminous masses with smooth outer surfaces. The inner lining, also similar to that of benign mucinous cystadenomas, is generally smooth, although papillary structures and solid thickening of the capsule have been observed in about 25% to 50% of lesions reported (Fig. 10.18). On microscopic examination, in contrast to benign mucinous cystadenoma, the epithelial lining of the borderline tumor is characterized by stratification of two or three layers. In the benign tumors, the cells show no atypia or pleomorphism, but the epithelium of the borderline lesions does demonstrate atypia, with irregular, hyperchromatic nuclei and enlarged nucleoli. Mitotic figures are also seen.

Trimble and Trimble reported an excellent review of epithelial ovarian tumors of low malignant potential in 1994. For serous and mucinous tumors of low malignant potential, the mean age at diagnosis falls close to 40 years, approximately 2 decades earlier than the mean age at diagnosis for invasive epithelial ovarian cancer. In a meta-analysis of 12 case-control studies conducted in the United States, Harris and colleagues found a mean age of 44 years for women with tumors of low malignant potential compared with a mean age of 52.9 years for women with invasive ovarian carcinoma. The meta-analysis conducted by the Collaborative Ovarian Cancer Group found protective factors against the development of tumors of low malignant potential to be pregnancy, breastfeeding, and use of oral contraceptives. A history of infertility increased the risk of tumors of low malignant potential (odds ratio [OR], 1.9), and the use of infertility drugs further increased the risk for development of a tumor of low malignant potential above that of women with no history of infertility (OR, 4.0).

FIGURE 10.18 A, Mucinous tumor with low malignant potential. Gross appearance. B, Photomicrograph of mucinous tumor seen in A.

Kurman and Trimble reviewed survival in 22 studies of serous tumors of low malignant potential, excluding those patients with invasive peritoneal implants. For 538 patients with stage I disease, the survival rate was 99%, with a mean follow-up of 7 years. Even in the series of 415 patients with stage II and stage III disease, the survival rate was 92% with a mean follow-up of 7 years. In review of the causes of death in this series, three patients died of radiation-associated complications, nine died of chemotherapy-associated complications, eight died of bowel obstruction, and eight died of invasive carcinoma; 18 patients were reported as "dying of disease" without additional information. In short, more patients seemed to die with disease than of disease. In addition, more patients died of treatment-related complications than of bowel obstruction from progressive disease. For treatment of borderline lesions, the physician should strive to completely extirpate all grossly visible tumor. If disease is unilateral, a salpingo-oophorectomy or a carefully performed ovarian cystectomy is appropriate, on condition that a thorough evaluation of the other ovary (biopsy if necessary) is done. Julian and Woodruff evaluated 65 patients who had low-grade papillary serous carcinoma of the ovary and found that 100% of the 50 patients who had unilateral adnexectomy and 90% of the 10 patients who had complete operation (total abdominal hysterectomy and bilateral salpingo-oophorectomy) were alive at 5 years. Lim-Tan and colleagues described 35 patients with ovarian serous borderline tumors treated by unilateral cystectomy or bilateral cystectomy. Tumor persisted or recurred only in the ovary that had been subjected to cystectomy in two (6%) of the 33 patients, with stage I tumors in both the ipsilateral and contralateral ovary in one patient (3%) and only in the contralateral ovary in the other patient (3%). All of the patients were alive without evidence of disease 3 to 18 years after initial operation, with the average follow-up period of 7.5 years. Scattered reports of similar smaller series suggest that these lesions may be managed with ovarian cystectomy alone in patients desirous of further childbearing when acceptance of a small risk is appropriate.

If there is bilateral ovarian involvement, especially when papillary projections are found on the external surface of the tumor, or if peritoneal spread is noted, a more radical surgical approach, such as total abdominal hysterectomy with bilateral salpingo-oophorectomy and radical excision of involved pelvic peritoneum, is advocated. Peritoneal cytologic examination, partial omentectomy, and selected pelvic and periaortic lymphadenectomy should also be done in these patients with more advanced disease. Advanced (stage III) borderline lesions can occur with metastases to lymph nodes. The survival rate even with these advanced lesions is appreciable.

Several authors have described patients with ovarian serous borderline tumors with peritoneal implants. Gershenson and Silva report a 95% disease-free survival rate at 5 years and a 91% disease-free survival rate at 10 years. However, Bell and coworkers reported that 13% of patients died of tumor, and one patient was alive with widespread progressive tumor. The mortality rate resulting from tumor was 4% at 5 years and 23% at 10 years. Drescher and coworkers studied the significance of the DNA content and nuclear morphology in these lesions. Their results suggest that measurement of DNA ploidy and nuclear morphology by image analysis can provide important prognostic information in patients with borderline ovarian tumors. Some extraovarian implants are associated with irregular glandular structures in immature, desmoplastic, or inflamed stroma, and these represent a difficult diagnostic problem. Many also have a clear pattern of invasion of subjacent tissues and cellular features of malignancy. They thus exhibit a capacity for invasion not seen in the ovarian lesion and may represent an independent or autochthonous origin. Other bland cellular nests of cells in desmoplastic reactive granulation tissue do not invade the underlying tissue and are termed noninvasive compared with the invasive implants. Russell and Merkur reported that invasive implants are associated with a poor clinical outcome compared with the noninvasive group.

Gershenson and colleagues described seven assessable patients with invasive implants who underwent chemotherapy and a second-look surgery. Four of the patients had a response. No clear conclusion could be drawn about which agents were most active. A total of 39 patients with invasive implants were identified at their institution, and 12 (31%) developed progressive disease or a recurrence.

Kurman and Trimble have identified an aggressive subgroup of proliferative serous lesions, which they call micropapillary serous carcinoma. Seidman and Kurman found 11 patients with micropapillary projections, and according to Seidman and Kurman, these lesions should be classified as carcinomas, as should serous borderline tumors with invasive implants. The poor prognosis for these patients has prompted some clinicians to prescribe chemotherapy as an adjuvant to surgery.

The role of adjuvant therapy, whether radiotherapy or chemotherapy, in tumors of low malignant potential has not yet been established. Several prospective, randomized studies of adjuvant therapy in patients with invasive ovarian carcinoma have included patients with tumors of low malignant potential. From 1983 to 1992, the Gynecologic Oncology Group (GOG) studied 414 patients with low malignant potential lesions of the ovary. The purpose of the protocol was to evaluate the biologic behavior of these tumors, the effectiveness of melphalan chemotherapy in patients with clinically detectable residual disease after surgical staging and in patients with recurrent disease, and the response rate to cisplatin in patients who failed to respond to melphalan therapy. The preliminary conclusions were that ovarian serous tumors of low malignant potential limited to the ovary rarely recur. Conservative management with unilateral salpingo-oophorectomy or ovarian cystectomy is adequate therapy for women of reproductive age. The effectiveness of melphalan and cisplatin has yet to be analyzed.

Perhaps the largest study to date of borderline ovarian tumors is the **R**etrospective/prospective multicenter **o**utcome survey in **b**orderline **o**varian **t**umors (ROBOT) study, which was conducted in Europe. Du Bois et al. reported that of 950 patients with a confirmed borderline tumor, 7.8% recurred and 4.5% died during the follow-up period. Upon multivariate analysis, higher stage, incomplete staging, residual tumor, and fertility preservation surgery were independent factors for recurrence. Neither microinvasion nor micropapillary pattern yielded significance. Most recurrences ($n = 74$) were in the form of borderline ovarian tumor ($n = 52$ or 70% of recurrences), but eight patients (11% of recurrences) developed high-grade serous ovarian cancer. Patients who recurred with invasive cancer had significantly poorer 5-year progression-free survival (PFS) (83% vs. 12%; P <0.0001) and overall survival (98% vs. 50%; P <0.0001) rates than those who recurred with borderline tumors.

It is clear that some patients with advanced disease will ultimately die of their tumor. It is not clear that adjuvant chemotherapy has any impact on survival. A strong clinical need currently exists to develop a mechanism for distinguishing lesions that are biologically aggressive from lesions that persist in a state of equilibrium, posing no threat to the patients' health and welfare.

Fertility Preservation

Operative treatment has traditionally been the mainstay of management in ovarian carcinoma. The technical aspects of the initial laparotomy have a greater bearing on outcome than do many subsequent therapeutic decisions. Hysterectomy with bilateral salpingo-oophorectomy continues to be the most cogent therapy for ovarian carcinoma. The opposite ovary is removed because of the frequency of bilateral synchronous tumors and the possibility of occult metastases, which in the normal-appearing opposite ovary have varied from 6% to 43%, depending on the report and stage of the disease. Because the uterine serosa and endometrium are often sites of occult metastasis and because the prevalence of synchronous endometrial carcinoma is relatively high, hysterectomy is also indicated. Because 3% to 17% of patients with ovarian cancer are younger than 40 years of age, some patients may consider options for fertility preservation in the setting of an adnexal mass.

Conservative therapy, designed by preservation of some ovarian tissue, appears to be safe, although no prospective trials have compared conservative surgery with bilateral salpingo-oophorectomy. Trimble and Trimble collected eight series (Table 10.9). In a study of these data, there were only 10 recurrences in 148 patients for an incidence of 6.8%. Zanetta and colleagues published their results with 99 women aged 40 years or younger with stage I ovarian carcinoma. Of the 99 women,

56 underwent fertility-sparing surgery, and 43 had more radical surgery with a median follow-up period of 7 years; they observed five recurrences (9%) of carcinoma in the women treated conservatively and five recurrences (12%) in those treated more radically. Two recurrences after conservative surgery involved the residual ovary (3.6%). These two women developed a borderline tumor in the contralateral ovary and were treated with surgery. More recent data from Schlaerth and colleagues from Memorial Sloan-Kettering Cancer Center evaluating 123 patients with stage I ovarian cancer, including 20 with preservation of the uterus and contralateral ovary, found no difference in 5-year PFS (84% vs. 78%) or survival (84% vs. 82%) for fertility-preserving versus standard surgical approaches. Wright and coworkers reviewed a large population database of patients with early-stage ovarian cancer and noted that neither ovarian nor uterine preservation had an effect on survival. Colombo and associates reported data of 99 patients younger than 40 years with stage I ovarian cancer. Conservative surgery was performed in 56 of the patients (36 stage Ia, 1 stage Ib, and 19 stage Ic). Relapses occurred in three patients assigned to stage Ia (grades I, II, and III). One recurrence was in the residual ovary, and the patient was rescued by surgery; the other two patients had relapses at distant sites and died as a result of the tumors. Seventeen patients who desired to become pregnant did so, for a total of 25 conceptions.

Some centers are studying the role of ovarian cystectomy alone for low-grade stage I epithelial neoplasms. Others have permitted patients with stage I lesions, grade II and III lesions, and stage Ic neoplasms to undergo ovarian tissue-sparing surgery followed by chemotherapy in an attempt to preserve fertility. These investigations await further observation and confirmation as to long-term safety. Chemotherapy administered after such ovarian tissue-sparing procedures may destroy the remaining ova, especially in patients older than 30 years.

It is estimated that 7% to 8% of stage I ovarian cancer cases occur in women younger than age 35 years. Considerations for conservative management of stage Ia ovarian cancer are listed in Table 10.10. Unilateral salpingo-oophorectomy may be the definitive treatment of a young woman of low parity found to

---

TABLE 10.9   Recurrence Rate in Patients With Low Malignant Potential Lesions With Conservative Surgery

Author	Incidence of Recurrence (%)
Casey et al.	0/7 (0)
Chambers et al.	2/20 (20)
Lim-Tan et al.	4/35 (11)
Manchul et al.	0/15 (0)
Rice et al.	0/32 (0)
Sawada et al.	1/5 (20)
Tazelaar et al.	3/20 (15)
Tropé et al.	0/14 (0)
Total	**10/148 (7)**

Modified from Trimble CL, Trimble EL. Management of epithelial ovarian tumors of low malignant potential. *Gynecol Oncol* 1994;55:S42.

TABLE 10.10   Optimal Requirements for Conservative Management in Stage Ia Epithelial Ovarian Cancer

1. Well differentiated
2. Young woman of low parity
3. Otherwise normal pelvis
4. Encapsulated and free of adhesions
5. No invasion of capsule, lymphatics, or mesovarium
6. Peritoneal washings negative
7. Adequate evaluation of opposite ovary and omental biopsy result negative
8. Close follow-up probable
9. Excision of residual ovary after completion of childbearing

Modified from DiSaia PJ, Townsend DE, Morrow CP. The rationale for less than radical treatment for gynecologic malignancy in early reproductive years. *Obstet Gynecol Surv* 1974;29:581. Copyright © 1974 by The Williams & Wilkins Co.

have a well-differentiated serous, mucinous, endometrioid, or mesonephric carcinoma of the ovary. The tumor must be unilateral, well encapsulated, free of adhesions, and not associated with ascites or evidence of extragonadal spread. Peritoneal washings for cytologic examination should be taken from the pelvis and upper abdomen, and the opposite ovary should be evaluated for disease. If the opposite ovary is of normal size, shape, and configuration, surgical evaluation is not routinely done. Munnell and others have calculated the incidence of microscopic metastases in the opposite ovary to be approximately 12%. The paraaortic and pelvic wall nodes must be carefully palpated and sampled, peritoneal staging biopsies must be performed, and an adequate sample of the omentum must be taken for biopsy. In addition, the preserved pelvic organs should be reasonably normal because there is little to be gained by retaining the opposite ovary in a patient who is not fertile. With the finding of carcinoma in any of these areas, conservative surgery must be abandoned. After the patient has completed childbearing, some consideration should be given to the removal of the other ovary to eliminate the risk of another ovarian malignant neoplasm. Because the incidence of epithelial cancer of the ovary increases when a woman reaches the sixth decade of life and because a patient with a history of such a lesion harbors the unfortunate milieu that could promote another epithelial lesion, it is reasonable to remove the vestigial ovarian tissue after childbearing.

Cyst Rupture or Spill of Tumor

The subject of tumor spill has been controversial in gynecologic oncology for some time. The Federation of International Gynecologists and Obstetricians (FIGO) staging system was updated in 2014 to reflect several changes. Stage IC is now subclassified by whether the mass was ruptured preoperatively versus intraoperatively or had capsule involvement or whether there were positive washings or malignant ascites. Traditionally, upstaging to IC leads to a recommendation for the use of postoperative chemotherapy also. It is logical to assume that implantation and germination of cancer cells are conceivable and probable when a malignant cyst ruptures at the time of surgery. The data to support the independent prognostic significance of intraoperative cyst rupture are mixed, however. Other changes in the 2014 updated FIGO staging system include division of stage IIIA into IIIA1 and IIIA2 to microscopic extrapelvic disease involving retroperitoneal lymph nodes or microscopic peritoneal involvement and division of stage IV into IVA and IVB with the former including only malignant pleural effusion and the latter including hepatic or splenic parenchymal metastases or other extraperitoneal metastases.

Analyses of older studies in which complete surgical staging was not performed and contemporary chemotherapy regimens were not used make it difficult to understand the relevance of cyst rupture as a single variable (Table 10.11). Sjöval and associates described 247 patients with stage I disease who were at risk of spill. There was no difference in survival between the patients whose tumors had intact capsules and the patients in whom rupture occurred during surgery (78% vs. 85%, respectively). However, a significant difference in survival was found

TABLE 10.11 Recurrence Rates as a Function of Cyst Rupture

Series (Year)	Ruptured Neoplasm (%)	Unruptured Neoplasm (%)
Purola and Nieminen (1968)	18/30 (60)	83/100 (83)
Williams et al. (1973)	3/7 (43)	57/58 (98)
Parker et al. (1970)	16/27 (59)	12/20 (60)
Dembo et al. (1989)	98/119 (82)	168/199 (84)
Sevelda et al. (1989)	23/30 (76)	23/30 (76)

between patients in whom rupture occurred before surgery and those with intraoperative rupture (59% vs. 85%, respectively). The conclusion was that manipulation during surgery that results in puncture or rupture does not have a negative influence on the outcome for patients. However, rupture occurring at some interval before surgery may lead to seeding in the peritoneal cavity. Vergote and colleagues assessed 1545 stage I ovarian cancer patients and found that tumor differentiation or grade and cyst rupture were the two most important predictors for disease-free survival. Cyst rupture occurring before definitive surgery heralded a poorer prognosis than that occurring intraoperatively. Bakkum-Gamez and associates reported on 161 patients with stage I ovarian cancer, all of whom underwent thorough surgical staging. In a multivariate analysis, capsular rupture and positive peritoneal cytology were independent predictors of poorer disease-free survival. It is noted that rupture may occur as a result of laparoscopic removal and drainage, may occur by cyst wall weakening (necrosis, tumor penetration), or may be associated with adhesions and adhesion lysis required to remove the cyst. The effect of these confounding variables is difficult to separate, however.

We believe that collection of cytology before the mass is manipulated provides important information. Cysts should be removed intact when possible, recognizing that coexisting conditions (endometriosis, adhesions, infection, inflammation) may make this impossible. In some cases, particularly with a large, simple cyst, aspiration by a needle attached to suction (with the ovary placed in a bag during MIS or the area draped off with dry laparotomy pads during open surgery) has been used to decompress a cyst. Our experience with this type of "controlled spill" is that it appears to be safe and has not adversely affected outcome. In cases of masses with solid components or a high suspicion for malignancy, we favor removing the mass intact. Most authors advocate platinum-based chemotherapy for at least three cycles in patients with stage IC disease secondary to tumor rupture. No prospective study comparing these different approaches has been reported.

Prophylactic versus Risk-Reducing Oophorectomy

The early diagnosis of ovarian carcinoma is as difficult and infrequent now as in the past. Although survival figures for this disease may be recently improving to a slight degree, the prognosis is still grave. The gynecologist frequently counsels women

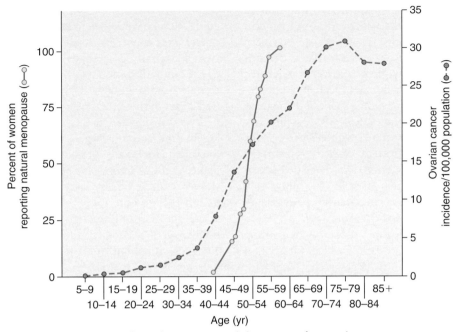

FIGURE 10.19 Incidence of ovarian cancer and the onset of natural menopause versus age.

with regard to strategies to reduce the risk of developing ovarian cancer. In one typical clinical scenario, a low-risk patient who is to undergo a hysterectomy for benign indications must be counseled as to the risk and benefits of removing the ovaries at the time of surgery (prophylactic oophorectomy).

At some time during their lives, 1% to 2% of all women develop ovarian carcinoma. The risk increases after 40 years of age, with a peak incidence between 55 and 60 years of age, closely paralleling the peak incidence of menopause in Western countries (Fig. 10.19). The function of the ovary lies in its role of ova production for procreation and as the primary site of estrogen production. After the need for ova has passed in a woman's life, only estrogen production remains an essential function. The adverse effects of oophorectomy on several metabolic parameters are well known; understanding of the endocrinology, sexuality, and psychology of postmenopausal patients (natural or surgical) has increased considerably during the past decade, and good methods of adequate substitution for the loss of ovarian function are now available.

In 1981, Grundsell and associates reported on a series of 352 women with ovarian carcinoma and studied the incidence of previous pelvic surgeries performed on these patients; 21 (6%) had undergone previous pelvic surgery, and 16 (4.6%) of these patients had surgery at some time after the age of 40 years. Others (Table 10.12) have reported similar results (Bloom, Gibbs, Grogan, Kofler, and Terz). McKenzie, Christ, and Paloucek reported that as many as 3.6% of women who have pelvic surgery with preservation of ovarian tissue will need subsequent surgery for benign lesions of the ovary, further influencing the argument for prophylactic oophorectomy.

Averette and Nguyen found that 18.2% of patients reported previous hysterectomy with ovarian conservation in a national survey of 12,316 ovarian cancer cases. Of these, hysterectomies

TABLE 10.12 Frequency of Prior Pelvic Surgery or Hysterectomy

Author (Year)	All Ages (%)	Age >40 Yr (%)
Bloom (1962)	10.6	
Grogan (1967)	8.2	
Terz (1967)	8.8	3.8
Gibbs (1971)	11.8	
Kofler (1972)	8.1	8.1
Grundsell (1980)	6.0	4.6
Averette and Nguyen (1994)	18.2	10.1

were abdominal in 7.2%, vaginal in 4.2%, and unspecified in another 6.8%. In a subsequent analysis, Boike and associates found that 57.4% of hysterectomies were performed after the age of 40 years. Thus, a potential 1286 ovarian cancer cases could have been prevented if prophylactic oophorectomy had been practiced in women undergoing hysterectomy at the age of 40 years or later. Assuming an annual incidence of 24,000 new ovarian cases and that 5% to 14% of these cases had previous hysterectomies with conserved ovaries, it is estimated that at least 1000 cases could have been prevented if prophylactic oophorectomy were diligently practiced after the age of 40 years.

We are obviously influenced by the frequent task of caring for patients with advanced ovarian carcinoma. The occurrence of this disease in patients who had previous pelvic surgery and in whom the ovaries could have been removed is certainly frustrating. Randall and coworkers have shown that unilateral oophorectomy does not influence the subsequent incidence of ovarian carcinoma.

Removal of the contralateral ovary in women with an adnexal mass requires careful thought and scrutiny. Although benefits are appreciable including reduction of ovarian cancer risk, a large dataset including the Women's Health Initiative demonstrated that elective oophorectomy increases overall mortality, largely because of coronary heart disease. Elective oophorectomy before age 55 years doubled a woman's risk of dying from coronary heart disease by age 80 years (15.95% vs. baseline risk of 7.57%). Other known risks associated with elective oophorectomy include cognitive impairment caused by estrogen deficiency, increased risk of hip fracture, and decreased sexual function (Erekson, 2013). Women should be thoroughly informed about the possible adverse effects and the advantages to enable them to make an informed decision.

A second clinical scenario is that in a patient with a strong family history of breast or ovarian cancer or who harbors a known mutation in the *BRCA1* or *BRCA2* gene. These high-risk patients frequently seek consultation to undergo surgery to remove the ovaries to reduce the risk of development of ovarian cancer. Risk-reducing salpingo-oophorectomy (RRSO) has been evaluated in several populations of women at high risk for developing ovarian cancer. Women with known *BRCA1* mutations are estimated to have a lifetime risk of developing ovarian cancer from 39% to 46%, and those with *BRCA2* mutations have a risk from 12% to 20%. Removing the ovaries in this high-risk group of patients reduces the risk of ovarian cancer, with 0.8% to 1% of women subsequently developing a primary peritoneal cancer. In addition, premenopausal women undergoing RRSO have a 50% to 80% reduction in the risk of breast cancer. In a consensus statement by the SGO, women at high risk of ovarian cancer based on family history or *BRCA1* or *BRCA2* mutation should be offered RRSO when childbearing is complete or by age 40 years, whichever occurs first. It should be noted that in the setting of RRSO, some patients will be identified with an incidental early-stage cancer of the ovary or fallopian tube, and thus serial 2- to 3-mm sectioning is mandated to evaluate for occult carcinoma. Although the original recommendation was removal of both fallopian tubes and ovaries in women with hereditary risk, in women who are not yet ready to undergo oophorectomy, salpingectomy has been shown to be a safe and cost-effective strategy if delayed oophorectomy is performed once deemed acceptable by the patient (Kwon et al., 2013). RRSO should not be offered routinely for women at average risk for ovarian cancer because there are no data to support improved survival in these patients. Patients undergoing hysterectomy for other reasons (fibroids, endometriosis) should be counseled as to the risk and benefits related to salpingo-oophorectomy with reference to age. Risk reduction must be balanced against changes in cardiovascular, bone, and sexual health.

For the bibliography list, log onto www.expertconsult.com ⟨http://www.expertconsult.com⟩

11

Epithelial Ovarian Cancer

Eric L. Eisenhauer, MD, Ritu Salani, MD, MBA, Larry J. Copeland, MD

OUTLINE

KEY POINTS

1. Ovarian cancer is the most lethal of all gynecologic cancers. Elderly women are more likely to develop ovarian cancer than young women.
2. Oral contraceptives decrease the incidence of ovarian cancer substantially.
3. Ovarian cancer may be inherited with increased risk being caused by a mutation in *BRCA1* or *BRCA2*, mismatch repair defect, or any number of other less common genes tested in the current panels.
4. A combination of surgery and chemotherapy is almost always recommended for treatment. The order depends on the extent of disease, volume, and location.
5. Significant strides have been made in survival as treatment and surgery have evolved.

Malignant neoplasms of the ovary are the cause of more deaths than any other female genital tract cancer. In the United States, there were approximately 21,290 new cases and 14,180 deaths in 2015 as a result of ovarian cancer. Ovarian cancer accounts for 5% of all cancers among women. In the United States, deaths from this cause occur at a rate of one every 44 minutes, and this disease will develop in one of every 68 women. Doctors and patients alike continue to be frustrated by our lack of understanding of the factors that lead to ovarian cancer and the failure to achieve a significant reduction in mortality.

CLASSIFICATION

The most practical classification scheme is based on the histogenesis of the normal ovary, shown in Table 11.1. The early development of the ovary is divided into four stages. During the first stage, undifferentiated germ cells (primordial germ cells) become segregated and migrate to the genital ridges, which are bilateral thickenings of coelomic epithelium. The second stage consists of proliferation of the coelomic epithelium and the underlying mesenchyme. During the third stage, the ovary becomes divided into a peripheral cortex and a central medulla. The fourth stage is characterized by the development of the cortex and involution of the medulla. The histogenetic classification categorizes ovarian neoplasms with regard to their derivation from coelomic epithelium (epithelial ovarian cancer), germ cells (germ cell tumors), and mesenchyme (sex cord-stromal tumors). The majority (85%–90%) of malignant ovarian tumors are epithelial. They can be grouped into predominant histologic types as follows:

Serous cystadenocarcinoma	42%
Mucinous cystadenocarcinoma	12%
Endometrioid carcinoma	15%
Undifferentiated carcinoma	17%
Clear cell carcinoma	6%

The specific malignant histologic type has less prognostic significance than clinical stage, extent of residual disease, and histologic grade. Histologic grade, however, is an important

TABLE 11.1 Histogenetic Classification of Ovarian Neoplasms

Neoplasms derived from the coelomic epithelium
- Serous tumor
- Mucinous tumor
- Endometrioid tumor
- Mesonephroid (clear cell) tumor
- Brenner tumor
- Undifferentiated carcinoma
- Carcinosarcoma and mixed mesodermal tumor

Neoplasms derived from germ cells
- Teratoma
  - Mature teratoma
    - Solid adult teratoma
    - Dermoid cyst
    - Struma ovarii
    - Malignant neoplasms secondarily arising from mature cystic teratoma
  - Immature teratoma (partially differentiated teratoma)
- Dysgerminoma
- Embryonal carcinoma
- Endodermal sinus tumor
- Choriocarcinoma
- Gonadoblastoma

Neoplasms derived from specialized gonadal stroma
- Granulosa–theca cell tumors
  - Granulosa tumor
  - Thecoma
- Sertoli–Leydig tumors
  - Arrhenoblastoma
  - Sertoli tumor
- Gynandroblastoma
- Lipid cell tumors

Neoplasms derived from nonspecific mesenchyme
- Fibroma, hemangioma, leiomyoma, lipoma
- Lymphoma
- Sarcoma

Neoplasms metastatic to the ovary
- Gastrointestinal tract (Krukenberg)
- Breast
- Endometrium
- Lymphoma

TABLE 11.2 Probability for Females at Birth Developing Cancer by Age 85 Years in the United States

Site	Probability
All sites	1 in 3
Breast	1 in 9
Cervix	1 in 154
Uterine corpus	1 in 41
Lung	1 in 18
Ovary	1 in 81
Colon–rectum	1 in 26

DevCan 6.6.0, National Cancer Institute 2011. http://surveillance.cancer.gov/devcan.

TABLE 11.3 Primary Ovarian Neoplasms Related to Age

Type	Age <20 Yr (%)	Age 20–50 Yr (%)	Age >50 Yr (%)
Coelomic epithelium	29	71	81
Germ cell	59	14	6
Specialized gonadal stroma	8	5	4
Nonspecific mesenchyme	4	10	9

independent prognostic factor in patients with epithelial tumors of the ovary (Fig. 11.1). Because survival for patients with grade II and III tumors is more closely related, research studies frequently stratify by low-grade (grade I) and high-grade (grade II and III) tumors.

INCIDENCE, EPIDEMIOLOGY, AND ETIOLOGY

Approximately 22% of gynecologic cancers are of ovarian origin (Fig. 11.2), but 47% of all gynecologic cancer deaths occur in women who have ovarian cancer. Cancer of the ovaries is the fifth most frequently occurring fatal cancer in women in the United States and also ranks high as a cause of cancer death in Canada, New Zealand, Israel, and countries of northern Europe.

Ovarian cancer will develop in approximately 14 of every 1000 women in the United States older than age 40 years (Table 11.2), but only four of the 14 will be cured. The remaining patients often develop repeated bouts of intestinal obstruction as the tumor spreads over the surface of the bowel, develop inanition and malnutrition, and quite literally starve. In a review of mortality trends in the United States, age-adjusted (to the 2000 US standard population) ovarian cancer mortality rates from 1975 to 2002 showed the absolute number of deaths increased, consistent with a growing and aging population. Over the past 30 years, mortality rates decreased for women younger than 65 years but increased for women older than 65 years, with some plateauing over the past 10 years. These changes may result from increased use of oral contraceptives in younger patients and a shifting of the survival curve to the right. Even when matched for stage, survival was worse in older women. In some cases, this may be a result of less aggressive treatment in the older woman and the higher percentage of low-grade disease in younger patients. Age-adjusted death rates were higher in whites than in blacks. Asians and Pacific Islanders, American Indian and Alaskan natives, and Hispanics have lower death rates than blacks.

Malignant neoplasms of the ovaries occur at all ages, including infancy and childhood (Fig. 11.3). Throughout childhood and adolescence, the rate of death from ovarian carcinoma in the United States is exceeded by those for leukemia; lymphomas; and neoplasms of the central nervous system, kidney, connective tissue, and bone. The major histologic types occur in

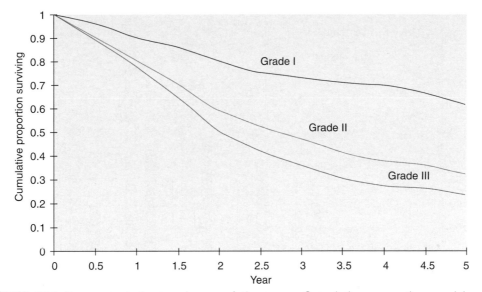

FIGURE 11.1 Serous cystadenocarcinoma of the ovary. Cumulative proportion surviving by degree of differentiation. (From International Federation of Gynecology and Obstetrics. *Annual Report on the Results of Treatment in Gynecological Cancer,* vol 22. Stockholm, 1994, Author.)

FIGURE 11.2 Leading sites of new cancer cases, 2016 estimates. Data from Cancer Facts and Figures 2016 estimates.

distinctive age ranges (Table 11.3). Whereas malignant germ cell tumors are most commonly seen in girls younger than age 20 years, epithelial cancers of the ovary are primarily seen in women older than age 50 years. Beginning at age 45 to 49 years, with a rate of 16.4 cases per 100,000, incidence increases progressively with age. The rate increases after the age of 60 years to 40 cases per 100,000 and then peaks at 61 cases per 100,000 in the age group 80 to 84 years. The largest absolute number of patients with ovarian cancer is found in the age group 60 to 64 years; more than one-third of the cases occur in patients 65 years or older. Elderly women are more likely than younger women to be in advanced stages of ovarian cancer at initial diagnosis, and the 5-year relative survival rate for elderly women is about half the rate (28.4%) observed in women younger than 65 years (56.6%).

Epidemiologic evidence strongly suggests that environmental factors play a major role in developing epithelial cancer of the human ovary. Highly industrial countries have the highest reported incidence, and physical or chemical products of industry may be causative factors. A notable exception is highly industrialized Japan, where rates for ovarian cancer have been among the lowest recorded in the world. Of interest, the incidence of ovarian cancer increases in Japanese immigrants to the United States and their offspring, eventually approaching that of Anglo-Saxon whites by the second and third generations. This suggests that causative carcinogens may be present in the immediate environment, such as food, personal customs, and other influences that change gradually during the cultural transition. To date, there are no firm clues as to which dietary items or other environmental contacts are specifically carcinogenic for the ovary.

A decreased incidence of ovarian cancer is related to less frequent ovulation. Danforth and coworkers prospectively examined risk of ovarian cancer in the Nurses' Health Studies and found that women who never breastfed faced a 1.5-fold risk of ovarian cancer compared with women who breastfed for longer than 18 months. These observations coincided with data illustrating a reduction in the disease incidence with the use of oral contraceptives (Table 11.4). The hypothesis that oral contraceptive use reduced the risk of epithelial ovarian cancer was suggested by Casagrande and associates in 1979. In 1982, Rosenberg and colleagues reported a case-control study in which combination oral contraceptives were used by 26% of the patients with ovarian cancer and 35% of the control participants. The relative risk estimate for combination oral contraceptive use was 0.6 (Table 11.5). The reduction in risk appeared to persist for as long as 10 years after use has ceased and to be greater for longer durations of use, but these results were not statistically significant. Their conclusion was that the use of combination oral contraceptives protects against epithelial ovarian cancer. The theory of "incessant ovulation" suggests that the epithelial lining of the ovary may be sensitive to the events of ovulation, which in turn can act as a promoting factor

FIGURE 11.3 Obviously malignant ovarian epithelial tumors: age distribution by stage. (From International Federation of Gynecology and Obstetrics. *Annual Report on the Results of Treatment in Gynecological Cancer,* vol 22. Stockholm, 1994, Author.)

TABLE 11.4   Odds Ratio for Invasive Epithelial Ovarian Cancer According to Parity

| Term Pregnancies (*n*) | Cases | % | Population Studies | | Odds Ratio |
			Controls	Percentage	
0	322	24	765	14	1.44
1	164	12	605	11	1.6
2	376	28	1515	27	1.53
3	265	19	1259	22	1.48
4	135	10	774	14	1.36
5	56	4	345	6	1.33
6	45	3	346	6	1.29

Modified from Whittemore AS, Harris R, Itnyre J. Characteristics relating to ovarian cancer risk: collaborative analysis of 12 US case-control studies. II. Invasive epithelial ovarian cancers in white women. Collaborative Ovarian Cancer Group. *Am J Epidemiol* 1992;136:1184.

TABLE 11.5   How Oral Contraceptive Use Affects the Risk of Ovarian Cancer

Duration of Oral Contraceptive Use	Women Who Developed Ovarian Cancer (*n*)	Controls (*n*)	Relative Risk
Never	242	1532	1.4
3–6 months	26	1280	0.6
7–11 months	14	1134	0.7
1–2 years	65	1602	0.7
3–4 years	40	1397	0.6
5–9 years	39	1594	0.4
≥10 years	13	1328	0.2

From The reduction in risk of ovarian cancer associated with oral-contraceptive use. The Cancer and Steroid Hormone Study of the Centers for Disease Control and the National Institute of Child Health and Human Development. *N Engl J Med* 1987;316:650. Reprinted by permission from the *New England Journal of Medicine.*

in the carcinogenic process. Gross and Schlesselman determined the effect of oral contraceptive use on the cumulative incidence of epithelial ovarian cancer from ages 20 to 40 years, 20 to 50 years, and 20 to 55 years and stratified these age categories by family history and parity. The number of epithelial ovarian cancer cases estimated to occur per 100,000 oral contraceptive users decreased with increasing duration of use. Their results suggest that 5 years of use by nulliparous women can reduce their ovarian cancer risk to the level seen in parous women who never use oral contraceptives, and 10 years of use by women with a positive family history can reduce their risk to a level below that of women whose family history is negative and who never use oral contraceptives. On the basis of these data, the recommendation is strongly made that premenopausal patients with risk factors for ovarian cancer use oral contraceptives when pregnancy is not being sought.

Over many years, studies have disagreed as to the association between fertility drug exposure and ovarian cancer. Whittemore and associates noted that infertile women treated with infertility drugs had a 2.8 times increased risk of ovarian cancer compared with women without infertility. The risk was higher among women who did not become pregnant compared with the parous women. Specific drug exposure was not documented. Subsequent studies by Franceschi, Rossing, Venn, Shishan and colleagues disagreed as to whether induction with clomiphene or gonadotropins were associated with increased risk. The largest reported cohort drew 126 women with invasive epithelial ovarian cancer from a cohort of 54,362 women treated at all Danish infertility clinics from 1963 to 1968. The effects of four separate groups of fertility drugs were evaluated individually and in combination (gonadotropins, clomiphene citrate, human chorionic gonadotropin, and gonadotropin-releasing hormone). No convincing associations were found between use of these fertility drugs and ovarian cancer risk. The published data suggest that there is probably little relationship between fertility drug use and ovarian cancer. Further investigations are underway to clarify this association. The concept is appealing when one considers the reduction in incidence noted with the use of oral contraceptives and parity.

Whittemore and associates, in a population-based study, noted protection against ovarian cancer with increasing parity (see Table 11.4). McGowan and colleagues, on the basis of a study of 197 women with ovarian cancer, estimated that nulligravidae were 2.5 times more likely to have malignant ovarian tumors and 2.9 times more likely to have ovarian carcinoma of low potential malignancy than were women who had been pregnant three or more times. The risk of ovarian cancer in their series was further reduced among women who had been pregnant at least once. One possible interpretation could be that the endocrine state of pregnancy protects against ovarian cancer and that the lack of this protection places infertile women at higher risk for ovarian cancer. A second explanation could be that infertility and ovarian cancer result from a similar genetically abnormal gonadal status. This theory would explain why infertile women are more at risk than never-married and never-pregnant women.

In the large prospective Cancer Prevention Study II, Rodriguez and coworkers evaluated the use of acetaminophen and a possible relationship to ovarian cancer mortality. Women who reported using acetaminophen daily had a death rate from ovarian cancer 45% lower than that of women reporting no use (relative risk = 0.55; confidence interval [CI] = 0.27–1.09). In a case-control study, Cramer and associates had previously reported that the odds ratio was 0.52 for development of ovarian cancer among women who used the drug at least once a week for at least 6 months; lowest risk was found in women who used the drug daily and for more than 10 years. Cramer et al. also noted that the odds ratio of ovarian cancer was 0.75 (CI 0.52–1.10) for aspirin and 1.03 for ibuprofen.

Parazzini and colleagues studied the influence of various menstrual factors on the risk of epithelial ovarian cancer. They reported that the risk rose with later age at menopause and with early menarche. Studies of dietary fat have been inconclusive, and other dietary factors are not well characterized. Although the Women's Health Initiative investigators reported a low-fat diet was associated with up to a 40% reduction in ovarian

cancer risk, several large cohort studies have not been able to demonstrate this. Because diet and exercise are potentially modifiable risk factors, continued investigation into their role is warranted.

Some have suggested that ovarian cancer may be initiated by a chemical carcinogen through the vagina, uterus, and fallopian tubes and that damaged ovarian surface epithelium from ovulation induces inflammation and mutation susceptibility. For years, Woodruff and coworkers suggested this hypothesis of migration of chemical carcinogens from the vagina to the pelvic peritoneum. Venter demonstrated with the use of radionuclides that upward migration is possible. Certainly, many different chemical substances could migrate to vulvovaginal areas and be implicated in carcinogenesis. The agent most extensively studied has been talc powder, but many of the studies that noted a slight increased risk of ovarian carcinoma in association with talc did not adjust for other factors (oral contraceptive use, family history) that are related to ovarian cancer. Others included low malignant potential tumors with their invasive cancers or did not correct for integrity of the female genital tract status. The relationship (if any) of talc to ovarian cancer would appear to be minimal at best.

No epidemiologic or experimental evidence exists to incriminate viruses in the development of neoplasms of the human ovary. Attempts to isolate viruses from cultures of human ovarian cancer cells have been unsuccessful to date. Because of its gonadotropic properties, mumps virus is an obvious candidate among known viruses for oncogenic activity in the ovary. At present, however, the evidence for mumps virus as an etiologic agent in ovarian cancer remains speculative.

Familial Ovarian Cancer

Familial hereditary ovarian cancer currently falls into three categories:

1. Site-specific familial ovarian cancer
2. Hereditary breast-ovarian cancer syndrome, in which there is an increased incidence of breast and ovarian carcinomas alone or in combination
3. Lynch syndrome type II, in which family members may develop a variety of cancers, including colorectal, endometrial, and ovarian cancer

Inherited genetic mutations are associated with approximately 10% of women who develop ovarian cancer. The mutation is inherited in an autosomal-dominant fashion (maternal or paternal transmission), and multiple family members are affected over several generations. First-degree relatives (mother or sister) are frequently involved.

True hereditary ovarian cancer and breast cancer mainly result from mutations of BRCA1 and BRCA2 genes. Individuals with these mutations (BRCA1 and BRCA2) generally have a germline mutation (inherited mutated copy of the gene) in contrast to the more common somatic mutation (noninherited, or acquired) in most patients with ovarian cancer. BRCA1 mutations are located on the long arm of chromosome 17q, and BRCA2 mutations are located on chromosome 13q12. Lynch II syndrome arises as a result of inherited mutation in a family of DNA repair genes (MSH2, MLH1, PMS1, PMS2); this group accounts for only a small number of inherited ovarian cancers. Initial evaluation of these germline mutations suggested an estimated risk of ovarian cancer of 39% to 46% for carriers of the *BRCA1* mutation but a lower rate of 10% to 20% for carriers of the *BRCA2* mutation. With more than 400 mutations identified in the *BRCA1* and *BRCA2* genes along with multiple polymorphisms, estimating risk is difficult. In most women with a strong family history who do develop ovarian cancer, the disease is sporadic in nature and not inherited. Houlston and colleagues evaluated 391 women who were self-referred to a screening clinic for familial ovarian cancer. Of these women, 290 (74%) appeared to have no clear inheritance pattern, and there was no increased risk of cancer in the first-degree relatives. There were 82 (21%) pedigrees compatible with multisite cancer family syndrome with a relative risk of about 6, or development of ovarian cancer in 1 of 16. In the 19 families with site-specific ovarian cancer, the relative risk for first-degree relatives was 39, with a lifetime risk of 1 in 2. Kerlikowske and associates reviewed published studies of familial ovarian cancers and used ovarian cancer incidence data from the Surveillance, Epidemiology, and End Results (SEER) database to estimate lifetime probabilities of ovarian cancer in these families. They noted that the lifetime probability of ovarian cancer for a 35-year-old woman was 1.6% in an individual without a family history of ovarian cancer. It increased to 5% if she had one relative and 7% if she had two relatives with ovarian cancer. These and other studies by Bourne and colleagues were based on family history pedigree and preceded *BRCA1* and *BRCA2* testing.

Claus and associates, using a previously fit autosomal-dominant genetic model, evaluated the Cancer and Steroid Hormone Study of 4730 patients with breast cancer aged 20 to 54 years and 4688 control subjects to estimate the proportions of breast and ovarian cases in the general population that are likely to result from breast and ovarian cancer susceptibility genes. About 10% of patients with ovarian cancer in the general population were estimated to be carriers of a breast or ovarian cancer susceptibility gene. The risks for ovarian cancer in carriers to the age of 60 years and 80 years were estimated to be about 10% and 27%, respectively. Carriers were predicted to have at least a 15-fold age-specific risk of ovarian cancer compared with noncarriers. Some ethnic groups appear to be at high risk for gene mutation, and the Ashkenazi Jews have been most extensively studied. In a large study by Struewing and associates, 5318 Jewish subjects had *BRCA1* and *BRCA2* evaluated, identifying 120 carriers. Carriers had a significantly elevated risk, with an estimated risk of 2% by age 50 years and 16% by age 70 years compared with the noncarrier risk of 0.4% by 50 years and 1.6% by 70 years. Metcalfe and colleagues performed *BRCA* testing for three founder mutations in 2080 self-identified Jewish women and found the *BRCA* mutation rate to be 1% (22 women) in an unselected population.

Frank and associates evaluated 283 women with breast cancer before age 50 years or ovarian cancer at any age and at least one first- or second-degree relative with either diagnosis for *BRCA1* followed by *BRCA2* analysis. Mutations were identified in 94 women (39%), including 59 of 117 (50%) from families with ovarian cancer and 35 of 121 (29%) from families without

ovarian cancer. In women with breast cancer, mutations in *BRCA1* and *BRCA2* were associated with a 10-fold increased risk of subsequent ovarian cancer. Mutations were noted in 24 of 38 women (63%) who had ovarian cancer. In women from breast–ovarian cancer families, 30 of the germline mutations occurred in *BRCA2*. Of note in this study, the authors did not find Ashkenazi ancestry significantly increased in the identification of *BRCA1* or *BRCA2* mutation, suggesting the importance of a strong family history.

In considering women at high risk, two questions should be addressed: (1) Who should be tested? and (2) Are there screening or prophylactic measures that can be applied to decrease the risk? A family history of breast or ovarian cancer, particularly before the age of 50 years in a first-order relative, and Ashkenazi Jewish ancestry, are risk factors for *BRCA1* or *BRCA2* mutations. Family history, both maternal and paternal, should be obtained (three generations is desired), and age at diagnosis should be noted. Pathology reports or death certificates verify accuracy of history; there can be considerable errors from history alone. Lifetime empirical risks can be determined from this information and may suggest that testing for a gene mutation is indicated. The extensive evaluation of family history and counseling should be done before genetic testing. Interpretation and plan of action that will influence medical management should be discussed in detail before genetic testing is performed. Testing of family members known to have cancer before testing of the cancer-free members is recommended. If a suspect mutation is found in the family member with cancer, the relatives without cancer can be tested for that specific mutation. If the family member with cancer does not have a mutation, other relatives probably will not benefit from testing. In one study, women sought DNA testing most commonly because of concern about the potential cancer risk to their children and secondly for their own cancer surveillance and prevention.

In a consensus statement of the Cancer Genetics Studies Consortium, annual or semiannual screening with transvaginal ultrasonography (TVS) and determination of serum carcinoma antigen 125 (CA-125) levels beginning at age 25 to 35 years are recommended for *BRCA1* mutation carriers. Both of these tests carry relatively high false-positive and false-negative rates with low positive predictive value. Narod and associates found that oral contraceptives protected against ovarian cancer in patients with mutation in either the *BRCA1* or *BRCA2* gene.

Risk-reducing salpingo-oophorectomy after completion of childbearing, or age 40 years, in women at high genetic risk is associated with a significant reduction in the risk of *BRCA1*- or *BRCA2*-associated ovarian cancer. A National Institutes of Health (NIH) Consensus Conference recommended that women with two or more first-degree relatives with ovarian carcinoma be offered prophylactic oophorectomy after completion of childbearing or age 35 years. Prophylactic oophorectomy does not prevent subsequent primary peritoneal cancer, in which failure rates of 4% to 5% at 20 years after risk-reducing salpingo-oophorectomy (RRSO) were reported by Finch and colleagues. Rebbeck and associates clarified risk reduction estimates in their 2009 meta-analysis. They found RRSO was associated with an 80% risk reduction in *BRCA1*- or

BRCA2-associated ovarian, fallopian tube and peritoneal cancer, and a 50% risk reduction in *BRCA1*- or *BRCA2*-associated breast cancer.

A 2005 study by Pal and colleagues suggested that previous studies may have underestimated the frequency of *BRCA1* and *BRCA2* mutations. Of 209 patients with invasive cancer, 32 patients (15%) had mutations of *BRCA1* ($n = 20$) or *BRCA2* ($n = 12$). Based on their data, they suggested it may be reasonable to offer genetic counseling to any woman with an invasive, nonmucinous epithelial ovarian cancer, and subsequent studies have supported this observation. A 2014 Society of Gynecologic Oncologists (SGO) Clinical Practice Statement on Genetic Testing for Ovarian Cancer recommended women diagnosed with epithelial ovarian, tubal, and peritoneal cancers receive genetic counseling and be offered genetic testing even in the absence of a family history.

The Gynecologic Oncology Group (GOG) has conducted a study (GOG 199) of 2605 women at increased risk for developing ovarian cancer, either by known *BRCA* mutation or family history risk factors. Patients were enrolled after choosing either prophylactic oophorectomy or screening, and both groups followed with CA-125 levels and Risk of Ovarian Cancer Algorithm (ROCA) assessment. The study was designed to evaluate both the prospective incidence of new and occult ovarian cancers and to assess the ROCA and quality of life. In 2014, Sherman and colleagues reported a portion of the analysis of high risk women older than 30 years of age who elected RRSO. Clinically occult cancers were detected in 2.6% of high risk women (*BRCA1* mutation carriers, 4.6%; *BRCA2* mutations carriers, 3.5%; noncarriers, 0.5%), and further results from this trial will be forthcoming.

SIGNS, SYMPTOMS, AND ATTEMPTS AT EARLY DETECTION (SCREENING)

Although the wide range of ovarian tumor types generally presents in a similar manner, the diagnosis of early ovarian cancer is often more a matter of chance than a triumph of the scientific method. As the ovary enlarges (Fig. 11.4), there may be progressive compression of the surrounding pelvic structures, producing vague abdominal discomfort, urinary frequency, and "pelvic pressure" (Table 11.6). The insidious onset of ovarian cancer needs no elaboration. As the neoplasm reaches a diameter of 10 to 15 cm, it may account for abdominal enlargement. The notions that the development of ovarian cancer is "silent" and there are no early symptoms of ovarian cancer are a focus of the patient advocacy "listen for the whisper" educational efforts. Vague symptoms may be present for several months before the diagnosis. Such complaints are usually not recognized as anything more than gas or indigestion. **A high index of suspicion is warranted in all women between the ages of 40 and 69 years who have persistent gastrointestinal (GI) symptoms that cannot be diagnosed.** The majority of such nonspecific complaints are nonmalignant, causing the primary care physician to dismiss the possibility of ovarian cancer in many cases. Too frequently, it is only when the patient has gross abdominal enlargement marking the occurrence of ascites and abdominal

FIGURE 11.4 Large bilateral ovarian neoplasms: low-grade mucinous adenocarcinoma.

TABLE 11.6 Most Frequent Presenting Symptoms of Ovarian Cancer (Goff BA et al., 2000)

Symptom	Relative Frequency
Abdominal swelling	60%
Abdominal pain	40%
Dyspepsia	30%
Urinary frequency	30%
Weight change	10%

carcinomatosis that appropriate diagnostic evaluation is undertaken.

Methods for early diagnosis have been investigated in limited studies using cul-de-sac aspiration for peritoneal cytologic assessment and frequent pelvic examinations. All of these endeavors have failed to show a significant impact on early diagnosis of this disease. Most ovarian neoplasms grow quickly and painlessly. A persistent ovarian enlargement should be an indication to consider surgery, and the diagnosis is made by the pathologist. The size of the tumor does not indicate the severity of disease; indeed, many of the largest neoplasms are histologically benign, most commonly mucinous cystadenoma. Moreover, many large adnexal masses may be of nonovarian etiology. Nonovarian causes of apparent adnexal masses are diverticulitis, tubo-ovarian abscess, carcinoma of the cecum or sigmoid, pelvic kidney, and uterine or intraligamentous myomas. At the time of surgery, it may be difficult to discern the malignant potential of a particular ovarian neoplasm (Table 11.7). There is sufficient overlap of morphologic criteria to cause confusion. The diagnosis rests with the histologic examination of the specimen, and the error rate of frozen section ranges from 5% to 15%.

Immunologic diagnosis of subclinical ovarian cancer by means of identification of specific tumor-associated antigens in the serum has yet to materialize. Several tumor-associated antigens, including CA-125, have been identified and purified.

TABLE 11.7   Surgical Findings

	Benign	Malignant
Surface papilla	Rare	Very common
Intracystic papilla	Uncommon	Very common
Solid areas	Rare	Very common
Bilaterality	Rare	Common
Adhesions	Uncommon	Common
Ascites (100 mL)	Rare	Common
Necrosis	Rare	Common
Peritoneal implants	Rare	Common
Capsule intact	Common	Infrequent
Totally cystic	Common	Rare

TABLE 11.8   Nonmalignant Conditions That May Elevate CA-125 Concentrations

Gynecologic	Nongynecologic
Acute pelvic inflammatory disease	Active hepatitis
Adenomyosis	Acute pancreatitis
Benign ovarian neoplasm	Chronic liver disease
Endometriosis	Cirrhosis
Functional ovarian cyst	Colitis
Meigs' syndrome	Congestive heart failure
Menstruation	Diabetes (poorly controlled)
Ovarian hyperstimulation	Diverticulitis
Unexplained infertility	Mesothelioma
Uterine myoma	Nonmalignant ascites
	Pericarditis
	Pneumonia
	Polyarteritis nodosa
	Postoperative period
	Renal disease
	Rodent exposure (HAMA response)
	Systemic lupus erythematosus

HAMA, Human antimouse antibody.

Research identifying patterns of protein fragments (proteomics) in patients with ovarian carcinoma requires validation in larger trials and a cost-effective way to implement.

It has been suggested that every woman should have a periodic pelvic examination, pelvic ultrasound examination, and CA-125 test to make sure she does not harbor an occult ovarian cancer. Enthusiasm for early detection of ovarian cancer is laudable. However, it has been calculated that 10,000 routine pelvic examinations would be required to detect one early ovarian cancer in a population of asymptomatic patients. For a low-incidence cancer such as ovarian cancer, cost-effective screening strategies require a positive predictive value (PPV) greater than 10%. This generally requires a technique specificity of greater than 99%, with a high sensitivity of greater than 75%. The majority of early trials of screening techniques did not meet this metric. Jacobs and colleagues studied 22,000 postmenopausal women screened with CA-125 determinations and have reported follow-up observed for a mean of 6.76 years; 767 women (3.5%) had elevated CA-125 values, of whom 49 (6%, or 0.0022% of the total screened) had cancer. One-third of these were early stage. Overall specificity was 97%, and sensitivity at 1 year and 7 years of follow-up was 75% and 57%, respectively. The PPV of 3% was not high enough to be an effective screening method, and there is no current role for screening with CA-125 levels in unselected women. Many conditions of a benign nature, and most GI tract malignant neoplasms may elevate the CA-125 concentration (Table 11.8). The value of ultrasonography in screening for early ovarian carcinoma has received much attention. Campbell and coworkers reported early detection of five primary ovarian cancers in approximately 5000 women screened by abdominal ultrasonography (Table 11.9). DePriest and associates studied postmenopausal women or women with a family history of ovarian cancer (24% of women) with TVS. They screened 6470 women with 14,829 scans; 90 women had persistent abnormalities on TVS and underwent surgery. Six primary ovarian cancers were found (five stage I and one stage

TABLE 11.9   Stage and Prevalence of Screen-Detected Primary Ovarian Cancer in 20 Prospective Screenings

	Screened	Prevalence of Detected Primary Cancer	Screen-Detected Cancers per 100,000	Stage I
GENERAL POPULATION				
Ultrasonography	15,834	8	51	6
Exclude LMP	6	38	4	
Multimodal*	27,560	14	51	7
Exclude LMP	13	47	6	
HIGH-RISK POPULATION				
Ultrasonography[†]	4551	21	461	12
With family history	3146	15	477	9
Exclude LMP		8	254	2

LMP, Low malignant potential.
*CA-125.
†With or without CA-125.
From Bell R, Petticrew M, Sheldon T. The performance of screening tests for ovarian cancer: results of a systematic review. Br J Obstet Gynaecol 1998;105:1136.

IIIb), and only four were epithelial. Sensitivity was 86%, and specificity was 99%, with a PPV of only 7% but with a negative predictive value (NPV) of 99.9%.

One strategy to improve the effectiveness of ovarian cancer screening would be to target populations at increased risk for the development of the disease, such as individuals with a positive family history of ovarian cancer. Bourne and colleagues reported the results of such a strategy in screening patients with TVS in combination with color-flow Doppler imaging and morphologic assessment. In the screening of 1601 patients, 57% required repeated TVS to confirm the presence of a mass. Six ovarian cancers were diagnosed (two stage I, three low malignant potential tumors, and one stage III). Karlan and associates reported screening of 597 patients with a family history of cancer by CA-125 measurement, TVS, and color-flow Doppler imaging. Initially, 115 patients had an abnormal finding on TVS, and 68 had abnormal CA-125 levels. After repeated TVS, because of abnormal findings of color-flow Doppler imaging, 19 patients underwent surgery. At the time of the report, one low malignant potential tumor had been diagnosed.

Bell and colleagues reviewed 25 studies on screening for ovarian cancer, 16 studies on women at average risk, and nine studies on women at higher risk. Many studies were limited by small numbers, imprecise methodology, scant follow-up, and single versus multimodality screening techniques. For women at average risk, 75% of primary cancers were stage I when they were detected with ultrasonography, and 50% were stage I when they were detected by multimodal screening (see Table 11.9). In women at higher risk, if low malignant potential tumors were excluded, only 25% were stage I. False-negative rates were also higher in the higher risk population than in the group at average risk. The false-negative data, when applied to a population with an annual incidence of 40 per 100,000, imply that 30 to 60 surgical procedures would be carried out for every cancer detected at annual gray-scale ultrasonography (assuming 100% sensitivity), and 2.5 to 15 surgical procedures would be carried out for every cancer detected by multimodal screening. Even if screening detects all ovarian cancers and these are treated with 100% success, the absolute reduction in mortality would be only 1 in about 2500 screened women per year. This is much smaller than the complication rate from unnecessary diagnostic surgery or recall for further tests.

Combining CA-125 levels with TVS has been explored as a means by which to improve predictive value. Skates and colleagues developed a risk of ovarian cancer (ROC) algorithm based on rising CA-125 that has been validated in a prospective cohort. Their initial validation PPV was high (19%); it has been applied to two large prospective trials. Buys and associates reported the ovarian portion of the Prostate, Lung, Colorectal and Ovarian Cancer (PLCO) trial, which randomized 78,216 women aged 55 to 74 years to annual screening with CA-125 and ultrasound versus usual care for up to 13 years. There was no reduction in the ovarian cancer mortality rate, and there was a 15% incidence of serious surgical complications in patients undergoing surgery for false-positive results. Retrospective application of the ROC algorithm by Pinsky and associates failed to show a survival benefit. Recently, Jacobs and colleagues

reported results from the UK Collaborative Trial of Ovarian Cancer Screening (UKCTOCS), which randomized 202,638 women aged 50 to 74 years to annual multimodality screening (MMS) with CA-125 interpreted with the ROC algorithm, annual ultrasound screening, or no screening. Although the incidence of ovarian cancer and mortality was similar in the primary analysis, there was a significant mortality reduction with MMS in patients who lived longer than 7 years, likely because of detection of earlier stage cancers. These results require further follow-up, cost-effectiveness strategies, and validation in daily practice but give some further insight into early detection strategies.

Currently, however, there are no reliable data that screening for ovarian cancer is effective in improving length and quality of life in women with ovarian cancer. Another strategy to improve sensitivity and specificity in screening for ovarian cancer involves the use of multiple serum tumor markers. Because fewer than 50% of patients with stage I ovarian cancer will have an elevated CA-125 concentration and because CA-125 can be elevated by benign and malignant conditions, the addition of other markers in the screening strategy could potentially improve predictive value. Yurkovetsky and colleagues reported the results of their screening panel of four biomarkers, with 86% sensitivity at 98% specificity for detecting early-stage disease, and additional studies looking at additional biomarkers are ongoing. These techniques may also offer useful guidelines for predicting therapeutic response and for treatment selection. The NIH Consensus Development Conference on ovarian cancer screening in 1994 reached the following conclusions: There is no evidence available yet that the current screening modalities of CA-125 measurement and TVS can be used effectively for widespread screening to reduce mortality from ovarian cancer or that their use will result in decreased rather than increased morbidity and mortality. Routine screening has resulted in unnecessary surgery with associated risks. Clearly, it is important to identify and validate effective screening modalities. Currently available technology for screening should be used in the context of clinical trials to determine the efficacy of these modalities and their effect on ovarian cancer mortality. In addition, research must be continued to identify additional markers and imaging techniques that will be useful. Although these same recommendations still hold, we may have better techniques for screening because the data from ongoing trials mature. If a woman has one first-degree relative with ovarian cancer (making her lifetime risk of developing the disease 5%) but no clinical trials are available to her, she may think that despite the absence of prospective data, this is sufficient risk for her to be screened. This opportunity for screening should be available to the woman and her physician.

If a woman were undergoing pelvic surgery, removal of the ovaries at that time would almost fully eliminate her risk of ovarian cancer (although there remains a small risk of peritoneal cancer). If the woman is premenopausal, discussion of estrogen replacement therapy is important before removal of the ovaries because the risk of premature menopause and the potential for osteoporosis may outweigh the risk of ovarian conservation and the potential for ovarian cancer.

DIAGNOSTIC TECHNIQUES AND STAGING

Routine pelvic examinations detect only one ovarian cancer in 10,000 asymptomatic women. However, pelvic examination remains the most practical means of detecting early disease. Pain is usually a late complication; it is seen with early disease only in association with a complication such as torsion; rupture; or, rarely, infection. The physician should have a high index of suspicion for an early ovarian neoplasm in any ovary palpated in a menopausal patient. These patients should be considered for immediate laparoscopy or laparotomy when ultrasound examination findings suggest malignant change (eg, complex mass, >5 cm, or intracystic papillations).

To help with evaluating a patient with a complex pelvic mass, the American College of Obstetricians and Gynecologists (ACOG), in conjunction with the SGO, published guidelines in 2002 that could help direct referral to or consultation with a gynecologic oncologist. Physicians should perform a pelvic examination and imaging as appropriate for the patient's symptoms or physical examination findings. For premenopausal women with a suspicious pelvic mass, referral to a gynecologic oncologist should be considered by at least one of the following: CA-125 level higher than 200 U/mL, ascites, abdominal or distant metastases, or one or more first-degree relatives with breast or ovarian cancer. For postmenopausal women with a concerning pelvic mass, consultation should be considered for any CA-125 elevation, ascites, nodularity or limited mobility, evidence of metastasis, or a first-degree relative with breast or ovarian cancer.

Routine laboratory tests are not of great value in the diagnosis of ovarian cancer but may help rule out other pelvic disorders. Pelvic ultrasonography may reveal calcifications consistent with myomas or benign teratomas. Colonoscopy and upper GI endoscopy may be helpful in patients who have lower or upper intestinal symptoms, respectively. Computed tomography (CT) with contrast enhancement may be helpful in identifying the extent of clinical disease. No imaging modality is conclusive, however, and suspicious pelvic masses, especially in postmenopausal women, should be evaluated surgically. In general, we recommend against needle biopsy of ovarian masses because such a procedure can result in spillage of malignant cells into the peritoneal cavity. Regardless of whether the fluid contains neoplastic cells, surgery will likely still be necessary to remove either the large benign neoplasm or to define the extent of the malignant process. In addition, up to 50% of ascitic fluid samples from patients with true ovarian malignant neoplasms will be negative for malignant cells on cell block analysis. Needle biopsy in a patient with a pelvic abdominal mass is therefore both unnecessary and potentially dangerous (Fig. 11.5).

The staging of ovarian cancer is surgical (Table 11.10) and based on the surgical and pathologic findings (Fig. 11.6). A longitudinal midline incision is recommended to remove the neoplasm and to visualize the entire abdominal cavity, including the undersurface of the diaphragm. A Pfannenstiel incision is ill advised in a patient suspected of having an ovarian malignancy. Ovarian cancer classically involves the entire peritoneal cavity (Fig. 11.7). Although lymphatic spread to retroperitoneal

FIGURE 11.5 Large cystic tumors, similar to the illustration, are at risk of perforation and leakage at the time of paracentesis.

nodes is common in ovarian cancer, the disease most often spreads intraperitoneally; free-floating cells shed from the primary tumor are capable of implanting on any peritoneal surface. Any peritoneal fluid (ascites) found when the peritoneal cavity is opened should be aspirated and submitted for cytologic examination. In the absence of peritoneal fluid, washings should be taken by lavage of the peritoneal surfaces, including the undersurface of the diaphragm (Fig. 11.8). Care should be taken to visualize and palpate all peritoneal surfaces, particularly the diaphragm, the surface of the liver, the lateral abdominal gutters, and the small and large bowel mesentery. The omentum should be removed because microscopic disease is often present in the omentum that is not obvious grossly. Recommended surgical therapy is presented in sequence in Table 11.11. If the disease is limited to the pelvis, the primary tumor should be removed intact. All suspicious surfaces in the peritoneal cavity should be removed as biopsy specimens. This includes adhesions, which should be excised, not incised, because they often contain microscopic disease. Several studies have been performed to investigate the efficacy of "blind" peritoneal biopsies and routine retroperitoneal node dissections in the proper staging of early epithelial cancer of the ovary (Table 11.12). Proper staging is important for treatment planning and for providing an accurate prognosis (Table 11.13).

THERAPEUTIC OPTIONS FOR PRIMARY TREATMENT

Borderline Malignant Epithelial Neoplasms

Over the past 4 decades, investigators have described a subset of epithelial ovarian tumors whose histologic and biologic features lie between those of clearly benign and frankly malignant ovarian neoplasms. These borderline malignant neoplasms account for approximately 15% of all epithelial ovarian cancers and share molecular characteristics with low-grade ovarian cancers. They have also been called proliferative cystadenomas

TABLE 11.10 Carcinoma of the Ovary: Staging Classification Using the Federation of International Gynecologists and Obstetricians (FIGO) Nomenclature

FIGO Stage	Description
I	Tumor confined to ovaries or fallopian tube(s)
IA	Tumor limited to one ovary (capsule intact) or fallopian tube; no tumor on ovarian or fallopian tube surface; no malignant cells in the ascites or peritoneal washings
IB	Tumor limited to both ovaries (capsules intact) or fallopian tubes; no tumor on ovarian or fallopian tube surface; no malignant cells in the ascites or peritoneal washings
IC	Tumor limited to one or both ovaries or fallopian tubes, with any of the following:
	IC1: Surgical spill
	IC2: Capsule ruptured before surgery or tumor on ovarian or fallopian tube surface
	IC3: Malignant cells in the ascites or peritoneal washings
II	Tumor involves one or both ovaries or fallopian tubes with pelvic extension (below pelvic brim) or primary peritoneal cancer
IIA	Extension and/or implants on uterus and/or fallopian tubes and/or ovaries
IIB	Extension to other pelvic intraperitoneal tissues
III	Tumor involves one or both ovaries or fallopian tubes or primary peritoneal cancer with cytologically or histologically confirmed spread to the peritoneum outside the pelvis and/or metastasis to the retroperitoneal lymph nodes
IIIA	IIIA1: Positive retroperitoneal lymph nodes only (cytologically or histologically proven):
	IIIA1(i) Metastasis ≤10 mm in greatest dimension
	IIIA1(ii) Metastasis >10 mm in greatest dimension
	IIIA2: Microscopic extrapelvic (above the pelvic brim) peritoneal involvement with or without positive retroperitoneal lymph nodes
IIIB	Macroscopic peritoneal metastasis beyond the pelvis ≤2 cm in greatest dimension, with or without metastasis to the retroperitoneal lymph nodes
IIIC	Macroscopic peritoneal metastasis beyond the pelvis >2 cm in greatest dimension, with or without metastasis to the retroperitoneal lymph nodes (includes extension of tumor to capsule of liver and spleen without parenchymal involvement of either organ)
IV	Distant metastasis excluding peritoneal metastases
	Stage IVA: Pleural effusion with positive cytology
	Stage IVB: Parenchymal metastases and metastases to extra-abdominal organs (including inguinal lymph nodes and lymph nodes outside of the abdominal cavity)

From International Federation of Gynecology and Obstetrics. Staging classification for cancer of the ovary, fallopian tube, and peritoneum. *Int J Gynecol Obstet* 2014;124:1.

TABLE 11.11 Surgical Therapy in Ovarian Cancer

Peritoneal cytologic examination
Determination of extent of disease
- Pelvis
- Peritoneal surfaces
- Diaphragms
- Omentum
- Lymph nodes
Removal of all tumor possible (total abdominal hysterectomy and bilateral salpingo-oophorectomy) plus node sampling and omentectomy

and tumors of low malignant potential and are more completely discussed in Chapter 10. Compared with invasive epithelial ovarian cancer, epithelial borderline tumors affect a younger population and may have a 10-year survival rate approaching 95% (see Chapter 10). Although symptomatic recurrence and death may rarely develop as late as 20 years after therapy, these neoplasms are correctly labeled as being of low malignant potential. Most gynecologic oncologists recommend conservative therapy, especially in patients who are desirous of further childbearing and have stage IA disease (see Chapter 10). We have found surgical excision of disease the most effective therapy and when necessary have used repeated explorations, reserving chemotherapy for patients who develop ascites or whose tumor changes histologic features or demonstrates rapid growth (Fig. 11.9).

Treatment of Malignant Epithelial Neoplasms

The most common epithelial cancers of the ovary are histologically categorized as serous, mucinous, endometrioid, and clear cell (mesonephroid) types (Figs. 11.10 to 11.13). Most large studies demonstrate that these different histologic types have similar outcomes with existing therapy, stage for stage and grade for grade. Mucinous and endometrioid subtypes are more commonly found in earlier stages. There are ongoing studies to investigate targeted therapies in certain cell types, most notably mucinous and clear cell cancers. Based on our current data, however, prognosis, survival, and therapy for these various forms of epithelial cancer will be considered collectively.

The unifocal theory of ovarian epithelial cancer growth suggests that the disease initially grows locally, invading the capsule and mesovarium, and then invades adjacent organs by local extension and lymphatic spread. Cells on the surface exfoliate into the peritoneal cavity, where they circulate and implant on free peritoneal surfaces. Local and regional lymphatic metastasis may involve the uterus, fallopian tubes, and pelvic and aortic lymph nodes.

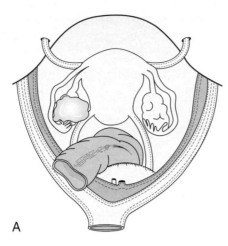

A

One ovary, capsule intact; no tumor on ovarian surface

B

Both ovaries, capsule intact; no tumor on ovarian surface

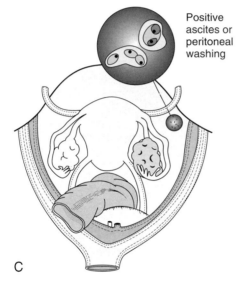

Positive ascites or peritoneal washing

C

One or both ovaries with capsule ruptured or tumor on ovarian surface; malignant cells in ascites or peritoneal washings

D

Extension and/or implants on uterus and/or tubes; adnexae

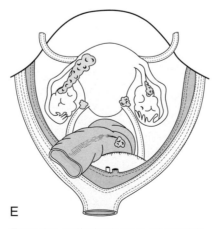

E

Extension and/or implants to other pelvic tissues; pelvic wall, broad ligament, adjacent peritoneum, mesovarium

FIGURE 11.6 Ovarian epithelial carcinoma. **A,** Stage Ia. **B,** Stage Ib. Ovarian epithelial carcinoma. **C,** Stage Ic. **D,** Stage IIa. **E,** Stage IIb. Ovarian epithelial carcinoma.

Positive ascites or peritoneal washing

Stage IIIa: microscopic peritoneal metastasis beyond pelvis, including peritoneal surface of liver

Stage IIIb: macroscopic peritoneal metastasis beyond pelvis <2 cm in greatest dimension, including peritoneal surface of liver

F

Extension and/or implants to other pelvic tissues with malignant cells in ascites or peritoneal washings

G

Tumor on liver capsule

Omental cake

Lymph node metastases

Pleural fluid (positive cytology)

Lung parenchymal metastases

Liver parenchymal metastases

H

Peritoneal metastasis beyond pelvis >2 cm in greatest dimension and/or regional lymph node metastasis

I

FIGURE 11.6, cont'd **F**, Stage IIc. **G**, Stages IIIa and IIIb. **H**, Stage IIIc. **I**, Stage IV.

Woodruff suggested a multifocal mechanism of disease spread, whereby the entire coelomic epithelium can give rise to this lesion after exposure to carcinogenic agents that enter the peritoneal cavity from the vagina through the fallopian tubes. Indeed, the lesion could then originate in a multifocal distribution, "like a measles rash," over large portions of the coelomic epithelium. Although the early precursors leading to advanced ovarian cancer are incompletely understood, more current molecular evidence favors the unifocal origin theory.

In the past decade, as risk-reducing salpingo-oophorectomy has become more common, a moderate body of literature suggests that a significant percentage of "ovarian cancers" may actually arise in the fallopian tube fimbria with metastasis to the ovaries. Kindelberger and colleagues have reported a potential causal relationship based on identification of tubal intraepithelial carcinomas (TIC) and analysis of p53 mutations therein. Regardless of origin, the most important prognostic variable for each patient is the extent, or "stage," of disease. A staging

TABLE 11.12 Aortic Lymph Node Metastases in Epithelial Ovarian Cancer

	Stage I		Stage II		Stages III and IV		
Series	Positive Lymphangiography	Positive Biopsy	Positive Lymphangiography	Positive Biopsy	Positive Lymphangiography	Positive Biopsy	Total
Hanks and Bagshaw (1969)	2/9	—	2/6	—	4/7	—	8/22
Parker et al. (1974)	3/13	—	2/29	—	12/27	—	17/69
Knapp and Friedman (1974)	—	5/26	—	—	—	—	—
Delgado et al. (1977)	1/5	—	1/5	—	—	3/5	2/10
Buchsbaum et al. (1989)*	—	4/95	—	8/41	—	7/46	—
Burghardt (1991)	—	1/20	—	4/7	—	51/78	—
Total	**10/141**	**12/48**	**61/129**				

*All patients had optimal carcinoma with metastatic lesions smaller than 3 cm.

TABLE 11.13 Carcinoma of the Ovary, Obviously Malignant Cases, All Histopathologic Classes: 5-Year Actuarial Survival by Stage

Stage	Patients (n)	5-Year Survival (%)
Ia	632	89
Ib	69	86
Ic	663	83
IIa	72	70
IIb	93	65
IIc	241	71
IIIa	128	46
IIIb	271	41
IIIc	2030	32
IV	626	18

From Heintz APM, Odicino F, Maisonneuve P, et al. Carcinoma of the ovary. FIGO 26th Annual Report on the Results of Treatment in Gynecological Cancer. *Int J Gynaecol Obstet* 2006;95(suppl 1): S161-192.

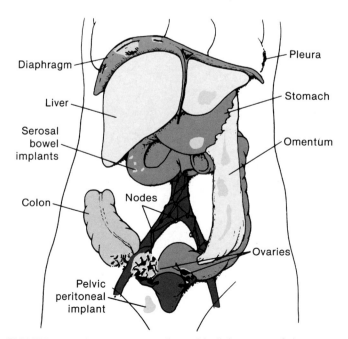

FIGURE 11.7 Spread pattern for epithelial cancer of the ovary. (From DiSaia PJ. Diagnosis and management of ovarian cancer. *Hosp Pract [Off Ed]* 1987;22:235.)

FIGURE 11.8 Technique of obtaining subdiaphragmatic cytologic washings at laparotomy. Saline lavage of the space between the diaphragm and the dome of the liver is easily accomplished; fluid pockets collecting in the lateral recesses are aspirated with a bulb syringe.

system has been devised that allows treatment results in patients with similar prognostic factors to be compared among different institutions. Survival is affected by the cancer stage, grade of differentiation, gross findings at surgery (Table 11.14), amount of residual tumor after surgery, and additional treatment required.

Stages IA, IB, and IC

Careful surgical staging is critical in the management of stage I invasive ovarian cancer and should include bilateral salpingo-oophorectomy, hysterectomy, omentectomy, and pelvic and aortic lymph node sampling, with peritoneal biopsies and washings. Accurate staging forms the cornerstone of clinical decision-making regarding the type and duration of adjuvant therapy.

Pelvic and aortic lymph nodes may be involved 10% to 20% of the time in apparent stage I disease, and lymphadenectomy

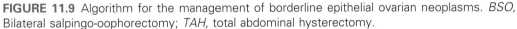

FIGURE 11.9 Algorithm for the management of borderline epithelial ovarian neoplasms. *BSO,* Bilateral salpingo-oophorectomy; *TAH,* total abdominal hysterectomy.

FIGURE 11.10 Papillary serous adenocarcinoma of ovary. Histologic appearance with prominent fibrous stalks and non–mucin-producing epithelial cells.

FIGURE 11.12 Endometrioid adenocarcinoma of the ovary. Histologic appearance with columnar and pseudostratified epithelial cells showing prominent elongated hyperchromatic nuclei.

FIGURE 11.11 Mucinous adenocarcinoma of ovary. Microscopic appearance. Note the tall, columnar, mucin-producing cells.

FIGURE 11.13 Clear cell adenocarcinoma of the ovary. Microscopic view showing hobnail or peg cells.

TABLE 11.14 Guidelines for Staging in Epithelial Ovarian Cancer

Four peritoneal washings (diaphragm, right and left abdomen, pelvis)
Careful inspection and palpation of all peritoneal surfaces
Biopsy or smear from undersurface of right hemidiaphragm
Biopsy of all suspicious lesions
Infracolic omentectomy
Biopsy or resection of any adhesions
Random biopsy of normal peritoneum of bladder reflection cul de sac, right and left paracolic recesses, and both pelvic sidewalls (in the absence of obvious implants)
Selected lymphadenectomy of pelvic and paraaortic nodes
Total abdominal hysterectomy, bilateral salpingo-oophorectomy, and excision of masses when prudent

TABLE 11.15 Lymph Node Metastasis in Stage I Ovarian Cancer

Author	Patients
Di Re	16/128
Benedetti–Panici	5/25
Wu	1/7
Burghardt et al.	9/37
Petru	9/40
Knapp and Friedman	5/26
Tsuruchi	1/51
Chen et al.	3/11
Lanza	3/11
Carnino	2/47
Baiocchi	32/242
	86/625 (13.7%)

TABLE 11.16 Frequency of Subclinical Metastasis in Patients With Presumed Early-Stage Ovarian Cancer (Based on 14 Studies)

Localization	Frequency (%)	Range (%)
Peritoneal cytology	22	10–46
Diaphragm	9	0–44
Omentum	5	0.7
Pelvic nodes	8	0–20
Paraaortic nodes	12	0–25
Pelvic peritoneum	9	6–10
Abdominal peritoneum	8	7–9
Bowel mesentery-serosa	6	3–13

is an important diagnostic and therapeutic procedure. Baiocchi and associates reviewed their experience in 242 women who had pelvic and aortic lymphadenectomy in whom cancer was apparently confined to the ovaries (stage I), and nodal metastasis was found in 32 patients (13%). Patients with serous adenocarcinoma had the highest incidence of node metastasis (25%). Those with grade III lesions had 39% metastasis compared with 6% with grade I and grade II cancers. There were 33 women with low malignant potential tumors, and seven (21%) had nodal metastasis. When only one to three nodes were involved, metastases were usually ipsilateral, but these patients could also have metastases to the common iliac or aortic nodes. Positive aortic nodes were also found in the absence of positive pelvic nodes. Accumulated reports of lymph node metastases in clinical stage I ovarian cancer patients are shown in Table 11.15. Without thorough surgical staging, occult metastasis may be present and missed, leading to inadequate subsequent therapy. Many studies have addressed this item (Table 11.16).

The use of adjuvant therapy and its role in stage I ovarian cancer continues to be investigated. Through three GOG studies in early-stage (I and II) ovarian cancer, the use of platinum combination therapy became the preferred regimen as it demonstrated better survival outcomes and an improved, although

not statistically significant, toxicity profile over intraperitoneal (IP) colloid 32P.

European investigators have also reported their experience with platinum-based therapy in early-stage ovarian cancer. The European gynecologic groups reported a combined analysis of the International Collaborative Ovarian Neoplasm (ICON) 1 and the Adjuvant Chemotherapy In Ovarian Neoplasm (ACTION) trials. More than 900 patients with early-stage ovarian cancer received either platinum-based adjuvant chemotherapy or observation until chemotherapy was indicated. After a median follow-up period of more than 4 years, the improved overall survival (OS) (82% chemotherapy vs. 74% observation) and recurrence-free survival (76% vs. 65%, respectively) rates at 5 years favored treatment with platinum-based therapy. Although not all patients had undergone comprehensive staging, a subgroup analysis of these patients was reported. In another European Organization for Research and Treatment of Cancer (EORTC)-ACTION trial of 448 patients, the authors noted that the benefit of chemotherapy was limited to patients who lacked comprehensive surgical staging, questioning the necessity of adjuvant therapy in the patient with well-staged early ovarian carcinoma.

The next evolution of GOG trials involved the addition of paclitaxel to a platinum-based regimen because the treatment protocols for advanced-stage disease had demonstrated improved survival by replacing cyclophosphamide with paclitaxel. GOG 157 evaluated carboplatin (AUC 7.5) and paclitaxel (175 mg/m^2) in high-risk, early-stage disease, randomly assigning patients to three versus six chemotherapy cycles. Over a 3-year interval, 457 patients were enrolled and evaluated after a median follow-up period of 6.8 years. Although the recurrence rate was 24% lower with the six cycles ($P = 0.18$), OS was similar for the two arms (hazard ratio [HR], 1.02). The study concluded that the additional three cycles contributed to increased toxicity (11% grade III/IV neurotoxicity vs. 2% with only three cycles) without an OS advantage. Building on the hypothesis that low-dose paclitaxel may have antiangiogenesis activity, GOG 175 tested whether the addition of 24 weekly paclitaxel treatments (60 mg/m^2) to the initial three cycles of carboplatin and paclitaxel would improve outcomes. Although the recurrence rate was 20% lower in patients receiving extended paclitaxel, the result was not statistically significant, and there was no appreciable difference in OS.

In the young woman with stage IA disease who is desirous of further childbearing, unilateral salpingo-oophorectomy may be associated with minimal increased risk of recurrence, provided a careful staging procedure is performed and due consideration is given to grade and apparent self-containment of the neoplasm. After conservative treatment for invasive ovarian cancer, term delivery rates have been reported as high as 30%, and successful pregnancy outcomes have been reported after adjuvant chemotherapy. Conservative surgery is generally not recommended for patients with clear cell or carcinosarcoma or grade III tumors and when disease is present outside the ovaries. A careful discussion regarding the risks and benefits of this approach is essential because Maltaris and colleagues reported that 12% of patients undergoing fertility-sparing ovarian cancer surgery experienced recurrence, and 4% of patients died from their disease.

In the management of stage I ovarian cancer, the physician must weigh the possible benefits of adjuvant chemotherapy against the risks. It appears reasonable to not recommend adjuvant therapy for patients with stage IA, IB, grade 1 and 2 lesions who have been comprehensively staged. Patients with stage I, grade 3 and stage IC disease present a more difficult problem because the incidence of recurrence in this group approaches 50% in some series. We favor treatment with platinum-based combination chemotherapy even though no clear data show a survival advantage over single-agent therapy. Because combination therapy is our best treatment for metastatic disease, it is difficult to withhold the apparent best therapy from a group of patients who may have the best situation for a chemotherapy "cure." In addition, this group is usually younger and better able to tolerate combination chemotherapy.

Stages IIA, IIB, and IIC

In most institutions, the therapy of choice for stage IIA and stage IIB disease is staging surgery followed by platinum-based combination chemotherapy. Although historically the role of pelvic and abdominal irradiation and IP 32P has been described, the radioisotope and irradiation treatment approaches have faded from frontline therapy for ovarian carcinoma. Careful surgical staging is essential to successful treatment planning. A combined analysis of GOG 95 and 157 revealed that the stage II patients represented a disproportionate percentage of the recurrences. The GOG now includes stage II patients in their clinical trials of patients with advanced-stage disease. Outside of a clinical trial, patients with stage II disease should be managed in a similar fashion to optimally debulked stage III disease.

Stage III

In addition to surgical staging, every reasonable effort should be made to remove all visible metastatic tumors. Retrospective studies have strongly suggested that the survival rate in patients with stage III disease is related to the amount of residual tumor after surgery, such that patients with no macroscopic residual tumor appear to have the best prognosis after primary chemotherapy (Table 11.17 and Fig. 11.14). Most centers prefer combination platinum-based chemotherapy for this group of patients because of the excellent response rates reported in the literature (see later section on combination chemotherapy and IP therapy).

The duration of multiple-agent therapy is usually six cycles. If after primary chemotherapy the patient has no clinical evidence of disease (clinical complete response), a second-look procedure was often considered in the past to ascertain the presence of subclinical residual disease. However, a secondary data analysis of GOG 158 suggested no apparent outcome advantage from second-look surgery. For the most part, second-look surgery is no longer recommended.

Stage IV

The ideal management of stage IV disease is to remove as much cancer as possible and to administer chemotherapy after

TABLE 11.17 Relationship of Residual Tumor Size and Median Survival (Months)

Author	Patients (n)	Optimal (<2 cm)	Suboptimal (>2 cm)
Griffiths et al.	102	28	11
Wharton et al.	104	27	15
Hacker et al.	47	22	6
Sutton et al.	56	39	22

FIGURE 11.14 Survival in patients with stage IIIc disease by completeness of surgery (n = 1059). (From International Federation of Gynecology and Obstetrics. *Annual Report on the Results of Treatment in Gynecological Cancer,* vol 23. Stockholm, 1998, Author.)

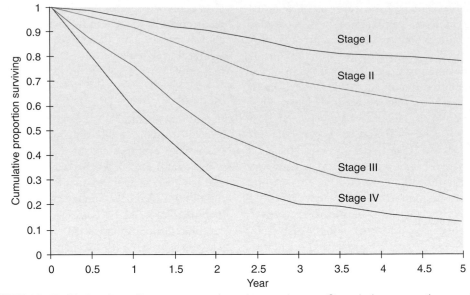

FIGURE 11.15 Obviously malignant cases of ovarian carcinoma. Cumulative proportion surviving by stage. (From International Federation of Gynecology and Obstetrics. *Annual Report on the Results of Treatment in Gynecological Cancer,* vol 22. Stockholm, 1994, Author.)

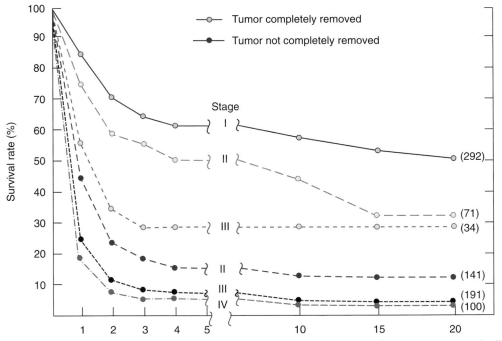

FIGURE 11.16 Survival rates stage for stage in patients in whom all tumor was surgically removed versus patients in whom not all tumor was completely removed. (From Aure JC, Hoeg K, Kolstad P. Clinical and histologic studies of ovarian carcinoma. Long-term follow-up of 990 cases. *Obstet Gynecol* 1971;37:1.)

surgery. The role and benefit of surgical cytoreduction in these patients is detailed in the next section. The OS is worse for this group of patients than for those of other stages, as expected (Fig. 11.15).

Maximal Surgical Effort

The goal of primary surgery for advanced ovarian cancer should be to remove all visible tumor and to use all reasonable surgical means to do so (Fig. 11.16). In the 1970s, Griffiths and coworkers evaluated the importance of postsurgical tumor residual by using a multiple linear regression equation with survival as the dependent variable to control simultaneously for the multiple therapeutic and biologic factors that contribute to the ultimate outcome in the individual patient. The most important factors proved to be histologic grade of the tumor and size of the largest residual mass after primary surgery. In Griffiths et al.'s original study, the operation itself contributed nothing to survival unless it effected reduction in the size of the largest residual tumor mass below the limit of 1.6 cm.

Cytoreductive or "debulking" procedures have gained considerable attention in the management of ovarian cancer. The concept is to reduce the residual tumor burden to a level at which subsequent chemotherapy can be most effective. A careful dissection by a well-trained gynecologic oncologist can often remove disease that on first impression appear to be unresectable (Fig. 11.17). Removal of large ovarian masses and omental involvement may reduce the tumor burden by 80% to 99%. The

theoretical value of debulking procedures lies in reducing the number of tumor cells and the advantage this affords to adjuvant therapy. This is especially relevant in bulky chemosensitive solid tumors such as ovarian cancer, in which removal of large numbers of cells in the resting phase (G0) may propel the residual cells into the more vulnerable proliferating phases. Several careful retrospective studies have repeatedly demonstrated improved survival rates in patients who can be surgically reduced to minimal tumor burden. The GOG has attempted to better define primary cytoreductive surgery with a detailed analysis of the results of surgery in patients with advanced disease. Their initial study compared survival of the patients with stage III disease who were found at surgery to have abdominal disease of 1 cm or smaller with that of patients found to have disease larger than 1 cm but whose tumors were surgically cytoreduced to 1 cm or less. If surgery was the only important factor, survival should have been equivalent in both groups. This was not the case. Patients found to have small-volume disease survived longer than did patients who had cytoreduction to small-volume disease at surgery, suggesting that the tumor biology also carries prognostic significance. In a second study, GOG investigators evaluated the effect of the diameter of the largest residual disease on survival in patients with suboptimal cytoreduction. They demonstrated that cytoreduction so that the largest residual mass was 2 cm or less resulted in a significant survival benefit, but all residual diameters larger than 2 cm had equivalent survival (Fig. 11.18). Therefore, unless the mass could be cytoreduced to 2 cm or less, residual diameter did not influence survival. In evaluating

FIGURE 11.17 A large omental cake of ovarian cancer exceeding 25 cm in greatest measurement.

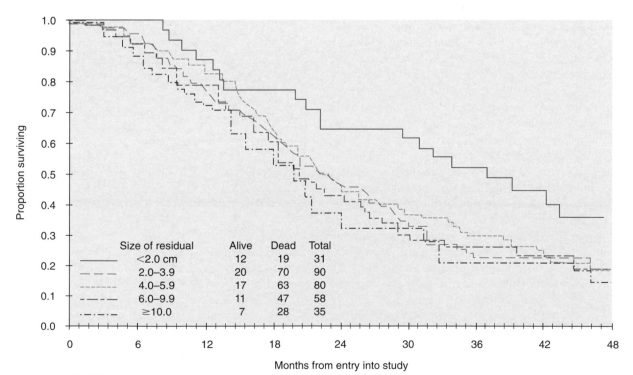

Size of residual	Alive	Dead	Total
<2.0 cm	12	19	31
2.0–3.9	20	70	90
4.0–5.9	17	63	80
6.0–9.9	11	47	58
≥10.0	7	28	35

FIGURE 11.18 Survival by maximal diameter of residual disease. (From Hoskins WJ, McGuire WP, Brady MF, et al. The effect of diameter of largest residual disease on survival after primary cytoreductive surgery in patients with suboptimal residual epithelial ovarian carcinoma. *Am J Obstet Gynecol* 1994;170:974.)

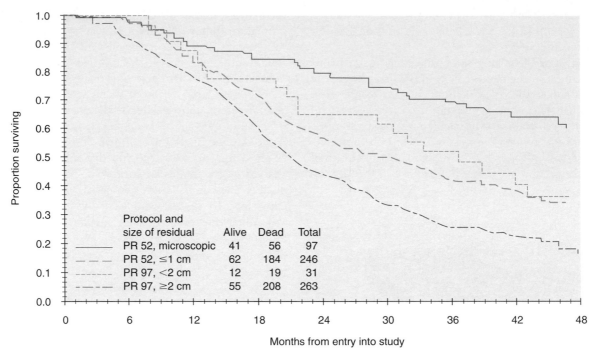

FIGURE 11.19 Survival by residual disease, Gynecologic Oncology Group protocols (PR) 52 and 97. (From Hoskins WJ, McGuire WP, Brady MF, et al. The effect of diameter of largest residual disease on survival after primary cytoreductive surgery in patients with suboptimal residual epithelial ovarian carcinoma. *Am J Obstet Gynecol* 1994;170:974.)

optimal and suboptimal cytoreduction, these GOG investigators showed that three distinct groups emerged: microscopic (no visible) residual, residual disease of less than 2 cm, and residual disease of greater than 2 cm (Fig. 11.19). It is clear from these studies that whereas patients with microscopic disease had a 4-year survival rate of about 60%, patients with gross disease 2 cm or less had a 4-year survival rate of 35%. However, patients whose disease could not be cytoreduced to 2 cm or less had a 4-year survival rate of less than 20%. Most striking, however, was the failure of cytoreductive surgery to improve survival unless the largest diameter of residual disease was 2 cm or less. The effect of maximal cytoreductive surgery can be seen in the percentage of negative second-look procedures (Table 11.18).

An inverse correlation between the amount of residual disease after surgery and OS has been consistently associated. In 2002, Bristow and associates published a meta-analysis of published studies at the time, in which the impact of cytoreduction was clearly demonstrated. By comparing currently available studies of advanced ovarian cancer patients undergoing surgical cytoreduction, they demonstrated that for each 10% increase in the proportion of patients undergoing optimal cytoreduction, the median survival rate increased by 5.5% to 6%. Although the current accepted definition of "optimal cytoreduction" is no visible residual tumor smaller than 1 cm in greatest dimension, the best reported outcomes occur in patients who have complete cytoreduction or no visible residual disease.

In an effort to remove visible tumor deposits and achieve optimal cytoreduction, gynecologic oncologists frequently perform radical surgical procedures beyond those required for

TABLE 11.18 **The Effect of Cytoreductive Surgery on Residual Disease as Found by Second-Assessment Surgery**

Author (Year)	Negative Second Look (%)		
	No Residual	Optimal Residual	Suboptimal Residual
Barnhill (1984)	67	61	14
Cain (1986)	76	50	28
Smirz (1985)	75	—	25
Webb (1982)	95	36	20
Podratz (1983)	82	44	33
Curry (1981)	79	45	22
Dauplat (1983)	100	100	40
Hoskins (1989)	75	45	25
Mean	**81**	**52**	**23**

standard staging. Eisenkop and associates described 163 consecutive patients assigned to stage IIIC and stage IV. Complete cytoreduction could be performed in 86% of patients using an array of radical procedures. The overall median survival time was 54 months, but it was 62 months in those whose tumors were optimally debulked. Aletti and colleagues reported that for patients cytoreduced to low-volume residual disease, their favorable survival was directly associated with the need for radical surgery. Two sites that often require radical operations to clear are tumor metastases to the bowel and to the upper abdomen. Multiple investigators have reported the utility and safety of large or small bowel resection, which may be necessary in up to 50% of cases to achieve optimal cytoreduction and has been associated with a subsequent improvement in survival. Upper abdominal cytoreduction has also been shown to be safe and effective but may require additional training or assistance. Cliby and colleagues reported procedures such as liver resection, splenectomy, and diaphragm resection to be possible and associated with an acceptable morbidity. Chi and coinvestigators demonstrated that the addition of upper abdominal procedures to achieve optimal cytoreduction resulted in a median survival time longer than 5 years, which was comparable to that of patients who did not require these extensive procedures for optimal cytoreduction. Improvements in surgical cytoreduction have developed in consort with additional advances in intensive care and postoperative care, allowing additional benefits for our ovarian cancer patients.

The role of cytoreductive surgery in stage IV cancers has been investigated. Several studies have suggested that optimal debulking can be performed in many of these patients with beneficial effect. Liu and associates described 47 patients with stage IV cancers, of which 14 (30%) were optimally debulked to less than 2 cm residual. The median survival time was 37 months in the patients in whom the cancer was optimally debulked compared with 17 months in the patients in whom the cancer was suboptimally debulked. A study by Chi and colleagues identified 92 patients; optimal debulking was achieved in 45% with a median survival time of 40 months compared with 18 months for suboptimal debulking. A recent ancillary study by the GOG demonstrated that the ability to achieve cytoreduction to less than 5 cm residual disease in stage IV patients rendered some survival advantage, although the most favorable subgroup was patients reduced to no visible residual disease. Aletti and colleagues also demonstrated that using radical procedures to perform cytoreduction to no visible residual disease resulted in median survival times longer than 3 years in stage IV patients. For patients known or suspected to have thoracic metastases, the use of video-assisted thoracic surgery (VATS) can be diagnostic, potentially therapeutic, or both. Positive findings on VATS may allow for intrathoracic cytoreduction in select cases or may indicate which patients are best served with neoadjuvant chemotherapy as a result of unresectable pleural disease.

Even though cytoreductive surgery consistently appears to have therapeutic value, controversy continues. The primary unresolved issue is whether the poor prognosis with bulky disease is caused by the presence of increased tumor burden (in which case cytoreductive surgery is of potential benefit) or whether it is associated with differences in tumor biology or a decreased sensitivity to chemotherapeutic regimens. (If these possibilities are indeed the case, cytoreductive surgery is not likely to have a major impact on survival.) The implication is that patients who have disease that can be cytoreduced are a select group with good prognoses on the basis of factors independent of the surgery. Furthermore, if chemotherapy is delayed because of complications of surgery, this may have a deleterious effect on long-term survival. The percentage of patients with advanced ovarian cancer who can effectively undergo cytoreductive surgery seems to range from 43% to 87%, depending on the investigators reporting. This difference may not only reflect the individual skills of the surgeons but also may be influenced by different referral patterns and other selection factors. Neoadjuvant chemotherapy has been investigated as a means by which to address this issue; these studies are described in the subsequent section.

The role of lymphadenectomy in patients with advanced disease continues to be debated. Lymph node involvement is common in patients with advanced disease (>50%); the question is whether lymphadenectomy improves survival. It has been suggested by some that metastases in lymph nodes do not respond well to chemotherapy, and therefore these potential metastatic sites should be removed. Opponents state that recurrence most frequently occurs in the peritoneal cavity, and therefore lymph node status has little impact on the overall disease course. Several studies have come to somewhat different conclusions. Parazzini and associates evaluated 456 women with stage III or IV disease entered in a prospective randomized chemotherapy trial. There were 161 patients with positive nodes. They noted grade 3 tumors to have a greater number with positive nodes compared with grade 1 or grade 2 tumors. This was also true of stage IV compared with stage III cancer. They did not find a difference in survival between those with positive nodes and those with negative nodes. Scarabelli and colleagues evaluated lymph node status in 98 patients with stage IIIC to IV disease who had no gross residual disease after surgery compared with 44 patients who did not undergo lymphadenectomy. Survival was significantly improved if lymphadenectomy was done (Cox analysis). In 2005, Panici and coinvestigators reported their prospective multicenter analysis of 427 advanced ovarian cancer patients randomly assigned to lymphadenectomy or removal of bulky nodes only. Although progression-free survival (PFS) was improved in patients undergoing lymphadenectomy, OS was not different. The 2005 retrospective analysis of 889 patients enrolled in the Scottish Randomised Trial in Ovarian Cancer (SCOTROC-1) was conducted. The analysis demonstrated that optimal debulking (<2 cm) was more commonly achieved in patients accrued from the United States, Europe, and Australia than in patients recruited from the United Kingdom (71% vs. 58%). Comparison of the UK and non-UK patients who had no visible residual disease demonstrated a better survival for the non-UK patients, and the authors attributed this to the fact that non-UK patients more commonly underwent primary lymphadenectomy, suggesting a potential therapeutic benefit. It has been our practice to do pelvic and aortic lymphadenectomy routinely if the patient's tumor can be optimally debulked. Benefits of lymphadenectomy in patients with bulky residual disease remain questionable. It currently seems appropriate that patients with a diagnosis of advanced ovarian cancer should undergo resection of all masses when technically feasible.

Because a suboptimal surgical effort confers no survival benefit and adds only postoperative morbidity, accurate methods to determine which patients could be successfully resected would be useful. Both preoperative imaging and initial laparoscopy have been investigated as methods to determine the likelihood of success. Most imaging series have used preoperative CT scan to assess factors that could predict an optimal cytoreduction. Although sets of radiographic risk factors have been described, these have had poor predictive value because the majority of patients (62%–86%) identified as having "poor prognostic indicators" have been able to undergo optimal cytoreduction. Similarly, laparoscopy in advanced ovarian cancer has limitations in terms of how complete an assessment of the IP space is possible, and metastases at port sites have been reported. Wang and associates reviewed the literature to determine risk factors that may contribute to early recurrence at the port site. Of the gynecologic cancers, ovarian cancer was the most common malignant neoplasm with subsequent port site metastasis. Metastasis to the port site was more common if ascites and IP carcinomatosis were present. The earliest time from laparoscopy to port site metastasis was 8 days; however, the clinical significance of port site metastases is unclear because they often clinically resolve with systemic therapy.

Whether a suboptimal primary surgery can be improved upon by subsequent surgical cytoreduction after chemotherapy is controversial. The EORTC group reported its initial experience with interval debulking surgery in patients with advanced ovarian carcinoma after unsuccessful primary cytoreductive surgery. Patients received three courses of cisplatin and cyclophosphamide and were then randomly assigned to receive interval debulking surgery or no further surgery. All patients received six courses of chemotherapy. There were 278 patients evaluated, and the median survival rate was 26% versus 20% (surgery vs. no surgery; *P* = 0.012). Debulking surgery was an independent prognostic factor in multivariate analysis. After adjustment for all prognostic factors, surgery reduced the risk of death by 33% (*P* = 0.008). GOG investigators conducted a similar study. This study (GOG 152) enrolled 550 patients, all of whom had initial primary surgery by a gynecologic oncologist. Patients who were suboptimally debulked (residual tumor >1 cm) received three cycles of paclitaxel plus cisplatin. Patients were randomized to continued chemotherapy or to a secondary surgical cytoreduction and then continued chemotherapy. Neither the PFS nor the relative risk of death was improved with the additional interval surgery. The authors speculate that the patients in the GOG study may also have undergone more aggressive primary surgery than the patients in the EORTC study, and this may have accounted for the difference in results. Most important, one could summarize these two studies by concluding that patients with advanced ovarian cancer are deserving of at least one maximal effort at cytoreduction, preferably by a gynecologic oncologist.

Although a maximal primary surgical effort appears to be a cornerstone of potential long-term survival, the timing of the surgical effort remains a focus of debate. In patients with borderline performance status, based on age, compromising medical disease, and extensive effusions (especially pleural or pericardial), and in patients with extensive abdominal disease, unlikely to be effectively debulked, strong consideration should be given to initiating therapy with neoadjuvant chemotherapy. After two to four cycles, a good clinical response to chemotherapy may provide an opportunity for an effective surgical debulking with an acceptably low complication

rate. Before initiating chemotherapy, the diagnosis of ovarian, tubal, or peritoneal cancer should be confirmed by cytology or minimally invasive surgery. Neoadjuvant chemotherapy treatment (followed by surgical debulking) results have been reported in small retrospective reports of between 20 and 90 patients and generally report survival outcomes similar to those of patients who have been suboptimally cytoreduced. A meta-analysis of these studies by Bristow et al. and Chi et al. demonstrated that the use of neoadjuvant chemotherapy was associated with a reduction in survival of approximately 4 months with every preoperative cycle, implying that surgical intervention should be performed as soon as is feasible. However, Vergote and colleagues have reported results from the large randomized EORTC noninferiority trial of patients with advanced ovarian cancer treated with primary surgery followed by chemotherapy versus neoadjuvant chemotherapy for three cycles followed by surgical cytoreduction and three additional cycles of chemotherapy. Complete resection of all macroscopic disease was the strongest predictor of OS. They demonstrated comparable survival outcomes (~29 months in both arms), and overall the results favored neoadjuvant chemotherapy given the lower surgical morbidity compared with the primary surgery group. Another trial evaluating the role of neoadjuvant chemotherapy, Chemotherapy Or Upfront Surgery in Ovarian Cancer Patients (CHORUS), randomized women with stage III or IV ovarian cancer to receive upfront surgery followed by six cycles of chemotherapy (carboplatin and paclitaxel) or three cycles of chemotherapy, surgery, and then three additional cycles of completion chemotherapy. A total of 550 women were evaluated, and the OS time was 22.6 months in the primary surgery group compared with 24.1 months in the primary chemotherapy group. The authors also reported a lower rate of grade 3 or 4 postoperative adverse events and deaths in the primary chemotherapy group, concluding that the primary chemotherapy approach is noninferior to the primary surgery approach. Although the neoadjuvant approach is a reasonable option for some patients, it is important to recognize several criticisms to the study. Both studies reported low rates of primary optimal cytoreduction (~40% in both studies) and low median OS compared with other contemporary ovarian cancer trials. Therefore, neoadjuvant chemotherapy has not been widely adopted as an equivalent primary treatment option in the United States, and further studies are ongoing.

Role of Radiation Therapy

With improvements in chemotherapy and surgery for ovarian cancer, radiation therapy rarely plays a role in primary therapy. The systemic pattern of spread makes effective radiation therapy difficult, and with bulky residual disease, radiation therapy is particularly ineffective. Studies by the GOG and others demonstrated the extent to which the addition of radiation did not improve outcomes even before the current era of highly active chemotherapy. Some special problems are listed in Table 11.19. The entire abdomen must be considered at risk; therefore, the volume that must be irradiated is large, resulting in multiple limitations for the radiotherapist. However, consideration of

TABLE 11.19 Special Problems in Ovarian Cancer
Limits of tumor spread often unknown
Variability of radiosensitivity
Total tumor burden usually large
Free mobility of tumor cells within the abdominal cavity
Radiation dosage restricted by neighboring organs
Infrequent detection of early disease

TABLE 11.20 Dose Restrictions
Tolerance of small intestine
Limited tolerance of kidneys
Bone marrow depression
Radiation enteritis caused by large volume of intestine irradiated
Adhesive peritonitis

radiotherapy for specific histologies and isolated recurrences is being further studied. Dose restrictions are listed in Table 11.20.

Radioisotopes

Numerous trials have been conducted comparing IP 32P with or without pelvic radiation with whole abdominal radiation or single-agent chemotherapy in various clinical settings of ovarian cancer. Because IP 32P has failed to demonstrate improved outcomes, can be associated with increased complications, and is "technique intensive," it is rarely considered for contemporary treatment planning.

Chemotherapy

The evolution of chemotherapy agents for advanced ovarian cancer over the past 30 years has been significant. Ovarian cancer was one of the first solid malignant tumors demonstrating responsiveness to chemotherapy. Effectiveness of the various chemotherapy treatments has been measured by response rates (usually complete plus partial responses), negative second-look rates, PFS, and OS. All of these outcome measures can be subject to error. Even survival outcomes can be compromised by the fact that many patients receive a number of variously active chemotherapy treatments over their treatment history.

The earliest agents used for the treatment of ovarian carcinoma (1970–1980) were predominantly the alkylating agents melphalan (also called phenylalanine mustard, Alkeran, L-PAM, and L-sarcolysin), cyclophosphamide, chlorambucil, and thiotepa. Response rates were usually reported in the 20% to 60% range, but median survival rates for patients with advanced ovarian cancer were often in the range of 10 to 18 months, quite inferior to most outcomes from today's clinical trials. Antimetabolites, such as 5-fluorouracil and methotrexate, were also used in many of the earlier trials, especially in combination with alkylating agents. The contemporary use of these agents in epithelial ovarian cancer is rare to nonexistent.

The late 1970s and 1980s saw the introduction of combination chemotherapy regimens, such as Hexa CAF (hexamethylmelamine, cyclophosphamide, doxorubicin, and 5-fluorouracil) and CAP (cyclophosphamide, doxorubicin, and cisplatin). By the early 1980s, combination therapy was the standard treatment for most patients. The 1980s also witnessed the introduction of cisplatin and later carboplatin. The introduction of these platinum compounds increased response rates to the 50% to 80% range and increased median survival periods to the 12- to 30-month range in most studies. The wide range was often attributable to select patient populations, with the "suboptimal" debulked patients having the 12- to 18-month survival times and the "optimal" debulked patients having the 18- to 30-month survival times. The platinum compounds have remained an integral component of treatment to this day.

The 1990s saw the introduction of paclitaxel, an agent first extracted from the stripped bark of the Pacific yew tree, *Taxus brevifolia*. Paclitaxel, now chemically synthesized, demonstrated a new mechanism of action by promoting microtubular assembly and stabilizing tubulin polymer formation, thus inhibiting rapidly dividing cells from completing the mitotic process. The initial single-agent paclitaxel response rates in patients with refractory ovarian cancer were in the 25% to 35% range. Contemporary drug development continues to look at new formulations of the taxane group. Docetaxel in several studies has shown equivalent efficacy to paclitaxel with a different side effect profile, and other modified taxanes such as Abraxane and CT-2103 have been evaluated.

The past 2 decades have also seen the introduction of additional cytotoxic agents with demonstrated activity in ovarian cancer, including topotecan, a topoisomerase I-inhibitor; a pegylated liposomal encapsulated form of doxorubicin; and gemcitabine. These three drugs were tested in the frontline setting by the GOG 182/ICON-5 clinical trials, discussed later.

For the past decade, there has been considerable interest in developing agents targeting specific molecular targets. Two important categories of targeted therapies in ovarian cancer have been angiogenesis inhibitors, of which bevacizumab has been most widely studied, and poly(ADP-ribose) polymerase (PARP) inhibitors. Immune therapies continue to be in development and will continue to be a therapeutic focus in the next decade.

Clinical Trials

The relatively low rates of response to most single agents stimulated investigators to search for combination schedules. In the "modern" era, platinum-based combinations have proved to be the most successful. Pertinent clinical trials relating to early-stage disease are discussed earlier in this chapter, and the following discussion focuses on trials for advanced ovarian cancer.

Development of ovarian cancer combination chemotherapy through the 1980s and 1990s saw transition from doxorubicin–cyclophosphamide (AC), to cyclophosphamide–doxorubicin–cisplatin (CAP), to cyclophosphamide-platinum, and finally to taxane–platinum as the evolving standard of care. The trials performed by the GOG as well as European investigators were primarily responsible to developing these standards. In 1986, GOG 47 reported results comparing CAP to AC, with improved response rate, response duration, and PFS but not OS in the whole cohort. Subgroup analysis of patients with measurable disease (227 of 440 assessable patients) did show improved OS, and the potential advantage of incorporating platinum therapy was recognized. GOG 52 evaluated CAP versus cyclophosphamide–cisplatin alone in optimally cyto-reduced patients and demonstrated equivalent PFS and OS endpoints. With less toxicity by withholding doxorubicin, cyclophosphamide–cisplatin became the "standard" arm for many clinical trials in the late 1980s and early 1990s. Before abandoning doxorubicin completely, four trials were considered in a meta-analysis that specifically evaluated the benefit of doxorubicin in ovarian cancer. Considering only pathologic complete responses, the study showed a constant small benefit for CAP, highest in the North-West Oncology Group (GONO) and Danish Ovarian Cancer Group (DACOVA) studies. By pulling together these data in a meta-analysis, it was possible to detect a statistically significant benefit of pathologic complete responses (6%) and OS (7%) with CAP. However, because in three trials the dose intensity was greater for CAP than for cyclophosphamide–cisplatin, to what extent the benefit of CAP is from greater dose intensity or from doxorubicin itself remains unsolved.

In the 1990s, paclitaxel became available on trial, and GOG 132 evaluated 614 patients with suboptimally debulked cancer who were treated in a three-arm protocol comparing cisplatin alone, paclitaxel alone, and a combination of the two drugs. Neither PFS nor OS was different among the three arms, but significant crossover to the other drug in the single-drug arms muddled somewhat the clarity of the outcome data. Some interpreted the results of this study to indicate that a platinum agent should be a component of primary therapy. With some evidence for efficacy, the paclitaxel–cisplatin combination was compared to the existing standard, cyclophosphamide–cisplatin. The GOG 111 study randomized 386 patients with large-volume disease to paclitaxel–cisplatin versus cyclophosphamide–cisplatin. In the paclitaxel arm, administration of paclitaxel before cisplatin was important to optimize response and minimize toxicity. In terms of therapeutic efficacy, the cisplatin–paclitaxel arm produced a significantly greater overall response rate (73% vs. 60%) and clinical complete response rate, but the frequency of pathologic complete response was similar between the two arms. The paclitaxel arm showed significant improvements in PFS (18 vs. 13 months) and OS (38 vs. 24 months). The risk of progression was 32% lower among those treated with the paclitaxel regimen, and the risk of death was 39% lower (Fig. 11.20). A European-Canadian Intergroup trial (OV-10) had a study design similar to GOG 111, testing the replacement of cyclophosphamide with paclitaxel. This study included patients with optimal and suboptimal stage IB, IIB, III, and IV. Again, the clinical response rate was superior for the paclitaxel arm (59% vs. 45%), with a subsequent 25% reduction in the rate of death. The combination of paclitaxel and cisplatin became the standard for combination first-line chemotherapy for the treatment of epithelial ovarian carcinoma.

When combined with cisplatin, paclitaxel requires an extended infusion interval (24 hours) to prevent unacceptable neuropathy. This administration schedule was inconvenient, prompting many community providers to replace cisplatin with carboplatin, with which paclitaxel did not require this extended

P + T = platin + taxol
P + C = platin + cytoxan

FIGURE 11.20 Survival by treatment group. (Modified from McGuire WP, Hoskins WJ, Brady MF, et al. Cyclophosphamide and cisplatin compared with paclitaxel and cisplatin in patients with stage III and stage IV ovarian cancer. *N Engl J Med* 1996;334:1. Copyright © 1996 Massachusetts Medical society. All rights reserved. Adapted 2006 with permission.)

infusion. Several groups conducted equivalency trials to compare paclitaxel (175–185 mg/m^2) and carboplatin (AUC 5–7.5) with the standard cisplatin–paclitaxel regimen. The GOG conducted GOG 158 on the optimal (<1 cm) patient population as a noninferiority trial. The relative risk (RR) of progression on the paclitaxel plus carboplatin arm was equivalent (RR = 0.88; 95% CI, 0.–1.03), and toxicity was greater on the paclitaxel plus cisplatin arm. Similar findings regarding therapeutic equivalence and toxicity preference for carboplatin over cisplatin were reported by the Arbeitsgemeinschaft Gynäkologische Onkologie (AGO) Ovarian Cancer Study Group. The combination of intravenous (IV) paclitaxel and carboplatin replaced paclitaxel and cisplatin as the standard first-line chemotherapy for ovarian cancer.

Care must always be taken in interpreting response rates as a correlate for survival rates. Too often a chemotherapeutic regimen will produce an excellent response rate but not affect the OS rate. Therefore, the clinician must await longer term studies of combination chemotherapy to accurately understand its impact on survival of patients. Omura and colleagues reported a sobering analysis of two large GOG studies of multiagent chemotherapy in epithelial ovarian cancer. In this analysis of 726 women with stage III or stage IV disease, excellent follow-up had been obtained. The authors concluded that the impact of chemotherapy to date had been modest. Fewer than 10% of their patients were progression free at 5 years, and late failures continued to occur, even beyond 7 years. Sutton and coworkers reported a 7% disease-free survival rate at 10 years. Unfortunately, the superiority of any particular combination of chemotherapeutic agents as reflected by statistically significant improvement in long-term survival remains unproved. Although carboplatin appears to be the most active agent in epithelial cancer of the ovary, there is still controversy that combining it with other agents improves outcome.

In vitro testing of chemotherapy resistance or sensitivity has been investigated for at least 3 decades without clarification of its role in either primary or recurrent disease. Multiple technologies are currently in use, and there is a need to identify the relative value of this testing modality.

Dose-intense Chemotherapy

Dose intensity refers to the amount of chemotherapy to which a cancer is exposed per unit of time; this is generally assumed to be reflected by the dose of drug in milligrams per square meter of body surface area per unit of time. The theory is well grounded in preclinical work showing that as the concentration of drug in culture medium increases, the fraction of surviving cancer cells decreases logarithmically. The cell kill for a particular drug frequently follows a sigmoidal curve, indicating a point at which continued dose escalation will yield little improvement in results. To determine whether dose intensity is important clinically, randomized trials are needed. The GOG did design such a trial in patients with large-volume, advanced disease. A total of 458 patients were entered into the study and were randomly assigned to low-dose cisplatin 50 mg/m^2 plus cyclophosphamide 500 mg/m^2 every 3 weeks for eight cycles or high-dose cisplatin 100 mg/m^2 plus cyclophosphamide 1000 mg/m^2 every 3 weeks for four cycles (same total dose in half the time). In patients with measurable disease, the overall response and clinical complete response rates were equivalent. There was no difference in PFS or OS in the subsets of patients with measurable or nonmeasurable disease. The results of this study did not support the concept that increased dose intensity will produce greater therapeutic effect of cisplatinum or cyclophosphamide. Colombo and associates reported a randomized trial in patients with advanced disease who were given cisplatin 75 mg/m^2 every 3 weeks for six cycles or cisplatin 50 mg/m^2 per week for 9 weeks (same total dose in half the time). Again, no significant differences were seen in clinical or pathologic complete response rates, PFS, or OS. Although neither of these randomized trials of pure dose intensity in cisplatin showed an advantage for a higher dose intensity across a clinically relevant range of doses, other lines of evidence have been cited to support the use of higher dose schedules.

In trials conducted by the National Cancer Institute (NCI) of the United States, even higher dose intensities of cisplatin in conjunction with hypertonic saline to protect the kidneys had been stated to yield higher response rates than more standard doses. A closer examination of these data reported by Rothenberg and coworkers shows confusing results. In patients with large-volume disease, the NCI regimen complete response rates were no different (11% vs. 12%) than the GOG results with CAP, as reported by Omura, regimens with a 3.3-fold difference in dose intensity of cisplatin. In patients with small-volume disease, the NCI regimen complete response rates were not statistically different (38% vs. 30%) from the GOG results with

a two-drug combination of cisplatin plus cyclophosphamide, as reported by Omura in 1989. There appears to be no evidence from these data to support the importance of dose intensity of cisplatin over a 3.3-fold range of doses. At least 11 randomized trials have compared standard doses of carboplatin- or cisplatin-based chemotherapy with double doses of the same platinum analogs. Most of these trials showed no advantage in most outcome parameters. A second meta-analysis of the Levin and Hryniuk meta-analysis (in which it appeared that dose intensity had a positive impact on response rate and survival) suggested that platinum dose intensity is unimportant, although intensity of all administered drugs is important, as is tumor residual volume at initiation of therapy.

Katsumata and colleagues from the Japan GOG reported their results of their phase III trial in advanced ovarian cancer evaluating IV carboplatin and paclitaxel dosed every 3 weeks versus IV carboplatin with weekly dose-dense paclitaxel. For each 3-week cycle of therapy, the weekly dose-dense arm received 240 mg/m^2 of paclitaxel versus 180 mg/m^2 of paclitaxel in the control arm. PFS and 3-year OS were significantly improved in the weekly paclitaxel arm (28 vs. 17 months, 72% vs. 65%), with a higher incidence of grade III and IV anemia. Pignata and colleagues reported results from the similar Multicentre Italian Trials in Ovarian Cancer 7 (MITO-7) trial but showed no difference in PFS or OS for weekly versus paclitaxel every 3 weeks. GOG investigators for GOG 262 investigated this question of carboplatin plus weekly paclitaxel versus paclitaxel every 3 weeks in a similar manner to the Japanese Gynecologic Oncology Group (JGOG), with the addition of with or without bevacizumab in each arm. Preliminary results reported no difference in PFS between the arms if bevacizumab was received, but without bevacizumab, the weekly paclitaxel arm had improved PFS.

For 2 decades, high-dose chemotherapy with autologous bone marrow transplantation (ABMT) or peripheral blood stem cell support has been reported for several solid tumors, and there has been a tendency for improved response rates but a relatively short period of disease-free survival in most of the reports reviewed. Many reports show that even in advanced cases, the most important factor for long-term survival after high-dose chemotherapy is the completeness of the primary cytoreductive surgery. Most of the reports in the literature with high-dose chemotherapy with ABMT have been phase II trials of patients with a mixed response to first-line chemotherapy. The best response and survival have been in patients who had had a complete response to pretransplantation chemotherapy. The MD Anderson group reported its experience of 96 patients undergoing transplantation, of whom 43% were in clinical remission. The overall 6-year survival rate was 38% and was 53% in the clinical remission group. Bengala and colleagues reported the results of the European Group for Blood and Marrow Transplantation (EBMT) for 91 patients in first complete remission treated with high-dose chemotherapy and ABMT. The median survival time was 44 months, and they were unable to identify a subgroup more likely to benefit. These reported median survival times are not significantly better than that with use of paclitaxel as second-line therapy. However, the toxicity of high-dose chemotherapy is a serious concern, as is the additional expense. Although interesting, it appears that targeting of patients for high-dose therapy with bone marrow support cannot be considered standard therapy and should only be done as part of an established national protocol so that information can be obtained to increase our knowledge of this therapy.

Immunotherapy

In the past 3 decades, there has been considerable interest in combining chemotherapy with immunotherapy for better results in patients with epithelial cancer of the ovary. The GOG and others have investigated immunomodulating agents such as *Corynebacterium parvum* and bacille Calmette-Guérin (BCG). Results have been conflicting as to whether nonspecific immunostimulation combined with chemotherapy improves survival.

The potential role of immune response modifiers in the treatment of ovarian cancer has been investigated. Ovarian cancer is a suitable model for biologic therapies because the peritoneal cavity is capable of mounting an inflammatory response to many stimuli, and this response has been shown to induce an antitumor effect. Early experimental observations confirmed that ovarian cancer is a suitable prototype tumor in which to evaluate novel immunotherapeutic and chemoimmunotherapeutic approaches. Berek and coworkers have reported that recombinant interferon alfa has clinical activity in patients with small-volume residual disease. Numerous phase II trials, using substances such as tumor necrosis factor, interleukin-2, and the like, along with other studies using combinations of cytokines have failed to demonstrate significantly improved outcomes. Combining biologic immune response modifiers with standard chemotherapy has proved to be more difficult than initially conceived because of overlapping toxicities. In view of this, it seems prudent to await proven efficacy before attempting to launch the phase III trials with biologic immune response modifiers.

Recent results from trials using programmed cell death protein 1 (PD-1) inhibitors, such as nivolumab and avelumab, have shown some promise. PD-1 is a T-cell "programmed cell death" receptor on T cells that can blocked by a tumor-secreted ligand, inactivating the T cell and allowing the cancer to evade the host immune system. Competitive blockade of this ligand should allow improved cancer immune regulation, and initial results reported by Brahmer and associates in melanoma, non–small cell lung cancer, renal cell cancer, and ovarian cancer were promising. Hamanishi and colleagues have reported their initial results with nivolumab in a cohort of patients with platinum-resistant ovarian cancer, with an encouraging safety profile and activity, including two durable responses. NRG Oncology and others have open trials investigating this mechanism in ovarian cancer. We await the results of these endeavors as to whether these novel treatments will show the same promise in ovarian cancer that has been demonstrated thus far in melanoma.

Intraperitoneal Chemotherapy

Ovarian cancer is predominantly a disease limited to the peritoneal cavity for most patients. For some chemotherapeutic agents, IP administration offers pharmacokinetic advantages, including high IP drug concentration and longer exposure in the peritoneal cavity. Although IP chemotherapy proposals date back decades, it has only been over recent years that the accumulated clinical trial data favor this approach.

Results from randomized trials, listed in Table 11.21, summarize the experience of clinical trials conducted since the mid-1980s. These studies, all primary therapy trials, compare IV chemotherapy with combined IV and IP chemotherapy. The initial IP study demonstrating that IP chemotherapy may represent a survival advantage was a combined Southwestern Oncology Group (SWOG)/GOG trial (SWOG 8501 and GOG 104). The study compared IV cisplatin and IV cyclophosphamide with IP cisplatin and IV cyclophosphamide in patients with less than 2-cm-diameter residual disease. The IP arm produced a median survival of 49 months compared with 41 months for the IV arm, with an HR of 0.77. However, critics pointed out that the subsequent introduction of paclitaxel to our frontline treatment may have neutralized this apparent advantage for IP therapy. The other concern is that accrual was extended beyond the initial study design for patients with 0- to 0.5-cm residual disease, and still this subgroup failed to demonstrate superior survival (51 months vs. 46 months; HR, 0.80). One would have expected the treatment difference to be most pronounced in this patient subgroup. Partly because of these issues, IP therapy was not uniformly supported as producing a survival advantage over the current IV standard, carboplatin-paclitaxel.

Another GOG study, GOG 114, reported in 2003, compared IV cisplatin and paclitaxel (six cycles) with high-dose (AUC, 9) carboplatin IV (two cycles) plus six cycles of IV paclitaxel and IP cisplatin in patients with stage III disease less than or equal to 1-cm diameter residual. The median survival for the IP arm was 67 months versus 51 months for the IV arm and was statistically significant. Because the patients in the IV arm did not receive the extra two cycles of the high-dose carboplatin, critics were hesitant to support IP delivery as the reason for the survival improvement.

The most recently reported GOG study, GOG 172, compared IV paclitaxel (135 mg/m^2/24 hours) followed by either IV cisplatin (75 mg/m^2) on day 2 or by IP cisplatin (100 mg/m^2) on day 2 and IP paclitaxel (60 mg/m^2) on day 8—each arm for six cycles at 21-day intervals. The patient population was similar to GOG 114—stage III, less than 1 cm diameter residual. The median survival for the IP arm was 66.9 months compared with 49.5 months for the IV arm (HR, 0.71), results remarkably similar to the preceding study, GOG 114 (Fig. 11.21). This survival advantage prompted an NCI alert that IP therapy should be considered for first-line treatment for women with optimally cytoreduced advanced ovarian cancer.

However, this study reported significant toxicity for the IP arm, with double-digit percentage grade III or IV toxicities. Additionally, 33% of patients experienced catheter-related complications, which may be decreased with the use of a venous catheter with a subcutaneous access port overlying the lower ribs (Fig. 11.22). Not surprisingly, in GOG 172, only 42% of patients on the IP treatment received the complete six of IP therapy, and 48% received three or fewer cycles of IP chemotherapy. However,

TABLE 11.21 Randomized Trials Comparing Intravenous Versus Intraperitoneal First-Line Treatment of Ovarian Cancer

Study Identifier (Author, Year Published)	Control Regimen	Experimental Regimen	Target Population	Patients (n)	Median Duration of Survival for Control Regimen (Months)	Median Duration of Survival for Experimental Regimen (Months)
SWOG/GOG-104 (Alberts et al., 1996)	Cisplatin 100 mg/m² IV, ctx 600 mg/m² IV q 3 weeks × 6	Cisplatin 100 mg/ m² IP, ctx 600 mg/m² IV q 3 weeks × 6	Stage III ≤2 cm residual	546	41	49
Greek (Polyzos et al., 1999)	Carboplatin 350 mg/m² IV, ctx 600 mg/m² IV q 3 weeks × 6	Carboplatin 350 mg/m² IV, ctx 600 mg/m² IV q 3 weeks × 6	Stage III ≤or >2 cm residual	90	52	63
GONO (Gadducci et al., 2000)	Cisplatin 50 mg/m² IV, ctx 600 mg/m² IV, epidox 60 mg/m² IV q 4 weeks × 6	Cisplatin 50 mg/m² IP, ctx 600 mg/m² IV, epidox 60 mg/m² IV q 4 weeks × 6	Stage II or IV <2 cm residual	113	25	26
GOG-114/SWOG (Markman et al., 2001)	Cisplatin 75 mg/m² IV, tax 135 mg/m² (24 hr) IV q 3 weeks × 6	Carboplatin AUC 9 IV q 28 days × 2, cisplatin 100 mg/m² IP, tax 135 mg/m² (24 hr) IV q 3 weeks × 6	Stage III ≤1 cm residual	462	51	67
Taiwan (Yen et al., 2001)	Cisplatin 50 mg/m² IV, ctx 500 mg/m² IV epi/adr 50 mg/m² IV q 3 weeks × 6	Cisplatin 100 mg/m² IV, ctx 500 mg/m² IV, epi/adr 50 mg/m² IV q 3 weeks × 6	Stage III ≤1 cm residual	118	48	43
GOG-172 (Armstrong et al., 2006)	Cisplatin 75 mg/m² IV, tax 135 mg/m² (24 hr) IV q 3 weeks × 6	Tax 135 mg/m² (24 hr) IV, cisplatin 100 mg/m² IP, tax 60 mg/m² IV on day 8q 3 weeks × 6	Stage III ≤1 cm residual	415	49	67

adr, doxorubicin; *crbpt,* carboplatin; *ctx,* cyclophosphamide; *epi,* epirubicin; *epidox,* epirubicin; *GOG,* Gynecologic Oncology Group; *GONO,* Gruppo Oncologico Nord Ovest; *IP,* intraperitoneal; *IV,* intravenous; *SWOG,* Southwestern Oncology Group; *tax,* paclitaxel.

Treatment	Censored	Failed	Total
IV	83	127	210
IP	104	101	205

FIGURE 11.21 Overall survival for Gynecologic Oncology Group 172: intraperitoneal (IP) therapy versus intravenous (IV) therapy for optimally debulked advanced ovarian carcinoma.

in total, 83% of the patients on the IP arm completed six cycles of chemotherapy (IP, IV, or both). An ancillary study of GOG 114 and 172 by Tewari and colleagues reported that the risk of death decreased by 12% for each cycle of IP chemotherapy completed. Although the IP-treated patients reported a significantly worse quality of life before cycle four and 3 to 6 weeks posttreatment, there was no difference in quality of life between the IP or IV arms 1 year after treatment, except for moderate neurotoxicity (paresthesias) being more common in the IP arm. Despite the evidence for a survival advantage from IP therapy

and the resultant NCI clinical alert, IP therapy has not been accepted universally as a result of issues with catheter placement and therapy-associated toxicities. GOG 252 was designed to address issues of toxicity in IP chemotherapy and includes the question of weekly paclitaxel therapy in advanced ovarian cancer. The trial included a modification of the winning arm in GOG 172 with IP cisplatin dose reduced to 75 mg/m² and paclitaxel given over 3 instead of 24 hours, a second arm with IP carboplatin AUC 5 replacing the IP cisplatin, and a third arm using carboplatin AUC 6 every 3 weeks with weekly paclitaxel 80 mg/m² for 3 weeks per cycle. Preliminary results indicate no difference in toxicity or PFS for the three arms. All three arms appear to be more toxic than standard carboplatin–paclitaxel therapy every 3 weeks but less toxic than the winning IP arm of GOG 172. No OS data are available at the current time, and no definitive recommendations for altering standard of care can be made (Fig. 11.23).

Extraovarian Peritoneal Serous Papillary Carcinoma

Extraovarian peritoneal serous papillary carcinoma, or "primary peritoneal carcinoma," is a recognized clinical-pathologic entity in which peritoneal carcinomatosis of ovarian serous type is found in the abdomen or pelvis. Similar tumor deposits may be found on the surface of the ovary, but histologic evidence of primary or in situ ovarian carcinoma is either absent or insignificant. The tumor deposits are rarely noninvasive (borderline). This entity was first reported as "mesothelioma resembling

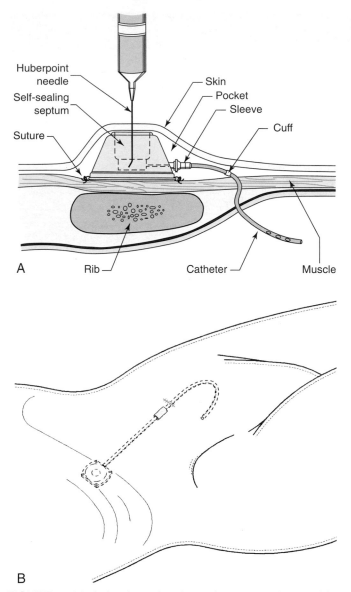

A, Huberpoint needle; Self-sealing septum; Suture; Rib; Skin; Pocket; Sleeve; Cuff; Catheter; Muscle

B

FIGURE 11.22 A, Implanted peritoneal access catheter with a subcutaneous self-sealing port providing a path for intraperitoneal therapy. **B,** Intraperitoneal chemotherapy.

TABLE 11.22	Gynecologic Oncology Group Criteria for Diagnosis of Extraovarian Peritoneal Carcinoma

Both ovaries must be either physiologically normal in size or enlarged by benign process.
Involvement in extraovarian sites must be greater than involvement on the surface of either ovary.
Microscopically, the ovarian involvement must be:
- Nonexistent
- Confined to ovarian surface epithelium or underlying cortical stromal involvement of no more than 5 mm
Histologic characteristics are primarily serous type, similar or identical to ovarian serous papillary adenocarcinoma.

papillary ovarian adenocarcinoma" by Swerdlow in 1959. Parmley and Woodruff, in 1974, demonstrated that pelvic peritoneum had the potential to differentiate into a Müllerian type of epithelium. This entity is different from mesothelioma. The malignant neoplasm spreads inside the peritoneal cavity, invading mostly the omentum, with minimal or no involvement of the ovary. Peritoneal studding is commonly present with psammoma bodies. Although usually serous, other cell types have been demonstrated. This entity has been identified in women who have had previous oophorectomies. The GOG has developed criteria for the diagnosis of extraovarian peritoneal carcinoma (Table 11.22).

Experience with extraovarian serous neoplasia of this type has been compared with clinical outcomes of homologous ovarian tumors of similar stage end grade. Fromm et al., Dalrymple et al, and others have reported series with generally similar outcomes when equivalent therapy regimens to ovarian cancer are given. A GOG trial of cisplatin and cyclophosphamide in these patients demonstrated a response similar to that in women with papillary serous ovarian cancer.

Our experience has been that these patients generally respond to therapy in a manner similar to patients with serous papillary carcinoma of the ovary. Because many characteristics of this entity and serous ovarian cancer are similar, the GOG accepts patients with extraovarian peritoneal carcinoma into its protocols of epithelial ovarian cancer. CA-125 measurements also appear similar in both groups of patients. There have been reports suggesting a higher incidence of polyclonal cell populations in peritoneal carcinoma than in the generally monoclonal ovarian cancers, which may lead to higher rates of chemoresistance. Although most reports show similar survival rates between ovarian and peritoneal cancers, this polyclonal nature has been suggested to explain those series showing a decreased survival rate in peritoneal cancer. There appears to be an increased incidence of extraovarian peritoneal cancers in patients with a hereditary predisposition for development of ovarian cancer. In Piver et al.'s report of women at high risk for hereditary ovarian cancer, extraovarian cancer developed after prophylactic oophorectomy in almost 2%, 10 times greater than the lifetime incidence in the general population. *BRCA1* mutations appear to arise in a similar number of women with extraovarian and primary ovarian cancers.

Small Cell Carcinoma of the Ovary

Small cell carcinoma of the ovary is a specific histopathologic entity that is rare, highly aggressive, and primarily affects children and young women between the ages of 10 and 40 years. The first 11 cases were documented by Dickersin and colleagues in 1982. Many, but not all, patients with this lesion have an associated hypercalcemia. Neuron-specific enolase may be both a histologic marker (immunohistochemistry) and a serum marker for this disease. Various chemotherapeutic agents have been suggested with minimal success. Young and associates reported on the poor prognosis of these patients, with only 33% of women with stage Ia tumors alive and no survivors with advanced stage disease. In general, similar chemotherapy regimens used for small cell lung carcinoma will be used to treat this

	Rel Haz	Var (in[HR])
SWOG/GOG–104 (1996)	0.760	0.013
GONO (2000)	0.670	0.077
GOG–114/SWOG (2001)	0.810	0.012
Talwan (2001)	1.130	0.064
EORTC–55875 (2003)	0.820	0.054
GOG–172 (2005)	0.710	0.020

χ^2 heterogeneity (5 d.f.) = 3.1, $P = 0.68$

Hazard ratio (HR) is not reported for the GONO study but it is calculated from the available data reported. HR is not reported for the Greek study.

FIGURE 11.23 Treatment hazard ratios for death intraperitoneal versus intravenous therapy. *EORTC,* European Organization for Research and Treatment of Cancer; *GOG,* Gynecologic Oncology Group; *GONO,* Gruppo Oncologico Nord Ovest; *IP,* intraperitoneal; *IV,* intravenous; *Rel Haz,* relative hazard; *SWOG,* Southwestern Oncology Group; *Var,* variability. (Adapted from National Cancer Institute Clinical Announcement, December, 2005.)

disease. Pautier and colleagues have reported the most promising regimen to date: a combination of cisplatin, doxorubicin, etoposide, and cyclophosphamide, with, if complete remission is achieved, high-dose chemotherapy with carboplatin, etoposide, cyclophosphamide, and stem cell support. Of 27 patients treated, 21 were stage II to IV and 18 complete responses were seen. Median duration of the 18 complete responses was 30 months, and 10 patients went on to receive high-dose chemotherapy. The OS rate at 3 years was 49%. Further study of this devastating group of tumors is necessary.

FOLLOW-UP TECHNIQUES AND TREATMENT OF RECURRENCES

Ovarian cancer is insidious in that it is late to cause symptoms, and thus follow-up examinations are imperative to detect early recurrence. The optimal follow-up strategy for asymptomatic patients who have advanced ovarian cancer after initial treatment remains undecided. Important considerations are divided between more passive and active approaches to follow-up. Currently, the National Comprehensive Cancer Network (NCCN) practice guidelines in oncology recommend surveillance of patients after the completion of primary therapy regardless of stage. This follow-up includes a comprehensive physical examination every 2 to 4 months for the first 2 years, every 6 months for the next 3 years, and then annually after 5 years. Laboratory studies, such as blood counts and chemistry profiles, should be done as indicated.

Use of CA-125 Levels and Other Tumor Markers

The oncology practice guidelines also recommend that the measurement of CA-125 level, or other relevant tumor markers, should be assessed at each follow-up evaluation if the level was initially elevated. CA-125 is an antigenic determinant of a murine immunoglobulin Ig1 monoclonal antibody that was raised against an epithelial ovarian carcinoma cell line and is

expressed in more than 80% of nonmucinous epithelial ovarian cancers.

Multiple CA-125 determinants are associated with a mucin-like glycoprotein of more than 200,000 daltons. Traces of the antigen are expressed in adult tissues derived from the coelomic epithelium, including mesothelial cells lining the pleura, pericardium, and peritoneum, and from the epithelial component of the female reproductive system. Thus, there are other causes of elevated CA-125 levels, which include both gynecologic and nongynecologic conditions. Acute inflammatory processes involving the pelvic area and other regions of the body may increase CA-125. These may include acute hepatitis or pancreatitis, chronic liver disease, colitis, congestive heart failure, diverticulitis, arthritis, and pneumonia, to name a few.

The radioimmune assay was developed to detect CA-125 in serum and body fluids. The day-to-day coefficient of variability for the assay is approximately 15%. Consequently, a doubling or halving of antigen levels has been considered significant. If a cut-off of 35 U/mL is chosen for the upper limit of normal, elevated CA-125 levels should be found in 1% of apparently normal blood bank donors, 6% of patients who have benign disease, 28% of individuals who have nongynecologic malignant neoplasms, and 82% of patients who have surgically demonstrable epithelial ovarian cancer. Niloff and coworkers reported detection of elevated CA-125 in sera from patients who have advanced fallopian tube, endometrial, and endocervical adenocarcinomas. In epithelial ovarian carcinoma, rising or falling levels of CA-125 have correlated with disease progression or regression in more than 90% of patients. In the report by Niloff et al., when CA-125 levels returned to less than 35 U/mL, findings of second-look surveillance procedures were in fact normal in 14 of 36 cases, but in no instance was a nodule larger than 1 cm found. Persistently elevated CA-125 levels have been associated consistently with persistence of disease. Recurrence of disease has been heralded by elevations of CA-125 in 85% of patients whose tumors shed the antigen. Elevated CA-125 levels preceded disease recurrence by 1 to 14 months with a mean of 5 months in one study reported by Knapp and Friedman. Elevation of CA-125 in hepatocellular disease and in chronic peritonitis is important to note but should not compromise the utility of CA-125 as a marker for monitoring ovarian cancer.

A rapid regression of the serum CA-125 level to normal limits shortly after commencement of chemotherapy has been shown to be associated with a higher frequency of negative results at second-assessment surgery. Levin reported that almost all patients who subsequently come to a negative second-look laparotomy have serum CA-125 levels within normal ranges within 3 months of primary cytoreductive surgery. Buller and colleagues have shown that a favorable outcome is associated with a steep regression curve of serum CA-125 levels after cytoreductive surgery and chemotherapy. These investigators demonstrated that patients in whom the CA-125 level reverts sharply to within the normal range by the third course of chemotherapy after surgery have a survival that is markedly improved over that of the patients who have an elevation of CA-125 levels before their fourth course of chemotherapy. Buller and coworkers described the regression curve of the serum CA-125 level as "S." Indeed, they have suggested that patients with a delayed "S" curve (regression of the elevated value) possibly should be considered for alternative therapy rather than persisting with the same chemotherapeutic regimens. Hogberg and Kagedal demonstrated that 23 patients with a serum CA-125 half-life shorter than 16 days during induction chemotherapy had an estimated survival of 68% at 59 months after second-look operation. This is compared with a survival rate of 18% in 49 patients with a serum CA-125 half-life longer than 16 days. However, one must be aware that normal levels may also accompany disease, with tumors up to 2 cm, in one-third or more of cases.

An elevation of CA-125 in the posttreatment surveillance period is usually related to recurrence of tumor, even if clinically otherwise undetectable. It remains controversial if patients should restart chemotherapy based on CA-125 elevation alone. The EORTC conducted a randomized study of early treatment for ovarian cancer relapse based on CA-125 level alone versus clinical or symptomatic recurrence. They evaluated 527 patients, approximately 265 in each group, and found no difference in OS rate between the two groups, even though patients in the arm evaluating CA-125 levels were treated earlier. Thus, they concluded that routine measurement of CA-125 may not be warranted. However, it is important to note that patients in this study were predominantly treated with second-line chemotherapy. Therefore, the role of secondary cytoreductive surgery, discussed in detail later, for asymptomatic recurrences may not have been accounted for, and the survival benefit of early detection based on CA-125 level may be underestimated for this group. Therefore, at this time, construction of the specific plan of follow-up should be individualized to each patient's needs.

In addition to CA-125, other tumor markers are being investigated for the detection of recurrent disease. Currently, the human epididymis protein 4 (HE4) has gained interest as a biomarker of recurrence. In a recent study, HE4 was shown to be elevated several months before CA-125 levels, implying a potential role for early detection of recurrent disease. Other studies have evaluated the markers including glycodelin, matrix metalloproteinase 7 (MMP7), in addition to HE4 and CA-125. The combination of these biomarkers was found to be useful for the detection of relapse before the onset of clinically detectable disease. However, these tests are in their infancy, and larger studies need to be conducted to confirm their efficacy.

Radiographic Imaging

For patients demonstrating a complete response to primary therapy, the NCCN guidelines recommend the use of radiographic imaging as clinically indicated. This may include the use of CT scan, magnetic resonance imaging (MRI) scan, or positron emission tomography (PET)/CT scan. The detection of recurrent disease on radiographic imaging varies dependent on modality and the size and location of disease. CT and MRI studies detected recurrent tumor in 66% to 95% of cases. However, most often failed to detect small-volume disease and disease located on visceral surfaces. Recently, PET/CT scan with F-18 fluorodeoxyglucose for the evaluation of recurrent ovarian cancer has been used. This modality has been shown to detect disease recurrence, particularly when patients presented with rising CA-125 levels and negative or equivocal CT scan or MRI. Although one must be aware of the limitations, namely physiologic uptake of the FDG (fluorodeoxyglucose), particularly in the GI and urinary systems, and misalignment with CT scan secondary to bowel peristalsis and respiratory movements, FDG-PET/CT has become a more common imaging choice.

FDG-PET/CT scan not only offers the benefit of functional and anatomic imaging but also allows for the ability to locate small-volume disease in locations not amenable to physical examination and the ability to differentiate metabolically active disease from inactive disease. In an effort to detect small lesions, PET/CT scan was performed for suspected recurrence and confirmed by surgical exploration or clinical follow-up. The investigators reported PET/CT scans had a sensitivity of 93% to 95% and specificity of 97% to 100%, suggesting that PET/CT may be used for posttherapy evaluation of recurrent ovarian cancer. Thus, PET/CT scan may provide valuable prognostic information, similar to second-look operations, without the associated morbidity.

However, the role of radiographic imaging for routine surveillance is less clear. In a retrospective case-control study, investigators evaluated survival impact based on the asymptomatic versus symptomatic detection of ovarian cancer. The common practice in this study was CT scanning of the abdomen and pelvis at 6-month intervals for the first 2 years followed by annually for the next 3 years. The authors reported a significant difference in postrecurrence survival favoring those detected asymptomatically on imaging (45 vs. 29.4 months). However, these tests are not without costs and should be evaluated in a prospective fashion to determine the true benefit. Until then, the decision to evaluate asymptomatic patients for recurrent disease with imaging should be individualized.

Maintenance Therapy

In addition to surveillance, patients with a complete response after primary therapy may be candidates for maintenance therapy, which is chemotherapy given with the intention of extending the disease-free interval and improving OS. Currently, the role of maintenance therapy, or consolidation therapy, is still under investigation, which includes identifying the ideal agent(s) and dosages, the treatment interval, and the length of treatment.

As one of the most active agents in the primary setting, platinum agents are a natural choice for maintenance therapy. In patients with advanced disease who achieved a complete response after six cycles of chemotherapy, Kim and colleagues evaluated the role of three additional cycles of platinum and paclitaxel compared with observation (control arm). The authors noted that both groups demonstrated similar survival outcomes. Additional studies have evaluated the efficacy of single-agent carboplatin and IP cisplatin for maintenance therapy; however, similar to the aforementioned study, no survival advantage was ascertained.

Several randomized studies have also been conducted studying the role of paclitaxel for maintenance therapy. In one randomized study, six additional cycles of paclitaxel were compared with observation. The investigators reported no difference in PFS or OS at 3 years. Weekly paclitaxel (80 mg/m^2) for 12 weeks was evaluated after primary therapy, and the investigators reported a 2-year survival rate of 94% and acceptable tolerability. In contrast, a study by the GOG (protocol 178) compared three cycles with 12 cycles of paclitaxel after a complete clinical response. The study was closed early by the Data Safety Monitoring Board when a planned interim analysis demonstrated a progression-free interval advantage of 7 months for the extra 9 months of treatment. However, a follow-up report failed to demonstrate any survival advantage, which was difficult to interpret because the early closure caused the trial to be underpowered for this endpoint. Currently, the GOG (protocol 212) is conducting a study randomly assigning patients to monthly paclitaxel, paclitaxel poliglumex, or observation for 12 months after the completion of primary therapy. Until the results of this trial are available, the role of paclitaxel for maintenance therapy remains to be determined.

Two trials evaluating the role of bevacizumab combined with carboplatin and paclitaxel and bevacizumab maintenance therapy in the first-line setting have recently been reported. Bevacizumab is a potent antitumor therapy that targets vascular endothelial growth factor (VEGF) and for which there are multiple phase II trials demonstrating efficacy in recurrent ovarian cancer. GOG 218 randomly assigned women with advanced ovarian cancer after initial debulking surgery to one of three treatment arms: (1) standard carboplatin and paclitaxel for six cycles, (2) carboplatin–paclitaxel plus bevacizumab for six cycles, and (3) carboplatin–paclitaxel plus bevacizumab for six cycles followed by bevacizumab for up to an additional 16 cycles. PFS was improved in the bevacizumab-throughout arm, with OS similar in all three groups. Oza and colleagues reported the results of a large European trial, ICON seven, evaluating chemotherapy (carboplatin–paclitaxel) versus chemotherapy plus bevacizumab plus bevacizumab maintenance in a similar patient population. PFS and OS were similar in both arms, but a predefined high-risk subgroup (stage IV or suboptimal) did

have improved OS. The demonstrated activity of bevacizumab against ovarian cancer may require more time to define how best to use this activity to improve survival.

In addition to platinum and paclitaxel, studies have been conducted evaluating the impact of numerous other chemotherapy agents, including topotecan, pegylated liposomal doxorubicin, and altretamine, which also failed to demonstrate a survival advantage. Over the past decade, biologic agents have also been investigated, such as oregovomab, a monoclonal antibody targeting CA-125 antigen; tanomastat, a matrix metalloproteinase inhibitor; and pazopanib, a multikinase inhibitor. However, none of these agents demonstrated a survival benefit. Additional trials are in progress to clarify the potential role for maintenance therapy.

Chemotherapy for Recurrent Disease and Targeted Therapies

Advanced epithelial ovarian cancer is a highly chemosensitive solid tumor with responses in the range of 70% to 80% to first-line chemotherapy, including a high proportion of complete responses. Most patients, however, eventually relapse and ultimately die of chemoresistant disease. Even with platinum-based chemotherapy, fewer than a quarter of the patients with an initial advanced disease diagnosis are alive at 5 years. In all forms of ovarian epithelial cancer, second-line chemotherapy has to date been disappointing. When effective drug combinations are initially used and fail, there is a very limited chance of inducing a sustained remission or cure with a second or third drug or combinations. Response and control of malignant effusions can frequently be achieved, but these are usually of progressively shorter duration. Most gynecologic oncologists attempt to treat these patients with use of a reasonable second-line regimen usually consisting of active chemotherapeutic agents that have not been used in the first treatment plan (Table 11.23). The selection of therapy is based on the following factors: (1) potential for platinum sensitivity, (2) number of previous regimens, (3) potential cumulative toxicities, (4) patient performance status and symptoms, and (5) patient choice.

Patients whose disease recurs within 6 months of achieving a complete clinical response to front-line platinum-based therapy are deemed "platinum resistant." In comparison, patients who respond and have a progression-free interval of more than 6 months off treatment are defined as "platinum sensitive" or, more appropriately, chemotherapy sensitive. The response rates to second-line therapy are strikingly different in these two groups of patients. Blackledge and associates, in an analysis of 92 patients receiving five different second-line regimens, found that the interval off platinum-based therapy was a strong predictor of response. This observation held for both platinum-based and non–platinum-based second-line regimens. A response rate of less than 10% was observed for patients with a treatment-free interval of less than 6 months compared with up to 90% for those with an interval more than 21 months (Table 11.24).

Seltzer and coworkers reported a 72% response rate, including a 36% complete response rate, to second-line therapy with cisplatin in 11 patients who had achieved complete response

TABLE 11.23 Agents Used in Epithelial Ovarian Cancer

Active Agents	Inactive Agents
Alkylating agents	BCNU
Bevacizumab	Vincristine
Hexamethylmelamine	6-Mercaptopurine (6-MP)
Doxorubicin	Dactinomycin
Cisplatin	Raltitrexed (Tomudex)
Carboplatin	CI-958
5-Fluorouracil	
Methotrexate	
Etoposide (VP-16)	
Paclitaxel (Taxol)	
Vinorelbine tartrate (Navelbine)	
Gemcitabine	
Topotecan	
Liposomal doxorubicin	
Docetaxel	

BCNU, bis-chloroethylnitrosourea.

TABLE 11.24 Response Rate Versus Interval From Previous Treatment With Platinum-Based Regimen

Interval (Months)	Total (n)	Responding (n)	Responding (%)
<3	39	4	10
4-6	11	1	9
7–9	11	4	36
10–12	6	1	17
13–15	4	2	50
16–18	4	3	75
19–21	1	1	100
>21	16	15	94

From Blackledge G, Lawton F, Redman C, Kelly K. Response of patients in phase II studies of chemotherapy in ovarian cancer: implications for patient treatment and the design of phase II trials. Br J Cancer 1989;59:650.

to platinum-based, first-line chemotherapy. Markman and coworkers reported a 77% response rate to cisplatin in patients who had received no treatment for more than 24 months compared with 27% in women whose treatment-free interval remained 5 to 12 months. Similarly, Eisenhauer and associates reported a 43% response rate to carboplatin in patients whose treatment-free interval was more than 12 months compared with 10% in those whose treatment-free interval was less than 12 months. These findings make it mandatory that we define the populations of patients in clinical trials of second-line therapy. Phase II trials should include multiple adequately sized cohorts, such as patients with platinum-sensitive disease and those with platinum-refractory disease. In addition, patients should probably be stratified by the length of their treatment-free interval. In general, in phase II trials, response rates of more than 25% to 30% are expected for active agents being tested in the platinum-sensitive population, and response rates

of greater than 10% to 15% are considered promising in the platinum-resistant population.

A current issue of debate is whether recurrent ovarian cancer is better managed by sequential single-agent therapy or combination chemotherapy. Two European reports suggest combination therapy is superior. One trial (ICON4/AGO-OVAR 2.2) reported on more than 800 patients. The patient population was "very platinum sensitive," with more than 75% of the patients having more than a 12-month platinum-free interval. After a median follow-up of 42 months, analysis showed the combination had a 2-year survival rate of 57% versus 50% for the platinum-only treated patients, and the median survival difference was 29 months versus 24 months. This study has been the subject of some criticisms. The study was an analysis of multiple parallel trials conducted by difference groups involving five countries and 119 hospitals. The platinum agent was either cisplatin or carboplatin. The treatments were given monthly. A number of the patients had not previously received a taxane, and there was no difference in outcome if the patient previously received a taxane in their primary therapy. Thus, considering most patients receive a taxane and carboplatin for primary therapy in the United States, the application of this experience to our US population is questioned. Other smaller studies, including a Spanish study (Grupo Español de Investigación en **Cáncer** de Ovario [**GEICO**]), also suggested the observation that combination therapy in the refractory setting may offer better outcomes. However, in general, in patients with disease-free intervals of longer than 12 months, the tendency is to retreat with taxane plus platinum combinations.

In addition to the rechallenge with platinum, single-agent paclitaxel is often used in the treatment of recurrent disease. In patients with platinum-sensitive disease, although rechallenge with platinum-based combination is favored, paclitaxel as a single agent has moderate response rates, ranging from 20% to 45%. Even in the platinum-resistant disease setting, standard-dose paclitaxel has been shown to produce response rates of 22% to 23%. Kohn and associates evaluated higher doses of paclitaxel, which required hematologic support, and observed a 48% response rate in platinum-refractory patients. As with other agents, these responses were generally of short duration. Nonetheless, paclitaxel should figure prominently in the consideration of second-line therapy for patients who have platinum-resistant disease. In a phase II GOG study, weekly paclitaxel (80 mg/m^2) in the platinum- and paclitaxel-resistant population demonstrated a response rate of more than 20% and was found to be well tolerated. The importance of dose intensity in this setting is being explored in randomized studies throughout the world. The results will have important implications for paclitaxel dose in combination regimens, which are being evaluated both as first- and second-line therapy.

Along with platinum and paclitaxel, three chemotherapeutic agents have received the most interest in evaluating their role in the treatment of recurrent ovarian cancer: gemcitabine, pegylated liposomal doxorubicin, and topotecan. In addition to activity in recurrent disease, these agents offer the strategy of extending the platinum-free interval. Discussed in detail later, these agents have been widely incorporated into clinical trials, in both primary (first-line), second-line recurrent, and third-line recurrent disease settings.

The GOG reported a positive phase II trial with a 5-day topotecan (1.5 mg/m^2) regimen (every 21 days), demonstrating a 33% response rate and median response duration of 11.2 months. Even in patients with platinum-resistant disease response rates range from 13% to 17%. Fatigue, anemia, and thrombocytopenia were the prominent toxicities. A weekly regimen of topotecan, administering 3.5 to 4 mg/m^2 on days 1, 8, and 15 on a 28-day cycle has also been used, and data comparing the weekly with 5-day regimen have shown improved efficacy with the 5-day regimen. In a phase II study, the use of 5-day topotecan (1.0 mg/m^2) with carboplatin (AUC, 5) in a platinum-sensitive group not only demonstrated a response rate of 40% but also was well tolerated. Thus, topotecan as part of a combination regimen seems to be a promising therapeutic choice for patients with recurrent ovarian cancer.

Gordon and coinvestigators reported a phase III trial in patients with refractory ovarian cancer comparing pegylated liposomal doxorubicin (Doxil), 50 mg/m^2 every 28 days, with topotecan, 1.5 mg/m^2 per day for 5 days every 21 days. In the platinum-refractory patient group, there was no survival difference. In the platinum-sensitive group, there was a 30% decrease in the risk of death for the pegylated liposomal doxorubicin-treated patients (median survival, 108 weeks vs. 70 weeks). Pegylated liposomal doxorubicin has demonstrated response rates up to 26% in the platinum-resistant group, making it an attractive option in this patient population. Recently, pegylated liposomal doxorubicin was studied as combination therapy in recurrent disease. In the CALYPSO (Caelyx in Platinum Sensitive Ovarian patients) trial, carboplatin in combination with either pegylated liposomal doxorubicin or paclitaxel was evaluated in a randomized trial for patients with relapsed, platinum-sensitive disease. PFS was 11.3 months for the pegylated liposomal doxorubicin arm compared with 9.4 months for the paclitaxel arm, resulting in an 18% reduction in risk of recurrence. Although generally well tolerated, dose-limiting toxicity includes palmar–plantar erythrodysesthesia.

Although gemcitabine has demonstrated modest activity as a single agent in the refractory setting, in combination with a platinum, most commonly cisplatin, the activity appears substantial. Nagourney and colleagues reported results of treatment with cisplatin (30 mg/m^2) plus gemcitabine (600–750 mg/m^2) on days 1 and 8 in a 21-day cycle. They reported 26% complete responses and 44% partial responses (70% overall response rate) with a median time to progression, for responders, of 7.9 months (range, 2.1–13.2 months). Neutropenia, anemia, thrombocytopenia, nausea and vomiting, and peripheral neuropathy were problematic toxicities. Additional studies suggest that gemcitabine may reverse cisplatin resistance and may be a useful combination for both platinum-sensitive and platinum-resistant groups.

Bevacizumab for the treatment of ovarian cancer in the recurrent setting has also demonstrated activity. In 62 patients, both platinum-sensitive and platinum-resistant patients, single-agent bevacizumab (15 mg/kg every 21 days) demonstrated a response rate of 21%. In a predominantly platinum-resistant group, bevacizumab (15 mg/kg every 21 days) resulted in a 16% overall response rate. Although GI perforation rates ranged from 0% to 11% in these studies, both cohorts were composed of patients who had received multiple chemotherapy regimens before the use of bevacizumab. Bevacizumab has also been studied in combination with other agents. The addition of bevacizumab to cytotoxic agents has also been shown to have activity in this setting. Response rates range from 15% to 43% and include combinations with gemcitabine, taxanes, cyclophosphamide, liposomal doxorubicin, 5-fluorouracil, and erlotinib. In platinum-sensitive disease, bevacizumab plus chemotherapy was evaluated in the multicenter OCEANS (Ovarian Cancer Study Comparing Efficacy and Safety of Chemotherapy and Anti-Angiogenic Therapy In Platinum-Sensitive Recurrent Disease) trial, reported by Aghajanian and colleagues. Patients were randomized to carboplatin–gemcitabine, with or without bevacizumab, and followed until progression. Response rate (79% vs. 57%) and PFS (12 vs. 8 months) were significantly improved with bevacizumab, although the later reported OS (not the primary endpoint) showed no difference. In platinum-resistant disease, Pujade-Lauraine and colleagues reported similar findings form the AURELIA (Avastin Use in Platinum-Resistant Epithelial Ovarian Cancer) trial. Patients with platinum-resistant disease were randomized to investigator's choice chemotherapy without or without bevacizumab, and the study powered to PFS as the primary endpoint. Significant improvements in response rate and PFS were seen in the patients receiving bevacizumab; the OS trend was not significant.

Intraperitoneal therapy (discussed elsewhere in this chapter) has been used with several antineoplastic agents as second-line therapy in ovarian cancer. Activity is essentially limited to patients with small-volume residual disease (<0.5 cm in maximal diameter) when the second-line therapy program is initiated. In the absence of a randomized phase III trial, the ultimate impact of these surgically documented responses on survival is difficult to evaluate. Although rare, long-term disease-free survival in patients with small-volume refractory disease has been reported after IP therapy.

There is limited evidence of sustained benefit from second-line therapy in patients with ovarian cancer. Overall, only modest response rates with short durations of response have been reported. In addition, there has been a lack of consistency in these studies with regard to key definitions, such as platinum sensitivity compared with platinum resistance. Future second-line trials should clearly define their patients in these two categories. It may also be necessary to discuss paclitaxel-sensitive versus paclitaxel-resistant lesions in the future. Platinum-sensitive patients are appropriate for pilot studies of platinum combinations incorporating different cytotoxic mechanisms of action and dose schedule investigations. Patients with platinum resistance are good candidates for novel investigational approaches and studies of drug resistance. Various other agents, such as hexamethylmelamine, 5-fluorouracil, etoposide, and others, rarely induce modest short-duration responses.

Radiation to the abdomen and pelvis has been used in select second-line situations. Whole-abdomen irradiation with a pelvic boost has been given in patients with minimal disease at second-look surgical reassessment for ovarian carcinoma. With limited follow-up, some studies report as many as 30% of such patients have remained in remission. However, our experience is that with longer follow-up periods, more than 90% of patients will have recurrence, even in this optimal group.

Targeted Therapy

The area with the most rapid development in regard to ovarian cancer treatment is in the area of targeted therapeutics. Secondary to the toxicities and emerging resistance, alternatives or additions to chemotherapy are coming to the forefront. This is best demonstrated with bevacizumab, described earlier, which has been studied in the primary and recurrent setting and in maintenance therapy. Multiple other agents are now under investigation.

Tyrosine kinase inhibitors, which target vascular endothelial growth factor receptors (VEGFR), inhibit an important target in ovarian cancer. The most studied agent in this group, cediranib, has demonstrated response rates of 41% and 29% in platinum-sensitive and platinum-resistant groups, respectively. As a result of this activity, cediranib is being further evaluated in the phase III randomized trial ICON-6 in conjunction with carboplatin and paclitaxel in the primary setting.

Poly(ADP-ribose) polymerase inhibitors have recently garnered interest in ovarian cancer treatment. PARP is an enzyme responsible for the repair of DNA single-strand breaks. Inhibition of the PARP repair mechanism is particularly effective in tumors in which homologous double-stranded repair mechanism is also deficient, such as in patients with *BRCA* mutations. Olaparib, a PARP-1 inhibitor, was not only well tolerated but demonstrated good response rates ranging in patients with a known *BRCA* mutation. Ledermann and colleagues reported the results from their randomized phase 2 "Study 19" evaluating olaparib maintenance therapy versus placebo in platinum-sensitive recurrent ovarian cancer patients. Patients enrolled had received a median of three prior therapies, and approximately 22% of patients in each arm had a germline *BRCA* mutation. Median PFS was significantly improved with olaparib maintenance (8.4 vs. 4.8 months), but an interim analysis showing no improvement in OS likely prevented US Food and Drug Administration (FDA) approval for this indication. Recently, Domchek and colleagues reported a 34% response rate for olaparib oral monotherapy in *BRCA1* or *BRCA2* mutation carriers with recurrent ovarian cancer and three or more lines of therapy, including a 30% response in platinum-resistant tumors, leading to FDA approval for this indication. Studies have shown that many sporadic epithelial cancers may be *BRCA* deficient as a result of inactivation of a *BRCA* allele despite intact BRCA gene status. Thus, the use of PARP inhibitors, alone or in combination, is now being studied in epithelial ovarian cancer irrespective of *BRCA* status.

Inhibition of the epidermal growth factor receptor (EGFR), which affects cell proliferation, angiogenesis, and apoptosis, has emerged as a possible therapeutic option for patients with ovarian cancer. Agents in this category may inhibit EGFR through tyrosine kinase inhibition (erlotinib, gefitinib, CI-1033) and monoclonal antibodies (trastuzumab, cetuximab). Patients

with refractory, recurrent ovarian cancer have demonstrated modest activity to EGFR inhibitors. Currently studies are evaluating the role of EGFR in the recurrent and maintenance setting, both as a single agent and in combination with other cytotoxic or biologic agents. A multitude of other molecular agents have also been evaluated in epithelial ovarian cancer. VEGF-trap, which inhibits VEGF and platelet growth factors, targets angiogenesis and has shown some activity in the platinum-resistant group and are under further investigation. The mTOR (mammalian target of rapamycin) inhibitors (temsirolimus, everolimus, deforolimus) target the PI3K/AKT/mTOR pathway and have recently been studied in phase II evaluations. The use of this agent in combination with other biologic and cytotoxic therapy is currently underway. Other agents being further evaluated include platelet-derived growth factor inhibitors, multikinase inhibitors (sorafenib, dasatinib), and folate receptor inhibitors.

The advent of molecular targets has been promising to date; however, it is still premature in understanding its true role. As information regarding the genetics of cancer and activity at the cellular level increases, this class of agents will have more applicability in cancer care. However, improving our understanding into these agents, providing selective use in specific populations, and maximizing efficiency in conjunction with cytotoxic therapies will be of continued importance.

Surgery for Recurrent Disease

Because recurrence is the rule than the exception for women with ovarian cancer, the role of surgery for recurrent disease both generally and selectively has been evaluated. The philosophy of secondary cytoreductive surgery is sometimes similar to that of primary cytoreductive surgery: Reduce disease burden to enhance the effectiveness of chemotherapy. However, surgery in the recurrent setting is also used selectively when it can make the most impact: a single remaining tumor mass resistant to multiple prior lines of chemotherapy or a single area of recurrence after years of treatment-free interval. To date, there are no prospective trials comparing secondary cytoreductive surgery with chemotherapy. Although several retrospective studies have shown benefit in specific groups of patients, the role of secondary cytoreductive surgery may be limited to select patients. Factors associated with a perceived survival benefit include patients with a good performance status; a longer disease-free interval, typically more than 12 months; and patients with disease localized to one or two sites. The most significant contributor to OS is the ability to resect all macroscopic disease at the time of recurrent disease. This has been demonstrated in a European multi-institutional review (Descriptive Evaluation of preoperative Selection KriTeria for OPerability in recurrent OVARian cancer [DESKTOP OVAR]) that showed that only patients who were able to undergo complete resection of recurrent disease benefit from surgical intervention. This finding was also reported in a meta-analysis, confirming that the only factor associated with survival benefit was complete resection of disease. Presently, the role of cytoreductive surgery in the recurrent setting is being evaluated in two prospective studies, DESKTOP II and a GOG study (protocol 213). Ideally, these studies will help elucidate the ideal patients and the true role of surgery for patients with recurrent ovarian cancer. Until the results are available, therapy should be individualized.

When the focus of care shifts from a curative intent to quality of life, surgery may play a role in the relief of symptoms. Although the risks and morbidity from invasive procedures must be considered, several situations during the terminal stages of the disease may be amenable by surgical intervention. Most commonly, this pertains to patients who develop an intestinal obstruction. Surgery may afford relief of symptoms by resecting the area followed by reanastomosis or performing an intestinal bypass. To decrease morbidity, patients with a distal obstruction may be excellent candidates for a diverting ostomy or intraluminal stent placement. For patients with a more proximal obstruction, endoscopic or percutaneous placement of a gastrostomy tube may provide symptomatic relief. Although occurring less frequently than GI blockage, malignant urologic obstructions may also occur with recurrent disease. To minimize morbidity, and depending on the location of the obstruction, treatment options include the placement of ureteral stents, percutaneous nephrostomy tubes, or a suprapubic catheter.

Patients with refractory disease may also develop ascites that significantly compromise their quality of life. This may result in a multitude of symptoms, including abdominal pain or discomfort and respiratory embarrassment. Unfortunately, some patients develop ascites that cannot be controlled by systemic chemotherapy, and they may require periodic aspiration. Although a palliative paracentesis may be adequate, patients with refractory, symptomatic ascites may benefit from the use of a long-term catheter. Patients may be found to have pleural effusions during the time of primary or recurrent disease diagnosis, which may present with symptoms of respiratory compromise. This may be a direct result of pleural disease or indirect result secondary to abdominal ascites. Similar techniques for the management of ascites can be used for pleural effusions. Thoracentesis (Fig. 11.24), which may be used for immediate relief of symptoms, is often used. When patients develop refractory reaccumulations, they may require insertion of an indwelling pleural catheter or chest tube drainage followed by pleurodesis. Pleurodesis can be performed with the instillation of bleomycin (60–120 mg) or talc into the pleural cavity and offers the highest probability of successful palliation.

REHABILITATION

The nature of ovarian cancer is such that the major vital organs (lungs, heart, liver, and kidneys) remain unaffected. The disease itself and its therapy appear primarily to attack the GI tract. Indeed, the terminal event for most patients who succumb to this disease is electrolyte imbalance caused by prolonged GI obstruction, malnutrition, and significant protein and electrolyte loss from repeated paracentesis and thoracentesis. It is necessary to support these patients with various forms of alimentation during therapy to sustain them sufficiently to tolerate the somewhat vigorous therapy often prescribed. The placement of semipermanent Silastic IV catheters (eg, Hickman, Broviac, or Groshong) greatly facilitates the ability to support these patients (Fig. 11.25). Some clinicians prefer to gain IV access by means of a device (Port-A-Cath) implanted in the subcutaneous tissue. Many centers can arrange IV alimentation at home for patients who are unable to take sufficient nourishment by mouth. Home pharmacy services are available in many areas, and IV medications, including analgesics, can be administered at home by pump infusion devices through these semipermanent IV catheters.

In general, the most discouraging aspect in the management of patients with ovarian cancer is the apathy of many physicians. In truth, these diseases are discouraging, but a determined attitude is medically sound and reassuring to the patient. Significant numbers of patients referred to oncologic centers as "unresectable" not only have had their tumor debulked but also have responded nicely to postoperative therapy. Still other patients have survived complicated combinations of multiple surgical and adjuvant therapies. A positive approach to the disease, which restores hope in the patient with this devastating illness, is justified on that basis alone.

CONCLUSIONS ON MANAGEMENT

Although adenocarcinoma of the ovary remains one of the solid tumors most sensitive to chemotherapeutic regimens, the mortality rate from this disease remains high. Progress over the past 30 years has been modest, and although there has been some improvement in survival, there is significant opportunity to do better (Table 11.25). There appears, however, to be great promise with newer developments in the management of this disease.

When treating a patient with ovarian cancer, the following general principles should be kept in mind. An optimal surgical procedure should be carried out whenever possible. This is defined as the removal of all visible tumor with the intent to leave no macroscopic residual disease. It is not possible to advocate any one operation for all patients, and the clinician must make a judgment at the time of surgery. Unquestionably, patients with small residual tumor volumes have a better prognosis with any postoperative therapy. Even when optimal debulking is not possible, bilateral salpingo-oophorectomy, total

FIGURE 11.24 Thoracentesis.

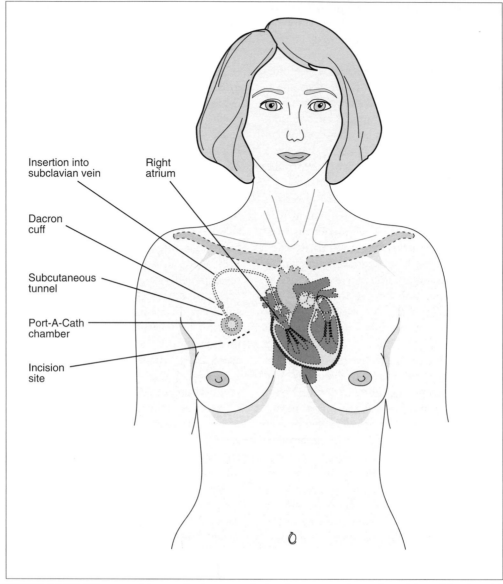

Insertion into
subclavian vein

Right
atrium

Dacron
cuff

Subcutaneous
tunnel

Port-A-Cath
chamber

Incision
site

FIGURE 11.25 Silicone rubber catheter tunneled subcutaneously and positioned in the right atrium.

TABLE 11.25 Relative Survival Percentage* for Women During Three Time Periods			
	Periods, by Cancer Site		
Site	**1974–1976**	**1984–1986**	**2001–2007**
All sites	56	58	67
Breast	75	80	90
Colon	50	57	68
Lung and bronchus	16	16	19
Ovary	36	39	44
Pancreas	2	3	6

*5-year relative survival rates based on follow-up of patients through 2008.
Source: SEER Program, 1975–2008, National Cancer Institute, 2011.

abdominal hysterectomy, and omentectomy can afford temporary improvement of symptoms for the patient. Second, the use of a chemotherapeutic regimen, containing platinum and taxane, plays an integral role in the care of patients with advanced disease. Recent advances in the route of administration (IP chemotherapy), use of dose-dense paclitaxel, and addition of bevacizumab are encouraging and further improvements need to be verified with ongoing clinical trials. Physicians should offer patients treatment on clinical trials whenever available.

Advances in genetics have helped increase our understanding regarding the natural history of ovarian cancer. Tumor suppressor genes such as *BRCA1*, *BRCA2*, and p53 and oncogenes including K-ras and erb-b2 are known to be altered in a fair number ovarian cancer cases. Developing specific targets for known genetic or cellular functions within tumors has become a popular area of interest and shows potential in early studies.

The role of continued surveillance for recurrent disease continues to evolve; thus, it is important to counsel patients on symptoms of recurrence, thus providing early intervention. When a recurrence is detected, multimodality treatment options, including surgery and chemotherapy, are available. Although, to date, therapies for recurrent disease have been short-lived with modest efficacy, promising new combinations of chemotherapy and biologic agents are being studied in hopes of improving outcomes.

CURRENT AREAS OF RESEARCH

Over the past several decades, the majority of advances in ovarian cancer treatment have resulted from phase III trial outcomes. These results include the combination of more effective chemotherapeutic agents, more effective route of administration, better understanding of drug resistance, and the addition of biologic response modifiers as a new modality, each strategy improving the outcome for this devastating group of malignant neoplasms.

Chemotherapy has proved curative in some types of advanced cancers and is useful as an adjunct to surgery and radiotherapy in many others. That 90% of the cures with chemotherapy occur in 10% of the tumors that affect humans is a perplexing biologic problem that appears to be related to the greater propensity of some tissue to develop specific and permanent resistance to chemotherapy of a broad nature. A discussion of tumor cell resistance is beyond the scope of this section; however, understanding and overcoming the mechanisms by which tumor resistance occurs will be necessary to improve treatment outcomes.

Although much has been learned about ovarian cancer and treatment modalities, the surface has just been scratched. With the explosion of new techniques to explore the genetic, immunologic, and molecular biology of this disease, many avenues for research are open and need exploration. The establishment of the NRG tumor and serum bank will continue to allow further investigation into these and many other aspects of molecular biology.

In addition to biologic targets, there are data supporting experimental therapies, such as gene therapy. Although gene therapy in its infancy, if the genetic defect is identified, the gene could be replaced. Many types of gene therapy are possible: immunogene, antioncogene, and tumor suppressor gene; anti–growth factor and cytokine gene drug resistance; and genes that are associated with apoptosis. All of these may be attractive, and preliminary studies have been started. Because of the emergence of chemotherapy resistance, new agents that have non–cross-resistance properties and novel approaches to modulations or targeting are sought. Many new drugs are in the pipeline to be evaluated in phase II studies.

More recently, receiving much deserved attention is a focus on patient's quality of life. Reliable and valid tools for measuring quality of life on multiple facets have been developed and are being incorporated into study protocols by the NRG and other cooperative group studies. These areas of study include symptoms related to cancer and surgical intervention, toxicities associated with therapy, and factors related to psychological stress. Other topics of interest include measurements of pain management, sexual function, and social support. This area is a challenge, and continuing studies will improve our ability to deliver optimal comprehensive care to our patients.

For the bibliography list, log onto www.expertconsult.com ⟨http://www.expertconsult.com⟩

12

Germ Cell, Stromal, and Other Ovarian Tumors

Emily R. Penick, MD, Chad A. Hamilton, MD, G. Larry Maxwell, MD, Charlotte S. Marcus, MD

KEY POINTS

1. Germ cell tumors are classified according to degree of differentiation. Two classes exist: undifferentiated germ cell tumors, which include dysgerminoma and gonadoblastomas, and differentiated tumors, which include all other germ cell tumors.
2. Most germ cell tumors are found in the second and third decades of life.
3. Surgery is the preferred initial approach in the treatment of germ cell cancers.
4. Recurrences usually occur within 2 years of initial diagnosis.
5. Granulosa cell tumors are typically ovarian cancers of low grade.

GERM CELL TUMORS

Classification

Ovarian germ cell tumors consist of several histologically different tumor types that arise from primordial germ cells of embryonic gonad and sex-stromal derivatives. This class of ovarian tumors is rare, accounting for 1% to 2% of all ovarian malignancies. The concept of germ cell tumors as a specific group of gonadal neoplasms evolved over the past 5 decades and has become generally accepted (Fig. 12.1). This theory is based primarily on the common histogenesis of these neoplasms and the frequent presence of histologically different tumor elements within the same mass. Additionally, histologically similar neoplasms occur in extragonadal locations along the line of migration of the primitive germ cells

from the wall of the yolk sac to the gonadal ridge, and there is remarkable homology between the various tumor types in men and women. In no other group of gonadal neoplasms has this homology been better illustrated. An example of this is the striking similarity between the testicular seminoma and its ovarian counterpart, the dysgerminoma. These were the first neoplasms to become accepted as originating from germ cells. A number of classifications of germ cell neoplasms of the ovary have been proposed over the past few decades. A modification of the classifications originally described by the pathologist Gunner Teilum in the 1950s is shown in Table 12.1. This schema is similar to that proposed by the World Health Organization (WHO), which divides the germ cell tumors into several groups, including neoplasms composed of germ cells and "sex" stroma derivatives.

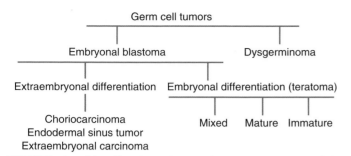

FIGURE 12.1 Classification schema of germ cell tumors of the ovary.

TABLE 12.2 Relative Frequency of Ovarian Neoplasms

Type	Frequency (%)
Coelomic epithelium	50–70
Germ cell	15–20
Specialized gonadal stroma	5–10
Nonspecific mesenchyme	5–10
Metastatic tumor	5–10

TABLE 12.1 Classification of Germ Cell Neoplasms of the Ovary

GERM CELL TUMORS

Dysgerminoma
Endodermal sinus tumor
Embryonal carcinoma
Polyembryoma
Choriocarcinomas
Mixed malignant germ cell tumor
Teratoma
- Immature (solid, cystic, or both)
- Mature
  - Solid
  - Cystic
    - Mature cystic teratoma (dermoid cyst)
    - Mature cystic teratoma (dermoid cyst) with malignant transformation
Monodermal or highly specialized
- Struma ovarii
- Carcinoid
- Neuroectodermal
- Others

TUMORS COMPOSED OF GERM CELLS AND SEX CORD–STROMAL DERIVATIVE

Gonadoblastoma
Mixed germ cell–sex cord stromal tumor

Germ cell tumors are classified according to the degree of differentiation. Two classes exist:
1. **Undifferentiated germ cell tumors, which include dysgerminoma and gonadoblastoma**
2. **Differentiated tumors, which include all other germ cell tumors.**

Differentiated tumors are further classified based on whether the tumor differentiates histologically into embryonic or extraembryonic structures. Extraembryonic tumors include choriocarcinoma and endodermal sinus tumors. Embryonal tumors include embryonal carcinoma, polyembryoma, and teratomas, the latter of which may be mature, immature, monodermal, or highly specialized. Dysgerminomas, immature teratoma, yolk sac tumors, and mixed tumors make up more than 90% of all malignant germ cell tumors. Finally, it is important to recognize that germ cell tumors clinically behave in part on whether they are histologically pure, consisting of only one cell type, or mixed. Tumors such as embryonal carcinoma, choriocarcinoma, and polyembryoma rarely exist in pure form and have a poorer prognosis. The clinical behavior of germ cell tumors typically conforms to the most aggressive histologic subtype present in mixed tumors. Treatment, therefore, should be predicated on this knowledge.

Clinical Profile

Germ cell tumors present at all stages of disease and are typically curable. **Germ cell tumors represent 20% of all ovarian** (Table 12.2) **neoplasms of which 97% are benign and only 3% are malignant.** There are no known risk factors predisposing women to germ cell tumors, **although most tumors occur in young women.** A Surveillance, Epidemiology and End Results (SEER) database review of malignant germ cell tumors from 1973 to 2002 revealed the highest incidence of disease in the 15- to 19-year-old age group. Because these tumors occur predominantly in reproductive age groups, it is not surprising that they are encountered commonly during pregnancy. **Dysgerminomas and teratomas are the most common germ cell tumors diagnosed during pregnancy or after delivery.** Surgical evaluation and treatment, including chemotherapy if necessary, can be safely performed in the second and third trimesters. Although rare reports of familial clustering of ovarian and testicular germ cell tumors have been described in the literature, there is no known syndrome or genetic abnormality conferring susceptibility to germ cell malignancies.

With respect to race, Asian and black women are affected by malignant germ cell tumors three times as frequently as white women and often have a worse prognosis. For example, SEER database results from 1988 to 2004 revealed improved survival in white women compared with black women, a finding attributable to a more favorable stage distribution and histology in whites. In this study, white patients were twice as likely as black patients to have dysgerminomas and one and a half times less likely to have immature teratomas. Advanced-stage tumors were also more common in black patients. Nevertheless, on multivariate analysis, race was not an independent predictor for survival after controlling for histology and stage of disease. Similarly, Smith et al. evaluated the incidence and survival rates of women with malignant germ cell tumors over a 30-year period from 1973 to 2002. In this study, malignant germ cell tumors were noted more often among Asians and Pacific Islanders and Hispanics compared with non-Hispanics. When women

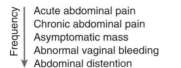

Acute abdominal pain
Chronic abdominal pain
Asymptomatic mass
Abnormal vaginal bleeding
Abdominal distention

FIGURE 12.2 Initial symptoms in young patients with malignant germ cell tumors.

were stratified by race and ethnicity, nonwhite women had a higher incidence of germ cell tumors than whites. The reasons for these racial differences in prevalence and outcomes are unknown.

According to SEER data, germ cell tumors are associated with excellent 5 and 10-year survival rates in excess of 91%. Survival rates are lower for older women and those with advanced-stage disease. Dysgerminomas have the most favorable survival rates among the histologic subtypes. A reduction in the number of women with distant and unstaged disease has been noted throughout the years, which suggests that these tumors are being diagnosed earlier.

Most of these lesions are found in the second and third decades of life and are frequently diagnosed by finding a palpable abdominal mass, often associated with pain (Fig. 12.2). Except for benign cystic teratoma, ovarian germ cell tumors are usually unilateral, rapidly enlarging abdominal masses that often cause considerable abdominal pain. At times, the pain is exacerbated by rupture or torsion of the neoplasm. One of the classic initial signs of a dysgerminoma, for example, is hemoperitoneum from capsular rupture of the tumor as it rapidly enlarges, although this may occur with any germ cell tumor. Asymptomatic abdominal distention, fever, or vaginal bleeding is occasionally the presenting complaint. Isosexual precocious puberty has also been described, occurring in young patients whose tumors express human chorionic gonadotropin (hCG).

The tumors typically present at an early stage and spread by direct extension, seeding abdominal and pelvic peritoneal surfaces, and by hematogenous and lymphatic spread. Hematogenous spread to the lungs and liver parenchyma is more common in germ cell malignancies than in epithelial ovarian cancer, as is lymphatic spread. Many germ cell tumors produce serum markers that are specific and sensitive enough to be used clinically in following disease progression. A detailed discussion of individual tumor markers is presented in the sections on specific tumor types.

Staging

Germ cell tumors should be staged surgically in the same manner as epithelial ovarian cancers and in accordance with the guidelines of the International Federation of Gynecologists and Obstetrician (FIGO). Because germ cell tumors occur more frequently in young patients, extirpation of the disease involves decisions concerning childbearing and probabilities of recurrence. Adjuvant chemotherapy is the standard of care for women with germ cell malignancies except for those with stage Ia dysgerminoma or stage Ia grade I immature teratoma. Comprehensive staging therefore allows patients to be appropriately risk stratified and selected for surveillance versus adjuvant

therapy. The recommended staging procedures for germ cell tumors consists of a laparotomy; a sampling of ascitic fluid if present; cell washings; a careful exploration of the abdomen and pelvic cavity; omentectomy; and random biopsies of the paracolic gutters, pelvic sidewalls, cul de sac, vesicouterine reflection, and diaphragm. If extensive disease is present in the abdominal cavity, omentectomy and cytoreduction to optimal residual disease should be performed if possible. Pelvic and paraaortic lymph node sampling should be performed, but a complete lymphadenectomy is not necessary. Bulky lymph nodes, if present, should be removed. Based on an analysis of SEER data, the prevalence of lymph node metastasis in germ cell malignancies is 18%. Dysgerminomas have the highest prevalence of nodal disease at 28% followed by mixed germ cell tumors at 16% and immature teratomas at 8%. After controlling for age, race, stage, and histology, positive lymph nodes remained an independent predictor of poor survival on multivariate analysis.

Despite the prognostic significance of positive lymph nodes and the obvious benefits of guiding adjuvant therapy, comprehensive surgical staging is frequently not performed. In a paper evaluating compliance with surgical staging guidelines, only three patients of 131 with germ cell malignancies had complete staging performed. Failure to perform recommended lymph node sampling was the most common reason for noncompliance (97%) followed by no omentectomy (36%) and no cytologic washings (21%). The decision to proceed with another operation for patients who have not been staged at their initial surgical procedure is controversial because patients with recurrences can often be salvaged with chemotherapy. According to a study from the Centre Léon Bérard in Lyon and the Institut Curie in Paris, the risk of recurrence was significantly higher (hazards ratio [HR], 4.5; 95% confidence interval [CI], 1.5–13.3) in unstaged patients who clinically appeared to have stage I disease and were observed after surgery versus another cohort treated with adjuvant chemotherapy. Among the unstaged patients, relapses occurred in five of 13 patients who underwent surveillance but none of the seven patients who received adjuvant treatment recurred. Data from the Pediatric Oncology Intergroup suggest that deviations from standard staging requirements do not adversely affect survival. In this study, the recommended surgical guidelines were seldom followed in this pediatric population, and the 6-year survival rate was 93.3% in girls with stage IV disease.

Laparoscopy is less common in patients with ovarian germ cell tumors given the larger size of these tumors, the solid components they contain, and the risk of tumor spillage and cyst rupture. Shim et al. evaluated laparoscopic management of early-stage malignant nonepithelial ovarian tumors to determine the feasibility and safety of a minimally invasive approach. This study included 20 patients with sex cord stromal tumors (SCSTs) and eight with malignant germ cell tumors. The median primary tumor diameter was 10.4 cm, and laparoscopic pelvic and paraaortic lymph node dissection was performed in nine cases. Tumors were removed through a 10-mm port using an endoscopic specimen retrieval system to prevent tumor spillage. For a mass that did not fit in the retrieval system, hand-assisted laparoscopic surgery was performed. All patients in this study had stage I disease. No intraoperative complications occurred. Five patients received adjuvant chemotherapy. The median follow-up period was 34.5 months during which time one patient recurred and was treated with chemotherapy. No patient died of the disease.

In patients with suspected early-stage disease, laparoscopy may represent a preferred surgical route and in several studies has been shown to be comparable with traditional open procedures. Prado et al. introduced guidelines to apply when considering a laparoscopic technique, such as careful case selection, adequately trained teams, use of an endobag for tumor removal, and minimizing tumor manipulation to decrease rupture of the mass. For advanced stage disease, it may not be feasible to attempt a laparoscopic procedure.

Treatment Options

Surgery is the preferred initial approach in patients with suspected germ cell tumors for both diagnostic and therapeutic intent. The extent of primary surgery is dictated by intraoperative findings and the reproductive desires of the patient. If childbearing has been completed, then a bilateral salpingo-oophorectomy and hysterectomy are performed in addition to a full staging procedure. However, if preservation of fertility is desired, then every attempt should be made to perform a unilateral salpingo-oophorectomy and staging while preserving the uterus and contralateral ovary. The safety of such an approach has been well established in the literature. **In select cases such as stage Ia dysgerminoma and stage Ia grade I immature teratoma, unilateral salpingo-oophorectomy is thought to be curative and is all that is required.** All other cases will likely require adjuvant therapy. In all cases of apparent unilateral disease confined to the ovary, the contralateral ovary should be carefully evaluated. Although **dysgerminoma is the only germ cell malignancy with a propensity for bilaterality (10%–20% of cases),** other histologic subtypes occasionally involve both ovaries. The contralateral ovary, if abnormal, should be biopsied or a cystectomy performed. If the frozen section confirms a diagnosis of malignancy, then the ovary should be removed. Frozen section is highly accurate for nonteratomatous sex cord stromal and germ cell tumors. If the contralateral ovary appears normal, then it should be left alone. Some clinicians have advocated performing a wedge biopsy of a normal-appearing contralateral ovary in cases of dysgerminoma to detect subclinical or microscopic disease. We recommend avoiding wedge biopsy of a normal-appearing ovary because of the potential for surgical complications such as hemorrhage or adhesion formation that may affect future fertility. Boran et al. evaluated pregnancy outcomes, menstrual function, and survival rates of patients after fertility sparing surgery for ovarian dysgerminomas. Twenty-three patients met inclusion criteria and underwent conservative surgical management with a median follow up time of 71 months. Regular menstruation after treatment resumed in 82% of the patients, and three primiparous patients had singleton live births after treatment.

The excellent response of germ cell malignancies to adjuvant chemotherapy has allowed a tailored approach to the surgical management of this disease in women desiring fertility preservation. Although **unilateral salpingo-oophorectomy should be considered the standard procedure** in such cases, recently, some clinicians have advocated ovarian cystectomy in select cases of immature teratoma. Beiner and colleagues reviewed eight cases of immature teratoma treated with ovarian cystectomy, including three with grade I, four with grade II, and one with grade III. Five of the eight patients received postoperative adjuvant chemotherapy. There were no recurrences in 4.7 years of follow-up, and three patients delivered a total of seven babies. The authors concluded that ovarian cystectomy with adjuvant chemotherapy appeared to be satisfactory therapy for early-stage immature teratoma if close follow-up was available, but more studies were needed to evaluate cystectomy alone as a surgical management option. This management strategy should be approached with caution, especially for other histologic germ cell subtypes, which may not share the same prognosis as early-stage immature teratoma.

Patients with bulky disease in the abdomen, pelvis, and retroperitoneum should undergo surgical cytoreduction to optimal residual disease. The literature to support this recommendation comes, primarily, from small retrospective studies. In a Gynecologic Oncology Group (GOG) study by Slayton and colleagues, patients with completely resected disease failed subsequent VAC (vincristine, dactinomycin, and cyclophosphamide) chemotherapy in 28% of the cases compared with 68% of cases with incomplete resection. In the same study, 82% of patients with bulky residual disease failed chemotherapy compared with 55% with minimal residual disease. Subsequently, the GOG published results showing that patients with clinically nonmeasurable disease after surgery treated with PVB (cisplatin, vinblastine, and bleomycin) remained progression free in 65% of cases compared with 34% of patients with measurable disease. Patients with optimal cytoreduction did better than those with unresectable bulky disease. This study also helped establish the efficacy of cisplatin-based chemotherapy for germ cell tumors. Finally, Williams and colleagues showed that patients with completely resected stage II or III disease treated with cisplatin, etoposide, and bleomycin had similar tumor-free recurrence rates as those with disease limited to the ovary. These studies provide the bulk of evidence to support cytoreductive surgery in germ cell cancers.

In patients with bulky metastatic disease, a normal-appearing uterus and contralateral ovary may be preserved, allowing for future fertility options if desired. Tangir and colleagues reviewed 64 patients with germ cell malignancies treated with fertility-preserving surgery. Ten patients had stage III disease (five IIIc, two IIIb, and three IIIa), and eight of the 10 women successfully conceived. Survival data were not included in the analysis. Zanetta and colleagues evaluated 138 women with germ cell malignancies of all stages treated with fertility-sparing surgery, 81 of whom received adjuvant chemotherapy. Survival was comparable between patients treated with radical surgery and fertility-sparing surgery after a mean follow-up period of 67 months. Similarly, Low and colleagues retrospectively reviewed 74 patients with germ cell malignancies of all cell types treated with conservative surgery. Forty-seven patients were treated with adjuvant chemotherapy. Fifteen patients had stage III to IV disease. After 52 months of follow-up, patients with advanced disease had a 94% survival rate, comparable to historical survival rates.

In summary, patients with germ cell malignancies should undergo operative evaluation, staging, and cytoreduction. If future fertility is not desired, surgical treatment should be identical to that for epithelial ovarian cancers. If preservation of fertility is desired, conservation of the uterus and contra-lateral ovary and maximal cytoreduction should be performed if possible. Despite the success of surgical management, surgeons should recognize the excellent response of these tumors to chemotherapy when aggressive and potentially morbid resections of metastatic and retroperitoneal disease are considered.

Surveillance for Stage I Tumors

As previously noted, **historically, in the gynecologic oncology literature, only patients with stage Ia dysgerminoma or stage Ia grade I immature teratoma of the ovary have been treated conservatively without adjuvant chemotherapy.** Although the recurrence rate approaches 20% for these patients, curative chemotherapy is administered after the recurrence. The recommendation for adjuvant treatment of any nondysgerminomatous histology is at odds with contemporary management practices of testicular germ cell tumors in which all patients with stage I disease are followed with observation only as standard practice. Rustin and Patterson published provocative data on their 37-year experience with a liberal surveillance policy for patients with stage I germ cell tumors of the ovary. In their first report, 24 patients with stage Ia germ cell tumor (nine dysgerminoma, nine pure immature teratoma, and six endodermal sinus tumor with or without immature teratoma) were followed without chemotherapy after surgery. The 5-year overall survival rate was 95%, and the disease-free survival rate was 68%. Eight patients had a recurrence or developed a second primary germ cell tumor and required chemotherapy. All but one who died of a pulmonary embolus were salvaged with chemotherapy. In their second publication, 37 patients with stage Ia germ cell malignancies were followed with surveillance only after surgery. Twenty-two percent of dysgerminoma and 36% of nondysgerminoma patients had a recurrence. All but one of these patients were successfully salvaged and cured with cisplatin-based chemotherapy at the time of recurrence. The overall disease-specific survival rate was 94%. It is unlikely that randomized trials addressing the safety of this approach in ovarian germ cell tumors will be performed. Given the potential serious toxicity associated with bleomycin, etoposide, and cisplatin (BEP) chemotherapy, managing patients with stage 1 germ cell tumors of the ovary with surveillance is a reasonable option if they have been adequately staged.

Second-Look Laparotomy

The role of the second-look laparotomy (SLL) in germ cell tumors of the ovary is unclear. Williams, when reporting the experience of the GOG, noted that in patients with complete tumor resection followed by BEP chemotherapy, 43 of 45 patients had no evidence of tumor or mature teratoma only at the time of the SLL, suggesting that there is no value of SLL in patients with completely resected disease. There were 72 patients with advanced, incompletely resected tumors who received chemotherapy followed by SLL. Of 48 patients who did not have teratomatous lesions in their primary surgery, 45 had no tumor. The three patients who had persistent tumors died of their disease despite aggressive therapy. **These authors think that the role of SLL is rarely, if ever, beneficial with an optimal cytoreduction followed by adequate chemotherapy.** However, patients in this series who had incompletely resected tumors at initial surgery and had teratomatous elements present may benefit from SLL. There were 24 patients who had teratomatous elements in the primary tumor and 16 who had progressive or bulky mature elements at SLL. Four patients had residual immature teratoma. Fourteen of the 16 with residual teratoma and six of the seven with bulky disease remained tumor free after secondary cytoreduction. Therefore, **the subgroup of patients that garner a survival benefit from SLL are those with incompletely resected disease with teratomatous elements at primary surgery.** The use of advanced imaging technologies such as positron emission tomography (PET) and computed tomography (CT) imaging may further reduce the impact of SLL. Preliminary studies suggest positive and negative predictive values of 100% and 96%, respectively, for PET imaging in seminomas looking for residual disease after chemotherapy, suggesting the possibility of similar results for germ cell malignancies.

Radiation Therapy

In the past, radiation therapy was traditionally used as adjuvant therapy for patients with germ cell malignancies and dysgerminomas in particular. Dysgerminomas are sensitive to radiation therapy with overall survival rates of between 70% and 100%. However, with the recent advances and success rates seen with combination chemotherapy, radiation therapy is rarely used today.

Chemotherapy

Current management strategies offer even patients with advanced malignancies an excellent chance at long-term control or cure. Because approximately 20% of patients with germ cell malignancies treated with surgery alone will be expected to recur, **patients, except those with stage Ia dysgerminoma and stage Ia grade I immature teratoma, should be treated with adjuvant chemotherapy to reduce the risk of recurrent disease.** VAC (vincristine, Adriamycin, and cyclophosphamide) was the first combination chemotherapy regimen widely used for treatment of these tumors. The GOG used VAC therapy to treat 76 patients with nondysgerminomatous germ cell tumors in the 1970s. Twenty-one percent of patients with stage I disease, 28% with completely resected disease, and 18% with immature teratomas failed VAC therapy, suggesting limited efficacy in these subgroups. However, 15 of 22 patients (68%) with advanced-stage or incompletely resected ovarian germ cell malignancies failed VAC therapy with a median progression-free survival (PFS) time of 8 months. VAC was also ineffective for approximately 50% of patients with endodermal sinus tumors (ESTs). Although the GOG subsequently treated 48 patients with stages I to III completely resected ESTs with VAC for six to nine courses. Thirty-five (73%) patients were free of disease with a median follow-up time of 4 years. Gershenson and associates also reported 18 of 26 (69%) patients with pure EST were free of tumors after VAC therapy. As a result of the success of cisplatin-based regimens in the treatment of testicular germ cell tumors, VAC was gradually replaced by VBP (vinblastine, bleomycin, and cisplatin). This transition resulted in an improvement in overall survival rate to 71%; however, failures still occurred even in patients with good prognosis at the conclusion of primary surgery. The GOG evaluated VBP in patients with stage III and IV or recurrent malignant germ cell tumors, many with measurable disease after surgery. Ninety-seven patients were treated, and this therapy produced a substantial number (43%) of durable complete responses. The overall progression-free interval at 24 months was approximately 51%.

In a landmark trial in testicular cancer in the 1980s, Williams et al. demonstrated improved survival and less neurotoxicity when etoposide was substituted for vinblastine. Subsequent smaller trials in ovarian germ cell tumors also demonstrated encouraging results. Williams reported the GOG experience with 93 patients who were given BEP as adjuvant treatment for malignant germ cell cancers of the ovary. Forty-two were immature teratomas, 25 were ESTs, and 24 were mixed germ cell tumors. At the time of Williams' report, 91 of 93 patients had no evidence of disease after three courses of BEP with a median follow-up time of 39 months. One patient developed acute myelomonocytic leukemia 22 months after diagnosis, and a second patient developed lymphoma 69 months after treatment. Dimopoulos and colleagues reported a similar result from the Hellenic Cooperative Oncology Group. Forty patients with nondysgerminomatous tumors were treated with BEP or PVB. With a median follow-up time of 39 months, five patients developed progressive disease and died. Only one of the five who failed received BEP. Most recently, de La Motte Rouge and associates reported on 52 women with endodermal sinus tumor, 35 of whom had stage I or II tumors and 17 with stage III or IV disease. All were treated with BEP. After a median follow-up time of 68 months, the 5-year overall survival and disease-free survival rates were 94% and 90%, respectively. In this series, fertility-sparing surgery was performed in 41 cases, and pregnancy was achieved in 12 of 16 (75%) women who attempted to conceive, demonstrating that conservative surgery plus chemotherapy resulted in an appreciable number of successful pregnancies after treatment.

The combination of bleomycin, etoposide, and cisplatin (BEP) has become the standard of care for ovarian germ cell tumors (Table 12.3). Treatment with BEP leads to cure in most women with malignant ovarian germ cell tumors and is well-tolerated. The BEP regimen consists of cisplatin 20 mg/m^2 and etoposide 100 mg/m^2 daily for 5 days and bleomycin 20 U/m^2 on day 1. The recommended treatment consists of three to four courses of BEP administered every 3 weeks in either inpatient or outpatient settings. Williams did demonstrate efficacy of

TABLE 12.3   VAC, VBP, and BEP Regimens

Regimen	Dosage Schedule
VAC	
Vincristine, 1.5 mg/m^2	Weekly IV administration for 12 wk (maximum dose 2.5 mg)
Dactinomycin, 0.5 mg	5-day IV course every 4 wk
Cyclophosphamide,	5-day IV course every 4 wk 5–7 mg/kg
VBP	
Vinblastine, 12 mg/m^2	IV every 3 wk for four courses
Bleomycin, 20 U/m^2	IV q wk for seven courses (maximum dose eighth course given in 30 U/m^2) wk 10
Cisplatin, 20 mg/m^2	Daily × 5 every 3 wk for three or four courses
BEP	
Bleomycin, 20 U/m^2	IV q wk × 9 (maximum dose, 30 U)
Etoposide, 100 mg/m^2	IV days 1–5 q 3 wk × 3
Cisplatin, 20 mg/m^2	IV days 1–5 q 3 wk × 3

BEP, Bleomycin, etoposide, and cisplatin; *IV,* intravenous; *q,* every; *VAC,* vincristine, actinomycin D (dactinomycin), and cyclophosphamide; *VBP,* vinblastine, bleomycin, and cisplatin.

carboplatin and etoposide in patients with stage IB to III dysgerminoma; none of the patients recurred after a median follow-up time of 7.62 years. However, contemporary data from studies with men with germ cell tumors showed cisplatin was superior to carboplatin, and the trial was closed early. Several investigators have also tried to determine if a 3-day BEP regimen is equally effective and decreases the occurrence of febrile neutropenia. Dimopoulos and colleagues demonstrated the safety and efficacy of outpatient BEP administered over 3 days using a lower dose of bleomycin in women with dysgerminoma or early-stage, optimally debulked nondysgerminoma malignancies. Likewise, the Taiwanese GOG investigated a 3-day BEP regimen. In this study, a regimen consisting of bleomycin (15mg/m^2; daily total dose <25 mg) and etoposide (100 mg/m^2) were administered on days 1 through 3, and cisplatin (100 mg/m^2) was administered on day 1 at 21-day intervals for 3 to 4 cycles. Among 239 patients, 159 had early-stage disease, and 53 had advanced-stage disease. When compared with early-stage disease, those with advanced disease had an approximately 20-fold increased risk of disease recurrence and a 19.2-fold increased risk of disease related mortality. Among patients with early-stage, optimally debulked tumors, the 3-day regimen did not adversely affect survival.

Controversy exists regarding the efficacy of high-dose cisplatin used in combination with etoposide and bleomycin (HDBEP). Several adult trials in testicular germ cell malignancies have suggested improved efficacy compared with standard-dose cisplatin, but other studies have not seen this association. Cushing and colleagues, however, evaluated HDBEP in 74 pediatric patients with ovarian germ cell malignancies. The HDBEP regimen consisted of high-dose cisplatin at 200 mg/m^2/d for 5 days with etoposide, 100 mg/m^2/d for 5 days, and bleomycin, 15 mg/m^2/d for 1 day per cycle. This study found no difference in overall survival and increased toxicity with the HDBEP regimen. These studies have not been replicated in adults with ovarian germ cell malignancies. Currently, there is no established role of high-dose therapy in ovarian germ cell tumors.

Current management strategies for germ cell malignancies use chemotherapy in an adjuvant setting and to treat recurrent disease. Completely resected disease treated in this fashion can be cured nearly 100% of the time. Metastatic or incompletely resected tumors, however, may fare worse but still have excellent long-term survival rates and should be treated aggressively with adjuvant chemotherapy.

Neoadjuvant Chemotherapy

Because the majority of patients with malignant ovarian germ cell tumors are diagnosed when the disease is in an early stage, most patients are treated with surgery followed by chemotherapy. In patients with widespread disease, neoadjuvant chemotherapy (NACT) may be warranted. Few trials, and certainly no randomized trials, are available to answer the question regarding utility in these patients. However, Talukdar et al. evaluated the use of NACT using four cycles of BEP followed by fertility-sparing surgery in 23 patients with bulky disease compared with 43 patients who underwent primary debulking surgery with FIGO stage III or IV disease during the same time period. The WHO criteria for response to chemotherapy were used, with a complete response defined as the complete disappearance of all clinically detectable disease and normalization of tumor markers. A partial response was defined as 50% or greater reduction in tumor size and decrease in tumor markers. After NACT, 21 patients showed a response to treatment with 16 achieving a complete response and five with a partial response. Eighteen of 21 patients in the NACT group were then able to undergo fertility-sparing surgery, and those with residual disease were given an additional two cycles of BEP. Of the evaluable patients, 21 of 23 patients survived with a median disease-free survival period of 211 months. Lu et al. also investigated the role of neoadjuvant treatment in a group of 127 women with yolk sac tumors. After a median follow-up period of 46 months, there was no significant difference in recurrence rate between the NACT and primary debulking group. For women presenting with advanced, bulky disease, or medical comorbidities, initial studies suggest a role for NACT.

Recurrences in Germ Cell Cancer

Even in cases of advanced-stage disease, the majority of patients with germ cell malignancies are cured with a combination of primary surgery and adjuvant combination platinum-based chemotherapy. All patients with germ cell malignancies, especially those with early-stage disease treated with conservative therapy for curative intent, warrant close follow-up. Patients with early-stage dysgerminoma treated with salpingo-oophorectomy alone, for example, have disease recurrence in 15% to 25% of cases. Studies evaluating surveillance strategies for ovarian germ cell tumors and SCSTs have not been performed; therefore, recommendations are based on expert opinion. Patients should be seen every 2 to 4 months for the first 2 years after treatment at which point they can transition to annual visits. Surveillance should include a thorough physical examination

and serum tumor markers. Radiologic scans should be reserved for elevations in tumor markers or concerning physical exam findings or symptoms, but for patients without elevated tumor markers, imaging within the first 2 years may be helpful.

Recurrences usually occur within 2 years of primary therapy and can be treated successfully. The value of secondary cytoreductive procedures in patients with germ cell malignancies has not been studied. Given the sensitivity of these malignancies to combination chemotherapy regimens, it is highly likely that metastatic lesions will respond to subsequent chemotherapy, limiting the value of secondary cytoreduction. Yet cytoreduction remains an effective management option for isolated lesions. The optimal chemotherapy regimen in recurrent disease is unknown. Historically, studies have included both patients with advanced primary disease and recurrent disease in the same trial. The recurrent cohorts in these trial are often very small, less than 10 patients, limiting significant conclusions about therapy. Recurrences after chemotherapy are defined as platinum resistant or platinum sensitive, a classification with clinical significance because platinum-resistant disease is not thought to be curable. For patients with platinum-resistant or platinum-refractory disease, optimal treatment has not been defined, and the prognosis overall is poor. The group at the MD Anderson Cancer Center noted 42 primary therapy failures in 160 patients with germ cell tumors. Vincristine, actinomycin-D, and cyclophosphamide were the principal agents used during the first 10 years of the study period. Cisplatin-based combination therapy was used more extensively in the late 1970s and 1980s. Salvage therapy varied with 24 patients receiving surgery and 34 patients receiving chemotherapy. Of patients receiving chemotherapy, 11 were treated with VAC and 11 with a platinum-based regimen. The median survival time for the entire group was 19 months. The PFS time was 6.8 months with a range of 0.9 to 24 months. No patient had disease recurrence longer than 2 years from initial diagnosis. More recently, male patients with platinum-resistant or platinum-refractory germ cell tumors have been treated with combination chemotherapy consisting of gemcitabine, oxaliplatin, and paclitaxel. This regimen has an acceptable toxicity profile, a 51% overall response rate, and a 39% complete or tumor marker–negative response rate. The median response duration was 8 months.

Treatment Toxicity

Given the favorable long-term outcomes associated with modern surgical management and combination platinum-based chemotherapy, the long-term effects of treatment must be considered carefully. Because many patients undergo conservative surgery for their disease, meticulous surgical technique is essential to avoid future infertility related to surgically induced pelvic adhesive disease. Equally important is avoiding unnecessary hysterectomies and biopsies of normal-appearing contralateral ovaries. Women with fertility-sparing surgery can be expected to have the same survival outcome as those patients treated with standard surgery. A review of SEER data from 1988 to 2001 involving 760 patients with germ cell malignancies concluded that the overall survival rate of patients treated with fertility-sparing surgery (*n* = 313) was not statistically different from those who underwent standard surgery. This study revealed that the use of fertility-sparing surgery also had increased over the study period. Two-thirds of the patients had stage I to II disease, and one third had stage III to IV disease. The most common histologic subtype was immature teratoma (55%) followed by dysgerminoma (32%).

Although successful, concern exists over potential toxicity of the BEP regimen. Namely, bleomycin is associated with acute and long-term pulmonary toxicity, etoposide with the risk of secondary malignancies, and cisplatin with nephro-toxicity. Controversy exists over whether baseline pulmonary function testing is required before initiating bleomycin. Data from retrospective trials and testicular cancer literature suggest carboplatin and etoposide is an acceptable regimen for patients who cannot tolerate BEP.

The long-term effect of combination chemotherapy in germ cell malignancies is less clear. **Of particular concern is the risk of development of acute myelogenous leukemia (AML) associated with etoposide use. This risk appears to be dose and schedule dependent.** AML rarely develops in patients receiving three cycles or less of etoposide or cumulative doses of less than 2000 mg/m². It is estimated that the risk of developing AML is 0.4% if these cutoff values are used. Leukemia, when it occurs, typically is seen within 2 to 3 years after treatment. An analysis of the risk-to-benefit ratio favors the use of etoposide in advanced germ cell malignancies, in which one case of etoposide-induced AML would be expected to occur for every 20 patients cured.

The long-term effects of chemotherapy on gonadal function appear to be minimal. Most younger patients can expect a return to normal ovarian function and reproductive potential with no additional risk of congenital malformations in their offspring. The most significant risk factor for impaired fertility is age and type of treatment administered. Although ovarian failure is a risk associated with chemotherapy, factors such as older age at treatment, higher drug doses, and long duration of therapy appear to confer higher risk. Childhood cancer patients treated with standard contemporary agents such as BEP have the greatest likelihood of preservation of fertility, resumption of normal menstrual cycles, and normal sexual development by virtue of the higher number of follicles present in young women compared with older women. Although normal menstrual cycles will likely resume in reproductive-age women, data suggest an increased risk of diminished ovarian reserve resulting in a significant reduction in the probability of pregnancy by 50%. Reproductive-aged women are likely to have reduced ovarian volume compared with control participants, fewer antral follicles on ultrasonography, and lower levels of inhibin B and estradiol on cycle days 2 to 5. Alkylating agents such as cyclophosphamide are far more likely to cause toxicity to the gonads than other chemotherapeutic agents. In one study, alkylating agents had an odds ratio (OR) of 4 for causing pre-mature ovarian failure compared with platinum agents (OR, 1.8) or plant alkaloids (OR 1.2).

There is some literature to suggest that gonadotropin-releasing hormone (GnRH) agonists may be cytoprotective for primordial follicles when given during chemotherapy.

Most of these data are retrospective; however, recently, Badawy and colleagues reported on a prospective randomized trial in 80 breast cancer patients younger than age 40 years who were randomly assigned to GnRH agonists with chemotherapy or chemotherapy alone. Ninety percent of study patients resumed menses, and 70% resumed spontaneous ovulation within 8 months of completing therapy compared with 33% and 26% of control patients, respectively. In the setting of germ cell malignancies, in which younger age at diagnosis is the norm, these patients should be counseled on the risks and benefits of GnRH agonists as well as consultation with a repro-ductive endocrinologist.

Dysgerminoma

Dysgerminoma is the most common germ cell malignancy, accounting for 1% to 2% of primary ovarian neoplasms and for 3% to 5% of ovarian malignancies. **Dysgerminoma may occur at any age from infancy to old age,** but most cases occur in adolescence and early adulthood (Fig. 12.3). They also present at a relatively early stage:

Stage Ia	65%–75%
Stage Ib	10%–15%
Stages II and III	15%
Stage IV	5%

Dysgerminoma consists of germ cells that have not dif-ferentiated to form embryonic or extraembryonic structures (Fig. 12.4). The stroma is almost always infiltrated with lym-phocytes and often contains granulomas similar to those seen in sarcoidosis. Occasionally, dysgerminoma contains isolated gonadotropin-producing syncytiotrophoblastic giant cells. An elevated serum lactate dehydrogenase or hCG level may be present in these patients. Grossly, the tumor may be firm, fleshy, cream colored, or pale tan; both its external and cut surfaces may be lobulated. **A few dysgerminomas arise in females with sex chromosome abnormalities, particularly those with pure (46,XY) or mixed (45,X, 46,XY) gonadal dysgenesis or testicular feminization (46,XY). In such cases, the dysgerminoma often develops in a previously existing**

FIGURE 12.3 Large (25-cm) solid mass of the right ovary in a 16-year-old girl with stage Ia dysgerminoma.

FIGURE 12.4 Dysgerminoma is characterized histologically by the presence of large, round, ovoid, or polygonal cells with stroma infiltrated by lymphocytes.

TABLE 12.4 Results of Conservative and Nonconservative Surgery in Stage Ia Dysgerminoma of the Ovary		
	10-Year Survival Rate	
	Conservative Surgery (%)	**Nonconservative Therapy* (%)**
Asadourian and Taylor	42/46 (91)[†]	21/25 (84)
Gordon et al.	68/72 (94)[†]	11/14 (79)
Malkasian and Symmonds	23/27 (85)[†]	13/14 (93)
Total	**133/145 (92)[†]**	**45/53 (85)**

*Surgery plus radiation.
[†]Includes those salvaged after a recurrence (23 or 25%–92%).

gonadoblastoma. The symptoms of dysgerminoma are similar to those observed in patients with other solid ovarian neoplasms. Large, rapidly growing tumors may lead to a relatively short duration of symptoms. **The most common initial symptoms are abdominal enlargement and the presence of a mass in the lower abdomen.** When the tumor is small and moves freely, its capsule is intact. Large lesions, however, may rupture or adhere to surrounding structures. Rupture can lead to peritoneal implantation, resulting in an increase in stage. Occasionally, menstrual and endocrine abnormalities may be the initial symptoms, but these symptoms tend to be more common in patients with dysgerminoma combined with other neoplastic germ cell elements, especially choriocarcinoma. In several cases, the tumor has been found incidentally at cesarean section or as a cause of dystocia. **Dysgerminoma is the most common malignant ovarian neoplasm observed in pregnancy.** The relatively common finding of dysgerminoma in pregnant patients is nonspecific and relates to the age of the patient rather than to the pregnant state. **Dysgerminoma is the only germ cell tumor in which the opposite ovary is frequently involved with the tumor process (10%–20% of cases).** Kurman and Norris reported a 20% incidence of disease in the serially sectioned normal appearing opposite ovary. **Dysgerminomas are notable by their predilection for lymphatic spread and their sensitivity to irradiation and chemotherapy.** The lymph nodes in the vicinity of the common iliac arteries and the terminal part of the abdominal aorta are typically the first to be affected. Occasionally, there may be marked enlargement of these lymph nodes, with a mass evident on abdominal examination. The lesion can spread from these abdominal nodes to the mediastinal and supraclavicular nodes. Hematogenous spread to other organs occurs later. Any organ can be affected, although involvement of the liver, lungs, and bones is most common.

Because 85% of all patients with dysgerminomas are younger than 30 years, conservative therapy and preservation of fertility are major considerations. In patients in whom unilateral salpingo-oophorectomy is performed, careful inspection of the contralateral ovary and exploration to rule out disseminated disease are mandatory. The authors' routine is not to wedge or bivalve the opposite ovary if it has a normal size, shape, and consistency. In a review of the literature, more than 400 cases of dysgerminoma were reported. Seventy percent of patients had stage I disease at diagnosis, and only 10% involved both ovaries. Schwartz and colleagues reported four patients with metastasis to the contralateral ovary and preservation of that ovary with subsequent chemotherapy. All patients were alive and had no disease 14 to 56 months after diagnosis. **Assessment of the retroperitoneal lymph nodes is an important part of the initial surgical therapy because these neoplasms tend to spread to the lymph nodes, particularly to the high para-aortic nodes.**

Conservative surgery without radiation or adjuvant chemotherapy in stage Ia lesions has resulted in excellent outcomes (Table 12.4). Several prognostic factors in dysgerminoma influence the decision to use adjuvant chemotherapy in early stages of the disease. Some authors suggest that in patients with large tumors (>10 cm), there is a greater chance of a recurrence; therefore, adjuvant therapy should be given. Today, most agree that tumor size is not prognostically important, and these patients do not require additional therapy. Although there is presently no good evidence that the behavior of an individual tumor can be assessed from its histologic appearance, we do know that the presence of other germ cell elements worsens prognosis. Data regarding the prognostic significance of age is inconsistent. **The long-term survival rate is almost 90% across all patients who have stage I lesions.**

De Palo and associates reported on 56 patients who had pure dysgerminomas. In their study, 44 patients underwent lymphangiography, and a positive study resulted in the restaging of 32% of patients. Diaphragmatic implants were not found in any patients, and positive cytologic findings were obtained in only three patients. The 5-year relapse-free survival rates were 91% in patients with stages Ia, Ib, and Ic; 74% in those with stage III retroperitoneal disease; and 24% in patients who had stage III peritoneal disease. Peritoneal involvement of any kind was associated with a poor prognosis if disease had extended to the abdominal cavity. All patients with stage III disease received postoperative radiation therapy.

These patients should be followed closely and have periodic examinations because approximately 90% of recurrences appear in the first 2 years after initial therapy. Fortunately, most recurrences can be successfully eradicated by salvage therapy including surgery, chemotherapy, and potentially radiation therapy. Recurrences should be treated aggressively with reexploration and cytoreductive surgery. The removed tissue should be examined carefully for evidence of germ cell elements other than dysgerminoma. Some presumed recurrent dysgerminomas have been found to be mixed germ cell tumors and should be treated accordingly.

Although radiation therapy has been successful in treating dysgerminomas, chemotherapy has become the treatment of choice because radiotherapy is associated with a high incidence of gonadal failure. The success rate of chemotherapy is as good as that of radiation, and preservation of fertility is possible in many patients, even those with bilateral ovarian disease. Weinblatt and Ortega reported on five children with extensive disease who were treated with chemotherapy as the primary therapeutic modality. Three of the five children were alive and free of disease at the time of the report, suggesting a therapeutic approach to extensive childhood dysgerminoma that spares pelvic and reproductive organs.

The common association of dysgerminoma with gonadoblastoma, a tumor that almost always occurs in patients with dysgenetic gonads, indicates that there is a relationship between dysgerminoma and genetic and somatosexual abnormalities. Patients with these genetic abnormalities should be offered gonadectomy after puberty to prevent the development of gonadoblastoma or dysgerminoma. Phenotypically normal females suspected of having a dysgerminoma should be evaluated with a karyotype, especially if ovarian conservation is desired. Patients with pathology reports that reveal streak gonads or gonadoblastomas should also be karyotyped. If a Y chromosome is present, the retained contralateral ovary should be removed to prevent neoplasia. Historically, fertility-sparing surgery has not been offered to patients with dysgerminoma associated with gonadoblastoma because of the frequent occurrence of bilateral tumors and the absence of normal gonadal function. Investigation of the genotypes and karyotypes of all patients with this neoplasm is recommended by some, especially if any history of virilization or other developmental abnormalities is elicited. In vitro fertilization can be used in patients without gonads. Therefore, it may be prudent to preserve the uterus in patients in whom the ovaries must be removed. In most cases, the authors leave the uterus. This is particularly important in prepubertal patients because in these patients, other signs of abnormal function (eg, primary amenorrhea, virilization, and absence of normal sexual development) are lacking.

Often lesions that consist primarily of dysgerminoma elements contain small areas of more malignant histology (eg, embryonal carcinoma or endodermal sinus tumor). If tumor markers such as alpha-fetoprotein (AFP) or hCG are elevated, a strong suspicion of mixed lesions should be entertained. When the dysgerminoma is not pure and these more malignant components are present, the prognosis and therapy are determined by the more malignant germ cell elements, and the dysgerminoma component is disregarded.

Endodermal Sinus Tumor (Yolk Sac Tumor)

Endodermal sinus tumors are the second most common form of malignant germ cell tumors of the ovary, accounting for 22% of malignant germ cell lesions in one large series. The median age at diagnosis is 19 years old, and three-fourths of the patients are initially seen with a combination of abdominal pain and abdominal or pelvic mass. Endodermal sinus tumors are characterized by extremely rapid growth and extensive intraabdominal spread; almost half the patients seen by a physician complain of symptoms of 1 week's duration or less.

Acute symptoms can alternatively be caused by torsion of the tumor and may lead to the diagnosis of acute appendicitis or a ruptured ectopic pregnancy. These yolk sac tumors are almost always unilateral. The tumor is usually large with most tumors measuring between 10 and 30 cm. On the cut surface, they appear gray-yellow with areas of hemorrhage and cystic, gelatinous changes. These neoplasms are highly malignant; they metastasize early and invade the surrounding structures. Intraabdominal spread leads to extensive involvement of abdominal structures with tumor deposits. Metastases also occur via the lymphatic system. AFP levels are often elevated.

Endodermal sinus tumors are thought to originate from germ cells that differentiate into the extra embryonal yolk sac because the tumor structure is similar to that found in the endodermal sinuses of the rat yolk sac. The tumors consist of scattered tubules or spaces lined by single layers of flattened cuboidal cells; loose reticular stroma; numerous scattered para-aminosalicylic–positive globules; and, within some spaces or clefts, a characteristic invaginated papillary structure with a central blood vessel (Schiller-Duval body) (Fig. 12.5). Frequently, intracellular and extracellular hyaline droplets that represent deposits of AFP can be identified throughout the tumor.

Historically, the prognosis for patients with endodermal sinus tumor of the ovary was unfavorable. Most patients died of the disease within 12 to 18 months of diagnosis. Until multiple-agent chemotherapy was developed, there were only a few known 5-year survivors, most of whom had tumors confined to the ovary. Kurman and Norris reported no long-term survivors in 17 patients with stage I tumors who were receiving adjunctive radiation or single alkylating agent, dactinomycin, or methotrexate. Gallion and colleagues reviewed the literature in 1979 and found that only 27% of 96 patients with stage I endodermal sinus tumors were alive at 2 years. The tumor is not sensitive to radiation therapy, although there may be an initial response. Optimal surgical extirpation of the disease has been advocated, but this alone is unsuccessful in producing a significant number of cures.

With surgery and multiagent chemotherapy, however, there have been optimistic reports of sustained remissions. In several cases, the tumor consisted of endodermal sinus tumors admixed with other neoplastic germ cell elements, frequently dysgerminoma. The clinical course in most patients with tumors composed of endodermal sinus tumor associated with dysgerminoma

FIGURE 12.5 Endodermal sinus tumor. **A,** Gross appearance with areas of hemorrhage and gelatinous necrosis. **B,** Microscopic appearance with isolated papillary projections containing single blood vessels and having peripheral lining of neoplastic cells (Schiller-Duval body).

FIGURE 12.6 Gross photograph of embryonal carcinoma of the ovary.

FIGURE 12.7 Microscopic appearance of large primitive cells with occasional papillary or glandlike formations characteristic of embryonal carcinoma.

or other neoplastic germ cell elements does not differ greatly from that in patients with pure endodermal sinus tumors. Mixed germ cell lesions often contain endodermal sinus tumors as one of the types present.

From a practical point of view, **serum AFP determination is considered to be a useful diagnostic tool in patients who have endodermal sinus tumors and should be considered an ideal tumor marker.** It can be useful when monitoring the results of therapy and for detecting metastasis and recurrences after therapy. As noted earlier, many investigators use AFP as a guide to the number of courses needed for an individual patient. In many cases, only three or four courses have placed patients into remission with long-term survival. Levels of hCG and its beta subunit (beta-hCG) have been found to be normal in patients with endodermal sinus tumor.

Embryonal Carcinoma

Embryonal carcinoma is one of the most aggressive ovarian malignancies (Fig. 12.6). The neoplasm closely resembles the

embryonal carcinoma of the adult testes, a relatively common tumor. However, it represents only 4% of malignant ovarian germ cell tumors in the ovary, and its confusion with choriocarcinoma and ESTs in the past accounts for its late identification as a distinct entity. It usually manifests as an abdominal mass or pelvic mass occurring at a mean age of 15 years. More than half of the patients have hormonal abnormalities, including precocious puberty, irregular uterine bleeding, amenorrhea, or hirsutism. The tumors consist of large primitive cells with occasional papillary or glandlike formations (Fig. 12.7). The cells have eosinophilic cytoplasms with distinct borders and round nuclei with prominent nucleoli. Numerous mitotic figures, many atypical, are seen; scattered throughout the tumor are multinucleated giant cells that resemble syncytial cells.

These tumors secrete hCG from syncytiotrophoblast-like cells and AFP from large primitive cells, and these tumor markers can be used to monitor progress during therapy. This

TABLE 12.5 Comparison of Embryonal Carcinoma With Endodermal Sinus Tumor

	Endodermal Sinus Tumor (n = 71)	Embryonal Carcinoma (n = 15)
Median age (yr)	19	15
Prepubertal status (%)	23	47
Precocious puberty (%)	0	43
Positive pregnancy test	None (0/15)	All (9/9)
Vaginal bleeding (%)	1	33
Amenorrhea (%)	0	7
Hirsutism (%)	0	7
Survival, stage I patients (%)	16	50
Human chorionic gonadotropin	Negative (0/15)	Positive (10/10)
α-Fetoprotein	Positive (15/15)	Positive (7/10)

From Kurman RJ, Norris HJ. Endodermal sinus tumor of the ovary: a clinical and pathological analysis of 71 cases. *Cancer* 1976;38:2404.

tumor probably arises from primordial germ cells, but it develops before there is much further differentiation toward either embryonic or extraembryonic tissue. In a review of 15 patients, Kurman and Norris reported an actuarial survival rate of 30% for the entire group; for those with stage I tumors, the survival rate was 50% (Table 12.5). This result is significantly better than the survival rate for endodermal sinus tumors for the same period of time and before the advent of multiple-agent adjuvant chemotherapy.

Polyembryoma

Polyembryoma is a rare ovarian germ cell neoplasm that consists of numerous embryoid bodies resembling morphologically normal embryos. Similar homologous neoplasms occur more frequently in the human testes. To date, only a few ovarian polyembryomas have been reported. In most cases, the polyembryoma has been associated with other neoplastic germ cell elements, mainly the immature teratoma. Polyembryoma is a highly malignant germ cell neoplasm. It is usually associated with invasion of adjacent structures and organs and metastases confined to the abdominal cavity. The tumor is not sensitive to radiotherapy, and its response to chemotherapy is unknown.

Choriocarcinoma

Choriocarcinoma, is a rare, highly malignant tumor that may be associated with sexual precocity. Gestational choriocarcinomas of the ovary contain paternal DNA and are further classified into primary gestational choriocarcinoma associated with ovarian pregnancy or metastatic choriocarcinoma arising in other parts of the genital tract, mainly the uterus. Nongestational choriocarcinomas are germ cell tumors that differentiate toward trophoblastic structures. Only nongestational choriocarcinoma of the ovary is discussed here. In most cases, the tumor is admixed with other neoplastic germ cell elements, and their presence is diagnostic of nongestational choriocarcinoma. The tumor, in common with other

malignant germ cell neoplasms, occurs in children and young adults. Its occurrence in children has been emphasized; in some series, 50% of cases occurred in prepubescent children. This high incidence in children may result from the previous reluctance of investigators to make the diagnosis in adults.

Choriocarcinomas secrete hCG, leading to manifestations of isosexual precocious puberty with mammary development, growth of pubic and axillary hair, and uterine bleeding. In adult patients, the increased production of hCG may cause signs of ectopic pregnancy. Estimation of urinary or plasma hCG levels is a useful diagnostic test in these cases. Historically, the prognosis of patients with choriocarcinoma of the ovary was unfavorable, but modern chemotherapy regimens have effectively improved survival.

Mixed Germ Cell Tumors

Mixed germ cell tumors contain at least two malignant germ cell elements. Dysgerminoma is the most common component, 80% in Kurman and Norris' report and 69% in material from the MD Anderson Hospital. Immature teratoma and EST are also frequently identified; embryonal carcinoma and choriocarcinoma are seen only occasionally. It is not unusual to see three or four different germ cell components. In 42 patients treated at the MD Anderson Hospital from 1944 through 1983, nine patients were treated with surgery alone, and another six patients received radiation therapy; all developed recurrences. To improve outcomes, the most malignant cell type should drive the selection of the adjuvant chemotherapy regimen.

Teratoma
Mature Cystic Teratoma

Accounting for more than 95% of all ovarian teratomas, the dermoid cyst, or mature cystic teratoma, is one of the most common ovarian neoplasms. Teratomas account for approximately 15% of all ovarian tumors. They are the most common ovarian tumors in women in the second and third decades of life. Most benign cystic lesions contain mature tissue of ectodermal, mesodermal, or endodermal origin. The most common elements are ectodermal derivatives such as skin, hair follicles, and sebaceous or sweat glands, accounting for the characteristic histologic and gross appearance of teratomas (Fig. 12.8). These tumors are usually multicystic and contain hair intermixed with foul-smelling, sticky, keratinous and sebaceous debris. Occasionally, well-formed teeth are seen along with cartilage or bone. If the tumor consists of only ectodermal derivatives of skin and skin appendages, it is a true dermoid cyst. A mixture of other, usually mature tissues (gastrointestinal, respiratory) may be present.

The clinical manifestation of this slow-growing lesion is usually related to its size, compression, or torsion or to a chemical peritonitis secondary to intraabdominal spill of the cholesterol-laden debris. The latter event tends to occur more commonly when the tumor is large. Torsion is the most frequent complication, observed in as many as 16% of the cases in one large series, and tends to occur more commonly during pregnancy, the puerperium, and in children and younger

FIGURE 12.8 Benign cystic teratoma. **A** and **B,** Gross appearance. **C,** Microscopic view of ectodermal elements (skin and skin appendages). **D,** Immature neural elements evident.

patients. **Severe acute abdominal pain is usually the initial symptom,** and the condition is considered to be an acute abdominal emergency. **Mature cystic teratomas are said to comprise 22% to 40% of ovarian tumors in pregnancy,** and 0.8% to 12.8% of reported cases of mature cystic teratomas have occurred in pregnancy. **Rupture of a mature cystic teratoma is an uncommon complication,** occurring in approximately 1% of cases, but it is much more common during pregnancy and may manifest during labor. **The immediate result of rupture may be shock or hemorrhage, especially during pregnancy or labor,** but the prognosis even in these cases is favorable. **Rupture of the tumor into the peritoneal cavity may be followed by a chemical peritonitis caused by the spill of the contents of the tumor.** This may result in a marked granulomatous reaction, leading to the formation of dense adhesions throughout the peritoneal cavity. Infection is an uncommon complication of mature cystic teratoma and occurs in approximately 1% of cases. The infecting organism is usually a coliform, but *Salmonella* spp. infection causing typhoid fever has also been reported. Removal of the neoplasm by ovarian cystectomy or, rarely, oophorectomy is adequate therapy. Malignant degeneration of mature teratomas is a rare occurrence. **When it occurs, the most common secondary tumor is a squamous cell carcinoma.** The prognosis and behavior of this secondary malignancy are similar to those of squamous cell cancers arising in other anatomic sites and appear to be highly dependent on stage. There is no consensus on treatment recommendations; however, patients with stage I to II disease treated with platinum-based chemotherapy and whole-pelvic radiation have a chance for long-term survival. Although squamous cell carcinoma in this setting is usually an incidental finding at pathology, preoperative risk factors include age older than 50 years, tumor size greater than 10 cm, and elevated concentrations of squamous cell carcinoma antigen and carcinoma antigen 125 (CA-125).

Mature Solid Teratoma

Mature solid teratoma is a rare ovarian neoplasm and a very uncommon type of ovarian teratoma. The histologic components in a mature solid teratoma are similar to those found in an immature solid teratoma, which occurs mainly in children and young adults. The presence of immature elements immediately excludes the tumor from this group; by definition, only tumors composed entirely of mature tissues may be included. The tumor is usually unilateral and is adequately treated by unilateral oophorectomy. Although this neoplasm is considered benign, mature solid teratomas may be associated occasionally with peritoneal implants that consist entirely of mature glial tissue. Despite the extensive involvement that may be present, the prognosis is excellent.

Immature Teratoma

Immature teratomas consist of tissue derived from the three germ layers—ectoderm, mesoderm, and endoderm—and, in contrast to the much more common mature teratoma, **they contain immature or embryonal structures.** These tumors have had a variety of names, including solid teratoma, malignant teratoma, teratoblastoma, teratocarcinoma, and embryonal teratoma. These names arose because immature teratomas have been incorrectly considered mixed germ cell tumors or secondary malignant tumors originating in mature benign teratomas. Mature tissues are frequently present and sometimes may predominate. **Immature teratoma of the ovary is an uncommon tumor, comprising less than 1% of ovarian teratomas.** In contrast to the mature cystic teratoma, which is encountered most frequently during the reproductive years but occurs at all ages, **the immature teratoma occurs most commonly in the first 2 decades of life and is almost unknown after menopause. By definition, an immature teratoma contains immature neural elements.** According to Norris and associates, **the quantity of immature neural tissue alone determines the grade.** Neuroblastoma elements, glial tissue, and immature cerebellar and cortical tissue may also be seen. **These tumors are graded histologically on the basis of the amount and degree of cellular immaturity.** The range is from grade I (mature teratoma containing only rare immature foci) through grade III (large portions of the tumor consist of embryonal tissue with atypia and mitotic activity). Generally, older patients tend to have lower grade primary tumors compared with younger patients. When the neoplasm is solid and all elements are well differentiated histologically (solid mature teratoma), a grade 0 designation is given (Table 12.6).

Immature teratomas are almost never bilateral, although occasionally a benign teratoma is found in the opposite ovary. These tumors may have multiple peritoneal implants at the time of initial surgery, and **the prognosis is closely correlated with the histologic grade of the primary tumor and the implants.** Norris and coworkers studied 58 patients with immature teratomas and reported an 82% survival rate for patients who had grade I primary lesions, 63% for grade II, and 30% for grade III (Table 12.7). These results antedate the use of multiple-agent chemotherapy.

Multiple sections of the primary lesion and wide sampling of the peritoneal implants are necessary to properly grade the tumor. In most cases, the implants are better differentiated than the primary tumors. Both the primary lesion and the implants should be graded according to the most immature tissue present. Patients with mature glial implants have an excellent prognosis; those with immature implants, however, do not.

To date, the histologic grade and fertility desires of the patient have been the determining factors regarding extent of surgical therapy and subsequent adjuvant therapy. Because the lesion is rarely bilateral in its ovarian involvement, the present method of **therapy consists of unilateral salpingo-oophorectomy with wide sampling of peritoneal implants. Total abdominal hysterectomy with bilateral salpingo-oophorectomy does not seem to be indicated because it does not influence the outcome for the patient.** Although some authors have advocated cystectomy alone for early-stage, low-grade disease, this management strategy should be approached with caution. Radiotherapy has also been shown to have little value. **If the primary tumor is grade I and all peritoneal implants are grade 0, no further therapy is recommended. However, if the primary tumor is grade II or III or if implants or recurrences are grade I, II, or III, triple-agent chemotherapy is frequently recommended.** The recommendation to use adjuvant chemotherapy in high-grade stage I disease is based on studies performed before meticulous surgical staging of germ cell malignancies was routine. Cushing and colleagues evaluated surgical therapy alone in 44 pediatric and adolescent patients younger than the age of 15 years who had completely resected immature teratomas of all grades. Thirty-one patients had pure immature teratomas, and 13 patients had immature teratomas with microscopic endodermal sinus tumor foci. The 4-year event-free and overall survival rates for both groups were 97% and 100%, respectively. The authors concluded that surgery alone was curative for most children and adolescents with completely resected ovarian immature teratomas of any grade and advocated avoiding adjuvant chemotherapy in this group.

In previous trials including SLL, these patients were free of immature elements but retained peritoneal implants containing exclusively mature elements. This was labeled chemotherapeutic retroconversion of immature teratoma of the ovary and is a similar if not identical syndrome as the "growing teratoma syndrome" described in testicular nonseminomatous germ cell tumors. All of these patients had uneventful follow-ups with the mature implants apparently remaining in static states. Growing teratoma syndrome (GTS) is characterized by the persistence or development of an enlarging mass during or after adjuvant chemotherapy. Normalization of tumor markers is also seen, and on pathologic analysis, only mature teratoma

TABLE 12.6 Immature Teratoma Grading System

Grade	Thurlbeck and Scully	Norris et al.
0	All cells well differentiated	All tissue mature; rare mitotic activity
1	Cells well differentiated; rare small foci of embryonal tissue	Some immaturity and neuroepithelium limited to low-magnification field in any slide (×40)
2	Moderate quantities of embryonal tissue; atypia and mitosis present	Immaturity and neuroepithelium does not exceed three low-power microscopic fields in any one slide
3	Large quantities of embryonal tissue; atypia and mitosis present	Immaturity and neuroepithelium occupying four or more low magnification fields on a single slide

TABLE 12.7 Immature (Malignant) Teratomas

Grade	Patients (n)	Tumor Deaths (%)
1	22	4 (18)
2	24	9 (37)
3	10	7 (70)

From Norris HJ, Zirkin HJ, Benson WL. Immature (malignant) teratoma of the ovary: a clinical and pathologic study of 58 cases. *Cancer* 1976;37:2359.

is noted in the specimen. Treatment of this syndrome is challenging, but surgery is diagnostic and is also the mainstay of therapy. Few cases of GTS are reported in the literature; thus, many current strategies are taken from reports of GTS after testicular nonseminomatous germ cell tumors. Byrd et al. reported on five cases of GTS in women undergoing treatment of early and advanced stage ovarian germ cell tumors. All women received BEP after surgery. GTS occurred 1 to 6 months after completion of chemotherapy in women with advanced disease and at 1 and 11 years in the two women with stage I disease. All patients in this cohort required extensive surgery but remain alive and well with no evidence of disease at last follow-up. For patients with this syndrome, maximal cytoreductive efforts should be undertaken because they offer optimal diagnostic and therapeutic benefit.

Monodermal or Highly Specialized Teratomas

Struma ovarii. Another tumor thought to represent the unilateral development of benign teratoma is **struma ovarii, which consists totally or predominantly of thyroid parenchyma.** This is an uncommon lesion and should not be confused with benign teratomas, which contain small foci of thyroid tissue. Between **25% and 35% of patients with strumal tumors will have clinical hyperthyroidism.** The gross and microscopic appearances of these lesions are similar to those of typical thyroid tissue, although the histologic pattern may resemble that in adenomatous thyroid. **These ovarian tumors may undergo malignant transformation, but they are usually benign and easily treated by simple surgical resection.**

Carcinoid tumors. **Primary ovarian carcinoid tumors usually arise in association with gastrointestinal or respiratory epithelium, which is present in mature cystic teratoma.** They may also be observed within a solid teratoma or a mucinous tumor, or they may occur in an apparently pure form. Primary ovarian carcinoid tumors are uncommon; approximately 50 cases have been reported. The age distribution of patients with ovarian carcinoid tumors is similar to that of patients with mature cystic teratoma, although the average age may be slightly higher in ovarian carcinoid tumors. Many patients are postmenopausal.

One-third of the reported cases have been associated with the typical carcinoid syndrome despite the absence of metastasis. This is in contrast to intestinal carcinoid tumors, which are associated with the syndrome only when there is metastatic spread to the liver. Excision of the tumor has been associated with the rapid remission of symptoms in all of the described cases and the disappearance of 5-hydroxyindoleacetic acid from the urine. The primary ovarian carcinoids are only occasionally associated with metastasis; metastasis was observed in only 3 of 47 reported cases in one review. The prognosis after excision of the primary tumor is favorable, and in most cases, a cure results.

Strumal carcinoid is an even rarer entity and represents a close admixture of the previously discussed struma ovarii and carcinoid tumors. Strumal carcinoids may actually represent medullary carcinoma, resulting in thyroid tissue. Most cases follow a benign course.

TUMORS OF GERM CELL AND SEX CORD DERIVATION

Tumors of germ cell and sex cord derivation are unique, rare tumors that are composed of two distinct populations of cells closely admixed but with different origins. The two histologic types of tumors that fall into this category are gonadoblastomas and mixed germ cell–SCSTs. Gonadoblastomas are benign tumors of the ovary that occur in dysgenetic gonads and are frequently associated with the development of a malignant germ cell component. The risk of developing a malignant germ cell component increases with age, such that prepubertal girls at the time of gonadectomy are very unlikely to have an associated malignant germ cell tumor, but the risk of malignancy approaches 100% for women in their 20s. Mixed germ cell–SCTSs occur in chromosomally normal gonads and are less frequently associated with malignant germ cell tumors than gonadoblastomas.

Gonadoblastoma

Gonadoblastoma is a rare ovarian lesion that consists of germ cells that resemble those of dysgerminoma and gonadal stroma cells that resemble those of a granulosa or Sertoli tumor. Sex chromatin studies usually show a negative nuclear pattern (45,X) or a sex chromosome mosaicism (45,X/46,XY). Gonadoblastomas usually arise in dysgenetic gonads, but the presence of dysgenetic gonads, a Y chromosome, or a Y fragment is not required; very rare cases of gonadoblastomas have been reported in normal women with normal ovaries and a normal karyotype. Because **patients with XY gonadal dysgenesis have a very high risk of gonadoblastoma and a nearly 100% risk of associated malignant germ cell tumor with advancing age, these patients are recommended to undergo prophylactic bilateral oophorectomy after puberty. Patients who have a gonadoblastoma usually have primary amenorrhea, virilization, or developmental abnormalities of the genitalia,** and the discovery of gonadoblastoma is made in the course of investigation of these conditions. It is poorly understood why some patients with these lesions become virilized and others do not. Although there is a correlation between the virilization of patients with gonadoblastoma and the presence of Leydig or lutein-like cells, this relationship is not consistent, and some virilized patients have tumors free of these cells. Another common initial sign is the presence of a pelvic tumor. **Most patients with gonadoblastoma (80%) are phenotypic women, and the remainder are phenotypic men with cryptorchidism, hypospadias, and internal female secondary sex organs.** Among the phenotypic women, 60% are virilized, and the remainder appear normal. **The prognosis of patients with gonadoblastoma is excellent if the tumor and the contralateral gonad, which may be harboring a macroscopically undetectable gonadoblastoma, are excised. Bilateral involvement is identified in approximately 50% of cases. The association with dysgerminoma is seen in 50% of cases and with other more malignant germ cell neoplasms in an additional 10%.** In view of this, the concept that these lesions represent an in-situ germ cell malignancy appears valid. When gonadoblastoma is associated with or overgrown by dysgerminoma, the prognosis is still excellent. **Metastases tend to occur later** and more infrequently than in dysgerminoma arising de novo. Complete or partial regression of virilization usually occurs after excision of the gonads. Exogenous estrogen therapy is given for periodic bleeding. The authors leave the uterus even after removing both gonads. Cyclic hormone therapy is indicated in these young women. Ovum transfer has been successful in patients who have had both ovaries removed. **Although gonadoblastomas themselves are benign, treatment should follow the usual tenets for surgical staging if a malignant component is identified.**

Mixed Germ Cell–sex Cord Stromal Tumors

Mixed germ cell–SCTSs are less common than gonadoblastomas **and occur in phenotypically normal women with normal karyotypes and normal gonads.** These tumors are usually identified in girls younger than age 10 years; however, they rarely may be seen in reproductive-age women. Although **clinically benign, these mixed tumors are associated with a malignant germ cell component in 10% of cases.** When this tumor is identified in postpubertal girls, the risk of a malignant germ cell tumor rises to 80%. **Isosexual precocity may be seen. Similar to gonadoblastoma, the most common germ cell tumor identified is dysgerminoma.** However, unlike gonadoblastoma, in which the sex cord element is usually mature, in mixed tumors, the sex cord element is usually less mature. Histologic features may resemble characteristics of multiple SCSTs such as retiform patterns or annular tubules and may not be characteristic of a single SCST type. They are usually large and unilateral tumors and metastasize or recur infrequently. **Because of the unilateral nature, unilateral oophorectomy and staging if a malignant germ cell component is identified is all that is required.** Because these patients are usually young and are phenotypically, anatomically, and karyotypically normal, surgical management should be guided by fertility preservation and appropriate staging if malignancy is identified.

TUMORS DERIVED FROM SPECIAL GONADAL STROMA

Classification, Clinical Profile, and Staging

This category of ovarian tumors includes all those that contain granulosa cells, theca cells and luteinized derivatives, Sertoli cells, Leydig cells, and fibroblasts of gonadal stromal origin. These tumors originate from the ovarian matrix and consist of cells from the embryonic sex cord and mesenchyme. **As a group, SCSTs are found in all age groups, with the age-related incidence increasing throughout the fifth, sixth, and seventh decades of life. These tumors account for approximately 5% of all ovarian tumors;** however, functioning neoplastic groups of this variety comprise only 2%. Approximately 90% of hormonally active ovarian tumors belong to this category and are associated with physiologic and pathologic signs of estrogen or androgen excess (or both), including isosexual precocity, hirsutism, abnormal bleeding, endometrial hyperplasia or carcinoma, and increased breast cancer risk. **Of ovarian**

cancers, 5% to 10% belong in the SCST group; most of these (70%) are granulosa cell tumors, which are low-grade malignancies with a relapse rate of 10% to 33%. Because SCSTs have a propensity for indolent growth, they tend to recur late. The average time to recurrence is between 5 and 10 years; some recur as late as 20 years after the initial diagnosis. Most authors report a 10-year survival rate of 90% for stage I disease and 0% to 22% for stage III. Prognostic factors shown to affect survival in multivariate analysis by Chan and colleagues include age younger than 50 years, tumor size smaller than 10 cm, and absence of residual disease. An analysis of SEER data from 1988 to 2001 including 376 women with SCST confirmed age younger than 50 and early-stage disease (I and II) as significant prognostic factors for improved survival. Observational studies have shown an improvement in relative and overall survival for SCST over time, likely attributable to the increased recognition of the importance of cytoreduction and residual disease on overall survival and accurate staging resulting in more favorable stage at diagnosis. SCSTs are staged surgically in accordance with FIGO guidelines and staging recommendations for ovarian epithelial tumors.

Treatment

The definitive treatment of SCST is based on findings encountered during complete surgical staging, the reproductive desires of the patient, and the histologic type of tumor. The majority of SCSTs are benign or low malignant potential tumors. As a result, surgical therapy is adequate in most cases and remains the cornerstone of treatment. **In patients who desire to retain fertility, unilateral salpingo-oophorectomy with preservation of the uterus and contralateral ovary and full surgical staging is appropriate therapy for patients with stage IA disease. Advanced-stage disease and disease in older women should be managed with complete staging and hysterectomy with bilateral salpingo-oophorectomy.** Although scientific evidence suggesting benefit is lacking, most authors recommend **aggressive attempts at complete cytoreduction if possible** when faced with advanced-stage, metastatic, or bulky disease. Secondary cytoreduction is controversial, although there may be a survival or palliative benefit for patients with focal recurrent disease.

Although **contemporary surgical practice mandates routine staging lymphadenectomy,** the therapeutic value of routine lymphadenectomy is uncertain. There is no doubt that staging lymphadenectomy is prognostic and is clinically useful in guiding adjuvant therapy decisions. Brown and colleagues recently reported on 262 patients with SCST of the ovary. Fifty-eight patients underwent lymphadenectomy as part of staging, and none were found to have positive lymph nodes. Of the 117 patients who eventually had a recurrence, six patients (5.1%) had nodal metastasis at the time of recurrence. Three of these patients had negative nodes at the time of initial staging. These authors concluded that lymphadenectomy could be omitted as part of surgical staging of ovarian SCST because lymph node metastasis at time of diagnosis is rare. Similar findings have been reported by Chi and colleagues, who noted no lymph node metastasis in 16 of 68 patients with granulosa cell tumors who underwent pelvic lymph node dissection as part of surgical staging or 13 of 68 patients who underwent paraaortic lymph-node sampling. Thirty-four patients ultimately experienced recurrence, 33 of which were incompletely staged at their initial operation. Only 15% of recurrences involved the retroperitoneum. In the context of these reports, it may be reasonable to omit routine pelvic and paraaortic lymphadenectomy. The surgeon should perform careful lymph node assessment and resect pathologically enlarged nodes. Similarly, the surgeon should perform standard staging lymphadenectomies in women in whom there is uncertainty regarding the precise histology of the ovarian neoplasm,

Two special clinical situations require additional surgical evaluation. **Because estrogen-secreting ovarian tumors are associated with endometrial hyperplasia or cancer in 25% to 50% and 5% to 10% of cases, respectively, surgical evaluation should include dilation and curettage of the uterine cavity, regardless of the benign or malignant nature of the ovarian primary. If malignancy in the uterus is encountered, it should be managed accordingly. Additionally, because sex cord tumors with annular tubules (SCTAT) associated with Peutz-Jegher syndrome (PJS; discussed later) can be associated with adenoma malignum of the cervix, it is imperative that the endocervix be evaluated with an endocervical curettage.** Although these ovarian tumors are benign, postoperative follow-up and surveillance of the cervix are required.

Patients with early-stage disease (IA or IB) may be treated with surgical therapy alone and expect an excellent prognosis. However, those with stage IC or greater disease should be counseled about adjuvant therapy despite strong evidence suggesting survival benefit. The most common chemotherapy regimen is BEP. **Brown and colleagues published results demonstrating taxane activity in patients with SCST as well.** In this study, a 42% response rate was noted in the setting of recurrent, measurable disease. In a subsequent study, Brown and colleagues directly compared BEP with taxanes in women with SCST. In this study, there was no difference in PFS, overall survival, or response rates in patients with newly diagnosed tumors treated with BEP compared with taxanes. In patients with recurrent measurable disease, BEP had a higher response rate compared with the taxane regimens (71% vs. 37%), a finding that is not statistically significant. In this study, the presence of a platinum compound in the taxane regimen correlated with response, suggesting that a **platinum and taxane combination is active in SCST tumors and may have equivalent efficacy but with lower toxicity compared with the standard BEP.**

The effectiveness of radiation therapy for SCST is controversial and unclear. There are small case series in the literature that would suggest that isolated incompletely resectable primary disease or pelvic recurrent disease may respond to radiation therapy. Because of the size and retrospective nature of these reports, no definitive conclusion can be drawn regarding the utility of radiation in this setting.

Granulosa–stromal Cell Tumors

Granulosa–stromal cell tumors include granulosa and theca cell tumors, and fibromas. They account for the majority of SCST.

TABLE 12.8　Granulosa Cell Tumor: Age Distribution of 118 Cases

Age	Patients (n)
Child	3
12–40 yr	27
41–50 yr	28
51–60 yr	32
60–79 yr	28
Total	**118**

Based on data from Evans AT 3rd, Gaffey TA, Malkasian GD Jr, Annegers JF. Clinicopathologic review of 118 granulosa and 82 theca cell tumors. *Obstet Gynecol* 1980;55:213.

They occur about as frequently in women in the reproductive age group as they do in women who are postmenopausal, with a peak incidence in perimenopausal women between ages 50 and 54 years. Only about 5% of granulosa cell tumors occur before puberty (Table 12.8). A number of risk factors have been associated with granulosa cell tumors, but most are not reproducible and have unknown clinical and biologic significance. A study by Boyce et al. evaluated risk factors for ovarian granulosa cell tumors and noted an independent association between nonwhite race and obesity as a hyperestrogenic state in the development of granulosa cell tumors; parity and oral contraceptive use had a protective effect.

Most granulosa and theca cells produce estrogen, but a few are androgenic. The exact proportion of these neoplasms that have function is not known because the endometrium is often not examined microscopically, and appropriate preoperative laboratory tests are not done. About 80% to 85% of granulosa cell and theca cell neoplasms are palpable on abdominal or pelvic examination, but occasionally an unsuspected tumor is found when a hysterectomy is done on a patient who has abnormal bleeding as a result of endometrial hyperplasia or endometrial carcinoma. Most patients present either with nonspecific symptoms such as awareness of an abdominal mass, abdominal pain, abdominal distention, or bloating. Some patients present with an acute abdomen as a result of internal tumor rupture and hemorrhage with resultant hemoperitoneum. **About 15% of patients with cystic granulosa cell tumors are first examined for an acute abdomen associated with hemoperitoneum.** In premenopausal women, menstrual irregularities or secondary amenorrhea may be the presenting symptom.

Granulosa cell tumors vary greatly in gross appearance (Fig. 12.9). Sometimes they are solid tumors that are soft or firm, depending on the relative amounts of neoplastic cells and fibrothecomatous stroma that they contain. They may be yellow or gray, depending on the amount of intracellular lipid in the lesion. **More commonly, the granulosa cell tumor is predominantly cystic and, on external examination, may resemble mucinous cystadenoma or cystadenocarcinoma. However, when sectioned, the cyst is generally found to be filled with serous fluid or clotted blood.**

FIGURE 12.9 Granulosa cell tumor of the ovary. **A,** Gross appearance. **B,** Microscopic appearance with Call-Exner bodies.

TABLE 12.9 Granulosa Cell Tumor in 76 Patients

Endometrial Histology	Patients (*n*)	Patients (%)
Proliferative endometrium	19	25
Atrophic endometrium	5	7
Hyperplastic endometrium	42	55
Adenocarcinoma	10	13

Based on data from Evans AT 3rd, Gaffey TA, Malkasian GD Jr, Annegers JF. Clinicopathologic review of 118 granulosa and 82 theca cell tumors. *Obstet Gynecol* 1980;55:213.

Granulosa cell tumors occur in two subtypes: adult and juvenile. **Adult granulosa cell tumors account for approximately 95% of all granulosa cell tumors.** They occur more commonly in postmenopausal patients and are the most common estrogen-producing tumor. Although uncommon, adult granulosa tumors can be found in children. Abnormal endometria in these patients, such as hyperplasia or even carcinoma of the endometrium, are not uncommon. A study by Evans and associates from the Mayo Clinic of 76 patients who had granulosa cell tumors and in whom endometrial tissue was available shows a **high incidence of endometrial stimulation** (Table 12.9). In another study, one-third of patients had atypical endometrial cells. In postmenopausal women, vaginal bleeding is common as a result of stimulation of the endometrium. **Approximately 10% of patients with this lesion will harbor an endometrial carcinoma, usually of the well-differentiated type.** Other estrogenic effects may also be noted (eg, tenderness or swelling of the breast), and vaginal cytology may show an increase in maturation of the squamous cells. Rarely, androgenic effects may be present in which hirsute changes occur, or progestational effects may be noted on histologic evaluation of the endometrium.

Histologically, fibrothecomatous components are common, and the cytoplasm is usually scanty. **The typical coffee-bean grooved cells are present.** Cells may be arranged in clusters or rosettes surrounding a central cavity and, when present, resemble primordial follicles called **Call-Exner bodies**. A high degree of tumor cell atypia or mitosis is uncommon. **Adult granulosa cell tumors are typically low-grade malignancies that demonstrate indolent growth and present as stage I disease in more than 90% of cases.** Unilateral disease is most common, but bilateral disease may be found in up to 10% of cases. **The most important prognostic factor is surgical stage.** A study by Kobel et al., in an attempt to understand the molecular pathogenesis of granulosa cell tumors, identified a somatic FOXL2 402C→G mutation, which was present in almost all adult-type granulosa cell tumors and may represent areas of future study for targeted treatments.

The majority of juvenile granulosa cell tumors are found in young adults, and most occur during the first 3 decades of life. Most juvenile granulosa cell tumors are hormonally active, producing estradiol, progesterone, or androgens. **Most of the juvenile granulosa cell tumors that occur in children result in sexual precocity with the development of breasts and pubic and axillary hair. Irregular uterine bleeding may also be present.** Thyromegaly may also occur. Juvenile tumors that are hormonally active may have a more favorable prognosis than inactive tumors, presumably resulting from earlier presentation as a result of the signs and symptoms associated with hormonal activity. Similar to the adult subtype, most of these tumors are limited to one ovary. Ninety-eight percent present with stage I disease. Histologically, thecomatous components are common; cytoplasm is abundant. Mitosis may be numerous; the nuclei are dark and do not usually have the grooved coffee-bean appearance. Pleomorphism may also be present. Juvenile tumors rarely demonstrate Call-Exner bodies. Even though these tumors appear to be less well differentiated than the adult type, the cure rate is quite high for early-stage disease. **In contrast to adult cell types that are typically indolent and recur late, juvenile types are aggressive in advanced-stage disease with recurrence and death occurring within 3 years after diagnosis.**

On the basis of their differentiation, granulosa cell tumors should be divided into two general categories: well differentiated and moderately differentiated. The former pattern may have various presentations, including microfollicular, macrofollicular, trabecular, solid tubular, and watered silk. Tumors in the moderately differentiated category have a diffuse pattern that has also been designated "sarcomatoid." Although many authors have made attempts, no distinct correlation between histologic structure and prognosis has yet been substantiated. It is important that undifferentiated carcinomas, adenocarcinomas, and carcinoids should not be misdiagnosed as granulosa cell tumors, which they may superficially resemble. Each of these tumors has a strikingly different prognosis.

True granulosa tumors are low-grade malignancies, the majority of which are confined to one ovary at the time of diagnosis. Only 5% to 10% of the stage I cases will subsequently recur, and they often appear more than 5 years after initial therapy. The prognosis for these patients is excellent: Long-term survival rates from 75% to 90% have been reported for all stages (Fig. 12.10). **These lesions are adequately managed during the reproductive years by removing the involved ovary and ipsilateral tube with full surgical staging. The uterus and uninvolved adnexa should be removed in the perimenopausal and postmenopausal age groups, which is the treatment for other benign or low malignant potential tumors.** In a series from the Mayo Clinic, 92% of the patients had survived 5 to 10 years (76 patients, 82% of whom had stage I lesions). The recurrence pattern in this same series (18.6% overall recurrence rate) revealed that 23% of the recurrences were more than 13 years after initial therapy. Most of the recurrences occurred in preserved genital tract structures. These kinds of data have prompted some authors to recommend that the preserved

FIGURE 12.10 Granulosa–theca cell tumors from the Emil Novak Ovarian Tumor Registry (1999). *GCT,* granulosa cell tumors; *GTCT,* granulosa-theca cell tumors; *TCT,* theca cell tumors. (Modified from Cronje HS, Niemand I, Bam RH, Woodruff JD. Review of the granulosa-theca cell tumors from the Emil Novak Ovarian Tumor Registry. *Am J Obstet Gynecol* 1999;180:323.)

internal genitalia be removed in perimenopausal patients in whom preservation may have been appropriate during the childbearing period.

Several studies address prognostic factors in granulosa cell tumors of the ovary. The most important prognostic factor is stage. Other than stage, mitotic activity, DNA ploidy, and S-phase fractions have been evaluated. In a study of 54 patients from Sweden, patients with mitotic rates of 4 of 10 high-power fields (hpf) had no deaths, but all patients with 10 of 10 hpf died, with the longest survival being 4 years. Patients with mitotic rate of 4 to 10/10 hpf had a median survival of 9 years. Fortunately, most patients had mitotic counts of 4 of 10 hpf. In another smaller study, among the two-thirds of the patients studied who were found to have euploid tumors, only one patient died of disease, but four of five patients with aneuploid tumors died of disease. S-phase fraction did not correlate with any clinical or histologic parameters. Recently the Hellenic Cooperative Oncology Group reported on 34 patients with adult granulosa cell tumors of the ovary. In this study, stage and the presence of residual disease were noted to have prognostic significance for overall survival on univariate analysis. Tumor rupture during surgery was also prognostic for disease-free survival. Thirteen patients with unresectable disease were evaluated for response to chemotherapy. Six of seven patients who responded to first-line platinum-based chemotherapy had complete responses to therapy, demonstrating the importance of platinum agents in treating this tumor type.

Inhibin is a nonsteroidal polypeptide hormone that is secreted by granulosa cells of the ovary. This hormone is secreted throughout the menstrual cycle and during pregnancy but not in postmenopausal women. A study by Mom et al. investigated the value of serum inhibin A and B for the assessment of disease status. Thirty patients with stage I to III granulosa cell tumors were included in the study with pre- and posttreatment measurements of inhibin A and B obtained. Inhibin A and B were elevated in these patients and negative in control participants. The sensitivity of inhibin A for diagnosis was 67% with a specificity of 100% compared with 89% and 100%, respectively, for inhibin B; therefore, inhibin B appears to reflect disease status more accurately than inhibin A.

In collective series, the relationship of tumor to the level of inhibin appears to be very good. However, there have been conflicting reports relative to specificity because inhibin may also be secreted by many other ovarian neoplasms, including mucinous ovarian epithelial neoplasms. Nevertheless, **serum inhibin levels have an important role as a marker for monitoring patients under therapy and for detection of tumor recurrence, and although both inhibin A and inhibin B have utility as tumor markers, inhibin B has increased sensitivity (89% vs. 67%) with equivalent specificity (100%) for the diagnosis of recurrent granulosa cell tumor and should be used preferentially when available.** Other tumor markers include Müllerian inhibiting substance (MIS) and estradiol. Estradiol is not used clinically because of poor sensitivity, and MIS, although demonstrating excellent specificity, is only used for research purposes. Tumor markers, when elevated in the surveillance setting, are typically followed by imaging to localize disease recurrence. In granulosa cell tumors, PET/CT has been shown to have variable F-18 fluorodeoxyglucose avidity, ranging from none to mild avidity, resulting in a potential false-negative study result.

Often, recurrent tumors have been treated effectively by means of reoperation, radiation therapy, chemotherapy, or a combination thereof. Although radiation therapy has been advocated for these tumors by many authors, careful search of the literature shows little evidence relating enhanced curability to the use of radiation therapy. A prospective study has never been done to compare one form of therapy with another for patients who have advanced or recurrent disease. The question of adjuvant radiotherapy in a postmenopausal woman found to have granulosa cell tumor is often an issue. Case reports are available and describe therapies used in recurrent granulosa cell tumors.

We recommend no further therapy for patients who have stage I lesions. Adverse prognostic factors that have been reported include large tumor size, bilateral involvement, intraabdominal rupture of the neoplasm, nuclear atypia, and a high mitotic rate. There appears to be agreement that the histologic pattern of the neoplasm has no predictive value. **Stage II or III or recurrent granulosa cell tumors are probably best treated with systemic chemotherapy.** Metastatic and suboptimally reduced disease should also be aggressively treated with combination chemotherapy because response rates as high as 83% have been reported. The GOG has evaluated BEP in a nonrandomized study of advanced or recurrent granulosa cell tumors of the ovary. Fifty-seven evaluable patients received four cycles of BEP followed by a reassessment laparotomy. Only 38 patients agreed to SLL, and 14 (37%) had negative results. Obviously, BEP is an active combination in these patients with advanced disease. Additionally, the following drugs have been used singly or in combination and appear to be effective: etoposide plus cisplatin; cyclophosphamide, doxorubicin, and cisplatin; paclitaxel and carboplatin; or a platinum agent alone. Reviews of the literature suggest that most granulosa cell tumors respond to hormonal therapy, and although data are sparse, aromatase inhibitors have been useful in the management of granulosa cell tumors in several reported cases. In a case report by Schwartz and Huang, a patient was identified with a recurrent granulosa cell tumor and was given anastrazole at the time of her third recurrence. This treatment caused rapid normalization of inhibin B. Ultimately, she showed partial response to therapy, but a later CT scan showed disease progression and she required further surgical resection. Subsequently, she later required external-beam radiation therapy and, on further monitoring, remained disease free for 3 years.

The natural history of patients with recurrences is prolonged, thus making analysis of any therapy very difficult in terms of overall survival. This is especially true of therapy used in an adjuvant setting. Although responses have been reported with paclitaxel alone, paclitaxel and carboplatin in combination, BEP, GnRH agonists, medroxyprogesterone acetate, megestrol, and alternating megestrol and tamoxifen, there are no good data to guide therapy in this setting. The role of biologic agents in the treatment of recurrence is unclear. Although some studies

have shown significant expression of platelet-derived growth factor receptor (PDGFR) alpha and beta in granulosa cell tumors, raising the possibility of response to drugs such as imatinib mesylate, other investigators have documented low levels of c-kit, c-Abl, and PDGFR, suggesting limited efficacy of this class of agent.

Thecomas

Thecomas are less common than granulosa cell tumors, but they have similar appearances. They **are solid fibromatous lesions that show varying degrees of yellow or orange coloration.** Whereas granulosa cell tumors are found to be bilateral in 2% to 5% of patients, **thecomas are almost always confined to one ovary.** On microscopic examination, most tumors in the granulosa–theca cell category are found to contain both cell types. If more than a very small component of granulosa cells is present, the term *granulosa cell tumor*, rather than *granulosa–theca cell tumor*, is generally applied. The designation *theca cell tumor* or *thecoma* should be reserved for neoplasms that consist entirely of benign theca cells.

Thecomas consist of neoplastic cells of ovarian stromal origin that have accumulated moderate to large amounts of lipid. Sometimes such tumors contain clusters of lutein cells, in which case the term *luteinized thecoma* is often used. Occasionally, tumors fall into a gray zone between thecomas and fibromas. Although the latter also arise from ovarian stromal cells, they differentiate predominantly in the direction of collagen-producing fibroblasts. Tumors in the gray zone may be designated as *thecoma-fibromas*. They are almost always unilateral and virtually never malignant. Several tumors have been reported in the literature as malignant thecomas, but at least some of these are better interpreted as fibrosarcomas or diffuse forms of granulosa cell tumors. **In cases in which preservation of fertility is important, a thecoma may be treated adequately by unilateral oophorectomy. However, total hysterectomy with bilateral salpingo-oophorectomy is recommended in most postmenopausal and perimenopausal women. Because thecomas are typically one of the most hormonally active SCSTs, 15% to 37% and 25% of cases are associated with endometrial hyperplasia and carcinoma, respectively,** and endometrial sampling should be performed. Patients typically present with abnormal bleeding and an abdominal or pelvic mass.

Fibromas and Sclerosing Stromal Cell Tumors

Fibromas are the most common SCST and occur primarily in postmenopausal women, although they can occur in any age group. **They are not hormonally active tumors. Fibromas are typically benign tumors;** however, recently, cellular fibromas have been described and are considered to be of low malignant potential. Fibrosarcomas, by contrast, are rare but considered highly aggressive tumors. The behavior of these tumors is correlated with mitotic activity and degree of anaplasia.

Fibromas may be associated with ascites or hydrothorax as a result of increased capillary permeability thought to be a result of vascular endothelial growth factor production. Meigs syndrome (ovarian fibromas, ascites, and hydrothorax)

is uncommon and usually resolves after surgical excision of the fibroma. Gorlin syndrome, or nevoid basal cell carcinoma syndrome, is a rare inherited predisposition to multisystem abnormalities, including ovarian fibromas. Because of the benign nature of fibromas, surgical excision is all that is required.

In contrast to most SCSTs, sclerosing stromal cell tumors typically present in the second and third decades of life, although they can occur in adolescents and premenarchal girls. They may be clinically undetectable or grow to a very large size. They are considered benign, occur unilaterally, and are hormonally inactive except in very rare cases. Clinical symptoms include premature menarche; menstrual irregularities; pain; and uncommonly, ascites. Imaging characteristics reveal predominately solid masses with hypervascularity, although complex cystic masses may be seen. Tumor markers are not elevated.

Sertoli-Leydig Cell Tumors

Sertoli-Leydig cell tumors contain Sertoli cells or Leydig cells in varying proportions and degrees of differentiation. The degree of differentiation contributes to the malignant potential of these tumors. Most well-differentiated tumors are clinically benign. Size greater than 5 cm, necrosis, nuclear atypia, vascular invasion, and high mitotic rate (>5 per 10 hpf) increase the likelihood of a malignant course. Because less well-differentiated neoplasms within this category may recapitulate the development of the testes, the terms *androblastoma and arrhenoblastoma* have been used as synonyms for *Sertoli-Leydig cell tumors.* However, their connotation of associated masculinization is misleading because some of these tumors have no endocrine manifestation, and others may even be accompanied by an estrogenic syndrome. Nevertheless, the WHO has selected *androblastoma* as an alternate term for *Sertoli-Leydig cell tumor.*

These neoplasms account for fewer than 0.5% of all ovarian tumors but are among the most fascinating from pathologic and clinical viewpoints. They are typically unilateral tumors and confined to the ovary in 97% of cases. **They occur in all age groups but are most often encountered in young women (between the ages of 20 and 30 years), who usually become virilized** (Fig. 12.11). Although rare in children, the clinical presentation is typically one of isosexual pseudoprecocity. **In immunocytochemical studies, testosterone appears to be localized predominantly within the Leydig cells, but estrogen and androstenedione are produced by many of the same cells.** Thus, one can appreciate the spectrum of the clinical presentation of this fascinating neoplasm. **Classically, there is progressive masculinization that is heralded by hirsutism, temporal balding, deepening of the voice, and enlargement of the clitoris. Other patients may manifest secondary amenorrhea, breast atrophy, and a marked increase in libido.**

Sertoli-Leydig cell tumors can be described in terms of differentiation and the presence or absence of heterologous elements, distinctions that have clinical relevance. Sertoli-Leydig cell tumors with heterologous elements may contain various unusual cell types, but the degree of differentiation of the tumors is probably of greater importance in determining its prognosis than is its content of unexpected tissue. Although these tumors have a distinctive histologic pattern that facilitates

FIGURE 12.11 Enlarged clitoris in a patient with a Sertoli-Leydig cell tumor (arrhenoblastoma).

diagnosis, antibody markers can aid in the differential diagnosis, such as inhibin.

In the report by Young and Scully, only 29 of 220 tumors of this type were clinically malignant. None of the 27 well-differentiated tumors and only four of 100 tumors of intermediate differentiation were known to be clinically malignant. A total of 59% of poorly differentiated tumors and 19% of heterologous tumors displayed malignant behavior. Zaloudek and Norris reported on **64 intermediate and poorly differentiated neoplasms. Only three of 50 patients with stage I disease developed a recurrence** (Table 12.10). The 5-year survival rate in all of their patients was 92%.

The overall 5-year survival rate of patients with Sertoli-Leydig cell tumors has been reported to range from 70% to more than 90%. Because these tumors occur predominantly in young women and are bilateral in fewer than 5% of cases, conservative removal of the tumor and adjacent fallopian tube is justifiable if preservation of fertility is an important consideration and if there is no evidence of extension beyond the involved ovary. Removal of the tumor will halt, but not fully reverse, the masculinizing process. Similar to granulosa cell tumors, they are considered to have low malignant potential. There are no solid data to suggest that adjuvant therapy has any value in preventing a recurrence in patients with stage I lesions. **Tumors with poor differentiation, heterologous elements, advanced stage, or recurrent lesions should be treated with adjuvant chemotherapy.** Again, **BEP chemotherapy is often recommended.** In the unusual patient who has an advanced or recurrent Sertoli-Leydig cell tumor, chemotherapy appears to be effective, although the experience is very limited.

TABLE 12.10	**Management of Germ Cell and Sex Cord Stromal Tumors**		
Neoplasms	**Suggested Surgery**	**Postoperative Chemotherapy**	**Reassessment Laparotomy**
Dysgerminoma	Unilateral S&O when confined to one ovary: preserve normal-appearing ovarian tissue	BEP for 3 cycles if the patient is not adequately staged or if stage II–IV	Not necessary unless a recurrence is suspected
Endodermal sinus	Debulk: attempt to preserve fertility	BEP for 3–4 cycles; follow with AFP titers	Same as above
Embryonal carcinoma	Same as above	BEP for 3–4 cycles; follow with β-hCG titers	Same as above
Malignant teratoma	Same as above	BEP or VAC for 3–4 cycles	Same as above
Granulosa cell	Unilateral S&O for young patients with stage Ia disease; otherwise TAH, BSO	BEP for 3–4 cycles; GnRH agonists for advanced disease	Same as above
Sertoli-Leydig cell	Same as above	BEP or VAC for 3–4 cycles for advanced disease	Same as above

AFP, Alpha-fetoprotein; *BEP,* bleomycin, etoposide, and cisplatin; *β-hCG,* β-human chorionic gonadotropin; *GnRH,* gonadotropin-releasing hormone; *S&O,* salpingo-oophorectomy; *VAC,* vincristine, dactinomycin, and cyclophosphamide.

Sex Cord Tumor With Annular Tubules

Sex cord tumor with annular tubules (SCTAT) represents a unique ovarian tumor that appears as a histologic intermediate between granulosa and Sertoli-Leydig cell tumors. SCTATs account for 6% of SCSTs. This tumor typically presents in the third to fourth decade of life and is usually unilateral. Presenting complaints are usually abnormal vaginal bleeding or postmenopausal bleeding, a testament to the endocrine activity of these tumors. Both estrogen and progesterone production have been reported. **Approximately 30% of SCTAT tumors are associated with PJS. Tumors associated with PJS are benign but are associated with adenoma malignum of the cervix in 15% of cases.** Because adenoma malignum has a relatively high mortality rate, these patients deserve careful evaluation and follow-up. **In contrast, SCTAT, which is not associated with PJS, has a 20% malignancy rate.** Malignant SCTAT seems to spread via the lymphatics with typical metastatic sites being the pelvic, paraaortic, and supraclavicular lymph nodes. There is limited experience in the literature with these tumors. Clinically, they should be managed in a similar manner to other SCSTs. Combination chemotherapy (BEP) may be helpful in patients with advanced disease. Because SCTAT represents an intermediate cell type between granulosa cell and Sertoli-Leydig cell tumors, SCTAT may express inhibin or MIS. Inhibin and MIS can be used as markers for recurrence, however, the utility of these tumor markers in this disease is uncertain.

Gynandroblastoma

Rarely, a gonadostromal tumor contains unequivocal granulosa cell elements combined with tubules and Leydig cells that are characteristic of arrhenoblastomas. Designated as gynandroblastomas, these mixed tumors may be associated with either androgen or estrogen production, and they can be expected to behave as low-grade malignancies similar to the individual components. The diagnosis of gynandroblastoma depends on histologic examination rather than the clinical and laboratory findings. The WHO definition of gynandroblastoma is very strict; therefore, tumors matching these exact specifications are rare.

Steroid Cell Neoplasms

Steroid cell neoplasms (also known as lipid cell neoplasms) are a heterologous group of tumors that have in common a parenchyma composed of polygonal cells that contain lipid. They include neoplasms that have been designated as hilus cell tumors, Leydig tumors, adrenal rest tumors, stromal luteomas, or masculinovoblastomas. Stromal luteomas are benign tumors, which account for 25% of steroid cell neoplasms and occur 80% of the time in postmenopausal women. They commonly present with postmenopausal bleeding, thought to result from a hyperestrogenic state from either direct secretion of estrogens by the tumor or secretion of androgens with subsequent conversion to estrogen. Estrogen secretion predominates, however. Leydig cell tumors are unilateral and are found commonly in the medulla or hilus regions of the ovaries. These tumors are androgen-secreting tumors and are not thought to be malignant. Reinke crystals, which normally occur in mature Leydig cells of the testes, are often found in these neoplasms, and their presence may be interpreted as signifying a benign lesion. **Steroid cell tumors (not otherwise specified)** are tumors that cannot be characterized as stromal luteomas or Leydig cell tumors. They **are androgenic tumors that may be associated with paraneoplastic manifestations such as hypercalcemia, erythrocytosis, or ascites. In 20% of cases, they will have spread to contiguous organs at the time of surgery. Tumors that have microscopic cellular pleomorphism with high mitotic activity or the presence of necrosis should be considered malignant.**

TUMORS DERIVED FROM NONSPECIFIC MESENCHYME

Benign and malignant tumors, including fibromas, hemangiomas, leiomyomas, soft tissue sarcomas, lymphomas, and rare neoplasms, may arise in the ovaries from nonspecific supporting tissues that are common to most organs. The most common and most important tumors in this category are fibroma and lymphoma.

MALIGNANT LYMPHOMA

Malignant lymphoid tumors of the genital tract are rare; however, the ovaries are the most common sites affected. Most commonly this represents ovarian involvement in overt systemic disease, almost always of the non-Hodgkin type. There has been debate as to whether lymphoma can arise de novo in the ovary; lymphoid aggregates do exist in normal ovarian tissue, which could give rise to such a lesion.

Patients with disease localized to one ovary usually do well with unilateral surgical resection followed by systemic chemotherapy. The use of chemotherapy is based on the principle that ovarian lymphoma must be considered a localized manifestation of systemic disease. The prognosis for such patients is much better than that of patients with obvious systemic disease.

METASTATIC TUMORS TO THE OVARY

The ovary is frequently the site of metastasis from certain primary carcinomas. Approximately 10% of ovarian tumors are not primary in origin. The most common source of metastatic disease is the endometrium. Many metastatic adenocarcinomas, particularly those that exhibit mucinous differentiation, can mimic primary ovarian adenocarcinomas. Immunohistochemistry (CK7 and CK20) staining has been widely used to aid in distinguishing primary from secondary ovarian adenocarcinoma. This is particularly true in the case of ovarian endometrioid carcinoma, which, according to Scully, is associated with a similar tumor in the endometrium in one-third of cases.

There are four possible pathways of spread to tumors to the ovary:
- Direct continuity
- Surface papillation
- Lymphatic metastasis
- Hematogenous spread

Lymphatic metastasis is undoubtedly the most common pathway for spread to the ovary. The rich network of lymph nodes and lymphatic channels in the pelvis readily explains the metastatic pathway of tumors in the uterus and contralateral ovary. The rare finding of clusters of tumor cells limited to lymphatics in the medulla of the ovary in cases of breast carcinoma confirms that this is the pathway of spread to the ovary. As yet, no one has convincingly described the pathway of metastasis to the ovaries from cancer of the stomach. It is known that the lymphatic channels that drain the upper gastrointestinal tract ultimately link up with the lumbar chain of lymph nodes. Ovarian lymphatics drain into the lumbar nodes. This could be the route of spread to the ovaries in these cases.

The latest reports confirm adenocarcinoma of the colon as the most frequent nongynecologic primary site of metastatic disease to the ovary, with breast cancer in second place. These lesions are characterized microscopically by the presence of large acini similar to those of primary intestinal carcinomas. Grossly, they may form solid metastases but more often appear as large, partly cystic tumors with areas of hemorrhage and necrosis (Fig. 12.12). In such cases, they are easily confused with cystic forms of primary ovarian cancers. Regarding labs, carcinoembryonic antigen (CEA) levels exceeding 5 ng/mL are often found in patients with gastrointestinal carcinomas. In particular, values above 20 ng/mL in the setting of colorectal cancer are often associated with metastatic disease. Buamah et al. published a study on 155 patients with elevated CA-125

FIGURE 12.12 Metastatic tumor to the ovary from adenocarcinoma of the colon. A, Gross appearance. B, Histologic appearance. Note the large acini similar to those of the intestinal carcinoma.

levels, 47 of whom had ovarian cancer and 38 with colorectal cancer. In this population, the ratio of CA-125 to CEA appeared to be excellent for differentiation between ovarian cancer and nonovarian cancers because all 47 patients with ovarian cancer had a ratio greater than 25.

Metastatic adenocarcinomas of large intestinal origin have become more common than Krukenberg tumors in the past 2 decades with the gradual decline in the incidence of carcinoma of the stomach. The term Krukenberg tumor should be reserved for metastases that contain significant numbers of signet-ring cells in a cellular stroma derived from the ovarian stroma. This restriction is important because tumors with these microscopic characteristics also have distinctive gross pathologic and clinical features. Almost all metastasize from the stomach, but some arise in the breast, intestine, or other mucous gland–containing organs. Krukenberg tumors form a solid, often uniform mass, the sectioned surface of which typically exhibits gelatinous necrosis and hemorrhage. Metastases from carcinomas of the breast are among the more common surgical specimens of the ovary, especially if one includes those found incidentally. They are almost always incidental findings in therapeutic oophorectomy and rarely form symptomatic masses that require surgical removal.

Cases of metastatic ovarian carcinoma have occurred in which the clinical presentation was consistent with hormonal activity. Both androgen and estrogen excretion have been described. Endometrial hyperplasia has been described in postmenopausal patients with metastatic ovarian carcinomas, presumably indicating estrogen activity within the metastatic lesion or its normal tissue capsule.

MALIGNANT OVARIAN TUMORS IN CHILDREN

The differential diagnosis of adnexal masses in children and adolescents is wide and encompasses a variety of ovarian and fallopian tube lesions. Ovarian tumors, cysts, and torsion are more frequent indications for surgical intervention in infancy and childhood than is commonly realized. The majority of patients in this age group with an adnexal mass can present with pelvic or abdominal pain, which is the most commonly reported symptom, accompanied by nausea, vomiting, and fever, symptoms that may mimic appendicitis.

In childhood, ovarian tumors are the most frequent neoplasms of the female genital tract and account for approximately 1% of all malignancies in patients from birth to 17 years of age. Tumors of germ cell origin constitute approximately 70% of ovarian tumors in children. The evaluation of an adnexal mass in a pediatric or adolescent patient is similar to that of an adult to include appropriate laboratory studies and inclusion of tumor markers. Pediatric ovarian malignancies are rare; therefore, only 36% to 63% of ovarian malignancy cases in adolescents and children are identified correctly before surgery.

The most common germ cell tumor in this patient population are dysgerminomas, constituting 9.5% to 11% of childhood ovarian tumors and 24.5% of pediatric ovarian malignancies. It is also important to examine for features of precocious puberty to include presence of axillary and pubic hair and breast and areolar development in children presenting with a pelvic mass. Isosexual precocious puberty is associated with ovarian tumors in 5% of patients; however, approximately 16% of children with ovarian tumors present with premature secondary sexual development. **Granulosa–theca cell tumors are by far the most common ovarian neoplasms found in these patients with isosexual precocity and adnexal enlargement.**

Treatment of adnexal masses must be balanced with the imperative to maintain the child's reproductive and developmental potential. A study by Park et al. reported on 42 pediatric and adolescent girls with malignant ovarian germ cell tumors. The median age of the patients was 12 years with immature teratoma as the most common tumor type. All patients underwent fertility-sparing surgery with the preservation of one adnexa and the uterus. Thirty-one patients received adjuvant chemotherapy with BEP. The 5-year disease-free survival rate for this patient population was 85%. Ablin reported on a study of 17 children with ovarian germ cell tumors treated with multiple-agent chemotherapy. Of the 17 patients, 13 showed complete responses to therapy, suggesting that survival rates in this group of patients have improved significantly with modern chemotherapy. Lack and coworkers reported that granulosa–theca cell tumors in the premenarche patient accounted for 4% of childhood ovarian tumors at their institution from 1928 to 1979. The average age of diagnosis of their 10 patients was 5 years, and precocious "pseudopuberty" was the most common presentation. These 10 lesions were solitary; five were on the right side, and five were on the left side, with an average diameter of 12 cm. All 10 patients survived at least 10 years, and salpingo-oophorectomy was curative despite tumor spillage in two patients. Fortunately, few ovarian masses are malignant and can be adequately treated using conservative surgery in combination with platinum-based chemotherapy.

For the bibliography list, log onto www.expertconsult.com ⟨http://www.expertconsult.com⟩.

13

Fallopian Tube Cancer

Erica R. Hope, MD, G. Larry Maxwell, MD, Chad A. Hamilton, MD

OUTLINE

KEY POINTS

1. Fallopian tube cancer (FTC) was historically thought to be a rare cancer. Now, most high-grade serous carcinomas are thought to arise from the fallopian tube as opposed to the ovary.
2. The triad of pain, metrorrhagia, and leukorrhea is considered pathognomonic for FTC.
3. *BRCA1* and *BRCA2* carriers are at increased risk for FTC and should undergo extensive sectioning

of the fallopian tubes during risk-reducing surgery.
4. Serous tubal intraepithelial carcinoma is a precursor lesion to high-grade serous carcinoma.
5. Early salpingectomy with delayed oophorectomy is currently being studied and may become an option in high-risk women to decrease mortality and maintain quality of life.

INTRODUCTION

Primary fallopian tube cancer (FTC) was traditionally considered an exceedingly rare gynecologic malignancy. Few pelvic serous tumors met rather strict diagnostic criteria for FTC, and the disease site was overshadowed by the clinicopathologically similar and far more common high-grade serous ovarian carcinoma (HGSOC). Over the past decade, mounting evidence implicates carcinogenic processes beginning in the fallopian tube as the true origin of the majority of extrauterine high-grade serous carcinomas (HGSCs) inclusive of both HGSOC and primary peritoneal carcinoma (PPC). Indeed, the most recent International Federation of Gynecologists and Obstetricians (FIGO) staging has recognized the commonality of these tumors in a unified staging system, and a broad international collaboration recommended fairly dramatic changes for assigning the site of origin for HGSC aligning with a paradigm of fallopian tube origin. This chapter describes FTC from what could be considered a historical perspective followed by a discussion of the precursor lesions and additional evidence leading to current models of carcinogenesis of FTC and by extension most extrauterine HGSCs.

TRADITIONAL CHARACTERISTICS

Epidemiology, Classification, and Etiology

Based on primary site classifications set forth by Hu and later modified by Sedlis, adenocarcinoma of the fallopian tube accounted for fewer than 0.2% of cancer diagnoses among women annually with an incidence of 0.41 per 100,000. The most complete systematic review to date comparing FTC versus HGSOC found few significant differences in FTC and HGSOC relative to risk factors, clinicopathology, and molecular biology. Notably, the reviewed studies defined FTC in traditional terms as set forth by Hu and later Sedlis.

In 1950, Hu and colleagues suggested diagnostic criteria for the diagnosis of tubal cancer: (1) the main tumor grossly should be in the fallopian tube; (2) histologically, the tubal mucosa should be involved with a papillary pattern; and (3) if the tubal wall is involved to a large extent, transition from benign to malignant tubal epithelium should be identified. Sedlis and colleagues modified these criteria in 1978: (1) the main tumor arises from the endosalpinx, (2) the histologic pattern reproduces the epithelium of tubal mucosa, (3) transition from the benign to malignant tubal epithelium is demonstrable, and

(4) the ovaries or endometrium are either normal or contain a tumor that is smaller than the tumor in the tube.

Using the above definitions, a few characteristics relative to both risk factors and presentation are uniquely associated with primary FTC. A number of investigators implicate chronic tubal inflammation in tubal carcinogenesis. The initial association was with tuberculosis, and sporadic reports of fallopian tube carcinoma with coexisting tubercular salpingitis continue. Although histologic features of old pelvic inflammatory disease or endometriosis are frequently noted on examination of the tube and changes consistent with chronic healed salpingitis have been found in the contralateral tube of patients with unilateral FTC, evidence supporting such inflammatory changes as precursors to the development of carcinoma is inconsistent.

Symptoms and Signs

Classic symptoms of FTC include vaginal bleeding or discharge or lower abdominal pain. In many cases, these symptoms are vague and nonspecific. Vaginal bleeding is the most commonly reported symptom of FTC and is present in approximately 50% of the patients. Vaginal bleeding is caused by blood that accumulates from the lesion in the fallopian tube, which subsequently passes into the uterine cavity and finally exits into the vagina. Because FTC occurs most frequently after menopause, postmenopausal bleeding is common. Although carcinoma of the endometrium is the first consideration, FTC should be considered if the results of dilation and curettage are negative and symptoms persist.

Pain, often colicky, is frequently a symptom in tubal carcinoma and often accompanies vaginal bleeding. The pain is caused by distension of the tubal wall and stimulation of peristaltic activity. This pain, in many cases, is relieved with the passage of blood or watery discharge. Vaginal discharge, which is usually clear, occurs in approximately 25% of patients with tubal carcinoma. The triad of pain, metrorrhagia, and leukorrhea is considered pathognomonic for tubal carcinoma, but it occurs infrequently. Pain combined with a profuse, watery vaginal discharge, referred to as hydrops tubae profluens, is reported to be present in fewer than 5% of cases. If a patient is examined during the time that hydrops tubae profluens is present, a palpable pelvic mass may be found. The mass can decrease during the examination while the watery discharge continues. With the cessation of watery discharge and decrease in pelvic mass, the pain also decreases. Hydrops tubae profluens is caused by the effusion produced by the tumor that accumulates within the tube and causes the distension, which in turn produces the colicky pain.

Delay of diagnosis appears to be common due to nonspecific findings and overlap with ovarian cancer features. In a study by Eddy and associates, symptoms had been present for as long as 48 months. Half of the patients had symptoms for 2 months or longer. Semrad and colleagues noted a delay from the onset of symptoms to the diagnosis of an average of 4 months in about half of their patients. Peters and colleagues reported that 14% of patients were asymptomatic in their series of 115 patients.

Malignant cells are found in 11% to 23% of cervical cytologic preparations in patients with tubal cancer. In patients with hydrops tubae profluens, the chance of obtaining malignant cells should be relatively high. The identification of psammoma bodies in cervical cytology of postmenopausal women is often a sign of uterine or clear cell carcinoma, with serous fallopian tube or ovarian cancer occasionally being identified as the source.

EMERGING PARADIGMS

As noted previously, until relatively recently, the prevailing view of extrauterine HGSC was that FTC was relatively rare and the majority of these cancers formed in the ovary, perhaps in cortical inclusion cysts. The major challenge to this theory was the lack of an identifiable precursor lesion despite decades of interrogation of the ovarian surface epithelium.

Fallopian Tube Cancer and *BRCA* Mutations

In the late 1990s, a number of reports emerged of FTCs associated with germline mutations in *BRCA*. Piek and colleagues, responding to these reports of FTC associated with *BRCA1* and *BRCA2* mutations and their own molecular evidence that FTC was part of the cancer spectrum in *BRCA* mutation carriers, began screening serial sections of fallopian tubes removed during risk-reducing surgeries of women determined to be at high genetic risk of ovarian cancer. In 2001, they published their findings of the presence of dysplasia in the fallopian tubes of six of 12 cases and hyperplastic changes in an additional five with no corresponding abnormalities in 13 control cases. The provocative findings provided evidence for hyperplastic or dysplastic changes occurring in the carcinogenesis sequence of FTC and recommendations that risk-reducing surgery include both the ovaries and fallopian tubes and furthermore that both should be examined in all such cases to "attain more insight into *BRCA1*-related oncogenesis."

Occult or Intraepithelial Fallopian Tube Cancer Found During Risk-Reducing Surgery

Accumulating evidence and Piek et al.'s initial report prompted increased pathologic scrutiny of the fallopian tubes at the time of risk-reducing surgeries. Investigators at Brigham and Women's Hospital and Dana Farber Cancer Institute developed the Sectioning and Extensively Examining the FIMbria (SEE-FIM) protocol in which the fallopian tubes are sectioned at 2- to 3-mm intervals and examined histologically with lengthwise sectioning of the fimbriated portion to maximize exposure of tubal plicae. When reviewing their series of 122 *BRCA*-positive patients undergoing risk-reducing surgery, these investigators found seven (5.7%) patients with occult malignancy, all of which originated in the distal fallopian tube. Additionally, six of the cancers were accompanied by a noninvasive component.

A number of other reports during this same decade corroborated the experience, although reported rates of occult malignancy varied because of differences in study populations, pathology processing, and diagnosis. The majority of occult lesions identified were invasive and noninvasive cancers in the fallopian tubes. The best estimate to date of invasive or intraepithelial ovarian, tubal, or peritoneal neoplasms in the genetically high-risk population is from the surgical intervention arm of Gynecologic Oncology Group (GOG) Protocol 0199 (GOG 0199), also known as the National Ovarian Cancer Prevention and Early Detection Study. This prospective trial found a 4.6% risk in *BRCA1* and 3.5% risk in *BRCA2* mutation carriers. The primary sites were assigned based on distribution and extent of tumor unless an intraepithelial lesion of the fallopian tube was identified, in which case it was designated as tubal cancer. Of the 25 (of 966) lesions identified, 10 were designated ovarian, 10 were designated tubal, and five were designated primary peritoneal. The authors acknowledge that the use of more sensitive sectioning protocols, combined with growing diagnostic acumen, may prove their estimates of tubal neoplasia low.

Serous Tubal Intraepithelial Carcinoma

The dysplastic tubal cells initially identified are now more commonly referred to as tubal intraepithelial carcinoma (TIC) or serous tubal intraepithelial carcinoma (STIC). TICs are distinguished from normal mucosa by variably stratified epithelium with nuclear enlargement and atypia, high nuclear-to-cytoplasmic ratio, prominent nucleoli, variable loss of cell polarity, and mitotic activity. Hyperchromasia, irregular nuclear membranes and chromatin distribution, and absence of cilia also characterize TICs.

Immunohistochemistry (IHC) may be useful adjuncts in diagnosis. An elevated Ki-67 labeling index (>10%) and either intense or absent p53 staining (both correlate closely with mutation) support the diagnosis of TIC. Somatic mutations of p53 are the most common mutations in HGSC and are detected in more than 90% of TICs. Whereas the majority are missense mutations that correlate with intense and diffuse p53 immunoreactivity, frameshift, nonsense, and splicing junction mutations are associated with complete loss of p53 staining.

Strongly p53-positive, benign-appearing epithelium, described by Lee and colleagues as "p53 signatures" may be an even earlier event in serous carcinogenesis than TICs. These investigators demonstrated that these signatures were equally common in nonneoplastic tubes from women with and without *BRCA* mutations but more frequently present and multifocal in fallopian tubes with STIC. These signatures were much more common in the secretory cells of the fimbriae similar to TICs and often represented reproducible p53 mutations. In laser-capture microdissected (LCM) specimens, they also demonstrated that TICs and their associated ovarian cancers shared identical mutations and in one case demonstrated an identical mutation between the p53 signature and a contiguous TIC.

Despite the characteristics of STICs noted, the recognition of these lesions remains challenging, and the spectrum of changes within the fallopian tube can be difficult to interpret. In an effort to establish a reproducible classification for STIC, Visvanathan led a group of six gynecologic pathologists from four academic institutions through serial independent reviews to establish a reproducible algorithm. Intraobserver reliability was only fair for STIC versus not STIC when classification was based on morphologic criteria alone. An algorithm incorporating morphology and IHC for p53 and Ki-67 resulted in substantial agreement and provided the basis for a standardized,

and later validated, classification of STIC for clinical diagnosis and future investigations.

Fallopian Tube Cancer and Serous Tubal Intraepithelial Carcinoma Beyond *BRCA*

Building on the findings from high-risk populations, in 2007, Kindelberger and colleagues published the first study extensively examining the fallopian tubes (SEE-FIM protocol) in a consecutive series of pelvic serous carcinoma from patient not necessarily known to be at high risk. Of 55 evaluable cases, 75% had endosalpingeal involvement, and of these, 71% (29 of 41) had a coexisting STIC. Tumors classified as HGSOC by conventional criteria based on disease distribution often involved the endosalpinx and contained TICs (71% and 48%, respectively, of 42 cases). Five of five cases of ovarian cancer with concurrent TICs contained identical p53 mutations, supporting their clonality.

Przybycin and colleagues similarly examined a series of 52 pelvic (nonuterine) gynecologic cancers in which fallopian tube tissue was available for extensive examination. TIC was identified in 28 (60%) of 47 HGSCs, and because TIC was associated exclusively with this histology, they suggested the more specific term *serous TIC* or *STIC*. STICs in the absence of invasive carcinoma in the same tube was identified in seven (30%) of cases. By including STIC as supplemental criteria for extrauterine HGSC, the rate of FTC increased from 13% by conventional criteria to 64%. More extensive LCM examinations of STICs by this same group confirmed the clonal relationships of p53 mutations in STICS and concurrent HGSOCs. Additionally, they demonstrated telomere shortening, an early change in carcinogenesis, in STICs compared with their concurrent ovarian cancers, further supporting the primary role of the fallopian tube in high-grade serous carcinogenesis.

In 2014, Singh and colleagues proposed new guidelines for assigning the primary site of HGSC intended as an evolutionary change based on current understanding of the state of the science. Their intent was to build on the 2014 FIGO staging revision, which unified staging but did not unify nomenclature under an umbrella term (eg, *pelvic serous carcinoma*) or provide specific guidance for primary site assignment. Indeed, there were numerous examples in which, depending on philosophy, different pathologists might assign the same clinical case as tubal, ovarian, primary peritoneal, tubo-ovarian, or undesignated in the new system. To avoid giving different diagnostic labels to the same disease in different centers, Singh et al. made a number of recommendations, offering a standard and systematic approach based on current knowledge. Among the most important recommendations was that the fallopian tubes should be sampled by a SEE-FIM–like protocol in all cases of HGSC and that any cases with STIC should be classified as tubal carcinoma.

The following year, this same group published an assessment of their system for primary site assignment in HGSC of the fallopian tube, ovary, and peritoneum. They retrospectively assessed 151 HGSC (both chemonaive and postneoadjuvant chemotherapy) of which 68% of cases were previously considered ovarian primaries. Using the new guidelines, they rendered

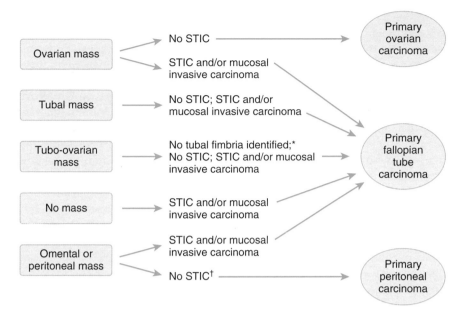

*Failure to detect the tubal fimbria implies overgrowth by tumor.
†Apply criteria as specified in the **Required Data Elements** (section iv: Tumour site) of the ICCR.

FIGURE 13.1 Flow chart for assigning the site of origin of extrauterine high-grade serous carcinoma from the International Collaboration on Cancer Reporting (ICCR). *STIC*, Serous tubal intraepithelial carcinoma. (Adapted from McCluggage WG, Judge MJ, Clarke BA, et al. Data set for reporting of ovary, fallopian tube and primary peritoneal carcinoma: recommendations from the International Collaboration on Cancer Reporting (ICCR). *Mod Pathol* 2015;28:1105.)

a revised diagnosis of fallopian tube primary in 74% of cases. In a prospective cohort of 111 HGSC cases, a majority of which were advanced stage, they classified 79% as fallopian tube primaries and only 14% as ovarian primaries. There were fewer cases of primary FTCs diagnosed after neoadjuvant chemotherapy and more diagnosed as primary peritoneal or undetermined potentially resulting from regression of small lesions in the fallopian tube. In chemonaive cases, ovarian involvement was bilateral in 62% of cases, but fallopian tube involvement was bilateral in only 16%, lending further evidence that ovarian disease is metastatic instead of primary. The proposed system combined with the revised FIGO staging system provided uniform and reproducible site assignment while classifying most HGSC as fallopian tube primaries.

Building on the above work, in 2015, the International Collaboration on Cancer Report (ICCR) published recommendations on the classification of peritoneal, ovarian, and fallopian tube carcinomas (Fig. 13.1). In this algorithm, any case with STIC and associated cancer involving the ovary, fallopian tube, or peritoneum should be classified as fallopian tube primary with classification using conventional criteria only if they lack STIC. The recommendations also conveyed that failure to identify fallopian tube fimbriae implied overgrowth by a fallopian tube carcinoma, and therefore careful attention to identify a fallopian tube in cases of an adnexal mass is important for accurate classification. Aberrant staining of p53 and Mindbomb E3 Ubiquitin Protein Ligase 1 (MIB1) is often found in association with STIC and therefore may prove helpful in confirming

the diagnostic presence of the preinvasive lesion in questionable cases.

CLINICAL IMPLICATIONS

Changes in classification of tumor origin will result in changes to the annual incidence of ovarian and FTCs. Because extrauterine HGSC are currently treated using the same platinum and taxane backbone, the immediate clinical implications reflective of this paradigm shift are limited in the setting of advanced disease. The management of STIC in the absence of other disease requires further study before evidence-based recommendations can be provided. Similar to precursors of serous uterine cancer, STIC, although intraepithelial, is capable of exfoliation and metastasis. The ICCR classifies such cases as stage IA tubal carcinoma with an annotation that there is no invasive carcinoma while also acknowledging that these lesions have a favorable prognosis based on limited data. Two series of isolated STIC with a total of 23 patients have recorded one recurrence to date. Although extremely limited, this initial signal calls into question whether isolated STIC warrants categorization as FIGO stage IA of the tube equivalent to other stage IA cancers. These data do provide hope that perhaps salpingectomy alone is sufficient for treatment, although further study is warranted before any utility of prophylactic cytotoxic therapy is ruled out.

The shifting paradigm of a fallopian tube origin for a substantial portion of HGSC has the potential to impact screening for HGSC. Preliminary investigations report that early genetic mutations, potentially of tubal origin, can be detected in cervical cytology specimens. Similarly, with a tubal precursor lesion for HGSC now identified, biomarkers, perhaps from proximal biofluids, may reveal early tubal pathogenesis.

For women at high risk for HGSC because of hereditary predisposition, risk-reducing bilateral salpingo-oophorectomy has proven effective. Given the impact on quality of life due to surgically induced menopause in addition to the potential risks of cardiovascular disease, osteoporosis, and cognitive impairment, the option of salpingectomy alone has become clinically relevant. This has been advocated by some as an alternative in women who are not prepared or who are unwilling to undergo oophorectomy. Similarly, it may be clinically prudent to recommend early salpingectomy with delayed oophorectomy in *BRCA* patients. The TUBA (TUbectomy in BRCA1/2 mutation carriers) study by Harmsen and colleagues is a prospective nonrandomized study evaluating early salpingectomy with delayed oophorectomy versus risk-reducing salpingo-oophorectomy for *BRCA1* and *BRCA2* mutation carriers. If patients elect to proceed with early salpingectomy, the completion oophorectomy will be postponed for 5 years compared with standard treatment for their *BRCA* status. The primary outcome is menopause-related quality of life with secondary measures including ovarian and breast cancer incidence, surgery-related morbidity, histopathology, cardiovascular risk factors and diseases, and cost effectiveness. This multicenter study, when completed, hopes to offer additional guidance for delayed oophorectomy in this high-risk population.

An American College of Obstetricians and Gynecologist (ACOG) Committee Opinion addresses salpingectomy for cancer prevention in women at population risk of extrauterine HGSC undergoing routine pelvic surgery. Highlighted in the opinion is that salpingectomy at the time of hysterectomy or as sterilization does not appear to increase complication rates (over hysterectomy or tubal ligation alone) nor does it impact ovarian function based on surrogate serum markers or in vitro fertilization response. The ACOG recommends that the surgeon and patient discuss the potential benefits of the removal of the fallopian tubes at the time of hysterectomy or as an option for sterilization and that prophylactic salpingectomy may offer clinicians the opportunity to prevent ovarian cancer in their patients.

CONCLUSION

Although the epidemiology of FTC is unclear, except a few idiosyncratic presentations, signs and symptoms largely mirror

---

TABLE 13.1   2014 International Federation of Gynecology and Obstetrics (FIGO) Staging Classification for Cancer of the Ovary, Fallopian Tube, and Peritoneum

I	Tumor confined to ovaries or fallopian tube(s)	T1
IA	Tumor limited to one ovary (capsule intact) or fallopian tube	T1a
	No tumor on ovarian or fallopian tube surface	
	No malignant cells in the ascites or peritoneal washings	
IB	Tumor limited to both ovaries (capsules intact) or fallopian tubes	T1b
	No tumor on ovarian or fallopian tube surface	
	No malignant cells in the ascites or peritoneal washings	
IC	Tumor limited to one or both ovaries or fallopian tubes, with any of the following:	T1c
	IC1 Surgical spill intraoperatively	
	IC2 Capsule ruptured before surgery or tumor on ovarian or fallopian tube surface	
	IC3 Malignant cells present in the ascites or peritoneal washings	
II	Tumor involves one or both ovaries or fallopian tubes with pelvic extension (below pelvic brim) or peritoneal cancer (Tp)	T2
IIA	Extension and/or implants on the uterus and/or fallopian tubes and/or ovaries	T2a
IIB	Extension to other pelvic intraoperative tissues	T2b
III	Tumor involves one or both ovaries or fallopian tubes or primary peritoneal cancer, with cytologically or histologically confirmed spread to the peritoneum outside the pelvis and/or metastasis to the retroperitoneal lymph nodes	T3
IIIA	Metastasis to the retroperitoneal lymph nodes with or without microscopic peritoneal involvement beyond the pelvis	T1, T2, T3aN1
IIIA1	Positive retroperitoneal lymph nodes only (cytologically or histologically proven)	
IIIA1(i)	Metastasis ≤10 mm in greatest dimension (note: this is tumor dimension and not lymph node dimension)	T3a/T3aN1
IIIA1(ii)	Metastasis > 10 mm in greatest dimension	
IIIA2	Microscopic extrapelvic (above the pelvic brim) peritoneal involvement with or without positive retroperitoneal lymph nodes	T3a/T3aN1
IIIB	Macroscopic peritoneal metastases beyond the pelvic brim ≤2 cm in greatest dimension, with or without metastasis to the retroperitoneal lymph nodes	T3b/T3bN1
IIIC	Macroscopic peritoneal metastases beyond the pelvic brim >2 cm in greatest dimension, with or without metastases to the retroperitoneal nodes*	T3c/T3cN1
IV	Distant metastasis excluding peritoneal metastases	Any T, any N, M1
	Stage IV A: Pleural effusion with positive cytology	
	Stage IV B: Metastases to extraabdominal organs (including inguinal lymph nodes and lymph nodes outside of abdominal cavity)†	

*Includes extension of tumor to capsule of liver and spleen without parenchymal involvement of either organ.
†Parenchymal metastases are stage IV B.
From Mutch DG, Prat J. 2014 FIGO staging for ovarian, fallopian tube and peritoneal cancer. *Gynecol Oncol* 2014;133:402.

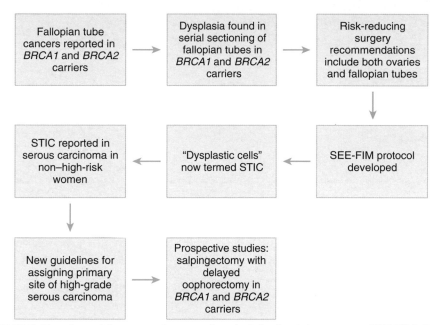

FIGURE 13.2 Timeline of the emerging paradigm in fallopian tube cancer. *SEE-FIM,* Sectioning and Extensively Examining the FIMbria; *STIC,* serous tubal intraepithelial carcinoma.

other HGSC. Similarly, the staging and treatment of FTC are identical to those of high-grade serous ovarian and primary peritoneal cancers (Table 13.1). The transition from FTC's relative rarity to the increasing number of cases diagnosed in high-risk women and discovery of a precursor lesion that is present in a majority of HGSCs has evolved dramatically over the past 2 decades (Fig. 13.2). It is likely that many HGSCs thought to be of ovarian origin will now be categorized as fallopian tube primary. Ongoing research will reveal whether salpingectomy is an effective risk-reducing strategy, especially in those at highest risk.

For the bibliography list, log onto www.expertconsult.com <http://www.expertconsult.com>.

14

Breast Diseases

Patricia A. Cronin, MD, Mary L. Gemignani, MD

OUTLINE

KEY POINTS

1. Appropriate investigation of symptomatic patients with a breast mass consists of triple assessment and is crucial to rule out an underlying breast malignancy. Triple assessment involves physical examination, breast imaging with mammography and ultrasonography, and pathologic or cytologic evaluation. Nonconcordant results should prompt further investigation or careful follow-up.

2. All women should undergo regular breast screening at the appropriate age, and high-risk patients should be identified

for elevated screening pathways dependent on individual risk assessment.

3. Surgical planning needs to be individualized to the patient with regards to suitability for breast conservation versus mastectomy. Adjuvant radiation is an essential treatment component after breast conservation. Reconstructive options should be offered and discussed with all patients undergoing mastectomy.

4. Clinically node-negative patients with invasive cancer should have SLNB for axillary staging. Having two or less positive sentinel nodes in the setting of breast conservation does not require completion axillary dissection. Axillary dissection is required with more extensive nodal positivity or in the setting of any positive sentinel node in patients having mastectomy.

5. *BRCA* genetic counseling and testing should be offered to women who meet testing criteria. Surveillance programs should include regular breast examination and imaging with mammography and magnetic resonance imaging for those who test positive. Risk-reduction options such as chemoprevention and surgery such as bilateral mastectomies and bilateral salpingo-oophorectomies should be discussed.

INTRODUCTION

Breast cancer remains the most common cancer in women and is second only to lung cancer as the leading cause of cancer-related death in the United States. In 2015, an estimated 231,840 new cases of invasive breast cancer were expected to be diagnosed in women in the United States along with 60,290 new cases of noninvasive (in situ) breast cancer. The lifetime risk among women of developing breast cancer is 12.5% (1 in 8); the lifetime risk of dying from breast cancer is 3.6% (1 in 28). About 40,290 women in the United States are expected to die in 2015 from breast cancer, though death rates have been decreasing since 1989. This decline is thought to be secondary to the increased use of mammographic screening with early detection of breast cancer and the use of effective adjuvant therapies. This chapter presents an overview of breast cancer screening, diagnosis, and treatment of benign and malignant conditions of the breast.

ANATOMY OF THE BREAST

The adult breast lies between the second and sixth ribs in the vertical plane and between the sternal edge (medially) and midaxillary line (laterally). The average breast measures 10 to 12 cm in diameter and 5 to 7 cm in thickness. It is concentric, with a lateral projection into the axilla named the axillary tail of Spence (Figs. 14.1 and 14.2).

The breast consists of three major structures: skin, subcutaneous fatty tissue, and breast tissue (parenchyma and stroma). The skin contains hair follicles, sebaceous glands, and eccrine sweat glands. The glandular breast is divided into 15 to 20 segments (lobes) that are separated by connective tissue and converge at the nipple in a radial arrangement. These lobes are made up of 20 to 40 lobules, which in turn consist of 10 to 100 alveoli (tubulosaccular secretory units). Five to 10 major milk-collecting ducts drain each segment and open at the nipple into subareolar lactiferous sinuses.

A superficial pectoral fascia envelops the breast; the undersurface of the breast lies on the deep pectoral fascia. The superficial pectoral fascia is continuous with the superficial abdominal fascia of Camper. Between these two fascial layers are fibrous bands called Cooper suspensory ligaments that provide support for the breast. The space between the deep layers of the superficial fascia of the breast and the deep investing fascia of the pectoralis is the retromammary bursa.

The epidermis of the nipple (mammary papilla) and areola is pigmented and wrinkled and consists of keratinized, stratified squamous epithelium that contains smooth muscle fibers in dense connective tissue. These fibers are responsible for the erection of the nipple. Two receptor-type nerve endings (Ruffini-like bodies and end bulb of Krause) are present on the nipple and associated with the tactile reception of stretch and pressure.

The areola has no hair follicles; it has sebaceous glands (at its margin), apocrine sweat glands, and accessory areolar glands (Montgomery glands) that open on the surface of the areola as small elevations called Morgagni tubercles. Montgomery glands are large sebaceous glands capable of secreting milk; they represent an intermediate stage between the sweat and the mammary glands.

The blood supply of the breast is mostly from superficial vessels. The principal blood supply is derived from the internal thoracic (mammary) and lateral thoracic artery and their tributaries. The posterior intercostal arteries of the second to fourth intercostal spaces also give off tributaries called the mammary branches. Approximately 60% of the breast, mainly the medial and central parts, is supplied by the anterior perforating branches of the internal mammary artery. About 30% of the breast, mainly the upper outer quadrant, is supplied by the lateral thoracic artery.

The superficial veins follow the arteries and drain through perforating branches of the internal thoracic vein, tributaries of the axillary vein, and perforating branches of posterior intercostal veins. The veins anastomose circumferentially around the nipple, which is called the circulus venosus.

Subepithelial or a papillary plexus of lymphatics of the breast are confluent with the subepithelial lymphatics over the surface of the body. These valveless lymphatic vessels communicate with subdermal lymphatic vessels and merge with Sappey's subareolar plexus. The subareolar plexus receives lymphatic vessels from the nipple and the areola and communicates by way of the vertical lymphatic vessels that are equivalent to those connecting the subepithelial and subdermal plexus elsewhere in the body. Lymph flows unidirectionally from the superficial to

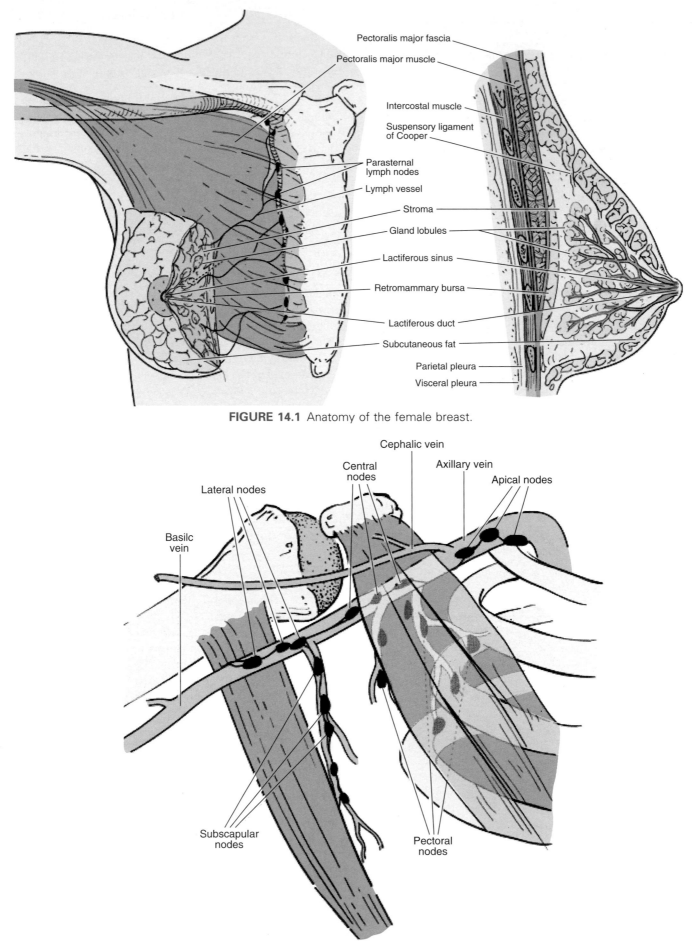

Pectoralis major fascia

Pectoralis major muscle

Intercostal muscle

Suspensory ligament of Cooper

Parasternal lymph nodes

Lymph vessel

Stroma

Gland lobules

Lactiferous sinus

Retromammary bursa

Lactiferous duct

Subcutaneous fat

Parietal pleura

Visceral pleura

FIGURE 14.1 Anatomy of the female breast.

Cephalic vein

Central nodes

Axillary vein

Apical nodes

Lateral nodes

Basilc vein

Subscapular nodes

Pectoral nodes

FIGURE 14.2 Axillary nodes.

the deep plexus and from the subareolar plexus through the lymphatic vessels of the lactiferous duct to the perilobular and deep subcutaneous plexus. Lymph flow from the deep subcutaneous and intramammary lymphatic vessels moves centrifugally toward the axillary and internal mammary lymph nodes. It is estimated that about 97% of the lymph flows to the axillary nodes and 3% to the internal mammary chain.

Axillary lymph nodes may be divided into three anatomic levels defined in reference to the pectoralis minor muscle. Level I nodes are the axillary vein lymph nodes that lie along the axillary vein from the lateral extent of the pectoralis minor muscle to the latissimus dorsi muscle. In this area, deep to the floor of the axilla, subscapular nodes that lie on the subscapularis muscle are identified.

Level II nodes are designated by their location underneath the pectoralis minor muscle. Medial to the pectoralis minor are level III nodes, which include apical or subclavicular nodes and are adjacent to Halstead's ligament.

Interpectoral nodes are called Rotter's nodes. They lie between the pectoralis major and minor muscle.

EMBRYOLOGY AND DEVELOPMENT OF THE BREAST

The mammary glands are highly specialized skin derivatives of ectodermal origin. The epithelial ridge that develops into breast tissue undergoes a series of proliferations to form the lactiferous ducts. Primitive breast tissue is under the gonadal control of fetal androgen production, which causes a suppression of breast growth during the period of gestation when the tissue is under the simultaneous influence of increasing levels of growth-promoting estrogen and progesterone. After birth, breast tissue remains dormant until adolescence, when estrogen produces a proliferation of ductal epithelium and progesterone produces rapid growth of the acini. However, breast growth and development are not totally dependent on estrogen and progesterone levels. Insulin, cortisol, thyroxine, growth hormone, and prolactin are also required for complete functional development. Minor deficiencies in any one of these hormones can be compensated for by an excess of prolactin.

PREGNANCY AND BREASTFEEDING

Increasing amounts of estrogen, progesterone, and human placental lactogen produce active growth of functional breast tissue during the course of pregnancy. Estrogen production is under the control of the fetus. Estrogen influences progesterone production, uteroplacental blood flow, mammary gland development, and fetal adrenal gland function. By the 20th week of pregnancy, most of the estrogen excreted in maternal urine comes from fetal androgens. About 90% of maternal estriol is derived from fetal precursors. Serum prolactin rises from nonpregnant levels of 10 ng/mL to term levels of 200 ng/mL. Amniotic fluid prolactin levels are more than 100 times greater than the levels in maternal or fetal blood early in pregnancy. It is not known whether the fetal pituitary gland or the trophoblast secretes the hormone into the amniotic fluid. Elevated levels of estradiol parallel those of prolactin and indicate that estriol may be responsible for increases in prolactin. Although estrogen may initiate prolactin secretion, high levels block its physiologic effects. Prolactin secretion is also controlled by the prolactin-inhibiting factor. A decrease in estrogen level after delivery and suppression of the prolactin-inhibiting factor by suckling increases prolactin levels. If breastfeeding does not occur, serum prolactin levels decrease to nonpregnant levels in about 1 week.

The release of oxytocin from the posterior pituitary gland affects contraction of the duct system, stimulating the delivery of milk to the nipples. However, after 3 to 4 months of breastfeeding, suckling appears to be the only stimulus required for lactation.

BENIGN BREAST CONDITIONS

Fibrocystic Changes

Fibrocystic change is the most common benign breast condition in women. It consists of no single entity and encompasses a histologic spectrum of changes in the breast, some of which are normal and some of which are abnormal. It is a result of fluctuating hormone levels and is most common in premenopausal women between the ages of 20 and 50 years. It is often associated with pain and tenderness (mastodynia) and tends to be bilateral. Most women report symptoms during the premenstrual phase of the cycle, which suggests that progesterone may play a role in the development and symptoms of cystic alterations in breast tissue. However, the proportional effect of both estrogen and progesterone on the cause of benign breast conditions is unclear.

Fibrocystic change is not a risk factor for cancer. In 1985, the Cancer Committee of the College of American Pathologists published a consensus statement and discouraged the use of the term *fibrocystic disease*; they prefer the terms *fibrocystic changes* or *fibrocystic condition*.

Mastodynia results from breast stromal edema, ductal dilation, and associated inflammatory response. An increase in breast size is also frequently reported. The differential diagnosis for breast pain includes other conditions affecting the anterior chest wall, such as intercostal neuralgia, myalgia, and chronic costochondritis. Women with large, pendulous breasts will have associated stretching of Cooper ligaments and associated breast pain.

The management of fibrocystic change in any patient presenting symptomatically first consists of ruling out any underlying breast cancer with appropriate imaging and workup. After that, advice can be given with respect to the patient's breast pain and tenderness. Symptomatic women may benefit from counseling regarding proper selection and fitting of a brassiere because improved mechanical support may relieve breast pain. The effectiveness of dietary interventions to reduce breast pain remains to be established. A low-fat diet was associated with a substantial improvement in mastalgia symptoms when 21 patients with severe mastopathy were randomized to a diet containing 15% fat intake or a general diet containing 36%

fat intake. Although many women report that a reduction in caffeine intake alleviates their breast pain, clinical studies have not shown consistent findings. In an uncontrolled study, 61% of women with breast pain who substantially decreased caffeine intake for 1 year had decreased pain or complete relief. Studies with small numbers of patients suggested a potential beneficial effect of vitamin E in fibrocystic change. Evening primrose oil (gammalinolenic acid) has been widely advocated as an option. Two small randomized, double-blind, placebo-controlled studies of evening primrose oil have shown efficacy in the treatment of breast pain. But this result has not been duplicated in other studies.

Hormonal manipulation may alleviate mastodynia but is associated with other side effects. There is no consensus with regards which of these is superior. Danazol is the only medication approved by the US Food and Drug Administration (FDA) for treatment of mastodynia. Overall, 59% to 92% of women treated with danazol experience relief of breast pain. Unfortunately, adverse effects occur in 30% of patients and result in discontinuation of treatment in 15% of patients, even when breast pain is improved. Adverse effects are dose related and are primarily androgenic, including acne, hair loss, decrease in voice pitch, weight gain, headache, nausea, rash, anxiety, and depression.

The selective estrogen receptor modulator (SERM) tamoxifen, which is commonly used to prevent and treat breast cancer, is effective in reducing pain in 71% to 96% of women with cyclic mastalgia and 56% of women with noncyclical mastalgia in controlled trials. In studies comparing tamoxifen dosages and duration for breast pain, the 10 mg/d dosage of tamoxifen was as effective as the 20 mg/d dosage with fewer adverse effects. Tamoxifen has a risk of potentially serious adverse effects, such increased risk of deep vein thrombosis and endometrial cancer. Menopausal symptoms such as hot flashes, nausea, menstrual irregularity, vaginal dryness or discharge, and weight gain have been associated with tamoxifen treatment and often lead to discontinuation.

Proliferative Changes

Proliferative changes include hyperplasia and adenosis. Hyperplasia is proliferation of ductal epithelium, which results in layering of the cells. Atypia may be associated with this proliferation. There are two types of atypical hyperplasia based on microscopic appearance: atypical ductal hyperplasia (ADH) and atypical lobular hyperplasia (ALH). Both are associated with an increased relative risk (RR) of approximately 4 for development of a later invasive breast cancer. Because there is an approximate 25% chance of finding a concurrent cancer with ADH found on core biopsy, surgical excision is recommended. In the case of ALH, recent studies have suggested the invasive cancer "upgrade" rate is lower (0%–6%) after surgical excision of ALH. Therefore, if radiologic findings are concordant or the findings are incidental, excision may not be warranted. All patients with atypical hyperplasia warrant careful clinical and radiologic follow-up.

Adenosis is also a proliferative lesion caused by changes in the acini in the distal mammary lobule. Sclerosing adenosis

refers to the dense, fibrotic tissue surrounding these small ducts. These lesions may present as a palpable mass in women in their 30s and 40s.

A papilloma can result from this ductal proliferation. Papillomas are papillary lesions with a branching fibrovascular core surrounded by epithelium. These lesions are associated with serosanguineous nipple discharge in 25% to 50% of presentations. Ninety percent of the time, there is a small palpable mass adjacent to the areola. Intraductal papillomas are rarely associated with carcinoma but require surgical excision to rule out the possibility of misdiagnosis of a malignancy.

Sclerosing Lesions

Sclerosing lesions have been described by a variety of names, including *sclerosing papillary proliferation, nonencapsulated sclerosing lesion, indurative mastopathy,* and *radial scar*. They are important because they may simulate carcinoma on mammographic, gross, and microscopic examinations. These lesions are typically less than 1 cm in diameter. On gross examination, they are irregular, gray or white, indurated with central retraction, and have an appearance identical to scirrhous carcinoma. On microscopic examination, the lesion has a stellate configuration and consists of a central, fibrotic core containing entrapped glandular elements. The surrounding breast tissue typically shows varying degrees of intraductal hyperplasia and adenosis. The significance of this lesion relative to subsequent development of carcinoma is controversial. Available evidence suggests that these lesions are part of the fibrocystic complex. It is likely that their premalignant potential is the same as that of the constituent parts. Local excision of these lesions is the treatment of choice.

Fibroadenoma

Fibroadenomas are benign fibroepithelial tumors and are the second most common benign lesion of the breast. They are the most common lesion found in women younger than age 25 years. They persist during the menstrual years of a woman's life, but regression after menopause has been reported. Patients typically present with a mobile, smooth, painless, palpable mass. Ultrasound examination along with physical examination can help in making the diagnosis.

Mammographically, fibroadenomas may appear as round, oval, or lobulated masses with circumscribed margins. In older women, they can have a rim of coarse calcifications. Fine-needle aspiration (FNA) will reveal benign ductal epithelial cells and elongated dense stromal cells. Microscopically, fibrous tissue comprises most of the fibroadenoma. Carcinoma arising in fibroadenomas is rare.

Fibroadenomas can be followed without the need for complete surgical excision. This can be achieved with physical examination or ultrasound examination if they are not palpable. However, surgical excision should be performed in the following situations:

- The mass continues to enlarge.
- The results of FNA or core biopsy are inconclusive or yield atypia.
- The patient desires surgical excision.

TABLE 14.1 Proliferative Breast Disease and Breast Cancer Risk

Characteristic	Relative Risk (Confidence Interval)
Proliferative disease, no atypia	1.3 (0.69–11.9)
Complex fibroadenoma*	1.46 (0.53–14.0)
Atypical hyperplasia	2.53 (1.01–6.3)
Neither proliferative disease nor complex fibroadenoma	1.27 (0.89–11.8)

*Contains cysts, sclerosing adenosis, epithelial calcification, or papillary apocrine changes.
Modified from Dupont WD, Page DL, Parl FF, et al. Estrogen replacement therapy in women with a history of proliferative breast disease. Cancer 1999;85:1277.

TABLE 14.2 Breast Diagnosis Grouped by Cancer Risk

Cancer Risk	Diagnosis
No increased risk	Adenosis, sclerosing or florid
	Apocrine metaplasia
	Cysts, macro or micro
	Duct ectasia
	Fibroadenoma
	Fibrosis
	Hyperplasia (mild)
	Mastitis
	Periductal mastitis
	Squamous metaplasia
Slightly increased	Hyperplasia, moderate or florid
	Papilloma, solid or papillary, with fibrovascular core
Moderately increased	Atypical hyperplasia
	Ductal
	Lobular

Table 14.1 lists proliferative breast disease and breast cancer risk. Table 14.2 shows breast diagnoses grouped by cancer risk.

Phyllodes Tumor

Phyllodes tumors are uncommon, slow-growing fibroepithelial tumors. Previously referred to as cystosarcoma phyllodes, this name contributed to confusion in understanding this entity. Although very similar to a fibroadenoma, the stromal component is hypercellular with increased pleomorphism and mitotic activity. Phyllodes tumors can occur in women of any age but more commonly occur in premenopausal women.

Malignant behavior in phyllodes tumors is rare in premenopausal women. Malignant phyllodes tumors are noted when there is a combination of increased mitotic activity, invasive borders, or marked pleomorphism. Incomplete excision is a major determinant for local recurrence. Treatment is total surgical excision with a wide margin of healthy tissue.

Adenoma

Adenoma of the breast is a well-circumscribed tumor composed of benign epithelial elements with sparse, inconspicuous stroma, a feature that differentiates this lesion from fibroadenoma, in which the stroma is an integral part of the tumor. For practical purposes, adenomas may be divided into two major groups: tubular adenomas and lactating adenomas. Tubular adenomas in young women are well-defined, freely movable nodules that clinically resemble fibroadenomas. Lactating adenomas manifest as one or more freely movable masses during pregnancy or the postpartum period. They are grossly well circumscribed and lobulated; on cut section, they appear tan and softer than tubular adenomas. On microscopic examination, these lesions have lobulated borders and are composed of glands lined by cuboid cells with secretory activity identical to the lactational changes normally observed in the breast tissue during pregnancy and the puerperium.

It should be noted that breast biopsy in a pregnant or lactating woman calls for meticulous hemostasis because of the increased vascularity and risk of postoperative hematoma formation. The lactating breast is predisposed to postoperative infection because milk is a good culture medium. Anesthesia by local injection may be difficult in the enlarged breast but is the method of choice. Incisional biopsy under local anesthesia is an option when excisional biopsy is a problem. Because of the significant risk of infection and milk fistula, the patient who is lactating should cease lactating before biopsy is performed.

Superficial Thrombophlebitis

Superficial thrombophlebitis is also known as Mondor disease of the breast. It is an uncommon benign inflammatory process. It can occur spontaneously but usually is associated with breast trauma, breast surgery, or pregnancy. It is a thrombophlebitis of the thoracoepigastric vein, which drains the upper-outer quadrant of the breast. Patients present with acute pain and a linear, tender fibrotic band with skin retraction over the distribution of the thoracoepigastric vein.

Treatment is conservative, with analgesics and application of heat. The condition resolves in 1 to 3 weeks. Skin retraction superficial to the area of inflammation can remain if the inflammation is extensive. Biopsy is not necessary.

Mastitis

Mastitis usually occurs in relation to lactation. It can occur in nonpuerperal periods in association with galactorrhea. Skin organisms, *Staphylococcus aureus,* and *Streptococcus* spp. may cause infection of the nipple and breast ducts. The presence of milk in the ducts can provide an excellent medium for infection.

Women with mastitis may continue to breastfeed. Antibiotic therapy with dicloxacillin sodium (250 mg qid) or penicillin G is indicated. If there is no response, an abscess that may require surgical drainage must be excluded. Inflammatory carcinomas can mimic mastitis, and if no resolution of infection is noted despite continued antibiotics, a skin biopsy may be indicated.

Galactoceles are milk-filled cysts. They are usually tender and present after the abrupt termination of breastfeeding. Aspiration of the cyst is often necessary for symptomatic relief. If reaccumulation occurs, however, surgical excision may be required to avoid infection.

Duct Ectasia

Duct ectasia is a condition that usually occurs in perimenopausal or postmenopausal women. Patients present with a tender, hard, erythematous mass adjacent to the areola in association with burning, itching, or a pulling sensation in the nipple area. A thick, greenish-black discharge may be present. The pathogenesis of this condition has not been fully established. Available evidence suggests, however, that the primary event is periductal inflammation and that ductal ectasia is the ultimate outcome of this disorder. The postulated sequence of events in the evolution of this disease is periductal inflammation leading to periductal fibrosis that subsequently results in ductal dilation. However, the etiology of the initial inflammatory response remains obscure. Histologic evaluation of the area shows dilated, distended terminal-collecting ducts obstructed with inspissated lipid-containing epithelial cells and phagocytic histiocytes. This process tends to occur in a segmental fashion extending from the involved nipple area to adjacent ducts. Occasionally, a small abscess forms at the base of the nipple. Treatment is excisional biopsy.

Younger women can present with inflammation of the ducts in the region of the nipple, which may produce fissures and fistulae with connection from the nipple ducts to the skin at the edges of the areola. Prior periductal mastitis leads to the squamous epithelium of the terminal dilated portion of the collecting ducts to undergo squamous metaplasia. Keratin is formed in the duct, accumulates, and can cause an abscess at the base of the nipple. Excision of the area usually is necessary.

Fat Necrosis

Fat necrosis is a relatively uncommon benign condition occurring as a response to breast trauma or surgery. Patients present with a hard mass that can mimic a carcinoma. The irregular mass is palpable and may involve skin retraction. Multiple calcifications can be seen on mammography.

The histology is active chronic inflammatory cells, with lymphocytes and histiocytes predominating. In the later stages, a collagenous scar is noted, with "oil cysts" or free lipid material released by lipocyte necrosis. Fat necrosis does not increase the risk of carcinoma, and its clinical importance is in the differential diagnosis of a carcinoma.

Nipple Discharge

Nipple discharge has been reported in 10.0% to 15.0% of women with benign breast disease and in 2.5% to 3.0% of those with carcinoma. Galactorrhea presents as bilateral milky nipple discharge consisting of lipid droplets; the condition is usually idiopathic but can be found after discontinuation of oral contraceptives or as a persistent discharge after pregnancy. Plasma prolactin levels should be determined because of the possibility of a prolactin-producing pituitary adenoma.

The discharge is classified according to its appearance as milky, green, bloody, serous, cloudy, or purulent. The drainage should be classified according to whether it is unilateral, bilateral, spontaneous, or recurrent. This information is obtained at the time of a thorough history and physical examination. For example, if the drainage first appeared in the patient's bra or nightgown on awakening, this finding is significant. The presence of a mass should also be investigated. The risk of cancer is increased when the discharge is unilateral from a single duct, when it occurs in a postmenopausal patient, or when a mass is present.

Unilateral, Spontaneous Nipple Discharge

In cases of unilateral, spontaneous nipple discharge, several causes are included in the differential diagnosis. The most common cause of nipple discharge is mammary-duct ectasia, which produces a multicolored (green, yellow, white, brown, gray, or reddish-brown) nipple discharge. The reddish-brown discharge is often mistaken for a blood discharge. It is thought to result from an increase in glandular secretions, with the production of an irritating lipid fluid that can produce a nipple discharge.

The next most common cause of a multicolored, sticky nipple discharge is nonpuerperal mastitis. The persistent type involves inflammation in deeper portions of the breast; the transient types are associated with periareolar inflammation. If the inflammation develops into an inflammatory mass, surgical excision and drainage are necessary. Medical management with local care, avoidance of all nipple manipulation, and administration of nonsteroidal antiinflammatory agents and an antistaphylococcal antibiotic are often successful when infection is suspected.

Bloody nipple discharge warrants surgical evaluation. Intraductal papillomas are the most common cause of bloody nipple discharge. During the breast examination, physicians should look for an associated periareolar mass. The examination consists of gently and carefully palpating the subareolar region to identify the pressure point that produces the discharge. It is important to reproduce the discharge and demonstrate the breast quadrant from which it emanates. All significant nipple discharges warrant referral for tissue biopsy. Although a mass is usually present when the discharge is a result of cancer, there is no palpable mass in 13% of cancers with nipple secretions. Bloody discharge occurring in the third trimester of pregnancy may be regarded as physiologic, however, and does not require intervention unless persistent for several months after delivery. There are no contraindications to breastfeeding in these patients. Cytology of the discharge is not routinely recommended because of a reported low sensitivity for detection of cancer ($\approx$27%). Galactography (injecting radiopaque contrast into the discharging duct and then performing mammography) offers better visualization of small intraductal papillomas but cannot differentiate between benign and malignant lesions. A surgical procedure is still necessary. Mammography has a 9.5% false-negative rate and a 1.6% false-positive rate for detecting cancer in patients with a nipple discharge. Table 14.3 reveals characteristics of nipple discharge.

HISTORY AND PHYSICAL EXAMINATION

Obtaining a thorough history, including a family history and information on menstrual status, pregnancies and lactation,

TABLE 14.3 Characteristics of Nipple Discharge

Color	Likely Cause	Percentage Caused by Cancer
Milky (galactorrhea)	Pituitary adenoma, pregnancy, oral contraceptives	Rare
Green, yellow, sticky	Ductal ectasia	Rare
Clear, watery	Ductal carcinoma	30–50
Bloody, sanguineous	Fibrocystic changes, ductal papillomas	25
Pink, serosanguineous	Fibrocystic changes, ductal papillomas	10
Yellow, serous	Fibrocystic changes, ductal papillomas	5
Purulent	Bacterial infection	Rare

hormone use, and prior breast surgeries and trauma, is essential. In addition, ascertaining whether the patient performs breast self-examinations (BSEs) and determining the presence and characterization of nipple discharge or a breast mass are important.

Bilateral breast examination is best performed after menstruation and before ovulation. At this time, breast engorgement and tenderness are less likely to be present.

A multipositional breast examination should be performed, including examination in the upright and supine positions. Breast retraction and subtle changes in the skin and nipple may be missed if the patient is examined in only one position.

The patient should be in the sitting position during the inception of the physical breast examination. In this position, asymmetry, skin or nipple retraction, and nipple ulceration should be most apparent (Fig. 14.3, A). When the patient's arms are raised (Fig. 14.3, B), skin changes in the lower half of the breast or in the inframammary fold become accentuated. Contraction of the pectoralis major muscle, affected by the patient pushing her hands against her hips (Fig. 14.3, C), may demonstrate an otherwise undetected skin retraction. Next, palpation of the breast with the patient still upright may allow detection of subtle lesions that would be more difficult to palpate if she were supine (Fig. 14.3, D). Examination of the supraclavicular areas and both sides of the neck for the purpose of detecting suspicious lymphadenopathy is also best done when the patient is in the upright position.

The axilla should be examined with the patient in the upright position. The patient's right arm should be fixed at the elbow and held there by the physician's right hand. This allows relaxation of the chest wall musculature (Fig. 14.3, E). Palpation with the left hand permits assessment of the lower axilla, and with extension higher toward the clavicle, the middle and upper portions of the axilla can be assessed. The left axilla is examined with the right hand after relaxation of the patient's left arm in the physician's left hand. If lymph nodes are palpable, the clinician must assess their level and size and whether they are suspicious, single or multiple, and mobile or fixed to underlying structures.

The second phase of the breast examination is conducted with the patient in the supine position and with the patient's arm raised above the head (Fig. 14.3, F). Digital palpation is carried out using the index and middle fingers and by applying varying amounts of pressure with the flats or pads of the fingers. A thorough examination systemically covers the entire breast and chest wall. The examination can be done in a clockwise direction or by rows (stripwise). It is important to carefully examine beneath the nipple–areolar complex and within the axilla.

An inflammatory appearance of the breast should raise suspicion of an inflammatory carcinoma. The classic appearance of inflammatory breast cancer includes a red, swollen breast with skin edema ("peau d'orange"). The breast is generally not tender. If the inflammation persists after a short course of antibiotics to rule out cellulitis, biopsy of the breast and skin is warranted. Inflammatory breast cancer is often a clinical diagnosis, and a benign skin biopsy should not dissuade the clinician from undertaking further evaluation and treatment. Any asymmetric skin changes or changes of the nipple–areolar complex should arouse suspicion. Paget disease of the nipple suggests the presence of intraductal or invasive cancer involving the nipple, and cancer should be excluded by a nipple biopsy of the abnormal area after a mammogram.

It is important to instruct patients in the technique of BSE. Physician-directed discussion on BSE is the most effective approach. Physicians have the opportunity to reinforce what is normal versus abnormal to patients during the examination. If no abnormal findings are noted on examination, it is critical to document negative findings. The date of the last mammogram, discussion of cancer screening, and plans for follow-up should also be recorded.

Hormones (hormone replacement therapy [HRT] or oral contraceptive pills [OCPs]) should not be renewed without a documented annual breast examination or mammography if indicated. A great deal of litigation results from failure to diagnose breast cancer. The Physician Insurers Association of America's breast cancer claims study, conducted in 1988, determined that 75% of successful malpractice lawsuits involved primary care physicians with practices in family medicine, internal medicine, or obstetrics and gynecology. It is important that the medical chart include careful documentation because approximately one-third of the cases reported in the Physician Insurers Association of America's study resulted from inadequate documentation.

Clinical breast examination (CBE) and BSE as methods for screening for breast cancer mainly aim at detection of palpable breast lesions. However, there are no published reports demonstrating these methods as being effective in breast cancer mortality risk reduction.

A Cochrane systematic review published in 2003 included two large population-based studies from Russia and Shanghai, China that compared BSE with no intervention. In both trials, almost twice as many biopsies with benign results were performed in the screening group compared with the control group (RR, 1.89; 95% confidence interval [CI] 1.79–2.00).

Three trials were designed to determine mortality outcomes by using CBE as the primary screening approach in countries

A

B

C

D

E

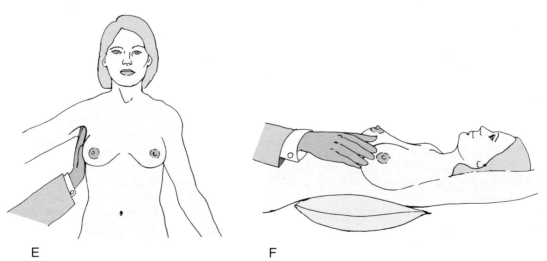

F

FIGURE 14.3 Physical examination of the breast. **A,** Upright position. **B,** Arms raised. **C,** Pushing hands against hips. **D,** Palpation in an upright position. **E,** Palpation of the axilla. **F,** Palpation in a supine position.

with limited health care resources and without mammography screening programs. The applicability of these trials to the United States is limited. One trial in the Philippines was discontinued because of poor acceptance, and the others are ongoing in India and Egypt.

In its most recent update, the United States Preventive Services Task Force (USPSTF) recommended against BSE based on a systematic review of published reports.

For breast cancer screening, the American Cancer Society (ACS) recommends CBE every 3 years for women aged 20 to 39 years and annually beginning at age 40 years.

TABLE 14.4   Randomized Population-Based Mammography Trials

Trial	Relative Risk (95% Confidence Interval)
Malmö	0.96 (0.68–1.35)
Canada	1.08 (0.84–1.40)
Göteborg	0.55 (0.31–0.95)
Stockholm	0.73 (0.50–1.06)
Kopparberg	0.58 (0.45–0.76)
Östergötland	0.76 (0.61–0.95)
New York	0.79 (0.64–0.98)
Edinburgh	0.87 (0.70–1.08)

MAMMOGRAPHY

The primary goal of mammography is to screen asymptomatic women to help detect breast cancer at an early stage. The goal of screening mammography is to find cancers before they are clinically palpable, more likely to be small, and less likely to have nodal involvement. Most studies of mammography use mortality as the endpoint, and the value of screening is often limited to mortality rates. Few studies factor the effects of early detection on quality of life or the fact that treatment at earlier stages carries less morbidity and has more treatment options.

In general, a routine screening mammogram consists of a mediolateral oblique (MLO) view and a craniocaudal (CC) view of each breast. With modern low-dose screening, the dose is less than 0.1 rad per study (for comparison, a chest radiograph delivers 0.025 rad per study). The effectiveness of screening depends on the density of the breast: The greater the breast density, the lower the sensitivity of the mammogram.

Breast composition may be one of four patterns of increasing density:
1. Almost entirely fat
2. Scattered fibroglandular densities
3. Heterogeneously dense
4. Extremely dense

It is important to note that the false-negative rate for mammograms is 10% to 15% and that a normal mammogram does not eliminate the need for further evaluation of a dominant mass in the breast. If the clinical examination is suspicious, a negative mammogram result should not delay further investigation. Breast density should be documented in the mammogram report, and many states require notification of the patients of their breast density in their results letter.

Mammographic screening in women 40 years or older has reduced mortality rates by 20% to 30%. The efficacy of screening mammography in decreasing breast cancer mortality rates has been demonstrated in numerous studies. In the 1960s, the Health Insurance Plan of Greater New York performed a study of physical examination and mammography in a study group of 30,756 women and a control group of 30,239 women between the ages of 40 and 64 years. At 10 years of follow-up, the study group had a 30% decrease in the breast cancer mortality rate compared with the control group.

A total of eight large randomized trials on mammographic screening have been conducted. Six of the eight trials revealed a statistically significant reduction in mortality with mammographic screening. The reduction in mortality rate was not as evident among women between the ages of 40 and 49 years compared with women older than 50 years of age. The relative mortality rate reduction appears later in women between the ages of 40 and 49 at randomization compared with women 50 years or older. It is also likely that the small numbers of women between 40 and 49 years of age in the existing randomized trials may have contributed to this difference.

In a meta-analysis of eight randomized controlled trials (RCTs) of mammographic screening, a statistically significant 18% reduction in mortality in women aged 40 to 49 years was noted. Combined data from five Swedish trials yielded a statistically significant mortality decrease of 29% (Table 14.4).

The updated Cochrane systematic review was published in 2013. Because of the inclusion criteria chosen for the review, they reported on six randomized trials. They concluded that screening is likely to reduce breast cancer mortality. The effect was lowest in the adequately randomized trials, and a reasonable estimate is an overall 15% reduction in mortality from breast cancer (RR, 0.81; 95% CI 0.74–0.87) after 13 years. However, it should be noted that there is a false-positive rate associated with screening.

Screening Interval

For several years, there has been a significant debate about the appropriate age at which to commence mammographic screening. Whereas the 2003 ACS guidelines for mammographic screening recommended a yearly mammogram starting at age 40 tears, the National Cancer Institute (NCI) recommended a mammogram every 1 or 2 years. The American College of Obstetricians and Gynecologists (ACOG) currently recommends annual mammography from 40 years of age. In October 2015, the ACS revised its guidelines with regards to screening mammography in average-risk women. The guidelines now advocate the commencement of annual mammography at age 45 years until age 54 years. Thereafter, from age 55 years onward, biennial mammograms are recommended while the patient's overall health is good or she has a life expectancy of 10 years or longer. The ACS falls short of recommending mammography from age 40 to 44 years but state that women should have the

TABLE 14.5 Recommendations for Mammographic Screening for Breast Cancer

Age (Years)	American College of Obstetricians and Gynecologists	American Cancer Society	National Cancer Institute	US Preventive Services Task Force
40–45	Annually	Not recommended but should have opportunity to begin	1–2 years	Individual decision
45–50	Annually	Annually	1–2 years	Individual decision
50–55	Annually	Annually	1–2 years	2 years
55–74	Annually	2 years	1–2 years	2 years

opportunity to commence screening. Table 14.5 lists recommendations by society.

Data from the Breast Cancer Surveillance Consortium, also recently published in October 2015, somewhat support this strategy. They reviewed screening mammography from 15,440 patients from ages 40 to 85 years who had either annual or biennial imaging. Premenopausal women diagnosed at the longer interval screening time point had more tumors with less favorable prognostic characteristics—that is, stage IIB or higher—than those screened annually. In those who were postmenopausal and not taking HRT, there was no difference in the proportions of stage IIB or higher tumors whether they were screened at 1 or 2 years. This would suggest that menopausal status rather than age may be a better factor to consider when determining mammographic screening interval. Biologically, this is plausible with the possibility that estrogen-exposed tumors may grow faster and thus have a decreased detectable preclinical phase combined with increased breast density premenopausally decreasing mammographic sensitivity.

The USPSTF published its screening recommendations in 2009 and currently has draft recommendations due for publication in 2015. After reviewing the evidence regarding the efficacy of BSE, CBE, and mammography in reducing breast cancer mortality, it recommends starting mammography at age 50 years and performing biennial screening. It does not recommend routine mammography in women younger than age 50 years but recommends that the decision is an individual one. They advise that, although there may be an improvement in the risk of dying from breast cancer with screening before age 50 years, that the advantage is not as big as in older women. They also note that it is associated with a higher false-positive rate in those younger than age 50 years; therefore, an individual can decide on her personal acceptability of the risk-to-benefit ratio. The task force cites the risk of false-positive mammography results (≤56%) as a potential harm and considers pain, anxiety, distress, and other psychologic responses as potential harms. However, the task force states that these harms are transient and thus do not represent a substantial deterrent to the continued use of mammography for screening. These recommendations have caused much controversy and debate in the medical community and lay press since they were announced in 2009. The majority of clinical societies did not change their recommendations after these guidelines were issued. Annual screening mammography may commence earlier than age 40 in a few special circumstances (Table 14.6).

TABLE 14.6 Screening Guidelines for Women Younger Than Age 40 Years

Condition	Timing of Annual Mammography
Lobular cancer in situ or breast cancer diagnosis	At time of diagnosis
First-degree relative with premenopausal breast cancer	10 years earlier than relative's age at diagnosis but not younger than 25 years
Mantle irradiation for Hodgkin disease	8 years after completion of radiation therapy
BRCA1 or BRCA2 mutation	Age 25–35 years; specific age chosen based on adequacy of mammography imaging in the first study and patient choice

Data from American College of Obstetricians and Gynecologists. *Primary and preventive care: periodic assessments.* ACOG Committee Opinion 246. Washington, DC, 2000, Author.

Breast Imaging Reporting and Data System

In the past, a lack of uniformity in mammography terminology and reporting often led to confusion as to the malignant nature of a lesion. In 1994, the Mammography Quality Standards Act was passed by Congress and is administered by the FDA. It requires that mammography facilities monitor the results of their breast cancer detection programs, including the number of recommended biopsies and the size, number, and stage of cancers detected. The American College of Radiology (ACR) uses a terminology and lexicon system called the Breast Imaging Reporting and Data System (BI-RADS) for reporting abnormalities seen on mammography (Table 14.7). This standardized reporting system was developed in 1995. Each category leads to a fixed assessment and specific management recommendations. In addition, associated findings, such as skin or nipple retraction, skin thickening, skin lesions, axillary adenopathy, and the presence of architectural distortion, should also be reported.

The predictors of malignancy for the BI-RADS categories are 0% to 2% for category 3 and approximately 98% or greater for category 5. Category 4 is less predictable. Liberman and colleagues and Orel and colleagues have placed the risk of malignancy for this category at around 30%.

The ACR Task Force has published a fifth edition of the BI-RADS classification system in the form of a *BI-RADS Atlas* that includes second edition BI-RADS classifications for ultrasonography and MRI. The new edition of BI-RADS

TABLE 14.7 American College of Radiology BI-RADS Assessment Categories

BI-RADS Category	Assessment
ASSESSMENT IS INCOMPLETE	
0	Need additional imaging evaluation and/or prior mammograms for comparison
ASSESSMENT IS COMPLETE: FINAL CATEGORIES	
1	Negative
2	Benign finding(s)
3	Probably benign finding; initial short-interval follow-up suggested
4*	Suspicious abnormality; biopsy should be considered
	Optional subdivisions:
	4A: Low suspicion for malignancy
	4B: Moderate suspicion of malignancy
	4C: High suspicion for malignancy
5	Highly suggestive of malignancy; appropriate action should be taken
6	Known biopsy; proven malignancy; appropriate action should be taken

BI-RADS, Breast Imaging Reporting and Data System.
*By subdividing category 4 into 4A, 4B, and 4C, it is encouraged that relevant probabilities for malignancy be indicated within this category so the patient and her physician can make an informed decision on the ultimate course of action.
Reprinted with permission of the American College of Radiology. No other representation of this material is authorized without expressed, written permission from the American College of Radiology.
D'Orsi CJ, Sickles EA, Mendelson EB, Morris EA, et al. *ACR BI-RADS® Atlas, Breast Imaging Reporting and Data System.* Reston, VA, 2013, American College of Radiology.

TABLE 14.8 Morphology of Microcalcifications and Associated Lesions

Morphology	Description and Associated Lesion
Typically benign	Includes skin (lucent centered)
	Vascular (parallel tracks)
	Coarse "popcorn-like" (fibroadenomas)
	Large rodlike (secretory disease)
	Eggshell or rim (fat necrosis)
	Milk of calcium (within tiny cysts)
	Dystrophic (after trauma or irradiation)
Suspicious	Amorphous
	Coarse heterogenous
	Fine pleomorphic
	Fine linear or fine linear branching
Distribution	Diffuse
	Regional
	Grouped
	Linear
	Segmental

includes the previously mentioned classification of patterns of breast density for uniform reporting in mammogram reports. Category 4 is divided into three parts based on the prebiopsy risk for malignancy of the lesion—4A (low suspicion), 4B (moderate), and 4C (high)—in an effort to better guide clinicians and to collect meaningful data about this category. By subdividing the category, the ACR hopes to provide better communication to the referring physician about the prebiopsy risk of malignancy. One recent retrospective study evaluated interobserver variability and positive predictive value of BI-RADS categories 4A, 4B, and 4C. The risk of malignancy was found to be 6%, 15%, and 53%, respectively. Table 14.7 shows BI-RADS reporting.

Diagnostic Mammography

Abnormalities found on mammographic screening may need further evaluation with additional mammography views or other imaging modalities, such as ultrasonography or magnetic resonance imaging (MRI). In some screening programs, the mammograms are reviewed by the radiologist as they are performed, and if additional views are needed, they are performed on the same day. In other programs, if additional studies are required, the patient is called back for them at a later date. In several studies, the frequency of "call-backs" has ranged from 5% to 11%.

Mammographic Lesions

A "mass" is defined as a space-occupying lesion seen in two different projections. If a possible mass is seen on only one view, it is called a "density" until its three dimensionality is confirmed. A description of the shape and the margins of the lesion are also necessary. The highest frequency of carcinoma is noted in masses that have an irregular shape or spiculated borders. These lesions are associated with pleomorphic calcifications that appear discontinuous and linear in distribution. This discontinuous linear pattern suggests irregular filling of a duct with abnormal cells.

Microcalcifications

The BI-RADS lexicon describes calcification morphology (shape) and distribution. Calcifications may be scattered or clustered, coarse or fine, and old or new. Comparison with prior mammograms is often necessary (Table 14.8).

Digital Mammography

The benefits of digital mammography over traditional film mammography concern image acquisition and facilitation of storage. In addition, digital-image processing allows manipulation of image contrast and may enhance subtle contrast differences. In January 2000, the General Electric Senographe 2000D was approved by the FDA. Since its introduction, population-based screening trials comparing screen-film and full-field digital mammography have been conducted. In the Oslo I Study conducted in Norway, full-field digital and screen-film mammography were performed in 3683 women aged 50 to 69 years. The investigators found no statistically significant difference in cancer detection rates between the two modalities. The Oslo II Study yielded similar results in cancer detection rates. Full-field digital mammography did yield higher cancer detection rates, but this difference between film and digital mammography was not statistically significant. In Canada and the United States,

49,528 women were enrolled in the Digital Mammographic Imaging Screening Trial (DMIST). All participants underwent both digital and film mammography in random order. The investigators noted that, although the diagnostic accuracy of digital and film mammography was similar, the accuracy of digital mammography was better in women younger than age 50 years, women with radiographically dense breasts, and premenopausal or perimenopausal women. Thus, in women who met those criteria, the investigators recommended digital mammography. Digital mammography is now available in most screening centers. It can be also combined with computer-aided detection (CAD), which is a process designed to analyze mammographic images for suspicious areas; it is in effect a "second pair of eyes" for the radiologist. The ACR believes that CAD, when used for screening or diagnostic film screen mammography, can be a valuable procedure to aid in the early detection of breast cancer.

Digital tomosynthesis, or three-dimensional mammography, is approved by the FDA but is not yet considered the standard of care for breast cancer screening. Other experimental methods of breast imaging are being investigated but are not in routine use such as contrast-enhanced digital mammography, which is a recent development of digital mammography using the intravenous injection of an iodinated contrast agent in conjunction with a mammography examination.

BREAST ULTRASONOGRAPHY AND MAGNETIC RESONANCE IMAGING

Breast ultrasonography can be used to distinguish between solid and cystic masses in the breast. It can be used to evaluate a focal mass identified on a mammogram or a palpable mass. It is also used as an adjuvant for biopsy. Because of its low specificity, it is not thought to be a good modality for screening. It cannot replace mammography because it has no ability to detect microcalcifications. Ultrasonography can complement mammography in young women with dense breasts because dense breasts limit the accuracy of the mammogram.

Magnetic resonance imaging has a high sensitivity for the detection of breast cancer, and it is not affected by breast density. Screening studies to date have been done in high-risk patients, primarily those at risk because of known or suspected BRCA mutations or a family history of breast cancer. A systematic review by Warner and colleagues in 2008 identified 11 prospective studies of MRI screening. In the systematic review, MRI's sensitivity was 75%. Combining mammography and MRI increased the sensitivity to 84%. The specificity of MRI (96·1%) was comparable but marginally lower than the specificity of mammography (98·5%). These studies on the use of MRI for surveillance of women at high risk for hereditary breast cancer have demonstrated a substantial benefit for breast cancer detection.

The ACS has issued guidelines about the use of annual MRI for screening in high-risk women. A guideline panel was assembled to review evidence and develop new recommendations for women at different levels of risk. Based on this panel

screening, MRI is recommended for women with an approximately 20% to 25% or greater lifetime risk of developing breast cancer. This includes women with strong family history of breast or ovarian cancer, untested first-degree relatives of BRCA mutation carriers, and women with a history of mantle radiation between ages 10 to 30 years. Screening MRI is also recommended for patients with Li-Fraumeni or Cowden syndrome and their first-degree relatives.

The optimal point in time to perform the MRI in relation to mammography has not currently been determined.

MRI can be useful in treatment selection for newly diagnosed breast cancers, particularly in evaluating tumor multifocality in women wanting to pursue breast conservation. However, it has not been shown to increase the likelihood of negative margins or the need to convert from lumpectomy to mastectomy. It is used to assess for residual disease after neoadjuvant chemotherapy. It is also a useful tool to assess for an occult primary breast tumor in patients presenting with axillary nodal metastases. There is insufficient evidence to recommend for or against screening with MRI for women with a personal history of breast cancer, atypical hyperplasia, or extremely dense breasts on mammography.

DIAGNOSTIC EVALUATION

Palpable Mass

The workup of a patient with a dominant mass should include bilateral mammography. In addition to gaining valuable information about the characteristics of the mass, a secondary purpose in this setting is to screen the normal surrounding breast and the contralateral breast for nonpalpable mammographic abnormalities (densities or calcifications). Evaluation of a palpable mass is important to determine whether the mass is cancerous even if the mammogram result is negative.

Fine-Needle Aspiration or Biopsy

Fine-needle aspiration can be extremely useful in providing a cytologic analysis of a palpable breast mass. Many palpable thickenings and all dominant masses should be considered for FNA because it can differentiate between solid and cystic masses. In addition, FNA can diagnose and treat simple cysts and provide cellular material for cytologic analysis. The FNA should be performed after radiologic examination because the resultant hematoma could mask an underlying abnormality.

The breast is prepped with alcohol; with the physician facing the patient, the lesion is stabilized with the physician's opposite hand. Usually, a 21- or 25-gauge needle on a 10-cc syringe is used. Approximately 3 cc of air is aspirated into the syringe to facilitate expulsion of the contents onto the slide after the procedure. The needle is introduced into the lesion, and suction is applied on the syringe. If the mass is cystic, the fluid is completely evacuated, and the lesion should completely disappear. The syringe is withdrawn, and the fluid is discarded if it is serous and nonbloody. The patient should return in 4 to 6 weeks for reexamination.

If the lesion encountered is not cystic or suspected to be solid, an FNA biopsy can be performed in the same manner.

After insertion into the lesion, multiple passes (10–15) through the lesion with changes in direction allow extensive sampling and create a "feel" for the mass (carcinomas are usually hard and gritty). The goal of sampling is to obtain material in the hub of the needle, not to fill the syringe. Care should be taken to release the suction before withdrawing the needle to prevent aspiration into the syringe. The sample is then ejected onto a glass slide, gently smeared with another slide, and placed in sterile jars containing 95% ethanol for transport to the cytology laboratory. Alternatively, it can be placed in a specimen jar containing cytofixative. The needle should be removed from the syringe, the medium aspirated into the syringe, the needle replaced, and the medium then ejected into the jar.

An FNA requires a cytopathologist experienced in breast pathology. The false-negative rate can range from 3% to 35% depending on the expertise of the aspirator and cytopathologist, the size of the lesion, the location within the breast, and the cellular composition of the lesion. Negative findings of an FNA sample in the presence of a suspicious mass should not preclude further diagnostic evaluation. A diagnosis of atypical cells after an FNA warrants a surgical biopsy. Any mass remaining after aspiration of a cyst should be excised. Similarly, a cyst that recurs in the same location after one or two aspirations should be excised.

The false-positive rate of an FNA sample is less than 1%, but in the United States most surgeons do not perform definitive surgery such as a mastectomy without a prior surgical biopsy, core-needle biopsy, or frozen-section diagnosis at the time of surgery. An FNA sample that is positive for adenocarcinoma could, however, provides a preliminary diagnosis and guides subsequent management.

Patients with palpable solid masses can have a biopsy of the mass in the office with use of a Tru-Cut 14.gauge biopsy device. The breast is prepped sterilely, and a local anesthetic is used to infiltrate the skin. A small nick is made in the skin with a scalpel to accommodate the biopsy instrument. A core biopsy of the solid mass is obtained. The instrument has a "firing range" and therefore should be kept parallel to the chest wall to avoid penetrating trauma. The specimen is placed in formalin and sent for pathologic examination. It is believed that if the specimen "floats" in the solution, it is likely nondiagnostic fat. Tumor specimens have a grayish appearance and typically "sink" in the solution.

Needle Localization and Excision

Needle localization is a technique that allows surgical excision of a lesion that is nonpalpable. The technique uses a hook and wire system to target the lesion, and image guidance can be provided by mammography; ultrasonography; and, in some cases, MRI. In mammography-guided needle localization, coordinates of the lesion are obtained by placing the breast in an alphanumeric grid. The needle is inserted and, when adequate placement is noted, the hook wire is deployed and the needle removed. Two mammographic views are then obtained.

The mammography films are available intraoperatively and show the relationship between the lesion and localizing hook. Excision with needle localization allows the surgeon to minimize the amount of breast tissue removed by following the needle to the targeted lesion. After removal, a specimen radiograph is obtained to ensure that successful removal of the lesion has been performed. Radiologists and surgeons experienced in needle localization and excisions report only 0.2% to 0.3% of lesions missed with this approach. The specimen radiograph helps to ascertain the lesion was not missed.

Another variation of this approach to excising nonpalpable lesions is the use of a radioactive seed, which involves a small titanium seed (4×0.8 mm) that is labeled with iodine-125 and placed in a similar fashion to the needle localization. Use of an intraoperative handheld gamma probe allows for accurate excision on the lesion, which is similarly radiographed to ensure retrieval of the lesion and the radioactive seed. It has advantages over needle localization because the placement of the radioactive can be performed several days before the procedure, which can improve flexibility with regards to scheduling.

Image-guided Percutaneous Breast Biopsy

With the current advancements available in breast imaging, percutaneous image-guided breast biopsy is increasingly being used as an alternative to surgical biopsy. Percutaneous biopsy methods differ with respect to the method of imaging guidance and the tissue-acquisition device used. The use of image-guided percutaneous biopsy has advantages over surgical excision for the diagnosis of breast lesions. It is less invasive, and because less tissue is removed, it will result in less scarring on subsequent mammograms. Regardless of whether the diagnosis is benign or malignant, the patients who have percutaneous biopsies will undergo fewer operations. In addition, in cases of malignancy, the discussion and surgical treatment plan can be streamlined. The choice of which image-guided modality to use depends on the lesion. Stereotactic biopsy is best for calcifications. If a lesion is seen on ultrasonography, it is best to use that modality because it is easier to use and has been reported to be less costly.

Stereotactic Biopsy

Stereotactic-guided core needle biopsy uses specialized mammography equipment to calculate the location of a lesion in three dimensions. Stereotactic biopsy can be performed with the patient prone on a dedicated table or with the patient sitting in an upright unit. Some patients may not be candidates for this approach. A patient may be too large to be accommodated by the system. The thickness of the breast must be adequate to accommodate to the automated biopsy device. Abnormalities just under the skin may also pose technical problems. A vague asymmetric density or diffuse group of widely separated calcifications may present difficulties. Patients who cannot remain prone or are unable to cooperate for the 20- to 40-minute duration of the procedure may not be candidates.

An automated core needle or directional vacuum-assisted biopsy probe is used to obtain the tissue specimens. Multiple tissue specimens are obtained for pathologic analysis. Many reports in the medical literature state the procedure has a sensitivity of 70% to 100% and a specificity of 85% to 100%. Studies have shown 99% accuracy with a 14-gauge needle obtaining five specimens. Radiography should be performed routinely on women with specimens of breast microcalcifications to determine whether calcifications were obtained.

Ultrasound-guided Biopsy

The use of ultrasound imaging for percutaneous biopsy of lesions seen on ultrasonography has certain advantages. For example, it requires no specialized equipment, requires no radiation exposure, and has the ability to sample areas that may be inaccessible with stereotactic biopsy (eg, the axilla). A 14-gauge automated needle is used, and real-time imaging allows accurate positioning. Multiple tissue core samples are sent for pathologic analysis. Consideration to placement of a clip to demarcate the area of biopsy is necessary, particularly in cases in which neoadjuvant chemotherapy will be considered.

Tissue-acquisition Devices

Available tissue-acquisition devices include fine needles, automated core needles, directional vacuum-assisted probes, and biopsy cannulas. Excellent results have been obtained using the 14-gauge automated needle for biopsy of masses under ultrasound or stereotactic guidance. Most centers use larger tissue-acquisition devices instead of fine needles because of accuracy of tissue diagnosis when a larger volume of tissue is obtained. Compared with the automated needle, the vacuum device acquires larger samples of tissue, has a higher frequency of retrieval of calcifications, and may provide more accurate lesion characterization. Accurate placement of a localizing clip through the biopsy probe is necessary to facilitate subsequent localization if needed.

Surgical Excision and Breast Biopsy

A biopsy can be performed on an outpatient basis under local anesthesia in the majority of patients. It is important to choose the appropriate incision and location. Unless the lesion is close to the nipple or suspected to be a fibroadenoma, the incision should be made in close proximity to the mass and not circumareolar. The surgeon should keep in mind the possibility of subsequent mastectomy when placing the incision. Many times, the biopsy is part of the treatment. The specimen should be adequately oriented for margin analysis by the pathologist and also sent for the appropriate markers such as estrogen-receptor (ER) and progesterone-receptor (PR) status and HER2/neu. Orientation of the specimen is important because a reexcision of an involved margin may need to be subsequently performed.

The incision should be closed with fine suture material with a subcuticular closure. Hemostasis needs to be ascertained before closing and is usually achieved with electrocautery. Weck clips can be placed in the cavity bed if a diagnosis of breast cancer is known and breast conservation is planned. No particular immobilization is required, but a good support bra is recommended to minimize hematoma, induration, and discomfort.

Certain benign lesions on core needle biopsy have a relatively high incidence of coexisting carcinoma found on subsequent surgical excision. The small volume of tissue obtained on core needle biopsy in these cases may not be adequate to rule out cancer. Atypical ductal hyperplasia is the most commonly encountered of these lesions. About 25% of atypical ductal hyperplasia on the core biopsy specimen will have carcinoma on excisional biopsy. Radial scars are reported to have a coexistent carcinoma in 20% and therefore also require surgical excision. The tissue obtained from a core needle biopsy may not be concordant with the imaging findings. In a study by Dershaw and colleagues, repeated biopsy for nonconcordance found carcinoma in 47% of cases. Lesions yielding ALH or lobular carcinoma in situ (LCIS) at core needle biopsy with imaging-histologic discordance warrant surgical excision because they have a high rate of cancer in these lesions (38%; 95% CI 9%–76%) on excision. Core needle biopsy with imaging-histologic concordance of ALH or LCIS, the cancer rate was significantly lower (3%; 95% CI 0%–9%); therefore, these do not always mandate surgical excision unless imaging is discordant with pathologic findings.

EPIDEMIOLOGY OF BREAST CANCER

Table 14.9 lists major risk factors for breast cancer.

RISK FACTORS AND ASSESSMENT

Age

The incidence of breast cancer increases with age. Age is the most significant risk factor for breast cancer.

Family History

Hereditary breast cancers account for 5% to 10% of all breast cancers and are thought to be attributable to highly penetrant mutations in breast cancer–susceptibility genes. Two such tumor-suppressor genes, *BRCA1* and *BRCA2*, have been well characterized. Breast cancer has also been noted to occur in association with other cancers, such as in Li-Fraumeni syndrome and Cowden syndrome.

Prospective data from the Nurses' Health Study noted that the risk of breast cancer doubled among women whose mother had breast cancer diagnosed before the age of 40 years or who

TABLE 14.9 Major Risk Factors for Breast Cancer
Older age
Family history of breast cancer
Benign breast disease
Proliferative changes
Atypical hyperplasia
Endogenous endocrine factors
Early menarche
Late menopause
Long menses duration
Nulliparity
Late maternal age at first pregnancy
Exogenous hormones?
Oral contraceptives
Estrogen replacement therapy

had a sister with breast cancer. The risk decreased with advanced maternal age; however, it remained elevated even with maternal diagnosis at age 70 years (RR 1.5; 95% CI 1.1–2.2). The data did show that the risk associated with a mother or sister with history of breast cancer is smaller than previously suggested. In the population of middle-aged women, the authors found that only 2.5% of breast cancer cases were attributed to a positive family history. In the large Cancer Prevention Study II by the ACS, the authors evaluated the association of fatal breast cancer and family history. They found that family history of breast cancer in a mother or sister was significantly related to fatal breast cancer risk after multivariate analysis. Association was significantly modified by age with a risk ratio of almost 5 in women younger than 40 years at enrollment compared with 1.28 in women aged 70 years or older.

Personal History

A patient's history of prior breast biopsy is important. Although the number of breast biopsies undergone does not increase a woman's risk of breast cancer, certain pathologic entities do play a role. Atypical ductal or lobular hyperplasia and LCIS are considered markers of increased risk of developing invasive breast cancer. A personal history of breast cancer increases the risk for development of another breast cancer. Women treated for breast cancer are at risk for the development of a contralateral breast cancer. Various studies have shown this risk to be between 0.5% and 1.0% per year. In addition, patients treated with breast conservation (lumpectomy and radiation therapy) are at risk for an ipsilateral recurrence. In these women, this risk could be 10% at 10 to 15 years posttreatment.

Reproductive History

Early menarche, late menopause, and nulliparity are thought to be risk factors for breast cancer. Age at first pregnancy is also thought to be an RR factor for breast cancer.

Early age at first pregnancy is often associated with a lower risk for breast cancer. For a woman younger than 19 years of age at first full-term birth, a 50% reduction in the risk of breast cancer compared with that of a nulliparous woman is predicted. If the first full-term pregnancy occurs at age 30 to 34 years, the risk of breast cancer is approximately the same as that noted in nulliparous women. Pregnancy in women after age 35 years is associated with an increased risk compared with that of a nulliparous woman. Pregnancies that are not full term do not show this protection.

Some have suggested that the time interval between the onset of menarche and the first full-term pregnancy is the important factor with regard to the endocrine milieu. This importance has a possible explanation in the "estrogen open window hypothesis." There is, however, some inconsistency in reported data in regard to relationship of age at first full-term pregnancy. The association depends somewhat on control subjects used, and later studies have suggested a less strong association.

Breastfeeding has been reported to reduce risk of breast cancer. Studies in the United States have suggested only a weak protective effect and do not demonstrate an association between reduction in risk and duration of breastfeeding.

The effect of menopause as it relates to breast cancer risk has been examined. Late menopause poses an increase in risk of breast cancer. Early exposure to the hormone milieu is thought by some to be an important etiologic factor. In one large international case-control study, it was noted that for each 2-year delay in the onset of menstruation, breast cancer risk was reduced by about 10%. The later a woman's menopause occurs, the higher her risk for breast cancer. For every 5-year difference in age at menopause, the risk for breast cancer changes about 17%. The effect of this later age at menopause in regard to increasing breast cancer is not seen for 10 to 20 years after menopause. It has been suggested that the total duration of menstruation may also be important because the risk increases in the woman who has menstruated more 30 years compared with those who have had less than 30 years of menstruation. Among women who have undergone a natural menopause, the risk among those whose menopause occurred at age 55 years is about twice that of women whose menopause occurred before age 44 years.

Data from observational studies demonstrate that bilateral oophorectomy before natural menopause has been reported to reduce risk of breast cancer compared with those who had a later natural or artificial menopause.

Exogenous Hormone Use

The role of exogenous estrogens in the promotion of breast cancer is still controversial. Studies of OCPs and HRT have yielded conflicting results. Studies of HRT and breast cancer risk indicate that women who are currently using HRT are at increased risk for breast cancer development. A meta-analysis of the largest studies, however, suggests that the increased risk is only about 10%. Women who have taken HRT in the past but are not currently using HRT are not at increased risk. Long-term use of HRT (>10 years) has been associated with a relative increase in breast cancer risk, and the highest risk was noted in those patients using HRT with progestins (RR, 1.41). Of note, multiple studies have shown that patients who develop breast cancer while taking HRT have smaller, less aggressive cancers and a lower risk of death from breast cancer.

Results from the Women's Health Initiative (WHI) RCT were reported. Between 1993 and 1998, 16,609 women with intact uteruses were randomly assigned to receive combination HRT (0.625 mg/day conjugated equine estrogens and 2.5 mg/day medroxyprogesterone acetate) or placebo. The planned duration of the trial was 8.5 years; however, the data and safety monitoring board of the committee recommended halting the trial because the incidence of invasive breast cancer had exceeded the stopping boundary that had been set at the initiation of the trial. This occurred after a mean of 5.2 years of follow-up. The increased risk of breast cancer reported hazard ratio (HR) was 1.25 (95% CI 1.00–1.59). There was also a reported increased risk of coronary heart disease (HR, 1.29; 95% CI 1.02–1.63) and stroke (HR, 1.41; 95% CI 1.39–3.25). Beneficial effects included decreased risk in colorectal cancer (HR, 0.63; 95% CI 0.43–0.92) and hip fracture (HR, 0.66; 95% CI 0.45–0.98). Based on the data, the safety monitoring board initially did not recommend stopping the estrogen-alone arm in women who had had a hysterectomy. Results of the estrogen-only arm and the WHI study have been reported. The study included 10,739 postmenopausal women (aged 50–79 years) with prior hysterectomy. These women were randomly assigned to receive 0.625 mg/day of conjugated equine estrogen or placebo. In February 2004, the National Institutes of Health decided to terminate the intervention phase of the estrogen-only study, which had been scheduled for a close-out interval of October 2004 to March 2005. With an average follow-up of 6.8 years, there was an increased risk of stroke (HR 1.39; 95% CI 1.10–1.77), a decreased risk of hip fracture (HR 0.61; 95% CI 0.41–0.91), and no effect on coronary heart disease incidence (HR 0.91; 95% CI 0.75–1.12). The investigators noted a possible reduction in breast cancer risk (HR 0.77; 95% CI 0.59–1.01) that warrants further investigation.

The annual increased risk for an individual woman is still relatively small. The increased risk for breast cancer is apparent after 4 years of HRT use. ACOG stresses the importance of addressing the reasons for initiating or continuing on HRT. It is no longer recommended to prevent heart disease in healthy women (primary prevention) or to protect women with preexisting heart disease (secondary prevention). In addition, it is no longer recommended solely for prevention of osteoporosis.

HRT is highly effective in treating vasomotor symptoms with limited effective alternative therapies. In this setting, short-term use (<5 years) can be considered because data on short-term use do not show an increased association with breast cancer. Attitudes of obstetricians and gynecologists toward hormone therapy after the WHI results were published were surveyed. Respondents to the survey remained skeptical of the results; 49.1% did not find them convincing. There was strong support for the use of HRT for vasomotor symptoms, vaginal dryness, and osteoporosis, but most of the physicians surveyed did not find it useful for prevention of cardiovascular disease or dementia.

In the past, most studies addressing OCP use and breast cancer risk concluded that there was a significant increase in risk associated with OCP use. However, the majority of studies regarding OCP use and breast cancer risk have demonstrated little association with breast cancer incidence rates. In women who have used OCPs for extended periods (>10 years), a minimal, nonsignificant increase in breast cancer cases has been reported, seen most commonly in the group of women who began using OCPs at a young age (<20 years). Past or present use of OCPs at the time of diagnosis of breast cancer does not affect mortality from breast cancer. The presence of a family history of breast cancer does not appear to further increase the risk of breast cancer associated with either OCP or HRT use.

Prior Exposure to Radiation Therapy

Exposure to ionizing radiation, such as that which occurs in treatment with mantle radiation for Hodgkin disease, poses a risk for breast cancer. This is noted 7 to 10 years after completion of radiation therapy. The cumulative probability of breast cancer at age 40 years approaches 35% in these women. The risk of breast cancer associated with radiation exposure decreases with increasing age at exposure.

Other Factors

Breast cancer is more frequent in Jewish women than in non-Jewish women and more frequent in black women than in white women. Women of Ashkenazi Jewish descent have a 1 in 40 (2.5%) risk of carrying a mutation in *BRCA1* and *BRCA2* genes, thus accounting for the increased risk in these women. Asian women have a low incidence of breast cancer. Japanese women show lower rates of breast cancer than white women. Although postmenopausal breast cancer is less common in Japanese women who have migrated to Western countries than among the general populations of these countries, after two or three generations, the incidences of breast cancer in these women approach that of white women. The Western diet, with its increased intake of animal fat, has been implicated in these studies.

Alcohol consumption has been reported to increase breast cancer risk in a dose-related manner. Women who drink approximately one drink per day have a slightly elevated risk of breast cancer over nondrinkers. This risk is significantly higher with moderate to high alcohol consumption (two to five drinks per day).

Relative Risk

Relative risk is a ratio that depicts the likelihood over time of an event's occurrence in a study population relative to that in a reference population. It is often used to quantify risk factors for breast cancer. Absolute risk is a percentage that depicts the likelihood over time of the occurrence of an event. For rare events, these two are the same, but for common events, they are not. It is best to discuss risk with patients in terms of absolute rather than RR.

Several models exist to estimate a woman's risk of breast cancer. The Gail model, developed for use in the National Surgical Adjuvant Breast and Bowel Project (NSABP P-1) Breast Cancer Prevention Trial, is available from the NCI and provides a measurement of absolute risk over time for breast cancer. However, in familial-type hereditary cases, it underestimates the risk of breast cancer by overlooking age at onset, bilaterality of disease among affected family members, and breast cancer in non-first–degree relatives (Table 14.10). The Tyrer-Cuzick (IBIS) model is another risk assessment tool that incorporates these aspects of family history, endogenous hormonal factors, benign disease, risk factors such as age and body mass index, as well as genetic factors (including *BRCA* mutations) into a single statistical model.

BRCA1 and BRCA2

BRCA1 and *BRCA2* are breast cancer-susceptibility genes that have expanded our knowledge of familial breast cancer. Linkage studies done in 1990 in early-onset breast cancer families led to cloning of the *BRCA1* gene at the University of Utah in Salt Lake City in 1994. The *BRCA1* gene consists of 22 coding exons distributed over approximately 100 kb of genomic DNA on chromosome 17q21. It is thought to be responsible for approximately 45% of early-onset hereditary breast cancers and nearly 90% of hereditary ovarian cancers in families with a high

TABLE 14.10   Breast Cancer Risk Factors

PERSONAL AND FAMILY HISTORY FACTORS WITH A RELATIVE RISK OF >4.0

Certain inherited genetic mutations for breast cancer

Two or more first-degree relatives with breast cancer diagnosed at an early age

Personal history of breast cancer

Age (≥65 years versus <65 years, although risk increases across all ages until age 80 years)

PERSONAL AND FAMILY HISTORY FACTORS WITH A RELATIVE RISK OF 2.1–4.0

One first-degree relative with breast cancer

Nodular densities seen on mammogram (>75% of breast volume)

Atypical hyperplasia

High-dose ionizing radiation administered to the chest

Ovaries not surgically removed before age 40 years

PERSONAL AND FAMILY HISTORY FACTORS WITH A RELATIVE RISK OF 1.1–2.0

High socioeconomic status

Urban residence

Northern US residence

REPRODUCTIVE FACTORS THAT INCREASE RELATIVE RISK

Early menarche (<12 years)

Late menopause (≥55 years)

No full-term pregnancies (for breast cancer diagnosed at age 40+ years)

Late age at first full-term pregnancy (≥30 years)

Never breastfed a child

OTHER FACTORS THAT AFFECT CIRCULATING HORMONES OR GENETIC SUSCEPTIBILITY

Postmenopausal obesity

Alcohol consumption

Recent hormone replacement therapy

Recent oral contraceptive use

Being tall

Personal history of cancer of endometrium, ovary, or colon

Jewish heritage

Data from American Cancer Society. *Breast cancer facts & figures 2001–2002.* Atlanta, 2001, Author; Hulka BS, Stark AT. Breast cancer: cause and prevention. *Lancet* 1995;346:883 and Kelsey JL. Breast cancer epidemiology: summary and future directions. *Epidemiol Rev* 1993;15:256.

TABLE 14.11   National Comprehensive Cancer Network (NCCN) Guidelines for Recommending Genetic Testing for *BRCA1* or *BRCA2* Mutations*

Personal history of breast cancer and one or more of the following:

- Diagnosed at age 45 years or younger
- Diagnosed with at least two breast cancer primaries (bilateral, separate ipsilateral), the first at age 50 years or younger
- Diagnosed at age 50 years or younger with one or more close relatives[†] with breast cancer (prostate or pancreatic) at any age
- Diagnosed with triple-negative breast cancer at age 60 years or younger
- Diagnosed at any age with one or more close relatives with breast cancer at age 50 years or younger
- Diagnosed at any age with two or more close relatives at any age
- Diagnosed at any age with one or more close relatives with invasive ovarian cancer (including fallopian tube and primary peritoneal) at any age
- Diagnosed at any age with two or more close relatives with pancreatic and/or prostate cancer
- Having a close male relative with breast cancer at any age

*Individuals with a limited or unknown family history may have an underestimated probability of a familial gene mutation detection.
†Close relative pertains to first-, second- or third degree blood relatives on the same side (either maternal or paternal) of the family.

incidence of breast and ovarian cancers. Two specific mutations, 185delAG and 5382insC, are present in approximately 1.00% and 0.25% of the Ashkenazi Jewish population, respectively. They are thought to be founder mutations (ie, an altered gene or genes seen with a high frequency in a population originating from a small ancestral group, one or more of whose founders were carriers of the mutant gene).

BRCA2 was isolated on chromosome 13q12-13 in 1995. The *BRCA2* gene is composed of 26 coding exons distributed over approximately 70 kb of genomic DNA. This gene appears to account for 35% of families with early-onset breast cancer. It confers a lower risk of ovarian cancer compared with breast cancer. A single mutation, 6174delT, is found in approximately 1.4% of the Ashkenazi Jewish population. Together, both *BRCA1* and *BRCA2* mutations are found in approximately 1 in 40 Ashkenazi Jewish individuals. For both genes, the estimated penetrance is 70% to 90% for breast cancer by age 70 years, but the risk of breast cancer by age 50 years may be lower for *BRCA2* mutations.

The likelihood of a patient having a *BRCA1* or *BRCA2* mutation depends on certain factors, such as age at the time of diagnosis of breast or ovarian cancer and the number and age of first- and second-degree relatives in the same parental lineage and ethnicity with breast or ovarian cancer. The parental lineage can be either maternal or paternal. The National Comprehensive Cancer Network (NCCN) guidelines recommend testing in patients with a personal history of breast cancer and one other risk factor such as bilaterality, other family members with breast or ovarian cancer, or any male breast cancers in the family (Table 14.11). In patients with a personal history of breast cancer and Ashkenazi Jewish heritage, no additional family history may be needed to meet testing criteria. The decision to undergo genetic testing is a complex one because it can affect an individual's personal, psychological, social, financial, and ethical well-being.

Women who have a negative genetic test result should still be considered at risk on the basis of age and environment and because of the possibility of other genetic factors or unknown mutations.

Natural History

The most common site of origin of breast cancer is the upper-outer quadrant (38.5%) followed by the central area (29%), upper-inner quadrant (14.2%), lower-outer quadrant (8.8%), and lower-inner quadrant (5%). These percentages correlate with the amount of tissue that is present in these quadrants. Metachronous bilateral carcinoma of the breast has been observed in 5% to 8% of patients.

Metastasis to the ipsilateral axilla is the most common route of spread. Metastasis to the internal mammary nodes is more frequent with inner-quadrant lesions and is more likely to occur when involvement of the axillary nodes is also present.

PATHOLOGY

Ductal Carcinoma In Situ

Ductal carcinoma in situ (DCIS) is an abnormal proliferation of malignant epithelial cells within the mammary ductal–lobular system without invasion into the surrounding stroma. It is classified as a heterogenous group of lesions with different growth patterns and cytologic features. Classification of DCIS has traditionally been based on architectural pattern. The most common types are comedo, cribriform, micropapillary, papillary, and solid. The increased use of screening mammography during the past 2 decades has led to a marked increase in the number of patients with a diagnosis of DCIS, and in many centers today, one DCIS is diagnosed for every two or three mammographically detected invasive breast cancers. **Today about 85% of all DCIS are detected solely based on mammography.** Age-specific time trends illustrate that the greatest increase has been in women older than 40 years who are more likely to have mammography. In 1980, only 2% of 10,000 cancer cases were DCIS. Between 1973 and 1992, age-adjusted DCIS incidence increased almost sixfold, but the incidence of invasive cancer has increased only by one-third. This increase is almost entirely a result of mammography screening. Indeed, autopsy series suggest that latent DCIS is relatively common, ranging from 6% to 18% of women who died of causes other than breast cancer. The natural history of DCIS is only partially understood, particularly for small, mammographically detected lesions. The microcalcifications in DCIS are most often secondary to calcification of necrotic cellular debris within the involved ducts, and their extent and characteristics are better defined with magnification views of the microcalcification.

The potential of DCIS to progress to invasive breast cancer is an unresolved issue. Because DCIS has historically been treated with mastectomy, little information on the risk of progression to invasive disease is available. The retrospective study by Page and colleagues of benign breast biopsy specimens revealed 25 patients who were subsequently identified with DCIS; seven (28%) had progressed to invasive disease during the period of observation. When recurrences occur after breast-conserving surgery for DCIS, half of the recurrences are invasive, and half are further in situ disease, suggesting that there is a progression pathway from DCIS to invasive disease.

Paget's Disease

Paget disease is involvement of the nipple with intraductal carcinoma. In the absence of a palpable mass, invasive carcinoma occurs in less than 40% of cases. The malignant cells are large and pale-staining, and are seen in the basal layer and upper portions of the epidermis. Diagnosis is made through a nipple biopsy.

Lobular Carcinoma In Situ

Foote and Stewart initially described LCIS in 1941 as a noninvasive lesion arising from the lobules and terminal ducts of the breast. LCIS is characterized by a solid proliferation of small cells with round to oval nuclei that distort the involved spaces in the terminal duct–lobular units. Three important features of LCIS are as follows:

1. It is usually an incidental microscopic finding that is not detected clinically or by gross pathologic examination.
2. It is multicentric, and the associated cancer may be ductal or lobular.
3. The risk for subsequent cancer is the same for both breasts.

It is unfortunate that Foote and Stewart chose the name they did because it has led to a great deal of confusion over the past several decades. LCIS is a marker for breast cancer risk and is not a malignant finding.

Pleomorphic LCIS or LCIS with necrosis, as opposed to classic LCIS, is of unknown clinical significance and is an area of clinical controversy. It is generally accepted to be a risk factor for invasive disease, as with classic-type LCIS. However, there is a suspicion that pleomorphic LCIS may carry a higher risk of progression to invasive disease because of its histopathologic similarities with those of DCIS. It is generally recommended that pleomorphic LCIS should be considered a nonobligate precursor to invasive disease and managed in a similar way to DCIS, although this is largely based on those histopathologic similarities rather than studies providing evidence on clinical outcomes. Excision to negative margins is usually recommended.

Invasive Duct Carcinoma

Invasive duct carcinoma is the most common group of malignant mammary tumors and comprises 65% to 80% of all mammary carcinomas. Included in this group are special subtypes: tubular, medullary, metaplastic, mucinous (colloid) papillary, and adenoid cystic carcinoma. Each subtype constitutes only 1% to 2% of all invasive breast cancers, except medullary carcinoma, which constitutes 7%, and the rare adenoid cystic carcinomas, which constitute less than 0.1%.

Many of these subtypes, such as tubular and medullary carcinomas, carry an excellent prognosis. Metaplastic carcinomas, however, often have aggressive behavior. These tumors are characterized by the presence of homologous (epithelial) or heterologous (mesenchymal) elements. Two types have been described: squamous and pseudosarcomatous metaplasia.

Invasive duct carcinoma not otherwise specified is a generic term that includes tumors that may express more than one element of the specific forms of duct carcinoma.

Infiltrating Lobular Carcinoma

Infiltrating lobular carcinoma has been reported to constitute 10% to 14% of invasive carcinomas. These carcinomas are characterized by uniform cells with small, round nuclei and limited cytoplasm. The presence of intracytoplasmic mucin vacuoles often gives the cells the appearance of signet-ring cells. The cells tend to grow circumferentially around ducts and lobules with a linear arrangement. This pattern is referred to as "single-file" or targetoid growth. There is often an associated desmoplastic stromal reaction.

Inflammatory Carcinoma

Inflammatory carcinoma is characterized by cutaneous findings present with an underlying invasive carcinoma. Usually the invasive tumor is a poorly differentiated infiltrating duct carcinoma. Upon microscopic evaluation, skin involvement often reveals tumor emboli in dermal lymphatics with an associated lymphocytic reaction in the dermis.

Metastases From Extramammary Tumors

The most common primary site of an occult extramammary tumor is the lung. Other primary sites include the ovaries, uterus, kidneys, and stomach. In those previously diagnosed, melanoma, prostate, cervix, uterus, and urinary bladder are the most common sites. Metastatic ovarian cancer may simulate papillary or mucinous carcinoma of the breast. A workup and history are often helpful in difficult cases. Often, identification of an in situ component helps to provide definitive evidence of a mammary origin.

BIOLOGIC MARKERS AND PROGNOSTIC FACTORS

Axillary Lymph Node Status

The most important prognostic factor is nodal status. The presence of metastasis and the number of lymph nodes involved is significant and correlates with local failure and distant metastases. It is predictive of overall survival.

Tumor Size

Tumor size correlates with the incidence of lymph node metastases. The size of the tumor is also important, even in the absence of lymph node involvement. Patients with tumors smaller than 1 cm in size, or with good histologic types measuring smaller than 3 cm, do very well.

Histologic Grade

Histologic grade also correlates with breast cancer outcome. Poorly differentiated tumors have been associated with more aggressive behavior.

Molecular Profiling

Molecular classification of breast cancer into different subtypes can be used to stratify breast cancers into different groups. The luminal subtype makes up the hormone receptor–expressing breast cancers. Generally, these have overall better prognosis than the other groups currently identified. The HER2/neu subtypes make up the tumors with HER2/neu overexpression. These subtypes confirm the clinical impression that tumors with HER2/neu overexpression are more aggressive tumors, are more likely to be grade III, and have a higher degree of

concomitant *TP53* mutations. The basal-like subtype of breast cancer was named because of the similarity in expression pattern of this subtype to that of basal epithelia cells. Basal subtypes lack estrogen-receptor expression, have low HER2/neu expression, and are more likely to be aggressive tumors. Patients with *BRCA1* mutations have preponderance to this subtype of tumor. Multiple studies have demonstrated that this subtype often carries a poor prognosis because this subtype is more likely than other subtypes to have tumors that are grade III and that have TP53 mutations.

Hormone Receptors

The estrogen and progesterone receptors can be measured by immunohistochemical (IHC) studies using monoclonal antibodies directed against the receptors. Positivity correlates with response to endocrine therapy and better prognosis.

HER2/neu

HER2/neu is an oncogene whose protein product may function as a growth factor receptor. It can be detected by IHC demonstration of the protein product or by gene amplifications. Overexpression or amplification has been shown to correlate with a poor prognosis; however, the studies differ with regard to the method of detection used and the interpretation of results. HER2/neu overexpression has been used as a predictor of response to certain chemotherapeutic agents. Particularly, increased response to doxorubicin-based therapy has been reported in the treatment of patients with positive nodes and overexpression of HER2/neu.

p53

A tumor-suppressor gene, p53 has a protein product that is a nuclear transcription factor with many functions, including regulation of the cell cycle and apoptosis. Most clinical studies have used IHC to study protein expression. Accumulation of p53 protein has been reported to correlate with reduced survival in some studies.

STAGING OF BREAST CANCER USING THE TUMOR–NODE–METASTASIS SYSTEM

The American Joint Committee on Cancer (AJCC) determines staging of breast cancer. The AJCC staging system is a clinical and pathologic staging system based on the tumor–node–metastasis (TNM) system. The 2009AJCC staging system incorporated sentinel node staging. It distinguishes micrometastasis from isolated tumor cells on the basis of size and histologic evidence of malignant activity. In the current AJCC staging system, supraclavicular lymph node metastasis is now classified as N3 disease rather than M1 disease, as in the old system (Tables 14.12 and 14.13).

TREATMENT OF BREAST CANCER

Most patients with intraductal carcinoma and stage I and stage II breast cancer have the options of breast-conservation therapy and mastectomy. For patients with invasive breast cancer, the

TABLE 14.12　American Joint Committee on Cancer Staging for Breast Cancer

DEFINITION OF TNM

Primary tumor (T): Definitions for classifying the primary tumor (T) are the same for clinical and for pathologic classification. If the measurement is made by physical examination, the examiner will use the major headings (T1, T2, or T3). If other measurements, such as mammographic or pathologic measurements, are used, the subsets of T1 can be used. Tumors should be measured to the nearest 0.1 cm increment.

TX	Primary tumor cannot be assessed
T0	No evidence of primary tumor
Tis	Carcinoma in situ
Tis (DCIS)	Ductal carcinoma in situ
Tis (LCIS)	Lobular carcinoma in situ
Tis (Paget)	Paget disease of the nipple NOT associated with invasive carcinoma and/or carcinoma in situ (DCIS and/or LCIS) in the underlying breast parenchyma. Carcinomas in the breast parenchyma associated with Paget disease are categorized based on the size and characteristics of the parenchymal disease, although the presence of Paget disease should still be noted.
T1	Tumor ≤20 mm in greatest dimension
T1mi	Tumor ≤1 mm in greatest dimension
T1a	Tumor >1 mm but ≤5 mm in greatest dimension
T1b	Tumor >5 mm but ≤10 mm in greatest dimension
T1c	Tumor >10 mm but ≤20 mm in greatest dimension
T2	Tumor >20 mm but ≤50 mm in greatest dimension
T3	Tumor >50 mm in greatest dimension
T4	Tumor of any size with direct extension to the chest wall and/or to skin (ulceration or skin nodules)
T4a	Extension to chest wall, not including only pectoralis muscle adherence or invasion
T4b	Ulceration and/or ipsilateral satellite nodules and/or edema (including peau d'orange) of the skin, which do not meet the criteria for inflammatory carcinoma
T4c	Both T4a and T4b
T4d	Inflammatory carcinoma

REGIONAL LYMPH NODES: CLINICAL

NX	Regional lymph nodes cannot be assessed (eg, previously removed)
N0	No regional lymph node metastasis
N1	Metastasis to movable ipsilateral level I, II axillary lymph nodes(s)
N2	Metastases in ipsilateral level I, II axillary lymph nodes that are clinically fixed or matted; or in clinically detected* ipsilateral internal mammary nodes in the absence of clinically evident lymph node metastases
N2a	Metastasis in ipsilateral level I, II axillary lymph nodes fixed to one another (matted) or to other structures
N2b	Metastasis only in clinically detected* ipsilateral internal mammary nodes and in the absence of clinically evident level I, II axillary lymph node metastasis
N3	Metastases in ipsilateral infraclavicular (level III axillary) lymph node(s) with or without level I, II axillary lymph node involvement or in clinically detected* ipsilateral internal mammary lymph node(s) with clinically evident level I, II axillary lymph node metastases; or metastases in ipsilateral supraclavicular lymph node(s) with or without axillary or internal mammary lymph node involvement
N3a	Metastasis in ipsilateral infraclavicular lymph node(s)
N3b	Metastasis in ipsilateral internal mammary lymph node(s) and axillary lymph node(s)
N3c	Metastasis in ipsilateral supraclavicular lymph node(s)

PATHOLOGIC (PN)[†]

pNX	Regional lymph nodes cannot be assessed (eg, previously removed, or not removed for pathologic study)
pN0	No regional lymph node metastasis identified histologically
	Note: Isolated tumor cells clusters (ITCs) are defined as small clusters of cells not greater than 0.2 mm, or single tumor cells, or a cluster of <200 cells in a single histologic cross-section. ITCs may be detected by routine histology or by immunohistochemical (IHC) methods. Nodes containing only ITCs are excluded from the total positive node count for purposes of N classification but should be included in the total number of nodes evaluated.
pN0(i−)	No regional lymph node metastasis histologically, negative IHC
pN0(i+)	Malignant cells in regional lymph node(s) no greater than 0.2 mm (detected by H&E or IHC including ITC
pN0(mol−)	No regional lymph node metastasis histologically, negative molecular findings (RT-PCR)
pN0(mol+)	Positive molecular findings (RT-PCR) but no regional lymph node metastases detected by histology or IHC
pN1	Micrometastases or metastases in 1–3 axillary lymph nodes and/or in internal mammary nodes with metastases detected by SLNB but not clinically detected[‡]
pN1mi	Micrometastases (>0.2 mm and/or > 200 cells but none greater than 2.0 mm)
pN1a	Metastases in 1–3 axillary lymph nodes, at least one metastasis >2.0 mm
pN1b	Metastases in internal mammary nodes with micrometastases or macrometastases detected by SLNB but not clinically detected[‡]
pN1c	Metastases in 1–3 axillary lymph nodes and in internal mammary lymph nodes with micrometastases or macrometastases detected by SLNB but not clinically detected
pN2	Metastases in 4–9 axillary lymph nodes or in clinically detected[§] internal mammary lymph nodes in the absence of axillary lymph node metastases
pN2a	Metastases in 4–9 axillary lymph nodes (at least one tumor deposit greater than 2.0 mm)
pN2b	Metastases in clinically detected[§] internal mammary lymph nodes in the absence of axillary lymph node metastases

TABLE 14.12 American Joint Committee on Cancer Staging for Breast Cancer—cont'd

pN3	Metastases in 10 or more axillary lymph nodes; or in infraclavicular (level III axillary) lymph nodes; or in clinically detected[§] ipsilateral internal mammary lymph nodes in the presence of one or more positive level I, II axillary lymph node(s); or in more than three axillary lymph nodes and in internal mammary lymph nodes with micrometastases or macrometastases detected by SLNB but not clinically detected[‡]; or in ipsilateral supraclavicular lymph nodes
pN3a	Metastases in 10 or more axillary lymph nodes (at least one tumor deposit >2.0 mm); or metastases to the infraclavicular (level III axillary) lymph nodes
pN3b	Metastases in clinically detected[§] ipsilateral internal mammary lymph nodes in the presence of one or more positive axillary lymph nodes or in more than three axillary lymph nodes and in internal mammary lymph nodes with micrometastases or macrometastases detected by sentinel lymph node biopsy but not clinically detected[§]
pN3c	Metastasis in ipsilateral supraclavicular lymph nodes

DISTANT METASTASIS (M)

M0	No clinical or radiographic evidence of distant metastases
cM0(i+)	No clinical or radiographic evidence of distant metastases but deposits of molecularly or microscopically detected tumor cells in circulating blood, bone marrow, or other nonregional nodal tissue that are no larger than 0.2 mm in a patient without symptoms or signs of metastases
M1	Distant detectable metastases as determined by classic clinical and radiographic means and/or histologically proven >0.2 mm

*Clinically detected is defined as detected by imaging studies (excluding lymphoscintigraphy) or by clinical examination and having characteristics highly suspicious for malignancy or a presumed pathologic macrometastasis based on fine-needle aspiration (FNA) biopsy with cytologic examination. Confirmation of clinically detected metastatic disease by FNA without excision biopsy is designated with an (f) suffix, for example, cN3a(f). Excisional biopsy of a lymph node or biopsy of a sentinel node, in the absence of assignment of a pT, is classified as a clinical N (eg, cN1). Information regarding the confirmation of the nodal status will be designated in site-specific factors as clinical, FNA, core biopsy, or sentinel lymph node biopsy (SLNB). Pathologic classification (pN) is used for excision or SLNB only in connection with a pathologic T assignment.

†Classification is based on axillary lymph node dissection with or without SLNB. Classification based solely on SLNB without subsequent axillary lymph node dissection is designated (sn) for "sentinel node," for example, pN0(sn).

‡"Not clinically detected" is defined as not detected by imaging studies (excluding lymphoscintigraphy) or by clinical examination.

§"Clinically detected" is defined as detected by imaging studies (excluding lymphoscintigraphy) or by clinical examination and having characteristics highly suspicious for malignancy or a presumed pathologic macrometastasis based on FNA biopsy with cytologic examination.

RT-PCR, Reverse transcriptase-polymerase chain reaction.

From Edge SB, Byrd DR, Compton CC, et al. *AJCC cancer staging manual*, 7th e. New York, 2009, Springer.

TABLE 14.13 Stage by Tumor, Node, Metastasis (TNM)

Stage	
Stage 0	Tis, N0, M0
Stage I	T1*, N0, M0
Stage IIA	T0, N1, M0
	T1*, N1, M0
	T2, N0, M0
Stage IIB	T2, N1, M0
	T3, N0, M0
Stage IIIA	T0, N2, M0
	T1*, N2, M0
	T2, N2, M0
	T3, N1, M0
	T3, N2, M0
Stage IIIB	T4, N0, M0
	T4, N1, M0
	T4, N2, M0
Stage IIIC[†]	Any T, N3, M0
Stage IV	Any T, Any N, M1

*T1 includes T1mic.

†Stage IIIC breast cancer includes patients with any T stage who have pN3 disease. Patients with pN3a and pN3b disease are considered operable and are managed as described in the section on stage I, II, IIIA, and operable IIIC breast cancer. Patients with pN3c disease are considered inoperable and are managed as described in the section on inoperable stage IIIB or IIIC or inflammatory breast cancer.

From Edge SB, Byrd DR, Compton CC, et al. *AJCC cancer staging manual*, 7th e. New York, 2009, Springer.

axillary nodes can be addressed with a sentinel lymph node (SLN) biopsy and, possibly, an axillary dissection. For patients with more extensive disease, a mastectomy may be necessary. The use of postmastectomy chest-wall irradiation in these patients may also be considered.

Surgery

Mastectomy

William Halsted performed a radical mastectomy in 1894. The guiding principle at this time was centered on the belief that cancer originates in the breast and spreads in a stepwise fashion to the regional lymph nodes first and then to distant sites. Removal of all the breast tissue, pectoral muscles, and axillary contents was the standard surgical treatment. Over the next several decades, two simultaneous trends existed. One involved less radical surgery, which included removal of the breast and axillary contents but preserved the pectoral muscles and more skin. This was described by Patey and Dyson in 1948 and is the modern-day modified radical mastectomy. The other trend involved more extensive surgery, the extended radical mastectomy, which included en-bloc removal of the internal mammary chain at the time of radical mastectomy. Retrospective studies found that survival rates were similar regardless of the extent of the operative procedure when the Halsted radical mastectomy was compared with any of the modified approaches; as a result, a modified approach was accepted in 1979 by the NCI Consensus Conference.

TABLE 14.14   Prospective Randomized Trials Comparing Conservative Surgery

	Patients (n)	Years	OVERALL SURVIVAL (%)	
			Conservative Surgery and Radiation	Mastectomy
Milan Cancer Institute	701	18	65	65
Institut Gustave-Roussy	179	15	73	65
National Surgical Adjuvant Breast Project B-06	1219	12	63	59
Project B-06 National Cancer Institute	237	10	77	75
European Organization for Research and Treatment of Cancer	874	8	54	61
Danish Breast Cancer	904	6	79	82

Modified from Winchester DP, Cox JD. Standards for diagnosis and management of invasive breast carcinoma. American College of Radiology. American College of Surgeons. College of American Pathologists. Society of Surgical Oncology. *CA Cancer J Clin* 1998;48:83.

TABLE 14.15   2015 National Comprehensive Cancer Network Guidelines Relating to Adjuvant Therapy

	ER/PR Positive Her2 Negative	ER/PR Positive Her2 Positive	ER/PR Negative Her2 Positive	ER/PR Negative Her2 Negative
T1a N0	± E	± E or ± C + Tr » E	± C + Tr	——
T1a N1mi	E ± C	E or C + Tr » E	± C + Tr	± C
T1b N0/N1mi	21 gene RT-PCR assay	E or C + Tr » E	± C + Tr	± C
T1c N0/N1mi	Low score <18: E	C + Tr » E	C + Tr ± P	C
T2 N0/N1mi	Inter score 18–30: E ± C	C + Tr ± P » E	C + Tr ± P	C
T3 N0/N1mi	High score ≥31: C » E	C + Tr ± P » E	C + Tr ± P	C
T1/2/3 N1	C » E	C + Tr ± P » E	C + Tr ± P	C

±, Use of this therapy optional ("consider"); », follow with; *C*, polychemotherapy; *E*, endocrine therapy; *ER*, estrogen receptor; *PR*, progesterone receptor; *RT-PCR*, reverse transcriptase-polymerase chain reaction; *Tr*, trastuzumab; P, pertuzumab.
From 2015 National Comprehensive Cancer Network guidelines relating to adjuvant therapy of breast cancer available at www.nccn.org/professionals/physician_gls/pdf/breast.pdf.

To facilitate immediate breast reconstruction, which is increasingly performed, the technique of skin-sparing mastectomy (SSM) is performed, and, more recently, nipple-sparing mastectomy (NSM) is also gaining favor. A recent meta-analysis looking at the oncologic safety of NSM as opposed to SSM or total mastectomy found no significant differences in overall survival, disease-free survival, and local recurrence between the two groups. Studies with follow-up periods longer than 5 years in patients undergoing NSM had mean overall local recurrence rate of 11.4% and nipple areolar recurrence rate of 3.4%. It should be noted, however, that there are no randomized data regarding the NSM approach.

Breast-conservation Therapy

The shift toward less radical surgery at the time of mastectomy occurred for several reasons. As earlier diagnosis of breast cancer with smaller tumors and less involvement of pectoral muscles occurred, the need for radical procedures decreased. In addition, even with radical mastectomy, not all patients were cured and, although regional recurrences were low, patients died of distant disease. The morbidity of the radical mastectomy was well documented, including lymphedema, immobility of the shoulder, and disfigurement. A shift to breast conservation followed the same trends. The initial trials with radiation therapy using radium implants at the Princess Margaret Hospital in Toronto had promising results.

This led to randomization studies comparing breast-conservation therapy with mastectomy. Table 14.14 lists randomized trials that compared radical and modified radical mastectomy in stage I and stage II carcinoma of the breast.

In breast-conserving surgery, a wide-local excision is performed with excision of the tumor and a 1- to 2-cm rim of normal tissue. This excision is referred to as "lumpectomy" or a "tumorectomy." This differs from a quadrantectomy, in which a resection of the tumor with the overlying skin and the involved quadrant of the breast is performed. The six randomized trials differed with respect to the type of wide-local excision performed and with respect to tumor size in the patients who were randomized. In the Milan trial, a quadrantectomy was performed. In the Insitut Gustave Roussy trial, the "tumorectomy" performed was removal of the tumor and a 2-cm margin of normal tissue. In the United States, the NSABP B-06 trial did not specify the margins on the lumpectomy specimen, providing they were grossly free of tumor. In the NCI study, there was a significantly higher local recurrence rate in the breast-conservation group, but only gross tumor removal was required for study entry. Whole-breast irradiation (45–50 Gy) was used in all trials, with a boost to the primary site given in five of the six trials.

In all trials, the authors noted comparable disease-free survival in both arms. The only difference noted was in local recurrence. In addition to the randomized trials, many nonrandomized reports have been published with similar results in survival between breast conservation and mastectomy.

In a meta-analysis of nine prospective randomized trials comparing conservative surgery and irradiation with mastectomy, no survival differences were found in seven of the trials. Local recurrence was reported in 6.2% of patients treated with mastectomy and in 5.9% of those treated with breast-conservation surgery. No difference was seen in the incidence of contralateral breast cancer or a second malignant neoplasm that was not breast cancer. The incidence of recurrence in the treated breast ranged from 3% to 19%. Most failures in the treated breast can be salvaged with mastectomy, which can result in 70% survival at 5 years. Mastectomy did not prevent local recurrences, which developed in 4% to 14% of patients after this treatment.

In 1992, the American Colleges of Surgeons, Radiologists, and Pathologists, along with the ACS and the Society of Surgical Oncology, began the process of describing standard practice for breast-conservation treatment. Many retrospective and prospective randomized trials suggested equally effective results in appropriately selected patients with early-stage breast cancer, regardless of whether they were treated with mastectomy or breast-conservation surgery. The results of these deliberations were published in 1998.

Radiation therapy is an important component of breast conservation. Adequate surgical margins are required to be negative on pathologic inspection. After healing, the radiation therapy is planned. Treatment to the entire breast should be at a dose of 1.8 to 2.0 Gy per day for a total of 45 to 50 Gy. A 10- to 15-Gy electron-therapy boost is often given to the lumpectomy bed. More recently, data on hypofractionation, which increases the daily dose and shortens the radiation therapy time, have been reported and demonstrate equivalence to standard radiation techniques.

Breast conservation depends on the use of radiation. The question of whether lumpectomy alone would yield similar results has been addressed through randomized trials. Local recurrence rates of 18% to 40% with lumpectomy alone have been reported compared with 2% to 14% with lumpectomy and radiation. In these studies, a significant reduction in relapse was noted in the lumpectomy and radiation arm.

The NSABP B-17 trial is the only prospective randomized trial of lumpectomy alone versus lumpectomy and radiation (50 Gy) in patients with DCIS. There were 818 women randomly assigned, and surgical margins were histologically tumor free. The mean follow-up time was 90 months (67–180 months). The incidence of noninvasive ipsilateral breast tumor was reduced from 13.4% to 8.2% ($P = 0.007$), and the incidence of invasive ipsilateral breast tumor was reduced from 13.4% to 3.9% ($P <0.001$). All women benefited from radiation therapy regardless of clinical or mammographic tumor characteristics. No difference in mortality was noted. Interest in partial-breast radiation for early-stage breast cancers has prompted single-institution studies to use brachytherapy catheters, the MammoSite balloon (Proxima Company, Alpharetta, GA), and three-dimensional external-beam partial-breast treatment. The FDA-approved MammoSite Radiation Therapy System is a means of administering brachytherapy internally in prescribed doses over a 5-day period. During the lumpectomy, a deflated balloon is placed inside the surgical cavity. A tube connects the balloon to the outside of the breast and may be inflated with saline to fill the cavity. Radiation is delivered within the inflated balloon over 1 to 5 days, after which the balloon is deflated and then removed.

These approaches are being studied as an alternative to the standard 5- to 6-week whole-breast radiation treatment. To shorten the radiation course, the proportion of breast tissue to be radiated is significantly less. Data on local recurrences after radiation show that the majority of recurrences after lumpectomy and whole-breast radiation occur in the same quadrant, hence the reason to consider partial-breast radiation. In this manner, a greater dose will be delivered to the lumpectomy site and the surrounding tissue in a shorter course of therapy. Currently, the National Surgical Adjuvant Breast and Bowel Project and Radiation Therapy Oncology Group (NSABP-RTOG) cooperative groups opened a phase III trial comparing whole-breast radiation therapy to some form of partial-breast radiation. The partial-breast treatment will be delivered using brachytherapy catheters, MammoSite balloon, or external three-dimensional conformal treatment. Randomization to either whole- or partial-breast radiation will occur at entry into the trial. Enrollment to this trial closed in 2013, and results are awaited.

Overall, it appears that clinicians can now be confident in recommending lumpectomy plus irradiation to patients because it seems to be equivalent to mastectomy in terms of survival and optimal local-regional control.

Breast-conserving surgery can also be combined with plastic surgery in a concept known as oncoplastic breast surgery. This combines the oncologic approach of wide-local resection with plastic surgery incisions and tissue transfer techniques aiming to preserve the natural shape of the breast and breast symmetry. Techniques range from volume displacement and redistribution techniques, such as mastopexy and mini-flaps, to more advanced techniques such as reduction mammoplasty and contralateral symmetry procedures.

Patient Selection

Possible contraindications can interfere with offering a patient breast-conservation therapy. Cosmetic result should be considered when deciding whether to offer breast-conserving surgery; tumor size in relation to breast size is an important consideration. In addition, other factors that may affect the ability to receive irradiation must be considered (ie, history of prior breast or chest irradiation, concurrent pregnancy, Li-Fraumeni syndrome, and autoimmune connective tissue disease). Particularly, with a history of systemic lupus erythematosus, radiation may not be a possibility. Women with multiple cancers in the breast are not candidates for this approach and require a mastectomy. In addition, patients with extensive calcifications on a mammogram suggesting a diffuse process may be better treated with mastectomy.

The American Society of Clinical Oncology, the Society of Surgical Oncology, and the American Society of Radiation

Oncology jointly published guidelines in 2014 after a meta-analysis of 33 studies and almost 30,000 patients, which recommended no tumor on ink as a satisfactory margin. **Patients with positive resected margins should undergo reexcision.** If resected margins remain positive on reexcision, mastectomy is the preferred treatment. Positive margins (ink on invasive carcinoma or DCIS) are associated with a twofold increase in the risk of recurrence compared with negative margins. This increased risk is not mitigated by favorable biology, endocrine therapy, or a radiation boost. There was no evidence that tumors with an extensive intraductal component (EIC), which were thought to be at more risk of recurrence benefited from a more widely clear margin. The status of surgical margins is probably the most important aspect of pathologic evaluation of breast tumor excision specimens in patients being considered for conservative surgery.

Extensive intraductal component is a condition that exists when more than 25% of the tumor is associated with DCIS. In these cases, the invasive component may be outside the area of the intraductal carcinoma. This has been reported to have a higher relapse rate with breast conservation; however, it is thought to be secondary to margin status because margin involvement may be an indication of residual intraductal carcinoma. In DCIS, Silverstein and associates developed the Van Nuys prognostic index (VNPI). The system combines the scores for histologic grade, tumor size, and margin status of a lesion to obtain an overall score. It considers margins of 1 cm to indicate a decreased rate of local relapse, even with no radiation. However, margin width has not been shown to be significant in other studies.

Management of the Axilla

The axilla is a pyramidal space between the arm and thoracic wall. It contains the axillary vessels and their branches, the brachial plexus and its branches, and lymph nodes embedded in fatty tissue. The primary route of lymphatic drainage of the breast is through the axillary lymph nodes. The lymph nodes are also divided into levels based on location relative to the pectoralis minor. Level 1 lymph nodes lie lateral to the lateral border of the pectoralis minor muscle, level 2 nodes lie behind the pectoralis minor muscle, and level 3 nodes are medial to the medial border of this muscle.

In an axillary dissection, nerve branches of the brachial plexus are encountered. The lateral and medial pectoral nerves supply the pectoralis muscles. The thoracodorsal nerve runs downward and innervates the latissimus dorsi. The long thoracic nerve is located on the medial wall of the axilla on the serratus anterior. It arises from the C5 to C7 roots, and injury to these nerves results in paralysis to part or all of the serratus anterior. The functional deficit is inability to raise the arm above the level of the shoulder.

At the time of Halsted's radical mastectomy procedure, a complete axillary dissection was performed. The status of the axilla is the most important prognostic factor for breast cancer. Clinical examination of the axilla is inaccurate because even in patients with a T1 lesion, there is a 10% risk of lymph node metastasis. Before the use of SLN biopsy (SLNB), there was no accurate method to adequately stage the axilla without an axillary dissection. Axillary lymph node sampling (ie, removal of only a few lymph nodes) was inadequate.

Metastatic involvement of lymph nodes usually occurs in a stepwise manner. Rosen and coworkers demonstrated the incidence of skip metastasis to be less than 2%. A complete level 1 and level 2 lymph node dissection provides excellent local control, and local recurrence after this procedure has been shown to be less than 1%.

The NSABP B-04 trial was begun in 1971, and the NSABP designed this trial to determine the value of prophylactic regional node dissection. Patients with clinically uninvolved axillary nodes (clinical stage I) were randomly assigned for treatment among radical mastectomy, total mastectomy plus irradiation of the chest wall and regional lymphatics, and total mastectomy alone. Women who had clinically involved axillary nodes (clinical stage II) were randomly assigned to treatment with either radical mastectomy or total mastectomy and irradiation to the chest wall and all lymph node drainage areas for the breast. If ignoring occult axillary metastases permitted continuing dissemination, the patients treated with total mastectomy alone should fare poorly; if having still-functioning nodes improves host defenses, the patients treated with total mastectomy alone should fare better than the others.

A total of 1665 patients were entered and observed for 72 months with no difference found among the three treatment arms in stage I. Overall, patients assigned stage II survived less well, but again, there was no difference between the two treatment alternatives. Only 60 (16%) of the 365 patients who did not undergo prophylactic axillary dissection developed progression in the axilla as a first sign of failure and underwent axillary dissections, predominantly in the first 30 months of follow-up but also as long as 112 months after surgery. In the group in which prophylactic axillary dissection was done, the incidence of positive nodes was 39%. More than half of the patients who should have had positive axillary nodes did not develop clinical evidence of such.

In 1985, Fisher and coworkers reported on this same group of 1665 women observed for a mean of 126 months. There were no significant differences between the two groups of patients who had clinically positive nodes treated by radical mastectomy or by total mastectomy without axillary dissection but with regional irradiation. Survival at 10 years was about 38% in both groups.

The morbidity associated with axillary lymphadenectomy is not inconsequential. About 10% to 15% of patients will develop lymphedema. In addition, numbness, pain, or weakness contributes to a significant decrease in the quality of life in these patients.

Sentinel Lymph Node Biopsy

Sentinel lymph node biopsy in breast cancer evolved out of efforts to minimize the morbidity associated with axillary lymph node dissection while still providing important staging information. Initial studies in melanoma carried out by Morton and colleagues in 1992 demonstrated the feasibility of the concept. Methods used include blue dye and radioisotope.

Several studies have confirmed the accuracy of SLNB. In the majority of the studies, successful identification of the SLN occurs between 92% and 98% of the time. The combination of blue dye and isotope has been reported to be better for identification of the SLN; when used in combination, the positive predictive value of the technique approaches 100%, with a negative predictive value close to 95%. The false-negative rate is about 5% to 10% in most studies.

The validity of the SLN concept lies in the ability of the SLN to predict the status of the regional lymphatic basin. Turner and colleagues performed IHC staining of all lymph nodes, sentinel and nonsentinel, in a series of patients undergoing standard axillary dissection with negative nodes. Of 157 SLNs, 10 (6%) demonstrated IHC positivity compared with 1 of 1087 (0.09%) of the non-SLNs. This provided validity to the SLN concept.

The SLNB procedure is widely used in invasive breast cancer and selectively in DCIS. In certain situations, however, a standard axillary dissection should still be considered, such as when bulky positive axillary nodes are present.

Previously, the presence of metastases in the SLNB prompted a completion axillary dissection. However, the results of the NSABP-B04 trial, in which some patients did not have their axilla dissected, called into question the value of the axillary dissection as a therapeutic instrument.

ACOSOG Z0011, a trial designed by The American College of Surgeons Oncology Group, investigated whether foregoing axillary dissection in patients undergoing breast-conserving therapy with 1 or 2 positive SLNs was safe. They reported no difference in local-regional failure, disease-free survival, or overall survival; the 5-year overall survival rates were 91.8% (95% CI 89.1%–94.5%) with axillary lymph node dissection (ALND) and 92.5% (95% CI 90.0%–95.1%) with SLNB alone; the 5-year disease-free survival rates were 82.2% (95% CI 78.3%–86.3%) with ALND and 83.9% (95% CI 80.2%–87.9%) with SLNB alone. Completion axillary dissection is still recommended in patients with T3 tumors, patients having partial breast irradiation, or those having a mastectomy for management of their primary tumor who are found to have a positive SLNB. In intraductal carcinoma, an SLNB or axillary dissection is generally not indicated. There are special circumstances of intraductal carcinoma, such as high-grade DCIS or extensive DCIS, in which a microinvasive component may be associated with the intraductal carcinoma. In these circumstances, and particularly if a mastectomy is being performed, an SLNB may be considered.

Adjuvant Therapy

Multiple randomized studies have demonstrated that the addition of chemotherapy improves overall survival in patients with breast cancer. The decision to use adjuvant chemotherapy or hormonal therapy depends on certain factors, such as the size of the primary tumor, the expression or lack of expression of ER or PR, lymph node status, HER2/neu status, tumor genomic profiling, and the presence or absence of metastatic disease.

Adjuvant treatment in breast cancer was first used more than 100 years ago. In 1894, Beatson reported on the results

of oophorectomy and response rate in the metastatic breast cancer setting. Initially, the use of systemic therapy involved the use of single-agent chemotherapy; later, multiagent chemotherapy was used. As in most breast cancer trials, the initial reports were of patients with metastatic disease. Adjuvant chemotherapy is standard treatment for patients with positive nodes or large tumors. The combination of CMF (cyclophosphamide, methotrexate, and 5-fluorouracil [5-FU]) has been used for many years in the treatment of patients with breast cancer. Anthracycline-based regimens and the possible addition of taxanes had been used in patients with high-risk factors for recurrence. The Early Breast Cancer Trialists' Collaborative Group (EBCTCG) was formed in 1985 to analyze all available, properly conducted randomized trials to examine which chemotherapy regimens gave the best results. In the 2012 EBCTCG meta-analysis, adjuvant chemotherapies using either an anthracycline-based regimen or CMF were compared with no treatment. The use of an anthracycline-containing regimen was associated a significant reduction in overall mortality (RR 0.84; 95% CI 0.78–0.91), which translated into an absolute gain of 5.0% at 10 years. Similarly, the use of CMF had a significant reduction in overall mortality (RR 0.84; 95% CI 0.76–0.93), which translated into an absolute gain of 4.7%. There was no improvement in the risk of recurrence, breast cancer, or overall mortality when CMF was compared with standard dose anthracycline-based regimens. However, the use of higher cumulative doses of anthracyclines compared with CMF did result in a reduction in the risk of recurrence (RR 0.89; 95% CI 0.82–0.96) with an absolute gain of 2.6%, breast cancer mortality rate (RR 0.80; 95% CI 0.72–0.88) with an absolute gain of 4.1 percent, and overall mortality rate (RR 0.84; 95% CI 0.76–0.92) with an absolute gain of 3.9%. They also assessed the role of taxanes when incorporated into the adjuvant chemotherapy for early breast cancer. In trials in which the **same control regimen** was used in both arms (*n* = 11,167 women), incorporation of taxanes into an anthracycline regimen resulted in a reduction in the risk of overall mortality (RR 0.86; 95% CI 0.79–0.93), which translated to a 3.2% improvement in overall survival at 8 years.

The NCCN recently published the 20th annual edition of its comprehensive breast cancer management practice guidelines, including recommendations for adjuvant therapy of breast cancer. The NCCN guidelines for chemotherapy are described in detail on its website (http://www.NCCN.org).

Since the demonstration of their superiority to other combination chemotherapy, anthracycline-based regimens have become the basis for the adjuvant treatment of high-risk patients with breast cancer. A variety of approaches have evolved regarding adjuvant polychemotherapy, including the addition of drugs such as taxanes and targeted agents and the establishment of dose-dense chemotherapy regimens that were based on modeling of human breast cancer growth.

Administration of dose-dense chemotherapy became possible with the introduction of granulocyte colony-stimulating factor, which allows the chemotherapy courses to be condensed without causing unacceptable toxicity. A dose-dense chemotherapy approach using concurrent doxorubicin and cyclophosphamide (AC) followed by paclitaxel (T) was assessed in the pivotal Cancer and Leukemia Group B (CALGB) 9741 trial, a phase III prospective randomized trial of adjuvant treatment of women with node-positive early-stage breast cancer. This trial showed a statistically significant improvement in disease-free survival and overall survival for dose-dense chemotherapy and has become one of the preferred regimens. Another preferred regimen is the combination of docetaxel and cyclophosphamide.

Estrogen Receptor–Positive Breast Cancer

Estrogen receptors are proteins found in hormonally dependent tissue, both malignant and nonmalignant. The amount of receptor present in the breast cancer specimen is predictive of the success or failure of endocrine therapy. The identification of the ER protein in certain human mammary cancers and the subsequent explanation of the role of estrogen in tumor growth clarified a clinical relationship that had been observed for a century. In 1896, Beatson produced regression of mammary cancer by oophorectomy. Huggins and Bergenstal demonstrated in 1952 that some mammary and prostatic cancers were not autonomous but under the partial control of the endocrine system. Regressions of mammary cancers were continually obtained by removing the source of endogenous circulating hormones by oophorectomy, adrenalectomy, and hypophysectomy. Alternatively, breast cancer regressions were also achieved by administering large doses of estrogen, androgen, progesterone, and glucocorticoids.

The choice of a particular endocrine therapy has been in large part empiric, guided by certain clinical features such as menopausal status, disease-free interval, site of the dominant lesion, and response to previous therapy. As a result of basic investigations by Jensen, Smith, and DeSombre of steroid hormone metabolism, there has been development of a series of assays that can identify with considerable accuracy breast cancers that are not autonomous and that will respond to endocrine manipulation. Such a method of predicting a priori those cancers that will be responsive to changes in the endocrine milieu greatly enhances the usefulness of hormone therapy and allows recommendation of such treatments on a plausible biochemical basis.

Knowledge of the ER content of either the primary or the recurrent mammary cancer must be viewed within the proper clinical perspective. This one determination is but a single piece in the mosaic of the subcellular biochemistry of breast cancer. To deprecate the clinical importance of this determination because some patients with significant ER content will not respond to hormone treatment (because of eventual escape from hormone regulation or because of lack of understanding of the role of other steroid or protein hormone receptors) begs the question. Knowledge of the ER content of either a primary or a metastatic tumor does not allow the physician to predict the hormone dependency of a tumor with enough accuracy for it to be rationally used in the selection of appropriate palliative treatment. It does, however, allow a good assessment of the likelihood that the patient with breast cancer would benefit from endocrine therapy.

HER2/neu–Positive Breast Cancer

In patients with HER2/neu–positive breast cancer, the use of trastuzumab (Herceptin) in addition to combination chemotherapy has been associated with a decrease in relapse. Trastuzumab is a humanized anti-HER2 antibody against the extracellular domain of the 2-neu oncoprotein.

Four major adjuvant trials—Herceptin Adjuvant (HERA), National Surgical Adjuvant Breast and Bowel Project (NSABP) B-31, North Central Cancer Treatment Group (NCCTG) N9831, and Breast Cancer International Research Group (BCIRG) 006—have investigated the use of trastuzumab in the adjuvant setting. These trials have shown that trastuzumab reduces the 3-year risk of recurrence by about 50% in this population. More than 13,000 women with HER2/neu–positive breast cancers were enrolled and received 1 year of adjuvant treatment with trastuzumab. These trials used different chemotherapy regimens but had similar improvements in recurrence-free survival. Cardiac events were at an acceptable level; however, they did note a slightly higher incidence (0.6%–3.3%) of congestive heart failure that was responsive to treatment. There was an overall survival benefit in the NSABP B-31 and NCCTG N9831 trials and a trend toward an overall survival benefit in the HERA and BCIRG trials.

Regimens using AC followed by a taxane are also one of the preferred regimens for HER2/neu–positive breast cancer with the addition of trastuzumab with or without pertuzumab with the taxane. Pertuzumab inhibits HER2 by binding to a different HER2 epitope than trastuzumab and represents a complementary mechanism of action to trastuzumab. The efficacy and safety of pertuzumab in combination with trastuzumab with or without chemotherapy have been demonstrated in both advanced and early stages of HER2-positive breast cancer.

Lapatinib (Tykerb) in combination with capecitabine is approved by the FDA for treatment of patients with advanced or metastatic breast cancer whose tumors overexpress HER2 and who have received previous therapy, including an anthracycline, a taxane, and trastuzumab.

Triple-Negative Breast Cancer

Triple-negative breast cancer accounts for approximately 10% to 15% of all breast cancers and accounts for a disproportionate share of breast cancer mortality. There is specific enrichment for triple-negative subtype in the breast cancers arising in *BRCA1* mutation carriers. By definition, triple-negative cancers do not have estrogen and progesterone receptors, and they are not HER2/neu receptor amplified. Therefore, the only available adjuvant treatment consists of chemotherapy. For patients with stage II and III triple-negative disease, regimens that contain anthracyclines and taxanes are the standard approach. Those with stage I disease are often treated with shorter and less toxic regimens. In general, chemotherapy reduces the overall risk of disease recurrence in the triple-negative setting by as much as 35% to 50%.

Ovarian Ablation

Ovarian suppression is one of the oldest methods for treating premenopausal metastatic breast cancer. This can be accomplished surgically by use of luteinizing hormone–releasing hormone analogs or radiation. In 1996, the EBCTCG published an overview of randomized trials concerning ovarian ablation in early breast cancer. There were 12 of 17 studies available for evaluation, all of which were begun before 1980. There were 2102 randomized women younger than 50 years and 1354 women aged 50 years and older. **In women younger than 50 years, there were six fewer recurrences or deaths per 100 women allocated to ovarian ablation (45% vs. 39% alive without recurrence) 15 years after randomization.**

The Suppression of Ovarian Function Trial (SOFT) and the Tamoxifen and Exemestane Trial (TEXT) were recent trials dedicated to premenopausal women with hormone-sensitive breast cancer and were developed to determine the role of ovarian ablation in women whose menses return after chemotherapy and are treated with tamoxifen and to test whether adjuvant aromatase inhibitor use improves outcomes in patients treated with ovarian ablation. Overall, in the SOFT trial, patients did not benefit from the addition of ovarian ablation. Nevertheless, for women at higher risk of recurrence who received adjuvant chemotherapy and remained premenopausal, addition of ovarian ablation to tamoxifen reduced the risk of recurrence. The effect was larger in younger patients. In the TEXT trial, adjuvant treatment with exemestane plus ovarian ablation, compared with tamoxifen plus ovarian ablation, significantly improved disease-free and distant disease-free survival, therefore representing a new treatment option. Tailored endocrine treatments should be considered in premenopausal patients with hormone-sensitive tumors.

In the joint analysis of the SOFT and TEXT trials, it should be noted that 13.7% had stopped all protocol assigned treatments early (16.1% of the patients in the exemestane–ovarian suppression group and 11.2% of those in the tamoxifen–ovarian suppression group). Nearly all women (98.3%) treated with ovarian suppression reported adverse events; in 30%, these were grade 3 or 4. The grade 3 or 4 events that were reported most frequently were hot flushes, musculoskeletal symptoms, and hypertension. Depression was reported in 50.2% of patients, with grade 3 or 4 depression in 4.1% of the patients.

Tamoxifen

Many prospective, double-blind, randomized studies have been performed to evaluate the role of adjuvant tamoxifen among women with early breast cancer. In 1998, the EBCTCG published an update on 55 such trials of 37,000 women. In the 18,000 women with ER-positive tumors, the reductions in the recurrence rate at 1, 2, and 5 years of tamoxifen use were 21%, 28%, and 50%, respectively. These figures are all highly significant. Women with ER-positive tumors with at least 100-fmol receptor per milligram of cytosol protein had a greater reduction in recurrence than those with positive receptors but less than 100 fmol (60% vs. 43% after 5 years of tamoxifen). The reduction in mortality was also greater in those with a higher receptor level (36% vs. 23%). Patients with ER-positive, PR-negative tumors had results (reduction of recurrences and mortality) similar to those of patients with ER-positive tumors (progesterone receptor status unknown). Among the 800

women with ER-poor tumors, the reduction in recurrence was only 10%, irrespective of length of time of tamoxifen treatment. Although this reduction is statistically significant, the apparent benefit is small, and the lower confidence limit is close to zero. Irrespective of the duration of tamoxifen use, the mortality rate reduction was only 6%. In the 2000 women with ER-poor, PR-poor tumors, tamoxifen had no apparent effect on recurrence or mortality rates (≈1%), but in the 602 women with ER-poor, PR-positive tumors, recurrence reduction was 23%, and mortality reduction was 9%. There were 12,000 women with unknown ER status. It can be estimated that about two-thirds of these women would have ER-positive tumors if measured. The data suggest highly significant benefits among women with unknown ER status.

Tamoxifen has been shown to reduce the risk of relapse and mortality in randomized trials of women with ER-positive breast cancer, with treatment for 5 years showing greater effectiveness than treatment for 2 years. Results of the Adjuvant Tamoxifen: Longer Against Shorter (ATLAS) trial showed that extending treatment to 10 years reduced the risk of relapse, breast cancer mortality ($P = 0.01$), and all-cause mortality ($P = 0.01$) compared with discontinuation. Most of this benefit seemed to accrue after completion of treatment with recurrence rates during the 5 extra years of tamoxifen (rate ratio, 0.90) and a more impressive carryover benefit during the 5 years of follow-up after completion of 10 years of tamoxifen (rate ratio, 0.75).

In addition, the reduced mortality rate was only apparent after completion of 10 years of treatment with tamoxifen. Previous trials of 5 years of tamoxifen have shown a similar carryover benefit more than 10 years after discontinuation. The benefit of continuing tamoxifen for a further 5 years gives rise to a total relapse risk reduction of 39% ($P < 0.0001$) and risk reduction of breast cancer mortality of 36% ($P < 0.0001$). After completion of 10 years of treatment, this estimated risk was reduced by 30% for relapse ($P = 0.01$) and 48% for mortality ($P < 0.0001$), continuing for at least 5 years. These carryover benefits contribute substantially to the cumulative benefits of treatment with tamoxifen because toxic effects only occur while on therapy. Overall, the benefits of extended tamoxifen seemed to outweigh the risks substantially.

There are well-described adverse effects with tamoxifen. Endometrial cancer is significantly more common among women who receive extended therapy with tamoxifen compared with those who did not. Five years of adjuvant tamoxifen is estimated to result in an absolute 15-year endometrial cancer risk of about 2% to 3%, and that use of 10 years rather than 5 years of tamoxifen would produce an additional risk by year 15 of about 2%. The numerical instances of death as a result of endometrial cancer were higher with extended tamoxifen treatment, although such events were rare. There was also a higher risk for pulmonary embolism with tamoxifen. There was a lower risk of ischemic heart disease in women who received extended tamoxifen therapy in ATLAS.

Following this and similar data, the American Society of Clinical Oncology guidelines now recommend that if women are pre- or perimenopausal and have received 5 years of adjuvant tamoxifen, they should be offered 10 years' total duration of tamoxifen. If women are postmenopausal and have received 5 years of adjuvant tamoxifen, they should be offered the choice of continuing tamoxifen or switching to an aromatase inhibitor for 10 years' total adjuvant endocrine therapy.

Aromatase Inhibitors

Aromatase inhibitors suppress estrogen levels by inactivating aromatase, the enzyme responsible for synthesizing estrogens from androgens. In contrast to tamoxifen, these compounds lack partial agonist activity. The Anastrozole, Tamoxifen Alone or in Combination (ATAC) trial compared 5 years of tamoxifen versus anastrozole versus the combination. Anastrozole was found to have a significantly better survival time, prolonged time to recurrence, reduced distant metastases, and lower incidence of contralateral breast cancer compared with tamoxifen. Letrozole, another aromatase inhibitor, was compared with tamoxifen in the multicenter Breast International Group (BIG) trial of 8028 postmenopausal women with metastatic breast cancer. Letrozole reduced significantly the risk of recurrent disease when compared with tamoxifen, especially at distant sites in these postmenopausal women. Another international study of 5187 women administered letrozole after completing 5 years of tamoxifen. The results from the data indicated a nearly 50% lower recurrence rate. As a result, letrozole is now an accepted treatment choice for postmenopausal women with hormone receptor–positive breast cancers who have used tamoxifen for a 5-year period. The American Society of Clinical Oncology now recommends aromatase inhibitors be used to lower the risk of recurrence in receptor-positive postmenopausal breast cancers as initial therapy or after treatment with tamoxifen.

Three double-blind, randomized, prospective studies—ATAC, the Intergroup Exemestane Study (EIS), and the BIG 1-98 trial—have confirmed the superiority of aromatase inhibitors over tamoxifen in early-stage cancers in postmenopausal women. All three studies have demonstrated an increase in disease-free survival. Short-term side effects were acceptable, but all had a negative impact on bone health. Based on the results of these trials, patients who are postmenopausal have the option of starting on anastrozole as first-line therapy after initial diagnosis. Patients who have been on tamoxifen for 2 to 3 years can be switched to an aromatase inhibitor to complete a total of 5 years of therapy.

The MA.17 trial, which examined whether extended endocrine therapy with letrozole after completion of 5 years of tamoxifen, found a significant increase in disease-free survival in postmenopausal patients with hormone-sensitive breast cancer irrespective of whether patients were node positive or node negative. The MA.17 trial was unblinded at the first planned interim analysis, after 171 events (median follow-up, 2.4 years), because of a significant difference in events that favored the letrozole arm and far exceeded predefined unblinding boundaries. The results of this pivotal trial led to the approval of letrozole as extended adjuvant treatment of early breast cancer in postmenopausal women who had received standard adjuvant tamoxifen therapy in the United States and in several European countries.

Gene Expression Assays

Two gene-expression assays used to determine the risk of breast cancer recurrence in patients with stage I or II node-negative breast cancer are currently available. Onco*type* DX (Genomic Health Institute, Redwood City, CA) is an assay performed on RNA extracted from paraffin-embedded tumor tissue. It analyzes the expression of 21 genes: 16 cancer-related genes and 5 reference genes. The results are used to calculate a recurrence score to identify the likelihood of cancer recurrence in patients treated with tamoxifen. The results of two studies evaluating the ability of Onco*type* DX to predict the risk of breast cancer recurrence suggest that patients with ER-positive, node-negative breast cancer, and a low recurrence score may need only adjuvant treatment with tamoxifen, but intermediate- and high-risk patients may require additional treatment with adjuvant chemotherapy. MammaPrint, an oligonucleotide microassay performed on fresh-frozen tumor samples, analyzes the expression of 70 genes. Studies have found that MammaPrint allows young patients (<61 years) with early-stage breast cancer to be categorized as having a high or low risk of distant metastasis. High-risk patients may then be managed with more aggressive therapy.

Metastatic Disease

The goal of therapy in metastatic disease is palliation of symptoms because cure is unlikely. The majority of patients with metastatic disease receive antihormonal therapy. First-line agents include tamoxifen or aromatase inhibitors such as letrozole or anastrozole. These agents offer a 20% response with ER- or PR-positive tumors. Disease stabilization is the goal of therapy, and because these therapies are less toxic than chemotherapy, most patients remain on them for prolonged periods. Upon failure of these agents, however, chemotherapy is the next step.

High-dose Chemotherapy

Five large randomized trials have been conducted addressing the use of high-dose chemotherapy with bone marrow or stem cell rescue in metastatic breast cancer. Only one trial, conducted in South Africa, showed a lower rate of relapse. The other four trials showed no increase in overall survival. The investigators of the trial conducted in South Africa subsequently admitted to fraud. Thus, it is believed that high-dose chemotherapy offers no survival advantage over conventional treatment approaches.

Neoadjuvant Chemotherapy

Neoadjuvant chemotherapy in patients with breast cancer has never demonstrated an improvement in overall survival compared with conventional adjuvant therapy; nevertheless, the downstaging of the primary tumor may increase the possibility for breast conservation and includes the potential to tailor systemic therapy based on responses observed in the neoadjuvant setting. This has led to increased utilization.

The surgical approach to the axilla in patients after neoadjuvant chemotherapy is still being elucidated. SLNB after neoadjuvant chemotherapy accurately stages the axilla and is associated with a low rate of nodal recurrence in patients presenting with clinically negative axillary lymph nodes. The

SENTINA (SENTinel NeoAdjuvant) trial investigated the appropriate timing and feasibility of SLNB in different settings of neoadjuvant chemotherapy. Patients who had clinically N1 nodal disease before chemotherapy who clinically downstaged to N0 underwent SLNB followed by axillary dissection. The false-negative rate was 24% with assessment of one node and 18.5% with two. The false-negative rate was less than 10% only when three or more sentinel nodes were identified. However, nodal recurrence rates after SLNB alone in this population are unknown. Boughey et al. reporting from a similar trial (ACOSOG Z1071) urged caution when they found a false-negative rate of 12.6% when two more nodes were assessed, which was greater than their predetermined upper limit of acceptable false-negative rate of 10%. However, their data also demonstrated a false-negative rate of 9.1% when three or more nodes were assessed. Therefore many believe that SLNB is safe after neoadjuvant chemotherapy if three or more nodes are assessed. Dual mapping with radioisotope and blue dye is recommended to ensure successful mapping. Patients who become clinically node negative after neoadjuvant chemotherapy (downstaging of axilla) may safely avoid axillary node dissection.

Radiation Therapy

As discussed, radiation therapy is used in conjunction with lumpectomy for patients opting for breast conservation. For whole-breast radiation, the dose used is 1.8 to 2.0 Gy in 25 fractions for a total of 45 to 50 Gy to the entire breast. A 10- to 15-Gy electron-therapy boost is often given to the lumpectomy bed. The Ontario Clinical Oncology Group and the UK START trials looked at hypofractionated schedules and have reported no difference in recurrence rates compared with standard radiation protocols with acceptable cosmetic outcomes. The Canadian protocol is a schedule of 42.5 Gy given in 16 fractions over a period of 22 days. The American Society of Radiation Oncology guidelines do support use of hypofractionated schedules but caution that these trials had a majority of patients in these trials who were older than 50 years of age, had small node-negative tumors, and did not receive adjuvant chemotherapy.

Postmastectomy chest-wall irradiation is used with increasing frequency. Women with a high risk of local recurrence benefit from radiation therapy after mastectomy. Patients with large tumors (T3 lesions) and more than three positive nodes or presence of extranodal extension are at risk for local-regional failure. Chest-wall radiation is 50 Gy over 5 weeks, with a 10-Gy boost to the mastectomy scar. In women with one to three positive nodes, the benefit of the use of postmastectomy irradiation is uncertain and is being tested in RCTs. For patients with a chest-wall recurrence, the option of surgical debulking followed by chest-wall irradiation is used.

Radiation therapy can also be used in the palliative setting. It can be used for metastatic lesions to the bone or brain and can help to alleviate the patient's symptoms.

Breast Reconstruction

Breast reconstruction represents a major advance in cancer rehabilitation for patients undergoing a mastectomy. Previously,

a 2-year surveillance period was recommended before reconstruction for detection of local disease recurrence. Immediate reconstruction has not interfered with disease detection, however, and it has the advantage of combining the two procedures into one. In addition, a greater amount of skin can be saved with planned immediate reconstruction, and the scar tissue that would be encountered with a delayed procedure can be avoided.

A delayed reconstruction can be performed if the patient is ambiguous about the reconstruction or if operative risk is increased with prolonged anesthesia. It is also considered in patients with locally advanced disease if a delay in adjuvant irradiation or chemotherapy is anticipated because of the reconstruction.

Reconstruction options include expandable breast prosthesis (implant) and autologous tissue transfer. Tissue-transfer operations may yield the greatest symmetry between breasts, especially with larger breasts; however, they take longer, require greater surgical expertise, involve a longer recovery, and result in another scar at the donor site. A variety of donor sites are possible such as free flap options (eg, deep inferior epigastric perforator [DIEP] flap, transverse/diagonal upper gracilis [TUG/DUG]) or pedicled flaps (eg, transverse rectus abdominis muscle [TRAM] or latissimus dorsi).

SPECIAL ISSUES

Breast Cancer in Older Women

The challenge in older patients is to balance effective treatment against potential comorbidities and to minimize both under- and overtreatment. However, patients older than the age of 70 years are underrepresented in clinical trials, and as such there is a paucity of data to guide our treatment decisions. Advanced age in itself should not be a limitation to treatment. In 2011, the average life expectancy of a 70-year-old woman in the United States, was 16 years and for an 80-year-old woman, it was almost 10 years. Trials have shown that surgery and tamoxifen in women older than 70 years are associated with both decreased risk of local recurrence and improved survival times than with tamoxifen alone. In the 2006 Cochrane review, data based on an estimated 869 deaths in 1571 women were unable to show a statistically significant difference in favor of either surgery or tamoxifen in respect of overall survival. However, there was a statistically significant difference in terms of progression-free survival (PFS), which favored surgery with or without tamoxifen. The HR for overall survival were 0.98 ($P = 0.9$) for surgery alone versus tamoxifen and 0.86 ($P = 0.06$) for surgery with tamoxifen versus tamoxifen alone. The HRs for PFS were 0.55 ($P = 0.0006$) for surgery alone versus tamoxifen alone and 0.65 ($P = 0.0001$) for surgery plus tamoxifen versus tamoxifen alone. For elderly patients, the 2015 St. Gallen expert consensus was very clear that for standard chemotherapy, there is no absolute age limit; rather, disease factors, comorbidities, life expectancy, and patient preferences should factor in the treatment decisions. Treatment-related mortality, however, is higher in women older than 65 years of age (1.5%) compared with those younger than age 50 years (0.2%).

Randomized trials strongly suggest that older women with small breast cancers on endocrine therapy after surgery may gain little or nothing from adjuvant radiotherapy. The EBCTCG published an updated analysis using individual patient data from 10,801 patients included in 17 randomized trials of radiation after breast-conserving surgery. This revealed that the addition of radiation therapy was associated with a highly significant absolute benefit of 15.7% in any first recurrence (local, regional, or distant recurrence) at 10 years (P <0.00001). The benefits of radiation therapy varied when adjusted for ER status, grade, and age. The absolute benefit of radiation therapy depended on the baseline risk of recurrence, which is a function of age. With increasing age, the baseline risk of recurrence is lower, leading to a smaller but still significant absolute benefit of radiation overall. In women older than age 70 years, the baseline risk of recurrence and therefore the benefit derived from radiation was about half—an 8.9% absolute reduction in a 10-year risk of a locoregional or distant recurrence. This analysis was based on chronologic age and included healthy older women as well as those with comorbidities.

Hereditary Breast Cancer

Approximately 10% of newly diagnosed breast cancers are likely to be hereditary. Most are ascribed to the *BRCA1* and *BRCA2* mutations, but increasingly, with genome-wide association studies, further mutations are being identified with possible increased risks of breast cancer. One of the most characteristic features of hereditary breast cancer is its tendency to manifest at a young age. In the Breast Cancer Consortium's study of *BRCA1*-linked families, more than 80% of breast cancers occurred in women younger than 50 years of age. *BRCA1*-associated cancers tend to occur at a younger age than their *BRCA2* counterparts.

Pathologic Features

There is a strong association between the type of *BRCA* mutation and the pathological features of the tumors they develop. About 70% to 90% of *BRCA1* mutation-associated breast cancers are triple negative, and approximately 80% of *BRCA2* mutation-associated cancers are hormone receptor positive.

Stage

Most studies demonstrate that *BRCA*-associated breast cancers are seen at a stage comparable to non–*BRCA*-associated breast cancers. The incidence of axillary metastasis does not appear to be significantly different in patients with *BRCA*-associated breast cancers. In the literature, conflicting study data exist regarding the prognosis of patients with *BRCA*-associated breast cancer. A recent meta-analysis has looked at the effect of *BRCA1* and *BRCA2* mutations on survival after a diagnosis of breast or ovarian cancer.

BRCA mutation-associated ovarian cancers (in particular *BRCA2*) have a better overall and PFS than their nonmutation carrier counterparts. In breast cancer outcomes, this positive effect was not seen. *BRCA1* mutation carriers had worse prognoses than noncarriers for overall survival but were not different from noncarriers in PFS. *BRCA2* mutation was not associated with breast cancer prognosis.

Treatment

The surgical management of hereditary breast cancer must take into account many variables that may be potentially different to sporadic breast cancers, namely, local recurrence risk and future contralateral breast cancer risk.

Studies comparing local recurrence risk after breast conservation between *BRCA* mutation carriers and noncarriers have conflicting results and have been generally retrospective. A meta-analysis that included 526 *BRCA* mutation carriers showed no difference in local recurrence in the first 7 years of follow-up. However, on longer follow-up, the rate of ipsilateral recurrence started to substantially increase in the *BRCA* mutation group, although this may be suggestive of new ipsilateral breast cancers rather than true recurrences. *BRCA1* or *BRCA2* mutations did not differ with respect to local recurrence risk. Adjuvant chemotherapy and oophorectomy were associated with lower rates of local recurrence.

There was a marked difference in *BRCA* carriers compared with noncarriers and between *BRCA* mutation types with respect to their risk of contralateral breast cancer development. Analyses of 807 carriers showed a pooled contralateral breast cancer rate of 23.7% versus 6.8% in noncarriers (P <0.001). A study of a larger pooled *BRCA* carrier population of more than 2000 patients analyzed by subtype showed a 21.1% contralateral breast cancer rate in the *BRCA1* group compared with a 15.1% rate in the *BRCA* patients ($\underline{P}$ = 0.04)

Factors that were shown to decrease contralateral breast cancer risk were oophorectomy, tamoxifen use, and increasing age. A study that looked more specifically at age and contralateral breast cancer risk showed that at 15 years, those younger than 50 years old at diagnosis had a much higher rate (37.6%) than those older than 50 years at diagnosis (16.8%) (P = 0.001). *BRCA2* mutation breast cancers, given their higher rate of hormone receptor positivity, are likely to be on endocrine treatment and to have stronger protective effect from oophorectomy.

Chemoprevention

Chemoprevention is the principle that cancer prevention can be achieved through pharmacologic intervention. It refers to the use of a medication in a healthy patient to reduce the risk of a particular cancer. It is an option for all women with significant risk for future breast cancer development. Currently, the only FDA-approved medication for prevention of breast cancer is tamoxifen. Tamoxifen is a SERM that acts as an antiestrogen in breast tissue. It has been used in the adjuvant setting in breast cancer since 1972 for both metastatic and early breast cancers. A reduction of 40% to 50% in contralateral breast cancer was seen in the adjuvant setting; thus, it was thought to be an ideal agent to use in a chemopreventive setting.

The trial to determine the role of tamoxifen in chemoprevention was performed by the NSABP. In this randomized, double-blinded trial, women with a projected risk of breast cancer of greater than 1.66% over a 5-year period received either tamoxifen or a placebo for a period of 5 years. The Gail model was used to assess the risk. This multivariate logistic regression model combines risk factors to estimate the probability of recurrence of breast cancer over time. Variables included in the model are age, number of first-degree relatives with breast cancer, nulliparity or age at first live birth, number of breast biopsies, pathologic diagnosis of atypia or hyperplasia, and age at menarche; the model then predicts the risk for breast cancer in 5 years or life expectancy. Participants eligible for this study were 60 years of age or older, between the ages of 35 and 59 years with a 5-year predicted risk of breast cancer of at least 1.66%, or had a history of LCIS. A total of 368 invasive and noninvasive breast cancers occurred, of which 244 were in the placebo group and 124 in the tamoxifen group. With invasive cancer, there was a 49% reduction in the overall risk (P <0.0001), with a cumulative incidence through 69 months of 43.4 per 1000 women and 22.0 per 1000 women in each of the two groups, respectively. For noninvasive breast cancer, the reduction was 50% (P <0.002). Reduction in noninvasive cancers was related to a decrease in the incidence of both DCIS and LCIS. Tamoxifen reduced the recurrence of ER-positive tumors by 69%, but there was no difference in recurrence of ER-negative tumors. There was, however, no survival difference between the two groups, with only nine deaths attributed to breast cancer, six in the placebo group, and three in the tamoxifen group.

Additionally, there was a 2.5-fold greater risk for development of endometrial cancer in the tamoxifen group compared with patients receiving placebo. There appeared to be no difference in ischemic heart disease or fatal myocardial infarction in the tamoxifen group versus the control group. Vascular events, including stroke, venous thrombosis, and pulmonary embolism, were greater in the tamoxifen-treated patients compared with those receiving placebo (91 vs. 52). There was a reduction in the risk of fracture of the hip, radius, and spine in the tamoxifen group compared with the placebo group, although the reduction was not statistically significant.

When an independent reviewing agency verified a 50% reduction in both invasive and noninvasive breast cancer cases in the population taking tamoxifen, the trial results were unblinded earlier than expected. Shortly thereafter, the use of tamoxifen was approved for chemoprevention. In patients who are desirous of tamoxifen for risk reduction, a discussion of the risks and benefits is important.

Two other chemoprevention trials using tamoxifen have been reported: the Italian tamoxifen-prevention study and the Royal Marsden Hospital tamoxifen trial in the United Kingdom. These two trials did not reveal a statistically significant reduction in breast cancer risk in women randomly assigned to tamoxifen. However, the studies differed in respect to subject numbers, median age, eligibility criteria, risk, and use of HRT.

Another SERM, raloxifene, is approved by the FDA for use in osteoporosis. In studies in which raloxifene was used for the treatment of osteoporosis, a secondary finding was a noted reduction in breast cancer risk of 50% to 70% in the population taking the medication. The women in the trials were at fairly low risk of breast cancer development. Results from the randomized double-blind trial to compare raloxifene with tamoxifen in a population of postmenopausal women at increased risk for breast cancer development, the Study of Tamoxifen and Raloxifene (STAR) trial/P-2 study, were recently reported.

The STAR trial randomized 19,747 postmenopausal women with an increased 5-year Gail risk to receive either tamoxifen or raloxifene. There were 163 and 168 invasive breast cancers in each group, respectively. The conclusion was that they were equivalent in reducing risks of breast cancer in postmenopausal women at high risk. Raloxifene had a better side effect profile, with fewer uterine cancers and thromboembolic events compared with tamoxifen. The risk reduction is thought to be about 50%, which is extrapolated from the P-1 study of tamoxifen and placebo. There was no placebo arm in this study; the conclusions were based on raloxifene having the same risk reduction as tamoxifen in the STAR trial.

In the NSABP P-1 study, there was an increased risk of developing endometrial cancer with tamoxifen use (annual risk, 2.3 of 1000 women versus 0.9 of 1000 women in the placebo group). All cases of endometrial cancer in the patients taking tamoxifen were early stage. Another important side effect noted was a higher incidence of thromboembolic phenomena. Raloxifene does not increase the risk of endometrial cancer and thus may prove to be an adequate alternative to tamoxifen in a chemopreventive role. An ideal SERM would have antiestrogenic effects on breast and uterine tissues but estrogenic effects on bone and the cardiovascular system, among others. Current investigations into other SERMs are being conducted.

Surveillance Versus Prophylactic Surgery in High-risk Patients

Patients with a genetic predisposition to breast cancer often ask about managing their risk. Many of these patients are young women. The diverse issues related to prophylactic mastectomy include both physical and psychologic factors. Appropriate counseling should encompass the extent of cancer risk reduction, surgical risks, and breast reconstruction options. Prophylactic mastectomy has been reported to have a risk reduction of approximately 90% in larger retrospective series with over 10 years of follow-up. Smaller prospective series with shorter follow-up suggest that this may be even higher. However, this reduction often relates to the type of mastectomy performed (eg, subcutaneous mastectomy may not remove all breast tissue).

Women with a genetic predisposition to breast cancer are also candidates for chemoprevention with tamoxifen. In the NSABP P-1 trial, women who had BRCA mutations were not protected by tamoxifen. However, because the number of such patients was small and CIs were wide, more data are needed. In addition, it is likely that chemoprevention may have no significant impact in women with BRCA1, in whom the tumors are predominantly ER negative. The data are still inconclusive regarding BRCA-predisposition genes and the use of tamoxifen for chemoprevention.

Participation in a screening program is another option. The NCCN screening recommendations in BRCA mutation carriers include a semiannual breast examination from the age of 25 years. Annual breast MRI from ages 25 to 29 is preferentially recommended but can be replaced with standard mammography if MRI is not available. From ages 30 to 75 years, both annual breast MRI and mammography are recommended.

These women are also at risk for developing ovarian cancer, and prophylactic oophorectomy at approximately age 40 years is an option. In addition, prophylactic oophorectomy before the age of 40 years has been reported to decrease the risk of breast cancer significantly (≈50%). But even prophylactic risk-reducing salpingo-oophorectomy does not exclude the risk of primary peritoneal cancer, which is estimated at 2%. Ovarian cancer screening programs currently use serum CA-125 and pelvic ultrasonography. Ovarian screening is not recommended for the general population, however, because of the low specificity of the tools currently available.

CONCLUSIONS

Screening for breast cancer is clearly indicated for all women at the appropriate age. Determining a woman's unique risk factors will help to determine both the age at which that screening should begin and the intensity of that screening. It will also help to identify women who need to be counseled regarding options for prevention of breast cancer. The hope is that by correctly identifying high-risk populations and then applying appropriate screening schedules and chemopreventive agents, many cases of breast cancers will be averted completely and that those that still occur will be found at the earliest stages. In addition, the understanding of breast disease, both benign and malignant, is crucial not only in the diagnosis of disease but also in helping to guide women in their treatment and follow-up.

For the bibliography list, log onto www.expertconsult.com ⟨http://www.expertconsult.com⟩.

15

Cancer in Pregnancy

Krishnansu S. Tewari, MD

OUTLINE

KEY POINTS

1. Data from the Surveillance, Epidemiology, and End Results database indicate that cancers during the reproductive ages, in order of decreasing frequency are breast, melanoma, thyroid, cervix, and lymphoma.

2. The most critical period for cancer treatment during pregnancy extends from the 3rd to 8th weeks of development (5th through 10th weeks of gestational age), when susceptibility to teratogenic agents is maximal. In the human fetus, the period of organogenesis usually ends by the 13th week of gestation.

3. Preterm babies have limited ability to metabolize drugs because of immaturity of the hepatic and renal systems. Neonates exposed to chemotherapy 3 weeks before delivery should be assessed for transient bone marrow suppression, and long-term neurologic and developmental follow-up is recommended.

4. As more women opt for conservative management of invasive cancers in an effort to preserve fertility, we may anticipate a larger number of referrals than what was seen previously for patients with persistent or even recurrent malignancy during pregnancy.

5. Many recommend that any child born to a mother with active or suspected malignancy should initially have a thorough physical examination with a complete blood count, comprehensive metabolic panel, liver function tests, coagulation battery, serum lactate dehydrogenase level, uric acid levels, and a urinalysis. In addition, the placenta should be macroscopically and microscopically examined for tumor involvement. It has been our practice to also obtain imaging studies, including magnetic resonance imaging of the brain and computed tomography scans of the chest, abdomen, and pelvis, when maternal breast cancer, hematopoietic malignancy, or melanoma is at issue or in the setting of confirmed placental metastases.

BACKGROUND AND EPIDEMIOLOGY OF CANCER IN PREGNANCY

Cancer in pregnancy poses significant challenges to both the clinician and the pregnant woman. This is undoubtedly the result of the trend to defer childbearing into the fourth decade of life, when the incidence of some of the more common malignant neoplasms begins to rise (Fig. 15.1). The tragedy of the presence of a malignant neoplasm discovered during pregnancy raises many issues (Table 15.1). Fortunately, the peak incidence years for most malignant diseases do not overlap the peak reproductive years (Table 15.2). Thus, as in any unusual situation that physicians rarely encounter, clear therapeutic decisions are not readily at hand. However, a significant number of well-studied reviews can provide some guidance in this dilemma. The largest series ever reported was that of Barber and Brunschwig in 1968, which consisted of 700 cases of cancer in pregnancy. The most common malignant neoplasms in that series were breast tumors and leukemias–lymphomas as a category, melanomas, gynecologic cancer, and bone tumors, in that order. Other authors suggest that gynecologic malignant neoplasms are second only to breast carcinoma and remind us that cancer of the colon and thyroid are also seen in pregnancy (Table 15.3).

The incidence of cancer in pregnancy is unclear but is estimated to be one in 1000. From historical case series collected at a variety of referral institutions, many commentators have concluded that cervical cancer is the most frequent malignancy

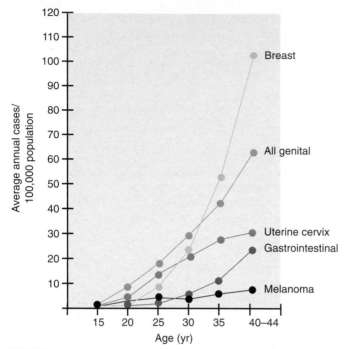

FIGURE 15.1 Incidence by age of the more common malignancies seen in pregnancy. (Data from the American Cancer Society Facts and Figures, 1995.)

TABLE 15.1 Cancer in Pregnancy: Issues to Consider

Oncologic Issues	Obstetric Issues	Ethical, Religious, Medicolegal, and Socioeconomic Issues
Timing of surgery	Fetal effects of therapy	Pregnancy termination
Type of therapy	Antepartum fetal surveillance	Independent advocate for the fetus
Maternal effects of therapy	Corticosteroid administration	Fetal viability
Maternal surveillance	Amniocentesis	Maternal risk
Fertility-sparing therapy	Timing of delivery	Healthcare costs
	Route of delivery	Principle of beneficence
	Neonatal effects of therapy	Right to autonomy
	Long-term effects of therapy	Mother's overall prognosis*

*It is important to take into account the estimated length of time the mother will realistically live to spend with the baby.

TABLE 15.2 Probability of Developing Invasive Cancers (%) Over Selected Age Intervals in Girls and Women, United States, 2003 to 2005

	Birth–39 Years	40–59 Years
All sites	2.07 (1 in 48)	8.97 (1 in 11)
Breast	0.48 (1 in 208)	3.79 (1 in 26)
Melanoma	0.27 (1 in 370)	0.58 (1 in 189)
Uterine cervix	0.15 (1 in 651)	0.27 (1 in 368)
Leukemia	0.12 (1 in 835)	0.14 (1 in 693)
Non-Hodgkin lymphoma	0.08 (1 in 1191)	0.32 (1 in 316)
Colon and rectum	0.07 (1 in 1343)	0.72 (1 in 138)
Uterine corpus	0.07 (1 in 1499)	0.72 (1 in 140)
Lung and bronchus	0.03 (1 in 2997)	0.81 (1 in 124)
Urinary bladder	0.01 (1 in 10,185)	0.12 (1 in 810)

Modified from The American Cancer Society, Surveillance and Health Policy Research, 2009.

TABLE 15.3 Distribution of Tumor Types Among 215 Women Diagnosed With Cancer in Pregnancy From 1998 to 2008 in Belgium, the Netherlands, and the Czech Republic

	Patients (n)	Patients (%)
Breast cancer	99	46
Hematologic malignancies	40	18
Dermatologic malignancies	21	10
Cervical cancer	17	8
Brain tumor	8	4
Ovarian cancer	8	4
Colorectal cancer	5	2
Other (eg, sarcoma, lung, liver, kidney, GI)	17	8

GI, Gastrointestinal.
Modified from Van Calsteren K1, Heyns L, De Smet F, et al. Cancer during pregnancy: an analysis of 215 patients emphasizing the obstetrical and the neonatal outcomes. *J Clin Oncol* 2010;28:683-689.

to complicate pregnancy. This finding is likely to be inaccurate because the incidence of cervical cancer in the United States and in most developed nations is steadily declining. In a 1984 population-based study, Haas reviewed the National Cancer Registry of the German Democratic Republic for the years between 1970 and 1979, and from a total of 31,353 cancer cases and 2,103,112 live births among women between the ages of 15 and 44 years, 355 pregnant women were diagnosed with a malignancy. Dinh and Warshal emphasized that in the Haas study, the incidence of cancer in pregnancy per 1000 live births

rose from 0.02 for women aged 15 to 19 years to 2.3 for women aged 40 to 44 years. In order of decreasing frequency, cancer of the cervix, breast cancer, ovarian cancer, lymphoma, melanoma, brain cancer, and leukemia were found to complicate pregnancy.

In a recent study using data from the Swedish Multi-Generation Register and the National Cancer Registry from 1963 to 2007, Andersson et al. noted that the three most common malignancies during pregnancy were melanoma (n = 232), breast cancer (n = 139), and cervical cancer (n = 139). Interestingly, with a slightly different rank order, these cancers are also the most common to occur in women of childbearing age. Overall the investigators believed that the number of observed cases during pregnancy was lower than expected for all cancers, the reasons of which were unclear. In this study, it was noteworthy that a rebound in the number of observed cases during the postpartum period was restricted to melanoma, nervous system malignancies, and breast and thyroid cancer.

Data from the Surveillance, Epidemiology, and End Results (SEER) program in the United States from 1992 to 1996 estimate that among women aged 15 to 44 years, in order of decreasing frequency, cancer of the breast, melanoma, thyroid cancer, cervical cancer, lymphoma, and ovarian cancer are coincident with pregnancy. The Centers for Disease Control and Prevention have highlighted pregnancy trends in the United States over the preceding 25 years. Although the birth rate for women younger than 30 years of age rose slowly until the early 1990s, it has steadily declined since then. In contrast, the birth rate for women older than 30 years of age has risen steadily over the past 2 decades by an average of 67%. Because of the changing attitudes regarding the role of women as part of the workforce, the delay in childbearing observed in this country will be associated with at least three considerations that are germane to the subject of this chapter.

1. Because many malignancies manifest with advancing age, it is reasonable to expect an increase in the occurrence of some specific types of cancers during pregnancy.
2. Theoretic concerns regarding possible effects of pregnancy-derived hormones among cancer survivors contemplating pregnancy will need to be addressed.
3. With the popularization of investigational fertility-sparing medical and surgical therapy for nulliparous patients with seemingly early lesions who strongly desire to retain childbearing capacity, there exists an increased potential for the oncologist to encounter recurrent disease irrespective of whether pregnancy occurs.

The enormous physiologic changes of pregnancy suggest many possible influences on the malignant state. First, it has been assumed by many that malignant neoplasms arising in tissues and organs influenced by the endocrine system are possibly subject to exacerbation with pregnancy, and this has often been erroneously extrapolated to a recommendation for "therapeutic" abortion. Second, the anatomic and physiologic changes of pregnancy may obscure the subtle changes of an early neoplasm. Third, the increased vascularity and lymphatic drainage may contribute to early dissemination of the malignant process. Although all these hypotheses are interesting, the validity of each is variable, even within the same organ.

Several additional points must be emphasized when caring for a pregnant patient with symptoms suggestive of cancer or in whom the diagnosis has been established. Although pregnancy is usually characterized by extensive medical observation, a delay in diagnosis can occur if attention is not paid to the subtle presentation of malignancies. Thus, although pregnancy has not been shown to increase the virulence of any tumor type, many pregnancy-associated cancers portend a poor prognosis for the woman. Even though many essayists have claimed that the conduct of the pregnancy is not affected by the cohabitation of malignancy, the oncologist must recognize that some tumor types have been shown to metastasize to the placenta and even to the fetus. In all cases of pregnancy complicated by malignancy, it is advisable to have a multidisciplinary team of specialists involved in the care of the patient.

When considering therapy in pregnancy, surgery is rarely contraindicated, with the optimal time being in the second trimester. Chemotherapy for the most part should have restricted use during the first trimester but can generally be safely administered thereafter. Certain diagnostic imaging procedures can be safely performed during pregnancy, but in most cases, radiation therapy should be postponed until after delivery. Aggressive nutritional support is a mandatory requirement for pregnant women with cancer. In the majority of cases, with a proper coordination of effort, the pregnancy need not be terminated to begin treatment.

Report From the European Society of Gynecological Oncology Cancer in Pregnancy Task Force

Amant et al. recently reported updated guidelines from the Second International Consensus Meeting arranged to disseminate experts' knowledge and form consensus guidelines for medical and oncologic intervention to address maternal malignancy diagnosed during pregnancy and the postpartum period. Protocols for management of pregnancy-associated cervical cancer, ovarian cancer, and vulvar cancer were reviewed. The guidelines developed advocate following standard treatment protocol as for nonpregnant patients to maximize maternal outcome but with the caveat that iatrogenic prematurity should be avoided. The experts committee stressed effective psychologic support throughout the pregnancy and endorsed diagnostic procedures including open or laparoscopic surgical staging examinations, as well as imaging being preferably performed using nonionizing radiation modalities such as magnetic resonance imaging (MRI) and ultrasonography. Importantly, most chemotherapy regimens were thought to be tolerable and safe from 14 weeks' gestational age onward. Although term delivery should be the goal, apart from cervical and vulvar cancer (with concomitant vulvar scarring), the mode of delivery should be based in most cases on obstetric indications.

THE MORE COMMON SOLID TUMORS IN PREGNANCY

Cervical Cancer

Cervical cancer complicates approximately 1 in 1200 pregnancies. As a consequence of widespread cytologic screening, the dramatic decrease in invasive cervical cancer observed in recent years has been paralleled by a rise in cervical intraepithelial neoplasia (CIN), especially in younger women. Because the peak incidence for both CIN and childbearing occurs during the third decade of life, abnormal Papanicolaou smears are common among gravid women, occurring at a rate of 0.5% to 5%. The diagnosis of cervical dysplasia in pregnancy may occur in up to 5% of some populations. For these reasons, screening for cervical neoplasia is an essential component of prenatal care. All pregnant women should have a cervical smear submitted for cytology. The ectocervix and endocervical canal should be sampled adequately. Patients noted to have a visible lesion should undergo cervical biopsy immediately because cervical smears taken directly from tumors often contain only inflammatory cells. A recent review from the

Magee Gynecologic Cancer Program in Pittsburgh noted that in some populations, up to 20% of pregnant women have an abnormal Pap result during pregnancy. Nearly 3% of newly diagnosed cervical cancer cases occur in pregnant women, probably because it is the one cancer that is screened for as part of routine prenatal care.

In concordance with the known risk factors for invasive cervical cancer, pregnant women who develop CIN tend to marry at an earlier age, have a higher parity, and are diagnosed at an earlier age than nonpregnant women with CIN. Hacker and colleagues compiled data from nine reports and noted that the average age of patients with carcinoma in situ (CIS) during pregnancy was 29.9 years, and the average parity was 4.0. Among nonpregnant women, the average age of CIS is 35 years. The investigators noted that the median age of patients diagnosed with invasive carcinoma of the cervix during pregnancy is 33.8 years (range, 17–47 years), and the average parity is 4.5. The average parity among pregnant women with cervical cancer was 5.4 in a study reported by Creasman and colleagues; in this group, increasing parity was not associated with a more advanced lesion, nor did it have an impact on prognosis.

Human Papillomavirus in Pregnancy

Although human papillomavirus virus (HPV) is strongly associated with cervical dysplasia and carcinoma in both nonpregnant and pregnant women, a significant relationship between pregnancy and HPV prevalence has not been established. Eversion of the endocervical epithelium results in exposure to the acidity of the vaginal environment, producing a high degree of squamous metaplasia. This metaplasia is important because HPV requires active cellular machinery to reproduce and transform cells. Schneider and colleagues examined the negative cervical smears of 92 pregnant and 96 nonpregnant, age-matched control participants for the presence of HPV DNA by Southern blot hybridization. The investigators demonstrated both an increased prevalence of HPV (preferentially the oncolytic HPV subtype 16) and a higher replication rate of viral DNA during pregnancy. Using the ViraPap/ViraType dot blot DNA hybridization procedure, Smith and coworkers detected an increase in HPV prevalence with advancing gestational age, suggesting that as estrogen levels increase, pregnant women may be more vulnerable to HPV infection. Using similar hybridization methods, however, Kemp and colleagues and Chang-Claude and colleagues were unable to demonstrate a higher prevalence of HPV infection during pregnancy.

Castellsague and colleagues performed a prospective study in Barcelona to quantitate the mother-to-child transmission of HPV subtypes. This study included 66 HPV-positive and 77 HPV-negative pregnant women and their offspring. To estimate HPV prevalence and genotypic distribution in pregnancy, the investigators also carried out a related screening survey of cervical HPV DNA detection among 828 pregnant women. Exfoliated cells from the mouth and external genitalia of the infants were collected at birth and at several intervals up to 2 years of age. At 418 infant visits and a mean follow-up time of 14 months, 19.7% of infants born to HPV-positive mothers and 16.9% of those born to HPV-negative mothers tested HPV

positive at some point during the infants' follow-up. The most frequently detected genotype both in infants and in mothers was HPV-16. Of note, there was a strong and statistically significant association between mother's and child's HPV status at the 6-week postpartum visit in that children of mothers who were HPV positive at the postpartum visit were five times more likely to test HPV positive than children of corresponding HPV-negative mothers ($P = 0.02$). The authors concluded that the risk of vertical transmission of HPV genotypes is relatively low and that vertical transmission may not be the sole source of HPV infections in infants. There exists the potential for horizontal mother-to-child transmission.

Evaluation of the Papanicolaou Smear in Pregnancy

The cytopathologist frequently encounters atypical cells when reviewing the cervical smear from a pregnant patient. Cells within the endocervical canal that undergo the Arias–Stella reaction may contain a vacuolated clear or oxyphilic cytoplasm, intraglandular tufts, hobnail patterns, delicate filiform papillae, intranuclear pseudoinclusions, cribriform intraglandular growth, and even occasional mitotic figures. Distinguishing features of dysplastic and frankly malignant cells would include an infiltrative pattern, spectrum of cytologic atypia, a high nuclear-to-cytoplasmic ratio, and increased mitotic activity. Other atypical cells exfoliated by the endocervix in pregnant women include small decidualized cells with sharp cytoplasmic borders and hypochromatic nuclei, but unlike dysplastic cells, decidualized cells contain regular chromatin and distinct nuclei. Finally, large, multinucleated trophoblastic cells may be discharged from the uterus. At this time, it is not clear if liquid-based cytology can decrease the false-positive rate. Nevertheless, careful inspection of the cervical smear maintains its reliability as a screening test for dysplasia among pregnant patients.

The Performance of Colposcopy in Pregnancy

Colposcopy is facilitated by the pregnancy-induced eversion of the normal cervical ectropion. **However, pregnancy results in dramatic alterations in the colposcopic appearance of the cervix, the most significant changes resulting from the elevated levels of circulating estrogen, which produces a significant increase in cervical volume through hypertrophy of the fibromuscular stroma.** The increased vascularity produces a bluish hue, which is then exaggerated with application of acetic acid to the metaplastic epithelium in pregnancy. Toward the end of the first trimester, eversion and metaplasia produce areas of fusion of columnar villa and distinct islands or fingers of immature metaplastic epithelium. Fine punctation and even mosaicism may accompany metaplasia, which in and of itself produces an acetowhite effect. Tenacious endocervical mucus develops, which further hinders colposcopic examination. Finally, stromal edema, enlargement of glandular structures, acute inflammatory responses, and stromal decidualization may occur in the second and third trimesters, which, although physiologic, may appear suspicious to the inexperienced colposcopist. For these reasons, colposcopy in pregnancy is difficult and should be reserved for an experienced gynecologist.

The aim of colposcopy in pregnancy is to exclude cancer, and only one directed biopsy of the site compatible with the most advanced area of dysplastic change should be performed to establish the histologic level of disease. Because of false-negative results ranging from 8% to 40%, random or nondirected biopsies should be avoided. **Great care must be exercised because the increased vascularity may lead to precipitous, heavy bleeding.** A Tischler or baby Tischler biopsy forceps should be used followed by immediate placement of a cotton-tipped applicator above the cervical epithelium. If bleeding occurs, it may be controlled with three silver nitrate sticks or with dehydrated Monsel's solution. An endocervical curettage, however, is best avoided during pregnancy.

Yoonessi and colleagues conducted a retrospective analysis of suspected CIN associated with pregnancy and concluded that colposcopic examination with or without directed biopsy eliminated the need for cervical conization in 104 of 107 patients. In their classic paper, Hacker and colleagues noted that serious morbidity, such as hemorrhage, preterm labor, miscarriage, or infection, only infrequently occurs when directed biopsies are performed. For 1064 reported colposcopic examinations during pregnancy, the diagnostic accuracy was 99.5%, and the complication rate was 0.6%. No case of frankly invasive carcinoma was missed, and the two cases of microinvasion missed on colposcopic biopsy both had a colposcopic pattern suggestive of microinvasion, which was confirmed by subsequent conization. Thus, in experienced hands, colposcopy reduces the need for cone biopsy in pregnancy, with a false-negative rate of less than 0.5%.

Recently, Wetta and colleagues presented the University of Alabama experience on 625 pregnant women with CIN. The most common referral cytology was low-grade squamous intraepithelial lesions (LSIL; 41%) followed by atypical squamous cells of undetermined significance (ASC-US; 34.1%) and high-grade squamous intraepithelial lesions (HSILs; 13.6%). Of the 269 patients with ASC-US and LSIL cytology, 20 of 78 patients who underwent cervical biopsy were diagnosed with CIN II or III. Of the 128 patients with HSIL, 31 of 60 patients who underwent cervical biopsy were diagnosed with CIN II or III. Repeat colposcopy in the third trimester was performed on 47 patients, and only three of 13 patients who had a repeat biopsy had CIN II or III. The authors concluded that pregnant patients with ASC-US or LSIL cytology rarely have colposcopically suspected CIN II or III at their initial colposcopy that warrants a cervical biopsy. The investigators consider it reasonable to defer the initial colposcopy in these cases until at least 6 weeks postpartum.

Onuma and colleagues have evaluated the diagnosis of ASC-H (atypical squamous cells with possible HSIL) in 60 patients. Among 30 who had histologic follow-up, three women (10%) had HSIL, and 13 (43%) had LSIL. Among 32 women who had cytologic follow-up, two (6%) had HSIL, three (9%) had LSIL, one (3%) had ASC-H, and three (9%) had ASC-US. High-risk HPV DNA was detected in 24 of 43 patients (56%). The authors suggest that ASC-H in pregnant women has a lower predictive value for an underlying HSIL compared with the general population. Although a positive high-risk HPV DNA test result was not a good indicator for underlying SIL, a negative result appeared useful for ruling out an underlying HSIL. The authors advocated for a more conservative follow-up for pregnant women with ASC-H and support using high-risk HPV DNA testing as an adjunctive test.

The Natural History of Cervical Intraepithelial Neoplasia in Pregnancy

It appears that in an immunocompetent host evaluated colposcopically and pathologically by experienced eyes, CIN rarely, if ever, progresses to microinvasive disease during pregnancy. In fact, there appears to be a subset of patients who will experience disease regression after delivery of the neonate. Postpartum regression rates for abnormal cervical cytology consistent with dysplasia (combining both LSIL and HSIL) have ranged from 25% to 77%. This wide range is hard to explain, with some authors postulating that regression occurs in at least one-third of patients as a consequence of resolution of pregnancy-induced changes in the maternal immunologic system. An Italian study published in 2008 detailed the natural history of CIN in 78 pregnant women. Among those with CIN II or III ($n = 36$; 46.2%), no invasion was suspected during pregnancy, and at the postpartum evaluation, no invasive or microinvasive cancer was diagnosed. Of note, there were 19 (52.7%) cases of persistent CIN II or III and 42 (53.8%) regressions. The authors noted that CIN I has a significantly higher tendency to spontaneous regression compared with nonpregnant women with CIN I. High-risk HPV testing may improve the follow-up of patients with SIL in pregnancy and postpartum to assist in the diagnosis of persistent infections.

Some authors have advanced the theory that vaginal birth trauma may result in the complete debridement of dysplastic tissues. This phenomenon was observed by Ahdoot and colleagues in a prospective collection of abnormal cytology during pregnancy and in the postpartum period. The investigators observed a 60% regression rate among women with HSILs who delivered vaginally versus 0% in those with HSILs who delivered by cesarean section ($P <0.0002$). A study by Siristatidis and colleagues demonstrated a 66.6% regression rate among women with HSILs who delivered vaginally versus 12.5% of those with HSILs who delivered by cesarean section ($P <0.002$). In direct contradistinction, the cytologic study by Murta and colleagues (LSILs in pregnancy) and the pregnancy-related histologic investigations by Murta and colleagues (CIN CIN II or III), Yost and colleagues (CIN II or III), and Coppola and colleagues (CIS) failed to show any statistically significant difference in postpartum regression rates for patients who delivered vaginally versus those who labored and went on to deliver by cesarean section versus those who underwent elective cesarean delivery.

A recent report by Ueda and colleagues describes the experience with CIN in pregnancy at Osaka University Hospital. The investigators observed regression of CIN in 34 (76%) of 45 cases of vaginal delivery and in six (50%) of 12 cases of cesarean delivery, indicating that the outcome of an initially diagnosed CIN and the delivery routes appear not to be significantly related. However, a different result was obtained when only patients whose CIN lesions persisted until the delivery were analyzed. Among the 35 such cases in the vaginal delivery group, 24 cases (69%) regressed after the delivery; in eight such cases from the cesarean delivery group, only two cases (25%) regressed after delivery. There was also significantly more frequent postpartum regression of biopsy-proven CIN lesions after vaginal delivery compared with cesarean section ($P = 0.042$; odds ratio [OR] 6.55; 95% confidence interval [CI], 1.13–37.8).

Conization and Related Procedures in Pregnancy

The performance of a cone biopsy during pregnancy is a formidable undertaking, and one must weigh the risks of the procedure against the anticipated yield of microinvasive carcinoma (MIC), which would remain otherwise undetected. **Maternal risk appears to be restricted to either immediate or delayed hemorrhage, occurring in up to 14% of cases and exceeding 400 mL when the procedure is performed during the third trimester.** Averette and colleagues reported the largest series of cold knife cervical conization biopsies in pregnancy and noted that 9.4% of the study group ($n = 180$) required a blood transfusion. Maternal death has not been reported. Injury to the pregnancy, resulting in spontaneous abortion, intrauterine infection, and preterm birth, however, places the fetus at considerable risk. Rogers and Williams presented a series of 72 pregnancy conizations and reported a perinatal complication rate of 19.4%. Across the literature, the risk of pregnancy loss when the procedure is performed during the first trimester ranges from 15.2% to 33%. **Overall, cone biopsy in pregnancy is associated with a 3% to 6% risk of perinatal death as a consequence of profuse hemorrhage or from delivery of a previable or extremely premature fetus through an incompetent cervix.** A further point that needs emphasizing is that 30% to 57% of pregnant cones will have dysplasia, microinvasive tumor, or both at the endocervical or ectocervical margins. For this reason, the procedure should not be considered therapeutic in the pregnant patient.

The large-loop electrosurgical excision of the transformation zone (LLETZ) may be used in the operating room to excise a shallow cone of sufficient breadth and depth to permit treatment decisions during pregnancy. Robinson and colleagues reported on 20 women who underwent LLETZ from 8 to 34 weeks of gestational age and noted significant morbidity in patients treated between 27 and 34 weeks of gestational age, including two blood transfusions, three preterm births, and one unexplained intrauterine fetal demise 4 weeks postprocedure. Mitsuhashi and Sekiya performed a LLETZ on nine women during the first 14 weeks of pregnancy, none of whom experienced spontaneous abortion, premature delivery, or excessive bleeding. These preliminary results suggest that LLETZ can be performed safely during the first trimester of pregnancy, but there are insufficient data to determine whether this procedure can replace the traditional cold knife cone biopsy. LLETZ is also associated with a significant proportion of patients left with residual disease.

Hacker and colleagues commented that most authors reserve conization for patients in whom the transformation zone was not fully visualized, microinvasion was shown on biopsy or

suspected colposcopically, or possible adenocarcinoma was found on biopsy. If colposcopy is unsatisfactory, one alternative to a full cone is a wedge resection of the cervix, removing only areas incompletely visualized colposcopically. **Another option is to place six hemostatic sutures, evenly distributed around the perimeter of the cervix close to the vaginal reflection (Fig. 15.2). These sutures reduce blood flow to the cone bed, evert the squamocolumnar junction, and facilitate performance of a shallow "coin" biopsy with little interruption of the endocervical canal (Fig. 15.3).**

To offset the risk of cervical incompetence, Goldberg and colleagues performed 17 cone cerclages between 12 and 27 weeks of gestation. All procedures were performed with the patient under general anesthesia. After injection of the entire ectocervix with vasopressin (20 units in 60 mL of normal saline), lateral hemostatic 2-0 polyglycolic acid sutures were

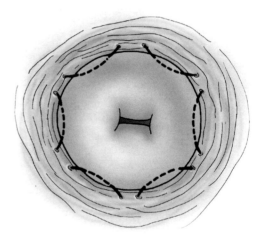

FIGURE 15.2 The locations of six hemostatic sutures. (From Creasy RK, Resnick R. *Maternal–Fetal Medicine: Principles and Practice.* Philadelphia, 1987, Saunders.)

FIGURE 15.3 Demonstration of shallow "coin" biopsy appropriate in pregnancy. (From Creasy RK, Resnick R. *Maternal–Fetal Medicine: Principles and Practice.* Philadelphia, 1987, Saunders.)

placed at the 10 and 2 o'clock positions on the cervix, and a standard McDonald cerclage using #1 nylon suture material was inserted as high and as close to the internal cervical os as technically possible without reflection of the bladder. After the cervical cone was excised, the McDonald suture was tied with the knot placed anteriorly, and an iodoform vaginal pack inserted for 24 hours. All 17 patients had uneventful pregnancies, delivering viable infants at or beyond 34 weeks of gestation.

Tsuritani and colleagues have reported on the safety and efficacy of CO_2 laser conization in pregnant women with CIN III or CIS ($n = 30$) and MIC ($n = 19$). The median gestational age was 17 weeks, and the median length of cervix resected was 14 mm. The median duration of surgery was 20 minutes, and median blood loss was 78 mL. Laser conization identified one case of International Federation of Gynecology and Obstetrics (FIGO) Ia2 carcinoma and three cases of FIGO IB1 disease. Of the 35 women who were able to be followed through until delivery, 27 (77.1%) delivered vaginally. Although eight (22.9%) had cesarean sections and six (17.1%) delivered preterm, no CO_2 conization–related obstetric complications were observed.

Fambrini and colleagues have performed CO_2 laser conization in 26 pregnant patients with biopsy-proven CIS or CIN III whose colposcopic evaluation was suspicious for invasion. The procedures were performed during the 18th week of gestation, and no major intraoperative or postoperative complications occurred. Two cases of occult FIGO stage IA1 carcinoma with free surgical margins were diagnosed. Twenty patients (76.9%) delivered vaginally, and six patients underwent cesarean section for indications not related to the prior conization. After a mean postpartum follow-up time of 18 months, 92.3% of patients were cytologically and colposcopically negative for persistent or recurrent disease. Two cases of persistent CIN were managed successfully by reconization.

Management of Cervical Intraepithelial Neoplasia in Pregnancy

An algorithm that illustrates several key points concerning the management of CIN in pregnancy is proposed in Fig. 15.4. The critical issue is to exclude the coexistence of microinvasive disease with pregnancy. This is because everything else,

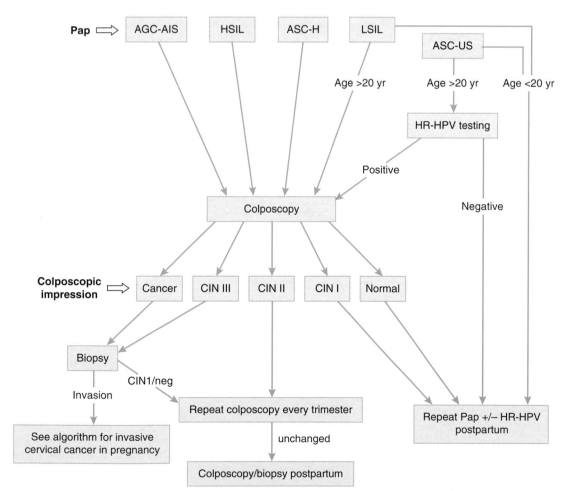

FIGURE 15.4 Management of abnormal cytologic findings in pregnancy. *AGC-AIS,* atypical glandular cells-adenocarcinoma in situ; *ASC-H,* atypical squamous cells with possible high-grade squamous intraepithelial lesion; *ASC-US,* atypical squamous cells of undetermined significance; *CIN,* cervical intraepithelial neoplasia; *ECC,* endocervical curettage; *HR-HPV,* high risk-human papillomavirus; *HSIL,* high-grade squamous intraepithelial lesion; *LSIL,* low-grade squamous intraepithelial lesion; *Pap,* Papanicolaou smear.

the gamut between cellular atypia and CIS, can be followed expectantly during pregnancy, with treatment deferred after its conclusion. We emphasize the following steps:

1. All abnormal cervical smears in pregnancy (excluding HPV-negative atypia) should prompt an evaluation by colposcopy.
2. An experienced colposcopist must accurately assess the disease to determine whether a directed biopsy is indicated.
3. In cases involving a CIS on directed biopsy, a coordinated effort between the gynecologist and the pathologist should be undertaken to determine whether an excisional biopsy is required to exclude invasion.

Management of Squamous Cell Abnormalities

In 2006, the American Society for Colposcopy and Cervical Pathology (ASCCP) updated its recommendations for cervical cancer screening in pregnancy and management of CIN and AIS in pregnancy. Highlights of these recommendations (which were published in 2007) include the following:

For squamous cell abnormalities:

1. Expectant management during pregnancy is acceptable for CIN I to III and CIS.
2. In patients for whom there is no concern for microinvasion, serial colposcopy during pregnancy (eg, every trimester) is not necessary.
3. Definitive management of CIN and CIS should be deferred to the postpartum period in most cases.

Pregnant women with normal prenatal cytologic screening traditionally undergo repeat screening during the postpartum period. Patients with a prenatal Papanicolaou test consistent with ASC-US may undergo reflex testing for oncolytic HPV subtypes if the Hybrid Capture II test (Digene Corporation) is available. Patients who test HPV negative may be reevaluated with cervical cytology 6 to 8 weeks after delivery. Pregnant women who are found to have cytology consistent with ASC-US and are high-risk HPV positive should be referred for colposcopic evaluation. Patients with cytology consistent with atypical squamous cells favoring a high-grade lesion, LSILs, HSILs, and squamous cell carcinoma (SCC) (and all Papanicolaou tests suggesting glandular cell abnormalities) should be referred for colposcopic evaluation. Because of the high prevalence of HPV in cytologic smears consistent with intraepithelial lesions and carcinoma, HPV testing is not indicated.

If the colposcopic impression is normal or consistent with CIN I, the Papanicolaou test with or without colposcopy can be repeated in the postpartum period provided that the original Papanicolaou test was not consistent with a high-grade lesion; if colposcopy was performed because of HSILs or SCC, the colposcopic evaluation should be repeated each trimester of the pregnancy, with a directed punch biopsy taken if the impression is consistent with progressive disease (above CIN II).

Patients for whom colposcopy is consistent with CIN II or greater should undergo a single directed biopsy. If this reveals CIN III or worse, the patient should undergo repeat colposcopic evaluation each trimester, with definitive treatment reserved for after delivery, provided there is no evidence for disease progression.

Patients whose biopsies are suspicious for microinvasion should undergo one of the excisional procedures described previously (ie, conization or LLETZ with or without cerclage, coin biopsy, or wedge biopsy). **If microinvasion is excluded, the patient should be observed during the pregnancy with colposcopy.** If microinvasion is established either by directed punch biopsy or by excisional biopsy, recommendations specific for malignant disease must be sought (see later).

In some circumstances, the colposcopic evaluation will be unsatisfactory, in that the entire transformation zone cannot be completely evaluated. If there is no evidence of a severe lesion in the evaluable areas and the original Papanicolaou test was not consistent with SCC or adenocarcinoma in situ (AIS), close observation with repeat colposcopy during each trimester of the pregnancy may be considered. Under more dire scenarios, a coin biopsy of the cervix or a wedge biopsy of the hidden part of the transformation zone may be necessary.

Management of Glandular Cell Abnormalities

Cervical smears containing glandular cell abnormalities may be reported as atypical cells not otherwise specified (AGC-NOS), atypical cells favor neoplasia, AIS, or even adenocarcinoma. **Of note, 40% of cervices associated with an atypical glandular cells of undetermined significance (AGUS) smear will have a significant tissue abnormality, with greater than 50% harboring an SIL.** The significance of an AGUS Papanicolaou result in pregnant and in postpartum women is not yet clear. In a recent manuscript by Chhieng and colleagues, 30 pregnant women and five within the immediate postpartum window were evaluated for a cytologic diagnosis of AGUS. Of 27 women for whom there was follow-up, 17 underwent colposcopic examination and biopsy. Five women (29.4%) had CIN, including three high-grade and two low-grade lesions on biopsy. It is interesting that the remaining patients (70.6%) had benign pathology, which included chronic cervicitis (*n* = 5), endocervical endometrial polyps (or both) (*n* = 4), Arias–Stella reaction (*n* = 2), and microglandular hyperplasia (*n* = 1); of the 10 patients who had repeat Papanicolaou tests, only two had persistent AGUS or ASC-US. Nevertheless, the finding that up to 30% of patients with pregnancy-associated AGUS had a significant preneoplastic lesion warrants careful evaluation.

The clinician's diagnostic armamentarium is limited during pregnancy. In the absence of a visible lesion or a significantly expanded cervix (ie, the barrel-shaped cervix), all patients with AGUS smears should undergo colposcopic evaluation with directed biopsy. Patients diagnosed with a squamous lesion or AIS should be evaluated by colposcopy during subsequent trimesters. It is not known whether a patient with AIS on directed biopsy should undergo wedge resection of that area to rule out invasion in a nearby "skip" lesion. A diagnostic LLETZ cold knife cervical conization (or both) during pregnancy is best reserved only for those few cases in which an AIS or squamous lesion suspicious for microinvasion is encountered on directed biopsy.

If colposcopy is unrevealing, however, the concern is raised that an endocervical lesion high in the canal or even within the endometrial compartment is being missed. Nevertheless, an endocervical curettage, cervical dilatation with fractional uterine curettage, or endometrial aspiration biopsy is best deferred until the postpartum period, when even a full cervical conization can be performed if needed. Therefore in these clinical scenarios, consultation with the cytopathologist should be arranged to determine if the original Papanicolaou slide contains troublesome features such as inflammatory cells, polyps, glandular hyperplasia, or the Arias–Stella reaction, any of which could confuse the picture, especially when dealing with an AGC-NOS Papanicolaou smear. Gravid women with a negative colposcopic survey for an atypical glandular cell (AGC) favoring neoplasia cervical smear can be evaluated safely in pregnancy with either endovaginal ultrasonography or MRI of the pelvis to search for a lesion within the endometrium or endocervical canal. In these latter circumstances, referral to a gynecologic oncologist should be contemplated.

The 2006 ASCCP management schema for AIS includes the following:

1. Expectant management during pregnancy is acceptable for AIS.
2. In patients for whom there is no concern for microinvasion, serial colposcopy during pregnancy (eg, every trimester) is not necessary.
3. Definitive management of AIS should be deferred to the postpartum period.

Intrapartum Hysterectomy

Some authors have described a program in which an intrapartum hysterectomy (after either vaginal or cesarean birth) is performed for patients with CIS or AIS who have completed childbearing or have proved to be noncompliant. Because there is not sufficient evidence to suggest that an immunocompetent patient is at risk for rapid progression of disease during pregnancy, the need to remove the diseased segment of the cervix is not urgent. Intrapartum hysterectomies, both elective and nonelective, can be associated with significant blood loss. Furthermore, among inexperienced obstetricians, the bladder is particularly at risk for injury. One must balance the noncompliance of a given patient with the possibility that microinvasion may not have been sufficiently excluded during pregnancy, especially in cases of CIS or AIS with positive margins. The observation that postpartum regression may also occur with even CIS argues against the routine performance of an intrapartum hysterectomy for the management of CIN in pregnancy.

Invasive Cervical Cancer

Presenting symptoms in order of frequency among pregnant women with cervical carcinoma include abnormal vaginal bleeding (63%), vaginal discharge (13%), postcoital bleeding (4%), and pelvic pain (2%). Of importance, in the review by Hacker and colleagues, 18% of patients were asymptomatic, as were 30% of the patients in the study by Creasman and colleagues. When bleeding occurs, this symptom must be investigated and not automatically attributed to the pregnancy. Examination during the first trimester will not lead to abortion. Third-trimester bleeding can be adequately assessed in the operating room as a double setup procedure. Many times, visual inspection is all that is needed for diagnosis of this malignant neoplasm. The FIGO staging system applies also in pregnancy.

To avoid the risks of radiation exposure to a developing fetus, the author recommends ultrasonography of the kidneys to evaluate for the presence of hydronephrosis and an MRI of the pelvis when there is concern for parametrial extension of the tumor. Chest radiography may be performed with appropriate abdominal shielding to exclude pulmonary metastases. An algorithm for the suggested management of invasive cervical cancer in pregnancy appears in Fig. 15.5.

A working group was set up in 2007 in France to propose national recommendations for the management of pregnant patients with invasive cervical cancer. The management of cervical cancer during pregnancy is affected by five factors:

1. FIGO stage (and tumor size)
2. Nodal status
3. Histologic subtype of the tumor
4. Gestational age at diagnosis
5. Patient's wishes regarding continuation of pregnancy

In patients with early-stage disease diagnosed during the first two trimesters of pregnancy, there is an increasing tendency to preserve the pregnancy while awaiting fetal maturity in patients with absence of nodal involvement.

Microinvasive Disease

The diagnosis of MIC in pregnancy is typically established with colposcopic directed biopsy, and in a minority of cases in which the colposcopic biopsy cannot exclude microinvasion, a shallow coin biopsy or the cervix or wedge excision of the area under suspicion as outlined earlier is suggested. This is the only absolute indication for conization during pregnancy. Conization distinguishes patients who have "early stromal invasion" and who can proceed to term without appreciable risk to their survival from those with frank invasion in whom consideration must be given to early interruption of the pregnancy. The author advises patients with early stromal invasion (ie, FIGO stage Ia1) that the pregnancy may continue safely to term, provided the surgical margins are free. Karrberg et al. recently published their 16-year experience from the Western Region of Sweden and emphasize that early detection of cytologic atypia and proper follow-up during pregnancy will likely lead to detection of a high proportion of stage 1 cases, many of which could be cured via cervical conization, thus preserving current and future fertility.

Cesarean section is not thought to be necessary for this group of patients, and the route of delivery should be determined by obstetric indications. Patients with FIGO stage Ia2 or occult Ib1 lesions should undergo cesarean delivery when fetal pulmonary maturation is demonstrable followed by an immediate modified radical abdominal hysterectomy with bilateral pelvic lymphadenectomies. The author advocates the deployment of a vertical uterine incision so as to leave the lower uterine segment undisturbed for subsequent detailed pathologic examination. It is interesting that the physiologic changes of pregnancy actually enhance the performance of radical surgery by providing the surgeon with multiple levels of distinct tissue planes.

Recently, reports of laser conization for microinvasive disease have originated from Japan. As described earlier, Tsuritani and

FIGURE 15.5 Suggested therapy for cervical cancer in pregnancy. *C/S,* cesarean section; *HDR BT,* high dose rate brachytherapy.

colleagues have included 19 women with MIC in their series of 49 women and considered CO_2 laser conization within 20 mm of length to be safe in pregnant patients. Yahata and colleagues have reported their experience with four patients diagnosed with stage IA1 cervical adenocarcinoma who underwent KTP (potassium titanyl phosphate) laser conization and vaporization from 16 to 23 weeks of gestation. All patients delivered at term, at which point they underwent radical hysterectomy with lymphadenectomy ($n = 3$) or cold knife conization ($n = 1$). None have developed recurrent disease during a 2- to 13-year follow-up period.

Cesarean–Radical Hysterectomy With Pelvic Lymphadenectomies

In deciding on therapy for frankly invasive cervical cancer in pregnancy, the physician must consider both the stage of disease and the duration of pregnancy. The decision can often be influenced by the religious convictions of the patient and family and the desire of the mother for the child. For FIGO stage I and FIGO stage IIa lesions, radical hysterectomy with bilateral lymphadenectomy is acceptable during any trimester (Fig. 15.6). **We prefer the surgical approach because of the overall result, which includes ovarian preservation, improved sexual function, and elimination of unnecessary delays for the patient.** The complication rate of radical surgery for cervical carcinoma in pregnant patients does not exceed that in non-pregnant patients when normal surgical principles are scrupulously followed.

Monk and Montz examined their institutional experience in treating invasive cervical cancer complicating intrauterine pregnancy with radical hysterectomy. They identified 13 patients treated with radical hysterectomy and bilateral pelvic

FIGURE 15.6 An 18-week-old fetus. Cervical cancer with a vaginal cuff and an extruding placenta are seen in a radical hysterectomy specimen from a 32-year-old patient.

lymphadenectomy with the fetus in situ and eight others treated with cesarean delivery followed by radical hysterectomy and bilateral pelvic lymph node dissection. The mean operative time was 281 minutes, and the mean blood loss was 777 mL for radical hysterectomy with the fetus in situ plus lymphadenectomy and

1750 mL when cesarean section preceded the cancer operation. The surgical morbidity was minimal for the whole group, and after documentation of fetal maturation, seven healthy infants were delivered. Twenty patients (95%) are alive and free of disease with a mean follow-up of 40 months. The authors concluded that radical surgery offers immediate treatment for early-stage cervical cancer during intrauterine pregnancy, with low associated morbidity, acceptable survival, and preservation of ovarian function.

Radical Trachelectomy With Lymphadenectomy

In recent years, several reports have appeared describing the successful performance of radical trachelectomy during pregnancy. Abu-Rustum and colleagues treated a 37-year-old pregnant woman at 15 weeks of gestational age for a FIGO stage IB1 poorly differentiated lymphoepithelioma-like cervical carcinoma found on conization. The procedure was performed abdominally and included bilateral pelvic lymphadenectomies and permanent cerclage placement. The final pathology revealed 7-mm (of 19-mm) invasion with no lymphovascular involvement, negative margins, and negative nodes. The pregnancy was delivered by elective planned cesarean hysterectomy at 39 weeks of gestational age. This procedure has also been safely performed during the 19th week of gestation by Mandic and colleagues. Again, the abdominal approach was used, and the patient underwent successful cesarean section at 36 weeks of gestation. At the time of manuscript acceptance, the patient was in the 15th week of a new pregnancy and had normal cytologic screening and no evidence of metastatic or recurrent carcinoma. Finally, Gurney and Blank have described a patient diagnosed with FIGO IB1 disease at 21 weeks of gestational age who underwent postpartum radical abdominal trachelectomy. Ungar and colleagues reported five cases of radical abdominal trachelectomy during pregnancy and the birth of two healthy term infants.

The first case of vaginal radical trachelectomy was reported by van de Nieuwenhof and colleagues to have occurred at 16 weeks of gestation for a FIGO stage IB1 lesion. This patient underwent an uneventful cesarean section followed by radical hysterectomy at 36 weeks of gestational age, and at 9 months of follow-up, both the mother and infant were doing well.

Alouini and colleagues reported laparoscopic pelvic (with and without aortic) lymphadenectomy during pregnancy in eight patients from 12 to 32 weeks of gestation. There were no surgical or general anesthetic maternal or fetal complications. The mean number of lymph nodes removed was 18 (range, 11–28), and in five patients (stage IB1, $n = 4$; stage IB1, $n = 1$), there was pathologic evidence of nodal metastases. One patient experienced a spontaneous abortion after radical trachelectomy, but the remaining seven reached fetal maturity and had healthy babies by cesarean section. Laparoscopic staging with retrieval of 19 negative nodes for a FIGO stage IB1 carcinoma complicating a twin pregnancy was safely performed at 17 weeks of gestation by Favero and colleagues.

Finally, Silva and colleagues explored the possibility of sentinel lymph node (SLN) mapping in pregnant patients with cervical cancer. They reported the first case of SLN detection using technetium-labeled radiocolloid. Histologic analysis of the operative specimen demonstrated a poorly differentiated squamous carcinoma with metastasis n the sentinel and a neoplastic embolus in a blood vessel of the placental bed.

Whole-Pelvis Radiotherapy With Intracavitary Brachytherapy

Radiation therapy is equally efficacious in treating patients with early-stage (ie, FIGO stage Ib1) cervical cancer in pregnancy and, together with radiosensitizing chemotherapy, is the treatment of choice in more advanced stages (FIGO stages Ib2–IVa). In the first and second trimesters when the pregnancy is to be disregarded, treatment should begin with whole-pelvis irradiation. Spontaneous abortion usually occurs during therapy, and the treatment is then completed with intracavitary radium or cesium applications. **Spontaneous abortion usually occurs at about 35 days in the first trimester and at 45 days in the second trimester after onset of radiotherapy.** Some second-trimester patients will go 60 to 70 days before abortion occurs. An alternative approach in the patient who has not aborted is to evacuate the uterus by means of a hysterotomy followed by conventional intracavitary irradiation delivered within 1 to 2 weeks.

If spontaneous abortion does not occur by completion of the external-beam therapy, as occurs commonly after the 16th week of gestation, a modified radical hysterectomy without pelvic lymphadenectomy should be done to excise the remaining central neoplasm. This strategy delivers potentially curative doses of radiation to pelvic lymph nodes with microscopic foci of metastatic tumor followed by surgical resection of the remaining central tumor because the gravid uterus is not suitable for intracavitary radium or cesium. Although some clinicians prefer an extrafascial hysterectomy after 5000 cGy of whole-pelvis irradiation in patients who have early lesions, the author prefers the more extensive modified radical hysterectomy. This approach accomplishes adequate excision of the cervix and accompanying medial parametria and upper vagina, which includes all the tissues that would have been effectively irradiated by the pear-shaped isodose distribution of a tandem and ovoid application of radium or cesium. Those who advocate an extrafascial hysterectomy centrally often advise further vaginal vault irradiation after the surgical procedure to treat the upper vagina and medial parametria more completely.

Sood and colleagues assessed the effects of pregnancy on tumor control, survival, and morbidity associated with radiation therapy administered to pregnant patients. They identified 26 women treated primarily with radiation therapy before the era of concurrent chemoirradiation and matched these patients with 26 control participants based on age, histology, stage, treatment, and year of treatment. Patients were treated with external-beam radiation (mean dose, 46.7 Gy) and intracavitary radiation (mean dose, 56.5 Gy to point A). Three patients diagnosed during the first trimester were treated with radiation with the fetus in situ, and all had spontaneous abortions 20 to 24 days after the start of radiation (mean dose, 34 Gy). In all of these cases, radiation was interrupted for only 3 days or less. There were no statistically significant differences in recurrence rates or survival between the pregnant group and the control participants.

Benhaim and colleagues have reported two patients with locally advanced disease who were treated with chemoradiation during the first trimester with the fetus in utero. The first patient (FIGO stage IVA) was treated at 12 weeks of gestation and experienced recurrence at 20 months. The second patient (FIGO stage IIB) was also treated at 12 weeks of gestation and underwent completion surgery (radical hysterectomy with lymphadenectomy) and has survived disease free for 2 years.

Episiotomy Site Recurrence

Patients in whom the diagnosis of invasive cervical cancer is made in the postpartum period may have undergone vaginal delivery. This group of patients warrants immediate therapy and specialized surveillance. Recurrence of cervical cancer at the episiotomy scar is a rare event and is thought to occur through implantation at the time of vaginal delivery from an occult tumor, with subsequent early, isolated recurrence as opposed to regional spread. At least 15 cases have appeared in the literature since 1986, including one patient who experienced relapse along a perineal laceration scar (Table 15.4). In the majority of these patients, the primary diagnosis of cervical cancer was made during the postpartum period, with recurrence at the episiotomy site typically occurring within 6 months of primary treatment.

In a matched case-control study of women with cervical cancer diagnosed during pregnancy ($n = 56$) or within 6 months of delivery ($n = 27$), Sood and colleagues noted that among the patients diagnosed postpartum, one of seven who was delivered by cesarean section developed a local and distant recurrence, but 10 of 17 (59%) of those who delivered vaginally developed recurrences ($P = 0.04$). In multivariate analysis, vaginal delivery was the most significant predictor of recurrence. **We recommend delivery by cesarean section when the diagnosis is known antenatally, and in patients diagnosed in the postpartum period, vigilant examination of the episiotomy and vaginal laceration sites is warranted.** Although the mode of delivery in the setting of known microinvasive disease may be based on obstetric indications, it should be pointed out that among the 14 cases of episiotomy site recurrences, there was one patient who had been diagnosed with a stage Ia endocervical adenocarcinoma.

Neither the time of diagnosis nor time to recurrence appears to affect survival after episiotomy site recurrence. Goldman and Goldberg noted that no patient who received chemotherapy or radiotherapy for recurrent disease without excision survived 1 year. The treatment policy should include wide local excision of the entire nodule with adjuvant external radiotherapy plus brachytherapy. Of seven patients treated by this method, 71% were without evidence of disease at longer than 1 year.

There have been at least two cases of cervical cancer with concomitant episiotomy metastasis in the literature. Baloglu

TABLE 15.4			**Treatment Modalities and Survival of Patients With Episiotomy Site Recurrence**							
Authors	**Year**	**Stage**	**Prenatal Cytology**	**Pathology**	**Time of Initial Diagnosis**	**Primary Treatment**	**Disease-Free Interval**	**Treatment of Recurrence**	**Status**
Burgess and Waymont	1987	Ib	SCCA	SCCA	7 mo pp	XRT, BT	17 mo	Exenteration	n/r
Copeland et al.	1987	Ib	Normal	Adenocarcinoma	3 mo pp	RH	3 mo	WE, XRT, BT	NED >5 yr
		Ib	Normal	Adenocarcinoma	Biopsy at delivery	RH	5 mo	WE, XRT	NED 10 mo
Gordon et al.	1989	Ib	Normal	SCCA	Biopsy at delivery	RH	1 mo	WE, XRT, BT	NED 3.5 yr
van Dam et al.	1992	IIIa	n/r	SCCA	6 wk pp	Chemotherapy, XRT, BT	0 mo	BT	n/r
		Ib	Normal	Adenocarcinoma	9 wk pp	XRT, BT	3 mo	WE, XRT, BT	NED >10 yr
Khalil et al.	1993	IIIb	Not done	SCCA	8 wk pp	XRT, BT	3 mo	Chemotherapy, XRT	DOD 4 mo
Cliby et al.	1994	Ib	HSIL	SCCA	Biopsy at delivery	RH	9 wk	Chemotherapy	DOD 6 mo
		Ib	Not done	SCCA	Biopsy at 36 wk	RH	24 mo	Chemotherapy, WE, XRT	NED 1 yr
		Ib	Not done	SCCA	Biopsy at delivery	RH	3 mo	XRT	DOD 3.5 yr
		Ib	Not done	SCCA	5 wk pp	RH	1 mo	WE, XRT	DOD 6 mo
van den Broek et al.	1995	Ia1	Normal	Adenocarcinoma	3 months pp	Total abdominal hysterectomy	6 wk	WE, interstitial implants	DOD 1 yr
Goldman and Goldberg	2003	Ib	Normal	SCCA	1 wk pp	RH	5.5 yr	WE, XRT, BT	DOD 4.5 yr
Heron et al.	2005	Ib	AGUS	Villoglandular	Biopsy at 31 wk	RH, BPLND	44 mo	XRT, WE	NED 10 mo
Baloglu et al.	2007	IIIA	Unknown	SCCA	8 mo pp	ChemoRT	NED 1 yr f/u		

AGUS, Atypical glandular cells of undetermined significance; *BPLND,* bilateral pelvic lymphadenectomy; *BT,* brachytherapy; *ChemoRT,* chemoradiation; *DOD,* died of disease; *f/u,* follow-up; *HSIL,* high-grade squamous intraepithelial lesion; *n/r,* not reported; *NED,* no evidence of disease; *pp,* postpartum; *RH,* radical hysterectomy; *SCCA,* squamous cell carcinoma; *WE,* wide excision; *XRT,* whole pelvic radiotherapy. (Modified from Goldman NA, Goldberg GL. Late recurrence of squamous cell cervical cancer in an episiotomy site after vaginal delivery. *Obstet Gynecol* 2003;101:1127.)

and colleagues reported one of these patients for whom the diagnosis was unknown antenatally. This patient was diagnosed with locally advanced disease and an episiotomy site metastasis and received primary chemoradiation. She was without evidence of recurrence at 1 year of follow-up when the report was published. Women diagnosed with cervical cancer in the postpartum period should have the episiotomy or vaginal laceration site carefully examined if they experience vaginal delivery.

Planned Delay of Therapy

Historically, when invasive carcinoma was diagnosed before 20 weeks of gestation, recommendations included immediate treatment of the tumor, either by radical hysterectomy or radiation therapy, leaving the fetus in utero in both instances. This dogma has been challenged during the preceding decade, with multiple reports of a safe outcome for mother and child with a deliberate delay in therapy to permit gestational advancement (Table 15.5). For example, Duggan and colleagues reported a mean diagnosis-to-treatment interval of 144 days (range, 53–212 days) in eight patients with FIGO stage Ia or FIGO stage Ib cervical cancer who postponed therapy to optimize fetal outcome. All of these women were rendered disease free after a median follow-up period of 23 months. Sorosky and colleagues

identified eight pregnant women with FIGO stage I squamous cell cervical carcinoma who declined immediate therapy to improve fetal outcome. They were observed prospectively until the late third trimester, with a mean diagnosis to treatment interval of 109 days (range, 21–210 days). No clinical progression of disease was detected, and after therapy, all were alive and disease free after a mean follow-up time of 37 months (range, 13–68 months). Takushi and colleagues reported a delay in treatment of 6 to 16 weeks for four women with FIGO stage Ia2, Ib1, or 1b2 lesions. No disease progression was documented, and after cesarean–radical hysterectomy, all patients have been disease free at a follow-up period of 70 to 156 months.

Although most patients with FIGO stage Ib disease have fared well with deliberate delays in therapy, four patients are noted in whom progression of disease was observed ($n = 2$) or in whom recurrence and death from disease occurred ($n = 2$). Five patients with FIGO stage II disease who opted to delay therapy were reported by Lee and colleagues, and although they did not progress during the pregnancy, it should be noted that their cancers were diagnosed in the third trimester, and the treatment delays were relatively limited. Long-term follow-up data were not presented for this subset of patients. **Thus, for patients with FIGO stage Ia1 to Ib1 squamous cell lesions**

TABLE 15.5 Deliberate Delay of Definitive Therapy for Frankly Invasive Cervical Carcinoma in Pregnancy

Authors	Year	Stage	Patients (n)	Delay	Maternal Outcome
Prem et al.	1966	I	4	6 wk	NED 5 yr
		I	5	11–17 wk	NED 3–5 yr
Dudan et al.	1973	Ib	2	2 and 6 mo	Progression
Lee et al.	1981	Ib	1	12 wk	NED 10 yr
		Ib	2	11 wk	No progression
		II	5	1–11 wk	No progression
Nisker and Shubat	1983	Ib	1	24 wk	DOD
Greer et al.	1989	Ib	5	6–17 wk	NED 1–3 yr (n = 4), DOD (n = 1)
Monk and Montz	1992	Ib	4	10–16 wk	NED 3.5 yr
Hopkins and Morley	1992	Ib	5	12 wk	NED 5 yr (n = 40)
Mack et al.	1981	Ib	3	10–16 wk	NED
Duggan et al.	1993	Ib1	5	7–24 wk	NED 3 yr
Sivanesaratnam et al.	1993	Ib	2	2 and 4 wk	NED 5 yr
Allen et al.	1995	Ib	2	18–19 wk	NED 5 yr
Sorosky et al.	1995	Ib1	7	7–29 wk	NED 1.5–5.5 yr
Sood et al.	1996	Ib	3	3–32 wk	NED 1–30 yr
Tewari et al.	1997	Ib2	1*	11 wk	NED 2 yr
		IIa	1*	18 wk	DOD 9 mo
van Vliet et al.	1998	Ib	5	2–10 wk	DOD (n = 1), NED 1.5–9 yr
		IIa	1	2 wk	NED 12 yr
Marana et al.	2001	IIb	1*	21 wk	DOD 18 mo*
Takushi et al.	2002	Ib1	2	13 and 15 wk	NED 8 and 9 yr
		Ib2	1	6 wk	NED 7 yr
Germann et al.	2005	Ib1	9	4 mo	NED 5 yr
Traen et al.	2006	IB1	1	19 wk	NED

*Treated with neoadjuvant chemotherapy during pregnancy.
DOD, Died of disease; *NED,* no evidence of disease.
Modified from Tewari K, Cappuccini F, Gambino A, et al. Neoadjuvant chemotherapy in the treatment of locally advanced cervical carcinoma in pregnancy: a report of two cases and review of issues specific to the management of cervical carcinoma in pregnancy including planned delay of therapy. *Cancer* 1998;82:1529.

diagnosed before and after 20 weeks of gestation, a limited treatment delay to await fetal maturity may be acceptable. The counseling in such situations should be analogous to obtaining an informed consent from the mother.

Neoadjuvant Chemotherapy in Pregnancy

Patients with advanced disease (ie, FIGO stage Ib2 and greater) should be offered immediate therapy. A novel approach to patients with locally advanced disease who refuse interruption of pregnancy was first reported by our group in 1998. Two women with FIGO stage Ib2 and FIGO stage IIa lesions refused interruption of their pregnancies and received neoadjuvant chemotherapy consisting of vincristine (1 mg/m^2) and cisplatin (50 mg/m^2) during the early second and third trimesters. Both patients experienced significant tumor regression, rendering radical hysterectomy feasible at the time of cesarean delivery after documentation of fetal pulmonary maturation at 32 weeks and 34 weeks of gestation. At the time of publication, one patient had remained without evidence of recurrence for more than 2 years; unfortunately, the second patient experienced a lethal relapse 5 months after primary therapy. Both children have experienced normal development. Another early report was by that of Marana and colleagues, who treated a pregnant woman with a FIGO stage IIb tumor with bleomycin (30 mg on day 1) and cisplatin (50 mg/m^2 on day 2 and day 3) from 17 weeks to 38 weeks of gestation and achieved both tumor regression and a healthy infant, who continued to thrive long after the mother succumbed to recurrent disease 13 months after delivery. Although such a treatment approach remains investigational, the use of neoadjuvant chemotherapy while awaiting gestational advancement may be entertained when the pregnant woman with cervical cancer, for whom a treatment delay is ill advised, refuses interruption of therapy.

Since these initial publications, there have been at least eight additional case reports of patients who received neoadjuvant chemotherapy during pregnancy for cervical cancer along with a recent 21-patient case series reported by Kohler et al. Most patients were treated for locally advanced disease (FIGO IB2–IIIB), but two patients received neoadjuvant chemotherapy for FIGO stage IB1 lesions. Neoadjuvant therapy was usually administered during the mid-second trimester to the early third trimester (range, 17–33 weeks of gestation) and single-agent cisplatin (eg, 75 mg/m^2 every 10 days) has been used most often. The combination of cisplatin (50 mg/m^2) plus vincristine (1 mg/m^2) every 21 days has also been of continued interest in some cases. Obstetric outcomes have been universally favorable, as have maternal outcomes, although there was one case of rapid tumor progression. It should be emphasized, however, that despite the good results, follow-up in several cases has been of short duration.

In the aforementioned study by Kohler et al., 21 pregnant women at a mean gestational age of 17 weeks (range, 13–23 weeks) received a median of three cycles (range, two to four cycles) of platinum-based chemotherapy with cesarean delivery carried out between 30.4 and 36.5 weeks of gestation, resulting in 22 healthy babies without renal, hepatic, auditory, or hematopoietic impairment. Platinum concentrations in the umbilical cord blood and amniotic fluid were 23% to 65% and 11% to 42%, respectively. Because the observed in vivo measurement of platinum was consistently lower in the fetoplacental unit, the authors suggest that a placental filtration mechanism of platinum may exist.

Neoadjuvant chemotherapy should be considered for patients with locally advanced disease diagnosed in the early to mid second trimester who are adamant about continuing the pregnancy. Again, these patients need to be counseled regarding the investigational nature of this treatment modality under the clinical circumstances in question.

Prognosis for Patients With Cervical Cancer in Pregnancy

The overall prognosis for all stages of cervical cancer in pregnancy is similar to that in nonpregnant women (Table 15.6). The favorable overall prognosis for pregnant patients is related to a greater proportion of pregnant patients with stage I disease. In a report by Allen and colleagues of 96 cases of cervical cancer occurring in pregnancy, the disease-free survival rates for 87 patients who were available for analysis were noted to be 92.3% for FIGO stage Ia1, 68.2% for FIGO stage Ib, 54.5% for FIGO stage II, and 37.5% for FIGO stage III. The overall survival rate was 65.5%, which is slightly better than that reported by Hacker and colleagues. They also observed an association of advanced clinical staging with diagnosis in the third trimester and postpartum. Of 49 cases of FIGO stage Ib cervical carcinoma, 64.5% were diagnosed in the third trimester and postpartum; of 22 cases of FIGO stage II cervical carcinoma, 77.3% were diagnosed in the third trimester and postpartum; and all nine cases of stage III cervical carcinoma were diagnosed in the third trimester and postpartum. Of the 32 patients who underwent pelvic lymphadenectomy, 10 were noted to have positive nodes. This increase in frequency has not been our experience.

Zemlickis and colleagues compared 40 women who had carcinoma of the cervix in pregnancy with 89 nonpregnant women matched for age, stage, and tumor type. Long-term

TABLE 15.6 Long-Term, Cause-Specific Actuarial Survival for Cervical Cancer in Pregnancy Treated From 1960 to 2004 Compared With Two Control Participants Matched for Age, Disease Stage, Histopathology, and Treatment Year

Year	Cases (n = 41)	Control Participants (n = 82)
0	1.0	1.0
2	0.89	0.87
4	0.86	0.79
6	0.82	0.75
8	0.81	0.73
10	0.79	0.73
12	0.77	0.73

Log-rank test ($P = 0.85$)

From Pettersson BF, Andersson S, Hellman K, Hellström AC. Invasive carcinoma of the uterine cervix associated with pregnancy: 90 years of experience. *Cancer* 2010;116:2343.

survival rates were similar between the two groups. When pregnant women were compared with a series of 1963 cervical cancers in women younger than 45 years treated during the same time, the pregnant women were three times more likely to have stage I disease and had a lower chance of having FIGO stage III to IV cancers.

In 1993, Sivanesaratnam and colleagues reported surgical management of early invasive cancer of the cervix in a series of 18 patients who underwent radical hysterectomy and pelvic lymphadenectomy, with a 5-year survival rate of 77.7%. A comparable group of nonpregnant patients who also underwent radical surgery had a survival rate of 92.3%. Nisker and Shubat also reported that there was a slightly better survival in the nonpregnant group than in the pregnant group. These reports are in contrast to the previous reports by Creasman and colleagues, Sablinska and colleagues, and Lee and colleagues, who found no appreciable difference in the 5-year survival rates of pregnant versus nonpregnant patients with cervical cancer.

A multicenter, retrospective study conducted by the Korean Gynecologic Oncology Group (KGOG-1006) contained 40 pregnant subjects treated from 1995 to 2003. Each case was matched to three control participants on the basis of age, stage, histology, and date of treatment. Among 12 patients who delayed treatment for fetal maturity, two died of disease. There was no difference in overall survival between pregnant and nonpregnant patients with stage IB lesions.

Pettersson and colleagues recently published a 90-year experience from the Radiumhemmet. The 10-year actuarial survival rate improved significantly during the study period from 27% (1914–2004) to 79% (1960–2004). The 10-year cause-specific cumulative actuarial survival rate for 41 pregnant women treated during 1960 to 2004 did not differ statistically from the rate for an age-matched, stage-matched, and histopathology-matched control series of nonpregnant women treated at the Radiumhemmet during the same period. The authors concluded that during the study period, the incidence of cervical cancer during pregnancy declined, the cases were discovered at earlier stages, and survival improved.

For more advanced disease, pregnancy may have an unfavorable effect on prognosis as a result of problems with radiation dosimetry in pregnancy and the need to interrupt radiation therapy more frequently because of genital tract sepsis. **Clinical stage remains the most important determinant of prognosis.**

Obstetric Outcomes

Dalrymple and colleagues analyzed the obstetric outcomes among women in California with pregnancy-associated cervical cancer. Using computer-linked infant birth and death certificates, discharge records, and cancer registry files, cases were identified and then assigned to a prenatal or postpartum cancer diagnosis group. Among 434 cases, those diagnosed prenatally ($n = 136$) had higher rates of cesarean section, hospitalization longer than 5 days, low birth weight, very low birth weight, prematurity, and fetal deaths compared with pregnant control participants without cancer. No neonatal deaths were attributable to elective premature delivery. Very low birth weight,

prematurity, and fetal death rates remained elevated among those diagnosed postpartum.

> **Key summary points for the management of invasive cervical cancer during pregnancy:**
> 1. Reports describing the successful performance of trachelectomy during pregnancy, occasionally using robotic surgical platforms, continue to appear in the literature for management of early-stage disease.
> 2. For patients with locally advanced disease who insist on a definitive treatment delay to allow gestational advancement with concomitant fetal maturation, platinum-based neoadjuvant chemotherapy has been reported in more than 30 cases without significant maternal or fetal sequelae despite the observation that platinum does cross the maternal–fetal placental interface.

Ovarian Cancer

Ovarian cancer is reported to occur in 1 per 10,000 to 1 per 25,000 pregnancies. Pregnancy does not alter the prognosis of most ovarian malignant neoplasms, but complications such as torsion and rupture may increase the incidence of spontaneous abortion or preterm delivery. In a survey by Kohler of the largest studies in the literature, about 1 in 600 pregnancies will be complicated by an adnexal mass. More contemporary accounts suggest that adnexal masses may complicate as many as 1 in 190 pregnancies. At least one-third of pregnant women are asymptomatic, with the adnexal mass often discovered during obstetric ultrasonography.

Most cysts in pregnant patients are follicular or corpus luteum cysts and are usually no more than 3 to 5 cm in diameter. Functional cysts as large as 11 cm in diameter have been reported but are rare. More than 90% of these functional cysts will disappear as pregnancy progresses and are undetectable by the 14th week of gestation. **It appears that the size of the adnexal mass at the time of diagnosis is inversely related to the likelihood of spontaneous regression. Only 6% of masses smaller than 6 cm persisted during serial examinations, but 39% of masses larger than 6 cm persisted.** The complication rate increases with increasing size of the mass. In addition, a solid or complex ultrasonographic appearance and the presence of bilateral adnexal or ovarian abnormalities may also be indications to proceed with laparotomy. Adnexal masses with blood flow characterized by a high resistive index by Doppler ultrasonography are less likely to be malignant, independent of size. MRI may be useful when ultrasonographic findings are equivocal.

The most pressing problems associated with ovarian tumors in pregnancy are the initial diagnosis and the differential diagnosis. When the tumor is palpable within the pelvis, it must be differentiated from a retroverted pregnant uterus, a pedunculated uterine fibroid, a carcinoma of the rectosigmoid, a pelvic kidney, and a congenital uterine abnormality (eg, rudimentary uterine horn). Analysis of serum tumor markers is a complex undertaking and can be misleading because the titers for each of the markers, especially α-fetoprotein and β-human chorionic gonadotropin (hCG), and even CA-125, are routinely elevated in pregnancy for reasons unrelated to malignancy.

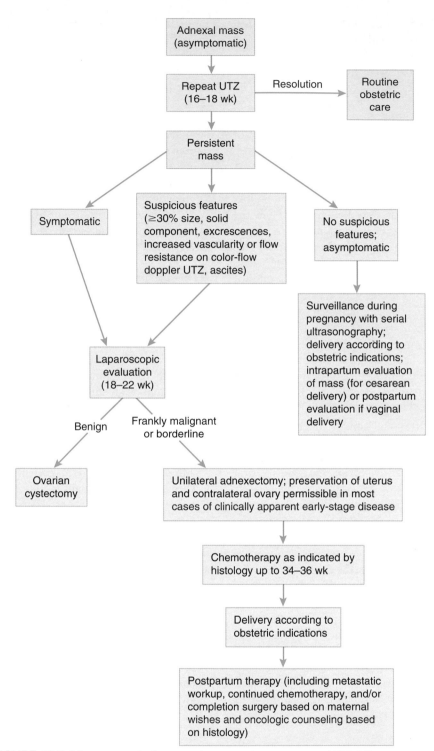

FIGURE 15.7 Management of an ovarian mass in pregnancy. UTZ, Ultrasonography.

A proposed management algorithm for the adnexal mass in pregnancy appears in Fig. 15.7. **Our experience has been that patients operated on around the 18th week of gestation have negligible fetal wastage associated with the exploration.** Therefore, 18 weeks of gestation appears to be a judicious period for laparotomy in terms of its safety both for the fetus and for the elimination of functional ovarian cysts. If the cyst is complex and suspicious for malignancy and increases in size, the patient should undergo exploration earlier than 18 weeks. **Whenever exploration is conducted, our recommendation is that the uterus not be manipulated during surgery (ie, the so-called hands-off-the-uterus approach) in an effort to minimize its irritability.**

Torsion is common in pregnancy, with 10% to 15% of ovarian tumors reportedly undergoing this complication. Most torsions (ie, 60%) occur when the uterus is rising at a rapid rate

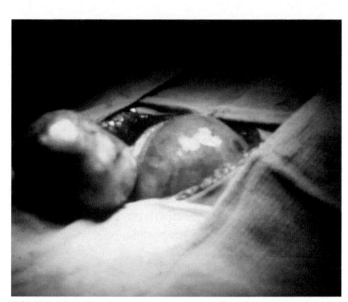

FIGURE 15.8 Benign cystic teratoma. Gross appearance at 18 weeks of gestation.

(8–16 weeks) or when the uterus is involuting (in the puerperium). The usual sequence of events is sudden lower abdominal pain; nausea; vomiting; and in some cases, shocklike symptoms. The abdomen is tense and tender, and there is rebound tenderness with guarding. If exploration must be undertaken during the first trimester and extraction of the ovary (or ovaries) is required, supplemental progesterone can be administered to decrease the likelihood of pregnancy loss.

In many instances, the presence of an ovarian tumor may not be suspected until delivery (Fig. 15.8). The large uterus obscures the growth of the ovarian neoplasm. The tumor may be growing in the abdomen behind the large uterus and may not fall back into the cul de sac until it is large. If there is a mechanical obstruction of the birth canal, exploratory laparotomy is indicated for both delivery of the baby and management of the ovarian neoplasm. Allowing labor to proceed when an ovarian neoplasm is causing obstruction of the birth canal may result in rupture of the ovarian cyst. Even if the cyst is not ruptured, the trauma of labor may cause hemorrhage into the tumor followed by necrosis and suppuration.

Asymptomatic Adnexal Masses

Before detailing the clinical approach to managing the different ovarian malignancies that may occur during pregnancy, some consideration should be given to asymptomatic adnexal masses. Admittedly, asymptomatic masses can be malignant; however, the vast majority are likely to be benign, particularly in the pregnant population. There has been a movement during the past decade that has challenged the dogma of operating on every asymptomatic mass larger than 5 cm that persists into the second trimester. Most of these masses can be followed conservatively in the absence of symptoms and in the absence of concerning sonographic ovarian and extraovarian findings (eg, ascites).

Endovaginal pelvic ultrasonography is essential in the evaluation of adnexal masses. Approximately 10% of masses are complex, and the examination should determine the origin of the mass and its location, size, and internal structure (eg, vegetations, septations). The mass should be classified unilocular, unilocular-solid, multilocular, multilocular-solid, or solid. Color Doppler imaging may be used to obtain a vascular road map of an ovarian mass. Pelvic MRI with gadolinium injection can be performed after the first trimester and should only be used during pregnancy to remove further doubt regarding possible malignancy or to provide additional information if ultrasonography is inconclusive.

Laparoscopic Management of the Ovarian Mass

Laparoscopy was previously thought to be contraindicated in pregnancy because of the unknown effect of the pneumoperitoneum on the gravid uterus, the possible injection of carbon dioxide into the amniotic cavity, and the potential for acidosis in the fetal environment as a result of maternal conversion of carbon dioxide into carbonic acid. Growing evidence, however, suggests that laparoscopy can be performed safely during pregnancy.

The recommended time for laparoscopic intervention mirrors that for open procedures and is between 16 and 20 weeks of gestation. There have been reports of laparoscopy up to the 28th week of gestation, but this appears to be the upper limit. Larger uteri increase surgical difficulty, and surgery after 23 weeks can be linked to adverse fetal outcomes and preterm labor. Intervention before the second trimester is not advisable because this does not give time for the ovarian mass to resolve on its own and could compromise ovarian hormone production before the placenta is fully functional.

The table should be tilted to the left or the right with the patient supine to move the uterus away from the site of trocal insertion. The left upper quadrant or subxiphoid insertion of the trocar should be used with at least 6 cm between the point of entry and the top of the fundus. The open Hasson technique is preferred over the Veress technique, although both have been used successfully in pregnancy. Ultrasound guidance may be used with the Veress technique together with elevation of the abdominal wall to reduce the risk of uterine injury.

Intraabdominal pressure should be kept below 15 mm Hg with the patient in the Trendelenburg position to ensure adequate venous return and uteroplacental blood flow during the operation. Positioning in this manner may require positive pressure ventilation to maintain adequate lung volumes. Depending on the circumstances and gestational age, fetal monitoring may be advisable.

Robotic-Assisted Laparoscopic Management of Adnexal Masses During Pregnancy

With widespread adoption of robotic surgical platforms for management of adnexal masses, cervical cancer, and endometrial cancer in the nonpregnant population, it is not surprising to see reports of robotic surgical applications applied to the pregnant patient. Eichelberger et al. evaluated their experience in planned robotic resection of adnexal masses in 19 pregnant women, all of which were performed without fetal or maternal complications. When compared with 50 consecutive laparoscopic cases from a recent historical database, the authors noted no differences in operative time, conversion to laparotomy, intraoperative or postoperative complications, or negative observed obstetric outcomes. Interestingly (and not altogether unexpected given the reported advantages of robotics in the nonpregnant population), in this study, the patients undergoing robotic surgery had a significantly shorter length of hospital stay and estimated blood loss. We anticipate surgeons continuing to report further experiences with robotic pelvic surgery in the coming years.

Ovarian Masses Specific to Pregnancy

Two adnexal conditions may specifically be associated with pregnancy. The operating surgeon must be cognizant of their possibility so that unnecessary oophorectomies will not be performed. **The luteoma of pregnancy can vary in size from microscopic to 20 cm in diameter and usually consists of multiple, well-circumscribed nodules that can be bilateral in one third of cases.** The luteoma may be associated with significant elevations in plasma testosterone and other androgens in about 25% of the cases. Maternal hirsutism or virilism may occur during the latter half of pregnancy, which may cause virilization in up to 70% of female infants born to masculinizing mothers. If the lesion is not recognized grossly, a biopsy may be taken for definitive diagnosis. Because these regress spontaneously postpartum, nothing further needs to be done. **Theca-lutein cysts may occur when hCG concentrations are abnormally elevated, such as in a molar pregnancy, fetal hydrops, or multiple gestations.** These are usually multiple and thin-walled cysts. Sometimes, massive bilateral theca-lutein cysts manifest that are considerably different from the solid nodules of the luteoma of pregnancy. These also regress postpartum and should not be resected unless acute complications develop.

Histologic Types of Ovarian Tumors

Struyk and Treffers reported on 90 pregnancies complicated by ovarian tumors. No functional cysts were noted in patients operated on after the 18th week. In eight patients, ovarian tumor enlargement was noted during a period of observation; two were malignant, one serous cystadenoma occurred, and five

were teratomas. Fifty-four percent of the tumors were diagnosed in the first trimester. Severe pain occurred in 26%, torsion in 12%, obstruction of labor in 17%, and rupture in 9%. Only 37% of the patients had no complications. Fetal wastage was high, with death in utero occurring in three cases and neonatal death in seven cases.

Thornton and Wells reviewed 131 ovarian enlargements in pregnancy, 81 of which were removed (including one carcinoma and six borderline lesions). Thirty-nine were greater than 5 cm in diameter and had simple internal echo patterns and smooth walls; three of these were borderline malignant neoplasms. Hoffman reviewed 13 reports of ovarian neoplasms removed in pregnancy and found benign cystadenomas or cystic teratomas most frequently diagnosed. The Hoffman review also included a summary of 127 malignant ovarian lesions found during pregnancy. A recent literature review by Kwon and colleagues describing the various histologies of ovarian tumors found in pregnancy appears in Table 15.7. Borderline and frankly malignant epithelial lesions were the most commonly encountered during pregnancy.

Borderline Ovarian Tumors

Adnexal masses larger than 6 cm that persist into the second trimester warrant removal at approximately 18 weeks of gestational age. Between 2% and 5% of these lesions will be malignant, with dysgerminoma being most common. Among epithelial tumors, serous carcinoma and serous tumors of low malignant potential are readily encountered. Thirty-five cases of serous ovarian tumors of low malignant potential in conjunction with pregnancy have been reported since 1988. In the 33 cases in which a FIGO stage was assigned, 30 were stage I (14 stage Ia, 1 stage Ib, 4 stage Ic, and 11 nonsubstaged I). All 33 patients for whom follow-up data were available were found to be alive without disease (range, 1 year to 20 years, 5 months). Recent evidence suggests that the hormonal influence of pregnancy can lead to histologic changes in serous low malignant potential tumors that, if not sorted out and characterized appropriately, could be mistaken for frankly invasive carcinoma. The group at the MD Anderson Hospital and Tumor Institute collected 10 cases from 1944 to 1993 and conducted a slide review, noting some very peculiar histologic features distinct from those seen in nonpregnant patients, including epithelial atypia and proliferation, eosinophilic cells, mucin production,

TABLE 15.7	Distribution of Ovarian Cancers in Pregnancy by Histology					
Histology	Dgani et al., 1989 (%)	Copeland and Landon, 1996 (%)	Zanotti et al., 2000 (%)	PUMCH, 2003 (%)	Behtash et al., 2008 (%)	Kwon et al., 2010 (%)
Epithelial—borderline	65	37.5	33–40	50	39.1	81.5
Epithelial—invasive	35	—	66	27.3	21.7	55.5
Germ cell	17	45	30-33	40.9	47.8	18.5
Sex cord–stromal	13	10	17–20	9.1	13	0
Other	5	7.5	12–13	0	0	0

PUMCH, Peking University Medical College Hospital.
Modified from Kwon YS, Mok JE, Lim KT, et al. Ovarian cancer during pregnancy: clinical and pregnancy outcome. *J Korean Med Sci* 2010;25:230.

decidual changes, and frequent microinvasion. Although these lesions remained within the spectrum of low malignant potential tumors, the histologic features were worrisome for a more aggressive clinical course, yet all 10 patients remained disease free after a variety of treatment modalities. We advise prompt recognition of these histologic findings after cystectomy or oophorectomy during pregnancy so as to classify them accordingly as being borderline rather than to confuse them with low-grade serous papillary carcinomas. Of additional interest is that in two cases, the tumor was resected both during pregnancy and after parturition (2 months and 3 years), and there was significant regression of the epithelial proliferation, the number of eosinophilic cells, and the amount of mucin production the second time around; this regression after parturition supports a hormonal etiology of these unusual histologic features. In contrast to frankly malignant ovarian carcinomas, unilateral adnexectomy is all that is required during pregnancy for the serous low malignant potential tumor.

Frankly Malignant Ovarian Tumors

Malignant ovarian tumors account for only 2% to 5% of all ovarian neoplasms found in pregnancy. The incidence for all pregnancies is 1 in 8000 to 1 in 20,000 deliveries. The diagnosis is usually fortuitous in that the patient undergoes laparotomy for an adnexal mass that is subsequently found to be malignant. In many instances, the close observation of the pregnant patient has led to the discovery of a lesion in the earlier stages. These include not only malignant germ cell tumors and sex cord–stromal cell cancers but also some epithelial malignancies. **If an ovarian malignant neoplasm is found at the time of abdominal exploration, the surgeon's first obligation is to properly stage the disease, as outlined in** Chapter 10. Although the gravid uterus hinders the surgeon's ability to access the retroperitoneum, every effort should be made to remove the tumor intact. The contralateral ovary should be carefully inspected and biopsied if anything suspicious is detected. In the scenario of a clinical stage I ovarian carcinoma, unilateral adnexectomy, omentectomy, unilateral pelvic and aortocaval lymph node sampling, peritoneal biopsies, and four-quadrant washings can be safely carried out during pregnancy, with chemotherapy reserved for those patients who are upstaged on histopathologic analysis. The chemotherapy regimen is similar to what is used for advanced disease (eg, a platinum compound and a taxane for the epithelial cancers); however, for patients with FIGO stage Ia or Ib, grade I non–clear cell tumors, no chemotherapy will be recommended.

Malignant Germ Cell Tumors in Pregnancy

Fortunately, ovarian germ cell neoplasms in pregnancy are usually benign. **Dermoid cysts are by far the most common neoplastic cysts found in pregnancy; however, malignant ovarian germ cell tumors such as the dysgerminoma, embryonal carcinoma, immature teratoma, and yolk sac tumor (formerly called "endodermal sinus tumor") have also been reported.** Although a considerable number of these cancers present with early-stage disease (in both pregnant and nonpregnant patients), there are several reports of advanced cancers

FIGURE 15.9 Immature teratoma in pregnancy.

associated with pregnancy. Combination chemotherapy during pregnancy has been given without deleterious effects on the fetus.

The management of malignant ovarian germ cell tumors is predicated on the histologic identity of the tumor (see Fig. 15.7). Patients with clinical stage Ia dysgerminoma and those with clinical stage Ia-Ib grade I immature teratoma require surgical staging to determine the need for adjuvant chemotherapy (Fig. 15.9). All other histologic types require adjuvant chemotherapy, and therefore unilateral adnexectomy is all that is typically accomplished at the time of laparotomy, along with removal of all gross metastatic disease. Because most malignant germ cell tumors are unilateral (the dysgerminoma is the exception in 10% of cases), it is inappropriate to remove both ovaries. Even when the opposite side may harbor an occult dysgerminoma, it is often not necessary to remove the entire contralateral ovary. If, however, both ovaries are grossly involved by malignancy and the pregnancy is in the second trimester and thus free from hormonal support by the corpus luteum, both ovaries should be extracted. The prognosis for this stage is not improved with more extensive surgery. Chemotherapy regimens currently used for this disease comprise bleomycin, etoposide, and cisplatin. This regimen has been used safely during pregnancy.

Combined chemotherapy has improved survival markedly for malignant germ cell ovarian tumors and can permit preservation of childbearing capacity and maintenance of the existing pregnancy if the disease is stage I. If the diagnosis is made during the first or second trimester, the patient must decide whether to permit the pregnancy to continue to viability before adjuvant chemotherapy is instituted. Because these tumors characteristically grow rapidly and often recur within months when therapy is withheld, delays in initiating systemic therapy can be harmful. Indeed, the high success rate obtained with adjuvant chemotherapy has been recorded with use of this modality in the immediate postoperative period. The effect of a treatment-free interval of several months before the commencement of adjuvant chemotherapy has not been tested adequately. Thus, a patient with a malignant ovarian germ cell tumor discovered early in pregnancy and in need of chemotherapy is faced with a dilemma for which no data are available. Malone and colleagues described a patient with stage Ic endodermal sinus tumor diagnosed in the 25th week of gestation who two cycles of combination chemotherapy consisting of vinblastine, bleomycin, and cisplatin and delivered a healthy boy by cesarean section at 32 weeks of gestation. She subsequently completed three more cycles of chemotherapy and remained well at the time of Malone and colleagues' report 18 months after initial diagnosis. To our knowledge, this was the first report of a case of a patient who had endodermal sinus tumor treated with combination chemotherapy during pregnancy that apparently had a successful outcome for both mother and infant. Subsequently, we and others have had similar experiences. Therapeutic decisions for patients who have more advanced stages of these tumors are also difficult and controversial. Many such patients can be cured with early adjuvant chemotherapy after surgery. As in earlier stages, the uterus and opposite ovary can be preserved if metastatic tumor is not found in these locations. Some clinicians preserve the uterus and opposite ovary under all conditions in the hope that postoperative chemotherapy will sterilize those organs also. No long-term follow-up of this approach is available. Delays in withholding chemotherapy are not warranted, and uterine evacuation is often requested because of fear of potential teratogenic effects when chemotherapy is required during the first trimester. The subject of adjuvant chemotherapy in pregnancy is discussed later, but we emphasize that all chemotherapeutic agents are theoretically teratogenic. Although retrospective studies have not shown frequent congenital abnormalities in patients treated in the second and third trimesters, many newer agents have not been used frequently in pregnancy.

Dysgerminoma in Pregnancy

Ovarian dysgerminomas are unique among the malignant germ cell tumors because of their overall good prognosis in FIGO stage Ia treated by surgery alone. **Dysgerminoma is particularly common and accounts for 30% of ovarian malignant neoplasms in pregnancy.** We believe that these tumors can be managed with a unilateral adnexectomy and continuation of the pregnancy without additional therapy in FIGO stage Ia. Optimal staging should include a pelvic and periaortic lymphadenectomy on the side of the tumor mass because dysgerminomas metastasize primarily through the lymphatic system to the ipsilateral pelvic and periaortic lymph nodes. Because lymphangiography and computed tomography (CT) are contraindicated when the pregnancy is to be continued, patients who have not had adequate exploration at initial surgery should be considered for reexploration before further therapy and continuation of the pregnancy are recommended. Appropriate diagnostic studies, including lymphangiography and CT scan of the abdomen and pelvis, may be performed in the postpartum period. A mass on scan or a suspicious lymph node on lymphangiography should be evaluated at reexploration.

Emergency surgical intervention and obstetric complications are common in patients with dysgerminomas. Karlen and associates reviewed 27 cases of dysgerminoma associated with pregnancy. Torsion and incarceration were found commonly in this group of patients who had rapidly enlarging neoplasms averaging 25 cm in diameter. Obstetric complications occurred in nearly half the patients, and fetal demise occurred in one-quarter of the reviewed cases. There were recurrences in 30% of 23 stage Ia tumors treated by unilateral oophorectomy, which calls into question the philosophy of treating these patients conservatively. The extent of exploration was not known in most cases, however, and therefore accuracy of staging cannot be assessed. This information is essential for appropriate interpretation of the findings. In our experience, lesions that are confined to one ovary have a 10% recurrence rate. Although most of these lesions recur in the first 2 years after surgery, we believe that this group of patients can continue their pregnancies safely with completion of their proper evaluation in the puerperium. Because radiation therapy and chemotherapy are successful in curing more than 75% of patients, even those with metastatic or recurrent dysgerminoma, and because there is a low incidence of recurrence in patients with FIGO stage Ia disease, we maintain a philosophy of conservatism for the treatment of these tumors.

Sex Cord–Stromal Tumors in Pregnancy

Granulosa and Sertoli–Leydig cell tumors together account for only 2% to 3% of all ovarian neoplasms. Although granulosa cell tumors are most commonly discovered in perimenopausal or postmenopausal women, 10% to 20% are encountered during the reproductive years. Sertoli–Leydig cell tumors occur in women in the reproductive age group in 74% of cases. Of note, sex cord–stromal tumors are rarely found in pregnancy. It is critical that these entities are distinguished from ovarian decidualization, luteoma of pregnancy, or even benign granulosa cell proliferations observed with pregnancy. **Typically, the sex cord–stromal ovarian tumors behave as they do in nonpregnant women, presenting with early-stage disease and having a slow, low-grade, and indolent course.** Thus, because their biologic behavior is akin to that of neoplasms of low malignant potential, it is recommended that they be managed conservatively (ie, unilateral adnexectomy without comprehensive surgical staging) as in young nonpregnant patients (see Fig. 15.7). It is important, however, to resect all visible tumor whenever possible.

Young and colleagues reported a series of 17 granulosa cell, 13 Sertoli–Leydig cell, and six unclassified sex cord–stromal tumors diagnosed during pregnancy or the puerperium. Eleven patients had abdominal pain or swelling when they were first seen by a physician, five were in shock, two had virilization, and one had vaginal bleeding. Three asymptomatic patients underwent exploration because of palpable masses, and one underwent exploration because of an adnexal mass found on ultrasound examination. In 13 patients, the tumors were discovered during cesarean sections; five patients had dystocia, and the tumors were incidental findings in eight patients. All of the tumors were FIGO stage I, but 13 of the tumors had ruptured. All but one were unilateral. Hemoperitoneum was present in seven cases.

Young and colleagues uncovered four major sources of difficulty in the interpretation of their series of 36 cases:

1. The young age of the patients
2. An alteration in the histologic appearance of the tumors during pregnancy
3. A decreased frequency of associated endocrine manifestations
4. Pregnancy-induced changes in other neoplastic and nonneoplastic lesions of the ovary that cause them to simulate sex cord–stromal tumors both morphologically and in terms of endocrine function.

Indeed, the pregnancy-associated tumors commonly exhibited alterations related to the pregnant state that tended to obscure characteristics and familiar features that are apparent in tumors removed from nonpregnant patients. The most striking changes included intercellular edema and increased extent of luteinization in the granulosa cell tumors and of Leydig cell maturation in the Sertoli–Leydig cell tumors. It is important to note that the edema often blurred the architectural patterns of the tumors and distorted the cytologic features of the neoplastic cells. The marked luteinization and Leydig cell maturation interfered with the recognition of these cells. The end result was that these pregnancy-associated changes made identification of the tumor type more difficult.

Granulosa cell tumors are clinically estrogenic in approximately two-thirds of cases, and Sertoli–Leydig cell tumors are virilizing in nearly 50% of cases. These hormonal manifestations often suggest the correct diagnosis to the gynecologist. However, during pregnancy, the hyperestrogenic clinical manifestations do not appear, with none of the 17 tumors in the series by Young and colleagues associated with estrogenic manifestations. It is quite probable, however, that many of these tumors were secreting estrogens in large quantities. Furthermore, only 16% (n = 5) of the 36 sex cord–stromal tumors were associated with clinical evidence of excess androgens (virilization in four cases and hirsutism in only one case). This low frequency may have been the result of the placenta's ability to aromatize androgens produced by the tumor. In fact, one of the masculinizing tumors was the largest in their series (32 cm in maximal diameter) and may have been secreting androgens in such great abundance that the aromatizing capacity of the placenta was exceeded.

Several other types of ovarian neoplasms and nonneoplastic disorders are more frequently associated with virilization during pregnancy than Sertoli–Leydig cell tumors. Tumors with functioning, proliferative ovarian stroma such as Krukenberg tumors and the mucinous cystic tumors may be confused morphologically with sex cord–stromal tumors. Other primary ovarian tumors that can cause virilization include luteinized thecomas and Leydig and lipid cell tumors. Finally, as described earlier, two nonneoplastic lesions of the ovary that develop during pregnancy and can be associated with virilization include the luteoma of pregnancy and the hyperreactio luteinalis (multiple luteinized follicle cysts). All of these virilizing tumors and lesions must be considered in the differential diagnosis when confronted with virilization of the pregnant mother so as to not make an erroneous clinical diagnosis of a sex cord–stromal tumor.

With one exception, the patients in the study by Young and colleagues were initially treated by conservative surgical procedures. Two of them received chemotherapy, and two received radiation therapy postoperatively. Hysterectomies and salpingo-oophorectomies were performed as second operations in eight cases; no residual tumor was found in any of these specimens. Only one patient had a recurrence, which was treated surgically. Follow-up for the average of 4.7 years was available for 30 of the 36 patients; all of them were free of disease at their last examination. Adjuvant therapy has not been demonstrated to improve the outcome in this group of patients and is not recommended during pregnancy.

Chemotherapy for Nonepithelial Ovarian Cancer During Pregnancy

A recent literature review by Azim and colleagues identified 18 cases of nonepithelial ovarian malignancies treated with systemic chemotherapy during pregnancy. Most patients had a yolk sac tumor (n = 10) and were treated after the first trimester with the bleomycin, etoposide, and cisplatin (BEP) regimen or the cisplatin, vinblastine, and bleomycin (PVB) regimen. Other histologies reported included three cases of dysgerminoma, three cases of immature teratoma, one mixed germ cell tumor, and one Sertoli–Leydig tumor. Fifteen of the 18 women completed their pregnancies without complications; there was one case of premature delivery after maternal dehydration at 28 weeks after BEP, there was one case of pregnancy-induced hypertension after three cycles of BEP, and a third patient developed oligohydramnios after three cycles of etoposide-platinum. Postnatal chemotherapy-induced adverse events were restricted to one baby who developed minor anemia and transient respiratory distress at delivery at the 35th week of gestation. This baby had been exposed to three cycles of carboplatin plus paclitaxel for a maternal dysgerminoma, and the condition resolved quickly, and the authors reported normal development at 20 months of follow-up.

Epithelial Ovarian Cancer in Pregnancy

Very few series of malignant ovarian carcinomas in pregnancy have been published. Reported in 2002, the most recent series contains nine ovarian cancers concurrent with pregnancy from Libya and Saudi Arabia. Among these cases were included seven epithelial cancers (four serous, two mucinous, one undifferentiated), one dysgerminoma, and one granulosa cell tumor. As expected, the latter two lesions occurred in younger women, aged 18 and 21 years, respectively. All seven women with epithelial cancers were multiparous (range, 3–10), which is of some interest given the epidemiologic data suggesting increasing parity to be inversely related to the risk of developing ovarian carcinoma. Four patients with FIGO stage Ia tumors, including two with epithelial lesions, underwent unilateral adnexectomy before 25 weeks of gestation. None of the patients with more advanced disease who went on to receive chemotherapy did so during pregnancy. The obstetric outcome was favorable for all patients except for one with a FIGO stage Ia serous cystadenocarcinoma whose infant died from complications of meconium aspiration. It is of sufficient interest that five of the epithelial tumors were early stage (three FIGO stage Ia and two FIGO stage Ic), and one was assigned FIGO stage IIa. The only death occurred in a patient with a FIGO stage III undifferentiated carcinoma. Thus, fully six of seven women with epithelial ovarian cancers were diagnosed with early or locally advanced disease only, which does not reflect what is typically observed in the general population. It is quite certain that antenatal care, including serial physical examinations and ultrasonography, contributed to these early pick-ups.

After the diagnosis of ovarian carcinoma is made during pregnancy, appropriate therapy should not be withheld (see Fig. 15.7). In patients who present with metastatic disease manifesting as malignant ascites and carcinomatosis, surgical exploration is warranted, with an attempt to remove as much of the tumor burden as is feasible. Depending on the degree of tumor involvement of the uterus and the mother's desire for the pregnancy, uterine preservation may be considered, and if so, the "hands-off" approach to the uterus and removal of mobile intraperitoneal deposits can be attempted. Certainly, the typical aggressive cytoreductive approach (eg, bowel resection, splenectomy) taken in nonpregnant women with advanced-stage ovarian carcinoma can result in significant morbidity, and if the pregnancy is to be continued, we advise against this approach unless the patient has presented with a bowel obstruction.

An untested option in this group of patients is measurement of the serum CA-125 and aspiration of ascites fluid under ultrasound guidance for cytologic analysis. After malignancy is confirmed and considered likely to be of ovarian origin, systemic chemotherapy during the second and third trimesters in a "neoadjuvant" fashion can be considered, with plans for interval cytoreductive surgery after delivery. The standard regimen for metastatic epithelial ovarian cancer in nonpregnant patients includes platinum-based chemotherapy. Regimens containing cisplatin alone and cisplatin plus paclitaxel and even administration of a full six cycles of carboplatin and paclitaxel (the current standard among nonpregnant women), have been used during the second and third trimesters of pregnancy. Because there does not appear to be any significant risk to the fetus when these drugs are used in the second and third trimesters, pregnant patients diagnosed during these periods should be offered the opportunity to receive platinum-based therapy without terminating their pregnancies. Postpartum, the patient may return to the operating room to undergo definitive surgical staging or comprehensive tumor debulking.

Patients remote from term (eg, during the first trimester) with metastatic disease should be advised to undergo hysterectomy with the fetus in situ in conjunction with tumor debulking. Because the prognosis for women with advanced carcinoma is poor, patients must be counseled regarding the realities of how much time they would have with their child when making decisions regarding pregnancy termination.

It should be noted that there are at least two reports of an advanced-stage epithelial carcinoma of the ovary in which the uterus and pregnancy were preserved at 15 and 20 weeks of gestation. Patients were treated with six cycles of single-agent cisplatin or four courses of carboplatin plus paclitaxel followed by cesarean section and completion hysterectomy. One patient

was disease free at a short follow-up of 6 months, but the other recurred in the pelvis at 24 months after delivery. This second patient underwent secondary cytoreduction and was retreated with platinum-based therapy and has remained disease free at 42 months. Although some have advocated sparing the uterus if it appears to be uninvolved and the pregnancy is remote from term, this approach should be used with extreme caution when dealing with advanced-stage epithelial ovarian cancer for which the outcome remains exceedingly poor irrespective of pregnancy status.

Chemotherapy for Epithelial Ovarian Cancer During Pregnancy

Azim and colleagues have collected 20 patients from the literature who were treated with chemotherapy during pregnancy for epithelial ovarian cancer. The histologic subtypes included serous ($n = 13$), mucinous ($n = 3$), endometrioid ($n = 2$), clear cell ($n = 1$), and undifferentiated ($n = 1$). The chemotherapy regimens used included cyclophosphamide plus cisplatin ($n = 5$); single-agent cisplatin ($n = 4$); single-agent carboplatin ($n = 3$); paclitaxel plus carboplatin ($n = 2$); and cyclophosphamide, doxorubicin, and cisplatin ($n = 2$). There also was one case each of the use of the following regimens: cisplatin plus paclitaxel, cisplatin plus docetaxel, carboplatin plus cyclophosphamide, and single-agent paclitaxel. Seventeen of the patients received their first cycle during the second trimester and three in the third trimester. Sixteen patients delivered at week 34 or after, and 16 had experienced no pregnancy-related complications. There was one case each of intrauterine growth restriction, premature rupture of the membranes, and preeclampsia. Nineteen fetuses had a normal outcome, with nine of these children reported to be normal at 1 year or longer follow-up. There was one neonatal death from multiorgan failure in a baby with congenital anomalies identified before starting cisplatin plus docetaxel at week 20.

Intravenous carboplatin plus paclitaxel is the most commonly used regimen for epithelial ovarian cancer. Although use of platinum derivatives appears to be feasible during the second and third trimesters, their administration does raise concern regarding the transplacental transfer of these drugs in late pregnancy, and the short- and long-term effects have not been well-studied. Intraperitoneal chemotherapy in combination with intravenous chemotherapy has been associated with higher survival rates for patients with epithelial ovarian cancer. In patients opting for this type of therapy, delivery should be induced as soon as fetal pulmonary maturation can be documented before starting intraperitoneal therapy. Catheters can be placed at the time of cesarean section or laparoscopically in the postpartum period if the pregnancy was delivered vaginally.

A recent trial by the Gynecologic Oncology Group demonstrated an improvement in progression-free survival among patients treated with intravenous carboplatin plus paclitaxel and the antiangiogenesis agent bevacizumab. To date, there are no reports of use of bevacizumab in pregnancy, and one cannot comment on its potential for maternal, fetal, and neonatal effects.

Targeted (biologic) therapy for ovarian cancer in pregnancy. After an 8-year drought beginning in 2006, during which time there were no new drug approvals for ovarian cancer (in nonpregnant patients), finally in 2014, the management of epithelial ovarian cancer entered the modern area of targeted therapy with two approvals by the US Food and Drug Administration. Bevacizumab, a fully humanized monoclonal antibody (mAb) that targets the vascular endothelial growth factor (VEGF) ligand and sequesters it to prevent binding to the VEGF receptor (VEGFR) and thereby prevent tumor angiogenesis was approved in combination with chemotherapy (physician's choice of pegylated liposomal doxorubicin or topotecan or weekly, dose-dense paclitaxel) for platinum-resistant recurrent ovarian carcinoma. For patients with recurrent ovarian carcinoma harboring germline *BRCA* mutations (*BRCA1* or *BRCA2*), the poly-ADP-ribose polymerase I (PARP) inhibitor was approved for fourth-line therapy and beyond.

It is unclear whether mAbs are safe when used to treat cancer in pregnancy. Sarno et al. performed a literature search encompassing the years 2000 through January 2013 and reviewed the safety of mAbs during pregnancy. As will be discussed later under the section concerning breast cancer in pregnancy, the anti-HER2 monoclonal antibody, trastuzumab, has been associated with oligohydramnios and poor neonatal outcomes. There are very few reports on the use of bevacizumab in pregnant women, but because its antiangiogenic effects may have possible negative consequences on fetal development, the consensus that has been reached is one in which this drug should be avoided during pregnancy. Not only has VEGF blockade during pregnancy been associated with maternal preeclampsia and fetal intrauterine growth restriction, but in murine models, administration of anti-VEGF receptor tyrosine kinase inhibitors (TKIs) has led to abnormal vascular patterning in the mouse retina. Another VEGF receptor TKI, sunitinib, has been associated with embryo and fetal developmental toxicity in rats and rabbits at clinically relevant dose levels. Parenthetically, there have been reports of intravitreal bevacizumab being given safely to pregnant women for choroidal neovascularization with resulting improvement in vision and no untoward fetal effects. However, given the significant potential for adverse fetal developmental outcome resulting from inhibition of the VEGF access, the use of mABs and oral TKIs in pregnancy should be avoided.

With respect to PARP inhibitors in pregnancy, as in the case of bevacizumab, there essentially are no data. It is known that PARP1 expression in the murine uterus is under regulation by estrogen and that successful embryo implantation requires upregulation of PARP1. This suggests that PARP inhibitors should be contraindicated during early pregnancy, and until reasonable data become available, the author does not recommend their use during the entire conduct of pregnancy.

Other Types of Malignant Ovarian Tumors

Some ovarian cancers are particularly aggressive, and chemotherapy should be started immediately upon diagnosis. These include small cell ovarian cancer and metastatic Krukenberg tumors. The only long-term survivor of an advanced-stage small cell ovarian cancer was reported by Tewari and colleagues,

who described a patient diagnosed with the disease during pregnancy. After the histology was confirmed, the patient returned to the operating room in the second trimester and underwent cytoreductive surgery with the fetus in situ and postoperatively was treated with a six-drug regimen that contained both epithelial-cell and germ-cell activity. Another patient diagnosed with small cell ovarian cancer with hypercalcemia underwent conservative surgery during pregnancy followed by chemotherapy and died of disease 10 months after diagnosis. Taylor and colleagues reported the surgical removal of a Krukenberg tumor at 15 weeks of gestation followed by treatment with 10 cycles of 5-fluorouracil (5-FU), folinic acid, and irinotecan every 2 weeks until the 36th week of pregnancy. The neonate was born without complications and at age 4 months showed normal development.

Summary of the Adnexal Mass and Ovarian Cancer in Pregnancy

The problem of an adnexal mass in pregnancy is simple: One must have a high index of suspicion for malignancy, make the diagnosis early, and treat promptly. The difficulty arises when both patient and physician resist abdominal exploration during pregnancy because of fear of precipitating fetal wastage. However, the potential danger to the mother far exceeds the imagined danger to the child. Most of the difficulties seen with ovarian tumors are those of omission rather than of commission. The probability of ovarian cancer must be kept foremost in the minds of physicians caring for these patients. At laparotomy, most malignant ovarian tumors apparently confined to one ovary will require complete surgical staging. A technique of "hands off the uterus," whenever possible, appears to reduce postoperative uterine contractions.

Breast Cancer

Pregnancy-associated breast cancer (PABC) is defined as breast cancer diagnosed during pregnancy or lactation up to 12 months postpartum. The disease is a disaster for all involved. Both the patient and physician find it difficult to accept this dreaded disease in a healthy young pregnant woman. Because breast cancer is rare in women younger than 35 years, this problem, fortunately, is a rare complication of pregnancy, with an incidence of approximately one case for every 3000 deliveries. Conversely, of all patients with breast cancer, 1% to 2% are pregnant at the time of diagnosis. PABC provides a challenging scenario for the mother and oncologist. **It is the second most common malignancy to complicate pregnancy, but unlike cervical cancer, it is not screened for during pregnancy, and because delays in diagnosis are common and the diagnosis itself is elusive, often patients are diagnosed with advanced tumors for which prognosis is poor.** Furthermore, the management of breast cancer often involves a coordination of surgery, radiotherapy, chemotherapy, and even hormonal therapy, all of which may affect the pregnancy. Finally, there are several distinct hormonal issues related to pregnancy that may have an influence on the course of breast cancer.

Recently, a group of specialists convened to review guidelines and provide guidance on how to implement recent advances in breast cancer diagnosis and treatment in the pregnant population. The consensus was that the majority of women with PABC will be considered for definitive treatment during pregnancy and that many treatments, including sentinel lymph node biopsy (SLNB) and systemic therapy with taxanes, platinum agents, and dose-dense regimens can be given safely after the first trimester of pregnancy. Radiation therapy and anti-HER2–directed therapy (eg, trastuzumab, lapatinib, trastuzumab emtansine [T-DM1], and pertuzumab) are best avoided during pregnancy but may be considered in some rare instances.

In a population-based cohort study using data from Swedish registries from 1963 to 2002 encompassing women aged 15 to 44 years at the date of breast cancer diagnosis, Andersson and colleagues noted that the incidence of PABC increased from 16.0 to 37.4 per 100,000 deliveries comparing the first and last calendar periods under study. The authors attributed the increasing incidence in Sweden partly to the trend of postponement of childbearing to an older age.

Historically, PABC has been associated with a poor prognosis, with accounts from the 19th century describing exceedingly rapid growth and a malignant course. In 1943, Haagensen and Stout reinforced this feeling of doom when they decided that the outcome for this group of patients was so poor that they recommended surgical treatment not be offered. Contemporary opinion for the most part maintains the dismal prognosis associated with PABC. It must be acknowledged that the literature comprises mainly single-institution retrospective experiences and case reports. The only series containing greater than 100 patients are four in number (White, Bunker and Peters, Ribeiro and Palmer, Clark and Reid), none of which were published after 1978.

Although the overall survival rate for breast cancer is greater than 60%, the overall survival rate in pregnancy is reported by some to have dropped to 15% or 20%. Pregnant patients tend to have a higher incidence of positive axillary lymph nodes. Locoregional spread of the tumor portends a poor prognosis and in all likelihood suggests that the neoplasm has metastasized at the time of the initiation of therapy. The advanced stage of the presentation of disease in pregnant patients has been attributed to multiple factors. First, the engorged breast can successfully obscure a lesion for a much longer period. Survival rates are lower for cases diagnosed late in pregnancy than for those recognized in the first trimester. Others emphasize the 30 to 50 multiples of increase in serum levels of estrogens and progesterone. In addition, there may be increased vascularity and lymphatic drainage from the pregnant breast, assisting the metastatic process to regional lymph nodes. If a lesion is detected early (present <3 months, smaller than 2 cm, and no positive nodes), the chance of survival (70%–80%) is the same for pregnant and nonpregnant patients. If, however, there is involvement of the subareolar region; diffuse inflammatory carcinoma; edema or ulceration of the skin; fixation of the tumor to the breast wall; or involvement of the high axillary, supraclavicular, or internal mammary nodes, the prognosis is poor for both pregnant and nonpregnant patients.

Presentation

At least 10% of patients with breast cancer who are younger than 40 years will be pregnant at diagnosis. PABC typically presents as a painless mass or thickening. In some cases, there may be an associated nipple discharge, and in the lactating breast, the infant may exhibit the "milk rejection sign," effectively refusing the breast that contains the cancer. The mean breast weight normally doubles in pregnancy from 200 to 400 g, resulting in breast firmness and increased breast density. Mammographic evaluation of the pregnant breast is difficult to interpret, and the clinical examination may be deceptive. This has profound implications in terms of delays in diagnosis and treatment, which, as discussed earlier, are common in PABC. Many patients with PABC will have a delay in diagnosis ranging from 1 to 2.5 months during pregnancy and up to 6 months during lactation. In a 1991 series from the Memorial Sloan-Kettering Cancer Center in New York, 44 of 56 patients did not have the diagnosis of cancer made until the postpartum period. **Overall, in a review of the literature by Puckridge and colleagues, a delay of 2 to 15 months longer from manifestation of the first symptoms to the diagnosis of cancer occurs in PABC.** Given the tumor-doubling time of 130 days, a 1-month delay in primary tumor treatment increases the risk of axillary metastases by 0.9%, and a 6-month delay increases the risk by 5.1%. **For this reason particularly, PABC has been considered an ominous diagnosis, but when age and stage are taken into account, there is no difference in the survival rate of PABC cases compared with non-PABC cases.** Pregnancy is not thought to be an independent risk factor.

Evaluation

A proposed management algorithm for PABC appears in Fig. 15.10. Early diagnosis has been associated with improved survival rates and relies on the liberal use of imaging strategies and the core and fine-needle biopsy techniques for this group of patients. Mammography in conjunction with abdominal lead shielding can be safely used during pregnancy, but as discussed earlier, the engorged and lactating breast increases tissue density and may mask abnormalities. Ultrasonography yields equivalent information with no known adverse effects to the fetus. Fine-needle aspiration (FNA) may be difficult to interpret cytologically secondary to cellular changes that take place during pregnancy and lactation and is often associated with an increase in the false-negative rate. Core biopsy remains the gold standard in making the diagnosis. When necessary, an open biopsy under local anesthesia is also appropriate. Stopping lactation with ice packs and breast binding or bromocriptine (2.5 mg three times daily for 1 week) beforehand will reduce the risk of a milk fistula. The breasts should be emptied of milk before the biopsy, and a pressure dressing will decrease the risk of hematoma that may develop from the hypervascularity of the pregnant breast.

Approximately 75% to 90% of PABCs are ductal carcinomas, mirroring what is observed in the nonpregnant population. Historically, there was a perceived increase in inflammatory carcinoma of the breast during pregnancy; however, this has since been refuted in contemporary series, in which the

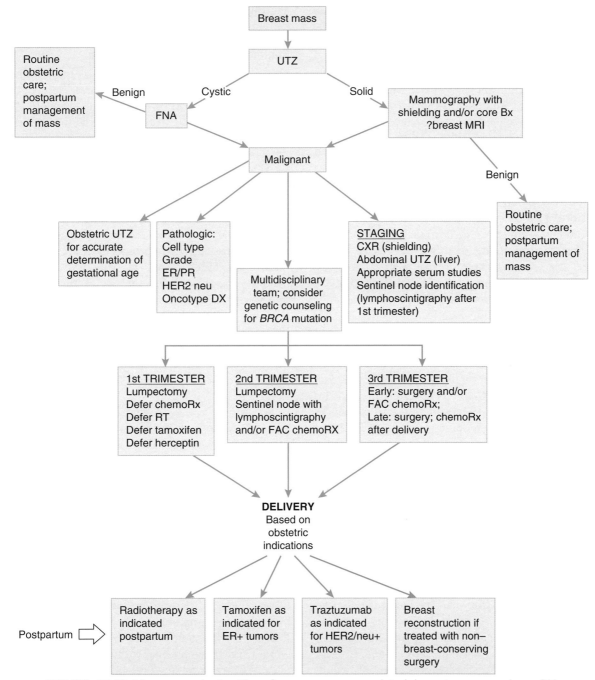

FIGURE 15.10 Management algorithm for pregnancy-associated breast cancer. *chemoRX,* chemotherapy; *CXR,* chest radiography; *ER,* estrogen receptor; *FAC,* 5-fluorouracil, doxorubicin (Adriamycin), and cyclophosphamide; *FNA,* fine-needle aspiration; *UTZ,* ultrasonography.

incidence ranges from 1.5% to 4.2% among pregnant and non-pregnant patients. Several studies have demonstrated adverse pathologic features in PABC. Most patients with PABC have estrogen receptor (ER)–negative and progesterone receptor (PR)–negative tumors. This may be a result of the production of false-negative results by the ligand-binding assay used for ER and PR when high circulating levels of estrogen and progesterone downregulate receptors. Immunohistochemistry has not been able to detect a difference in the number of hormone receptor–positive tumors when PABC cases are compared with cases of breast cancer in nonpregnant patients of similar ages. Additionally, higher levels of c-ERBB-2 overexpression and p53 mutations have been reported in lactational carcinomas but not in tumors diagnosed during pregnancy. Furthermore, there have been reports of increased HER-2/neu–positive tumors compared with nonpregnant control participant. It is interesting that the HER-2/neu oncogene product p105 is overexpressed not only in ductal carcinomas but also in fetal epithelial cells and the placenta and that toward the end of the third trimester of pregnancy, serum levels of p105 normally rise.

It is known from epidemiologic studies that there is an increased incidence of breast cancers in certain families; the risk increases 5 to 10 times if a patient's mother or sister has had the disease. It is interesting that women with a genetic predisposition to breast cancer may be overrepresented among cases of PABC, with a significant family history of breast cancer being three times more common in women with PABC than among nonpregnant patients with breast cancer. Along these lines, PABC has been associated with a higher rate of *BRCA2* allelic mutation compared with sporadic breast cancer. Indeed, a Swedish report of 292 women with breast cancer before the age of 40 years demonstrated a greater likelihood of known *BRCA1* and *BRCA2* carriers to develop cancer during pregnancy.

Staging of breast cancer currently uses a complicated system jointly recommended by the International Union Against Cancer and the American Joint Committee on Cancer (AJCC) (see Table 14.12). The Haagensen clinical staging for breast cancer is more useful in pointing out the unfavorable prognostic indicators in this disease process. Lateral and posteroanterior chest radiographs in conjunction with lead shielding are considered safe during pregnancy, with an estimated fetal dose of only 0.6 mGy. Provided a catheter is placed to allow rapid drainage of radioactive material from the bladder, a low-dose labeled technetium-99 bone scan is also safe. The low-dose bone scan exposes the fetus to 0.0008 Gy instead of the standard 0.0019 Gy. The higher radiation exposure to the fetus excludes the use of CT in planning a metastatic workup, but MRI may be used to study the thorax and abdomen and to image the skeleton. **MRI is preferred to ultrasonography for hepatic imaging and is also the safest and most sensitive way to study the brain.**

Surgical Management

Surgery is the definitive treatment for PABC (see Fig. 15.10). The extent of surgery in the treatment of breast cancer is being debated throughout the world, and this issue cannot be adequately addressed here. Lumpectomy or partial mastectomy is more commonly used, especially when the lesion is not large, although the preferred surgical treatment for stage I, stage II, and some stage III tumors involves mastectomy, thus avoiding the need for adjuvant radiotherapy in most cases (ie, early-stage breast cancer). Because nodal metastases are commonly identified in PABC and nodal status dictates the choice of adjuvant chemotherapy, axillary dissection has been routinely recommended, especially in light of the potential risk to the fetus from radioisotope if SLNB was attempted.

The timing of surgery for cancer diagnosed late in pregnancy is another source of debate. Some reports suggest that patients treated postpartum survive longer than those treated in the second and third trimesters. This suggests that postponement of therapy for patients near term may be of benefit. These reports fail to consider the possibility that patients selected for postponed treatment might have been those with small, more favorable cancers discovered late in pregnancy, but larger, aggressive, anaplastic cancers with rapid progression received immediate treatment. If such treatment bias exists, prompt treatment would not be expected to correlate with good results,

and treatment after delivery would appear favorable because of a preponderance of favorable patients in that group.

Sentinel Lymph Node Identification

Keleher and colleagues assessed the risk to the embryo or fetus associated with SLNB and lymphoscintigraphy of the breast in pregnant patients. After peritumoral injection of 92.5 MBq (2.5 mCi) of filtered ^{99m}Tc sulfur colloid the day before surgery in two nonpregnant women with breast cancer, they calculated the absorbed dose to the embryo or fetus for three theoretic extreme scenarios of biodistribution and pharmacokinetics and described the maximum absorbed dose to the fetus being 4.3 mGy calculated for the worst-case scenario. The authors concluded that breast lymphoscintigraphy during pregnancy presents a very low risk to the embryo or fetus. In 2008, Khera and colleagues searched a prospectively accrued breast database for cases of SLNB in patients with PABC and identified 10 patients. The mean gestational age at the time of biopsy was 15.8 weeks. All patients were successfully mapped, and a positive SLN was identified in five patients (50%). Nine patients (90%) delivered healthy babies without reported complications, and one patient elected to terminate the pregnancy in the first trimester to start chemotherapy. The authors concluded that SLNB can be safely performed in pregnancy with minimal risk to the fetus.

Spanheimer and colleagues measured abdominal, perineal, and urinary radiation in 14 women with breast cancer and total uterine doses were calculated. The average dose to the uterus from bladder radioactivity determined from voided urine was 0.44 ± 0.44 microGy. The average radiation dose to the uterus of 1.14 ± 0.76 microGy was derived through an average of abdominal and perineal doses plus contribution from the bladder dose. One patient was 16 weeks' pregnant at the time of SLNB, and the total calculated uterine dose was 1.67 microGy, suggesting that pregnancy does not significantly alter measured uterine radiation. When compared with average background radiation (ie, 3,000 microGy per year or 8.2 microGy per day), it was concluded that the measured uterine dose of radiation from lymphoscintigraphy for SLN biopsy was significantly less than the average daily background radiation.

In a recent report by Gentilni and colleagues, 12 patients with PABC received low-dose (10 MBq on average) lymphoscintigraphy using ^{99m}Tc human serum albumin nanocolloids. The SLN was identified in all patients. In 10 patients, the SLN was pathologically negative. One patient had a micrometastasis in an SLN, and another who had a metastasis in the SLN underwent axillary clearance. Eleven healthy babies were born with no malformations and appropriate birth weight. One baby who underwent lymphatic mapping during the 26th week of gestation was operated on at the age of 3 months for a ventricular septal defect and at 43 months was in good health. The malformation was suspected at the anatomy scan performed during the 21st week of gestation, well before lymphoscintigraphy. At a median follow-up period of 32 months, no overt axillary recurrence appeared in the patients with negative SLNs. This experience, together with those described earlier, supports the safety and efficacy of SLN identification in women with

PABC when performed with a low-dose lymphoscintigraphic technique.

Breast Reconstruction

Although the performance of a transverse myocutaneous flap of the rectus abdominis muscle (TRAM flap) is a satisfying, one-step, immediate reconstruction of good aesthetic quality without need for prosthetic materials, it is not recommended in patients with PABC who undergo mastectomy. The procedure should be deferred to the postpartum period. The problem of residual functional capacities of the abdominal wall deprived of a part or of all its rectus muscle also has important implications for future pregnancies. In fact, for some authors in the past, the desire for future childbearing was a contraindication to TRAM flap breast reconstruction because it was thought that the abdominal wall, weakened by rotation of one or both of its rectus muscles, would not be capable of withstanding the stress induced by pregnancy. **To avoid the development of a hernia in the abdominal wall at the donor site, an interval of at least 12 months between breast reconstruction with a TRAM flap and pregnancy is recommended.**

Adjuvant Therapy

Women with early lesions may opt for a tissue-sparing procedure. In these cases, local irradiation is often required. Radiotherapy to the breast, chest wall, or axillary lymph nodes, even with shielding, results in a significant fetal dose because of scatter in excess of that which is considered safe. The doses of internal scatter of radiation have been calculated. Embryonic exposure resulting from breast radiotherapy with a dose of 0.1 Gy during organogenesis in the first trimester not only increases the risk of malformations but can also cause mental retardation. Using anthropomorphic phantoms simulating the geometry of a pregnant woman, the dose to the fetus resulting from tangential breast irradiation in each trimester has been well-summarized by Toesca et al. in their review of locoregional treatment of PABC. With fetal shielding and x-ray energies from 4 to 10 MV as used for breast radiotherapy, the fetal irradiation dose in the first and second trimesters is lower than the threshold values associated with organ malformations. However, during the third trimester when the fetus moves out of the pelvis and into the abdomen, the dose exceeds this threshold. For example, at 12 weeks of gestation, the fetus would receive 10 to 15 cGy. In the third trimester, this dose can be as high as 200 cGy. This is because, although during the first trimester, the fetus is in a safer position and can be better shielded, it is more sensitive to the effects of radiation. In contrast, as the fetus enlarges and is less sensitive to radiation, it moves upward out of the pelvis, where it is less readily shielded and exposed to higher levels of ionizing radiation. Local irradiation should be deferred until after delivery of the fetus (see Fig. 15.10). **Women treated with adjuvant radiation during the postpartum period will not be able to lactate from the irradiated breast.**

Locally advanced disease is difficult to manage with the pregnancy in place. Chemotherapy or local radiotherapy, followed in 6 weeks by mastectomy, is the usual treatment plan for these lesions. For advanced disease, chemotherapy has been used after the first trimester when the mother is reluctant to terminate the pregnancy and the disease appears to be progressing at an alarming rate. The issue of whether chemotherapy should be administered to patients with node-positive breast cancer in pregnancy is complicated by reports suggesting that both single-agent and combination chemotherapy may significantly improve survival rates in premenopausal patients in an adjuvant setting. Follow-ups of 10 and 15 years are always necessary in breast cancer, but it appears that premenopausal patients are the best candidates for aggressive adjuvant chemotherapy and a resulting improved survival rate. This is especially pertinent to patients in whom positive nodes are discovered at the time of the initial procedure.

Table 15.8 contains reports of chemotherapy use during pregnancy, with favorable neonatal outcomes noted when treatment was administered only after the first trimester.

In a recent review by Azim and colleagues, the authors identified 56 different reports that have described the systemic treatment of PABC and separated them into four groups, as described in the following discussion.

Neoadjuvant and Adjuvant Chemotherapy for Pregnancy-Associated Breast Cancer

The FAC regimen (5-FU, doxorubicin, and cyclophosphamide) is the most commonly administered regimen in the neoadjuvant or adjuvant setting. The safety of this regimen was prospectively examined by Hahn and colleagues at the MD Anderson Hospital and Tumor Institute in Houston. Fifty-seven patients were treated, and the regimen was well tolerated and did not adversely affect the pregnancy. All women had live births, with three congenital defects reported, including Down syndrome, clubfoot, and congenital bilateral ureteral reflux. The investigators did not consider these anomalies to have resulted directly from chemotherapy exposure when the incidences were compared with those in the general population. Eighteen of the children have been followed until school age, and only two required special attention schools (including the child with Down syndrome).

Peccatori and colleagues from the European Institute of Oncology in Milan prospectively evaluated the safety of weekly epirubicin (35 mg/m^2) starting in the second trimester in 20 women with PABC. The schedule was selected to potentially allow lower peak plasma concentration of the drug, thus lowering the risk of maternal myelotoxicity and possible placental transfer of the drug. There were no grade III or IV toxicities and only one congenital anomaly (polycystic kidney). All children have had normal development at 2 years' median follow-up.

Based on these two studies and other retrospective series and case reports from the literature, Azim and colleagues suggested that anthracycline-based regimens are probably safe starting in the second trimester. FAC is the most commonly studied regimen, but offering epirubicin instead of doxorubicin is an option.

In recent years, taxanes have been incorporated into the adjuvant and neoadjuvant settings to improve outcomes. There have been seven reports of docetaxel treatment and two reports of paclitaxel therapy for PABC. In six of these cases, the taxane

TABLE 15.8	Congenital Anomalies After in Utero Exposure to Breast Cancer Chemotherapy				
Authors	**Year**	**Patients (n)**	**Treatment**	**Trimester**	**Outcome**
Tobias and Bloom	1980	1	AV, prednisone	2	No anomaly
Murray et al.	1984	1	AC, radiation	1	Imperforate anus, rectovaginal fistula
Mulvihill et al.	1987	1	CMF, melphalan	n/s	Spontaneous abortion
Zemlickis et al.	1992	2	CMF, melphalan (both cases)	1	Spontaneous abortion
		1	CAFV, tamoxifen	1	No anomaly
		1	CAF, tamoxifen	3	No anomaly
		1	CMF	3	No anomaly
Cullins et al.	1980	1	Tamoxifen	1, 2, 3	Goldenhar syndrome
Tewari et al.	1997	1	Tamoxifen	1, 2	Ambiguous genitalia
Turchi and Villasis.	1988	1	CAMF	1	No anomaly
Berry et al.	1999	24	CAF	2, 3	No anomaly
Isaacs et al.	2001	1	Tamoxifen, 0.0017 Gy RT	1, 2, 3	Preauricular skin tags
Andreadis et al.	2004	1	FEC,* 28 Gy RT,† tamoxifen,‡ zoledronic acid‡	1, 2, 3	No anomalies
Gonzalez-Angulo et al.	2004	1	Neoadjuvant paclitaxel	2, 3	No anomalies
Warraich and Smith	2009	1	T, tamoxifen	1, 2, 3	Pulmonary hypoplasia
Baele et al.	2009	1	T, tamoxifen	1, 2	Respiratory failure
Azim et al.	2009	1	T	Preconception	No anomaly

*First trimester only.
†Second trimester.
‡Second and third trimesters.
A, Doxorubicin (Adriamycin); C, cyclophosphamide; E, epirubicin; F, 5-fluorouracil; M, methotrexate; T, trastuzumab; n/s, not specified; RT, radiotherapy; V, vincristine.
Modified from Woo JC, Yu T, Hurd TC: Breast cancer in pregnancy: a literature review. *Arch Surg* 2003;138:91.

was given as a single agent. None of the nine cases were associated with a poor obstetric or fetal outcome. Although the experience using taxanes in PABC is clearly limited, this early evidence is reassuring.

The CMF regimen (cyclophosphamide, methotrexate, 5-FU) has been used for many years as standard adjuvant therapy in breast cancer. As a result of the potential for teratogenicity by methotrexate (after first-trimester exposure), this regimen is not recommended for PABC.

Chemotherapy for Metastatic Breast Cancer

In contrast to early PABC for which neoadjuvant or adjuvant therapy is administered in a good-prognosis setting, patients with metastatic disease have fewer options because treatment of the mother must take priority, especially in pregnancies remote from term. Anthracyclines remain the most studied agents for management of metastatic breast cancer, but data are extremely limited in PABC. Patients with bone metastases are frequently treated with bisphosphonates to decrease the risk of skeletal events. There has been some concern for the development of genital and skeletal defects with bisphosphonate use in pregnancy. In addition, the potential for hypocalcemia exists with bisphosphonate therapy, which may lead to stimulation of uterine contractions. There has been very limited experience in PABC, but no adverse events associated with bisphosphonate use have been reported. Among 21 pregnant women exposed to bisphosphonates for osteoporosis during the first trimester, there were no adverse events for the fetus or to the conduct of the pregnancy.

HER2/Neu–Targeted Agents in Pregnancy

Trastuzumab and lapatinib are two HER2/neu–targeted agents that have been used increasingly in recent years for the management of breast cancer. Azim and colleagues identified 13 cases of trastuzumab use for PABC and one report of lapatinib therapy for a patient with metastatic breast cancer who inadvertently became pregnant during therapy. For this patient, lapatinib was discontinued at 11 weeks of gestation, and the pregnancy continued with a normal outcome.

For the 13 patients exposed to trastuzumab, only one patient elected to undergo therapeutic abortion. Eight patients received the drug as a single agent; the others were treated in combination with taxanes, vinorelbine, or tamoxifen. Metastatic disease was the setting for three patients, and seven patients received the drug during the preconception period and the first trimester. There were five cases of anhydramnios, one case of oligohydramnios, one case of intrauterine growth restriction, and one case of preterm premature rupture of the membranes. Four neonatal deaths were reported secondary to respiratory and renal failure. Three additional babies developed transient respiratory or renal failure but recovered. None of the reports described any fetal or maternal serious cardiac events despite the pivotal role of HER2/neu in cardiogenesis and cardiac repair pathways.

The increased risk of oligo- or anhydramnios is thought to result from the effect of trastuzumab on the fetal renal epithelium in which HER2/neu is strongly expressed. Some have correlated the effect of trastuzumab to an inhibition of the VEGF, which regulates the production and reabsorption of amniotic fluid. Prolonged exposure to trastuzumab was consistently associated with serious adverse events both on the pregnancy and on the fetus in these cases. Azim and colleagues have advised that in the case of accidental pregnancy, the drug should be discontinued, and the patient should be counseled that brief exposure to the drug is unlikely to be detrimental to the fetus and pregnancy. Elective administration of trastuzumab during pregnancy is not advisable.

Hormonal Treatments for Pregnancy-Associated Breast Cancer

Preclinical models have shown that in utero exposure to tamoxifen increases the incidence of genital abnormalities. Tewari and colleagues reported the first case of fetal teratogenicity developing from maternal exposure to tamoxifen. The drug was discontinued at 20 weeks of gestation, but the fetus developed ambiguous genitalia with labial fusion and clitoromegaly. A second case has been reported in which tamoxifen was stopped at 26 weeks of gestation, and the fetus developed Goldenhar syndrome. A third patient had the drug discontinued during the first trimester, and the pregnancy outcome was normal; at 27 months' follow-up, the baby's development was without sequela. The literature contains only one patient who elected to receive tamoxifen as a therapeutic intervention for metastatic PABC; the pregnancy resulted in a normal baby. There are also two cases in which tamoxifen was administered in conjunction with trastuzumab, and pregnancy was accidentally discovered at 20 weeks of gestational age. In both cases, fetal mortality was reported, but this was likely secondary to trastuzumab exposure. Finally, normal outcomes have been reported in two cases in which tamoxifen was given together with FAC and with CMF plus vincristine.

As with trastuzumab, we recommend active contraception use during tamoxifen therapy, and in those cases in which pregnancy inadvertently occurs, the drug should be discontinued. Although 85 pregnancies with normal fetal outcomes are contained in a tamoxifen chemoprevention study, women should be counseled regarding the possibility of genital or more complex malformations associated with in utero exposure to this drug.

Prognosis of Pregnancy-Associated Breast Cancer

Thirty-two women with PABC referred to two European Union oncology centers between 1995 and 2007 were analyzed by Halaska and colleagues. Sixteen cases were diagnosed during pregnancy, and 16 were diagnosed within 1 year after delivery. The investigators matched each patient for age at diagnosis, tumor size, and stage to a control group of 32 nonpregnant patients. Overall survival was similar in the PABC and non-PABC patients ($P = 0.449$). The subgroup of patients with PABC diagnosed within 1 year after delivery showed a shorter time to relapse than controls or patients in whom PABC was diagnosed during pregnancy ($P = 0.0178$). Such findings concerning poorer prognosis among postpartum diagnoses had not been identified in previous series and warrant continued attention.

Cardonic and Iacobucci analyzed the maternal and fetal outcomes of 130 women with PABC that were reported to the voluntary Cancer and Pregnancy Registry and followed prospectively. Among the 130 patients, 120 were diagnosed with a primary tumor, eight with recurrent disease, and two with a new primary malignancy. The mean maternal age at diagnosis was 34.8 years, and the mean gestational age at diagnosis was 13.2 weeks. For 113 women who were followed for a mean of 3.14 years, recurrence was reported in 30 women at a mean of 16.2 months from delivery. Twenty-one patients are deceased at a mean interval of 24.71 months from delivery to death. Only 42% were diagnosed with an ER-positive tumor, and 35% of cases had PR-positive disease. Human epidermal growth factor receptor 2 was positive in 25% of patients. Survival rates by stage for a primary diagnosis in pregnancy included stage I, 100%; stage II, 86%; stage III, 86%; and stage IV, 0%. These survival rates are similar to what is observed in the nonpregnant breast cancer population.

A very large study was conducted by Rodriguez and colleagues evaluating 797 PBAC cases identified by linking the California Cancer Registry (1991–1997) with the California Patient Discharge Data Set; 4177 age-matched, non-PBAC breast cancer control participants were also identified. PABC cases were significantly more likely to have more advanced-stage, larger primary tumor, hormone receptor–negative tumor, and mastectomy as a component of their treatment. In survival analysis, PABC had a higher death rate than non-PABC (39.2% vs. 33.4%; $P = 0.002$). In multivariable analysis, advancing stage, African American ethnicity (68% increased risk over non-Hispanic whites), hormone receptor–negative tumors (20% increased risk), and pregnancy (14% increased risk) were all significant predictors of death.

Lactation

Whether breastfeeding is safe or possible has also been debated. Many have postulated that breast cancer is at least in part of viral origin, and the possibility exists that the contralateral breast will be contaminated with the causative agent, which will be passed to the fetus. This theory has never been borne out in fact, but most surgeons recommend artificial feeding of the infant, ostensibly to avoid vascular enrichment in the opposite breast, which may also contain a neoplasm.

Reports by Higgins and Haffty and by Tralins suggest that successful lactation in the breast treated by lumpectomy and irradiation is possible. Apparently, the location of the breast incision is important. **It is not surprising that circumareolar incisions were associated with diminished ability to lactate because such incisions interrupt a large number of major milk ducts. Radial incisions in the breast interrupt fewer ducts but may be cosmetically inferior.** In addition, the size, shape, and orientation of the nipple are important to allow its normal mechanical function. Patients whose nipples did not extend sufficiently, were not oriented properly, or were not supple found that the infant would not nurse from the treated breast. Finally, concerns have been expressed by some clinicians that attempts to breastfeed after conservative surgery may lead to a greater incidence of mastitis secondary to disruptions of the ductal system.

FIGURE 15.11 Hormonal considerations in breast cancer. *ER,* Estrogen receptor; *hCG,* human chorionic gonadotropin; *PR,* progesterone receptor.

Hormonal Considerations: Pregnancy Preceding Breast Cancer

Protective effect of human chorionic gonadotropin. **The hormonal issues specific to breast cancer appear in** Fig. 15.11. Epidemiologic data have demonstrated a 50% reduction in the risk of breast cancer in women who complete full-term pregnancies before 20 years of age. The benefit is seen among all ethnic groups worldwide and increases with increasing parity. There is a declination in risk reduction beyond the age of 30 years. Both human and animal breast tissues and human breast cell lines contain low levels of receptors that bind hCG and its structural and functional homolog luteinizing hormone. These gonadotropins exert numerous anticancer effects in breast cancer models and cells, prompting some investigators to speculate that the elevated levels of hCG associated with full-term pregnancies may exert a protective effect against the later development of breast cancer.

Recent antecedent pregnancy. The previous discussion notwithstanding, concerns have been raised that the protective benefit of pregnancy on the risk of later breast cancer may be biphasic, with a transient increase in the risk of breast cancer shortly after pregnancy followed by a greater long-term reduction in risk. Russo and colleagues have postulated that this may occur via the short-term stimulation of any existing malignant clones under the influence of the hormonal milieu of pregnancy, but longer term inhibition of breast carcinogenesis is a consequence of induction of differentiation of normal mammary stem cells in the later stages of pregnancy that otherwise have the potential for neoplastic change.

Further extrapolation leads to the possibility that a recent childbirth before the diagnosis of breast cancer may increase a woman's risk of dying from the disease. Whiteman and colleagues observed 4299 US women ages 20 to 54 years enrolled between 1980 and 1982 as incident breast cancer patients in the population-based, case-control study known as the Cancer and Steroid Hormone Study. The 15-year survival rates were 38%, 51%, and 60% among women aged 20 to 45 years whose last birth was 12 months or less, 13 to 48 months, and more than

48 months before diagnosis, respectively, compared with 65% among nulliparous women. Phillips and colleagues prospectively studied 750 women diagnosed with breast cancer before age 45 years who were part of the population-based Australian Breast Cancer Family Study and demonstrated that the proximity of last childbirth to subsequent breast cancer diagnosis was a predictor of mortality independent of histopathologic tumor characteristics. Specifically, compared with nulliparous women, the investigators found that women who gave birth within 2 years before diagnosis were more likely to have axillary node–positive (58% vs 41%; $P = 0.01$) and ER-negative (58% vs 39%; $P = 0.005$) tumors. The unadjusted hazard ratios for death were 2.3, 1.7, and 0.9 for patients who gave birth less than 2 years, 2 to 5 years, and 5 or more years before diagnosis, respectively.

Breastfeeding. In an effort to determine what contribution (if any) breastfeeding has on the subsequent development of breast cancer, the Collaborative Group on Hormonal Factors in Breast Cancer examined the individual data from 47 epidemiologic studies in 30 countries that included information on breastfeeding patterns. In total, 50,302 women with invasive breast cancer were compared with 96,973 control participants. The investigators noted that women with breast cancer had fewer births than did control participants (2.2 vs. 2.6) and that fewer parous women with cancer than parous control participants had ever breastfed (71% vs. 79%), with their average lifetime duration of breastfeeding being shorter (9.8 vs. 15.6 months). The relative risk for breast cancer decreased by 4.3% for every 12 months of breastfeeding, and a relative risk reduction of 7.0% was seen for each birth. Thus, the longer women breastfed, the more they were protected against breast cancer. The lack of or short lifetime duration of breastfeeding typical of women in developed countries may contribute greatly to the high incidence of breast cancer in industrialized nations.

Hormonal Considerations: Pregnancy Coincident With Breast Cancer

Although there is no clear evidence that pregnancy adversely affects the course of this disease, the suspicion persists. It has been established that after the diagnosis is made, stage for stage, pregnant patients do as well as nonpregnant patients. However, the low incidence of stage I lesions in pregnancy strongly suggests an acceleration of the disease process in the preclinical period. Many cell kinetic studies of breast cancer suggest that lesions are harbored within the breast for 5 to 8 years before becoming clinical entities. Because the period of gestation is no longer than 9 months, it is difficult to believe that the sole explanation for the high incidence of advanced disease in pregnancy is related to late diagnosis caused by the engorged breast.

The massive endogenous hormone production in pregnancy may adversely affect the course of breast cancer. Urinary excretion of all three major fractions—estrone, estradiol, and estriol—rises progressively after the eighth week of gestation, although there is a disproportionate rise in estriol production by the placenta. Serum concentrations of total estrogens rise nearly 2000-fold, from $4\,\mu g/dL$ early in pregnancy to mean values of 8 to 22 mg/dL at term. The ability of estrogens to promote growth of breast cancer in animals and humans has been amply illustrated. Whether the stimulatory effect of increased estrogen production has an adverse effect on prognosis or whether the disproportionate rise of estriol, a relatively weak estrogen and a possible antagonist of estrone and estradiol, confers some measure of protection is unknown.

Additional hormone substances secreted in increased quantities in pregnancy that might influence neoplastic growths in the breast include the glucocorticoids and prolactin. Elevated corticosteroid levels are a regular accompaniment of pregnancy and might influence the outcome of breast cancer. Mean production of 17-hydroxycorticosteroids increases from 12 mg/24 hours to approximately 18 mg/24 hours in late pregnancy. Because glucocorticoids can reduce cellular immunity and perhaps promote the implantation and growth of malignant neoplasms, this increased production has grave clinical implications.

Similarly, elevated levels of prolactin produced by the hypophysis and of human placental lactogen by the placenta late in pregnancy and during milk production might affect breast cancer adversely. Prolactin promotes the growth of dimethylanthracene-induced mammary tumors in mice. Its role is not established in humans, but it is a subject of current investigation. The levels of prolactin in patients with breast cancer are not appreciably different from those in control subjects, and prolactin suppression with ergot compounds or with L-dopa has not proved to be of therapeutic value. However, the observation that women with bone pain from metastatic breast cancer sometimes obtain relief from prolactin suppression implicates prolactin as a possible promoter of breast cancer in humans.

Estrogen-Receptor and Progesterone-Receptor Status

A recent paper by Middleton and colleagues detected ER positivity in seven and PR positivity in six of 25 patients with PABC whose tumors were studied by immunohistochemistry. Although most tumors associated with PABC are ER and PR negative, a proportion will be ER positive, thus bringing to the discussion the possibility of tamoxifen use during pregnancy

(see later). There has been one report of acquired resistance to tamoxifen during the treatment of a patient with PABC, in which the investigators suggest that the changing expression of ER isoforms in pregnancy may have contributed to drug resistance.

Pregnancy Termination

Historically, pregnancy was of concern to surgeons primarily because the risk of excess hemorrhage and shock with mastectomy was increased greatly in the gravid state. Billroth advocated premature induction of labor for this reason but did not find that abortion contributed to cure. More contemporary commentators have argued that the striking rise in estrogen production during pregnancy is of sufficient concern to warrant pregnancy termination and that future pregnancy avoidance should be an important principle of continuing care. Indeed, although many clinicians think that localized breast cancer in the first trimester is a valid reason to recommend termination, reports by Peters and Rosemond illustrate that therapeutic abortion has no effect on survival, and the presence of a fetus does not compromise proper therapy in early stages. Similarly, therapy for localized disease in later pregnancy can be carried out when the diagnosis is made without pregnancy termination. Of interest, in an updated presentation of 413 patients with PABC referred to the Princess Margaret Hospital in Canada between 1931 and 1985, Clark and Chua observed that therapeutic abortion in breast cancer with coincident, lactational, and subsequent pregnancies is associated with decreased survival. The reasons for this remain unclear. **Therapeutic abortion is not currently believed to be an essential component of effective treatment of early disease despite the theoretic advantage of removing the source of massive estrogen production.**

It is critically important to emphasize that treatment of breast cancer should not be delayed provided there are no major obstetric issues. In advanced breast cancer, therapeutic abortion is usually a necessity to achieve effective palliation. In the first trimester of pregnancy, the termination can be accomplished by suction curettage of the uterus; later in pregnancy, termination is accomplished by dinoprostone (Prostin) suppositories, oxytocin (Pitocin) administration, hysterotomy, or hysterectomy. When pregnancy enters the third trimester, the decision for preterm delivery depends heavily on the patient's wishes and the urgency for palliation. A short wait until a viable fetus can be obtained might not be accompanied by significant progress of the neoplasm. Continued gestation represents no threat to the fetus, and the risk of transplacental metastases to the fetus is negligible.

Tamoxifen

Tamoxifen citrate is a nonsteroidal weak estrogen that has found successful applications for each stage of breast cancer in the treatment of selected patients. Tamoxifen was originally introduced for the treatment of advanced disease in postmenopausal women; however, the drug is now also available for the palliative treatment of premenopausal women with ER-positive disease. The proven efficacy of tamoxifen and the low incidence of side effects made the drug an ideal agent to test as an adjuvant therapy for ER-positive women with axillary lymph node–positive breast cancer. Tamoxifen is a selective ER modulator that is often prescribed for up to 5 years after completion of primary therapy.

The long-term effects of tamoxifen use and whether it may increase gynecologic cancers in daughters are unknown. In pregnant rats, tamoxifen administration has been associated with breast cancer in the female offspring. Cunha and colleagues examined 54 genital tracts isolated from 4- to 19-week-old human female fetuses and grown for 1 to 2 months in untreated athymic nude mice or host mice treated by subcutaneous pellet with the antiestrogen clomiphene, tamoxifen, or the synthetic estrogen diethylstilbestrol. The investigators noted that condensation and segregation of the uterine mesenchyme were greatly impaired and that the fallopian tube epithelium was hyperplastic and disorganized with distortion of the complex mucosal plications in drug-treated specimens as compared with untreated age-matched control participant.

Table 15.8 also summarizes six reports of tamoxifen use during pregnancy. In 1997, Tewari and colleagues described the first patient to have given birth to a child with congenital anomalies after systemic tamoxifen therapy through 20 weeks of gestation. This 46,XX child had ambiguous genitalia, including labial fusion and clitoromegaly; her internal genitalia were normal according to ultrasonography. Another fetus exposed to tamoxifen during all the first, second, and early part of the third trimesters was born at 26 weeks' gestation with oculoauriculovertebral dysplasia (ie, Goldenhar syndrome). A third case appeared in 2001 and involved a fetus delivered at 31 weeks of gestation whose mother was given tamoxifen as the sole systemic therapy and locoregional irradiation before pregnancy was determined. In addition to moderate hyaline membrane disease and necrotizing enterocolitis that was attributable to prematurity, the child had preauricular skin tags but an appropriate birth weight and no major malformations. At 2 years of follow-up, this last child was meeting all developmental milestones. The presentation of these three cases has prompted the creation of a tamoxifen registry. It is not clear whether women with ER-positive tumors receiving tamoxifen should temporarily discontinue the medication if and when they become pregnant.

Hormonal Considerations: Pregnancy After Breast Cancer

It has been estimated that only 7% of fertile women go on to conceive after the diagnosis and treatment of breast cancer. Nevertheless, a patient with breast cancer may have several concerns regarding future fertility, not least of which is whether she will remain fertile after treatment. In addition, the risk of recurrence conferred by subsequent pregnancy needs to be addressed because several authors have postulated that the immunosuppressant and hormonal effects of pregnancy so close to diagnosis may have a significant deleterious effect. Finally, a patient may express fear that a child may inherit a genetic predisposition toward the later development of breast cancer. The recommendations given to such patients should be influenced by two major considerations:

1. Whether pregnancy promotes recurrence of cancer
2. The probability of having been cured

Thirty percent of women younger than age 40 years will become amenorrheic after chemotherapy for breast cancer, and 90% of women older than age 40 years will cease menstruating. For those who continue to ovulate and who are desirous of future childbearing, it has been common practice to recommend a waiting period of 2 years after the diagnosis of breast cancer before attempting to conceive because most recurrences occur within the first 2 years of diagnosis. In 1985, Nugent and O'Connell described a poor prognosis for women with early subsequent pregnancy, but many investigators have since refuted this. Of note, women who have a subsequent pregnancy have equivalent or possibly better survival when matched for stage. Gelber and colleagues evaluated 94 patients from the International Breast Cancer Study Group who became pregnant after the diagnosis of early-stage breast cancer and compared them with 188 control participants (ie, no subsequent pregnancy) matched for nodal status, tumor size, age, and year of diagnosis. Whereas the overall 5- and 10-year survival rates from the diagnosis of early-stage breast cancer among the study group were 92% and 86%, respectively, that of the comparison group was 85% and 74%, respectively. Some have speculated an antitumor effect of the pregnancy, but of course this could reflect the "healthy mother" bias in that only select women who feel healthy will go on to conceive. Although it may be presumptuous to conclude on the basis of retrospective studies that pregnancy protects against recurrence after mastectomy, it is reasonably safe to conclude that it does not promote it. In summary, therefore, it appears that future pregnancies are safe for the mother unless she has an ER-positive tumor and has not been placed into remission. Consequently, if a pregnancy occurs, there appears to be no justification for recommending its termination in patients without evidence of recurrence. The converse, that pregnancy with recurrence should be terminated in most instances and that an uneventful pregnancy in no way guarantees against a subsequent recurrence, is also true. Indeed, there are cases on record in which multiple pregnancies have eventually been followed by recurrence.

Prophylactic Oophorectomy

Surgical castration for patients with early-stage breast cancer has been advocated to prevent further pregnancy, which might cause recrudescence of the disease through hormone stimulation. Oophorectomy also serves to eliminate the ovarian source of estrogen production, ideally preventing or delaying subsequent recurrence. Neither argument is substantiated by data to support a role for "prophylactic castration." In many patients, chemotherapy will cause a cessation of ovarian hormone production. As discussed earlier, pregnancy after treatment for breast cancer has no influence on the disease, and a few reports even suggest that future pregnancies might be protective. The rationale for eliminating the ovarian source of estrogens in the primary treatment of early disease is based on an observation that castration in the presence of observable recurrent disease results in partial or complete temporary tumor regression in approximately one-third of cases. This argument has been refuted by two large clinical trials conducted in the United

States that failed to demonstrate a significant benefit from castration and adjuvant therapy. For example, the National Surgical Adjuvant Breast and Bowel Project (NSABP) conducted a randomized trial of prophylactic castration in premenopausal women involving 129 women who were castrated and 70 control women. After an observation period of 10 years, there was no evidence that those who were castrated derived any benefit from the procedure.

Survival Among Patients With Pregnancy-Associated Breast Cancer

Most of the datasets from the preceding few decades show that women with PABC have the same survival stage for stage as nonpregnant women with breast cancer. Women with PABC may do poorly in the aggregate because these patients tend to present with advanced disease. Table 15.9 is adapted from Keleher and colleagues and shows selected 5-year survival data by axillary nodal status for women with PABC. Holleb and Farrow reported a series of 283 patients with carcinomas of the breast in pregnancy, including 73 who had inoperable disease and 210 who underwent surgery with or without postoperative radiation. Of patients with inoperable disease, 93% died within 2 years of the diagnosis, including all seven of those who had interruption of pregnancy. The majority of the remaining 210 patients underwent radical mastectomy and were given

postoperative radiation therapy. Of 28 patients with a diagnosis in the first trimester, seven survived for 5 years. Peters and Meakin described 70 patients with breast cancer in pregnancy, all of whom were treated with preoperative, postoperative, or palliative radiotherapy in conjunction with radical mastectomy. The overall survival rates in this series were 32.9% at 5 years and 19.5% at 10 years. Of 12 patients treated during the first and second trimesters, three survived 5 years; only one of the nine patients treated during the third trimester survived 5 years, and she had active disease at the time of the report. The remaining 49 patients who were treated postpartum had a 39% 5-year survival rate, prompting the author to suggest that a delay in the treatment of breast carcinoma until after delivery should be considered.

It is now recognized that the independent variable of youth results in an unfavorable prognosis in patients with breast cancer, presumably because of the likelihood of more aggressive tumors in these young women. Previously, only young patients had an opportunity of having breast cancer coincident with pregnancy, but as women postpone childbearing, pregnancy coincident with breast cancer will become more common. Physicians must treat patients with breast cancer in pregnancy aggressively and with curative intent.

EVALUATION AND THERAPEUTIC MODALITIES

Anesthesia and Surgery in Pregnant Patients
Anesthesia
Anesthetic considerations in pregnant patients must take into account both the potential teratogenicity of the anesthetic agents and the maternal physiologic changes that result from both the pregnancy and the use of anesthetic agents. The vast majority of analgesics and anesthetics are category C drugs (Table 15.10). When a drug has demonstrated teratogenicity in animals, it is likely to have the same effect in humans. Therefore, although category C drugs lack human studies, the existing animal studies may be useful in predicting risk to the fetus. A consensus statement published in 1998 in the pages of *The New England Journal of Medicine* did not list any anesthetic agents as definitive causes of fetal anomalies. **Inhalational and local anesthetics, muscle relaxants, narcotic analgesics, and benzodiazepines are known to be safe in pregnancy.**

The hyperdynamic cardiovascular system of pregnancy is characterized by an increased cardiac output and increased

TABLE 15.9   Literature Review of Case-Control Series of Patients With Pregnancy-Associated Breast Cancer

Authors	Years	PABC	Matched Patients	Outcome
Petrek et al., 1991	1960–1980	56	166	No survival difference
Zemlickis et al., 1992	1958–1987	118	269	No survival difference
Ishida et al., 1992	1970–1988	192	192	Worse prognosis in PABC group
Chang, 1994	1979–1988	21	199	No survival difference
Nugent, 1985	1970–1979	19	157	No survival difference
Lethaby, 1996	1976–1985	20	362	Worse survival when diagnosed during lactation; no difference when diagnosed during pregnancy
Bonnier et al., 1997	1960–1993	154	308	Worse prognosis in PABC group
Ibrahim et al., 2000	1992–1996	72	216	No survival difference
Zhang et al., 2003	1957–1990	88	176	No survival difference
Halaska, 2009	1995–2007	32	32	No survival difference

PABC, Pregnancy-associated breast cancer.
Modified from Halaska MJ, Pentheroudakis G, Strnad P, et al. Presentation, management and outcome of 32 patients with pregnancy-associated breast cancer: a matched controlled study. *Breast J* 2009;15:461.

TABLE 15.10   Drug Safety Categories in Pregnancy

Category	Description
A	Safety established using human studies
B	Presumed safety based on animal studies
C	Uncertain safety; no human studies; animal studies show adverse effect
D	Unsafe; evidence of risk that may in certain clinical circumstances be justifiable
X	Highly unsafe

resting heart rate. **The total blood volume is increased by 40% and that of the red blood cells by 25%, resulting in the physiologic anemia of pregnancy that decreases the hematocrit by approximately 30%.** As the pregnancy progresses, a decrease in blood return to the heart from the inferior vena cava occurs via increasing intraabdominal pressures caused by the enlarging uterus.

A 30% to 40% increase in the tidal volume occurs during normal pregnancy as oxygen consumption increases and the abdominal organs undergo mechanical displacement by the gravid uterus. Anesthesiologists may expect a compensatory respiratory alkalosis in pregnancy with a P_aCO_2 of 30 to 35 mm Hg. Cricoid pressure should be applied during intubation to prevent aspiration, the risk of which is increased as a result of the pregnancy-associated decrease in lower esophageal sphincter pressure and delayed gastric emptying. Small-diameter endotracheal tubes are recommended to facilitate intubation later in pregnancy when airway edema is increased. Intraoperatively, the end-tidal CO_2 is monitored.

Surgery

With the improvements in neonatal care, fetal survival rates continue to increase, and although actual figures vary between different neonatal intensive care units, survival rates greater than 90% can be expected beyond 28 weeks of gestation. Table 15.11 contains neonatal intensive care unit survival statistics based on gestational age and birth weight. Patients in need of surgery during the second trimester can be permitted a short delay to attain fetal viability in many cases. When the clinical suspicion for malignancy is high or the diagnosis is established by biopsy, it is recommended that surgery not be delayed in the first or third trimesters. If an asymptomatic and clinically isolated adnexal mass is discovered during the first trimester, as

TABLE 15.11 Survival With Selected Neonatal Morbidity for Very-Low-Birth-Weight Infants Born in the NICHD Neonatal Research Network Between January 1, 1997, and December 31, 2002

	501–750 g (n = 4046)	751–1000 g (n = 4266)	1001–1250 g (n = 4557)	1251–1500 g (n = 5284)
Survived	55	88	94	96
Overall survival with morbidity	65	43	22	4
BPD alone	42	25	11	4
Severe IVH	5	6	5	4
NEC alone	3	3	3	2

BPD, Bronchopulmonary dysplasia; *IVH,* intraventricular hemorrhage; *NEC,* necrotizing enterocolitis; *NICHD,* National Institute of Child Health and Human Development.
Modified from Fanaroff AA, Stoll BJ, Wright LL, et al; NICHD Neonatal Research Network. Trends in neonatal morbidity and mortality for very low birthweight infants. *Am J Obstet Gynecol* 2007;196:147.e1-147.e8.

discussed earlier, it is reasonable to repeat an imaging study around 17 to 18 weeks of gestation to determine the need for surgery.

Pregnant patients undergoing surgery during the second trimester before fetal viability ($\approx$23–24 weeks of gestation) should have the fetal heart tones documented by Doppler preoperatively and postoperatively. Later in pregnancy, continuous fetal heart rate monitoring can be used perioperatively. After documentation of an adequate amniotic fluid volume of approximately 10 to 18 mL via ultrasonography, preoperative and postoperative prophylactic indomethacin at a rectal dose of 25 to 50 mg can be used to minimize uterine contractions in patients undergoing surgery before 30 weeks of gestation. The use of indomethacin is not advisable beyond this period because of concerns of premature closure of the patent ductus arteriosus. It must be recognized that, although prophylactic tocolytic agents can decrease uterine irritability, they have not been shown to decrease the incidence of preterm birth in patients undergoing surgery. The liberal use of lower extremity sequential compression devices intraoperatively and during periods of bed rest is advisable. Finally, an external tocodynamometer can be used in the postoperative period to monitor uterine irritability and preterm uterine contractions.

Laparotomy

Historically, laparotomy during pregnancy was a frequent cause of fetal wastage. A 17% loss rate was reported by Brant in 1967 after appendectomy during pregnancy. In 1973, Saunders and Milton observed a 23% rate of fetal wastage after laparotomy. In modern hospitals, however, loss of the fetus as a consequence of laparotomy is uncommon. For example, Kort and colleagues reported in 1993 that for 78 women who underwent nonobstetric operations, the perinatal mortality rate was not increased provided that fetal viability was established preoperatively. The most common indications for surgical treatment in their series were appendicitis, adnexal mass, and cholecystitis. Nonobstetric surgery was associated with an increased risk of preterm labor, and the authors identified no measurable benefit from the use of perioperative prophylactic tocolytic agents. The premature delivery rate was 21.8% after major surgery, which was twice the rate in pregnant control participants.

With rare exceptions, when laparotomy is required to evaluate a pregnant woman for suspected or known malignancy, the author uses the midline, vertical approach. This permits excellent visualization and inspection of the entire pelvis and upper abdomen and, perhaps as important, facilitates the "hands-off-the-uterus" approach the author has toward surgery in gravid patients.

Laparoscopy

Laparoscopy can be used to evaluate adnexal masses during pregnancy and has been shown to be well tolerated by both the mother and the fetus. By the end of the second trimester, the enlarging uterus interferes with the laparoscopic view, and a celiotomy is generally required. Two million deliveries in Sweden from 1973 to 1993 were the subject of a review by Reedy and colleagues, who evaluated 2233 laparoscopic and

TABLE 15.12 Recommendations for Laparoscopy in Pregnancy

16–20 wk of gestational age
Tilting table to left or right
Left upper quadrant or subxiphoid insertion (6 cm between point of entry and top of fundus)
Open Hasson technique preferable
Ultrasound guidance with elevation of abdominal wall if Veress technique used
Intraabdominal pressure 15 mm Hg
Trendelenburg position
Fetal monitoring as indicated

2491 open laparotomy cases. The outcome measures included gestational age at delivery, birth weight, intrauterine growth restriction, congenital malformations, stillbirths, and neonatal deaths. Although both groups were at increased risk for preterm delivery and neonatal birth weights less than 2500 g, there were no statistically significant differences between the two. Highlights from the Society of American Gastrointestinal Endoscopic Surgeons recommendations for the conduct of laparoscopy in pregnancy appear in Table 15.12.

For seemingly isolated 6- to 10-cm adnexal masses that persist into the second trimester, we defer laparoscopic evaluation until 18 weeks of gestation and typically use pelviscopy to determine which direction (ie, transverse or midline-vertical) to make the laparotomy incision. For persistent masses larger than 10 cm, we recommend proceeding directly to laparotomy via a vertical incision in an effort to maximize exposure and allow surgical removal of the mass without any manipulation of the uterus.

Diagnostic and Therapeutic Radiation in Pregnancy

The primary concern of both the oncologist and the obstetrician regarding radiation therapy during pregnancy is its possible effect on the baby. The embryo undoubtedly represents the most radiosensitive stage of human life because many of the cells are differentiating and thus relatively more sensitive to radiation injury. In addition, the high rate of mitotic activity in the cells of the embryo contributes to its radiosensitivity because the mitotic phase of the cell is the most radiosensitive period in the life cycle of the cell. Of note, if the embryonic cell is genetically altered or killed during development, the fetus will be deformed or will not survive. Finally, there is the concern that irradiation of the fetal and maternal gonads may contribute to reproductive difficulties in the future, of both the mother and her offspring.

Radiobiology

For the fetus, the most sensitive period is day 18 through day 38. After day 40, the primary organ systems have developed, and much larger doses of x-rays or gamma rays are necessary to produce serious abnormalities. Three periods of fetal development are highly significant from a radiologic point of view.

1. Preimplantation: In this phase, radiation produces an all-or-none effect, in that it either destroys the fertilized egg or does not affect it significantly.
2. Organ system formation: This is the period from day 18 through day 38, when doses of 10 to 40 cGy may cause visceral organ or somatic damage. Microcephaly, anencephaly, eye damage, growth restriction, spina bifida, and foot damage are reported with doses of 4 cGy or less. Cause and effect have not been proved with these lower doses.
3. Period of fetal development after day 40, when larger doses are likely to produce external malformations but organ systems, especially the nervous system, may still be undamaged

The dose to the fetus is related to internal scatter of radiation after it enters the supradiaphragmatic tissues. Some scatter may also come from the treatment head of the machine and the collimator. Zucali and colleagues used a tissue-equivalent phantom to measure scatter dose to the uterus. In this study, doses of 1.5% of the total dose were measured at the estimated top of the uterus, with less than 1% being measurable in the true pelvis. This occurs even with abdominal shielding.

It is estimated that 1 cGy of radiation produces five mutations in every 1 million genes exposed. Fortunately, most mutants are recessive. Mutant effects are not seen in the first generation and may not be expressed for many generations until two people with the same mutation mate. Most estimates of genetic damage are empiric, but it is estimated that to double the rate of gene mutation, 25 to 150 cGy must be given from birth to the end of reproductive age.

Constant changes are being made in what is considered the permissible body dose of radiation. Some authorities cite 14 cGy in the first 30 years of life; others cite 10 cGy or less as the maximum. This includes medical and background sources. Radiation doses in excess of 200 cGy during the first 20 weeks of gestation will result in congenital malformations in the majority of fetuses exposed (frequently microcephaly and mental retardation). With doses above 300 cGy, there is increasing risk of abortion. If therapeutic irradiation is necessary for a pregnant patient and therapeutic abortion is refused, delay in the initiation of treatment until at least the mid-second trimester is recommended. Irradiation of even supradiaphragmatic structures during pregnancy will deliver fetal doses ranging from 1.2% to 7.1% of the total treatment dose.

Radiation-induced Anomalies

There are varying sensitivities within the tissues in human embryos. Various abnormalities have been attributed to irradiation of embryos; microcephaly and associated conditions are most common. Other abnormalities of the central nervous system (CNS), the eye, and the skeleton have also been ascribed to irradiation. However, an accurate prediction of incidence with regard to dose has not been possible. It is widely accepted that irradiation of human beings, especially of their gonads, has certain undesirable effects. Any irradiation of gonadal tissue involves possible genetic damage because the photons can cause gene mutation or chromosome breakage with subsequent translocation, loss, deletion, and abnormal fusion of chromosome material. The effect is basically additive and cumulative;

the changes are generally in direct proportion to the total dose. Unfortunately, there is no threshold for genetic damage, and even relatively small doses of irradiation can cause gene mutations, most of which can be harmful.

Doses greater than 50 cGy may produce significant mental retardation and microcephaly, even in the second trimester (Fig. 15.12). An analysis of children exposed in utero to the atomic bomb in Hiroshima and Nagasaki shows a 30 in 1600 incidence of severe mental retardation. Most of the mentally retarded children were exposed at 8 to 15 weeks of life; no cases were reported before the eighth week of gestation. A rough linear relationship is suggested, with a probability of mental retardation occurring at 0.4% per cGy (rad).

As noted previously, the exposure dose that is associated with developmental abnormalities remains controversial. Hammer-Jacobsen suggests that 10 cGy received in the first 6 weeks of gestation should be considered a threshold for therapeutic abortion. Others disagree and suggest that the minimal level increases as the pregnancy progresses. Low-dose exposure (<100 cGy) seems acceptable only in the third trimester. Evidence suggests that an exposure of even 3 to 5 cGy can result in an increase in benign or malignant tumors in the child after birth.

Most of the data to date on the effects of irradiation on the fetus are from single-dose exposure; few data are available concerning the effects of fractionated irradiation. Reported cases of fractionated irradiation during pregnancy show a low incidence of fetal anomalies.

Diagnostic Radiology

The metastatic evaluation using diagnostic imaging and the treatment of malignancy by radiotherapy in the pregnant woman underscores an inherent maternal–fetal conflict in that the mother would be the major beneficiary, but the fetus could be at substantial risk. Several recommendations have been widely applied in this scenario, including delaying radiation therapy for breast cancer until after delivery, avoidance of SLN identification procedures during pregnancy, and termination of pregnancy when doses greater than 0.05 to 0.1 Gy are received by the fetus. It must be recognized that these recommendations are not based on sufficient knowledge of the radiation risks to the unborn child. Although individual doses are highest in association with radiation therapy, the greatest risk to both the general population and the cancer patient comes from diagnostic procedures. Most radiologic diagnostic procedures should be avoided during the first and second trimesters of pregnancy. The exposure to the fetus and gonads will vary with the procedure performed and the precautions taken. A chest radiograph will result in an exposure of 300 mcGy per plate, and a barium enema study will result in a total dose to the gonads and pelvis of 6 cGy. In a pregnant patient, the barium enema study is obviously a greater threat because of the greater dose and the area irradiated.

The International Commission on Radiological Protection prepared two reports on medical irradiation in pregnant women. The biologic effects of prenatal irradiation of the embryo and fetus were derived from animal studies, data from survivors of nuclear explosions, data from children exposed in utero to diagnostic radiographs, and data on children who were exposed to radiation from the Chernobyl accident in utero. As outlined in Table 15.13, lethality, malformations, mental retardation, and

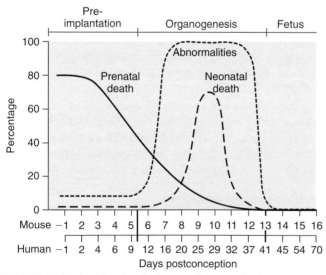

FIGURE 15.12 Incidence of abnormalities and of prenatal and neonatal death in mice given a dose of 200 cGy at various times after fertilization. The lower scale consists of Rugh's estimates of the equivalent stages for the human embryo. (From Hall EJ. *Radiobiology for the Radiologist.* New York, 1973, Harper & Row; after Russell LB, Russell WL. An analysis of the changing radiation response of the developing mouse embryo. *J Cell Physiol Suppl* 1954;43(suppl 1):103-149 and Rugh R. Low levels of x-irradiation and the early mammalian embryo. *AJR Am J Roentgenol* 1962;87:559.)

TABLE 15.13 **Effects and Risks After Exposure to Ionizing Radiation in Utero and Spontaneous Frequency (Without Exposure)**			
Time After Conception (wk)	Effect(s)	Risk Per 0.01 Gy	Spontaneous Frequency
0–2	Prenatal death*	0.01–0.001	0.3–0.6
3–8	Malformation	0.005†	0.06
8–15	Mental retardation, IQ decrease‡	0.004	0.005
16–25	Mental retardation, IQ decrease§	0.001	0.005
0–38	Leukemia, solid tumors in childhood	0.003–0.004	0.002–0.003

*Based on experimental data.
†Above threshold dose of 0.1 to 0.2 Gy.
‡Reduction of 21 IQ points per 1 Gy above the threshold of about 0.05 Gy; the threshold dose for mental retardation is about 0.06 Gy.
§Reduction of 13 IQ points per 0.1 Gy above the threshold dose of about 0.05 Gy; the threshold dose for mental retardation is about 0.25 Gy.
From Kal HB, Struikmans H. Radiotherapy during pregnancy: fact and fiction. *Lancet Oncol* 2005;6:328.

cancer induction comprise the expected effects of radiation exposure of fetuses.

Ionizing Radiation

In diagnostic radiograph or CT, ionizing radiation passes through the body to create an image, and ionizing radiation from radiopharmaceuticals used in nuclear medicine procedures are retained in the tissues for a period of time and are subsequently removed by elimination from the body and by radioactive decay.

Nonionizing Radiation

Both ultrasonography imaging and MRI form images using nonionizing radiation; however, theoretic risks to fetuses exist. Thermal effects occur in tissues with the absorption of ultrasonic energy, but cavitation (ie, mechanical) effects may occur through motion initiated by the ultrasonic. Both thermal and cavitation effects occur only with very high-intensity ultrasonography, and no confirmed biologic effects associated with the use of diagnostic ultrasonography with standard power levels have been reported. Potential injury at the cellular level in MRI may result from exposure to high static magnetic fields. In addition, heating can result from energy deposited by radiofrequencies used to generate the pulse sequences. The diagnostic magnets create static magnetic fields from 0.1 to 1.5T, and no adverse behavioral or physiologic effects are anticipated with fields up to 2T. Of note, there have been no immediately observable adverse effects or delayed sequelae encountered among fetuses from an MRI examination. Table 15.14 lists the imaging modalities used to diagnose metastatic disease.

Ionic or nonionic iodinated intravenous contrast media used in CT appear to be safe for fetuses; however, only animal studies have been performed using iodinated contrast agents. These agents are pregnancy category B drugs. Gadolinium-based contrast medium is not advisable during pregnancy because the gadolinium crosses the placenta, is filtered through the fetal kidneys, and is then reingested through the amniotic fluid. Gadolinium is a category C drug. The accuracy of bone scans is improved through the addition of single-photon emission computed tomography imaging. Whereas MRI is the most sensitive for studying the bone marrow, CT is highly sensitive for cortical destruction. Positron emission tomography scanning with 2-[fluorine-18]fluoro-2-deoxy-D-glucose is being used with increasing frequency in the metastatic workup, although the potential dose to the fetus precludes its use when the pregnancy is to be preserved.

Radionuclides

Most diagnostic nuclear medicine procedures use short-lived radionuclides (eg, ^{99m}Tc), resulting in a dose to the fetus generally less than 0.01 Gy. Special mention should be made regarding whole-body radionuclide scanning using iodine-131 for the metastatic workup of thyroid carcinoma. It is well established that oral administration of radioactive iodine to a mother will have deleterious effects on the thyroid gland of the fetus, with placental transfer of radioactive iodine occurring as early as 8

weeks after conception. The fetal thyroid gland will concentrate iodine and synthesize thyroxine by 11 to 12 weeks of gestation. The radiation dose delivered by 2 μCi of ^{131}I to the fetal thyroid gland ranges from 10,000 to 40,000 cGy. Stoffer and Hamburger studied 237 cases in which radioactive ^{131}I at doses from 10 to 150 μCi was administered during pregnancy. In 55 patients, therapeutic abortion was performed on medical recommendation, and among the remaining 182 pregnancies, there were two spontaneous abortions, two stillborn infants, and two infants born with abdominal or chest anomalies. Of note, there were six infants with hypothyroidism (3%), four of whom exhibited mental deficiencies. Pregnancy is a contraindication to the administration of ^{131}I.

TABLE 15.14	Imaging Modalities Used for Treatment Planning in Oncology	
Site of Anatomic Interest	Imaging Modality	Type of Radiation
Brain	CT scan	Ionizing
	MRI	Nonionizing
	FDG-PET	Ionizing
Chest	Chest radiograph	Ionizing
	CT scan	Ionizing
	MRI	Nonionizing
	FDG-PET scan	Ionizing
	Gallium scan	Ionizing
	Mammography	Ionizing
Abdomen	Ultrasonography	Nonionizing
	CT scan	Ionizing
	MRI	Nonionizing
	FDG-PET	Ionizing
	IVP	Ionizing
	Upper GI with small bowel follow-through	Ionizing
Pelvis (not bony pelvis)	Ultrasonography	Nonionizing
	CT scan	Ionizing
	MRI	Nonionizing
	FDG PET	Ionizing
	Barium enema	Ionizing
	Cystography	Ionizing
Skeletal	Radiograph	Ionizing
	Bone scan or SPECT	Ionizing
	CT scan	Ionizing
	MRI	Nonionizing
	FDG-PET	Ionizing
Lymph nodes	Lymphangiography	Ionizing
	CT scan	Ionizing
	MRI	Nonionizing
	Lymphoscintigraphy	Ionizing
	Sentinel node examination	Nonionizing and ionizing

CT, Computed tomography; FDG-PET, 2-[fluorine-18]fluoro-2-deoxy-D-glucose positron emission tomography; GI, gastrointestinal; IV, intravenous; IVP, intravenous pyelography; MRI, magnetic resonance imaging; SPECT, single-photon emission computed tomography.
Modified from Nicklas AH, Baker ME. Imaging strategies in the pregnant cancer patient. Semin Oncol 2000;27:623.

Radiation Therapy

When the patient wishes to continue her pregnancy, delay of initiation of therapeutic radiation as long as possible without compromising cure is recommended. Fortunately, most cancers in pregnant women that require radiation therapy are remote from the pelvis. Any radiation therapy to the abdomen should be postponed until after delivery, if at all possible. Therefore, with the exception of a locally advanced cervical tumor, radiation therapy can be used during pregnancy provided that the fetal dose is precisely estimated during the radiation planning sessions. **The dose to the fetus can be calculated from the internal scatter, which largely depends on the source of irradiation and on the size of the treatment fields and their proximity to the fetus.** Leakage radiation from the tube head of the linear accelerator, scatter from the collimator, and blocks also contribute to the fetal dose. Leakage and scatter can be reduced by proper shielding with four to five half-value layers of lead stacked over the patient's uterus.

Kal and Struikmans tabulated the dosimetry data and pregnancy outcomes of women who received radiation therapy during pregnancy for breast cancer (Fig. 15.13), Hodgkin disease, and brain or head and neck tumors (Table 15.15). Successful radiotherapy of breast cancers during pregnancy with fetal doses below the deterministic threshold (0.039-0.18 Gy) have resulted in the birth of healthy children. Similarly, several healthy children, some who have been observed for up to 11 years, have been delivered after radiation therapy for Hodgkin disease during pregnancy with fetal doses ranging from 0.014 to 0.136 Gy. Radiation treatment portals are now more restricted in size, and patients with stage I and II Hodgkin disease currently receive polychemotherapy followed by involved field radiotherapy, thus resulting in potentially less harm to the unborn child. Finally, the successful radiotherapeutic management of neck and cranial tumors in pregnancy suggests that high doses can be achieved with fetal exposures of less than 0.1 Gy, a dose below the deterministic threshold.

Radiation-induced Carcinogenesis

The subject of the carcinogenic effects of x-ray radiation was first raised nearly half a century ago by Stewart and Webb from Oxford University in the United Kingdom. Monson and Macmahon summarized the bulk of the data accumulated before the 1980s in their monograph that focused on prenatal x-ray exposure and cancer in children. Most of the available information on radiation-induced embryonic damage during the preceding 2 decades is derived from animal studies, extended follow-up of individuals exposed to atomic bomb explosions in Japan, and statistical analyses.

Of interest is a paper by Chen and colleagues, who studied the records of 37 women radiated for Hodgkin disease around the time of pregnancy and of 345 women who were not pregnant. They detected a higher risk of breast cancer after irradiation around the time of pregnancy, suggesting that pregnancy represents a time of increased sensitivity of breast tissue to the carcinogenic effects of radiation.

Genetic Damage and Infertility

In addition, the possibility that human exposure to ionizing radiation might have a detrimental genetic consequence remains a matter of concern and uncertainty. There is concern because recessive mutations may not become apparent for several generations, and there is uncertainty because, although

FIGURE 15.13 Irradiation of a pregnant woman after breast-conserving treatment. Shielding of leakage radiation is done with a mobile lead screen usually used for shielding of personnel in the brachytherapy room. (From Kal HB, Struikmans H. Radiotherapy during pregnancy: fact and fiction. *Lancet Oncol* 2005;6:328.)

TABLE 15.15	Radiotherapy During Pregnancy					
Malignancy	Patients (n)	Median Dose (Gy)	Shielding Used (N)	Median Estimated Fetal Dose (Gy)	Mean Gestational Age (Weeks)	No. Reported Cases With Adverse Outcomes in Offspring
Breast	23	41	2	0.15	17.5	2
Hodgkin lymphoma	58	36	31	0.085	20	3
Brain	7	42	2	0.03	21	1
Melanoma	2	43.5	2	0.05	23	2

Modified from Luis SA, Christie DR, Kaminski A, et al. Pregnancy and radiotherapy: management options for minimising risk, case series and comprehensive literature review. *J Med Imaging Radiation Oncol* 2009;53:559.

no human data are available, experimental animal studies have demonstrated significant radiation-induced genetic effects. There appears to be no apparent threshold dose for genetic damage, but the effect of any particular radiation dose is considerably reduced if that dose is administered during a prolonged period. Of importance also for patients planning childbearing after significant exposure of gonadal tissue to irradiation is that the genetic effect of radiation on the gonad may be minimized by delaying conception after exposure. **In humans, pregnancy should be delayed 12 to 14 months after significant exposure.**

Chemotherapy

Because nearly all antineoplastic drugs have been shown to be teratogenic in animal studies, the available data suggest endangerment to human fetuses even for drugs for which no human data are available. Their use often evokes moral, philosophic, and emotional decisions. Both the mother and fetus are at risk, with abortion, intrauterine fetal demise, malformations, and growth restriction being foremost considerations. These potential dangers to the fetus must be weighed against the possible detrimental effect to the mother of withholding these agents. The long-term effect on the fetus is unknown. The problem of long-term observation has been dramatically emphasized by the occurrence of adenosis of the vagina in young women exposed to diethylstilbestrol in utero during the first trimester of pregnancy. A similar long-term effect is possible when chemotherapeutic agents are used in pregnancy.

All chemotherapeutic agents profoundly affect rapidly growing tissues, and a high rate of cell division is characteristic of the fetus. Following this reasoning, one would expect a much greater effect than is actually observed. Unquestionably, the first trimester of pregnancy is when fetuses are most vulnerable to cancer chemotherapeutic agents. The two aspects to the problem of fetal damage are as follows:

- Death of the fetus
- Induction of fetal abnormalities inadequate to cause fetal death

Most of the available data suggesting the teratogenicity and mutagenicity of chemotherapeutic agents have been derived from experiments in laboratory animals. Rats, mice, and rabbits have placentas very similar to human placentas, and because the teratogenic effects of a drug are species specific, these animals provide models in which to study chemotherapy exposure in utero. These experiments indicate potential danger to human fetuses only. Teratogenic properties of chemotherapeutic agents also are predicated on the type, dose, and threshold dose of the drug. When considering an extrapolation of animal data to humans, it is important to note that the therapeutic doses used in humans are often lower than the minimum teratogenic dose studied in animal models. Thus, teratogenic data are useful only if the dose resulting in injury to the model does not also cause maternal toxic effects. Another important caveat is that many antineoplastic exposures in pregnancy that have resulted in malformations or even fetal deaths have typically been associated with multiagent therapy, sometimes also with

concomitant radiation therapy, so that it is difficult to single out one specific agent as the cause of an adverse outcome. It is important to note that in the majority of exposures, even during the first trimester, the outcome of the fetus is unremarkable. **Still, unless the mother's life is in grave danger, we do not recommend chemotherapy use during the first trimester.**

Teratology and Embryology

Teratology is the study of the causes, mechanisms, and manifestations of abnormal fetal development. Environmental factors, such as infectious diseases, drugs, chemicals, and radiation, have been shown to cause abnormal development by inducing chromosome abnormalities, specific gene changes, vascular changes, or mechanical disruption. In many instances, the exact cause of a fetal abnormality is unknown. Although different classes of teratogens have been established, certain general principles apply to all. There are three stages of embryonic development. In the first 2 weeks of life, the blastocyst is resistant to teratogens. It is during this period that a large insult is necessary to kill the blastocyst. A surviving blastocyst will not manifest any organ's specific abnormalities as a result of that teratogen. Early embryonic cells have not differentiated sufficiently, so if one cell dies, another can take over. The second stage is organogenesis, or the process of organ differentiation. **The most critical period extends from the third to eighth weeks of development (fifth through tenth weeks of gestational age), when susceptibility to teratogenic agents is maximal. In human fetuses, the period of organogenesis usually ends by the 13th week of gestation.** The third and final period of growth, organ development, is characterized by an increase in fetal and organ size. However, brain and gonadal tissue are exceptions because they continue to differentiate beyond the second period. Exposure to the teratogenic agent beyond the third period can affect general fetal growth but will not produce organ-specific morphologic malformations.

Fig. 15.14 depicts prenatal development from implantation through embryonic progression and into the fetal period. Drug responses vary among individuals because of differences in absorption, protein binding, and excretion rate and differences in placental transfer and fetal metabolism of the teratogen. Both polygenic and mendelian factors can be responsible for different responses to identical doses of a teratogen in two fetuses of the same species. Administration of small intermittent doses of a teratogen may enable a system to safely metabolize the teratogen and prevent malformation. The effect would be different if the total dose were administered at one time. However, small constant doses of a teratogen may interfere with cellular metabolism and cause more serious malformations than might be expected.

Transplacental Studies

Antineoplastic agents and their metabolites can be detected in placental tissue, amniotic fluid, umbilical cord blood, and breast milk. By enzyme-linked immunosorbent assay and spectrometry, Henderson and colleagues measured cisplatin–DNA adducts in placental tissues but were unable to do so in the

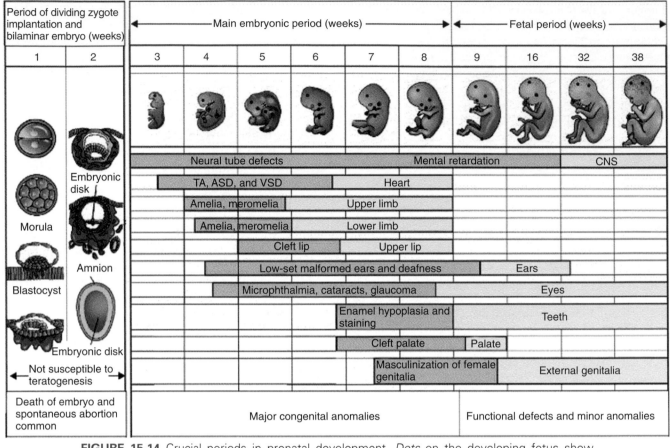

Period of dividing zygote implantation and bilaminar embryo (weeks)		Main embryonic period (weeks)						Fetal period (weeks)			
1	2	3	4	5	6	7	8	9	16	32	38

Morula
Blastocyst
Embryonic disk
Embryonic disk
Amnion
Not susceptible to teratogenesis
Death of embryo and spontaneous abortion common

Neural tube defects — Mental retardation — CNS
TA, ASD, and VSD — Heart
Amelia, meromelia — Upper limb
Amelia, meromelia — Lower limb
Cleft lip — Upper lip
Low-set malformed ears and deafness — Ears
Microphthalmia, cataracts, glaucoma — Eyes
Enamel hypoplasia and staining — Teeth
Cleft palate — Palate
Masculinization of female genitalia — External genitalia

Major congenital anomalies   Functional defects and minor anomalies

FIGURE 15.14 Crucial periods in prenatal development. *Dots* on the developing fetus show common sites of action of teratogens. *Horizontal bars* indicate fetal development during a highly sensitive period *(purple)* and a less sensitive period *(green).* *ASD,* Atrial septal defect; *CNS,* central nervous system; *TA,* truncus arteriosus; *VSD,* ventricular septal defect. (From Moore P, ed. *The Developing Human*, 6th ed. Philadelphia, 1998, Saunders.)

umbilical cord tissues or in amniotic cells. Karp and colleagues reported high levels of doxorubicin in placental tissue; the drug was absent in umbilical cord tissue or in the blood of a healthy child born 48 hours after maternal treatment. Separately, Roboz and colleagues and Barni and colleagues were unable to identify doxorubicin in the amniotic fluid after maternal administration. Transplacental conduct of antineoplastic drugs may occur. Although doxorubicin was not detected by liquid chromatography in the amniotic fluid, fetal brain, or fetal gastrointestinal tract 15 hours after its administration to the mother, d'Incalci and colleagues found the drug in the fetal liver, kidney, and lungs after elective termination. It would have been interesting to have had data from the fetal myocardial tissue. A metabolite of doxorubicin was present in the umbilical cord, placental tissue, and neonatal spleen of a stillborn baby delivered 36 hours after maternal treatment. Egan and colleagues reported a case in which milk and plasma concentrations of doxorubicin and cisplatin were measured after intravenous administration of these agents to a lactating patient who had ovarian cancer. Although the concentrations of doxorubicin in milk at times exceeded those detected in concomitant plasma samples, the total amount of drug delivered in the milk was negligible. However, the authors concluded that

it is prudent to advise lactating women who are receiving these antineoplastic drugs to refrain from breastfeeding.

Classes of Antineoplastic Agents

Antimetabolites. Antimetabolites are small, weakly acidic molecules that are cell cycle nonspecific, inhibiting cellular metabolism by acting as false substrates during RNA and DNA synthesis. Examples of these agents include methotrexate, 5-FU, aminopterin, cytarabine, thioguanine, and mercaptopurine. **The aminopterin syndrome has been reported after in utero exposure during the first trimester and is characterized by cranial dysostosis with delayed ossification, hypertelorism, wide nasal bridge, micrognathia, and ear anomalies.** Similar malformations have been associated with methotrexate administration when doses greater than 10 mg per week are used during the first trimester. There have been 53 reported cases of exposure to 5-FU during human pregnancy; when used after the first trimester (usually in combination with other agents), the development of intrauterine growth restriction without anomalies manifested in 11% of cases (*n* = 6). There have been four reports of limb malformations after cytarabine administration during the first trimester; among 89 additional cases in which the drug was given during all trimesters (usually in combination with other agents), adverse fetal events included transient cytopenia (5%), intrauterine fetal demise (6%), intrauterine growth restriction (13%), and two neonatal deaths from sepsis and gastroenteritis. Finally, 49 women have been treated with mercaptopurine during pregnancy, including 29 who were exposed to the drug during the first trimester, none of whom gave birth to an anomalous neonate.

There is no doubt that the antifolics aminopterin and methotrexate almost invariably result in spontaneous abortion or an abnormal fetus when they are given in the first trimester of pregnancy. These drugs should not be given to pregnant women in the first trimester unless there is life-threatening disease that can be counteracted by the drug. If an antifolic is used and the mother does not have a spontaneous abortion, therapeutic abortion should be seriously considered. A small amount of data seems to indicate that aminopterin and methotrexate do not cause harm when they are given after the first trimester of pregnancy.

Alkylators. Alkylating agents are an integral component of many combination chemotherapy regimens and include cyclophosphamide, busulfan, ifosfamide, chlorambucil, carmustine, and dacarbazine. First-trimester use of cyclophosphamide has resulted in absent toes, eye abnormalities, low-set ears, and cleft palate. When used during the second and third trimesters, cyclophosphamide appears to be safe, although from a combined experience involving 92 cases, there have been two fetal demises, seven cases of growth restriction, and one neonatal death. A very interesting case involves the twins reported by Reynoso and colleagues who were exposed to cyclophosphamide throughout the pregnancy. The girl had no abnormalities, but the twin boy was born with esophageal atresia, right-arm deformity, abnormal inferior vena cava, and growth restriction and went on to develop thyroid cancer at 11 years of age. There have been 19 reported cases of combined regimens containing dacarbazine in pregnancy, resulting in one case of growth restriction and possibly one minor malformation. Of interest, although there have been eight reports of busulfan use during the first trimester without anomalies, two patients who received the drug during the second trimester delivered anomalous neonates (one case each of pyloric stenosis and unilateral renal agenesis with liver calcifications).

Anthracycline and Antitumor Antibiotics

These high-molecular weight antibiotics interpose between DNA strands and include doxorubicin (Adriamycin), idarubicin, epirubicin, dactinomycin, bleomycin, and mitoxantrone. Turchi and Villasis collected 28 cases of doxorubicin and daunorubicin treatment after the first trimester. After one elective termination, two spontaneous abortions, and two maternal deaths from malignancy with the fetus in utero, 21 pregnancies were delivered without complications. Two of three limb abnormalities seen after doxorubicin exposure during the first trimester ($n = 25$) may be confounded by concomitant radiation or cytarabine treatment.

It has been recognized for a number of years that children and adults receiving anthracyclines are at risk of developing dose-related cardiotoxicity as a result of free radical damage that results in myocardial apoptosis and hypertrophy. It is not known whether in utero exposure to these agents places fetuses at risk for this complication. Meyer-Wittkopf and colleagues performed serial fetal echocardiograms on a pregnant patient receiving doxorubicin and on unexposed fetuses and were unable to detect any significant differences in systolic function. Postnatal echocardiograms revealed no evidence of myocardial damage up to 2 years after birth. There have been at least two cases of transient right-sided cardiomyopathy after second-trimester exposure to anthracyclines, including one case involving idarubicin, which is more lipophilic and favors increased placental transfer. **Until more information becomes available, we suggest that pregnant women requiring an anthracycline be given doxorubicin. Although the cardiac profile of fetuses exposed to anthracyclines appears to be safe in the majority of cases, because cancer treatment advances at a faster pace than the accumulation of safety data in human pregnancy, caution is always warranted before new agents are given to pregnant women.**

Plant Alkaloids

The vinca alkaloids are highly protein bound and include vincristine, vinblastine, and vinorelbine. They have been regarded as less potent teratogens than the antimetabolites. One of 29 patients treated with a four-drug regimen containing vincristine during organogenesis was delivered with malformations, including an atrial septal defect and no radii or fifth digits. There have been a total of 11 exposures to either vincristine or vinblastine during pregnancy, and excluding those malformations found only in first-trimester use, there have been nine cases of growth restriction, two fetal demises, and two neonatal deaths.

Taxanes

Paclitaxel and docetaxel inhibit microtubule disassembly, a process that is important for cell division and intracellular and intercellular functions. Because of their unique mechanism of action, many commentators have been concerned that taxanes may be detrimental to the fetus in many aspects. Animal studies have demonstrated lethality of paclitaxel to chick, rat, and rabbit embryos. Of note, when administered during the period of organogenesis, few malformations have been recorded. There have been only a handful of scattered reports of paclitaxel use during pregnancy in which the drug, when administered after the first trimester, has been shown to be safe for the fetus. As experience with these relatively newer chemotherapeutic agents increases, we anticipate an increase in the reporting of taxane use during pregnancy.

Platinum Analogs

The precise mechanism by which the platinum agents exert their antineoplastic effect has not been fully elucidated but may be similar to that of the classic alkylators. Drugs in this group include cisplatin, carboplatin, and oxaliplatin. There have been reports of exposure to single-agent cisplatin or cisplatin-based regimens, which have resulted in sensorineural hearing loss and cerebral atrophy resulting from impaired anterior cerebral circulation, respectively. In both of these cases, the babies were born before 30 weeks' gestation, so the complications associated with extreme prematurity may be confounding the clinical picture. Nevertheless, close assessment of the fetal CNS may be advisable when cisplatin is used during pregnancy. Among 24 cases of cisplatin exposure, five have been complicated by growth restriction, fetal demise, hearing loss, and ventriculomegaly. The two reports that have appeared in the literature describing carboplatin use during pregnancy have been associated with unremarkable neonatal outcomes at up to 30 months of age.

Pharmacokinetics, Sublethal Fetal Effects, and Maternal Risks

The increased blood volume and increased renal clearance of pregnancy should be considered when treating a pregnant woman for life-threatening disease. Together, these physiologic changes, along with the more rapid turnover of the hepatic mixed function oxidase system, may lead to a decrease in active maternal drug concentration. For example, because pregnant women receive similar weight-based dosages (adjusted with the continuing weight gain of pregnancy) as nonpregnant women, the increased drug clearance from the body may lead to a reduced area under the concentration versus time curve. In addition, changes in gastrointestinal function may have an impact on drug absorption of some agents. Fortunately, with the pregnancy-associated decrease in plasma albumin, the unbound active drug concentration should rise, and thus the efficacy of the drug should not be compromised when administered during pregnancy. As long as the increase in drug balances potential decrease in serum levels, toxicity should not be increased. This may indeed be the case because Zemlickis and colleagues have noted higher concentrations of free cisplatin in pregnant women compared with those who were not pregnant, but all were asymptomatic. Countering this is the argument that estrogens are known to increase other plasma proteins and thereby decrease active drug fractions. Accordingly, Cardonic and Iacobucci have reported more frequent nausea, vomiting, fatigue, alopecia, and neutropenia during postpartum chemotherapy compared with identical antenatal treatment. The volume of distribution, peak drug concentrations, and half-life of administration are likely to be changed during pregnancy, although to date we do not have pharmacokinetic data on pregnant patients receiving chemotherapy.

Concerns regarding sublethal fetal effects of maternally administered chemotherapy have been raised. When a multidrug regimen was used in a pregnant woman with leukemia, Morishita and colleagues reported consistently normal fetal hematopoiesis via percutaneous umbilical cord blood sampling 2 and 5 weeks after treatment. Chemotherapy-induced neonatal alopecia is also a reasonable concern parents may have, but this condition has been reported only in three newborns and involved administration of bleomycin, etoposide, and cisplatin or doxorubicin, cyclophosphamide, and 5-FU. Microscopic scanning of the hair of neonates exposed to chemotherapy for maternal acute monocytic leukemia by Gokal and colleagues did not reveal any cytotoxic damage.

Attention must also be directed to specific maternal risks associated with chemotherapy administration during pregnancy. The safe use of recombinant erythropoietin in pregnancy has been reported to offset the triple insult of pregnancy-associated dilutional anemia, iron-deficiency anemia, and chemotherapy-induced marrow suppression. Along similar lines, granulocyte-colony stimulating factor has been used without adverse sequelae during human pregnancy to counter the maternal and fetal susceptibilities to infection brought about by the generalized immunosuppression of pregnancy and chemotherapy-induced neutropenia. **Finally, because the pulmonary damage associated with bleomycin use is exacerbated by oxygen therapy, we do not advise the administration of oxygen during labor in women who have received bleomycin during pregnancy.**

Estimating the Stillbirth Rate

The background stillbirth rate associated with chemotherapy administration throughout pregnancy can be estimated. In 1992, Zemlickis and colleagues reported their experience with 21 pregnancies after in utero exposure to chemotherapy. Of the 13 women exposed during the first trimester, two of five whose pregnancies continued to term had major malformations in their infants, four had spontaneous abortions, and four had therapeutic abortions. Of four women with second-trimester exposure to chemotherapy, two had normal live births, one had a stillbirth, and one had a therapeutic abortion. All four pregnancies exposed to chemotherapy during the third trimester resulted in healthy live births. However, infants exposed to chemotherapy had statistically significantly lower birth weights than did matched-control infants, owing to significantly lower gestational age and substantial intrauterine growth restriction. The rate of stillbirth was 1 per 11; this was too small a series for comparison with matched control participants. However, the authors analyzed 223 births in their community occurring to women who had any form of cancer in the same 30-year period and found 10 stillbirths among the 223 deliveries, significantly more than in the general population ($P < 0.0005$); this stillbirth rate was calculated at a relative risk of 4.23 (95% CI 2.0–7.8).

Occupational Exposure

In a 1985 case-control study, Selevan and colleagues examined the relationship between fetal loss and occupational exposure to antineoplastic drugs in nurses in 17 Finnish hospitals. The pregnancies studied occurred in 1973 through 1980 and were identified using national sources. Each nurse with fetal loss was matched with three nurses who gave birth. A statistically significant association was observed between fetal loss and occupational exposure to antineoplastic drugs during the first trimester of pregnancy, with an odds ratio equaling 2.30 (95% CI 1.20–4.39). Analyses suggested associations between fetal loss and cyclophosphamide, doxorubicin, and vincristine, although the independent effect of each individual drug could not be specifically identified because many nurses reported handling more than one of these agents.

Recommendations on the Use of Chemotherapy During Pregnancy

In summary, the administration of chemotherapy during the first trimester can be associated with morphologic abnormalities and fetal loss. Although first-trimester use of chemotherapy is inadvisable, if a pregnant patient has an aggressive hematologic malignancy, chemotherapy at full doses can often be safely administered, even during the first trimester, if cure of the hematologic malignancy is considered reasonable.

Chemotherapy administered in the second and third trimesters appears not to be associated with a significant risk of structural anomalies, but some reports suggest an association with preterm delivery, fetal death in utero, and intrauterine growth restriction. The background incidence of growth restriction varies according to the population, geographic location, and standard growth curves used as a reference. We must also keep in mind that the pregnant woman's underlying illness may affect perinatal complications. When more than one regimen is available and effective for a particular cancer, clearly the agents for which the most extensive investigation during pregnancy has been conducted should be selected. Some form of antepartum fetal surveillance is advisable, and close coordination with a perinatologist can determine the need and schedule for serial ultrasonography and fetal heart rate monitoring (Table 15.16). Placental pathology is mandatory in all cases after delivery or termination.

Timing of Delivery

We recommend withholding chemotherapy after 35 weeks of gestation so as to avoid the maternal nadir period because spontaneous labor may occur before the bone marrow has recovered. Chemotherapy administered to the mother within 3 weeks of delivery may not be adequately excreted by the fetus and therefore persist in the newborn.

Preterm pregnancies are also problematic. Iatrogenic preterm delivery is not advisable, and impending preterm delivery should be treated aggressively. In pregnant patients for whom preterm delivery seems inevitable, it is important to withhold chemotherapy 3 weeks before delivery when possible. **Preterm babies have limited ability to metabolize drugs because of immaturity of the hepatic and renal systems. Neonates exposed to chemotherapy 3 weeks before delivery should be assessed for transient bone marrow suppression, and long-term neurologic and developmental follow-up is recommended.**

Breastfeeding

Durodola reported one case of neonatal neutropenia occurring in a breastfed infant whose mother was treated with cyclophosphamide during late pregnancy and early lactation. As described earlier, some drugs have been detected in the placental tissues and the breast milk. The ability of a drug to cross the placenta, however, has not correlated with its ability to pass into breast milk. Drug concentrations in breast milk are related to the dose and timing of therapy. **Because there are no breastfeeding data available for most agents, the author considers breastfeeding to be contraindicated during therapy.**

Long-term Neonatal Follow-up

Although children and adults treated for lymphoma are at risk for secondary leukemia within 10 years, the risk of secondary malignant disease after in utero exposure to chemotherapy is unknown. No cases of secondary leukemia in exposed fetuses have been reported. As described elsewhere, only one case of malignant disease (ie, thyroid cancer at age 11 years and neuroblastoma at age 14 years) in an anomalous child exposed to chemotherapy in utero has been published. It must be acknowledged, however, that there is a paucity of satisfactory long-term results among children exposed to chemotherapy in utero.

In one of the few studies to address this important subject, Aviles and Neri reported the outcomes of 84 children born to mothers with hematologic malignancies who received chemotherapy during pregnancy, including 38 during the first trimester (acute leukemia, $n = 29$; Hodgkin disease, $n = 26$; malignant lymphoma, $n = 29$). These children were examined for physical health, growth, and development and for hematologic, cytogenetic, neurologic, psychologic, and learning disorders. The occurrence of cancer or acute leukemia in these children was also considered by the investigators. In addition, some of their subjects had become parents, and their children were also considered in the analysis. In all the children studied, including the 12 second-generation children, the birth weight was normal, as was the learning and educational performance. Specifically, school performance and standardized intelligence testing did not differ significantly from unrelated matched children and unexposed siblings. No congenital, neurologic, laboratory, or psychologic abnormalities were observed. Tolerance of infections was also normal, as was secondary sexual development among the older children. With a median follow-up of 18.7 years (range, 6–29 years), no cancer or acute leukemia was detected.

The lack of adequate observation of the long-term status of the fetus or infant prevents any definite conclusions as to the relative safety or danger of anticancer chemotherapy during pregnancy, even in the second and third trimesters. It is surprising how often the detailed status of the fetus is not mentioned in available reports. The infant is often described as "normal," with few if any details on the physical or laboratory profile of the baby. **Long-term observation is necessary to establish normalcy because many of the defects may not be obvious on inspection and may emerge as derangements of growth, development, function, reproduction, and heredity.**

Supportive Therapy

Granulocyte-colony stimulating factors (G-CSFs), recombinant erythropoietin, and antibiotics are associated with very limited data sets in the medical literature. Among seven reports of G-CSF use during pregnancy (all after the first trimester), there were no adverse pregnancy- or neonatal-related events. Use of G-CSF appears to be reasonable for patients in desperate need of this drug. Although recombinant human erythropoietin (rhEPO) does not cross the placenta, evidence for its safety remains scarce, and blood transfusion should remain the first line of therapy for pregnant patients with severe anemia,

TABLE 15.16 Examples of Tests Used in the Antepartum Fetal Surveillance of Pregnant Patients With Cancer

Category	Details
Biochemical parameters	Progesterone; E3; hCG; Triple screen (E3, hCG, α-fetoprotein); Human placental lactogen
Fetal movements	Kick counting after 25 wk of gestation
Electronic fetal heart rate monitoring	Nonstress test; Contraction stress test; Sinusoidal rhythms (correlate with fetal anemia)
Ultrasonography	Accurate pregnancy dating; Confirm fetal well-being (viability); Uterine and adnexal abnormalities; Cervical length; Serial growth assessment; Assessment of the placenta; Assessment of fetal anomalies; Four-dimensional imaging
Fetal echocardiography	Evaluation for fetal cardiac defects
Color Doppler	Systolic-to-diastolic ratio in the umbilical cord artery; Systolic-to-diastolic ratio in the fetal middle cerebral artery ultrasonography
Fetal biophysical profile	Fetal breathing movements; Gross body movement; Fetal tone; Qualitative amniotic fluid volume; Reactive fetal heart rate
Chorionic villus sampling	9 wk
Amniocentesis	Genetic: 16–20 wk; Pulmonary maturation: third trimester
Percutaneous umbilical blood sampling	Fetal hematocrit; Fetal infection
Fetal fibronectin	22–34 wk
Fetal pulse oximetry	Acidemia with $P_aO_2 <30\%$

E3, Estriol; *hCG*, human chorionic gonadotropin.

particularly during the first trimester. Among the multitude of antibiotics available, penicillins are able to cross the placenta freely, but harmful fetal effects have not been reported. The combination of amoxicillin plus clavulanate is a regimen used frequently in patients receiving chemotherapy, but it is associated with an increased incidence of necrotizing enterocolitis in newborns and therefore should be avoided during pregnancy. Cephalosporins and metronidazole can be safely used during pregnancy; however, aminoglycosides, quinolones, trimethoprim, and tetracycline should not be administered. Aminoglycosides can cause eighth cranial nerve damage, and quinolones have been linked to congenital arthropathy in animal models. Similar to methotrexate, trimethoprim is a folate antagonist and is therefore contraindicated during pregnancy. Finally, tetracyclines are hepatotoxic to the mother and inhibit fetal bone growth. Although no adverse events have been reported with imipenem and meropenem, available data in human pregnancy are even more limited.

Serum Tumor Markers in Pregnancy

Table 15.17 lists serum tumor marker ranges for pregnant and nonpregnant women. Although the serum CA-125 has been found to fluctuate during pregnancy, comprehension of the established trends may assist in following pregnant women with a history of epithelial ovarian cancer and those being evaluated during pregnancy for a pelvic mass. Specifically, the CA-125 values are highest during the first trimester, with levels as high as 1250 U reported. The values decrease during the late first trimester and should remain below 35 U/mL of serum until delivery, at which point the CA-125 transiently increases 1 hour postpartum. It should be mentioned that Jacobs and Bast have reviewed the literature and found cases in which the maternal serum CA-125 remained within normal limits throughout uncomplicated pregnancies.

Bon and colleagues evaluated the concentrations of maternal CA-125 and CA-15-3 (a breast cancer tumor marker) in normal and 120 pathologic pregnancies (eg, spontaneous abortion, fetal death, growth restriction, chromosomal and structural abnormalities, and preeclampsia). The maternal CA-125 serum values were higher during the first and third trimesters during pregnancy, and the CA-15-3 serum levels were higher only during the third trimester. Neither antigen showed any relation with a pathologic outcome of pregnancy.

Of interest, Kiran and colleagues performed simultaneous measurements of CA-125, CA-15-3, CA-19-9, and carcinoembryonic antigen (CEA) in the maternal serum and umbilical cord blood in 53 pregnancies that were terminated by cesarean section. CA-19-9 is a pancreatic cancer tumor marker, and CEA is a marker of mucinous adenocarcinomas with levels that are normal or marginally elevated in normal pregnancy. With the exception of CEA, which was more elevated in the multigravida, all marker levels in maternal serum were significantly different than those of the umbilical cord, irrespective of fetal sex, fetal weight, and maternal parity.

Mammalian α-fetoprotein is classified as a member of the albuminoid gene superfamily. Molecular variants and genetic variants of α-fetoprotein differing in messenger ribonucleic acid (mRNA) kilobase length have been extensively described in the biomedical literature. After the discovery of the molten globule form in 1981, the existence of transitory, intermediate forms of α-fetoprotein was acknowledged, and their physiologic significance was realized. The maternal serum α-fetoprotein is a useful marker for women harboring a malignant germ cell tumor containing an endodermal sinus tumor or embryonal component. Initially produced by the yolk sac and later by the fetal liver and gastrointestinal tract, α-fetoprotein is also the predominant protein synthesized during fetal development. Maternal serum α-fetoprotein levels are routinely measured

TABLE 15.17 Serum Tumor Markers in Nonpregnant and Pregnant Patients

Marker	Malignancy	Normal Level	Effect of Pregnancy
CA-125	Serous papillary ovarian carcinoma and tumors of low malignant potential	<35 U/mL	Elevated during the first trimester
Human chorionic gonadotropin	Gestational trophoblastic neoplasia, malignant germ cell tumors of the ovary	<5 IU/L	Peak at 14–16 wk: 12,000–270,000 IU/L
α-Fetoprotein	Malignant germ cell tumors of the ovary, hepatocellular carcinoma	<15 ng/mL	Peaks at 200–300 mg/dL at 13 wk
Lactate dehydrogenase	Dysgerminoma, tumors of the liver	45–90 U/L	Fluctuates minimally
Inhibin	Granulosa cell tumors of the ovary	33–45 pg/mL	Increased with preeclampsia
Testosterone	Sertoli cell tumors of the ovary	30–95 ng/dL	May rise four- to ninefold over nonpregnant levels during normal pregnancy
DHEA-S	Tumors of the adrenal gland	35–430 mcg/dL	Can be increased (usually not >700 mcg/dL)
Carcinoembryonic antigen	Colorectal carcinoma, mucinous cystadenocarcinoma of the ovary, pseudomyxoma peritonei	<5 ng/mL	Normal or marginally elevated levels
CA-27.29	Breast cancer	≤38 U/mL	Not well studied
CA-15-3	Breast cancer	<40 U/mL	Elevated during third trimester in one study
CA-19-9	Pancreatic cancer	<40 U/mL	Not well studied
Prolactin	Pituitary tumor (prolactinoma)	<20 ng/mL	20–400 ng/mL
Total thyroxine	Thyroid carcinoma	5–12 mcg/dL	Increased because of increases in serum thyroxine-binding globulin

CA, Cancer antigen; *DHEA-S,* dehydroepiandrosterone sulfate.

between 16 and 20 weeks of gestation to screen for neural tube defects. **Pregnant women with marked elevations of serum α-fetoprotein should have a germ cell cancer or liver tumor included in the differential diagnosis.**

As Boulay and Podczaski point out in their excellent review on ovarian cancer complicating pregnancy, the use of α-fetoprotein levels to monitor women with a history of endodermal sinus tumor who subsequently become pregnant poses a distinct clinical dilemma. One way to distinguish between ovarian (ie, yolk sac) α-fetoprotein and fetal (ie, liver) α-fetoprotein is to divide the heterogeneous human α-fetoprotein into various subfractions stratified by differential reactivity with lectins, such as concanavalin A. Assay chromatography with concanavalin sepharose A will separate the α-fetoprotein into either the yolk sac or liver variant because the yolk sac form of α-fetoprotein contains the carbonal sugar and is the type produced by the endodermal sinus tumor.

The use of the hCG level to monitor pregnant women in remission after treatment for gestational trophoblastic disease is also problematic. **The hCG steadily increases during the first trimester of pregnancy and may reach levels beyond 100,000 U at 10 weeks of gestation.** Accordingly, women with a history of trophoblastic neoplasia must undergo transvaginal ultrasonography to document intrauterine pregnancy, and a metastatic workup should be conducted if the hCG remains markedly elevated during pregnancy or if focal symptoms manifest.

The glycolytic enzyme lactate dehydrogenase (LDH) is involved in the conversion of pyruvate to lactate. LDH is also a marker for gonadal and extragonadal dysgerminomas. Because the enzyme is ubiquitous, the heterogeneity afforded its multiple molecular forms permits electrophoretic separation into five isoenzymes. Isoenzyme fractions 1 and 2 are specifically elevated in women with dysgerminomas. **During pregnancy and the puerperium, LDH values fluctuate very little unless the patient has preeclampsia.** In 1992, our group used the LDH level to observe two women with dysgerminoma diagnosed during pregnancy; in both cases, the LDH value was correlated to disease activity.

Inhibin is a glycoprotein hormone produced by normal ovarian granulosa cells and testicular Sertoli cells. In the ovary, it inhibits the secretion of follicle-stimulating hormone. Patients with granulosa cell tumors have elevated serum levels of inhibin, and this finding has been used to detect recurrent tumor. In pregnancy, serum levels of inhibin do not rise significantly unless the patient has preeclampsia or gestational hypertension. The use of an inhibin mAb can preferentially mark inhibin secreted from granulosa cell tumors and Sertoli–Leydig cell tumors.

HEMATOLOGIC MALIGNANCIES IN PREGNANCY

Leukemia

Arising from bone marrow progenitor cells that have arrested along a line of differentiation, the leukemias manifest clinically when the arrested cells proliferate, overtake the bone marrow, and spill out into the peripheral blood. Without immediate

TABLE 15.18 Classification of the Leukemias

Acute	Chronic
Acute myelogenous leukemia	Chronic myelogenous leukemia
Acute promyelocytic leukemia	Chronic myelomonocytic leukemia
Acute myelomonocytic leukemia	Chronic lymphatic leukemia
Acute monoblastic leukemia	T cell
Acute erythroleukemia	B cell
Acute megakaryoblastic leukemia	Prolymphocytic leukemia
Acute lymphatic leukemia	Sézary syndrome
Common	Hairy cell leukemia
T cell	
B cell	
Pre–B cell	
Acute mast cell leukemia	

From Jandi JH. *Blood: Textbook of Hematology*, 2nd ed. Boston, 1996, Little, Brown.

therapy, patients with acute leukemia, particularly acute myelogenous leukemia (AML), survive a median of 3 months. In the United States, there are 30,000 new cases of leukemia and 20,000 deaths are attributable to the disease each year. Table 15.18 summarizes a classification scheme for the leukemias, with the major subtypes being AML (comprising 46% of all leukemias), chronic lymphatic leukemia (29%), chronic myelocytic leukemia (CML, 14%), and acute lymphatic leukemia (11%). **Leukemia is estimated to occur in 1 in 75,000 pregnancies, with AML accounting for more than 60% of reported cases, of which there are approximately 500.**

The attainment of a morphologic normal bone marrow containing less than 5% blasts, the absence of any signs of extramedullary leukemia, and the return of normal neutrophil counts (>1500/μL) and platelet counts (>150,000/μL) is the treatment goal of acute leukemia. Auer rods must not appear in the peripheral blood, and anemia, if present, does not preclude complete remission because this is often slow to recover. Bone marrow aspiration is performed weekly during the induction phase.

Because of severe myelosuppression caused by intensive chemotherapy, the achievement of complete remission is predicated on supportive care and the necessary maintenance of more than 500/μL circulating neutrophils and more than 20,000 circulating platelets to prevent infectious and hemorrhagic deaths. Cytosine arabinoside and daunorubicin are used to induce remission in AML, with postremission therapy requiring maintenances doses of cytosine arabinoside. When the analysis of the cerebrospinal fluid establishes CNS involvement, intrathecal chemotherapy with or without cranial radiation is administered. Finally, the treatment and maintenance of acute lymphatic leukemia uses multiagent regimens involving vincristine and CNS prophylaxis.

The ability to enter into complete remission is age dependent, with the overall rate for acute leukemia being 65%. The median survival time is approximately 2 years, with 25% of patients becoming long-term, disease-free survivors. The prognosis for patients undergoing treatment of leukemia after therapy for another disease, or in the recurrent setting, is very poor. Indeed, the majority of adult patients who achieve remission subsequently experience recurrence. The long-term survival rate seen in children is not obtained in adults.

Leukemia in Pregnancy

In pregnant patients, persistent fever, weight loss, lymphadenopathy, or an abnormal differential on the complete blood count should prompt an investigation and raise the clinician's suspicion for leukemia. As in the case of non-Hodgkin lymphoma (NHL) in pregnancy, patients with acute leukemia are often very ill, and the primary concern is to save the pregnant woman's life through induction chemotherapy or radiotherapy. Therefore, if the patient is remote from delivery, appropriate treatment will place the fetus at risk of exposure to chemotherapeutic agents, radiation therapy, or both. Chronic myelogenous leukemia in pregnancy, however, can be managed similar to Hodgkin disease, with a justifiable delay in definitive treatment of several weeks if indicated. The outcome of pregnancy-associated acute leukemia is only worse when compared with nonpregnant cases when therapy is delayed. Regardless of gestational age, the induction of remission with combination chemotherapy is the primary objective. Seventy-five percent of pregnant women enter into complete remission after therapy for acute leukemia, owing to their favorable age. During the first and early second trimesters, termination of pregnancy should be seriously considered, especially in acutely ill pregnant women. When the diagnosis is made later in pregnancy, it should be recognized that there are obvious advantages of delivery before the onset of chemotherapy, and this should be encouraged, if possible.

The average age of the patient with acute leukemia in pregnancy is 28 years. Premature labor is common in these women, and the average period of gestation is approximately 8 months. Postpartum hemorrhage occurs in 10% to 15% of cases. The fibrinogen level in patients with acute leukemia in pregnancy may be reduced from the level anticipated at that stage of gestation. Frenkel and Meyers stated that pregnancy exerts no specific effect on the course of acute leukemia except that early gestation poses an obstacle to vigorous treatment of leukemia. Other authors have observed that infants born of mothers with leukemia are as well as normal control participants. Lilleyman and colleagues and Bitran and Roth have written comprehensive reports on this subject.

The following factors are associated with the delivery of a normal baby:
1. Antimetabolite drugs not administered
2. Radiotherapy to the uterus not given
3. The fetus reaches the age of viability

The decision to interrupt a pregnancy in patients discovered to have leukemia is primarily based on the desires of the patient. Prompt therapy is always advisable for the possibility of obtaining remission. However, the physician's advice to the patient should be influenced by the aggressiveness of the disease process. For instance, patients with CML are less likely to be harmed by deferring termination of pregnancy than are patients with acute myelocytic leukemia demonstrating symptoms and having a somewhat fulminating course.

Chemotherapy for Acute Leukemia in Pregnancy

There are many reports of successful chemotherapy for patients who have acute leukemia in pregnancy, and there has been little, if any, significant increase in fetal wastage or congenital anomalies. In 1984, Catanzarite and Ferguson published a review of management and outcome of acute leukemia in pregnancy for the years 1972 to 1982. The investigators collected 14 pregnancies reported in patients cured of acute lymphocytic leukemia, of which there was one early spontaneous abortion and 13 term infants. All mothers survived. They also collected 47 reports of pregnancy in association with acute leukemia. In 40 pregnancies in which acute leukemia was treated, there were five abortions, three perinatal demises, one infant "live-born in grave condition," and 31 surviving infants. Median maternal survival was at least 6 months and possibly longer than 12 months from delivery. In the remaining seven cases, the leukemia was untreated. Despite this, there were two perinatal deaths, one abortion, and four living infants.

During the years of Catanzarite and Ferguson's study, effective combination chemotherapy was in widespread use. Previous reviews covered cases reported before the introduction of effective combination chemotherapy. There were fewer than 300 reported pregnancies, with a 36% to 69% perinatal mortality rate and a median maternal survival period from diagnosis of shorter than 6 months. Advances in the fields of hematology and oncology, maternal and fetal medicine, and neonatology have resulted in marked improvements in both perinatal survival statistics and median maternal survival time.

In women who refuse pregnancy termination or in whom delivery is not expected imminently, induction of remission should be attempted. When combination therapy is used during the first trimester (and for acute leukemia in pregnancy, this is not a contraindication), the stillbirth rate is 25%—this decreases to 13% in the second and third trimesters. A combination of cytarabine, doxorubicin, and etoposide has been used with good results for both mother and fetus, and when possible, we recommend this regimen. Delivery should be timed to precede the next course of chemotherapy; however, the majority of patients should be counseled to expect preterm delivery, either spontaneous or induced. It is mandatory to perform a hematologic evaluation of the newborn because the drugs used cross the placenta and can result in pancytopenia. Although no growth or developmental abnormalities have been demonstrated, the follow-up of children exposed to in utero chemotherapy for the management of acute leukemia has been limited.

Acute Myelogenous Leukemia

Acute myelogenous leukemia is the most common leukemia diagnosed during pregnancy. Azim and colleagues identified 87 patients (88 pregnancies) treated with systemic therapy during pregnancy in their literature review. Among those treated during the first trimester, nearly 50% had poor fetal outcomes. Among those treated after the first trimester, the combination of cytarabine and daunorubicin was most commonly used during the induction phase. Of 32 patients exposed to these two agents starting from the second trimester, only 15 had normal pregnancy outcomes. It is unclear whether this is secondary to cytarabine or daunorubicin. Whereas previous reports of single-agent cytarabine have been associated with normal pregnancy outcomes, single-agent daunorubicin has been associated with one case of maternal–fetal death. Idarubicin is also used for AML induction therapy and is more lipophilic compared with other anthracyclines; therefore, placental transfer of this drug is more likely to occur. There have been seven pregnant women exposed to idarubicin and cytarabine after the first trimester from which reports of stillbirth, limb deformities, and cardiomyopathy have appeared. It is of significant concern that the combination of cytarabine with daunorubicin or idarubicin is associated with significant fetal morbidity and mortality, even if administered after the first trimester. However, doxorubicin is an active agent in AML and has been associated with normal pregnancy outcomes both in AML and in PABC. Given the poor safety data of daunorubicin and idarubicin and probably noninferiority of doxorubicin when compared with other anthracyclines, Azim and colleagues consider it the treatment of choice for gestational AML for patients wishing to preserve the pregnancy.

Acute Lymphoblastic Leukemia

Approximately one-third of gestational leukemia is of acute lymphoblastic leukemia (ALL). Many of the patients in the literature treated with chemotherapy during the first trimester were unintentionally exposed. The expected findings of limb, ear, and lung deformities along with a case of esophageal atresia and even stillbirth emphasize the importance of active contraception in patients with ALL during the maintenance phase. Azim and colleagues have identified 21 patients treated after the first trimester. As was observed with daunorubicin and idarubicin exposure during the second trimester in patients with AML, these agents have also been associated with adverse fetal outcomes when given for ALL. Acute cardiac failure, premature delivery, and intrauterine fetal demise have been reported. Fortunately, data on doxorubicin in ALL is reassuring and again Azim and colleagues consider this agent as the anthracycline of choice during pregnancy after the first trimester.

Acute Promyelocytic Leukemia

Acute promyelocytic leukemia (APL) accounts for 13% of AML cases and commonly occurs in young adults. The specific chromosomal translocation, t(15/17), is found in the neoplastic promyelocytic proliferation that characterizes this disease. Disseminated intravascular coagulation (DIC) is a lethal complication of AML. All-trans retinoic acid (ATRA) targets t(15/17) and reduces the incidence of DIC and consequently increases the likelihood of achieving long-term remission. Azim and colleagues collected 22 cases of ATRA treatment during pregnancy, in which 14 patients received single-agent therapy and eight were treated with a combination of ATRA plus idarubicin or daunorubicin. No congenital anomalies or spontaneous abortions have been reported to have occurred among newborns

exposed to single-agent ATRA in utero. One baby who had been diagnosed earlier with Potter syndrome during the first trimester before exposure to ATRA died after the mother went into spontaneous labor; this newborn had been exposed to ATRA for 1 day during week 29 of gestation. Although two patients exposed to ATRA during the first trimester have been reported to have had normal outcomes, there are data that link first-trimester retinoic acid ingestion to craniofacial, cardiac, and brain malformations (ie, retinoic acid embryopathy).

Among patients treated with combined therapy, atrial septal defects were reported in two newborns exposed to ATRA plus idarubicin. Postnatal fetal death secondary to pulmonary hemorrhage was reported in a newborn exposed to ATRA plus daunorubicin and cytarabine. In patients with APL who received chemotherapy alone, again, daunorubicin has been associated with a high incidence of complications, including intrauterine fetal demise, spontaneous abortion, bone marrow aplasia, cerebral bleeding, and child maceration.

Management of Chronic Leukemia

Chronic myelocytic leukemia represents approximately 90% of all chronic leukemias in pregnancy. An additional 5% of the chronic leukemias in pregnancy are chronic lymphocytic leukemias. Several reports show that pregnant patients with chronic granulocytic leukemia treated during the first trimester with chemotherapy and radiation therapy to the spleen usually deliver apparently healthy, viable babies if the uterus is protected with lead shields. Lee and coworkers reported 12 cases of leukemia associated with pregnancy. Using lead shields to protect the uterus from radiation therapy to the spleen, six of seven women with chronic leukemia who also received chemotherapy went on to deliver six apparently healthy infants. The prognosis for these patients is poor; the median survival time is 45 months.

There has been some experience in treating CML during pregnancy with interferon-α. Mubarak and colleagues reported the outcomes of three women, ages 23 to 32 years, with Philadelphia chromosome–positive CML who received interferon-α during the first trimester of pregnancy. No maternal complications occurred, and three normal-appearing babies were delivered, one of whom had a transient mild thrombocytopenia. Subsequently, these children were followed for 4, 12, and 30 months, and all had normal growth and development.

Chronic Myelocytic Leukemia

Chronic myelocytic leukemia is rare among pregnant women. The disease accounts for only 15% of adult leukemias, with only 10% occurring during the childbearing years. The main driving force for development and maintenance of the leukemic clone is the BCR/ABL fusion gene, which is a target of imatinib mesylate. Complete responses with this agent are dependent on the continuous administration of this drug. Pye and colleagues have identified 55 pregnant women exposed to imatinib, 40 of whom (72%) delivered live births without any congenital anomalies. Seventy-five percent of the congenital anomalies encountered in this series ($n = 9$) were in fetuses exposed to imatinib during the first trimester. Exomphalos occurred in three neonates; renal agenesis or malformation in two; hypospadias in two; cleft palate, hydrocephalus, meningocele, pyloric stenosis and premature closure of skull bones in one; and warfarin syndrome in one. Among the 38 patients (21%) exposed to imatinib throughout the course of pregnancy, seven had a spontaneous abortion, and one developed the previously mentioned warfarin syndrome secondary to warfarin exposure. Azim and colleagues identified 26 additional cases of gestational imatinib exposure. Sixty percent were exposed during the first trimester and discontinued the drug when pregnancy was diagnosed. In these patients, one preterm delivery, two cases of newborn hypospadias, and one child with a fatal meningocele were reported. Nine patients became pregnant while taking imatinib and continued the pregnancy to term with no adverse events. Four patients who started imatinib therapy during the second and third trimesters were able to control their disease without affecting the pregnancy outcome. A total of 11 newborns have been followed for more than 1 year with no delayed adverse effects reported. It appears that early exposure to imatinib is associated with a high risk of spontaneous abortion and congenital anomalies. Imatinib therapy during the second and third trimester does not appear to add significantly to the risk associated with first-trimester exposure.

In the pre-imatinib era, both interferon (IFN) alpha and hydroxyurea (HU) were used to treat patients with CML. IFN was considered the standard of care for patients not eligible for bone marrow transplantation. Because of its high molecular weight, IFN is unlikely to cross the placenta. Approximately 15 patients have been exposed during the first trimester with no congenital anomalies reported. Preclinical data also support the safe use of IFN throughout the course of pregnancy.

Preclinical models have been less favorable for HU with significant evidence for teratogenicity in all animal species. Congenital anomalies of the heart, CNS, and skeleton as well as neural tube defects have been described. Among the 49 pregnant patients with CML exposed to HU in the literature review by Azim and colleagues, there was one neonatal death on day 10 of life secondary to intracranial bleeding not associated with congenital anomalies. Three intrauterine fetal deaths were reported, two cases of hip dysplasia, and one case each of pilonidal sinus and unilateral renal dilatation. Although chromosomal anomalies have not been reported in humans after HU exposure in utero, this drug should not be the treatment of choice for CML during pregnancy, particularly in light of its nonsuperiority to other agents used to treat this disease.

Hairy Cell Leukemia, Multiple Myeloma, and Chronic Lymphocytic Leukemia

Hairy cell leukemia (HCL), multiple myeloma (MM), and chronic lymphocytic leukemia (CLL) are among the rarest hematologic malignancies encountered during pregnancy. A few cases of IFN therapy for HCL and MM have been reported with normal outcomes. The standard of care for HCL is cladribine, but its use during pregnancy has not yet been reported. For the rare patient of childbearing age who develops CLL during pregnancy, a watch-and-wait approach is advisable in the absence of symptoms. Chlorambucil has been associated with normal pregnancy outcomes for patients with symptomatic CLL.

Hodgkin Disease

The importance of staging in Hodgkin disease was recognized by Peters as early as 1950, when she devised the first clinical staging classification. Lymphangiography then made possible the earlier detection of retroperitoneal lymph node involvement, and it became important to distinguish two subgroups: those with widespread disease confined to lymphatic organs and those with spread of disease beyond the lymph nodes, thymus, spleen, and Waldeyer ring to one or more extralymphatic organs or tissues, which is now recognized as stage IV disease. The subtype classification scheme for Hodgkin lymphoma appears in Table 15.19. The staging system as proposed by the Cotswolds meeting appears in Table 15.20. **Surgical staging has gained popularity in Hodgkin disease, and when evaluating young women in whom preservation of ovarian function is desired and pelvic irradiation is planned, surgical oophoropexy can be performed at the time of staging laparotomy.**

TABLE 15.19   Classification of Hodgkin Disease

Subtype	Frequency (%)	Characteristics
Nodular sclerosis	40	Mediastinal and pulmonary involvement
Mixed cellularity	30	Often advanced at presentation
Lymphocyte predominance	15	Rare classic Reed-Sternberg cells
Lymphocyte depletion	15	Oldest median age, worst prognosis

TABLE 15.20   Staging of Hodgkin Disease as Proposed in the Cotswolds, England, 1990

Stage*	Characteristics
I	Involvement of a single lymph node or lymphoid region (eg, spleen, thymus, Waldeyer ring) or a single extralymphatic site (Ie)
II	Involvement of two or more lymph node regions on the same side of the diaphragm; localized contiguous involvement of only one extranodal organ or site and lymph node region(s) on the same side of the diaphragm (IIe)
III	Involvement of lymph node regions on both sides of the diaphragm, which may also include spleen (IIIs) or one extranodal localized contiguous site (IIIe), or both (IIIes)
III1	With or without involvement of splenic, hilar, celiac, or portal nodes
III2	With involvement of paraaortic, iliac, and mesenteric nodes
IV	Diffuse or disseminated involvement of one or more extranodal organs or tissues

*Applicable designations: a, no symptoms; b, night sweats, fever, weight loss; cs, clinical staging; e, involvement of a single extranodal site contiguous or proximal to a known nodal site; ps, pathologic staging (by laparotomy); x, bulky disease (diameter >one-third of the mediastinum).

From Peleg D, Ben-Ami M. Lymphoma and leukemia complicating pregnancy. *Obstet Gynecol Clin North Am* 1998;25:365.

The feature of the disease most helpful in selecting therapy and estimating the prognosis at the time of onset is its clinical extent. In general, the more widespread the disease, the poorer the prognosis, even if all apparent disease is confined to the lymphoid regions. The poorer prognosis of patients who have involvement of sites beyond the usual lymphoid tissues is well known. Five-year survival rates of 50% are often reported for patients who have widespread lymph node disease, and rates of 8% are reported for those who have involvement of extranodal sites such as the lung, liver, bone, and bone marrow. Survival depends more on the patient's age and stage than on the subtype. Overall, 36% survive for 20 years, and about 70% do not have a relapse after primary treatment. Patients 17 to 34 years old have an 80% long-term survival rate compared with 35% for those 60 years or older.

The treatment of Hodgkin disease has undergone radical changes in the past 40 years. Present recommendations are based on the assumptions that radiotherapy is the mainstay of treatment of early-stage disease, combination chemotherapy is the primary treatment of advanced-stage disease with parenchymal organ involvement, and a combination of the two is required for patients with bulky disease (eg, a large mediastinal mass) or generalized abdominal lymph node involvement. Aggressive therapy has resulted in considerable improvement in overall survival rates for patients with Hodgkin disease. The most successful and widely tested combination of drugs has been developed at the National Cancer Institute (DeVita and colleagues) and consists of six 2-week cycles of therapy with nitrogen mustard, vincristine, procarbazine, and prednisone, the so-called MOPP program, although other combinations have been used successfully.

The major technical factors that determine the efficacy of radiation therapy in Hodgkin disease are the total radiation dose per field; the size, shape, and number of treatment fields; and the beam energy. Permanent eradication of any given site of involvement can be achieved consistently with doses of 3500 to 4500 cGy delivered at a rate of 1000 cGy/week. The desirability of irradiating apparently uninvolved lymph node regions has long been advocated by experienced radiotherapists. This approach is based on the knowledge of the clinical behavior of Hodgkin disease, the inadequacies of our diagnostic techniques to discover minute or microscopic foci of the disease, the advantage and efficacy of avoiding patchwork and overlapping fields, and the possible reseeding of previously irradiated regions from unrecognized and untreated sites. Extended-field irradiation, so-called total lymphoid or total radial therapy, is technically demanding and potentially hazardous.

Hodgkin Disease in Pregnancy

With a peak incidence between the ages of 18 and 30 years, Hodgkin disease commonly affects young people. It is now being cured and controlled for long periods with irradiation and chemotherapy. Hodgkin disease in pregnancy occurs in approximately 1 in 6000 deliveries. Young women diagnosed with Hodgkin disease are usually asymptomatic. **The nodular sclerosis subtype of Hodgkin disease is the most common subtype encountered in pregnancy and carries a favorable prognosis.**

Most reports suggest that the onset of Hodgkin disease during pregnancy does not adversely affect survival. Chemotherapy and radiation therapy to the abdomen can usually be postponed until the pregnancy is terminated. The drugs commonly used for Hodgkin disease are contraindicated in the first trimester of pregnancy and are preferably withheld until the postpartum period. The amazing successes achieved with early stages of this disease allow much more flexibility and improved regard for the fetus. **Pregnancy itself does not appear to adversely affect the course of the disease, and interruption of pregnancy during the course of the disease is not definitely indicated.** The management of the pregnant patient with Hodgkin disease should be individualized and should involve a multidisciplinary team of physicians and other professionals. Three of four patients diagnosed with Hodgkin disease will be cured.

Management of Hodgkin Disease in Pregnancy

Hodgkin lymphoma is the second most commonly diagnosed cancer in people aged 15 to 29 years and is the most common lymphoma diagnosed during pregnancy. The literature contains 68 pregnancies in 67 women with Hodgkin lymphoma who received systemic chemotherapy, immunotherapy, or both. Twenty-six of these cases were published by Aviles and colleagues, and an additional 42 were identified in the review by Azim and colleagues. In the former study, most patients had advanced disease and nodular sclerosis histology. More than one-third of patients were treated during the first trimester without sequelae (ie, no low birth weight or anomalies). These results are challenged by the finding of six congenital anomalies and three spontaneous abortions occurring in the 17 patients exposed to chemotherapy during the first trimester in the report by Azim and colleagues. The standard Hodgkin lymphoma regimen ABVD (doxorubicin, bleomycin, vinblastine, and dacarbazine) was given to 16 of the 42 patients. Those treated after the first trimester had normal pregnancy outcome with no adverse fetal events with the exception on one case of intrauterine fetal demise in the third trimester, one case of atrial septal defect, and one case of hemolytic anemia with jaundice at birth. It seems reasonable to start treating patients with the standard ABVD regimen in the second trimester.

For patients with localized disease in the cervical, occipital, or axillary regions, radiotherapy has been reported to be safe because the average embryo dose does not exceed 0.1 to 0.2 Gy in such sites. This represents the threshold dose at which stochastic effects (eg, mental retardation, organ malformation) could manifest.

The complexity of the management of Hodgkin disease during pregnancy cannot be overstressed. Thorough staging of the pregnant patient is significantly compromised without termination of the pregnancy by one means or another. Surgical staging of the pregnant patient after the 18th week of pregnancy is feasible and often avoids the necessity of many of the diagnostic techniques that might be harmful to the fetus, such as lower extremity lymphangiography, intravenous

pyelography, and bone and liver scans. **Splenectomy is often performed during these staging procedures, and no contraindication in pregnancy is known.** The purpose of staging with this disease is to achieve the best differentiation between those curable with local therapy (radiation) and those who require systemic therapy (chemotherapy or radiation) for cure. After a criterion for systemic therapy has been uncovered, no additional diagnostic procedures are required.

Treatment is obviously easier if the pregnancy is terminated, but that may not be an option. Current data suggest that the course of Hodgkin disease does not seem to be affected by an ongoing pregnancy. Other studies have also noted a survival rate of pregnant women with Hodgkin disease comparable with that of nonpregnant patients with Hodgkin disease. Hodgkin lymphoma is not associated with an increase in miscarriage, stillbirths, or congenital anomalies unless treatment is started in the first trimester. Metastasis to the placenta has been reported, although it is rare.

Hodgkin lymphoma is a potentially curable disease, and stage I and II disease typically are treated with megavolt radiotherapy unless bulky disease is present. Given in fractions over 3.5 to 4.5 weeks, a dose of 3500 to 4500 cGy is prescribed. In early-stage disease, the lymphoid areas that need to be irradiated include the mediastinum, Waldeyer ring and axilla (ie, mantle field), and the paraaortic area and splenic pedicle (spade field). When necessary, total nodal irradiation includes the pelvis (inverted Y field), as illustrated in Fig. 15.15.

Pregnant women with Hodgkin lymphoma present with typical manifestations, with painless enlargement of lymph nodes above the diaphragm, usually the cervical, submaxillary, or axillary nodes. In patients without obvious lymphadenopathy, a delay in diagnosis is common because symptoms of fatigue, weight loss, chest discomfort, and anemia may be overlooked and considered "normal" during pregnancy. The role of staging laparotomy in Hodgkin disease is diminishing, and if necessary, it should be delayed until after delivery, at which time bilateral oophoropexy can be performed. **It has been our practice to bring the ovaries as close to the midline as possible behind the uterus, where they can be shielded underneath a protective block placed between the two arms of the Y.**

Pohlman and Macklis carefully reviewed previously published guidelines for Hodgkin disease associated with pregnancy and have proposed the following management scheme, which the author of this chapter has endorsed (Fig. 15.16). The earlier the pregnancy, the stronger the recommendation for pregnancy termination so that proper staging and treatment can begin. Patients diagnosed during the first trimester of pregnancy may be observed until the second trimester, when therapy can commence. Those first-trimester patients with B symptoms, bulky or advanced-stage disease, or rapid progression have an indication to initiate treatment immediately and should undergo therapeutic abortion. **If the mother does not wish to sacrifice the pregnancy, single-agent vinblastine, which has a 7% anomaly rate when used in the first trimester, should be administered until the second trimester or until significant disease progression.** If combination chemotherapy is required, the ABVD regimen without dacarbazine during the first trimester should be given and then standard ABVD subsequently.

Patients presenting in the second or third trimester can be closely observed, and the fetus should be delivered as soon as viability and pulmonary maturation are demonstrable. **Delivery should be delayed as long as possible after the last dose of chemotherapy (before the next dose) to decrease the risk of marrow suppression in the neonate.** It may be worthwhile to consider a cesarean section so that surgical staging can be performed at the same time. **Umbilical cord blood should be collected and stored as a possible source of human leukocyte antigen–compatible stem cells.** Because the drugs used in Hodgkin disease can reach significant levels in breast milk, mothers receiving chemotherapy must avoid breastfeeding.

If treatment is necessary during the second and third trimesters of pregnancy, the standard ABVD regimen should be used. Postchemotherapy-involved field radiation therapy can be postponed until after delivery but should be initiated within 9 weeks after the last cycle of chemotherapy. Mantle and spade field radiotherapy with extensive abdominal shielding is also an acceptable alternative until the third trimester, when the uterus starts to impinge on the field. **The inverted Y field is not an option at any time during pregnancy.**

Among women with refractory or relapsed Hodgkin disease for whom the ABVD regimen and radiotherapy are not treatment options, MOPP and MOPP-like regimens have demonstrable efficacy with limited adverse effect on the fetus if administered after the first trimester.

Several older series that predate modern therapy suggest that Hodgkin disease has no biologic effect on pregnancy and vice versa. More contemporary reports have substantiated these claims. Investigators from the Hospital for Sick Children and Princess Margaret Hospital in Toronto identified 48 women

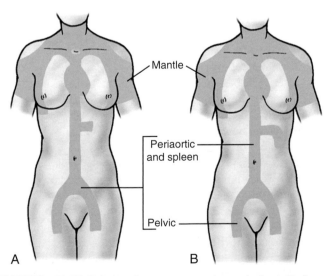

FIGURE 15.15 Schematic representation of "mantle" and "inverted Y" fields for total lymphoid irradiation. **A,** Two-field technique, with a small extension to include the splenic pedicle, used in splenectomized patients. **B,** Three-field technique usually used when the spleen is still present. (From.)

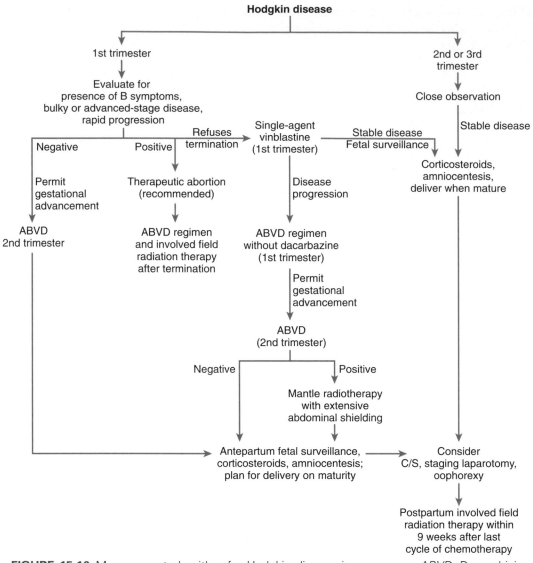

FIGURE 15.16 Management algorithm for Hodgkin disease in pregnancy. *ABVD,* Doxorubicin (Adriamycin), bleomycin, vinblastine, and dacarbazine; *C/S,* cesarean section.

with 50 pregnancies from 1958 to 1984 and matched them with three nonpregnant control subjects of similar age, stage, and year of diagnosis. Twelve women were diagnosed with Hodgkin disease before conception, 10 during pregnancy, and 27 after delivery or pregnancy termination. No statistically significant difference in stage at diagnosis, maternal outcome, or pregnancy outcome was identified between any of these subgroups and the similar control group. It should be noted that 16 patients received radiotherapy while pregnant, and five received combination chemotherapy and radiotherapy while pregnant.

In an investigation focusing on fetal effects of therapy, Ebert and colleagues identified 24 cases in the literature between 1983 and 1995. Among 15 women who received cyclophosphamide, vincristine, procarbazine, and prednisone (COPP; $n = 1$); mechlorethamine, vincristine, procarbazine, and prednisone (MOPP; $n = 4$); ABVD; ($n = 7$); or MOPP/ABVD ($n = 3$) beginning in the first ($n = 5$), second ($n = 8$), and third ($n = 2$) trimesters, all had healthy infants who went on to develop normally

during a median follow-up period of 9 years (range, 0–17 years) after delivery. Of the remaining nine women, most received one of the aforementioned regimens during the first trimester and either had therapeutic abortions or experienced spontaneous abortions, delivering fetuses with multiple anomalies.

In a study from Stanford University, the outcome of 17 pregnancies associated with Hodgkin disease between 1987 and 1993 was reported. Patients received radiation therapy ($n = 6$), chemotherapy ($n = 4$), or combined modality therapy ($n = 5$), although the specific timings of therapy in relation to pregnancy were not stated. Excluding four women who had a therapeutic or spontaneous abortion, no congenital anomalies were noted at delivery, and all children were reported to be healthy at the time of last follow-up. With a median follow-up time of 35 months (range, 6–79 months), 15 of the 17 mothers remain in complete remission.

A final report of interest was provided by Sutcliffe, who describes three women with stage II nodular sclerosing Hodgkin disease who received ABVD chemotherapy during the second and third trimesters of pregnancy. Two of these patients also received mantle-field radiation therapy after delivery. All three delivered healthy infants between 32 and 35 weeks of gestation. The chromosomal analyses of all three children were normal, and at more than 1 year, 5 years, and 7 years of follow-up, all three mothers and children remain healthy.

Non-Hodgkin Lymphoma

A total of 45,000 new cases of NHL are diagnosed in the United States each year. The mean age at diagnosis is 42 years. NHLs comprise a mixed family of diseases characterized by clonal neoplasms arising from one of the cellular constituents of the lymph node. Approximately 85% of NHLs are B-cell tumors; 15% are T-cell tumors; and a small percentage arise from other cells, primarily macrophages. A multitude of infectious agents (eg, the Epstein–Barr virus, the human T-cell leukemia/lymphoma virus), noninfectious agents (eg, radiation, radiation therapy, chemotherapy), and diseases (eg, ataxia telangiectasia, Sjögren syndrome, systemic lupus erythematosus) are associated with NHLs. Most patients present with painless lymphadenopathy, but NHLs may arise outside the lymphoid system in any tissue accessible to lymphocytes, most commonly in the gastrointestinal tract, pharynx, CNS, skin, and bone. Because the disease is usually widespread when peripheral lymph nodes have become involved, staging laparotomy is not used. The prognosis of NHL has been divided into favorable, intermediate, and poor. The Working Formulation is a classification scheme for NHL that is used in determining prognosis and treatment (Table 15.21). Unfortunately, NHLs are cured in fewer than 25% of the general population, although women of reproductive age have a 50% cure rate.

Early-stage (stage I or II), low-grade NHL is treated with extended-field or total lymphoid irradiation, with 5-year survival rates of 84%. Intermediate-grade tumors are managed with combination chemotherapy (prednisone, methotrexate, doxorubicin, cyclophosphamide, etoposide, cytosine arabinoside, bleomycin, vincristine, and leucovorin [ProMACE-CytaBOM]) with or without radiotherapy, resulting in sustained remissions at 4 years in approximately 45% of patients.

Non-Hodgkin Lymphoma in Pregnancy

Most women with NHL in association with pregnancy have an aggressive histologic subtype and advanced-stage disease, possibly as a result of a delay in diagnosis in many cases. **An unexpectedly high incidence of breast, uterine, cervical, and ovarian involvement among pregnant women has been noted when NHL is associated with pregnancy, with the predilection for these organs attributed to hormonal influences and increased blood flow to these organs.** In a review of 96 women with pregnancy-associated NHL, Pohlman and colleagues reported fully 50% of women presenting with stage IV disease. Seven percent of pregnancies ended in therapeutic abortion, and 4% of women experienced a spontaneous abortion. Eleven percent of infants were born prematurely, and 7% died. Only 31 mothers were known to have achieved a complete remission, and for 90 subjects in whom their long-term outcome was

TABLE 15.21 Working Formulation for Classification of Non-Hodgkin Lymphoma

	Histologic Type	Description	Prognosis
I	Low grade	Small lymphocytic cell Follicular (nodular) small cleaved cell Follicular mixed small cleaved cell	Favorable
II	Intermediate grade	Follicular large cell Diffuse small cleaved cell Diffuse mixed small and large cell Diffuse large cell cleaved or noncleaved	Intermediate
III	High grade	Diffuse large cell, immunoblastic Small noncleaved cell (Burkitt or non-Burkitt) Lymphoblastic (convoluted or nonconvoluted)	Unfavorable
IV	Miscellaneous	Composite Mycosis fungoides Extramedullary plasmacytoma Histiocytic Unclassified	—

From Peleg D, Ben-Ami M. Lymphoma and leukemia complicating pregnancy. *Obstet Gynecol Clin North Am* 1998;25:365.

known, only 39 were alive and disease free a median of 21 months (range, 2–132 months) after delivery, four were alive with disease, and 47 had died with a median of 6 months (range, <1–36 months) after delivery. Women who were diagnosed during the third trimester of pregnancy appeared to have a better outcome than those diagnosed earlier. Seventy-one of 96 children were reported alive, although the follow-up period for the majority was either less than 1 month or unknown.

Aviles and colleagues reviewed the outcome of both the mother and fetus in 19 pregnancies between 1975 and 1986. All patients received doxorubicin-based combination chemotherapy during pregnancy, including eight who received chemotherapy during the first trimester. Three mothers and their fetuses died during induction, and the 16 remaining women delivered healthy infants between 35 and 39 weeks of gestation. Eight of 12 mothers remained in complete remission 4 to 9 years after delivery, seven mothers died of lymphoma, and one was lost to follow-up.

Overall, the prognosis for all patients with NHL is worse than the prognosis for patients with Hodgkin disease. This is explained, in part, by the dissemination of disease at presentation. For this reason, although many dispute the claims that NHL arising in pregnancy is more virulent, the management of NHL in pregnancy needs to be aggressive. **A delay in treatment cannot be justified, and a woman who has not completed the first half of pregnancy should be advised to undergo therapeutic abortion unless she is willing to expose herself and** her fetus to the risks of combination chemotherapy. After 24 weeks of gestation, premature delivery may be necessary, depending on the mother's medical condition.

Patients with localized disease should receive three to eight cycles of cyclophosphamide, doxorubicin, vincristine, and prednisolone (CHOP) chemotherapy and then, after delivery but within 9 weeks of the last dose of chemotherapy, involved field radiation therapy should be prescribed. Patients with advanced-stage disease should be treated with six to eight cycles of CHOP chemotherapy. **Because high-dose methotrexate is an integral component of most effective regimens for Burkitt lymphoma, therapeutic abortion for women diagnosed in the first trimester is essential.** Finally, for women with relapsing NHL associated with pregnancy, treatment should not be compromised because the disease is highly aggressive, and therapeutic abortion is generally advisable during the first half of pregnancy because the fetal effects of standard salvage chemotherapy regimens are unknown.

A special consideration can be made for pregnant patients with indolent or low-grade NHLs. These patients may be safely observed until delivery or significant disease progression, provided they are asymptomatic, have a relatively normal complete blood count, and show no impending organ compromise. Such a profile has not yet been reported for NHL associated with pregnancy.

Ward and Weiss reviewed the cases of 42 patients with NHL during pregnancy. Twenty-four of the cases were reported from 1976 to 1985. Three first-trimester cases resulted in two surviving infants. Twenty-one second- and third-trimester cases resulted in 15 surviving infants. Whereas infants who were born to mothers who were untreated or treated with surgery had a 38% prenatal mortality rate, 87.5% of infants of mothers treated with chemotherapy survived. Eight of the 21 second- and third-trimester patients received single-agent or combination chemotherapy. Four of these patients survived. Spitzer and coworkers reported that radiotherapy treatments given to six women in the second or third trimester of pregnancy resulted in no harm to the fetus, yet four of the mothers died of their disease. Of the four cases with a successful delivery and maternal survival, two were treated with combination chemotherapy, one with chemotherapy and radiotherapy, and one with radiotherapy alone. High-grade lymphomas have a particularly poor outcome. In the review by Ward and Weiss, none of the patients diagnosed with Burkitt lymphoma during pregnancy ($n = 18$) survived; however, only five of the patients were treated with chemotherapy. Only five cases ended with fetal survival. The most important factor influencing the well-being of the fetus is the health of the mother.

Seventy-five cases of pregnant women receiving systemic therapy for NHL have appeared in the literature. The majority of patients have had diffuse large B-cell lymphomas, and the CHOP regimen is the most widely used. Most patients have been treated after the first trimester, although at least four were exposed to CHOP unintentionally during the first trimester. All patients have had a normal course and outcome of pregnancy with no fetal mortality or congenital anomalies encountered. It appears that CHOP is a safe regimen in pregnancy. The combination of CHOP plus bleomycin has also been used safely during pregnancy.

For patients with indolent and aggressive NHL, rituximab (an anti-CD20 mAb) has been shown to improve outcomes. There have been seven patients exposed to rituximab during pregnancy, six in combination with chemotherapy. One patient was exposed to rituximab during the first trimester, and the remaining six had the drug initiated during the second trimester. Five patients had normal pregnancy outcomes, including the patient who had first-trimester exposure. There was one case of postnatal B-cell depletion and one case of transient pulmonary insufficiency secondary to prematurity, which resolved after 46 days.

In summary, if the hematologic malignant disease is early stage or low grade, treatment can be deferred, or nontoxic therapy can be used. However, many NHLs present with dissemination or aggressive histologic features, for which the most effective therapy is chemotherapy. The pregnant patient deserves the most effective chemotherapeutic regimen despite its teratogenic potential.

OTHER TUMORS IN PREGNANCY

Melanoma

Melanoma accounts for 1 of every 50 cancer-related deaths in the United States. **The incidence is rising, with approximately 10,000 cases occurring annually among women aged 20 to 40 years.** Congenital nevi may be found within the first 6 months of life and have the highest chance of all nevi for malignant degeneration. Congenital melanocytic nevi may be found in up to 2% of newborns, and giant congenital nevi may cover large areas of the body. Nevi arising later in life are known as the common mole or acquired melanocytic nevi.

The common mole represents more than 95% of nevi and may be subdivided into junctional nevi, compound nevi, and dermal nevi. The blue nevus is another type that usually appears on the dorsal aspects of the extremities and has a very low tendency to become malignant. Nevertheless, any nevi, whether congenital, acquired, or blue, that undergoes suspicious changes should be biopsied. The "ABCD" warning signs that herald changes in nevi that are associated with melanoma are asymmetry, irregular borders, color changes, and moles that increase in diameter. All melanomas masquerade as nevi before diagnosis. The average individual has 15 to 20 nevi, and removal of all these lesions prophylactically is hardly practical. Lesions on the feet, palms, genitals, and areas of persistent irritation from clothing are potentially dangerous nevi and should be removed during childhood.

There are five main types of melanoma, the most common of which is the superficial spreading melanoma, which accounts for 70% to 75% and tends toward horizontal growth before becoming invasive. Approximately 15% of melanomas are nodular and become invasive early. In sun-damaged areas, a lentigo maligna may develop, and in darker-skinned persons, the acral-lentiginous melanoma can be found on the palms and

Level	Clark et al.	Breslow et al.
I	All tumor cells above basement membrane (in situ)	<0.75-mm depth of invasion
II	Tumor extends to papillary dermis	0.76- to 1.5-mm depth of invasion
III	Tumor extends to interface between papillary and reticular dermis	1.51- to 2.25-mm depth of invasion
IV	Tumor extends between bundles of collagen of reticular dermis	2.26- to 3.0-mm depth of invasion
V	Tumor invasion of subcutaneous tissue	>3-mm depth of invasion

TABLE 15.22 Microstaging Systems for Melanoma

From Tewari KS. Cancer of the vulva. In Manetta A, ed. *Cancer Prevention and Early Diagnosis in Women.* Philadelphia, 2004, Mosby.

soles. Finally, the least common are the amelanotic melanomas, which are difficult to diagnose.

Staging of Melanoma

Reference may be made to the final version of the AJCC staging system for cutaneous melanoma that was published in 2001. Both depth of penetration of the lesion and the extent to which the lesion has involved local and regional tissues are brought into the staging system. This new system is a blend of the Clark and Breslow microstaging classifications (Table 15.22). **The Clark microstaging classification provides a histologic staging scheme for classifying melanomas on the basis of level of penetration of the melanoma under the epidermis and dermis.** Prognosis for the patient relates well to this microstaging system. Data indicate that a Clark level I melanoma should be viewed as an in situ lesion requiring no lymph node dissection. Clark's level II indicates superficial dermal penetration, with lymph node metastases in 1% to 5% of patients not justifying an elective lymph node dissection. At the other end of this pathologic spectrum are melanomas of Clark's level IV and level V, which metastasize to regional lymph nodes in approximately 40% and 70% of patients, respectively, necessitating lymphadenectomy as part of initial therapy.

An alternative classification suggested by Breslow (see Fig. 8.28) and used by some clinicians is a simple micrometer measurement of lesion thickness. Lesions larger than 4 mm have a high incidence of distant metastasis. Lesions 1.5 to 4 mm have a 57% incidence of regional node involvement and 15% incidence of distant metastasis. Lesions between 0.76 and 1.5 mm have a 25% incidence of regional node involvement and an 8% incidence of distant metastasis. Lesions 0.75 mm or less are usually not associated with any spread.

Melanoma in Pregnancy

It is rare that pregnancy adversely affects a malignant process, but for many years, melanoma was placed in this category. The average age of patients with melanoma is 45 years, and 35% of women will be diagnosed during childbearing years. This is suggested by many case reports in which pregnancy has been

incriminated in the induction or exacerbation of a melanoma. Partial or complete regressions of melanoma after delivery have been reported. In contrast, Stewart describes a case in which a tumor recurred three times; each recurrence was a few weeks after the patient delivered a child. Female patients have improved survival compared with male control participants matched for age and tumor thickness. This suggests that some hormonally based mechanisms are operational in the biologic behavior of melanoma. Contemporary studies fail to substantiate any effect previously attributed to pregnancy.

After the second month of pregnancy, the pituitary gland increases production of melanocyte-stimulating hormone. Melanocyte-stimulating hormone activity is also increased by the pregnancy-associated increase in adrenocorticotropic hormone. This results in the increased pigmentation that is characteristic of pregnancy and often found in the nipples, vulva, linea nigra, and preexisting nevi. In animal studies, the high circulating levels of estrogens in pregnancy have been shown to control melanocyte activity. These observations have led some to believe that pregnancy can have an inciting influence or a deleterious impact on the course of melanoma and have given rise to several myths about this disease in relationship to pregnancy, including the following:

1. Pregnancy increases the risk of developing malignant melanoma.
2. Pregnancy worsens the prognosis.
3. Future pregnancies have an adverse effect both on prognosis and on recurrence.
4. Oral contraceptives and hormone replacement therapy are contraindicated in women with a history of melanoma because of theoretic stimulatory effects of hormones on melanocytes.

None of these claims are substantiated by the medical literature.

Historical Series of Melanoma in Pregnancy

The original report published by Pack and Scharnagel in 1951 contained 1050 patients with melanoma. Ten of these patients were pregnant, five of whom died within 3 years of diagnosis. Later authors would cite these observations, which suggested that melanomas in pregnancy grow with unusual rapidity and metastasize widely. Subsequently, many series have challenged the findings of Pack and Scharnagel.

In 1960, George and coworkers gave a comprehensive report of 115 patients with melanoma in pregnancy compared with 330 control participants from the same institution. In disagreement with an earlier report from their institution, they found that spread to regional nodes appeared to be more rapid in pregnant patients but that there was no significant difference stage for stage in the outcome for the patient. This was directly contradictory to the earlier philosophy popularized by Pack and Scharnagel that melanoma is indeed aggravated by the pregnant state.

In 1961, White and coworkers reported a study of 71 young women (aged 15–39 years), 30 of whom had melanoma during pregnancy. The 5-year survival rate in the pregnant group was 73%, and for the 41 nonpregnant patients, the survival rate was

54%. They concluded that on the basis of the 5-year survival rates in pregnant and nonpregnant women with age and stage of disease taken into account, survival was equal in the two groups. No deleterious effect of pregnancy on survival of women with melanoma was demonstrated in this series.

Reintgen and colleagues described 58 women who were pregnant when the disease was diagnosed and another 43 patients who became pregnant within 5 years of diagnosis. Control groups were extracted from a total of 1424 women who were registered at the Duke University Melanoma Clinic. The mean age of patients in the series was 28 years. Both actuarial disease-free intervals and survivals were calculated for the study populations and their respective control groups. There was no statistical difference in survival between patients who had mole changes and diagnosis of melanomas during pregnancy and the control population. The results of the study also indicated no difference in survival for women who became pregnant within 5 years of diagnosis.

Despite these equivalency studies, many authorities continue to recommend survivors of melanoma to avoid pregnancy for approximately 3 years after complete surgical excision because this is the period of highest risk of relapse. Obviously, each case must be individualized, and the recommendation should be heavily influenced by the size, depth of invasion, and any detected dissemination. The role of previous pregnancy as a protective factor in melanomas has been suggested by some but also remains controversial. Patients surviving disease free for 5 years have a 95% chance of long-term cure. Conversely, after a woman has had a diagnosis of having a cutaneous melanoma, subsequent pregnancy has no effect on recurrence rates or survival.

Contemporary Studies of Melanoma in Pregnancy

Contemporary studies also note no survival difference in patients with melanoma who are pregnant compared with nonpregnant patients. MacKie and associates evaluated 388 women with stage I melanoma divided into four groups: 85 treated before pregnancy, 92 treated while pregnant, 143 treated after completion of all pregnancies, and 68 treated between pregnancies. Of interest, poor prognostic factors (eg, tumor thickness and tumor occurring at a poor prognostic site, such as the head, neck, and trunk) occurred more frequently in pregnant patients than in nonpregnant patients. However, in multivariate analysis, pregnancy status was not significantly related to prognosis.

In 1998, Grin and colleagues critically reviewed controlled clinical trials to assess the effect of pregnancy on the prognosis of melanoma and examined the available epidemiologic data to evaluate the risk of melanoma after exposure to oral contraceptives and hormone replacement therapy. The investigators concluded that pregnancy before, during, or after the diagnosis of melanoma did not influence 5-year survival rates, and exposure to oral contraceptives and hormone replacement therapy did not appear to increase the risk of melanoma.

In a recent paper retrospectively evaluating a cohort of 185 women diagnosed with melanoma during pregnancy and 5348 women of the same childbearing age with melanoma not

TABLE 15.23   Multivariable Cox Regression Analysis for the 2101 Women With Melanoma With Known Breslow Thickness, Clark's Level, and Tumor Site

Variable	Hazard Ratio	95% Confidence Interval	P
Pregnancy at the time of diagnosis of primary melanoma*	1.08	0.60–1.93	0.804
Breslow thickness (per additional category)	2.16	1.80–2.58	<0.0001
Axial site vs. limb site of primary melanoma	2.51	1.78–3.56	<0.0001
Clark's level (>3 vs. <3)	1.39	0.92–2.14	0.12
Age (per year increase)	1.02	0.99–1.05	0.06

*Pregnant women at the time of diagnosis of melanoma ($n = 185$) vs. nonpregnant women at the time of diagnosis of melanoma ($n = 5348$).
From Lens MB, Rosdahl I, Ahlbom A, et al. Effect of pregnancy on survival in women with cutaneous malignant melanoma. *J Clin Oncol* 2004;22:4369.

associated with pregnancy, Lens and colleagues noted no statistically significant difference in overall survival between pregnant and nonpregnant groups (Table 15.23). Women with higher Breslow tumor thickness categories had a significantly higher risk of death than those with lower Breslow categories. Also, women with axial tumors (ie, head and neck, trunk) had a poorer prognosis than those with tumors localized on the extremities. Neither pregnancy status at the time of diagnosis of melanoma nor pregnancy status after the diagnosis of melanoma was a significant predictor of survival.

The cumulative retrospective case-controlled studies have involved more than 450 pregnant women with melanoma. The anatomic location of the primary tumor does not differ between pregnant and nonpregnant women, and no analysis identified any differences in survival from nonpregnant women. **Multivariate analyses have been performed and have revealed that the stage of disease at diagnosis, and not the pregnancy,** is the only consistent finding that influences prognosis. Thus, we conclude that pregnancy does not confer a worse prognosis for this diagnosis when matched for stage of disease.

Management of Melanoma in Pregnancy

It is essential that all physicians and midwives conduct a full examination of the skin of their patients. **A changing skin lesion should be subjected to an excisional biopsy. Early diagnosis of stage I disease often leads to curative therapy. Irrespective of pregnancy, treatment of melanoma is related to depth and stage. Lesions smaller than 1 mm in thickness usually require a wide, deep local excision with a 1-cm margin, and those between 1 mm and 4 mm need a 2-cm margin of excision.** Whereas a wide excision is curative for stage I lesions, the role of IFN-α for stage II and stage III disease is currently under investigation. Although the use of IFN-α in pregnancy has been reported for the management of chronic leukemia, there has been no published experience using this drug for melanoma in pregnancy.

A changing skin lesion should be subjected to excisional biopsy. Early diagnosis of stage I disease often leads to curative therapy. Irrespective of pregnancy, treatment of melanoma is related to depth of invasion and stage. Lesions less than 1 mm in thickness usually require a wide, deep excision with a 1-cm margin, and those between 1 mm and 4 mm need a 2-cm margin. Wide, deep local excision can be performed safely before 30 weeks of gestation, and for those beyond 30 weeks of gestation SLN identification can be offered after delivery.

Melanomas constitute nearly 50% of all tumors that metastasize to the placenta and account for nearly 90% of those that metastasize to the fetus. Although there have been no reported adverse fetal effects associated with IFN therapy for melanoma during the second trimester, experience with this drug in pregnancy is limited. Pregnant women with advanced or recurrent disease should undergo ultrasound examination during pregnancy for assessment of any obvious fetal tumor masses. Attention should be directed to placental thickness, the fetal liver, and the size of the fetal spleen.

Contemporary studies note no survival difference in patients with melanoma who are pregnant compared with nonpregnant patients. Multivariate analyses demonstrated that the stage of diseased at diagnosis, and not the pregnancy, is the only consistent finding that influences prognosis. In a recent series by Pages and colleagues, 22 patients were included: 10 with AJCC stage III and 12 with AJCC stage IV melanoma. Three patients elected to withhold therapy during pregnancy, 14 underwent surgery, four received chemotherapy, and one was treated with brain radiotherapy. The median gestational age was 36 weeks. Neither neonatal metastases nor deformities were observed, although placental metastases were found in one case. Among 18 newborns, 17 are currently alive at a median follow-up at 17 months; one experienced sudden infant death. The 2-year maternal survival rates were 56% for stage III and 17% for stage IV.

Pregnancy does not confer a worse prognosis for melanoma when matched for stage of disease. At delivery, cord blood should be examined for malignant cells, and the placental tissue should be sent for detailed pathologic evaluation.

The value of regional lymphadenectomy in clinically negative nodes has been controversial. The debate has been defused to some degree with the development of lymphatic mapping to identify the SLN. Pathologic evaluation of the SLN is predictive of regional lymph node metastasis in 96% to 98% of cases. Thus SLN identification and evaluation are indicated for lesions penetrating beyond 1 mm. Lloyd and colleagues emphasize that data regarding the effect of radioactive colloid on the fetus are insufficient to permit its use in pregnant women. The dose to the patient from lymphoscintigraphy is 0.4 mSv, with a dose to the uterus of 0.5 mGy. Most of the injected radioactivity stays at the injection site or moves to the SLNs, which are resected the following day during surgery. Despite the small amounts of injected activity, the local dose rate at the injection site is high, and injection sites close to the fetus (over the lower abdomen or back) combined with next-day rather than same-day resection may result in greater doses to the fetus at any stage of the pregnancy.

It is the author's practice to perform a wide, deep local excision only in women at less than 30 weeks of gestation; for those beyond 30 weeks of gestation, we offer SLN identification after delivery. Because small quantities of radioactivity can be excreted into the breast milk, breastfeeding is contraindicated if SLN identification is performed postpartum.

Melanoma Metastatic to the Products of Conception

The reported low incidence of metastasis of malignant neoplasms to products of conception is probably caused by several factors. One factor is the unexplained resistance of the placenta to invasion by maternal cancer, as demonstrated in many animal studies. Metastasis of maternal cancer to products of conception is rare despite the sizable number of pregnancies at risk. However, although melanoma accounts for only a small number of all cancers associated with pregnancy, almost half of all tumors metastasizing to the placenta and nearly 90% metastasizing to the fetus are melanomas.

A few cases of transplacental transmission of melanomas with subsequent death of the fetus or newborn child from disseminated melanoma have been described, but this situation is extremely rare and occurs only when the mother has widespread bloodborne metastatic disease during pregnancy. Schneiderman and colleagues reported a case of a primary fetal melanoma fatal to a newborn. Microscopic metastases were present in the lungs and liver, and the placenta showed widespread metastases to the chorionic villi but no evidence of invasion of the intervillous spaces. The mother had no evidence of disease 1 year after delivery. To date, no instances of metastasis from fetus to mother have been documented. Moller and associates reported a case of maternal melanoma with metastasis to the placental intervillous sinuses. Tumor cells were also present in the fetal cord blood. The mother died postpartum, and the infant survived. Cord blood should be examined for malignant cells, and placental tissue should be carefully inspected. A further discussion on the predilection of melanoma to metastasize to placentas and fetuses is presented in a separate section of this chapter.

Thyroid Cancer

Papillary, follicular, and anaplastic carcinomas are the most common primary thyroid malignant neoplasms, with medullary carcinoma accounting for only 5%. The disease usually manifests as a relatively asymptomatic nodular mass in the thyroid gland. The lesion is multifocal, as seen on careful sectioning in approximately 30% to 40% of patients, but in only 5% do these become clinically evident if thyroid tissue remains after surgery. Laboratory indices of thyroid function are contributory only if they indicate a hyperthyroid state, thus supporting the diagnosis of a toxic adenoma. Although studies show that these tumors involve regional lymphatics microscopically in 50% to 70% of patients, this subclinical involvement does not affect the prognosis. The growth of papillary carcinoma may depend on thyroid-stimulating hormone (TSH); therefore, thyroid hormone administration to suppress TSH is used routinely as an adjuvant in all patients. The prognosis for patients who have this cancer is favorable, especially in the younger age group. Specifically, in women younger than 49 years, a 90% to 95% survival rate at 15 years is consistently reported.

Papillary and follicular thyroid carcinomas are two to three times more common in women than in men (5.5 vs. 2.4 per 100,000, respectively). This female predominance is especially notable during the reproductive years, such that the diagnosis of thyroid carcinoma in pregnancy does occur. **In fact, approximately 10% of differentiated thyroid carcinomas in women of reproductive age are diagnosed during pregnancy or within the first year after delivery.** The actual incidence of thyroid cancer in pregnancy has not been established.

During pregnancy, nonpathologic enlargement of the thyroid gland to twice its normal size is common. Histologic examination shows this enlargement to be caused by an apparent hyperplasia of the follicular cells and abundant colloid formation. A mild suppression of TSH and slight elevation of free thyroxine is common in early pregnancy as a result of the stimulation of the TSH receptor by hCG. A rise in thyroxine-binding globulin during pregnancy results in elevated levels of total thyroid hormone.

Thyroid Cancer in Pregnancy

Because papillary carcinomas are the most common lesions to occur in the reproductive age group, a solitary nodule in an otherwise normal gland is the most common presentation of thyroid carcinoma in pregnancy. Sam and Molitch noted that the incidence of thyroid nodules during pregnancy may be increased, with some data suggesting a higher incidence of malignancy in these nodules. In a 1986 series of 30 pregnant women with thyroid nodules, Rosen and Walfish observed a 43% incidence of malignancy. In 1995, Doherty and colleagues reported the incidence of malignancy to be 39% among 23 women with pregnancy-associated thyroid nodules. In contrast, the incidence of malignancy of thyroid nodules in the nonpregnant population ranges from 8% to 17%. hCG may stimulate the growth of thyroid nodules by cross-reacting with the thyrotropin-stimulating hormone receptor.

Thyroid function tests and a FNA should be performed in pregnant patients with newly discovered thyroid nodules. The latter procedure is especially important when the nodule is larger than 2 cm in size. If the results of cytologic examination are benign, a course of thyroid suppression using 0.2 mg of L-thyroxine daily is indicated for the duration of the pregnancy. Repeated cytologic evaluation may be necessary if the nodule does not diminish on suppression or if it enlarges during pregnancy because 6% of needle aspirations give a false-negative result. The theoretic risk of two false-negative diagnoses is about 0.05%, thus providing excellent confirmation of a conservative approach if the aspirate is repeatedly negative.

If the FNA reveals a papillary or follicular carcinoma, the author advises patients to undergo surgery in the second trimester (Fig. 15.17). If the carcinoma has been discovered in the third trimester, the workup and treatment can be delayed until after delivery. Rapidly growing tumors and medullary carcinomas should be removed on discovery regardless of gestational age. Short treatment delays to permit gestational advancement may be acceptable for some patients with medullary carcinomas, but as soon as fetal maturity can be demonstrated, labor should be induced or a cesarean section should be performed. Surgery is the only known effective therapy for medullary carcinomas and results in a 50% survival rate at 5 years. A prophylactic lymph node dissection on the site of the lesion is indicated. Fetal loss associated with surgery has been reported only with extensive neck exploration. **After tumor resection, suppressive doses of thyroid hormone should be administered, keeping in mind that thyroid hormone requirements may be higher in pregnancy.**

Radioactive iodine is contraindicated during pregnancy and lactation. Even though trace doses are used in these uptake studies, there is still a theoretic risk of a destructive effect on the fetal thyroid and a concern for teratogenesis within the fetus. A whole-body[131] I can be performed 3 months after discontinuation of lactation, and if necessary,[131] I ablation is recommended.

Undifferentiated Lesions

In the uncommon situation of an anaplastic carcinoma of the thyroid, the main concern is to keep the pregnant woman alive until the pregnancy has come to term because these tumors are almost uniformly lethal lesions. Between 90% and 95% of patients are dead within 1 year of diagnosis. The standard treatment in these patients is radical thyroidectomy followed by radiation therapy. This obviously presents a difficult situation for the patient in the first or second trimester, and one must carefully discuss the situation with the patient and the family. Treatment of pregnant patients who have progressive, local, unresectable, or metastatic thyroid carcinoma has to be individualized and tailored to the wishes of the patient. Surgical removal of these poorly differentiated lesions will achieve the best local control. The role of radiation therapy and chemotherapy remains investigational.

Prognosis Among Pregnant Women With Thyroid Cancer

Pregnancy does not negatively influence the prognosis of patients with well-differentiated thyroid carcinoma. For example, Moosa and Mazzaferri found no difference in the outcome between 61 pregnant women with thyroid cancer and a group of age-matched, nonpregnant control participants. In addition, pregnancy has not been shown to increase the recurrence rate of women previously treated for thyroid cancer. Hill and coworkers described 70 women who conceived after the diagnosis of thyroid cancer and compared them with 109 women who remained childless. There was no difference in the overall recurrence rate. The authors concluded that subsequent pregnancy did not alter the course of the disease. Rosvoll and Winship reviewed the cases of 60 women treated for thyroid carcinoma who subsequently became pregnant and concluded that a history of thyroid cancer is not an indication for avoidance of pregnancy or for therapeutic abortion. Friedman suggested that pregnancy was not contraindicated if the disease-free interval was at least 3 to 5 years. However, even in patients who

Thyroid nodule

Thyroid function tests

Ultrasound

Cystic   Solid

Fine-needle   Core biopsy
aspiration

Benign ←——————→ **Malignant** ←——————→ Benign

Thyroid suppression   Thyroid suppression

Increase size or   Increase size or
no change   no change

Anaplastic carcinoma   **Medullary carcinoma**   **Papillary or follicular
                                                                  carcinoma**

- Diagnosis <20 weeks: - Radical thyroidectomy with   - 1st or 2nd trimester diagnosis:
  consider immediate therapy   ipsilateral lymphadenectomy   2nd trimester thyroidectomy
- Diagnosis >20 weeks: - Early 2nd trimester diagnosis: - 3rd trimester diagnosis:
  consider induction of   short treatment delay to   workup and surgery after
  delivery at viability followed achieve viability acceptable   delivery
  by immediate therapy   - Late 2nd to early 3rd trimester
                                  diagnosis: corticosteroids,
                                  amniocentesis, delivery 32–34
                                  weeks followed by surgery

FIGURE 15.17 Management algorithm for the thyroid nodule and thyroid cancer in pregnancy.

had residual or recurrent disease, the prognosis did not appear to be altered by the pregnancy.

Thyroid cancer is among the fastest-rising types of cancer among women in North America. In 2010, Holt summarized the Endocrine Society Guidelines for the management of thyroid dysfunction during pregnancy and postpartum. With respect to thyroid nodules or thyroid cancer, the guidelines stipulate the following:

1. Thyroid nodules measuring 1 cm or larger should be evaluated by FNA biopsy.
2. Individuals with nodules that are malignant or show rapid growth should be offered surgery in the second trimester of pregnancy.
3. It may be appropriate for patients with follicular neoplasia or early-stage papillary thyroid cancers to wait until postpartum for thyroidectomy because these lesions are not expected to progress rapidly and the risk of surgery may outweigh the benefits of immediate intervention.
4. Patients with known thyroid cancer should maintain a low but measurable TSH and normal thyroxine (T_4) values on levothyroxine while pregnant.
5. RAI (radioactive iodine) therapy should not be provided to women who are breastfeeding.
6. After RAI therapy, women should wait 6 to 12 months before becoming pregnant.

Recently, the risk of complications of thyroid and parathyroid surgery during pregnancy was evaluated in a retrospective,

US cross-sectional analysis of hospital discharge data from the Healthcare Utilization Project National Inpatient Sample (HCUP-NIS). A total of 201 pregnant and 31,155 age-matched nonpregnant women control participants who had undergone thyroid or parathyroid surgery were identified. Of the 201 pregnant women, 45.8% underwent surgery for thyroid cancer. Thyroidectomy during pregnancy was associated with a higher risk of complications from surgery for malignant (21% vs. 8%) or benign (27% vs. 14%) disease. After controlling for other risk factors associated with adverse outcomes, pregnant patients remained twice as likely to have surgical complications as their nonpregnant counterparts. Among the pregnant patients who had thyroid or parathyroid surgery, 5.5% had fetal complications (eg, fetal distress, abortion), and 4.5% had maternal complications (cesarean section, hysterectomy).

Rare Gynecologic Malignancies in Pregnancy
Vulvar Cancer

Fewer than 50 cases of invasive cancer of the vulva associated with pregnancy have been reported in the literature. Lutz and colleagues estimated an incidence of 1 case per 8000 deliveries at his institution; our experience has been less frequent, at about 1 per 20,000 deliveries. The most common of these are invasive epidermoid carcinomas followed by melanomas, sarcomas, and adenoid cystic adenocarcinomas. In recent years, reports of pregnancies complicated by recurrent vulvar carcinoma, metastatic vulvar melanoma, a rapidly enlarging myxoid leiomyosarcoma of the vulva, and primary choriocarcinoma of the vulva have also appeared. The majority of patients have been between 25 and 35 years of age; the youngest patient was 17 years old. **With the increasing frequency of the diagnosis of CIS of the vulva, the occurrence of preinvasive disease with pregnancy is common today.** As is the practice with CIN, therapy for the vulvar counterpart is delayed until the postpartum period. Adequate biopsies of the most suspicious areas are essential to rule out invasive disease. The presence of intraepithelial neoplasia should not prohibit vaginal delivery but should prompt a careful colposcopic evaluation of the lower genital tract to exclude other preinvasive or invasive foci.

Historical series of vulvar cancer in pregnancy. Gitsch and colleagues presented a concise review of therapy and outcome for this group of patients, correctly noting that the reports have been inhomogeneous. In a review of the literature, Barclay found 31 women with vulvar cancers associated with pregnancy. The vulvar cancers were actually diagnosed and treated during pregnancy in only 12 of these women; another two were treated after termination of pregnancy. In 1974, Barclay furnished further details on nine patients, one of whom was treated with radiation therapy during pregnancy. Five patients were treated surgically before delivery, and three women underwent vulvectomy in the postpartum period. With extended follow-up, none of the patients experienced recurrent disease, although one woman developed a cervical carcinoma that was irradiated. Lutz and colleagues reported three cases diagnosed during pregnancy but treated postpartum. Although no one survived, details concerning the stage, treatment, and survival time were not provided.

Management of vulvar cancer in pregnancy. **Invasive vulvar malignant disease diagnosed during the first, second, and early third trimesters is usually treated as indicated in nonpregnant patients some time after the 18th week of pregnancy.** T1 lesions should be managed by radical wide excision with ipsilateral groin dissection if the depth of invasion is larger than 1 mm. Larger and more deeply invasive tumors require a radical vulvectomy and bilateral inguinofemoral lymphadenectomy. Patients with palpable inguinofemoral nodes undergoing surgery early in pregnancy present a unique challenge because skin bridge metastases are more likely to occur in patients with bulky positive nodes. Such patients are advised to have the groin dissected using an en bloc approach because of the need to delay radiation therapy for many months. When the diagnosis is made after 36 weeks of gestation, we recommend a wide local excision with definitive surgery postponed until the postpartum period. This avoids the greatly enhanced vascularity in vulvar tissues during the later months of gestation and into the immediate postpartum period. A short delay does not appear to seriously prejudice the course of the disease. **Women treated during pregnancy may be allowed to attempt vaginal delivery provided the vulvar wounds are well healed and there are no indications for additional therapy.** Patients with high-risk surgicopathologic features warranting adjuvant radiation should undergo cesarean delivery as soon as fetal pulmonary maturation can be documented. After delivery of the baby, the ovaries should be transposed to the paracolic

gutters, and pelvic or groin irradiation (or both) can be administered postpartum.

Because this disease occurs more frequently in women of lower socioeconomic groups, who often do not seek prenatal care, many of these cases are diagnosed at the time of delivery or later. In this group of patients, definitive therapy should be started within 1 week after delivery during the same hospitalization. The pregnant state does not appear to significantly alter the course of the malignant process; survival of these patients stage for stage is similar to that of nonpregnant patients.

Bakour and colleagues have carefully considered the subject of future pregnancies in this group of patients and have found no contraindications after surveying the literature. In fact, they believe that these young patients who have undergone such extensive surgery obtain a great boost psychologically when they realize this possibility. There have been several reports of patients treated for carcinoma of the vulva with radical vulvectomy and bilateral inguinal lymphadenectomy who subsequently became pregnant and had normal deliveries. Whether the patient should deliver vaginally or by cesarean section is a decision that rests with the obstetrician, but it is heavily influenced by the state of the postsurgical vulva. In most instances, the vulva is soft and does not impede a vaginal delivery. In other instances, there may be a high degree of vaginal stenosis or other fibrosis, which makes cesarean section the more appropriate means of delivery.

Primary Invasive Vaginal Tumors

Cancer of the vagina has been found mainly in women older than 50 years. The diagnosis of vaginal cancer during pregnancy is exceptionally uncommon, even with the clear cell adenocarcinoma of the vagina alleged to be associated with the diethylstilbestrol-exposed offspring. Although all these clear cell adenocarcinomas have occurred in women younger than 34 years, the incidence in association with pregnancy has fortunately been rare.

Senekjian and colleagues described 24 women who were pregnant when clear cell adenocarcinoma of the vagina or cervix was diagnosed; 14 were in the first trimester, six in the second, and four in the third. Among the stage I and stage II tumors, 16 (73%) were vaginal, and six (27%) were cervical. Thirteen long-term survivors were reported among the 16 early vaginal lesions. No significant differences were observed when the group of 24 patients with pregnancy-associated tumors and 408 never-pregnant (age-corrected) patients were compared with regard to maternal hormone history, symptoms, stage, location, predominant histologic or cell type, greatest tumor diameter, surface area, depth of invasion, grade, and number of mitoses. The overall 5- and 10-year actuarial survival rates (86% and 68%, respectively) for the group pregnant at diagnosis did not differ significantly from the rates for the never-pregnant group analyzed concomitantly ($n = 408$). Pregnancy did not seem to adversely affect the outcome of clear cell adenocarcinoma of the vagina and cervix. Jones and colleagues reported a diethylstilbestrol-related clear cell carcinoma of the vagina in a patient whose tumor, observed directly over an extended period, did not appear to be influenced by elevated plasma estrogen levels during the period when the pregnancy was carried to term.

Primary SCC of the vagina discovered during pregnancy is exceedingly rare. In 1963, Collins and Barclay identified 10 patients from the literature and, although three responded well to radiation therapy, a rapidly progressive downhill course was described for four patients available for detailed analysis. In 1977, Lutz and colleagues reported a 24-year-old patient diagnosed at 24 weeks of gestation with a stage II SCC of the vagina, who despite immediate radiotherapy after preterm delivery, suffered a fatal recurrence 7 months later. Three additional cases have been reported by Palumbo and colleagues, Beck and Clayton, and Baruah and Sangupta, manifesting between 8 and 24 weeks of gestation and all resulting in maternal death within 18 months of diagnosis; in two of the cases, pregnancy termination had been performed so as to not delay radiotherapy.

Finally, Steed and colleagues reported a 28-year-old patient with antepartum bleeding at 20 weeks of gestation who was found to have a 6-cm diameter anterior vaginal wall SCC extending to the right lateral fornix. This patient opted to continue the pregnancy and received corticosteroids followed by cesarean delivery at 32 weeks of gestation. Before delivery, gold seeds were placed transvaginally to demarcate the tumor edges. Amazingly, although the patient was debulked of multiple, enlarged, positive pelvic lymph nodes, after treatment with chemoirradiation and brachytherapy, she had remained disease-free for 3 years at the time of publication. This report brings the total to 15 cases of primary invasive SCC of the vulva complicating pregnancy, with an overall survivorship rate of 38%, similar to what is observed in nonpregnant patients.

Both cervical cancer and vaginal cancer are staged clinically, and the management principles to be discussed in detail when cervical carcinoma complicates pregnancy also may be applied to vaginal tumors. Treatment of clear cell adenocarcinoma of the cervix and upper vagina is surgically similar to that of SCCs. Specifically, very early lesions involving the upper vagina may be treated by radical abdominal hysterectomy with pelvic lymphadenectomy, but all others are best managed radiotherapeutically. The pregnancy should be disregarded if the diagnosis is made in the first or early second trimester. If the pregnancy is further along, the decision for appropriate time of intervention depends on the preferences of the patient and the oncologist. Patients early in pregnancy who resist termination should be given corticosteroids and delivered as soon as fetal pulmonary maturation is demonstrable. The impact of a delay in therapy on the prognosis is impossible to predict. When there is extensive involvement of the vagina by any lesion, one should seriously consider evacuation of the uterus by a hysterotomy or cesarean section and institution of appropriate radiation therapy.

A few scattered reports of sarcoma botryoides of the cervix and vagina in pregnancy were recorded in the 1960s by Roddick and Honig and Schwartz and colleagues. When these sarcomatous lesions occur in the upper half of the vagina with or without cervical involvement, the most appropriate therapy has been a radical abdominal hysterectomy, upper vaginectomy,

and bilateral pelvic lymphadenectomy followed by postoperative adjuvant chemotherapy. In 2003, the first primary vaginal leiomyosarcoma diagnosed during pregnancy was reported by Behzatoglu and colleagues in a 21-year-old woman who presented during the third trimester with a 1.5-cm firm, fleshy, pedunculated mass arising from a short stalk on the right vaginal wall. Previously, female genital tract leiomyosarcomas that have been associated with pregnancy had originated from the uterus or vulva ($n = 10$). Finally, some malignancies have been reported in pregnancy to involve the vagina secondarily by direct extension (eg, tumors of the cervix), via lymphatic spread (eg, endometrial carcinoma), or through hematogenous dissemination (eg, gestational choriocarcinoma and placental site trophoblastic tumor). **In fact, secondary involvement from an extravaginal site is more common than the development of a primary vaginal neoplasm, irrespective of pregnancy.** Although pregnancy-associated vaginal cancer is rare, the entity must remain part of the differential diagnosis of bleeding in pregnancy. Steed and colleagues emphasize that visualization of the entire vagina and cervix is necessary during speculum examination, and the procedure should be performed in every pelvic examination and for all investigations carried out for antepartum bleeding.

Endometrial Cancer

Endometrial carcinoma in conjunction with pregnancy is extremely rare. Most of the reported cases have been diagnosed at examination of uterine contents obtained by curettage for elective pregnancy termination or spontaneous abortion. Leiomyosarcoma (including a myxoid leiomyosarcoma), endometrial stromal sarcoma, and carcinosarcoma have also been reported during pregnancy. They are usually incidental findings noted in surgical specimens. The recommended therapy for endometrioid adenocarcinomas associated with pregnancy is total hysterectomy with bilateral salpingo-oophorectomy and adjuvant radiotherapy when indicated.

In 1972, Karlen and associates reviewed the literature since 1900, summarized five acceptable cases, and added a sixth. In 2004, Itoh and colleagues collected a total of 29 patients (including one of their own), 11 of whom were older than 35 years. Twenty-one of the 29 cases had no or minimal myometrial invasion, 18 of which were histologically FIGO grade I, and three were FIGO grade II. This group includes a 28-year-old patient who received conservative treatment with high-dose medroxyprogesterone acetate after a uterine curettage that had revealed diffuse complex hyperplasia with atypia and a focus of well-differentiated adenocarcinoma showing stromal invasion. This patient subsequently conceived, and after delivery at term, she underwent a total abdominal hysterectomy. Pathologic examination of the uterus revealed a persistent well-differentiated endometrioid adenocarcinoma limited to the endometrium. This case serves to illustrate a very important point: **As more women opt for conservative management of invasive cancers in an effort to preserve fertility, we may anticipate a larger number of referrals than what was seen previously for patients with persistent or even recurrent malignancy during pregnancy.**

All 21 patients with favorable histopathologic features were alive at the time of their report, ranging from 3 months to 10 years after treatment. **Therefore, most cases of endometrial carcinoma associated with pregnancy are characterized by well-differentiated tumors, an endometrioid histology with no or minimal myometrial invasion, and favorable outcome, consistent with the typical clinicopathologic features of type I endometrial carcinoma that develops in obese women.** It has been hypothesized that the elevated serum progesterone level during pregnancy inhibits the growth of endometrial carcinoma cells, and this may contribute to the good outcomes observed among these 21 patients. This has prompted several authorities to argue that adenocarcinoma in pregnancy does not occur and that the reported cases were misdiagnosed Arias–Stella reactions.

However, the remaining eight of the 29 reported patients have had well-documented deep myometrial invasion or extrauterine extension. The FIGO grade distribution included grade I ($n = 3$), grade II ($n = 2$), and grade III ($n = 3$, including one serous papillary carcinoma), and the FIGO stage ranged from Ic to IV. Two of these eight patients died of disease, and it is notable that the patient submitted by Itoh and colleagues had deep myometrial invasion and negative expression of ER and PR. Of note, higher grade tumors or nonendometrioid adenocarcinomas are often negative for ER or PR expression, and this group of endometrial carcinomas associated with pregnancy is characterized by high-grade histology, including nonendometrioid type, deep myometrial invasion, advanced stage, and poor outcome consistent with the type II carcinoma manifesting in nonobese patients. Thus, not all endometrial carcinomas associated with pregnancy have a favorable prognosis.

Fallopian Tube Cancer

The fallopian tube can become secondarily involved by malignancy through direct extension of an ovarian tumor or from an endometrial carcinoma. Primary fallopian tube carcinoma was described by Starr and colleagues as a disease of recent vintage, having been first reported in 1847 by Raymond and later, in 1861, by Rokitansky. The disease is the least common gynecologic tumor. The mean age ranges from 50 to 55 years. Thus, the possibility of its presence in pregnancy is extremely remote. Cases have been reported to be associated with pregnancy; in these instances, the neoplasm is usually unilateral and most often adenocarcinoma.

The clinical presentation of carcinoma of the tube is variable and nonspecific even without an associated pregnancy. **The usual watery, blood-tinged vaginal discharge would be obviated in pregnancy because at 12 weeks of gestation, the communication between the uterine cavity and the fallopian tube is blocked.** In most instances, the diagnosis is established at laparotomy, and the treatment is total abdominal hysterectomy with bilateral salpingo-oophorectomy and postoperative radiotherapy or chemotherapy, depending on the operative findings and the residual disease after surgery. Several instances are reported in the literature of incidental findings of CIS of the tube noted in specimens submitted after postpartum tubal ligation. In these instances, a total abdominal hysterectomy with bilateral salpingo-oophorectomy has been recommended; however, simple removal of the fallopian tubes may be a reasonable alternative.

Adolph and colleagues reported the first case of a recurrent fallopian tube carcinoma associated with pregnancy in 2001. The patient originally underwent a limited surgical procedure to preserve fertility followed by chemotherapy and subsequently experienced an intraperitoneal recurrence 1 year later during her 16th week of pregnancy. After a cesarean section at term, she underwent optimal cytoreductive surgery and was alive with stable disease 6 months after salvage chemotherapy when the paper was published. This case is included with some detail to emphasize a point made earlier, in that as fertility-preserving oncologic procedures become more widely accepted for certain early-stage malignancies, the probabilities increase for having to manage recurrent disease in pregnancy. The criteria through which surgeons determine candidacy for fertility preservation must be carefully devised and rigorously adhered to.

Trophoblastic Tumors of the Fallopian Tube: "Ectopic" Pregnancy

Although choriocarcinoma most frequently arises in the uterus, a primary choriocarcinoma of the fallopian tube may be associated with ectopic pregnancy. In these scenarios, the biologic behavior is very aggressive, with distant metastases manifesting in 75% of cases. A review of the world literature of 93 reported cases by Ober and Maier in 1981 yielded 58 acceptable cases, to which the authors added 18 from the files of the Armed Forces Institute of Pathology. Since that time, there have been approximately 15 additional reports, bringing the total to 91 cases of primary choriocarcinoma of the fallopian tube. **The mean age is 33 years, with 66% of patients presenting with acute symptoms consistent with a ruptured ectopic pregnancy.** The remainder typically have presented with a gradually expanding adnexal mass clinically indistinguishable from an ovarian tumor. Endovaginal ultrasonography may offer an image compatible with an extrauterine pregnancy in the left appendages, and the quantitative serum β-hCG is elevated. Grossly, the tumor appears as a hemorrhagic friable mass, occasionally containing spongy tissue resembling the placenta. Smaller tubal choriocarcinomas are difficult to distinguish on gross inspection from the common ectopic pregnancy. Histopathologic features and the distribution of metastases are similar to gestational choriocarcinoma arising in the uterus.

The surgical approach has not been uniform, with some women undergoing unilateral salpingectomy only or unilateral adnexectomy or total abdominal hysterectomy with bilateral salpingo-oophorectomy. Most patients have gone on to receive polychemotherapy. In the review by Ober and Maier, it was noted that of 47 acceptable cases treated before modern chemotherapy, the mortality rate was 87% ($n = 41$). Of 16 cases treated with modern chemotherapy, the salvage rate was 94% ($n = 15$). Fewer than 10 patients have been cured by unilateral salpingectomy or unilateral salpingo-oophorectomy alone. Whenever possible, a histologic examination of the tubes should be performed in all cases of ectopic pregnancies. Serial measurements of the β-hCG is an essential component of the surveillance of all patients treated for ectopic pregnancy and especially for those treated with methotrexate or by salpingotomy alone.

Primary choriocarcinoma of the fallopian tube coexistent with a viable intrauterine pregnancy was first reported by Lee and colleagues in 2005, and a heterotopic pregnancy of a primary placental site trophoblastic tumor of the fallopian tube and an intrauterine pregnancy was first reported by Su and colleagues in 1999.

Placental and Fetal Tumors

The placenta may be the site of origin of gestational trophoblastic neoplasia (GTN) or can be secondarily involved by other malignancies. The disease spectrum of GTN encompasses molar pregnancies (eg, complete, partial, invasive), nonmetastatic GTN, gestational choriocarcinoma (ie, metastatic GTN), and placental site trophoblastic tumors. These entities are discussed in a separate chapter. The occurrence of gestational choriocarcinoma and placental site trophoblastic tumors in the fallopian tube has been addressed earlier in this chapter under the section concerning tumors of the fallopian tube in pregnancy. The following sections have as their focus the occurrence of a twin pregnancy complicated by a complete mole and a normal fetus, placental and fetal metastases, and primary fetal cancers that may manifest in utero.

Complete Hydatidiform Mole With Coexistent Fetus

Ultrasonography depicting the combination of a live fetus and a molar-appearing placenta suggests three distinct possibilities:
1. A singleton pregnancy consisting of a partial mole with a live fetus
2. A twin pregnancy comprising one placenta exhibiting a complete mole (no fetus) and the other placenta sustaining a normal twin
3. A twin pregnancy with a partial mole and fetus in one sac and a normal twin in the other sac

The first possibility involves a triploid fetus that usually dies during the first trimester. The third possibility is easily eliminated by the presence of two fetuses.

The incidence of complete hydatidiform mole with coexistent fetus (CMCF) ranges from 1 in 10,000 to 1 in 100,000 pregnancies. The true incidence is difficult to establish, and the observed increased incidence of iatrogenic multiple gestations in recent years is expected to result in a higher incidence of CMCF. Vaisbuch and colleagues have conducted a comprehensive review of the literature, and after exclusion of duplicate publications they have identified 130 cases, some of which include higher-order gestations (eg, triplets and quadruplets). Fifty-three elected to terminate. Thirty-three live births (25%) occurred. The calculated incidences of specific complications included 30% preeclampsia, 33% persistent GTN, and 22% metastatic GTN.

Steller and colleagues discovered eight well-documented cases of twin pregnancy with CMCF. They compared the clinical features of these eight patients with 71 women with singleton complete hydatidiform mole. **Although the presenting symptoms were similar in both groups, a twin pregnancy with**

CMCF was diagnosed at a later gestational age (20.1 weeks vs. 13 weeks), had higher preevacuation β-hCG levels, and had a greater propensity to develop persistent GTN (55% vs. 14%).

Bristow and colleagues reported 25 cases from the literature and one of their own, of whom 19 were evacuated before fetal viability and only seven resulted in a live-born infant. Although the previable and viable group were unremarkable with respect to mean age, gravidity, parity, uterine size, and presence of theca-lutein cysts, significant differences in gestational age at diagnosis (17.4 weeks vs. 29.4 weeks) and preevacuation serum hCG levels (>1,000,000 mIU/mL vs. 170,000 mIU/mL) were observed. In addition, previable cases were also associated with higher frequencies of preeclampsia (31.6% vs. 14.3%) and persistent GTN (68.4% vs. 28.6%). Clinical factors that required termination of the pregnancy might have been surrogates for aggressive trophoblastic growth and therefore persistent disease and the subsequent need for adjuvant systemic therapy. Bruchim and colleagues reported a 53.3% incidence of persistent GTN (including four patients with pulmonary metastasis) when they analyzed 15 cases of CMCF that had resulted in a live neonate delivered at a mean age of 34.3 weeks of gestation. Although CMCF is associated with a higher risk of persistent GTN compared with the risk attributable to a singleton complete hydatidiform mole, the issues regarding pregnancy termination are unclear. It does not appear that advanced gestational age is an independent risk factor for developing persistent GTN in the setting of a CMCF. **After fetal anomalies and an abnormal karyotype are excluded, with some degree of caution, the literature supports continuing the pregnancy provided there is no evidence of preeclampsia and the pregnant woman strongly wishes to do so.** A declination in serum levels of hCG may also be included in the criteria through which expectant management can be offered. Patients should be informed that only 25% of such pregnancies will result in a live birth and that there may be some serious consequences of premature delivery and prematurity.

The overall risk of developing persistent GTN ranges from 19% to 57% (Table 15.24), **irrespective of whether the**

TABLE 15.24   **Evolution to Gestational Trophoblastic Neoplasia After Twin Pregnancy With Complete Hydatidiform Mole and Coexistent Fetus**

Reference	Pregnancies (*n*)	Gestational Trophoblastic Neoplasia (%)
Steller et al., 1994	22	12 (55)
Fishman et al., 1998	7	4 (57)
Matsui et al., 2000	18	9 (50)
Sebire et al., 2002	77	15 (19)
Hancock et al., 2006	9	3 (33)
Niemann et al., 2007	8	2 (25)
Massardier et al., 2009	14	7 (50)

From Massardier J, Golfier F, Journet D, et al. Twin pregnancy with complete hydatidiform mole and coexistent fetus: obstetrical and oncological outcomes in a series of 14 cases. *Eur J Obstet Gynecol Reprod Biol* 2009;143:84.

pregnancy is terminated or carried to viability or term. Therefore, the major obstacles to continuing the pregnancy are the development of a paraneoplastic medical complication, catastrophic vaginal hemorrhage, and formation of metastatic foci antenatally. In the exceedingly rare situation in which metastatic GTN coexists with a normal gestation, intravenous systemic chemotherapy is necessary during pregnancy unless the disease is discovered when the baby is of advanced gestational age, in which case delivery followed by immediate systemic therapy might be an option.

Presenting symptoms of a complete hydatidiform mole with coexisting fetus are similar to those seen with complete hydatidiform moles alone (ie, size greater than dates, abnormal vaginal bleeding). A twin pregnancy with a complete hydatiform mole and coexisting fetus may be diagnosed later in gestational age (eg, 20 weeks vs. 13 weeks), have a higher preevacuation β-hCG level, and have a greater propensity to develop persistent GTN necessitating chemotherapy.

After fetal anomalies and an abnormal karyotype are excluded, the literature supports continuing the pregnancy provided there is no evidence of preeclampsia and the mother strongly wishes to do so. In cases of twin pregnancy with a complete hydatidiform mole and coexisting live fetus, continuation of pregnancy is acceptable with a normal fetal karyotype, no anomalies, no early preeclampsia, and declination of hCG levels (Table 15.25); the risk of persistent trophoblastic disease may rise to 57%. The overall risk of developing persistent GTN is 33% irrespective of whether the pregnancy is terminated or carried to viability or term. The major obstacles to continuing the pregnancy are the development of a paraneoplastic medical complication, catastrophic vaginal hemorrhage, and formation of metastatic foci antenatally.

A series of 14 cases were recently reported by Massardier and colleagues. In 10 cases (71%) the diagnosis was made by ultrasonography, with the differential diagnoses including partial hydatidiform mole and mesenchymal dysplasia. Eight patients elected to terminate their pregnancies, and six chose to continue. Of the latter, there were three intrauterine deaths or spontaneous abortions and three (21%) normal live births. Only one patient delivered after 37 weeks of gestational age. Seven patients (50%) were diagnosed with GTN, and none of the 14 had a fatal evolution. Of note, vaginal bleeding, preeclampsia, and hyperthyroidism did not have an impact on the risk of persistent GTN, nor did continuation of the pregnancy increase that risk.

TABLE 15.25 Recommendations for Continuation of Pregnancy in the Setting of a Twin Pregnancy With Complete Hydatidiform Mole and Coexisting Fetus

Normal fetal karyotype
No anomalies
No early preeclampsia
No observance of decrease in levels of human chorionic gonadotropin

Placental and Fetal Metastases

Patients diagnosed with cancer in pregnancy commonly ask whether the disease can spread to their children. Although cancer during pregnancy is not uncommon, metastases to the placental tissue or the fetus rarely occur. Most malignancies, when matched stage for stage, portend the same prognosis for the woman whether she is pregnant or not. Exceptions include hepatocellular cancer, lymphoma, thyroid cancer, colon cancer, and nasopharyngeal cancer. In addition to the primary cancer sites, metastatic disease to the products of conception predicts an ominous course for the mother. Metastatic lesions to the fetus or placenta remain a poorly understood subject.

The first report of metastases to the placenta or fetus appeared in 1866. In this case, Friedreich observed a mother with disseminated "hepatic" carcinoma that spread to and killed the fetus. There have been no other reports of "hepatic" metastases to the products of conception, and we suspect that Friedreich's patient had a melanoma, which is most likely to behave in this clinical manner. Indeed, melanoma is the most common cancer to metastasize to placentas and fetuses. Rothman and associates reported 35 cases of disseminated maternal malignant disease with either placental or fetal involvement. In only two instances was tumor demonstrated on both the maternal and fetal sides of the placenta and in the fetus. It is rare for the fetus to be involved if there is invasion only of the maternal side of the placenta. Of six cases in the literature when the villus itself was invaded, there was only one case of demonstrable fetal disease. In another report by Potter and Schoeneman, 24 cases of maternal cancer metastasizing to the fetus or placenta were reviewed. Melanoma, by far the most common tumor to spread to fetuses or placentas, was found in 11 cases. Breast cancer was found in four cases. Eight infants were found to have cancer at birth, and six of them subsequently died of their malignant neoplasms. Two infants with metastatic melanoma were noted to have complete tumor regression and ultimately survived. Seven of eight occurrences of metastasis to the fetus were found in cases of maternal melanoma, and there was one case of lymphosarcoma. Finally, Holland reported a case in which maternal, placental, and fetal disease was documented.

Since Friedreich's initial report, there have been fewer than 90 cases of maternal malignancy metastatic to the gestation (Table 15.26). Because of its generous blood flow, large surface area, and favorable biologic environment for growth, one would consider a placenta to be an ideal site for metastases, and therefore the relative paucity of such events remains unclear. Why have the products of conception been privileged in this way? Perhaps immunologic rejection of tumor cells, uteroplacental circulatory mechanisms, or even a protective role of the trophoblast limits the establishment of metastatic foci. Cancers that have been reported to metastasize to the intervillous space or to the placenta proper include sarcomas, carcinomas, lymphomas, leukemias, and melanomas. Of note, 30% of the cases are melanomas followed by breast cancer (18%) and then the hematopoietic malignancies (13%).

Nearly half of the reports contain cases of known malignancy diagnosed before the onset of pregnancy. Unfortunately, 93% of such women died of their disease, sometimes within hours

TABLE 15.26 Most Common Cancers in Pregnancy to Affect Placentas or Fetuses

Cancer Type	Cases Reporting Placental Involvement	Cases Reporting Only Fetal Metastasis	Cases Reporting Both Placental and Fetal Metastasis	Total Cases Affecting Placenta and/or Fetus	Percentage of Total Cases
All cancers	72	10	6	88	100
Melanoma	21	3	3	27	31
Breast	15	0	0	15	17
Lung	8	1	1	10	11
Leukemia	6	0	0	9	10
Lymphoma	3	2	2	7	8

From Alexander A, Samlowski WE, Grossman D, et al. Metastatic melanoma in pregnancy: risk of transplacental metastases in the infant. *J Clin Oncol* 2003;21:2179.

of delivery. Gestational reactivation of malignancy has been reported in women who had been disease free for 5 years before becoming pregnant. **Contrasting with the unfavorable prognosis for mothers with placental metastases, the prognosis for the infant has been excellent, with 53 of the reported cases revealing no evidence of disease in the baby.** In addition, since 1966, no infant has succumbed to metastatic disease, although several reports contained fetal demises as a consequence of complications of prematurity. More recently, the first case of maternal pulmonary adenocarcinoma metastatic to the fetus has been reported; the involved scalp was widely excised, and skin graft coverage was applied at 3 months of life. At the time of publication, the child was 5 years old and disease free.

Another unusual scenario is that of GTN metastatic to the fetus, with 15 to 20 cases reported to date. It is interesting that widely metastatic disease in the delivered neonate can occur in the absence of metastatic GTN in the mother. There are also reports of acute leukemia developing postnatally in the child of a mother with acute leukemia. In one report by Cramblett and associates, the child developed acute leukemia 9 months after delivery; in another report by Bernard, disease manifestation occurred 5 months after delivery. Transplacental transmission of maternal B-cell lymphoma was reported by Maruko and colleagues when a 29-year-old mother developed the disease at 29 weeks and her infant developed malignant lymphoma at 8 months of life. Hypotheses relating to familial, hereditary, environmental, and viral factors can be advanced in these circumstances, but the weight of evidence suggests that acquisition of maternal malignant disease by fetuses is extremely unlikely.

Guidelines for the evaluation of children born to women with cancer are sparse in the literature. **Tolar and Neglia recommend that any child born to a mother with active or suspected malignancy should initially have a thorough physical examination with a complete blood count, comprehensive metabolic panel, liver function tests, coagulation battery, serum LDH level, uric acid levels, and a urinalysis. In addition, the placenta should be macroscopically and microscopically examined for tumor involvement. It has been the author's practice to also obtain imaging studies, including an MRI of the brain and CT scans of the chest, abdomen, and pelvis, when maternal breast cancer, hematopoietic malignancy, or melanoma is at issue or in the setting of confirmed placental metastases.**

Continued surveillance should be ongoing during the first year of a child's life because some cases of maternal to fetal metastases have not presented until several months after birth. Because not all cases with documented placental involvement have corresponding fetal metastases, infants with an initially negative workup should not be prophylactically treated but should be closely observed with frequent physical examinations, laboratory tests, and imaging studies as clinically indicated.

Primary Fetal Tumors

Benign tumors such as teratomas or lymphangiomas may progress rapidly in utero, distorting the fetal anatomy and resulting in intrauterine fetal and obstetric complications and morbidity. In addition, several developmental tumors, including hamartomas and vaginal adenosis, are not malignant in utero but may undergo malignant degeneration after delivery. Benign and malignant tumors present diagnostic problems and therapeutic challenges. Both typically appear as heterogeneous masses with solid and cystic components when viewed by ultrasonography. The extent and tissue characteristics of these lesions may be further evaluated by MRI, and the diagnosis can occasionally be guided by a cytologic analysis of fluid aspirated from a cystic lesion. **Jauniaux and Ogle maintain that expectant management should be the rule in the initial phase, with serial ultrasound evaluations to detect rapid enlargement, metastasis, or secondary fetal complications such as nonimmune hydrops.**

The sacrococcygeal teratoma is a tumor arising from totipotential embryonic cells of the coccyx and has an incidence of 1 in 35,000 to 40,000 deliveries. There is a four to one female to male predominance, although the sex ratio in the incidence of malignant tumors is equal. With routine prenatal ultrasonography, these lesions are being diagnosed increasingly when views of the spine to rule out neural tube defects are obtained. The advent of antenatal ultrasonography has shifted the management focus from birth to the antenatal period, in which the fetal mortality rate ranges from 30% to 50%. The most common cause of perinatal loss is premature labor secondary to polyhydramnios, with one series reporting the combination of hydrops and placentomegaly as a very ominous sign with 100% mortality. On this basis, fetal surgery with tumor resection has been advocated in selected cases if the hydrops appears before 28 weeks and the tumor is deemed resectable. Because of the risk of dystocia and traumatic hemorrhage, cesarean section has been the rule for tumors larger than 5 cm. After birth, complete excision of the tumor should not be delayed, and those who survive surgery should have a favorable prognosis. Residual tumor, however, may lead to malignant change, and although the recurrence risk is extremely low, isolated cases have been reported.

Congenital neuroblastoma is a cancer of neuronal lineage that may occur along the sites of the sympathetic ganglia from the neck to the presacral region, including the adrenal medulla. They typically contain Schwann cells and are the most common malignant tumor of newborns, representing 30% to 40% of all congenital tumors. The genetic defect is characterized by the loss of locus p36 on chromosome 1. The clinical features are a function of the size, location, and humoral activity of the neuroblastoma, with catecholamine or vasoactive intestinal polypeptide characterizing their biologic behavior. Fetal neuroblastomas are well encapsulated and may displace the kidney inferiorly and laterally, with a predilection for the right side. The presence of calcification by ultrasonography has been associated with improved survival. Of note, neuroblastoma cells may infiltrate the placenta beyond the fetal capillaries and villous trophoblast, with metastasis to maternal tissue. Postpartum symptoms attributable to catecholamine production may be observed in the mother and include sweating, flushing, palpitations, and hypertension.

Concordance for neuroblastoma in monozygotic twins has been rarely reported, with the cause for the shared pathology unestablished. In 2001, Anderson and colleagues described a case of infant monozygotic twins developing neuroblastomas that were morphologically, clinically, and molecularly indistinguishable but with a delay of 6 months between times of presentation. Both tumors had metastasized and had amplification of MYCN and deletion at 1p36. The twin who developed neuroblastoma first had constitutional karyotype abnormalities in at least 5% of peripheral blood mononuclear cells. The second twin had a normal constitutional karyotype and lacked rearrangements or deletions. The authors proposed an acquired neuroblastoma predisposition specific for the first twin and in utero metastatic spread of tumor cells to the second twin (ie, twin-to-twin metastasis) via the shared placental circulation.

Acute congenital leukemia is the second most common fetal cancer, occurring at an incidence of 1 in 4.7 million live births per year. The diagnosis requires the proliferation of blast cells together with anemia, thrombocytopenia, and leukocytosis. Important congenital infections, including cytomegalovirus, rubella, and toxoplasmosis, must be excluded. In utero, hepatosplenomegaly and nonimmune hydrops are common at presentation.

Sporadic heritable retinoblastoma is a malignant tumor of the retina that is inherited in an autosomal-dominant manner. The mutant retinoblastoma gene is mainly derived from the father and may be related to exposure of paternal germ cells to carcinogens. Primary hepatic malignant tumors of the fetus may present with an abdominal mass, and in cases of hepatoblastoma, the serum levels of α-fetoprotein are markedly elevated and reflect the tumor burden. Finally, rhabdomyosarcoma is the most common soft tissue sarcoma in children and is commonly located at the level of the head and neck. It is associated with a loss of heterozygosity of the short arm of chromosome 11. Only a few cases have been described during pregnancy, during which time the tumors manifested as rapidly growing masses of irregular contour.

For the bibliography list, log onto www.expertconsult.com ⟨http://www.expertconsult.com⟩.

16

Complications of Disease and Therapy

Kemi M. Doll, MD, MSCR, Daniel L. Clarke-Pearson, MD

KEY POINTS

1. Women with gynecologic cancers can have significant complications from treatment.
2. Vaginal bleeding is usually controlled with packing.
3. Ureteral obstruction can be treated by diversion either with surgery or stent placement.
4. Bowel complications are treated with conservative management or surgery depending on the patient's disease status and overall condition.
5. Deep vein thrombosis always needs to be considered for prophylaxis and treatment if necessary.
6. Infectious complications always need to be considered and managed appropriately.
7. The risk of complications always needs to be considered and the patient counseled appropriately.

Women with gynecologic cancers often experience complications associated with their primary disease process or from the cancer-directed treatment modalities. In addition, many women have medical comorbidities, are obese, or are elderly, all of which further complicate therapy and treatment decisions. Minimizing these problems requires the clinician to astutely evaluate the patient, be proactive in prevention strategies, and provide early intervention.

Complications of disease are, in fact, commonly the primary presenting symptom (chief complaint) of a gynecologic cancer. Common symptoms of disease include hemorrhage (cervical and endometrial cancers), urinary tract obstruction or fistulae (cervical cancer), and intestinal obstruction or weight loss (ovarian cancer). Although some complications have been discussed previously in this text, it seems appropriate to devote a chapter exclusively to complications of disease and therapy. Not all possible complications can be covered, and readers are referred to texts that expand on them. However, the most common complications and management are discussed.

DISEASE–ORIENTED COMPLICATIONS

Symptoms caused by cancer, such as bleeding, urinary tract obstruction, fistula, and intestinal obstruction, are complications of the primary gynecologic cancer that usually need to be managed coincidentally with the cancer itself.

Hemorrhage

Bleeding from cervical or endometrial cancer is a common presenting symptom. Although bleeding is rarely severe, the acute management of hemorrhage may be required before cancer therapy can be undertaken. Patients who are bleeding should be initially assessed for hemodynamic stability. On rare occasions, the bleeding is so severe that the patient may be in hypovolemic shock. Immediate management should include venous access, blood volume replacement, and supportive care. When stabilized, the patient should be examined, and the source of the bleeding should be determined. Most commonly, massive hemorrhage results from an exophytic cervical cancer eroding into a small cervical or vaginal artery. Prolonged slow vaginal bleeding from an endometrial cancer or sarcoma may also result in a patient presenting with profound chronic anemia. Because the bleeding has been slow over a longer period, the patient has often adapted to the anemia and may be hemodynamically stable despite profound anemia. Biopsy should be performed to document the pathology, and the patient should be evaluated to make a clinical estimation of the extent (stage) of disease.

Control of an actively bleeding cervical lesion is usually accomplished with a vaginal pack applied firmly to the cervix, filling the entire vagina. Monsel's solution (ferric subsulfate) may be put on the portion of the pack abutting the tumor. Soaking of the entire pack with Monsel's solution should be avoided because it will desiccate the normal vaginal mucosa, making removal of the pack and subsequent pelvic examinations difficult. **Application of acetone to the pack adjacent to the tumor has also been helpful,** although acetone is often difficult to acquire in today's medical environment. An indwelling Foley catheter should be placed in the bladder because pressure from the pack will usually obstruct the urethra. The pack should be removed slowly 24 to 48 hours later, and the patient should be observed. Removal of the pack under anesthesia may provide a level of safety if immediate cautery or repacking was necessary. This would also provide the opportunity to perform an examination under anesthesia and cystoscopy or proctoscopy if indicated. Suturing bleeding points in a cervical cancer is rarely successful because the suture will tear through the tumor.

Pelvic radiation therapy for a patient with locally advanced cervical cancer who is actively bleeding should be initiated immediately. Alternatively, if the patient's cancer is an operable lesion, surgery should be performed expeditiously. In either event, if the patient has received more than 4 units of packed red blood cells (PRBCs), it is prudent to assess coagulation factors because the patient may have developed a "dilutional" coagulopathy and require fresh-frozen plasma (FFP), cryoprecipitate, or platelets.

If bleeding cannot be controlled with packing, other measures must be considered. Consultation with an interventional radiologist should be obtained to **consider arteriographic embolization of the hypogastric or uterine arteries. Arteriographic evaluation will usually identify the specific bleeding vessel, and selective embolization can be accomplished.** Arterial access is usually obtained through the femoral artery, and the catheter is advanced to the aortic bifurcation. Using contrast injected into the artery, the arterial vascular supply of the pelvis can be investigated to identify the specific bleeding site. Both sides of the pelvis should be evaluated. Intravascular contrast can be nephrotoxic and therefore must be used cautiously in patients who have an element of renal failure or who have diabetes. Control of the bleeding site can be accomplished by continuous vasopressin infusion, by embolization using synthetic materials (Gelfoam) or Gianturco springs imbedded with Dacron or with a balloon catheter (Fig. 16.1). Embolization is usually the procedure primarily chosen because the vasopressin infusion and balloon catheters require that the artery remain cannulated for a longer duration.

Hypogastric (internal iliac) artery ligation is usually the procedure of last resort for bleeding from a primary gynecologic cancer and is most commonly performed to control intraoperative hemorrhage. Details of hypogastric artery ligation are discussed later in this chapter.

Urinary Tract Complications
Ureteral Obstruction
Ureteral obstruction may be the primary presenting symptom of a locally advanced cervical cancer and less commonly other gynecologic cancers, including endometrial and ovarian cancers. **The most common evidence of ureteral obstruction is an elevated serum creatinine level** (rather than complaints of anuria or symptoms of uremia). Of course, acute renal failure

FIGURE 16.1 A patient who is postoperative from a vaginal hysterectomy with significant vaginal bleeding requiring multiple blood transfusions. The patient also has von Willebrand disease. *Arrowheads* represent areas of hemorrhage, resolved after embolization. **A,** Hemorrhage from the internal pudendal artery on the right. **B,** After embolization, no hemorrhage is seen from the internal pudendal artery. Dye in the pelvis is localized to the bladder, and the left ureter can be visualized. (Courtesy of Ivan Vujic, MD, and Keeling Warburton, MD, Medical University of South Carolina.)

may arise from a number of causes, which should be investigated (Table 16.1). **The ureters may be obstructed as a result of local extension of the cancer, by metastases to retroperitoneal lymph nodes, or by extrinsic compression of the ureter by large masses.** Uremia secondary to bilateral ureteral obstruction is rarely encountered today but warrants immediate recognition and treatment. Given evidence of an elevated creatinine, evaluation of the ureters should avoid the use of nephrotoxic

TABLE 16.1   Major Causes of Acute Renal Failure

Disorder	Example
PRERENAL FAILURE	
Hypovolemia	Skin, gastrointestinal, or renal volume loss; hemorrhage, sequestration of extracellular fluid (pancreatitis, peritonitis)
Cardiovascular failure	Impaired cardiac output (infarction, tamponade); vascular pooling (anaphylaxis, sepsis, drugs)
POSTRENAL FAILURE	
Extrarenal obstruction	Urethral occlusion; bladder, pelvic, or retroperitoneal neoplasms; surgical accident; calculi
Intrarenal obstruction	Crystals (uric acid, oxalic acid, sulfonamides, methotrexate)
Bladder rupture	Trauma
ACUTE TUBULAR NECROSIS	
Postischemic	All conditions listed above for prerenal failure
Pigment induced	Hemolysis (transfusion reaction); rhabdomyolysis (trauma, coma, heatstroke, severe exercise, potassium or phosphate depletion)
Toxin induced	Antibiotics; contrast material; anesthetic agents; heavy metals; organic solvents
Pregnancy related	Septic abortion; uterine hemorrhage; eclampsia

FIGURE 16.2 A double-J stent has been inserted into the right kidney, ureter, and bladder through a percutaneous nephrostomy.

intravenous (IV) contrast dyes. A noncontrasted computed tomography (CT) scan of the abdomen and pelvis can demonstrate suspected hydronephrosis and provides the additional benefit of evaluating disease burden. Alternative imaging methods may include ultrasonography of the kidneys or a Lasix-renal scan to access if the kidney remains viable. If bilateral ureteral obstruction is diagnosed, the patient should be rapidly evaluated to determine the true extent of the cancer before any intervention is undertaken. If the cancer appears to be locally advanced and not widely metastatic, **relief of the ureteral obstruction should be attempted by cystoscopy and placement of retrograde ureteral stents. If stent placement is unsuccessful, then percutaneous nephrostomy (PCN) tubes should be inserted.** Dialysis may be necessary in extreme circumstances until the obstruction can be relieved. Postobstructive diuresis and correction of electrolytes should be carefully evaluated in the several days after relief of the ureteral obstruction.

Complications of PCN placement include a high frequency of urinary tract infections (UTIs) and pyelonephritis (70%), catheter occlusion (65%), and bleeding (28%). Seventy percent of the patients will have recovery of renal function after PCN placement (Dudley).

Comment needs to be made on two sets of circumstances in which the physician, patient, and family must seriously consider the possibility that relief of the obstruction may not be in the patient's best interest. These clinical situations include the following:

- A patient who presents with a widely metastatic malignancy for which there is little significant opportunity to provide effective therapy

- A patient who has previously been treated for cervical cancer and has bilateral obstruction secondary to recurrent pelvic disease. This is a situation in which there is no therapy available that would significantly prolong the patient's life. Careful evaluation should be made to be certain that the obstruction is not a result of retroperitoneal fibrosis caused by prior radiation therapy or from a lymphocyst.

Often, patients with bilateral ureteral obstruction are uremic and comatose. Decisions regarding intervention and care then fall to the next of kin, who must make the difficult decisions regarding intervention that may reverse the uremia but cause the patient to succumb from other complications of the cancer versus allowing the patient to expire peacefully in a uremic coma. Compassionate and knowledgeable consultation and advice with an experienced gynecologic oncologist are crucial in these difficult circumstances.

Unilateral ureteral obstruction at the time of initial presentation may not require stent or PCN placement if the patient's renal function is normal and therapy (eg, pelvic radiation therapy) is expected to control the cancer and relieve the obstruction. Placement of a PCN or stent in these circumstances must be balanced against the potential complications that might delay or interrupt therapy (Fig. 16.2). A Lasix renal scan

can aid in evaluating the function of the obstructed kidney. If the organ is still viable, placement of a stent to avoid loss of function while awaiting tumor shrinkage from therapy can be helpful.

Urinary outlet obstruction (obstruction of the urethra) by a cancer that has invaded the anterior vaginal wall (vaginal, vulvar, or cervical cancers) may usually be corrected by placement of a Foley catheter. If a Foley catheter cannot be placed, either a suprapubic catheter or PCNs should be considered.

Urinary Tract Fistulas

Vesicovaginal fistula caused by a primary gynecologic cancer is relatively rare and is more commonly caused by therapy. Nonetheless, some patients will present with tumor that has eroded into the bladder, and subsequent loss of integrity between the bladder and vagina results in urinary leakage. Correction of the fistula caused by a cancer cannot be considered until the cancer has been eradicated. In the interim, while cancer therapy is initiated, the patient may be very uncomfortable from the continued loss of urine. Attempts to diminish the leakage should be undertaken. Placement of a Foley catheter will often partially divert urine from the fistula into the catheter. Modified menstrual cups or external appliances to collect urine have been used on occasion with success. Urinary diversion (ileal or transverse colon conduit) may be the only complete solution to profuse vaginal urinary leakage. Performing this major surgery should be weighed against the delay in primary cancer therapy, which would be required while the patient recovers from surgical diversion.

Gastrointestinal Complications
Gastrointestinal Obstruction

Intestinal obstruction as a presenting symptom of a gynecologic cancer is most commonly caused by advanced ovarian cancer. In cases of small intestinal obstruction, initial therapy should include correction of fluid volume and electrolytes, nutritional assessment, and bowel rest. If nausea and emesis continue despite antiemetics, a nasogastric (NG) tube decompression should be placed. Alternatively, an NG tube may be placed immediately if there is significant stomach distention requiring decompression. Assessment of intestinal patency a CT scan with oral contrast should be performed to have a better understanding of the location and extent of obstruction. The colon should also be evaluated to exclude the possibility of colonic obstruction, which would need to be relieved at the same surgical procedure. **In most cases, surgical exploration is necessary to establish and stage the cancer diagnosis, debulk the tumor, and relieve the obstruction.** Small bowel or colonic resection performed to relieve obstruction and to debulk the primary tumor is commonly done. Although patients presenting with gastrointestinal (GI) obstruction may be severely malnourished, the role of preoperative total parental nutrition is debatable. The highest quality evidence suggests that at least 10 days of total parenteral nutrition (TPN) administration is necessary to provide a benefit of reduced postoperative complications.

Short bowel syndrome may result from extensive resection of the small bowel, colon, or both. The syndrome is characterized by frequent diarrhea, fluid and electrolyte depletion, malabsorption, and weight loss. Depending on the extent and location of the intestinal segment(s) resected, malabsorption of nutrients may include copper, zinc, chromium, selenium, essential fatty acids, vitamins A and E, biotin, thiamine, and vitamin B_{12}. Over time, the remaining small bowel often adapts, and fluid and nutrient absorption is improved. However, in the interim, attempts to relieve short bowel syndrome should be directed at decreasing transit time by the use of an "elemental" diet and Imodium or Lomotil, cholestyramine (to decrease irritation of bile salts on the colonic mucosa), and somatostatin (to decrease intestinal digestive fluid production). In extreme cases, support with IV fluids and TPN may be necessary for several months.

On occasion, the preoperative assessment (usually with a CT scan) discovers far advanced disease (extensive carcinomatosis), which would be unlikely to be successfully debulked. In these patients, neoadjuvant chemotherapy, rather than surgical intervention, may be the best option. If this therapeutic strategy is taken, GI decompression (NG tube or gastrostomy) and parenteral nutritional support (TPN) will be required for several weeks while the neoadjuvant chemotherapy has the opportunity to result in a tumor response and relief of the intestinal obstruction. Fortunately, many patients with ovarian cancer will regain intestinal function after two or three cycles of chemotherapy.

Even in the setting of neoadjuvant treatment route, correction of a colonic obstruction is necessary to prevent colonic perforation, peritonitis, sepsis, and death. Management options include placement of an intraluminal stent or surgical intervention. In a recently published experience with gynecologic oncology patients, rates of technical success of stent placement ranged from 75% to 88%; however, clinical success was lower, with more than one-third (33%–38%) of patients with stent placements requiring further intervention for either stent complication or failure. Advantages of stents include the avoidance of major surgery and a stoma. Systematic review of large patient populations beyond gynecologic oncology demonstrate median placement success rates of 96%, with associated risks of perforation (4.5%), stent migration (11%), and reobstruction (12%). In a palliative population, the median duration of patency was 106 days. Alternatively, surgical correction of the colonic obstruction may be considered, with colostomy as a frequent outcome given the disease burden in a neoadjuvant patient. If the patient has an excellent response to subsequent chemotherapy, colostomy take-down in the future is reasonable to consider.

Intestinal obstruction often occurs late in the course of progressive ovarian cancer. In these situations, superb clinical judgment is required to obtain an optimal palliative outcome because not all patients with recurrent ovarian cancer and intestinal obstruction benefit from surgical intervention. It does seem intuitive that patients with colonic obstruction should be either offered a self-expanding stent or undergo surgery to create colostomy, ileostomy, or cecostomy. A patient with a small bowel obstruction requires careful thought and triage. Initially, conservative management with IV fluid and electrolyte replacement and NG tube decompression should be instituted. Some patients may reestablish bowel function with a few days of "bowel rest." However, if the obstruction persists, the decision to place a gastrostomy tube (which can often be placed percutaneously) or to attempt to surgically relieve the intestinal obstruction must be made. (Of course, a patient who has a small bowel obstruction caused by adhesions should undergo surgery in all cases.) The problem in decision making comes when it is clear that the patient has recurrent ovarian cancer. Many investigators have attempted to identify factors that would predict successful outcome (often defined as surviving 30 days or being discharged from the hospital and able to take oral fluids) or postoperative complications and death. These factors include presence of ascites, poor nutritional status, amount of prior chemotherapy regimens, availability of therapy with some potential for response, prior use of radiation therapy, length of time since prior therapy, and potential for being "platin sensitive." If surgical intervention is deemed appropriate, surgical procedures might include bypass of involved segments of small bowel (entero-enterostomy), bowel resection with anastomosis, or ileostomy. Unfortunately, in every investigator's experience, there are patients who undergo laparotomy only to find such extensive carcinomatosis that they are deemed inoperable. The decision to operate, then, should be based on a clear communication between the surgeon and patient regarding expectations and definitions of "success." In the authors' experience, which is reasonably representative of the general literature, the median survival time after small bowel obstruction surgery was 88 days, and only 14% of patients were alive at 12 months. In addition, 49% of patients had at least one significant postoperative complication, including wound infections, enterocutaneous fistula, sepsis, and recurrent obstruction.

If the decision is made not to operate, further decisions regarding management are also complex, including methods to palliate vomiting (percutaneous gastrostomy is recommended) and whether to continue IV fluids or even consider TPN in a hospice setting.

Gastrointestinal Fistulas

Rectovaginal fistula may be discovered at the time of primary diagnosis of cervical, vaginal, or vulvar cancers. Involuntary loss of feces, flatus, and mucous discharge are the most common symptoms. If the patient has vulvar pain and excoriation, a fistula from the small intestine must be suspected. In this instance, a fistulogram can be helpful if definitive diagnosis of a fistulae is in question, and a CT scan with oral contrast should be performed to define the exact anatomic structures involved. If a rectovaginal fistula is found, diversion with a loop colostomy or end-colostomy is suggested to divert the fecal stream and allow prompt treatment of the cancer (usually radiation therapy). If vulvar cancer is so advanced as to cause a rectovaginal fistula, some surgeons manage the cancer and the fistula in the same surgical procedure (eg, a posterior pelvic exenteration and modified radical vulvectomy). Others have had excellent results treating locally advanced vulvar cancer with radiation therapy and concurrent radiosensitizing chemotherapy, thereby preserving the rectal sphincter. Colostomy diversion is still suggested for patient comfort and hygiene. If the cancer treatment is successful, attempts to close the fistula are

reasonable, and if successful, the colostomy may ultimately be reversed.

Enterovaginal fistulas are rare to complicate the initial cancer diagnosis and more often occur as a result of complications of therapy (radiation) or at the time of cancer recurrence. The flow of intestinal contents out of the vagina is usually liquid and caustic to vulvar skin. Thorough evaluation of the upper and lower GI tracts and the urinary tract is mandatory because many of these fistula are "complex," involving more than one viscus and more than one defect. Surgical intervention is necessary in most cases to either resect or isolate the involved bowel. If resection is not possible, the fistulized bowel will need to be isolated and excluded from the intestinal stream. Because the isolated bowel will continue to create succus entericus and subsequent continued vaginal drainage, resection is generally preferred.

Venous Thromboembolic Complications

Venous thromboembolic complications may precede the diagnosis of gynecologic cancer or may be the result of cancer treatments, especially surgery and chemotherapy. Most women with gynecologic cancers have several risk factors that increase the probability of developing a venous thromboembolic event during their course of therapy.

Risk Factors

The causal factors of venous thrombosis were first proposed by Virchow in 1858 and include a hypercoagulable state, venous stasis, and vessel endothelial injury. In addition to the increased risk of venous thromboembolism (VTE) resulting from cancer, other clinical risk factors include advanced age; major surgery; nonwhite race; a history of deep vein thrombosis (DVT) or pulmonary embolism; lower extremity edema or venous stasis changes; presence of varicose veins; being overweight; a history of radiation therapy; and hypercoagulable states, such as factor V Leiden, pregnancy, or use of oral contraceptives, estrogens, or tamoxifen. Intraoperative factors associated with postoperative DVT included increased anesthesia time, increased blood loss, and the need for transfusion in the operating room. It is important to recognize these risk factors in order to provide the appropriate level of venous thrombosis prophylaxis. The modified Caprini risk assessment model for VTE has been widely adopted as a predictive tool for surgical patients. This tool has limited use in the gynecologic oncology population, however. Importantly, nearly all gynecologic oncology patients, by virtue of having a malignancy, being older than 40 years old, with an operative time of more than 45 minutes are in the highest risk group, with a VTE risk of 6% in the absence of prophylaxis.

Prophylactic Methods

Deep vein thrombosis and pulmonary embolism, although largely preventable, are significant complications in women with gynecologic cancers and especially those who are postoperative. The magnitude of this problem is relevant to gynecologic oncologists because 40% of all deaths after gynecologic surgery are directly attributed to pulmonary emboli, which is also the most common cause of postoperative death in patients with uterine or cervical carcinoma.

A number of prophylactic methods have been shown to significantly reduce the incidence of DVT in women with gynecologic cancers, and a few studies have included a large enough patient population to demonstrate a reduction in fatal pulmonary emboli. The ideal prophylactic method would be effective, free of significant side effects, well accepted by the patient and nursing staff, widely applicable to most patients, and inexpensive. Available prophylactic methods may be divided into pharmacologic agents that reduce hypercoagulable states and mechanical methods that reduce stasis and may also enhance fibrinolysis. A key to the successful use of prophylactic methods is the understanding that women with gynecologic cancers are at very high risk and that more intense prophylactic measures are necessary to achieve maximal success. Based on the American College of Chest Physician Guidelines, all high-risk patients should receive either pharmacologic anticoagulation or combination pharmacologic anticoagulation and mechanical device prophylaxis. In addition, extended prophylaxis after surgery is recommended for patients undergoing major abdominal or pelvic surgery for cancer.

Low-dose heparin. The use of small doses of subcutaneously administered heparin for the prevention of DVT and pulmonary embolism is the most widely studied of all prophylactic methods. More than 25 controlled trials have demonstrated that heparin given subcutaneously 2 hours preoperatively and every 8 to 12 hours postoperatively is effective in reducing the incidence of DVT. The value of low-dose heparin in preventing fatal pulmonary emboli was established by a randomized, controlled, multicenter international trial, which demonstrated a significant reduction in fatal postoperative pulmonary emboli in general surgery patients receiving low-dose heparin every 8 hours postoperatively. In gynecologic oncology patients, a randomized trial of heparin given either in a regimen of 5000 units subcutaneously 2 hours preoperatively and every 8 hours postoperatively or 5000 units subcutaneously every 8 hours preoperatively (a minimum of three preoperative doses) and every 8 hours postoperatively was performed. Both of these prophylaxis regimens were effective in significantly reducing the incidence of postoperative DVT in patients with gynecologic cancers. The authors conclude that in women undergoing surgery for gynecologic malignancy, a regimen of low-dose heparin 5000 units every 8 hours is necessary to provide effective prophylaxis.

The benefits of unfractionated heparin (UFH) are its rapid onset of action and ability for quick reversal; ability for frequent monitoring with activated partial thromboplastin time (aPTT) levels; and lack of renal metabolism, making it ideal in cases of renal insufficiency or renal failure. The most serious adverse risk of UFH use is the occurrence of heparin-induced thrombocytopenia (HIT). HIT has been found to be associated with low-dose heparin use in 6% of patients after gynecologic surgery, although its overall postoperative risk is considered to be around 1%. If patients remain on low-dose heparin for more than 4 days, it is reasonable to check a daily platelet count for 14 days or until heparin is stopped, whichever comes first.

Low-dose heparin is also limited by a narrow therapeutic range, requiring frequent monitoring.

Low-molecular-weight heparins. Low-molecular-weight heparins (LMWHs) are the preferred choice in perioperative pharmacologic prophylaxis. LMWHs are fragments of heparin that vary in size from 4500 to 6500 daltons. When compared with UFH, LMWHs have more anti-Xa and less antithrombin activity, leading to less effect on partial thromboplastin time (PTT) and possibly to fewer bleeding complications. An increased half-life of 4 hours results in increased bioavailability when compared with UFH. The increase in half-life of LMWHs also allows the convenience of once or twice-a-day dosing at 30 to 40 mg/day and can be used in the outpatient setting.

Randomized controlled trials (RCTs) have compared LMWH with UFH in patients undergoing gynecologic surgery. In all studies, there was a similar incidence of DVT. Bleeding complications were similar between the UFH and LMWH groups, and meta-analysis of all studies comparing the incidence of HIT confirmed that HIT is significantly less common with LMWH. A meta-analysis of general surgery and gynecologic surgery patients from 32 trials likewise indicated that daily LMWH administration is as effective as UFH in DVT prophylaxis without any difference in hemorrhagic complications, and these results have been confirmed in cancer surgery populations. Finally, prolonged prophylaxis for 4 weeks postoperatively has resulted in improved outcomes in high-risk surgical populations. In one randomized study of 1113 patients, 4 weeks of treatment after abdominal or pelvic cancer surgery reduced VTE rate from 4.6% to 0.8%, without increased bleeding complications. This extended prophylaxis has been adopted as the standard of care by the American College of Chest Physicians (ACCP), the National Comprehensive Cancer Network, and the American Society of Clinical Oncology.

Oral agents. Investigations into the use of oral agents, specifically vitamin K antagonist warfarin, and a host of newly developed factor Xa inhibitors is ongoing. High-quality randomized trials and investigations in cancer populations have been limited to date, so the agents are not recommended in perioperative VTE prophylaxis at this time.

Mechanical Methods

Stasis in the veins of the legs has been clearly demonstrated while the patient is undergoing surgery and continues postoperatively for varying lengths of time. Stasis occurring in the capacitance veins of the calf during surgery plus the hypercoagulable state induced by cancer and surgery are the primary factors contributing to the development of acute postoperative DVT. Prospective studies of the natural history of postoperative venous thrombosis have shown that the calf veins are the predominant site of thrombi and that most thrombi develop within 24 hours of surgery.

Although probably of only modest benefit, reduction of stasis by short preoperative hospital stays and early postoperative ambulation should be encouraged for all patients. Elevation of the foot of the bed, raising the calf above heart level, allows gravity to drain the calf veins and should further reduce stasis.

Graduated compression stockings. Controlled studies of graduated pressure stockings are limited but do suggest modest benefit when they are carefully fitted. **Poorly fitted stockings may be hazardous to some obese patients who develop a tourniquet effect at the knee or midthigh.** Variations in human anatomy do not allow perfect fit of all patients to available stocking sizes. There is no therapeutic advantage of thigh-length stockings as compared with calf-length stocking. The simplicity of elastic stockings and the absence of significant side effects are probably the two most important reasons that they are often included in routine postoperative care.

External pneumatic compression. The largest body of literature dealing with the reduction of postoperative venous stasis deals with intermittent external compression of the leg by pneumatically inflated sleeves placed around the calf or leg during intraoperative and postoperative periods. **Calf compression during and after gynecologic surgery significantly reduces the incidence of DVT on a level similar to that of low-dose heparin.** In addition to increasing venous flow and pulsatile emptying of the calf veins, external pneumatic compression (EPC) also appears to augment endogenous fibrinolysis, which may result in lysis of very early thrombi before they become clinically significant.

The duration of postoperative EPC has differed in various trials.

External pneumatic compression used in patients undergoing major surgery for gynecologic malignancy has been found to reduce the incidence of postoperative venous thromboembolic complications by nearly threefold but only if calf compression is applied intraoperatively and for the first 5 postoperative days. Patients with gynecologic malignancies may remain at risk because of stasis and hypercoagulable states for a longer period than general surgical patients and therefore appear to benefit from longer use of EPC.

External pneumatic leg compression has no significant side effects or risks and is considered slightly more cost effective compared with pharmacologic methods of prophylaxis. Of course, compliance to wearing the leg compression while in bed is of utmost importance, and the patient and nursing staff should be educated to the proper regimen for maximum benefit. We have investigated the risk factors associated with the failure of external compression to prevent DVT in a retrospective analysis of 1862 consecutive gynecologic surgery patients who received postoperative intermittent pneumatic compression. **A history of prior VTE, diagnosis of cancer, and age older than 60 years were factors independently associated with the development of VTE despite EPC prophylaxis** ($P <0.05$). Patients having two or more of these factors had a 16-fold increased risk of postoperative VTE despite prophylaxis. In these extremely high-risk patients, of which the majority of gynecologic oncology patients would be categorized, combined methods of prophylaxis (eg, EPC plus low-dose UFH or LMWH) is recommended by the guidelines written by the ACCP. Although there have be no randomized trials on ECP alone versus combination prophylaxis specifically within gynecologic oncology populations, high-quality data from other cancer surgical populations have led to consensus recommendations that we follow. **Mechanical prophylaxis alone should be reserved for perioperative gynecologic oncology patients with unacceptably high bleeding risk.**

Postoperative Prophylaxis

Patients undergoing abdominal or pelvic surgery for malignancy remain at increased risk for development of VTE for an extended period of time after surgery. The administration of LMWH for 4 weeks postoperatively has been consistently shown to decrease development of VTE in this high-risk population. **For all patients undergoing laparotomy for gynecologic cancer surgery, we recommend extended (4 weeks) chemoprophylaxis with LMWH.** Evidence for extended treatment for patients undergoing minimally invasive procedures is less clear. Minimally invasive approaches to hysterectomy are associated with a threefold decreased incidence of VTE. In several retrospective reviews of large ($n \geq 400$) institutional studies, rate of VTE after laparoscopic or robotic hysterectomy has been reported at 0.5% to 1.2%, on par with the risk associated with open benign hysterectomy (0.6%). This suggests extended prophylaxis may not be required for this patient population. Importantly, in one study of 573 cases in which the VTE rate was highest (1.2%), the authors identified a high-risk group of women with a body mass index (BMI) greater than 40 and operative time longer than 180 minutes, who had a VTE rate of 9.5% (4 of 42) compared with 0.6% (3 of 531) of the remaining population. At this time, the authors recommend extended prophylaxis after minimally invasive surgery only for patients with other conferring risk factors (ie, limited mobility, super morbid obesity, history of VTE).

Management of Deep Vein Thrombosis and Pulmonary Embolism

Diagnosis of deep vein thrombosis. Because pulmonary embolism is the leading cause of death after gynecologic surgical procedures, identification of high-risk patients and the use of prophylactic VTE regimens is an essential part of management. In addition, the early recognition of DVT and pulmonary embolism and immediate treatment are critical. **Most pulmonary emboli arise from the deep venous system of the leg, although after gynecologic surgery the pelvic veins are a known source of fatal pulmonary emboli also.**

The signs and symptoms of DVT of the lower extremities include pain, edema, erythema, and prominent vascular pattern of the superficial veins. These signs and symptoms are relatively nonspecific; 50% to 80% of patients with these symptoms do not actually have DVT. Conversely, approximately 80% of patients with symptomatic pulmonary emboli have no signs or symptoms of thrombosis in the lower extremities. Because of the lack of specificity when signs and symptoms are recognized, additional diagnostic tests should be performed to establish the diagnosis of DVT.

Doppler ultrasonography. **B-mode duplex Doppler imaging is currently the most common technique for the diagnosis of symptomatic venous thrombosis, especially when it arises in the proximal lower extremity.** With duplex Doppler imaging, the femoral vein can be visualized, and clots may be seen directly. Compression of the vein with the ultrasound probe tip allows assessment of venous collapsibility and the presence of a thrombus diminishes vein wall collapsibility. Abnormal Doppler color flow is an additional sign of DVT. It should be recognized that Doppler imaging does not detect isolated iliac vein or proximal femoral thrombosis. In addition, 2% of patients with initially negative studies will develop DVT in the next 7 days. Repeat testing is warranted on any patient where a high suspicion or risk of DVT is present.

Venography. Although contrast venography has been the "gold standard" for diagnosis of DVT, other diagnostic studies have nearly equivalent accuracy when performed by a skilled technologist and, in most patients, may replace the need for this study. Venography is moderately uncomfortable, requires the injection of a contrast material that may cause allergic reaction or renal injury, and may result in phlebitis in approximately 5% of patients. However, if noninvasive imaging is normal or inconclusive and the clinician remains concerned given clinical symptoms, venography should be obtained to obtain a definitive answer.

Magnetic resonance venography. Magnetic resonance venography (MRV) has a sensitivity and specificity comparable to those of venography. In addition, MRV may detect thrombi in pelvic veins that are not imaged by venography. The primary drawback to MRV is the time involved in examining the lower extremity and pelvis and the expense of this technology.

Impedance plethysmography. Impedance plethysmography measures the change in blood volume in the calf from the impedance of a blood pressure cuff after rapid deflation. The measurements are determined by electrodes placed on the calf. When performed appropriately, it has high sensitivity (91%) and specificity (96%) for proximal vein thromboses. However, patients must lie still for 2 minutes for accurate measurements, and skilled personnel are required for performance of the test. For these reasons, this method is not routinely used.

Treatment of deep vein thrombosis. **The treatment of postoperative DVT requires the immediate institution of anticoagulant therapy.** Untreated, symptomatic DVT is associated with a 50% risk of pulmonary embolism, and untreated pulmonary embolism carries a 30% risk of mortality. Treatment may be with either UFH or LMWHs followed by 6 months of oral or subcutaneous anticoagulant therapy. Prolonged anticoagulation (lifetime) is recommended for women who continue to have active cancer (ie, those not in remission after treatment) because they remain at very high risk to rethrombose.

Low-molecular-weight heparin. Low-molecular-weight heparins (eg, enoxaparin, dalteparin) have been shown to be effective in the treatment of VTE and have a cost-effectiveness advantage over IV heparin in that they may be administered in the outpatient setting. The dosages used in treatment of thromboembolism are unique and weight adjusted according to each LMWH preparation. Because LMWH have a minimal effect on activated PTT, serial laboratory monitoring of PTT levels is not necessary. Similarly, monitoring of anti-Xa activity (except in difficult cases or those with renal impairment) has not been shown to be of significant benefit in a dose adjustment of LMWH. The increased bioavailability associated with LMWH

allows for twice-a-day dosing, potentially making outpatient management for a subset of patients an option. A metaanalysis involving more than 1000 patients from 19 trials suggests that LMWH is more effective, safer, and less costly compared with UFH in preventing recurrent thromboembolism.

Unfractionated heparin. Unfractionated heparin may be the initial treatment of choice in a recent postoperative patient or other clinical settings in which a significant bleeding risk is appreciated and the need for immediate reversal may be evident. An initial bolus is given intravenously followed by a continuous infusion adjusted to therapeutic aPTT levels. Weight-based nomograms to aid in appropriate dosing are widely available and often embedded in hospital pharmacy administration processes.

Long-term anticoagulation. Traditionally, oral anticoagulation with warfarin was used in the long-term treatment of DVT in cancer patients. Warfarin may be a difficult drug to administer to some patients, however, especially if their nutrition is inadequate, their oral intake is variable, or they require prolonged use of antibiotics or other drugs that might alter the metabolism of warfarin. This is particularly common in women with advanced ovarian cancer. Given the wide variation in the international normalized ratio (INR) in many of these patients who are then predisposed to either bleeding complications or rethrombosis, we have found that it is safer to use subcutaneous LMWH (at therapeutic doses) for prolonged therapy. This clinical experience has been confirmed in a number of large, high-quality, RCTs that have demonstrated the superiority of LMWH over warfarin in the clinical setting. In each study, LMWH resulted in equal or reduced risk of recurrent DVT, with no increase in bleeding events, major or minor. In addition, two trials demonstrated a mortality benefit with LMWH over warfarin. Meta-analyses including these studies have supported these results, including one study with seven RCTs and 1908 cancer patients that demonstrated a hazards ratio of 0.47 (95% confidence interval [CI] 0.3–0.7) for reduction of recurrent DVT. The authors therefore recommend LMWH as the first-line therapy for long-term treatment of DVT in gynecologic cancer patients.

Oral anticoagulants. If oral anticoagulation must be used (eg, patient refuses daily injections, previous history of HIT), a vitamin K antagonist such as warfarin is preferred over no therapy. The conversion from parenteral heparin or LMWH to oral warfarin may start on the initial day of therapy. The change in INR resulting from warfarin administration often precedes the anticoagulant effect by approximately 2 days, during which time low protein C levels are associated with a transient hypercoagulable state. Therefore, both heparin and warfarin are given, and the heparin is discontinued when the warfarin has reached a therapeutic INR of 2 to 3 for 2 consecutive days. Patients should be cautioned to avoid the use of drugs and dietary products that might alter the metabolism or absorption of warfarin.

New agents such as direct thrombin or factor Xa inhibitors that have been approved for the treatment of acute DVT have not been well tested in cancer populations. Given the significant impact of surgery, chemotherapy, and radiation on a patient's nutrition, performance status, and comorbid conditions, the authors do not believe there is sufficient data to support the use of the medications over warfarin. Their use is best restricted to scenarios when co-management with a hematologic specialists is available.

Inferior vena cava filter. In the gynecologic oncology population, acute DVT may often be diagnosed in the immediate pre- or postoperative setting, when pharmacologic anticoagulation is contraindicated because of bleeding risks. In these cases, placement of a retrievable (ie, temporary) inferior vena cava (IVC) filter is an alternative strategy to reducing the risks associated with DVT. The filter can remain in place until bleeding risks decrease, at which time the patient should be started on an appropriate anticoagulation regimen. Filter retrieval is associated with a high technical success rate (85%) and should be pursued given that long-term filter placement is associated with IVC thrombosis, increased recurrent DVT, and the potential for filter migration.

Diagnosis of pulmonary embolism. Many of the signs and symptoms of pulmonary embolism are associated with other, more commonly occurring pulmonary complications after surgery. The classic findings of pleuritic chest pain, hemoptysis, shortness of breath, tachycardia, and tachypnea should alert the physician to the possibility of a pulmonary embolism. Many times, however, the signs are much more subtle and may be suggested only by a persistent tachycardia or a slight elevation in the respiratory rate. Several diagnostic algorithms have been devised to aid in estimating the likelihood of pulmonary embolism before definitive imaging, such as the Wells or Geneva scoring systems. Interestingly, these algorithms have been compared against physician clinical estimations in a meta-analysis of 52 studies including 55,268 patients. Clinical acumen indeed has comparable sensitivity (0.85 vs. 0.84–0.91) to structured diagnostic algorithms when both are combined with D-dimer testing. Patients with suspected pulmonary embolism can be evaluated initially by chest radiography, electrocardiography, and arterial blood gas assessment. However, a high clinical suspicion or high likelihood based on diagnostic algorithms should prompt immediate spiral CT scan of the chest for definitive diagnosis. **Any evidence of abnormality should be further evaluated by spiral CT scan of the chest if renal function permits. Ventilation-perfusion lung scan is an option in the setting of renal insufficiency or failure,** although, a high percentage of lung scans may be interpreted as "indeterminate." In this setting, careful clinical evaluation and judgment are required to decide whether pulmonary arteriography should be obtained to document or exclude the presence of a pulmonary embolism.

The treatment of pulmonary embolism is similar to that of acute DVT in the hemodynamically stable patient. UFH, LMWH, or fondaparinux are all initial parental anticoagulation treatment options. Recommendations from the ACCP currently favor LMWH or fondaparinux for initial treatment, although UFH may be more prudent for the gynecologic oncology patient for whom a perioperative status or high disease burden often confers a bleeding risk requiring easy reversal of anticoagulation method. Hemodynamically unstable patients require immediate care in an intensive care unit (ICU) and assessment for thrombolytic therapy (eg, recombinant tissue type plasminogen activator, streptokinase) or embolectomy if thrombolysis is contraindicated.

Superior vena cava syndrome. **Superior vena cava syndrome is caused by advanced cancers arising in or invading the mediastinum, subsequently obstructing the venous drainage of the head, neck, and upper thoracic regions.** Primary tumors are most commonly the cause of this syndrome (bronchogenic carcinomas), although metastasis to the mediastinum from gynecologic cancers can also present in this manner. **The vena cava has a low intravascular pressure and is easily compressed by adjacent masses.** Most commonly, the symptoms caused by venous obstruction are dramatic swelling and plethora of the head, neck, upper extremities, and chest. Pleural and pericardial effusions can occur with decreased venous return to the heart and a resultant decrease in cardiac output. Patients also commonly complain of a severe headache. A similar clinical syndrome is also seen associated with thrombosis of the subclavian vein and superior vena cava, which is induced by central venous catheters. The diagnosis of the cause of superior vena cava syndrome is critical to selecting proper management. **If a localized primary or metastatic neoplasm is identified, immediate radiation therapy is usually the most effective method to achieve resolution.** Radiation therapy to the mediastinum in doses of 400 cGy for 3 days and then 150 to 180 cGy per day for a total dose of 3000 to 5000 cGy has been successful in relieving the vascular obstruction. **Responses are commonly recognized in 3 to 4 days.** Chemotherapy may also play a role, although the resolution of symptoms is usually much slower. Expandable wire stents across the constricted portion of the vena cava have also been used successfully.

In patients in whom thrombosis is the etiology of venous obstruction, immediate anticoagulant therapy should be instituted (Fig. 16.3). The edema and plethora will usually diminish in 1 to 3 days. In many instances, the central venous catheter may be left in place and used. However, if the condition persists or recurs, the catheter should be removed.

Biliary Obstruction

Obstruction of the biliary tree by gynecologic cancers is rare and is usually associated with far advanced cancers and limited life expectancy. Nonetheless, the resulting jaundice and pruritus caused by the obstruction is distressing to the patient and her family. Surgical relief of the obstruction is usually impossible because of the extent of cancer involvement in the region. However, **endoscopic placement of a stent in the common duct often will resolve the symptoms and provide a better quality of life.** If a stent cannot be placed as a result of extreme compression or other technical reasons, percutaneous placement of a drainage tube into the dilated biliary tree will also resolve symptoms.

Metastatic adenopathy high in the paraaortic chain resulting in biliary obstruction can commonly obstruct the duodenum, leading to gastric outlet obstruction. Although surgical intervention (gastrojejunostomy) or self-expanding metal stents may correct the anatomic problem, careful consideration should

FIGURE 16.3 Extensive thrombosis of large vessels in the thorax. Multiple collaterals are present. The subclavian catheter is evident *(arrow)*.

be given to the patient's life expectancy. These are similar considerations to those made in women with small intestinal obstructions and recurrent ovarian cancer discussed previously. In women with just days or weeks to live, placement of a gastrostomy tube may be more prudent.

TREATMENT-RELATED COMPLICATIONS

Surgical

Intraoperative and Postoperative Hemorrhage

Intraoperative management of vascular complications. Surgery for gynecologic cancer often requires extensive dissection in the retroperitoneal space, which may be distorted by cancer metastatic to lymph nodes or invading adjacent structures. It is not surprising, then, that injury to pelvic veins and arteries is common and may result in significant intraoperative blood loss and hemorrhage. Surgeons must be prepared for this eventuality and have in their armamentarium the tools and skills to bring a stop to the bleeding.

Before attempting to bring final control to a significant bleeding area, a few basic principles should be used. First, the patient's blood volume and coagulation factors must be maintained at all times. Poor communication between the surgeon and the anesthesiologist can lead to significant hypovolemia and cardiovascular instability. Frequent serial laboratory assessments are critical in this setting. Loss of coagulation factors during intraoperative hemorrhage results in continued bleeding that cannot be controlled by surgical means. The surgeon should pack the involved area to allow replacement of blood volume (PRBCs), coagulation factors (FFP, platelets, and cryoprecipitate), and acquisition of appropriate assistance. When the patient is stable and the team is fully prepared, the packed

area should be exposed a small area at a time to identify the specific bleeding site.

Before attempting to control the bleeding point, the adjacent anatomy should be identified and protected. In particular, the ureter, adjacent vessels, and viscera must be recognized to avoid further injury. **In most cases of arterial bleeding, the artery can be isolated and controlled with sutures. Small arteries may be best controlled by vascular clips, but larger arteries may require sutures with 4-0 or 5-0 vascular suture** (Prolene). This holds for injury to the aorta and common and external iliac arteries. Injury to the internal iliac (hypogastric) artery may be controlled with total ligation of the artery. Patency of distal arteries should be confirmed throughout the remainder of the procedure and postoperatively. In rare instances, arterial injuries must be managed by vascular grafting.

Venous bleeding in the pelvis is probably more common given the fragility of the thin vein wall and the extensive network of pelvic venous plexus. **Often a specific bleeding point cannot be identified but, after several minutes of direct pressure on the bleeding area, a clot will form over the low-pressure veins, and the bleeding will resolve. If it does not, control will have to be achieved with vascular clips, clamps, and suture ligature.** Slow but persistent oozing from unidentified vessels can often be controlled by products that either serve as a matrix for clotting (Avitene, Surgicel, Gelfoam) or supply clotting factors that complete the clotting cascade (CoSeal, TISSEEL, FLOSEAL). After application of any of these products, pressure should be applied to the site for 5 minutes and then the site should be reevaluated. If bleeding has not been controlled, it may be necessary to place a pack and transfer the patient to an ICU. In all cases, **it should be emphasized that prompt replacement of clotting factors provided by transfusion of FFP and platelets is critical to achieve hemostasis in the face of hemorrhage.**

Replacement of platelets and clotting factors in patients with massive transfusion and microvascular bleeding is dependent on clinical and surgical assessments. Guidelines have been provided by the American Society of Anesthesiologists task force regarding replacement of these products. In general, platelet transfusion is rarely indicated for counts greater than 100,000/μL and usually indicated for counts less than 50,000/μL (with intermediate platelet counts 50,000/μL to 100,000/μL, transfusion should be based on the risk of bleeding). FFP therapy is indicated in massively transfused patients with microvascular bleeding or hemorrhage if the prothrombin time (PT) or aPTT values exceed 1.5 times the normal values. In cases of massive intraoperative blood loss, it may be prudent to administer FFP empirically. This strategy is aimed at preventing the patient from becoming hypocoagulable while awaiting the laboratory results (PT and PTT), which may take nearly an hour and another hour to thaw the FFP before it is available to be administered. Cryoprecipitate transfusions are recommended for correction of microvascular bleeding in massively transfused patients with fibrinogen concentrations less than 80 to 100 mg/dL. **For trauma patients with massive blood loss, on the order of 30% to 40% of their blood volume, a transfusion ratio of 1:1:1 for PRBCs, FFP, and platelets has been consistently reported to be associated with decrease in death** caused by hemorrhage. **If surgical bleeding has taken on this level of severity, such a massive transfusion protocol should be initiated.**

Bleeding from the sacrum is usually not encountered except in the course of performing a total pelvic exenteration or rectosigmoid resection or during a sacral-colpopexy. **If bleeding from the sacrum cannot be controlled by suture ligatures or vascular clips, placement of sterile thumbtacks pushed into the sacral bone will usually compress veins exiting the sacrum and achieve hemostasis.**

Hypogastric (internal iliac) artery ligation. When the usual steps to control hemorrhage have failed, hypogastric artery ligation should be performed. Although the arterial blood supply to the pelvis is rich with anastomosis, ligation of the hypogastric arteries will usually decrease the arterial and venous pressure to the point at which (in a patient who is not hypocoagulable) venous bleeding will slow and can either be controlled by ligature or will clot with prolonged packing.

To safely perform hypogastric artery ligation, the vascular anatomy must be exposed, and adjacent structures, especially the ureter, must be identified. A retroperitoneal approach should be taken. The peritoneum overlying the psoas muscle (lateral to the external iliac artery) should be incised parallel to the artery. As the peritoneum is mobilized medially, the external iliac artery will first be identified. Dissection cephalad along the external iliac artery will identify the common iliac artery and the bifurcation of the internal iliac artery. **Invariably, the ureter crosses the pelvic brim at the bifurcation of the common iliac artery.** At this location, the ureter will be identified attached to the medial peritoneum. Further opening of the retroperitoneal space keeping the iliac vessels lateral and the ureter medial will create the pararectal space and further expose the internal iliac artery. Be aware that the common external and internal iliac veins lie just beneath their respective arteries. Without clear identification of these veins, injury can occur, which will further complicate the procedure. The hypogastric artery bifurcates into an anterior and posterior branch 2 to 3 cm from its origin from the common iliac artery. Because most bleeding arises from the blood supply from the anterior division, the anterior branch should be ligated if at all possible. (Ligation of the posterior branch increases the risk of buttock pain and potential necrosis of the gluteus.) A right angle clamp should be carefully passed from lateral to medial beneath the hypogastric artery. A heavy suture (eg, 0-silk) should be used to ligate the artery (Fig. 16.4). There is no reason to transect the artery between two ligatures. It is usually best to perform bilateral hypogastric artery ligation as the collateral blood supply crosses over the midline.

Finally, if all methods to control hemorrhage have been unsuccessful, the bleeding site should be packed firmly, and the abdomen should be closed. The patient should be taken to the surgical ICU and stabilized. Central monitoring and blood product replacement should be the primary focus of management. After the patient is stabilized, attempts at angiographic embolization should be considered. Ultimately, after 24 to 48 hours, the patient should be returned to the operating room and reexplored and the pack removed carefully. Surprisingly,

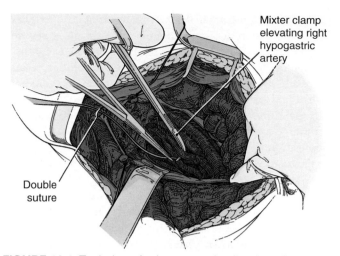

FIGURE 16.4 Technique for intraoperative ligation of the hypogastric artery. The ligature is placed 2 to 3 cm below the bifurcation so that the posterior branch will not be ligated. The clamp is passed lateral to medial to prevent trauma to the internal iliac vein. (From Nichols DH, Clarke-Pearson DL, eds. *Gynecologic, Obstetric and Related Surgery*, 2nd ed. St. Louis, 2000, Mosby.)

many times the bleeding will have stopped as a result of compression of the injured veins and correction of the hypocoagulable state.

Management of shock. During and after gynecologic surgery, blood-volume deficit that results from intraoperative blood loss or postoperative hemorrhage is the most common cause of shock. **This shock usually is manifested by arterial hypotension, tachycardia, a weak pulse, anxiety, skin pallor, diminished urinary output, and peripheral vasoconstriction.** In addition to hemorrhage (hypovolemic shock), the differential diagnosis of shock must include many other causes, such as cardiogenic (myocardial infarction) and cardiac compressive conditions (cardiac tamponade or pneumothorax), sepsis, drug overdose, and pulmonary embolism. Appropriate studies are dictated by the patient's signs and symptoms.

Consideration should be given to obtaining arterial blood gas analysis, an electrocardiogram, a chest radiograph, blood chemistry studies, and blood cultures. The patient should be prepared for blood transfusion. The degree and duration of postoperative shock determine the need for resuscitation, central venous pressure monitoring, and Swan-Ganz pulmonary artery catheterization.

Resuscitation of a hemorrhaging patient during or after gynecologic surgery involves stabilization of the hemodynamic status and correction of the cause of the blood loss. When the hemorrhage is massive, fluid, electrolyte, and hemodynamic shifts are likewise massive. Central to stabilization efforts are the replacement and maintenance of adequate intravascular volume.

Central monitoring. Invasive cardiovascular monitoring may be lifesaving for patients with massive hemorrhage or patients who are at additional risk because of preexisting cardiopulmonary disorders. The monitoring allows the rational use of fluids and cardioactive medications while avoiding their complications.

In patients with marked hemodynamic instability, peripheral artery cannulation allows continuous monitoring of systemic arterial pressure and ready access to obtain repeated analysis of arterial blood gases. The radial artery is usually chosen because of accessibility and has good collateral circulation, although the brachial and femoral arteries may be used. The complications of arterial cannulation include catheter-related septicemia (4% in one large study), local infection (as high as 18%), and arterial embolization (0.2%–0.6%).

In patients without cardiopulmonary disease, monitoring of central venous pressure along with monitoring of the vital signs, urine output, and other clinical signs usually provide sufficient information for appropriate fluid resuscitation. In addition, central venous pressure monitoring avoids several of the complications of a pulmonary artery (Swan-Ganz) catheter.

A central venous catheter may be introduced into the great intrathoracic veins by way of the antecubital, external or internal jugular, or subclavian veins. Cannulation of the right internal jugular vein, which provides a straight course to the right atrium, has the lowest overall complication rate. In all cases, a chest radiograph should be obtained immediately after catheter insertion to confirm proper location and to assess for possible pneumothorax.

The usefulness of the Swan-Ganz catheter in critically ill patients (even those without heart disease) who do not respond to therapy based on an initial noninvasive assessment is primarily limited to its use as a diagnostic monitoring tool. Several randomized trials, including those of high-risk surgical patients, have confirmed that there is no mortality benefit to use of the Swan-Ganz catheter. It does provide additional diagnostic information concerning unsuspected cardiac dysfunction, pulmonary artery embolization, or sepsis. Patients without primary myocardial insult but with hypotension and evidence of inadequate perfusion of vital organs (eg, oliguria, acidosis, mental obtundation) can be managed with more information (Table 16.2).

In patients with cardiac or pulmonary disease, cardiac output and resistance measurements allow the proper use of pressors, afterload and preload reducers, and fluids. In addition, if sepsis

TABLE 16.2	**Hemodynamic Calculations***	
Parameter	**Formula**	**Normal Range**
MAP	$\frac{1}{3}$ (SBP − DBP) + DBP	0.70–105 mm Hg
CO	Heart rate × Stroke volume	1.4–8 L/min
Cardiac index	CO/body surface area (m²)	2.5–4 L/min/m²
SVR	MAP − (Right arterial pressure/CO)	0.10–20 U
Pulmonary vascular resistance	PAP† − (PCWP/CO)	1.1–3 U

*Stroke volume can be derived from cardiac output (CO) and heart rate. Resistance is derived from a relative change in pressure on each side of the circuit from which resistance is to be measured.
†PAP = (2 [Pulmonary SBP] + Pulmonary DBP)/3.
DBP, Diastolic blood pressure; *MAP,* mean arterial pressure; *PAP,* mean pulmonary artery pressure; *PCWP,* pulmonary capillary wedge pressure; *SBP,* systolic blood pressure; *SVR,* systemic vascular resistance.

is part of the clinical picture, careful monitoring of pulmonary capillary wedge pressures may be necessary to prevent pulmonary edema, which is seen with even mild increases in left atrial pressures as a result of the increased permeability of the pulmonary vascular bed. This increased permeability also may be seen in patients in hypovolemic shock, again leading to pulmonary edema at relatively normal wedge pressures. Finally, invasive monitoring not only provides a direct measurement of cardiac function but also provides information within minutes about the effects of therapy.

These catheters may be placed from the antecubital fossa, although the percutaneous subclavian or internal or external jugular vein approaches are more commonly used. Complications of pulmonary artery catheters include pulmonary infarction distal to the catheter (1%–2% of cases), pulmonary artery rupture (0.2% of cases), balloon rupture (3% of cases), and sepsis (2% of cases), all of which are made more likely by prolonged use of the catheter.

Intraoperative Genitourinary Injuries

Given the close anatomic relationships of the gynecologic organs and the urinary tract, ureteral and bladder injury are to be anticipated, even in the hands of the most skilled surgeon. Prevention of urinary tract injury is predicated on the identification of the key urinary tract structures before embarking on radical or extended surgery for gynecologic cancers. Retroperitoneal exploration by opening the lateral retroperitoneal spaces (pararectal and paravesical spaces) allows for identification of the ureter and lateral bladder (and key vascular structures). If the medial pelvic peritoneum requires resection, the ureter must be detached from the peritoneum and mobilized laterally (ureterolysis). The ureter may be dissected throughout its entire pelvic course to the bladder, although between the uterine artery crossing the ureter and the insertion of the ureter into the bladder, techniques similar to those required for a type II or III radical hysterectomy will need to be used. Identification of the bladder is usually not a problem; however, because of anatomic distortion by advanced cancer, radiation therapy, or extensive adhesions from prior surgery, the bladder sometimes is not easily recognized. One simple method to identify the bladder is to fill it retrograde through the indwelling Foley catheter. With the bladder distended, dissection of the uterus or tumor from the bladder may be facilitated. Opening the retropubic space (space of Retzius) and the paravesical space also facilitates identification and protection of the bladder.

Injury to the bladder is usually easily corrected at the time of surgery. Incisions in the dome of the bladder should be closed in two layers with 3-0 or 2-0 delayed absorbable suture. The bladder should be allowed to heal by leaving the Foley catheter to dependent drainage for approximately 5 days. Cystotomies at the base of the bladder have a higher risk of fistula formation and ureteral occlusion. Furthermore, they may be more difficult to recognize. **Whenever there is concern about potential bladder injury, the bladder should be filled in a retrograde fashion with either sterile infant formula or indigo carmine–dyed saline.** The authors prefer infant formula because the formula does not stain tissues and potentially obscure the site of injury. After the cystotomy in the base of the bladder is identified, it is important to assess the location of the ureteral orifices. This may be accomplished by cystoscopy or by opening the dome of the bladder and directly visualizing the orifices. The administration of IV indigo carmine may aid in the identification of the orifices. Closure of the cystotomy should again be accomplished using two layers of delayed absorbable suture. **If the cystotomy is near the ureteral orifice, retrograde placement of a stent is prudent to ensure that there is no occlusion or narrowing of the ureter.** If the pelvis has been previously radiated, the authors recommend placement of an omental J-flap between the bladder and the vaginal cuff to bring a new, nonirradiated blood supply into this area. The Foley catheter should be left to drain for several weeks, and a cystogram should be obtained before the decision to remove the catheter.

Injury to the ureter as it passes through the pelvis may be managed by several methods depending on the location and extent of the injury. Ureteral injury above the pelvic brim is usually best managed by end-to-end anastomosis over a ureteral stent (Fig. 16.5). Injury below the pelvic brim may be best corrected by a ureteroneocystostomy with psoas hitch or a Boari

FIGURE 16.5 Ureteral injury at the pelvic brim repaired with an ureteroureterostomy using interrupted 4-0 delayed absorbance sutures. The ureter is spatulated to achieve a larger lumen at the anastomosis. The anastomosis is done over a ureteral stent, and the area is drained with a suction drain. (From Nichols DH, Clarke-Pearson DL, eds. *Gynecologic, Obstetric and Related Surgery*, 2nd ed. St. Louis, 2000, Mosby.)

flap (Fig. 16.6). In either method of repair placement, a closed suction drain in the pelvis is advised to prevent a urinoma from a leak of the anastomosis.

In cases of suspected injury to the ureter, IV indigo carmine should be injected, and the pelvis should be inspected for spill of dye-colored urine. If the extent of ureteral injury is a clamp crush or ligature, placement of a ureteral double-J stent left in place for 6 weeks will usually allow the injured ureter to recover and at the same time prevent ureteral stricture.

Postoperative Urinary Tract Injury

Unless bilateral ureteral obstruction has been caused by surgery, most patients with postoperative anuria or severe oliguria will have these findings secondary to prerenal hypovolemia, which will resolve with hydration and diuresis. **However, unilateral ureteral injury may not be recognized until several days postoperatively, manifest by flank pain, pyelonephritis, or a slight rise in serum creatinine.** The volume of urinary output is rarely altered. When postoperative ureteral obstruction is suspected, evaluation may include intravenous pyelography (IVP) or CT scan with contrast (when the serum creatinine level is normal) or with a renal ultrasound or Lasix renal scan. **If ureteral obstruction is discovered, initial management should include cystoscopy with retrograde stent placement.** If successful, the obstruction is likely a result of tethering from nearby sutures or extrinsic compression from a mass (hematoma, lymphocyst, tumor). Leaving the stent in place for 6 weeks and then reevaluating with follow-up IVP is recommended. If a stent cannot be placed, however, consideration should be given to reexploration to correct the obstruction. If reoperation is not reasonable, a PCN tube should be placed.

Urinary tract fistulae are recognized complications of radical hysterectomy for the primary treatment of cervical cancer, with recent estimates at just over 1% incidence. It is thought that the extensive dissection of the distal ureter and base of the bladder may lead to ischemic necrosis and the development of a vesicovaginal or ureterovaginal fistula. In contemporary reports, these fistulas occur in only 1% to 3% of cases. The risk of fistula is increased when surgery is performed after prior pelvic radiation therapy.

Vaginal leakage of fluid during the first 10 weeks postoperatively is an ominous finding and requires evaluation for a urinary tract fistula. Confirming the presence of a fistula and, if present, identifying the location are the next priorities. Clinic-based examinations include retrograde filling of the bladder with dyed (eg, indigo carmine) saline and inspection of the vaginal vault for vesicovaginal fistula and administration of IV indigo carmine or oral pyridium with vaginal inspection for ureterovaginal fistula. Both of these methods do carry false-negative risks, and even if negative, in cases of continued vaginal leakage, a definitive CT scan with IV contrast (CT urogram or CT of the abdomen and pelvis with delayed phase contrast) should be obtained. Acute vesicovaginal fistula should be managed by decompression of the bladder by placement of an indwelling Foley catheter to allow continuous drainage. This management often allows the fistula to close spontaneously. If a ureterovaginal fistula is discovered, a ureteral stent should be

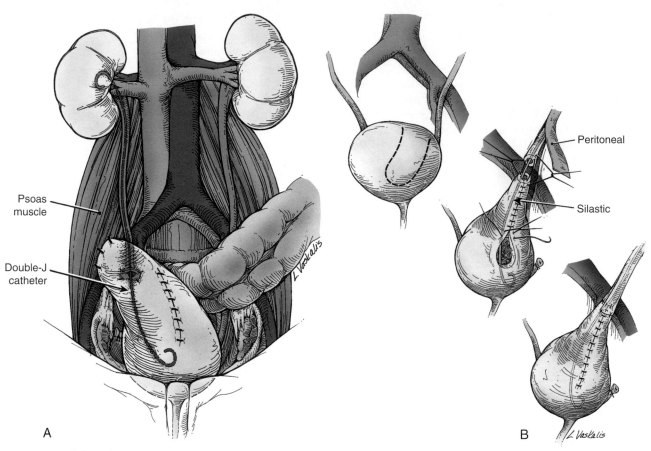

FIGURE 16.6 A, Ureteroneocystostomy with psoas hitch. The bladder is mobilized and sutured to the psoas muscle at the pelvic brim near the site of planned ureterovesical anastomosis. **B,** Boari flap. A flap from the dome of the bladder is created and "rolled" into a tube to substitute for the absent distal ureter and to reach the proximal ureter, which is reanastomosed. In either procedure, the area should be drained by closed suction. (From Nichols DH, Clarke-Pearson DL, eds. *Gynecologic, Obstetric and Related Surgery*, 2nd ed. St. Louis, 2000, Mosby.)

placed across the section of ureter that is fistualized. The stent may be placed retrograde at the time of cystoscopy or antegrade via a PCN. This usually allows the ureteral injury to heal "over" the stent. Throughout attempts at conservative management, prevention of UTI is an important priority. If after 6 weeks of conservative management the vesicovaginal or ureteral fistula has not resolved, surgical correction will be required.

Bladder Dysfunction After Radical Surgery

Voiding dysfunction after radical hysterectomy is commonly recognized and should be discussed in the preoperative informed consent. The exact frequency of occurrence depends on how the problem is diagnosed (patient report vs. prospective urodynamic testing) but occurs to a greater or lesser degree in nearly all patients. It is clear that a less radical hysterectomy (type I or II) is associated with a significantly lower incidence of bladder dysfunction as compared with the traditional radical (type III) hysterectomy.

Serial cystometric studies of patients undergoing radical hysterectomy have defined the natural history of bladder function in the perioperative period. **There is a nearly uniform development of detrusor hypertonia characterized by low capacity, high resting tone, and high filling pressure in the immediate postoperative phase.** Bladder insensitivity to filling is also present. The patient often has difficulty initiating her stream and may have overflow incontinence when the capacity is exceeded. **Hypertonia generally subsides within 3 to 6 months,** but other abnormalities often persist for years. The duration of bladder dysfunction is also variable, with extremes recognized as full recovery of bladder function to the rare patient who will require lifetime intermittent self-catheterization to achieve adequate bladder drainage. Many patients have persistent decrease in bladder sensation or prolonged urinary hesitancy.

The pathophysiologic mechanism of voiding dysfunction after radical hysterectomy is still not clearly understood. Some investigators have proposed that incomplete innervation of the bladder produced a temporary parasympathomimetic predominance that usually resolves with nerve regeneration. The use of parasympatholytic drugs, however, has been ineffective in altering the detrusor muscle function in this circumstance. Forney and colleagues have suggested that disruption of the sympathetic fibers that travel through the paracervical web results in loss of inhibition for the detrusor and trigone, leaving an uncoordinated parasympathetic dominance. This is supported by the observation that incomplete division of the cardinal ligament results in decreased postoperative detrusor hypertonia compared with complete division.

It also seems clear that overdistention of the bladder aggravates bladder dysfunction. Therefore, a variety of techniques have been proposed to avoid overdistention, including short- or long-term use of a urethral Foley catheter, suprapubic catheter, or intermittent self-catheterization. All techniques have their proponents and varying degrees of success, but none has been proven to be superior.

Intraoperative Gastrointestinal Injuries

A mechanical bowel preparation with preoperative oral antibiotics (eg, erythromycin and neomycin) should be planned for all patients undergoing major abdominal surgery for which bowel surgery is anticipated. Several retrospective and prospective cohort studies of patients undergoing colorectal resection for colon cancer consistently demonstrate decreases in surgical site infection, anastomotic leak, and ileus in patients receiving both mechanical and antibiotic preparation. In a prospective cohort study of over 1500 patients, mechanical preparation plus oral antibiotics resulted in lower infection (4.6% vs. 12.4%; $P <0.001$) and lower rate of ileus (3.8% vs. 8.9%; $P = 0.006$) compared with mechanical preparation alone. Additionally, researchers using a national surgical quality database of more than 8000 patients found that surgical site infection (6.1% vs. 12.0% vs. 14.3%), anastomotic leak (2.0% vs. 3.6% vs. 4.5%), postoperative ileus (9.1% vs. 12.1% vs. 15.1%), and 30-day mortality rate (0.4% vs. 0.6% vs. 1.5%) were all reduced in the dual prep method versus mechanical preparation alone versus no preparation. It should be noted that all patients in these studies also received parenteral antibiotics, confirming the additional benefit of the dual preparation. Bowel preparation may also reduce the risk of intraoperative intestinal injury, and if injury does occur, spill of GI contents can be minimized. Mechanical methods to prepare the bowel include the use of cathartics such as magnesium citrate or the ingestion of 4 L of polyethylene glycol (GoLYTELY).

Prior abdominal surgery and radiation therapy increase the probability of intraoperative injury to the small intestine. Adhesions to the anterior abdominal wall or small intestines adherent to the pelvic peritoneum increase the risk of entry into the intestines as adhesions are lysed. Interruption of the serosal and superficial muscular layers should be repaired with interrupted 2-0 or 3-0 sutures. Care should be taken to avoid narrowing of the intestinal caliber (Fig. 16.7). If the entire thickness of the intestine is entered, the segment of bowel must be assessed to decide whether primary closure should be undertaken or whether bowel resection and anastomosis should be performed. Primary closure is usually safely accomplished if the closure can reapproximate well-perfused bowel under no tension on the suture line and the bowel lumen is not narrowed. If these conditions cannot be met, resection and anastomosis will be necessary.

Primary closure of an enterotomy should be in two layers, the first being an interrupted layer of 2-0 or 3-0 polyglycolic

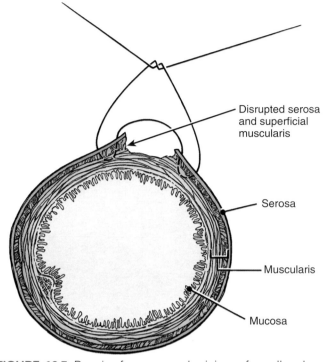

FIGURE 16.7 Repair of seromuscular injury of small or larger bowel. Interrupted imbricating sutures are used to reapproximate the injured seromuscular layer. (From Nichols DH, Clarke-Pearson DL, eds. *Gynecologic, Obstetric and Related Surgery*, 2nd ed. St. Louis, 2000, Mosby.)

Disrupted serosa and superficial muscularis

Serosa

Muscularis

Mucosa

acid suture incorporating the mucosa and muscularis, with the knot tied into the intestinal lumen. A second imbricating layer may be of either absorbable or nonabsorbable suture and incorporates the serosa and superficial muscularis (Fig. 16.8). Attention to the direction of closure of the enterotomy should ensure that the lumen is not narrowed.

Injury to the colon most commonly occurs in the pelvis, and the risk is increased in the face of prior pelvic surgery, cancer involving the colon, or prior radiation therapy. If colonic injury occurs, the decision must be made as to whether a primary closure is sufficiently safe or whether the fecal stream should be temporarily diverted by performing a transverse loop colostomy or ileostomy. **In most cases, primary closure without diversion may be performed; especially if the patient has had a mechanical bowel preparation.** The principles for closure require viable tissue and no tension on the closure. In patients who have had prior pelvic radiation, the risk of perforation of the colostomy closure is significantly increased, and diversion is usually advised. After a two-layered closure of a rectosigmoid injury, the authors routinely perform proctoscopy and a "bubble test" (Fig. 16.9). If either test suggests a defect in the reanastomosis, a diverting ostomy is again recommended.

Postoperative Gastrointestinal Complications

Ileus. After abdominal or pelvic surgery, most patients experience some degree of intestinal ileus. The exact mechanism by which this arrest and disorganization of GI motility occurs

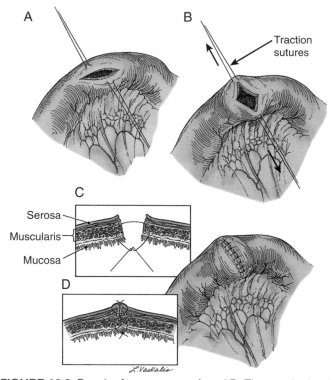

FIGURE 16.8 Repair of enterotomy. **A** and **B**, The repair should be performed so that the closure is perpendicular to the axis of the small bowel. **C** and **D**, Two-layer closure incorporating the mucosa and muscularis in the inner layer and the serosa and muscularis on the outer layer. (From Nichols DH, Clarke-Pearson DL, eds. *Gynecologic, Obstetric and Related Surgery*, 2nd ed. St. Louis, 2000, Mosby.)

is unknown, but it appears to be associated with the opening of the peritoneal cavity and is aggravated by manipulation of the intestinal tract and prolonged surgical procedures. (Ileus is much less commonly associated with minimally invasive surgical procedures. If ileus were to occur after laparoscopy or robotic surgery, the surgeon should strongly consider a more serious bowel injury and evaluate the patient accordingly.) Infection, peritonitis, postoperative hypervolemia causing bowel wall edema, and electrolyte disturbances may also result in ileus. For most patients undergoing gynecologic cancer operations, the degree of ileus is minimal and GI function returns relatively rapidly, allowing the resumption of oral intake within a few days of surgery. Patients who have persistently diminished bowel sounds, abdominal distention, and nausea and vomiting require further evaluation and more aggressive management.

Ileus is usually manifest by abdominal distention and should be evaluated initially by physical examination assessing the quality of bowel sounds and searching for tenderness or rebound on palpation. The possibility that the patient's signs and symptoms may be associated with a more serious intestinal obstruction or other intestinal complication must be considered. Pelvic examination should be performed to evaluate the possibility of a pelvic abscess or hematoma that may contribute to the ileus. Abdominal radiography to evaluate the abdomen in the supine position and in the upright position usually will aid in the diagnosis of an ileus. The most common radiographic findings include dilated loops of small and large bowel and air–fluid levels in the upright position. In postoperative patients, especially in the upright position, the flat plate of the abdomen may also show evidence of free air. This is a common finding

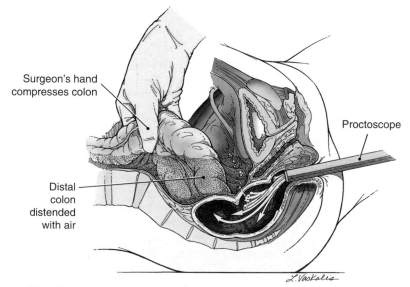

FIGURE 16.9 "Bubble test" to evaluate for rectosigmoid injury and to ensure a "watertight" closure of a colostomy or rectosigmoid anastomosis. The pelvis is filled with saline, and the proximal sigmoid or descending colon is occluded above the segment to be tested. Insert a proctoscope into the anus and inflate with air. Distend the occluded rectosigmoid colon with air and observe for bubbles, which would indicate a bowel defect. (From Nichols DH, Clarke-Pearson DL, eds. *Gynecologic, Obstetric and Related Surgery*, 2nd ed. St. Louis, 2000, Mosby.)

after surgery; it lasts 7 to 10 days in some instances and is not indicative of a perforated viscus in most patients. The remote possibility of distal colonic obstruction or pseudoobstruction (Ogilvie syndrome) suggested by a dilated cecum should be excluded by rectal examination, proctosigmoidoscopy, or barium enema.

The initial management of a postoperative ileus is aimed at GI tract decompression and maintenance of appropriate IV replacement fluids and electrolytes.

1. If a patient has moderate to severe vomiting, not improved with bowel rest and antiemetics, an NG tube should be placed to evacuate the stomach of its fluid and gaseous contents. Prolonged NG suction continues to remove swallowed air, which is the most common source of air in the small bowel.

2. Fluid and electrolyte replacement must be adequate to keep the patient well perfused. Significant amounts of third-space fluid loss occur in the bowel wall, the bowel lumen, and the peritoneal cavity during the acute episode. GI fluid losses from the stomach may also lead to a metabolic alkalosis and depletion of other electrolytes. Careful monitoring of serum chemistries and appropriate replacement are necessary.

3. Most cases of severe ileus begin to improve over a period of several days. In general, this is recognized by reduction in the abdominal distention, return of normal bowel sounds, and passage of flatus or stool. Follow-up abdominal radiographs should be obtained as necessary for further monitoring.

   • When the GI tract function appears to have returned to normal, the NG tube may be removed, and a liquid diet may be instituted.
   • If a patient shows no evidence of improvement during the first 48 to 72 hours of medical management, other causes of ileus should be sought. Such cases may include ureteral injury, peritonitis from pelvic infection, unrecognized GI tract injury with peritoneal spill, or fluid and electrolyte abnormalities such as hypokalemia. In the evaluation of persistent ileus, the use of water-soluble upper GI contrast studies may assist in the resolution of the ileus, the recognition of a small bowel obstruction, or injury (leak) of the GI tract.

Small bowel obstruction. Obstruction of the small bowel after abdominal surgery occurs in approximately 1% to 2% of patients, but it may be more common after radical gynecologic oncology procedures as a result of the extensive dissection and manipulation of the small bowel. (Again, this complication is less common in patients who have undergone minimally invasive surgery.) **The most common cause of small bowel obstruction is adhesions to the operative site.** If the small bowel becomes adherent in a twisted position, partial or complete obstruction may result from distention, ileus, or bowel wall edema. Less common causes of postoperative small bowel obstruction include entrapment of the small bowel into an incisional hernia and an unrecognized defect in the small bowel or large bowel mesentery. Early in its clinical course, a postoperative small bowel obstruction may exhibit signs and symptoms identical to those of ileus. **Initial conservative management as outlined for the treatment of ileus is appropriate.** Because of

the potential for mesenteric vascular occlusion and resulting ischemia or perforation, worsening symptoms of abdominal pain, progressive distention, fever, leukocytosis, or acidosis should be evaluated carefully because immediate surgery may be required.

However, in most cases of postoperative small bowel obstruction, the obstruction is only partial, and the problem usually resolves with conservative management.

   • After several days of conservative management (NG tube drainage, fluid and electrolyte replacement), further investigation may be necessary. Evaluation of the GI tract with barium enema and an upper GI series with small bowel follow-through is appropriate. Alternatively, an abdominal and pelvic CT scan with GI contrast may be useful in identifying the location of obstruction ("transition point") and evaluates for the presence of an abscess, lymphocele, or ureteral injury. In most cases, complete obstruction is not documented, although a narrowing or tethering of the segment of small bowel may indicate the site of the problem.
   • Further conservative management with NG decompression and IV fluid replacement may allow time for bowel wall edema or torsion of the mesentery to resolve.
   • If resolution is prolonged and the patient's nutritional status is marginal, the use of TPN may be necessary.

4. Conservative medical management of postoperative small bowel obstruction usually results in complete resolution. However, if persistent evidence of small bowel obstruction remains after full evaluation and an adequate trial of medical management, exploratory laparotomy may be necessary to surgically evaluate and manage the obstruction. In most cases, lysis of adhesions is all that is required, although a segment of small bowel that is badly damaged or extensively sclerosed from adhesions may require resection and reanastomosis.

Colonic obstruction. Postoperative colonic obstruction after gynecologic oncology surgery is exceedingly rare. Advanced ovarian carcinoma is the most common cause of colonic obstruction in postoperative gynecologic surgery patients and is caused by extrinsic impingement on the colon by the pelvic malignancy. Occult intrinsic colonic lesions (eg, colon cancer) also may cause obstruction. When colonic obstruction is manifest by abdominal distention and abdominal radiographs reveal a dilated colon and enlarging cecum, further evaluation of the large bowel is required by barium enema or colonoscopy. **Dilation of the cecum to more than 10 cm to 12 cm in diameter as viewed by abdominal radiography requires immediate evaluation because there is a higher probability of colonic perforation.** When there is no logical cause for a mechanical obstruction, Ogilvie syndrome should be considered. Colonoscopy should be performed, and the colonic gas should be evacuated. If a true mechanical obstruction is documented, surgical decompression by performing a colectomy, colostomy, or cecostomy may be required on an urgent basis. In some circumstances, an intraluminal stent may be placed endoscopically. Surgery should be performed as soon as the obstruction is documented. **Conservative management of colonic** obstruction is not appropriate because the complication of colonic perforation has an exceedingly high mortality rate.

Diarrhea. Episodes of diarrhea often occur after abdominal and pelvic surgery as the GI tract returns to its normal function and motility. However, prolonged and multiple episodes may represent a pathologic process such as impending small bowel obstruction, colonic obstruction, or pseudomembranous colitis. Excessive amounts of diarrhea should be evaluated by abdominal radiographs and stool samples tested for the presence of ova and parasites, bacterial culture, and *Clostridium difficile* toxin. Proctoscopy and colonoscopy may also be advisable in severe cases. Evidence of intestinal obstruction should be managed as outlined previously. Infectious causes of diarrhea should be managed with the appropriate antibiotics and fluid and electrolyte replacement. *C. difficile*–associated pseudomembranous colitis may result from recent exposure to any antibiotic. Discontinuation of these antibiotics (unless they are needed for another severe infection) is advisable, along with the institution of appropriate therapy. Because of the expense of vancomycin, the authors usually institute therapy with oral metronidazole for mild to moderate cases. Because of rising resistance to oral metronidazole, initiation of treatment with oral vancomycin may be necessary because clinical success (resolution of diarrhea) is lower (73% vs. 81%; *P* = 0.02) with metronidazole. Therapy should be continued until the diarrhea abates, and several weeks of oral therapy may be required to obtain complete resolution of the pseudomembranous colitis.

Fistula. Gastrointestinal fistulas are relatively rare after gynecologic surgery. They are most often associated with malignancy, prior radiation therapy, or surgical injury to the large or small bowel that was unrecognized or a leak from an anastomosis. Signs and symptoms of GI fistula are often similar to those of small bowel obstruction or ileus except that a fever is usually a more prominent component of the patient's symptoms. When fever is associated with GI dysfunction postoperatively, evaluation should include early assessment of the GI tract for its continuity. When fistula is suspected, the use of water-soluble GI contrast material is advised to avoid the complication of barium peritonitis. Evaluation with abdominal pelvic CT scan may also assist in identification of a fistula and associated abscess. Recognition of an intraperitoneal GI leak or fistula formation usually requires immediate surgery unless the fistula has drained spontaneously through the abdominal wall or vaginal cuff.

An enterocutaneous fistula arising from the small bowel and draining spontaneously through the abdominal incision may be managed successfully with medical therapy. Therapy should include NG decompression, replacement of IV fluids, TPN, and appropriate antibiotics to treat an associated mixed bacterial infection. If the infection is under control and there are no other signs of peritonitis, the surgeon may consider allowing potential resolution of the fistula over a period of up to 6 weeks. Some authors have suggested the use of somatostatin to decrease intestinal tract secretion and allow earlier healing of the fistula. In many cases, especially if the bowel was not radiated, the fistula will close spontaneously with this mode of management. If the enterocutaneous fistula does not close with conservative medical management, surgical correction with resection, bypass, or reanastomosis will be necessary in most cases.

A rectovaginal fistula that occurs after gynecologic surgery is usually the result of surgical trauma that may have been aggravated by the presence of extensive adhesions or tumor involvement of the rectosigmoid colon and cul de sac. Low rectal anastomoses are also at risk to breakdown and lead to a rectovaginal fistula. Perforation of a colonic diverticulum is another possible cause for a colovaginal fistula. A small rectovaginal fistula may be managed with a conservative medical approach in the hope that decreasing the fecal stream will allow closure of the fistula. A small fistula that allows continence except for an occasional leak of flatus may be managed conservatively until the inflammatory process in the pelvis resolves. At that point, usually several months later, correction of the fistula is appropriate. Larger rectovaginal fistulas that have no hope of closing spontaneously are best managed by performing an initial diverting colostomy followed by repair of the fistula after inflammation has resolved. After the fistula closure is healed and deemed successful, the colostomy may be taken down and closed.

Lymphedema

Lower extremity lymphedema can occur after pelvic, paraaortic, or inguinal lymph node dissections that are commonly part of comprehensive surgical staging for gynecologic cancers. In addition to swelling, patients may report sensations of heaviness, numbness, aching, and pain. When defined as early accumulation of fluid that resides with limb elevation, the rate of lymphedema has been reported as high as 35%, although symptomatic rate of occurrence may be lower (5%–15%). This discrepancy is secondary to both a lack of a consensus definition of lymphedema and a paucity of studies. Patients presenting with lymphedema postoperatively should have early referral to physical therapy services specializing in lymphedema to reduce long-term swelling and improve quality of life.

Lymphocysts

The occurrence of lymphocysts after pelvic and paraaortic lymphadenectomy occurs in approximately 20% of cases, but it symptomatic in as few as 2% to 6%. It has been suggested that prevention requires the ligation of the ascending lymphatics at the time of lymphadenectomy. Furthermore, there is evidence that the use of low-dose heparin increases lymphatic drainage and lymphocyst formation. In years past, the parietal peritoneum was closed after lymphadenectomy, and a closed-suction drain was placed in the retroperitoneal space to aspirate any lymphatic fluid. Certainly, a suction drain is reasonable and likely does prevent lymphocysts whenever the retroperitoneum is closed. Currently, most gynecologic oncologists do not close the peritoneum, allowing the lymphatic fluid to drain into the peritoneal cavity and be reabsorbed. Retrospective reports indicate that there is no increase in lymphocyst formation using this strategy. However, the problem of lymphocyst formation has not been entirely eliminated.

Lymphocysts may be recognized clinically by palpation of a mass along the pelvic sidewall or in the iliac fossa on abdominal examination. **Most will be asymptomatic.** However, when a lymphocyst is found, investigation should be undertaken to evaluate for the possibility of ureteral or venous obstruction. **If hydroureter is found, the lymphocyst should be drained.** This may usually be accomplished by an interventional radiologist who can place a percutaneous drain in the lymphocyst. Suction drainage will collapse the lymphocyst and allow the cyst walls to sclerose together. If percutaneous drainage is not feasible or is unsuccessful, surgical exploration may be required to excise a wall of the lymphocyst and allow the lymphatic fluid to drain into the peritoneal cavity. There are reports of successfully performing this surgery laparoscopically. Placing an omental J flap into the cavity of the lymphocyst has been suggested to provide additional routes of lymphatic drainage. When extrinsic venous compression is discovered to be associated with a lymphocyst, the patient should be evaluated for the possibility of a venous thrombosis. If a venous thrombosis is found, the authors advise anticoagulation in order to stop propagation and allow stabilization of the thrombus. Thereafter the lymphocyst should be drained. Drainage of the lymphocyst before anticoagulation may result in venous decompression and subsequent embolization of the thrombus. Rarely, lymphocysts will become infected and require drainage and antibiotic therapy.

Lymphocysts can also occur in the inguinal region after inguinofemoral lymphadenectomy performed as part of the staging and treatment of vulvar carcinoma. **Small, asymptomatic lymphocysts may be managed by observation.** However, larger lymphocysts usually cause pain or lymphedema and require drainage with placement of a closed-suction drain. If repeated aspiration is required, sclerotherapy should be considered.

Postoperative Infections

Infections are a major source of morbidity in the postoperative period. Risk factors for infectious morbidity in gynecologic oncology patients include a lack of perioperative antibiotic prophylaxis, contamination of the surgical field from infected tissues or from spillage of large bowel contents, an immunocompromised host, diabetes, poor nutrition, chronic and debilitating severe illness, poor surgical technique, and preexisting focal or systemic infection. Sources of postoperative infection can include the lung, urinary tract, surgical site, pelvic sidewall, vaginal cuff, abdominal wound, and sites of indwelling IV catheters. Early identification and treatment of any infections will result in the best outcome from these potentially serious complications.

Although infectious morbidity is an inevitable complication of surgery, the incidence of infections can be decreased by the appropriate use of simple preventive measures. In cases that involve transection of the large bowel, spillage of fecal contents also inevitably occurs. Preoperative mechanical preparation in combination with oral and systemic antibiotic prophylaxis will help decrease the incidence of postoperative pelvic and abdominal infections in these patients. The surgeon can further decrease the risk of postoperative infections by using meticulous surgical technique. Blood and necrotic tissue are excellent media for the growth of aerobic and anaerobic organisms. When there is higher-than-usual potential for serum and blood to collect in spaces that have been contaminated by bacterial spill, closed-suction drainage may reduce the risk of infection. Elective surgical procedures should be postponed in patients who have an infection preoperatively.

Historically, the standard definition of febrile morbidity for surgical patients has been the presence of a temperature of 100.4°F (38°C) or higher on two occasions at least 4 hours apart in the postoperative period, excluding the first 24 hours. However, other sources have defined fever as two consecutive temperature elevations greater than 101.0°F (38.3°C). Febrile morbidity has been estimated to occur in as many as half of patients; however, it is often self-limited, resolves without therapy, and is usually noninfectious in origin.

The assessment of febrile surgical patients should include a review of the patient's history with regard to risk factors. Both the history and the physical examination should focus on the potential sites of infection. The examination should include inspection of the pharynx, a thorough pulmonary examination, percussion of the kidneys to assess for costovertebral angle tenderness, inspection and palpation of the abdominal incision, examination of sites of IV catheters, and an examination of the extremities for evidence of DVT or thrombophlebitis. In gynecologic surgery patients, an appropriate workup may also include inspection and palpation of the vaginal cuff for signs of induration, tenderness, or purulent drainage. **A pelvic examination should also be performed to identify a mass suggesting a pelvic hematoma or abscess and to recognize signs of pelvic cellulitis.**

Patients with a fever in the early postoperative period should have an aggressive pulmonary toilet, including incentive spirometry. If the fever persists beyond 72 hours postoperatively, additional laboratory and radiologic data may be obtained. The evaluation may include complete and differential white blood cell counts and a urinalysis. A routine urine culture has a yield of only 9%; therefore, one should not be sent unless indicated by the urinalysis results or symptoms. Routine chest radiographs have a yield of 6% to 12.5% and should be obtained in patients with and without signs and symptoms localizing to the lung. Blood cultures can also be obtained but will most likely be of little benefit unless the patient has a high fever (102°F). In patients with costovertebral angle tenderness, CT scan, renal ultrasonography, or IVP may be indicated to rule out the presence of ureteral damage or obstruction from surgery, particularly in the absence of laboratory evidence of UTI. Patients who have persistent fevers without a clear localizing source should undergo CT scanning of the abdomen and pelvis to rule out the presence of an intraabdominal abscess. Finally, in patients who have had GI surgery, a CT scan with oral contrast, a barium enema, or an upper GI series with small bowel follow-through may be indicated late in the course of the first postoperative week if fever persists to rule out an anastomotic leak or fistula.

Urinary tract infections. Historically, the urinary tract has been the most common site of infection in surgical patients.

However, the incidence reported in the more recent gynecologic literature has been less than 4%. This decrease in UTIs is most likely the result of increased perioperative use of prophylactic antibiotics.

Symptoms of a UTI may include urinary frequency, urgency, and dysuria. In patients with pyelonephritis, other symptoms include flank pain, headache, malaise, nausea, and vomiting. A UTI is diagnosed on the basis of microbiology and has been defined as the growth of 10^5 organisms/mL urine cultured. Most infections are caused by coliform bacteria, with *Escherichia coli* being the most common pathogen. Other pathogens include *Klebsiella*, *Proteus*, and *Enterobacter* spp. *Staphylococcus* organisms are the causative bacteria in fewer than 10% of cases.

Despite the high incidence of UTIs in the postoperative period, few of these infections are serious. Most are confined to the lower urinary tract, and pyelonephritis is a rare complication. Catheterization of the urinary tract, either intermittently or continuously with the use of an indwelling catheter, has been implicated as a main cause of urinary tract contamination.

The treatment of UTI includes hydration and antibiotic therapy. Commonly prescribed and effective antibiotics include sulfonamide, cephalosporins, fluoroquinolones, and nitrofurantoin. The choice of antibiotic should be based on knowledge of the susceptibility of organisms cultured at a particular institution. In some institutions, for example, more than 40% of *E. coli* strains are resistant to ampicillin. For uncomplicated UTIs, an antibiotic that has good activity against *E. coli* should be given in the interim while awaiting the urine culture and sensitivity data.

Patients who have a history of recurrent UTIs, those with chronic indwelling catheters (Foley catheters or ureteral stents), and those who have urinary conduits should be treated with antibiotics that will be effective against the less common urinary pathogens such as *Klebsiella* and *Pseudomonas* spp. Chronic use of the fluoroquinolones for prophylaxis is not advised because these agents are notorious for inducing antibiotic-resistant strains of bacteria.

Pulmonary infections. The respiratory tract is a relatively common site for complications after surgery for gynecologic cancer. Risk factors include extensive or prolonged atelectasis, preexistent chronic obstructive pulmonary disease, severe or debilitating illness, central neurologic disease causing an inability to clear oropharyngeal secretions effectively, and NG suction. In surgical patients, early ambulation and aggressive management of atelectasis are the most important preventive measures.

A significant proportion (40%–50%) of hospital-acquired pneumonias are caused by Gram-negative organisms. These organisms gain access to the respiratory tract from the oral pharynx. Gram-negative colonization of the oral pharynx has been shown to be increased in patients in acute care facilities and has been associated with the presence of NG tubes, preexisting respiratory disease, mechanical ventilation, tracheal intubation, and paralytic ileus (which is associated with microbial overgrowth in the stomach).

A thorough lung examination should be included in the assessment of all febrile surgical patients. In the absence of significant lung findings, chest radiography should nonetheless be obtained in patients at high risk for pulmonary complications. A sputum sample should also be obtained for Gram stain and culture. The treatment should include postural drainage, aggressive pulmonary toilet, and antibiotics. The antibiotic chosen should be effective against both Gram-positive and Gram-negative organisms, and in patients who are receiving assisted ventilation, the antibiotic spectrum should include drugs that are active against *Pseudomonas* organisms.

Wound infections. The results of a prospective study of more than 62,000 wounds are revealing in regard to the epidemiology of wound infections. The wound infection rate varied markedly, depending on the extent of contamination of the surgical field. The wound infection rate for clean surgical cases (infection not present in the surgical field, no break in aseptic technique, no viscus entered) was lower than 2%, but the incidence of wound infections with dirty, infected cases was 40% or higher. Preoperative showers with hexachlorophene slightly lowered the infection rate for clean wounds, but preoperative shaving of the wound site with a razor (but not clippers) increased the infection rate. A 5-minute wound preparation immediately before surgery was as effective as preparation 10 minutes before surgery. The wound infection rate increased with the duration of the preoperative hospital stay and with the duration of the surgical procedure. (Prophylactic antibiotics should be readministered if the surgical procedure lasts longer than 4 hours.) In addition, incidental appendectomy increased the risk of wound infection in patients undergoing clean surgical procedures. The study concluded that the incidence of wound infections could be decreased by short preoperative hospital stays, hexachlorophene showers before surgery, clipping hair (not shaving) of the wound site immediately before incision, use of meticulous surgical technique, decreasing operative time as much as possible, bringing drains out through sites other than the wound, and dissemination of information to surgeons regarding their wound infection rates. A program instituting these conclusions led to a fall in the clean wound infection rate from 2.5% to 0.6% over an 8-year period. Although the wound infection rate in most gynecologic services has been lower than 5%, reflective of the "clean" nature of most gynecologic operations, it is higher in gynecologic oncology patients.

The symptoms of wound infection often occur late in the postoperative period, usually after the fourth postoperative day, and may include the presence of fever, erythema, tenderness, induration, and purulent wound drainage. Wound infections that occur on postoperative days 1 through 3 are generally caused by streptococcal and clostridial infections. The management of wound infections is mostly mechanical and involves opening the infected portion of the wound above the fascia, with cleansing and débridement of the wound edges as necessary. Wound care, consisting of débridement and dressing changes two to three times daily with mesh gauze, will promote growth of granulation tissue, with gradual filling in of the wound defect by secondary intention. **The application of a Wound-Vac (negative pressure wound therapy) to larger wounds speeds recovery and minimizes dressing changes.**

In a gynecologic oncology population, the median number of days of wound vac therapy was 32 days (range, 3–88 days) with a 96% reduction in the median size of the wounds. Clean, granulating wounds can often be secondarily closed with good success, shortening the time required for complete wound healing.

The technique of delayed primary wound closure can be used in contaminated surgical cases to reduce the incidence of wound infection. Briefly, this technique involves leaving the wound open above the fascia at the time of the initial surgical procedure. Vertical interrupted mattress sutures though the skin and subcutaneous layers are placed 3 cm apart but are not tied. Wound care is instituted immediately after surgery and continued until the wound is noted to be granulating well. Sutures may then be tied, and the skin edges can be further approximated using sutures or staples. Using this technique of delayed primary wound closure, the overall wound infection rate has been shown to be decreased from 23% to 2.1% in high-risk patients.

Vaginal cuff infection after hysterectomy is characterized by erythema, induration, and tenderness at the vaginal cuff. Occasionally, a purulent discharge from the apex of the vagina may also be present. The cellulitis is often self-limited and does not require any treatment. Fever, leukocytosis, and pain localized to the pelvis may accompany severe cuff cellulitis and most often signifies extension of the cellulitis to adjacent pelvic tissues. In such cases, broad-spectrum antibiotic therapy should be instituted with coverage for Gram-negative, Gram-positive, and anaerobic organisms. If purulence at the vaginal cuff is excessive or if there is a fluctuant mass noted at the vaginal cuff, the vaginal cuff should be gently probed and opened with a blunt instrument. The cuff can then be left open for dependent drainage.

Intraabdominal and pelvic abscess. The development of an abscess in the surgical field or elsewhere in the abdominal cavity is most likely to occur in contaminated cases in which the surgical site is not adequately drained or as a secondary complication of hematoma that becomes infected. The causative pathogens in patients who have intraabdominal abscess are usually polymicrobial in nature. The aerobes most commonly identified include *E. coli* and *Klebsiella, Streptococcus, Proteus,* and *Enterobacter* spp. Anaerobic isolates are also common, usually from the *Bacteroides* group. These pathogens are mainly from the vagina but also can be derived from the GI tract, particularly when the colon has been entered at the time of surgery.

An intraabdominal abscess is sometimes difficult to diagnose. The evolving clinical picture is often one of persistent febrile episodes with a rising white blood cell count. Findings on abdominal examination may be equivocal. If an abscess is located deep in the pelvis, it may be palpable by pelvic or rectal examination. For abscesses above the pelvis, diagnosis will depend on radiologic confirmation.

Ultrasonography can occasionally delineate fluid collections in the upper abdomen and the pelvis. However, bowel gas interference makes visualization of fluid collections or abscesses in the mid-abdomen difficult to distinguish. CT scanning with oral and IV contrast is much more sensitive and specific for diagnosing intraabdominal abscesses and is the radiologic procedure of choice.

Standard therapy for an intraabdominal abscess is drainage combined with appropriate parenteral administration of antibiotics. Abscesses located low in the pelvis, particularly in the area of the vaginal cuff, can often be reached through a vaginal approach. In many patients, the ability to drain an abscess by placement of a drain percutaneously under CT guidance has obviated the need for surgical exploration. With CT guidance, a pigtail catheter is placed into an abscess cavity via percutaneous, transperineal, transrectal, or transvaginal approaches. The catheter is left in place and irrigated daily until drainage decreases. Transperineal and transrectal drainage of deep pelvic abscesses has been successful in 90% to 93% of patients, obviating the need for surgical management. However, for patients in whom radiologic drainage is not successful, surgical exploration and evacuation are indicated. The gold standard of initial antibiotic therapy has been the combination of ampicillin, gentamycin, and clindamycin. Adequate treatment can also be achieved with currently available broad-spectrum single agents (including the broad-spectrum penicillin), second- and third-generation cephalosporins, levofloxacin and metronidazole, and the sulbactam/clavulanic acid–containing preparations.

Necrotizing fasciitis. Necrotizing fasciitis is an uncommon infectious disorder; approximately 1000 cases occur annually in the United States. **The disorder is characterized by a rapidly progressive bacterial infection involving the subcutaneous tissues and fascia while characteristically sparing underlying muscle.** Systemic toxicity is a common feature of this disease, as manifested by the presence of dehydration, septic shock, disseminated intravascular coagulation, and multiorgan system failure.

The pathogenesis of necrotizing fasciitis involves a polymicrobial infection of the dermis and subcutaneous tissue. Historically, hemolytic streptococcus was believed to be the primary pathogen responsible for necrotizing fasciitis. However, it is now evident that numerous other organisms are present in addition to streptococcus, including other Gram-positive organisms, coliforms, and anaerobes. Bacterial enzymes such as hyaluronidase and lipase released in the subcutaneous space destroy the fascia and adipose tissue and induce a liquefactive necrosis. In addition, noninflammatory intravascular coagulation or thrombosis subsequently occurs. Intravascular coagulation results in ischemia and necrosis of the subcutaneous tissues and skin. Late in the course of the infection, destruction of the superficial nerves produces anesthesia in the involved skin. The release of bacteria and bacterial toxins into the systemic circulation results in septic shock, acid–base disturbances, and multiorgan impairment.

The diagnostic criteria for necrotizing fasciitis include extensive necrosis of the superficial fascia and subcutaneous tissue with peripheral undermining of the normal skin, a moderate to severe systemic toxic reaction, the absence of muscle involvement, the absence of clostridia in wound and blood culture, the absence of major vascular occlusion, intensive leukocytic infiltration, and necrosis of subcutaneous tissue.

Most patients with necrotizing fasciitis suffer pain, which in the early stages of the disease is often disproportionately greater than that expected from the degree of cellulitis present. Late in the course of the infection, the involved skin may actually be anesthetized secondary to necrosis of superficial nerves. Temperature abnormalities, both hyperthermia and hypothermia, are concomitant with the release of bacterial toxins and with bacterial sepsis, which is present in up to 40% of patients. The involved skin is initially tender, erythematous, and warm. Edema develops, and the erythema spreads diffusely, fading into normal skin, characteristically without distinct margins or induration. Subcutaneous microvascular thrombosis induces ischemia in the skin, which becomes cyanotic and blistered. **As necrosis progresses, the skin becomes gangrenous and may slough spontaneously.** Most patients will have leukocytosis and acid–base abnormalities. **Finally, subcutaneous gas may develop, which can be identified by palpation (crepitus) and by radiograph.** The finding of subcutaneous gas by radiograph is often indicative of clostridial infection, although it is not a specific finding and may be caused by other organisms. These organisms include *Enterobacter* spp., *Pseudomonas* spp., anaerobic streptococci, and *Bacteroides* spp., which, unlike clostridial infections, spare the muscles underlying the affected area. A tissue biopsy specimen for Gram stain and aerobic and anaerobic culture should be obtained from the necrotic center of the lesion to identify the causative organisms.

Predisposing risk factors for necrotizing fasciitis include diabetes mellitus, alcoholism, an immunocompromised state, hypertension, peripheral vascular disease, IV drug abuse, and obesity. Increased age, delay in diagnosis, inadequate debridement during initial surgery, extent of disease on initial presentation, and the presence of diabetes mellitus are all factors that have been associated with an increased likelihood of mortality from necrotizing fasciitis.

Early diagnosis and aggressive management of this lethal disease have led to improved survival. In an earlier series, the mortality rate was consistently higher than 30%, but in more recent series, the mortality rate has decreased to less than 10%.

Successful management of necrotizing fasciitis involves early recognition, immediate initiation of resuscitative measures (including correction of fluid, acid–base, electrolyte, and hematologic abnormalities), **aggressive surgical debridement (and redebridement as necessary), and broad-spectrum antibiotic therapy.** Many patients benefit from central venous monitoring and high caloric nutritional support.

During surgery, the incision should be made through the infected tissue down to the fascia. An ability to undermine the skin and subcutaneous tissues with digital palpation often confirms the diagnosis. Multiple incisions can be made sequentially toward the periphery of the affected tissue until well-vascularized, healthy, resistant tissue is reached at all margins. The remaining affected tissue must be excised. The wound can then be packed and sequentially debrided on a daily basis as necessary until healthy tissue is displayed at all margins.

Hyperbaric oxygen therapy historically was considered to benefit, particularly in patients for whom culture results are positive for anaerobic organisms. Retrospective studies demonstrated that the addition of hyperbaric oxygen therapy to surgical debridement and antimicrobial therapy appears to significantly decrease both wound morbidity and overall mortality in patients with necrotizing fasciitis. However, more contemporary, large-scale studies have failed to show a benefit of this treatment. **Given the technical difficulty with its administration, hyperbaric oxygen treatment should only be considered in hemodynamically stable patients for whom the treatment will not delay surgical management.**

After the initial resuscitative efforts and surgical debridement, the primary concern is the management of the open wound. Allograft and xenograft skin can be used to cover open wounds, thus decreasing heat and evaporative water loss. Interestingly, temporary biologic closure of open wounds also seems to decrease bacterial growth. Application of a wound vacuum-assisted closure (VAC) device will also promote wound healing. When spontaneous closure is not likely, the VAC device may allow for the development of a suitable granulation bed and prepare the tissue for graft placement, thereby increasing the probability of graft survival. Finally, skin flaps can be mobilized to help cover open wounds after the wound infections have resolved and granulation has begun.

Special Populations

Obesity

Incidence and definition. Obesity (BMI ≥30) is an epidemic in the United States and is commonly encountered as a risk factor for complications associated with gynecologic oncology surgery. Centers for Disease Control and Prevention statistics from the year 2014 indicate that 34.9% of US adults (and 36.1% of women) older than age 20 years are obese. Current American Gastroenterology Association Guidelines use BMI to define classes of obesity (overweight, 25–29.9; class I, 30–34.9; class II, 35–39.9; and class III, >40.0). Of importance to the gynecologic oncologists are the further classes of morbid obesity (BMI >40) and super morbid obesity (BMI >50).

Postoperative complications and management. Obese patients are at much higher risk for postoperative complications because of the more common occurrence of comorbidities, including diabetes, hypertension, coronary artery disease, sleep apnea, obesity hypoventilation syndrome (OHS), and osteoarthritis of the knees and hips. These underlying alterations in physiology result in increased surgical risks and complications, including respiratory failure, cardiac failure, DVT and pulmonary embolism, aspiration, wound infection and dehiscence, postoperative asphyxia, and misdiagnosed intraabdominal catastrophe.

Control of the airway is critical in the immediate postoperative period. Extubation may not be prudent or possible at the end of the case as a result of tracheal edema resulting from a difficult intubation. Alternatively, the patient may not have the physical capacity to adequately ventilate as a result of suppression of the respiratory drive from anesthetics and excess chest wall weight. Many obese patients have OHS, which increases their baseline hypercarbia and may also delay extubation. It is may be necessary to plan immediate postoperative admission to a surgical ICU with mechanical ventilation and serial arterial blood sampling to aid in the proper timing for extubation.

After extubation, ventilation of the obese patient during sleep may be aided by the use of noninvasive positive-pressure ventilation units, particularly if the patient has a history of sleep apnea and uses a continuous positive airway pressure (CPAP) machine at home. Respiratory therapists can be of assistance in patient instruction and management of CPAP machinery in addition to other respiratory toilet. Monitoring with continuous pulse oximetry assists in the detection of impending respiratory failure.

There is a higher risk of aspiration in obese patients due to increased gastric residual volumes, a higher rate of gastroesophageal reflux disease (GERD), and increased intraabdominal pressure from mass effect. Neutralization of the stomach contents with a proton pump inhibitor can minimize the chemical burn potential of aspirated stomach contents. GI motility agents such as metoclopramide may decrease residual volume by increasing intestinal transit. It is also prudent to raise the head of the bed to prevent aspiration.

Prophylaxis for postoperative venous thrombosis and pulmonary embolism (as detailed earlier) should be ordered for obese patients because they are at higher risk for these complications.

Venous access poses another problem. Extreme obesity obliterates anatomic landmarks and makes insertion of peripheral lines and central lines problematic. Adjunctive visualization technology such as Doppler ultrasonography or fluoroscopy should increase the accuracy and safety of line placement. Arterial line placement facilitates monitoring of pressures and blood gas parameters. Ideally, central venous lines and arterial lines should be placed intraoperatively by the anesthesia team to ensure adequate access in the postoperative period. The intraoperative placement of central lines should be verified for position postoperatively by chest radiography in the postanesthesia care unit.

Medication administration must consider the concepts of total body weight and ideal body weight. Certain medications are dosed on ideal body weight (corticosteroids, penicillin, cephalosporins, beta-blockers). Others are dosed on total body weight (heparin), and still others are based on a calculated "dosing weight" (aminoglycosides, fluoroquinolones, vancomycin). An inpatient pharmacist should be consulted for assistance with proper dosing and monitoring of pharmacotherapy.

Minimally invasive surgical techniques decrease the morbidity of surgery in obese patients. In particular, wound complications are greatly reduced, and patients are able to ambulate sooner and have a faster return to full levels of activity. This is particularly important in the endometrial cancer population, for whom obesity is such a strong driver of disease. Concerns regarding longer operating times and the feasibility of steep Trendelenburg positioning were initially raised in this population. A recent multi-institution retrospective cohort study of 1032 obese (BMI >30) patients who all underwent robotic endometrial cancer staging reported a pulmonary complication rate of just 3% ($n = 33$) and overall complication rate of 14% ($n = 146$), both significantly less than that of laparotomy. Several more large studies have consistently reported decreased complication rates with equal or improved comprehensive surgical staging rates for obese patients undergoing minimally invasive surgery. Minimally invasive surgery has been endorsed by the Society of Gynecologic Oncology as the preferred surgical approach for all, including obese, patients with endometrial cancer.

Elderly patients. The life expectancy of American women continues to increase. In addition, as the baby boomer generation ages, we will see an increasingly larger population of older women who will develop gynecologic cancers. **Elderly women are at higher risk of developing gynecologic cancer in that 57% of vulvar cancers, 55% of epithelial ovarian cancers, 41% of endometrial cancers, and 20% of cervical cancers occur in women older than 65 years of age.** Although many of these cancers are managed with radical surgery, careful consideration must be given in selection of surgical procedures in women who may be at high risk for surgical complications. In addition to patient's chronological age, preoperative evaluations that include measurements of frailty, performance status, quality of life, and geriatric assessments can aid greatly in appropriate patient selection for radical surgery. In fact, complications of radiation therapy and chemotherapy are more likely to occur in older patients, so selection of any therapy requires consideration of patient tolerance. In past years, radical surgery was avoided in elderly women. We now know that surgery can be safely and successfully accomplished, despite a patient's age, if the patient is fully evaluated and determined to be a surgical candidate. There is no doubt that **older patients present with more advanced disease and have poorer preoperative performance status and more comorbid conditions than younger patients.** Retrospective review of elderly patients with gynecologic cancers demonstrates that 90% of women older than age 65 years can undergo radical surgery as definitive therapy for their gynecologic cancers. Compared with women younger than 65 years, the postoperative mortality rate was 1.5%, and the minor complications and length of stay were similar in the two groups. In women older than 65 years of age who underwent radical hysterectomy for early-stage cervical cancer, there was no perioperative mortality or ureteral fistula. Transfusion requirements and lymphedema were also similar. Febrile morbidity was less common in the older patients, although postoperative small bowel obstruction, bladder dysfunction, and pulmonary emboli were more commonly encountered in the older patients. In a population-based evaluation of 28,651 women undergoing cytoreductive surgery for ovarian cancer across the country, age was significantly associated with increased complication rate (<50 years, 17%; >70 years, ≥30%), including surgical site, medical, and infectious complications. With regard to minimally invasive surgery, in contrast, there is minimal increase in morbidity associated with age. Elderly cohorts of patients undergoing robotic surgery for endometrial cancer have been reported to have equivalent outcomes of blood transfusions, surgical complications, and length of hospital stay while preserving surgical comprehensive staging.

Perioperative management is the key to success when managing elderly women. Cardiac and pulmonary complications are the two most common serious problems encountered postoperatively. Careful preoperative assessment of cardiac status should include assessment for underlying coronary artery disease, valvular heart disease, and chronic congestive heart failure. Several risk-assessment algorithms may be applied to estimate cardiac risk of major noncardiac surgery. Because more than 40% of elderly women have hypertension, optimal blood pressure control should be achieved preoperatively; intraoperative hypotension is one of the most common causes of myocardial ischemia and infarction. Pulmonary complications occur in nearly 40% of elderly women after major abdominal surgery. Because physiologic changes of aging diminish vital capacity, lung compliance, reduced expiratory flow rates, and increased residual volume, elderly patients are more likely to have pulmonary complications after general anesthesia. These women may be at even higher risk if they have chronic obstructive pulmonary disease or asthma. Preoperative assessment may include assessment of pulmonary function by performing spirometry and obtaining an arterial blood gas measurement. Patients with underlying pulmonary disease should have their medical regimen maximized preoperatively, including the use of bronchodilators and corticosteroids. Conduction anesthesia should be considered in consultation with an anesthesiologist to avoid the pulmonary complications more often encountered with general anesthesia.

Avoiding perioperative hypothermia and hypoxemia are extremely important to avoid additional cardiac oxygen consumption. Invasive monitoring and planned ICU admission should be considered in any circumstance when there is an increased risk of cardiac or pulmonary complications. Care must also be taken when ordering pharmacologic agents because elderly patients may have altered GI absorption and decreased renal or hepatic clearance of specific drugs. Consultation with a clinical pharmacist is advised to establish the correct dose of drug for patients with altered renal or hepatic function.

Radiation complications in elderly patients are also increased. **Thin, hypertensive patients appear to be at greater risk for radiation therapy complications to both the GI and genitourinary tracts.** It appears that elderly women tolerate initial therapy poorly and often require delays in treatment or discontinuation of treatment because of acute toxicity such as diarrhea, dehydration, or neutropenia. This observation, then, requires carefully planned treatment decisions as to whether the patient would be best treated with surgery or radiation therapy. Neither is without risk, and it cannot be assumed that radiation therapy is necessarily less toxic.

Radiation Therapy

Radiation therapy serves as a primary treatment modality for cervical and vaginal cancers (and occasionally advanced vulvar cancers) and as an adjuvant therapy for patients with high-risk endometrial cancers. Furthermore, individualized radiation therapy may be used in nearly all gynecologic cancers to achieve palliation under specific circumstances. Morbidity resulting from properly conducted radiation therapy in patients with carcinoma of the cervix and vagina is usually minimal. However, there are unfortunate misconceptions about the magnitude of radiation morbidity because of issues regarding failure to distinguish between adverse effects from poor techniques, failure to recognize that poorer outcomes of patients with inoperable extensive tumors, and lack of recognition that morbidity attributed to irradiation may actually result from uncontrolled tumor (ie, rectovaginal and vesicovaginal fistulas). As in the case of surgery, the treatment-related morbidity can be minimized by good application, but it cannot be eliminated.

Because the small bowel, bladder, and rectum are adjacent to the female genital tract, most of the side effects and complications of radiation involve these adjacent organs. Radiation complications are related to the dose, field size, and type of radiation equipment used. **The larger the field, the greater the risk of problems if the dose remains constant. Usually, as the fields enlarge, the dose must be decreased.** Conversely, as the fields become smaller, a larger dose can be tolerated. The use of brachytherapy also increases the risk of local complications. Finally, the use of combined chemoradiation therapy seems to increase slightly some complications during therapy (eg, neutropenia) but does not seem to lead to serious long-term sequelae.

The pathogenesis of radiation-induced injury may be divided into acute and delayed complications. **Complications during therapy are caused by ionizing radiation injury to cells that are mitotically active such as the GI epithelium.** Damage of the mucosal cells results in mucosal thinning and denudation followed by malabsorption and fluid and electrolyte loss (resulting from diarrhea). The GI mucosal stem cells generally recover totally, and the acute symptoms resolve. **Late complications involve a different mechanism of tissue injury based on vascular endothelial damage.** Radiation results in an endarteritis and the gradual occlusion of small vessels. Subsequent tissue hypoxia leads to fibrosis of the affected tissue. These changes are progressive and may be aggravated further by other vascular compromise such as diabetes, hypertension, and aging. In severe cases, ulceration, stricture, perforation, and fistula formation may occur.

Gastrointestinal Complications

Acute complications. **Nearly all patients receiving external radiation to the pelvis will develop radiation proctitis or enteritis with associated diarrhea.** This problem commonly begins after 2 weeks of radiation therapy and is **usually easily managed by dietary modification and antidiarrheal medications (diphenoxylate; Lomotil). As a rule, the diarrhea resolves within 7 to 10 days of completing radiation.** Some of the transitory symptoms are tenesmus and the passage of mucus and even blood per the rectum. **Diarrhea and abdominal cramping characterize small intestinal irritation (radiation enteritis). This problem is more common and more severe when a portion of the small intestine is fixed in the pelvis as a result of adhesions or other pathologic conditions.** Anorexia may also occur during radiation therapy. If nausea and vomiting occur, the patient should be evaluated for dehydration. This is more common when concurrent chemotherapy is being given along with the radiation. IV hydration and correction of electrolytes is occasionally required. If dehydration is severe, radiation should be interrupted until these acute side effects are corrected.

The patient should have a complete blood count weekly during radiation therapy. If the hemoglobin decreases below 10 g/dL, PRBC transfusion is advised to achieve improved tumor kill. Occasionally, radiation of the pelvic bone marrow will result in neutropenia or thrombocytopenia. In severe cases, radiation will need to be temporarily interrupted. **In nearly all cases, the acute side effects of radiation therapy will resolve after the radiation course is completed.**

Chronic conditions. Radiation injury to the small intestine may manifest itself at any time after therapy and may vary from chronic diarrhea to small bowel obstruction or fistula. A typical patient with small bowel injury will initially present with postprandial abdominal cramps and pain, anorexia, and diarrhea. About half of small bowel injuries occur within 1 year after radiation, and three-fourths occur within 2 years. These symptoms are more common in patients who have had a prior laparotomy. Initial conservative management focuses on dietary modification (avoiding green leafy vegetables, milk products, and fried foods). Antidiarrheal drugs and oral cholestyramine (which binds bile salts) are often useful in managing symptoms.

As small bowel injury progresses, fibrosis of the injured bowel wall develops, leading to stricture and partial or complete obstruction. Patients usually present with worsening abdominal pain, cramps, diarrhea, and vomiting. Sometimes the intermittent obstruction goes unrecognized until a significant weight loss is recorded. If medical management of a partial small bowel obstruction fails, surgical intervention is the course of last resort. The decision to proceed with surgical intervention in cases of intermittent obstruction is a difficult one and should be undertaken with proper preoperative preparation. Often, patients have developed a significant degree of malnutrition and should have their nutritional status corrected with preoperative TPN. Mechanical bowel preparation is mandatory, although sometimes it must be limited to enemas because the patient's small bowel obstruction will not allow the ingestion of oral cathartics. Dilated loops of bowel should be decompressed preoperatively with NG suction. Surgical correction depends on the situation encountered at the time of surgical exploration. **The obstruction is usually found to be bowel adherent in the pelvis that has been radiated.** The bowel usually is thickened, edematous, and fibrotic. **The two primary surgical options are resection of the obstructed loops with either reanastomosis or small bowel bypass. In either event, it is preferable to make anastomoses to intestinal segments that have not been radiated in order to have maximum opportunity for healing.** Care should be taken to have adequate perfusion and no tension on the anastomosis. Perforation or fistula, if present, must be isolated and diverted; more extensive surgery (resection and anastomosis) must be done only if it is technically feasible (Fig. 16.10).

Radiation injury to the rectum is more common after treatment for cervical cancer because of the high rectal doses from the intracavitary brachytherapy. **Injury to the rectum may manifest as proctitis, rectal ulcer, stricture, or fistula.** Complete colonic obstruction from radiation injury is extremely rare. The symptoms of radiation proctitis may develop after an asymptomatic interval of many months to years after radiation

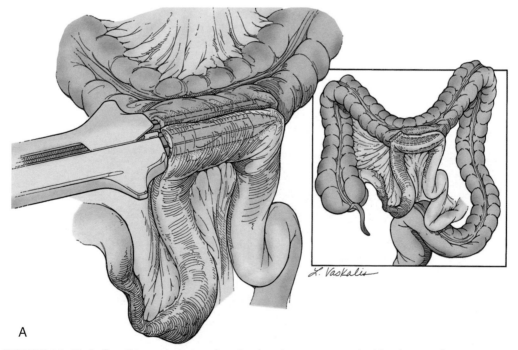

A

FIGURE 16.10 A, Small bowel obstruction that has been managed with a bypass ileotransverse enteroenterostomy.

Continued

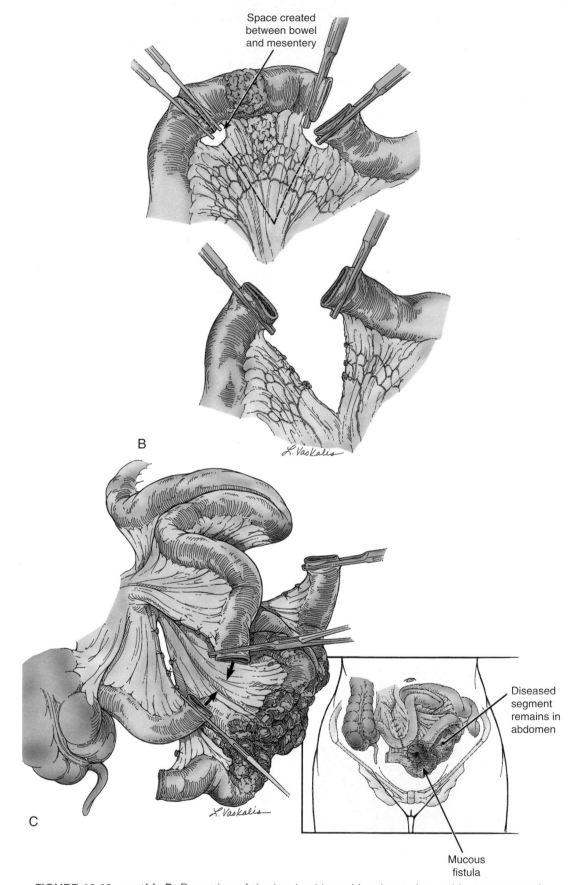

FIGURE 16.10, cont'd **B,** Resection of the involved bowel has been done with reanastomosis of the small bowel. Sufficient terminal ileum must be present for this procedure to be accomplished. **C,** The obstructed bowel has been isolated with formation of a mucous fistula. An end-to-side anastomosis has also been done. (From Nichols DH, Clarke-Pearson DL, eds. *Gynecologic, Obstetric and Related Surgery*, 2nd ed. St. Louis, 2000, Mosby.)

therapy is completed. Diarrhea with or without rectal bleeding is the most common presenting symptom. Cramping abdominal pain may be associated with the diarrhea. The injury is most often located on the anterior rectal wall that received the maximal dose from the brachytherapy application and range from thickened, fragile mucosa to thin, atrophic mucosa or mucosal ulceration. These changes usually heal with conservative measures, including low-residue diet, anticholinergic drugs, stool softeners, and corticosteroid enemas. Hyperbaric oxygen treatments also appear to enhance healing of a rectal ulcer. If there is excessive bleeding from the rectal ulcer or proctitis, diversion of the fecal stream (colostomy) may be necessary to allow healing. Obviously, when bleeding is encountered, full evaluation of the rectosigmoid colon with flexible sigmoidoscopy is mandatory to exclude recurrent cancer, rectal cancer, polyps, diverticula, or hemorrhoids as the cause of bleeding.

Rectovaginal fistula is the most common significant radiation injury to the large bowel and is often preceded by radiation proctitis and rectal ulceration. All patients with rectovaginal fistulas should have a diverting colostomy. It is rare that diversion will result in spontaneous healing of radiated colon, and it is often necessary to decide as to whether repair of the fistula may be subsequently undertaken. Whenever surgical correction is considered, endovascular flaps are used to bring a new blood supply to the repair (Fig. 16.11). **Only after the fistula repair has completely healed and absence of obstruction of the bowel has been documented should the colostomy be reversed.**

Radiation-induced strictures or obstruction of the rectosigmoid colon appear at approximately 24 months from the completion of the radiation therapy. Again, the initial step in management is a diverting colostomy. Correction requires a

FIGURE 16.11 A, Barium enema demonstrating a rectovaginal fistula after irradiation. B, Repair of the rectovaginal fistula has been strengthened by interposition of the bulbocavernosus fat pad. C, The cross-section shows placement of the neovascular fat pad.

rectosigmoid resection with low rectal anastomosis. Harris and Wheeless reported their experience with the end-to-end stapler device in low colorectal anastomosis associated with rectal injury. This was accomplished in 49 patients, 17 of whom had prior radiation therapy. All five postoperative complications (two strictures, two anastomosis breakdowns, and one fecal incontinence after colostomy closure) occurred in the patients who had prior radiation. In a more recent series by Mirhashemi et al., prior pelvic radiation remained a significant risk factor for anastomotic breakdown and fistula (35% vs. 7.5%, N = 77).

Complex fistulas may include a variety of communications between the small bowel, colon, vagina, bladder, and skin. Thorough evaluation of the anatomy involved is mandatory and should include all organ systems that are possibly involved. The evaluation may include barium enema, proctosigmoidoscopy, upper GI series with small bowel follow-through, IVP, cystography, cystoscopy, and a "fistulogram" (injection of contrast directly into the fistula and imaging the retrograde flow of the contrast dye). These complex fistulas are often very difficult to repair, and the patients should be in optimal medical condition before surgery is performed. This usually includes antibiotics to control infection, TPN, and mechanical bowel preparation. If a fistula can be resected, it should be; however, many times the fistula must be isolated and the intestinal stream diverted around the lesion.

Prior pelvic radiation to the ileum (or resection or bypass surgery of the ileum) may lead to the malabsorption of vitamin B_{12} and result in a megaloblastic anemia. Because the liver usually has significant stores of vitamin B_{12}, it may be several years after radiation or surgery before the anemia is recognized. It is therefore advised that patients have annual complete blood counts indefinitely. A Shilling test can differentiate between vitamin B_{12} and folic acid deficiency. Treatment of vitamin B_{12} deficiency requires weekly vitamin B_{12} injections until the hemoglobin level returns to normal (usually 4–6 weeks) and then monthly injections to prevent recurrent anemia.

Urologic Complications

Acute radiation cystitis is occasionally encountered during radiation therapy or in the period immediately after completion of therapy. Typical symptoms of cystitis are usually present, but urine cultures show no significant bacterial growth. Management includes increased oral liquid intake and urinary analgesics and anticholinergics to relieve symptoms. Chronic radiation cystitis commonly presents with symptoms of urinary frequency, suprapubic pain, and hematuria. The patient should have an immediate urine culture because a UTI further aggravates bladder mucosa damaged by radiation therapy. **Gross hematuria (rather than microscopic hematuria) usually can be relieved by continuous bladder irrigation using 0.5% or 1% acetic acid, a 1:1000 potassium permanganate, or an alum solution.** Clots may need to be evacuated by cystoscopic irrigation to relieve bladder spasms. Cystoscopy may also be needed to identify bleeding points that may be fulgurated. An experienced urologist should be consulted because **excessive fulguration or unnecessary biopsies may lead to an iatrogenic vesicovaginal fistula. As a last resort, the bladder may be sclerosed with formaldehyde irrigation.** In the most extreme cases, cystectomy and urinary diversion may be required to control bleeding.

Vesicovaginal fistulas are more common when the patient has had intensive radiation therapy and are increased by brachytherapy. Improper placement of the tandem and ovoids may result in an excessive dose to the base of the bladder and speaks to the importance of careful placement of intracavitary devices and attention to bladder doses delivered. Surgery after radiation therapy, such as a "completion" hysterectomy for bulky stage IB2 or "barrel" lesions of the cervix, further increases the risk of vesicovaginal fistula. In many cases, upper vaginal radiation necrosis is recognized months before the occurrence of the fistula. **Treatment of the necrosis may prevent the progression to a fistula. Therapy includes half-strength hydrogen peroxide douches, intravaginal estrogen, and hyperbaric oxygen therapy.**

Evaluation of an apparent vesicovaginal fistula should include a complete evaluation of the bladder and the upper tracts. **It is common to discover an associated ureterovaginal fistula or ureteral stricture or stenosis, which must be addressed at the time of fistula repair.** Furthermore, given the proximity of the upper vagina to the bladder and rectum, proctosigmoidoscopy is advised because the rectosigmoid colon may also communicate with the fistula.

Repair of a radiation-induced vesicovaginal fistula is difficult and less successful than fistula repair in nonirradiated areas. **The primary complicating matter is diminished blood supply to the radiated tissues. Therefore, techniques of repair often use the mobilization of a nonirradiated tissue with a good blood supply into the surgical repair.** If an intraabdominal, transvesical approach is taken to repair the vesicovaginal fistula, the omentum and its blood supply may be mobilized and used to cover the repair of the fistula, often being interposed between the closed bladder and vagina. Vaginal approaches to vesicovaginal fistula repair may include repair combined with colpocleisis or the use of the bulbocavernosus labial flap (Martius flap), which is mobilized and interposed between the repaired bladder and vagina (Figs. 16.12 and 16.13). Ureteral injury after radiation therapy may require reimplantation of the distal ureter into the bladder (ureteroneocystostomy) or permanent diversion (urinary conduit).

Sexual Function and Vaginal Stenosis

Vaginal stenosis results from fibrosis and narrowing of the upper vagina after vaginal brachytherapy in both cervical and endometrial cancer treatment. Given the dose-rate response, vaginal toxicity is more common in definitive chemoradiation management of cervical cancer (89%) than adjuvant pelvic or vaginal radiation for endometrial cancer (widely ranging from 1% to 55% in published reports). Vaginal dilator use can significantly prevent the severity of vaginal stenosis and should be encouraged both during and after therapy. One recent study examined risk factors for vaginal stenosis after adjuvant brachytherapy in endometrial cancer patients. Of 101 patients examined, 33 (33%) had either mild or severe vaginal stenosis, and multivariate analysis revealed that factors of having more than

Interposition of
bulbocavernosus
and vestibular bulb

A

Flap of muscle
sutured over
fistula

B

FIGURE 16.12 A, Vesicovaginal fistula repair using the bulbocavernosus fat pad as a source of neovascularization. **B,** Repair using an omental J flap for neovascularization. (From Nichols DH, Clarke-Pearson DL, eds. *Gynecologic, Obstetric and Related Surgery*, 2nd ed. St. Louis, 2000, Mosby.)

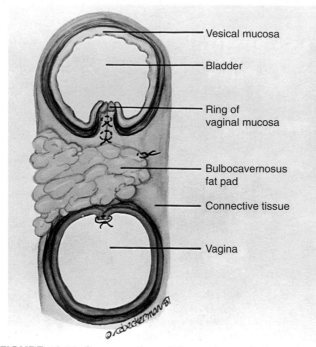

Vesical mucosa

Bladder

Ring of vaginal mucosa

Bulbocavernosus fat pad

Connective tissue

Vagina

FIGURE 16.13 Cross-section of the vesicovaginal repair using the bulbocavernosus fat pad as a source of neovascularization.

60% of the vagina treated and a total dose larger than 14 Gy were significantly associated with greater odds of vaginal stenosis. It should be noted that the Common Terminology Criteria for Adverse Events (CTCAE), version 4.03 criteria for vaginal stricture was used to grade vaginal stenosis, and 26 of the 33 women with stenosis had grade 1 severity.

For the bibliography list, log onto www.expertconsult.com ⟨http://www.expertconsult.com⟩.

17

Basic Principles of Chemotherapy

Christina S. Chu, MD, Stephen C. Rubin, MD

OUTLINE

KEY POINTS

1. In malignant tumors, unregulated growth appears to result from a combination of loss of normal cell cycle controls and a failure of normal apoptotic mechanisms. Despite uncontrolled growth, malignant cell division does not appear to be more rapid than normal cell division.
2. In general, as tumors grow, they display gompertzian growth characteristics: As the tumor mass increases in size, the time necessary to double its size also becomes progressively longer. Metastases generally have a shorter doubling time than the primary lesion.
3. In late stages of tumor growth, only a few doublings in tumor mass may make a dramatic impact on the size of the tumor and the status of the patient.
4. Chemotherapeutic agents work by first-order kinetics—that is, they kill a constant fraction of cells rather than a constant number.
5. The effectiveness of any cancer treatment is limited by drug resistance, which may be intrinsic or acquired and may develop to one drug or to multiple drugs.
6. Alkylating agents, such as the platinum compounds and cyclophosphamide, prevent cell division primarily by cross-linking strands of DNA.
7. Antimetabolites, such as 5-flurouracil and methotrexate, act by inhibiting essential metabolic processes that are required for synthesis of purines, pyrimidines, and nucleic acids. These agents are typically S phase specific.
8. Antitumor antibiotics, such as bleomycin and doxorubicin, generally work via DNA intercalation.
9. Several chemotherapeutic agents, such as the taxanes, work via inhibition of normal microtubule function.
10. Antiangiogenesis therapies, such as bevacizumab, are among the most common targeted agents.
11. Hematologic toxicity and nausea and vomiting are the most frequently observed side effects in patients undergoing chemotherapy.
12. Common antiemetic regimens include use of a 5-HT3 receptor antagonist with dexamethasone or aprepitant, a substance P/NK1 antagonist.
13. The taxanes and platinum compounds are the most likely to cause hypersensitivity.
14. Unlike reactions to taxanes, which typically occur within minutes of starting the initial dose, reactions to platinum agents typically do not manifest until several cycles have already been administered.

HISTORICAL OVERVIEW

The era of modern chemotherapy began in the 1940s with the Nobel Prize–winning work of Huggins and Hodges on the antitumor effect of estrogens in prostate cancer. This observation was followed in the mid-1940s by the investigation of nitrogen mustard, a byproduct of nitrogen gas used in World War I, for its effects against lymphomas and solid tumors. Between 1945 and 1965, a wide variety of chemotherapeutic agents was identified and studied, including actinomycin D, cyclophosphamide, the vinca alkaloids, 5-fluorouracil (5-FU), and the progesterones. In the 1970s, cisplatin was noted to exert significant antitumor effects against ovarian and testicular cancers, and tamoxifen was found to have activity against breast cancer for both adjuvant therapy and treatment of advanced disease. In the same decade, bleomycin, etoposide, and doxorubicin came into clinical use, and derivative compounds such as carboplatin, vinorelbine, and idarubicin were developed for their ability to achieve similar antitumor effects but with less hematologic toxicity. The 1980s and 1990s led to the widespread use of a host of new drugs, such as the taxanes (paclitaxel and docetaxel), ifosfamide, the topoisomerase inhibitors (topotecan and irinotecan), and nucleoside analogs (gemcitabine and capecitabine).

The growing number of agents in the chemotherapeutic armamentarium has been accompanied by advances in alternative dosing regimens; differing formulations using liposomal or polymer-based encapsulation; and varying schedules, sequences, and routes of administration. Fortunately, supportive therapies for gastrointestinal (GI) and hematologic toxicities have also evolved to include routine usage of 5-HT3 receptor antagonists (eg, ondansetron and granisetron) for antiemetic prophylaxis and colony-stimulating factors (eg, sargramostim and filgrastim) to allow for greater chemotherapeutic dose intensity.

GENERAL PRINCIPLES

Chemotherapeutic agents are a crucial part of physicians' armamentarium in the ever-broadening fight against cancer. Physicians can, with use of these drugs, ameliorate and sometimes even cure diseases that were usually fatal in the past. Until recently, in most cases, chemotherapy has been reserved for relatively late stages of the disease, but its increasingly successful use, particularly in the treatment of hematologic malignancies, suggests that chemotherapy should be administered earlier. All physicians and surgeons must understand the nature and use of cancer chemotherapy so they can make rational decisions about when it may be indicated. The outcome of cancer chemotherapy is not fully predictable, but the chances of remission can be improved by judicious selection of patients, careful assessment of the tumor's growth pattern, and treatment of the neoplasm with the drug or drugs most likely to be effective. **The clinical response to chemotherapy may be assessed using standard Response Evaluation Criteria in Solid Tumors defined by the National Cancer Institute** (Table 17.1).

TABLE 17.1 National Cancer Institute Response Evaluation Criteria in Solid Tumors

Evaluation	
TARGET LESIONS	
Complete response	Disappearance of all target lesions
Partial response	At least a 30% decrease in the sum of the longest diameter of target lesions, taking as reference the baseline sum longest diameter
Progressive disease	At least a 20% increase in the sum of the longest diameter of target lesions, taking as reference the smallest sum longest diameter recorded since the treatment started or the appearance of one or more new lesions
Stable disease	Neither sufficient shrinkage to qualify for partial response nor sufficient increase to qualify for progressive disease, taking as reference the smallest sum longest diameter since the treatment started
NONTARGET LESIONS	
Complete response	Disappearance of all nontarget lesions and normalization of tumor marker level
Incomplete response or stable disease	Persistence of one or more nontarget lesion(s) or maintenance of tumor marker level above the normal limits
Progressive disease	Appearance of one or more new lesions or unequivocal progression of existing nontarget lesions*

*Although a clear progression of "nontarget" lesions only is exceptional, in such circumstances, the opinion of the treating physician should prevail, and the progression status should be confirmed later on by the review panel (or study chair).

Unfortunately, not all patients with cancer are amenable to chemotherapy. The suitability of a patient for treatment depends on at least three critical criteria:
1. The nature of the neoplasm
2. Its extent of spread or stage
3. The patient's clinical condition

Not all cancers are equally sensitive to drugs. Factors that determine a given tumor's susceptibility include how the drug is distributed to the tumor, drug transport into the cell, whether a drug-sensitive biochemical pathway is present in the tumor cell, and the relative rates of intracellular activation and inactivation of the drug. A thorough knowledge of the cell cycle and growth kinetics is fundamental to understanding of the appropriate uses of chemotherapy.

CELL CYCLE CONTROL AND GROWTH KINETICS

All living things have an inherent capacity to multiply, and they cease multiplication for various reasons. Control appears to be mediated by an unknown feedback mechanism, probably resulting from contact phenomena when cells are crowded together. Knowledge of growth patterns has aided in the derivation of chemotherapeutic principles. Strategies for therapy have evolved to take advantage of these differences in growth characteristics between normal and malignant tissues.

Normal tissues fall into three predominant categories: static, expanding, and renewing. Static populations of cells are generally well differentiated and after a period of proliferation in fetal life rarely undergo division during adult life. Examples of static tissues include neurons and skeletal muscle. Because of the rare incidence of cell division, these cells are unlikely to be injured by chemotherapies that target rapidly dividing cells. Expanding tissue populations are also usually inactive in adult life, but unlike static populations, they retain the ability to proliferate rapidly in response to stress or injury. Typical examples of expanding cells include hepatocytes and vascular endothelium. Last, the renewing cell populations are those that are constantly undergoing division, such as bone marrow and GI epithelium. Renewing tissues are most sensitive to injury by chemotherapeutic agents (Table 17.2).

In malignant growth, cells do not cease multiplying when they reach a critical mass. This unregulated growth appears to result from a combination of loss of normal cell cycle controls and a failure of normal apoptotic mechanisms. Despite uncontrolled growth, malignant cell division does not appear to be more rapid than normal cell division.

In general, as tumors grow, they display gompertzian growth characteristics (Fig. 17.1): As the tumor mass increases in size, the time necessary to double its size also becomes progressively longer. Thus, in the early phases of growth, tumor cells appear to grow exponentially, but as tumor mass increases, there is a progressive increase in the doubling time, although doubling times in humans may vary greatly. For example, whereas embryonal tumors and some lymphomas have relatively short doubling times (20–40 days), adenocarcinomas and squamous cell carcinomas have relatively long doubling times (50–150 days). Three explanations have been given for this prolonged volume-doubling time:

1. An increase in cell cycle time (the time from one mitosis to the next)
2. A decrease in the growth fraction (cells participating in cell division in the tumor)
3. An increase in cell loss from tumor cells with insufficient nutrients and vascular supply

The gompertzian model has several important implications for cancer progression. First, metastases generally have a shorter doubling time than the primary lesion. If it is assumed that an exponential growth occurs early in the malignancy's history and that the malignancy starts from a single cell, then a 1-mm mass will have undergone approximately 20 tumor doublings. A 5-mm mass (a size that is first recognizable on a radiograph) may have undergone 27 doublings. It follows that a 1-cm mass will have undergone 30 doublings, and a clinician will be pleased to have detected such an "early" lesion. Unfortunately, this "early" lesion has already undergone 30 doublings, with significant DNA change being possible. Using this rationale, clinical techniques that are currently available tend to recognize malignancies late in their growth, and metastatic disease may well have occurred long before there was obvious clinical manifestation of the primary lesion. **Another implication from this kinetic information is that in late stages of tumor growth, a few doublings in tumor mass make a dramatic impact on the size of the tumor and the status of the patient.** When a tumor becomes palpable (1 cm in diameter—30 doublings), only three more doublings will produce a very large tumor mass (8 cm in diameter).

The gompertzian model also has clinical implications that have guided a good deal of clinical chemotherapy research. **As a mass responds to treatment (ie, gets smaller), the doubling time has been assumed to decrease as a consequence of a greater number of cells moving into cycle. This larger percentage of metabolically active cells would therefore increase the sensitivity of the neoplastic population of cell cycle–specific agents. This has led to the sequential use of cell cycle–nonspecific agents (eg, cyclophosphamide) to bring down the mass to be followed by cell cycle–specific agents (eg, methotrexate).** Although these sequential combinations have been theoretically attractive, none has shown clear superiority in clinical trials. Another implication of the gompertzian growth concept is that metastases can be expected to be more sensitive to chemotherapy in general, and to cell cycle–specific agents in particular, than the primary tumor from which they arise. The smaller the size of the metastatic focus, the greater is the differential sensitivity. Therefore, the insensitivity of a primary tumor to a given drug regimen might not necessarily predict the response of metastasis to the same regimen.

TABLE 17.2   Classification of Normal Tissues by Rate of Proliferation

Renewing (Rapid Proliferation)	Expanding (Slow Proliferation)	Static (Rare Proliferation)
Bone marrow	Lung	Muscle
Gastrointestinal mucosa	Liver	Bone
Ovary	Kidney	Cartilage
Testis	Endocrine glands	Nerve
Hair follicles	Vascular endothelium	

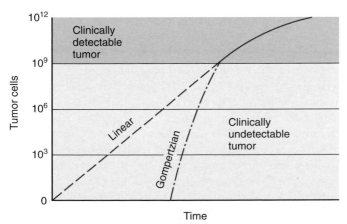

FIGURE 17.1 Tumor growth. As tumors grow, they display gompertzian characteristics. As tumor mass increases, doubling time becomes longer. However, a palpable tumor needs relatively few doublings to achieve a large mass.

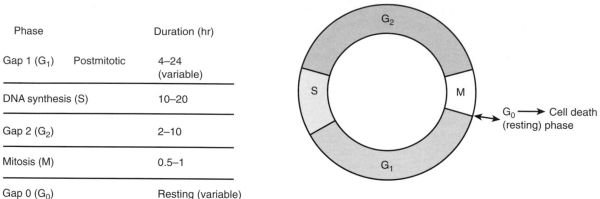

Phase		Duration (hr)
Gap 1 (G₁)	Postmitotic	4–24 (variable)
DNA synthesis (S)		10–20
Gap 2 (G₂)		2–10
Mitosis (M)		0.5–1
Gap 0 (G₀)		Resting (variable)

FIGURE 17.2 Cell generation time and sequence are similar for all mammalian cells. Tumor cells do not have faster generation times but do have more cells in the active phases of replication.

The rationale for the use of drugs in the treatment of cancer is to achieve the selective killing of tumor cells. Underlying this rationale are the basic principles of the "cell kill" hypothesis first described by Skipper and associates. The following four principles were worked out in the L1210 leukemia model.

1. The survival of an animal with cancer is inversely related to the number of cancer cells.
2. A single cell is capable of multiplying and eventually killing the host.
3. For most drugs, a clear relationship exists between the dose of the drug and its ability to eradicate tumor cells.
4. A given dose of a drug kills a constant fraction of cells, not a constant number, regardless of the cell numbers present.

This fourth and most important principle implies that chemotherapeutic agents work by first-order kinetics—that is, they kill a constant fraction of cells rather than a constant number. This concept has important implications in cancer treatment. A single exposure of tumor cells to an antineoplastic drug may be capable of producing two to four logs of cell kill. With a common tumor burden of 1012 cells (1 kg), a single dose of chemotherapy will destroy a large number of cells but not be curative. Thus, there is a need for intermittent courses of chemotherapy to achieve the magnitude of cell kill necessary to eradicate the lesion. Clinically, first-order cell kinetics dictate that to eradicate a tumor population effectively it is necessary to either:

• Increase the total dose of the drug or drugs to the maximal limits tolerated by the host, or
• Start treatment when the number of cells is small enough to allow the destruction of the tumor at total doses of the drug that are reasonably tolerated.

The logical conclusion derived from this hypothesis is that the maximal opportunity for achieving cure exists during the early stage of disease. In the past, chemotherapy was generally reserved for the treatment of disseminated cancer; surgery and radiotherapy were treatments of choice for localized disease. However, this concept of "log kill hypothesis" provides a rationale for the philosophy of adjuvant chemotherapy, which assumes the presence of undetectable cell masses of 101 to 104

cells after the initial surgical therapy that are capable of producing tumor relapse. This small tumor burden is particularly vulnerable to effective chemotherapy.

To better understand cell kinetics, it is imperative to visualize cell cycling. All dividing cells follow a predictable pattern for replication. The time that it takes a cell to complete one cycle of growth and division is termed its *generation time*. There are five basic phases (Fig. 17.2). The G1 phase (G stands for gap and uncertainty as to purpose) lasts for a variable amount of time—usually between 4 and 24 hours. If this phase is prolonged, the cell is usually referred to as being in the G0, or resting, phase. The S phase is the phase of DNA synthesis and usually lasts between 10 and 20 hours. The G2 phase is a premitotic phase that lasts from 2 to 10 hours, and the M phase, when actual mitosis takes place, lasts between 0.5 and 1 hours. Tumors do not have faster generation times but have more cells in the active phases of replication than normal tissues. Normal tissues have a large number of cells in the G0 phase, wherein the cell is not actively committed to division or is "out of cycle."

Some chemotherapeutic agents appear to act at several phases of the cell cycle (Fig. 17.3). Alkylating agents appear to act in all phases from G0 to mitosis. They are called cycle-nonspecific agents. Drugs such as hydroxyurea, doxorubicin (Adriamycin), and methotrexate appear to act primarily in the S phase. Bleomycin appears to act in the G2 phase, and vincristine appears to act in the M phase. These drugs are called cycle-specific agents (Table 17.3) because they act chemotherapeutically only on cells that are in a specific phase of a cell generation cycle. Steroids, 5-FU, and cisplatin have rather uniform activity around the cell generation cycle. **In theory, if certain cancer therapeutic agents attack only cells that are dividing and more tumor cells are dividing than normal tissue cells, then by properly spacing the chemotherapeutic agent and combining agents that act in different phases of the cell cycle, one should be able to kill tumor cells in much greater numbers than normal cells.** Kinetic studies in humans and animals suggest that tumors that have been cured by chemotherapy are those with large fractions of cells in the proliferative phase (eg, gestational choriocarcinoma and Burkitt

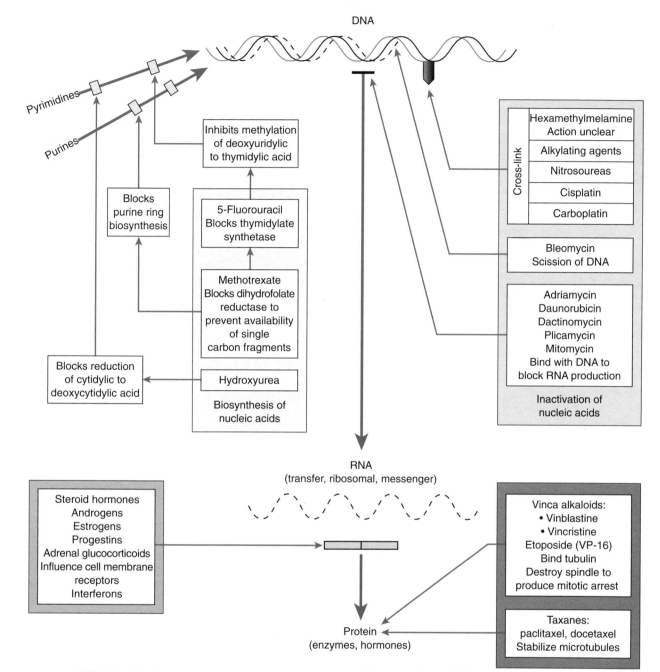

FIGURE 17.3 Cancer chemotherapeutic agents. (Modified from Krakoff IH. Cancer chemotherapeutic agents. *CA Cancer J Clin* 1987;37:93.)

lymphoma). The extent of the disease rather than the total mass of tumor is the most important factor when considering curative radiation or surgery, but in using chemotherapy, the total mass is most important. When tumor volume is reduced, the remaining tumor cells can begin to divide actively (they are propelled from the G0 phase into the more vulnerable cell generation cycle), thus rendering them susceptible to chemotherapy. These chemotherapeutic agents, as in radiation therapy, kill by first-order kinetics—that is, there is a reduction of the tumor population by a characteristic percentage, regardless of the actual number of tumor cells initially present (Fig. 17.4). If the tumor burden is small, fewer cycles of chemotherapy may

be necessary. One milligram of tumor usually consists of 106 cells. One cubic centimeter of tumor usually consists of 109 cells. Patient death usually occurs at 1012 cells.

DYNAMICS OF CHEMOTHERAPY

The doubling time of a tumor depends on both generation time and cell death rate (Fig. 17.5). One cannot assume a long generation time simply because a tumor enlarges slowly. Slow tumor growth can result from rapid generation time combined with a high cell death rate. For similar reasons, a small tumor discovered on radiographic or physical examination is not

TABLE 17.3   Cell Cycle (Phase)–Specific Drugs

Phase Dependence	Type	Drugs
S phase dependent	Antimetabolite	Cytarabine
		Doxorubicin
		5-Fluorouracil
		6-Mercaptopurine
		Methotrexate
		Hydroxyurea
		Prednisone
M phase dependent	Vinca alkaloids	Vincristine
		Vinblastine
	Taxanes	Paclitaxel
		Docetaxel
	Podophyllotoxins	Etoposide
		Teniposide
	Epothilones	Ixabepilone
G2 phase dependent	—	Bleomycin
G1 phase dependent	—	Corticosteroids

cycle-specific agents. Thus, there is some flexibility in the interplay of chemotherapeutic agents.

The phenomenon of increased susceptibility of tumor cells during recovery from alkylating agents is the rationale for sequentially combining cycle-nonspecific and cycle-specific agents in many new regimens. If, in addition, drugs with different mechanisms of toxicity are combined, each drug can be given safely in the dose used when it is given alone. Each drug chosen for combination therapy should have antitumor activity when used alone. Whenever possible, intermittent courses of chemotherapy are used to allow restoration of normal cells if they were reduced in number by treatment. In cases in which an antidote to the chemotherapeutic agent is known—for example, leucovorin (citrovorum factor, folinic acid) for methotrexate—the antidote can also be given to hasten normal cell recovery. Of course, the danger of revitalizing sublethally injured tumor cells also exists and must be evaluated with each new treatment regimen. Although careful studies are needed to compare each new combination with the single agents concerned, the trend in chemotherapy is unquestionably toward exploitation of drug combinations used simultaneously and sequentially.

PHARMACOLOGIC PRINCIPLES

Several general pharmacologic factors significantly affect the appropriate use of chemotherapeutic agents, including drug absorption, distribution, transport, metabolism, and excretion. These principles not only impinge on drug effectiveness but also dictate drug dose and schedule and how drugs are selected for use in combination. The effectiveness of a given regimen depends on optimizing the *concentration x time* (also known as the area under the curve [AUC]) at the site of tumor. Drug absorption influences route of administration, which in turn affects the AUC. Whether a drug is given orally, intravenously, intraarterially, intramuscularly, or intraperitoneally is also determined by patient acceptance, feasibility, and toxicity. Drug distribution and delivery to the tumor site also affects AUC. Factors such as drug binding (to albumin or to plastic catheters), lipid solubility, and membrane transport are critical in determining effectiveness of a given agent. Certain sites in the body, such as the brain and testes, represent pharmacologic sanctuaries where drug delivery is limited. Similarly, poor tumor perfusion because of necrosis or hypoxia may also impair drug delivery and concentration. Understanding of membrane transport mechanisms is also key: Certain drugs, such as 5-FU and mitomycin C, may enter cells through passive diffusion, but others, such as cisplatin and melphalan, require active transport.

Drug metabolism is often necessary to convert an inactive prodrug into the active form. One example is cyclophosphamide, which requires cytochrome P-450 activation before antitumor effects are possible. Agents requiring hepatic metabolism to active forms are not amenable to intraperitoneal or intraarterial administration. Conversely, metabolism and excretion of the active drug also affects AUC. The liver and the kidneys are responsible for the majority of drug elimination,

necessarily an early tumor; only serial studies to judge its growth rate will help establish its age. Bulky tumors (diameters >2–3 cm) enlarge more slowly than small ones because their cells, especially those of the inner core (farthest from the blood supply), have a long generation time. Competition for nutrients and other less-defined competitive pressures reduce the activity of the entire mass.

Successful chemotherapy of cancer requires a physiologic edge that can be exploited to differentially kill cancer cells but spare normal cells as much as possible. The more rapid growth rate of tumors and the increased synchronicity of tumor cells compared with normal tissues may be taken advantage of when designing therapeutic regimens. At any given time, comparatively large numbers of cancer cells will be in the DNA synthesis phase (S phase) of the cell cycle, the only time during which cycle-dependent agents (those inhibiting DNA synthesis) can act. Thus, short-term high-dose chemotherapy with agents affecting DNA synthesis, such as methotrexate, is most effective in killing rapidly dividing tumor cells with relative sparing of normal bone marrow elements. Unfortunately, bone marrow cells, the epithelial cells that line the GI tract, and hair follicles all have generation times comparable with those of tumors, and they are therefore vulnerable to compounds that inhibit DNA synthesis (see Table 17.2). However, compared with the more synchronously growing tumor cell population, only a few of the bone marrow cells are in their S phase at any given time, and this accounts for the selective toxicity of phase-dependent compounds. A course of therapy extending over a period of several days or even weeks may be required to kill a slow-growing tumor in which only a few cells are in the stage of DNA synthesis at any one time. Agents that do not depend on DNA synthesis for their effects (ie, cycle-nonspecific agents), such as alkylating agents, are most effective against bulky, slow-growing tumors. The cells remaining after treatment tend to divide more rapidly and are more susceptible to attack by

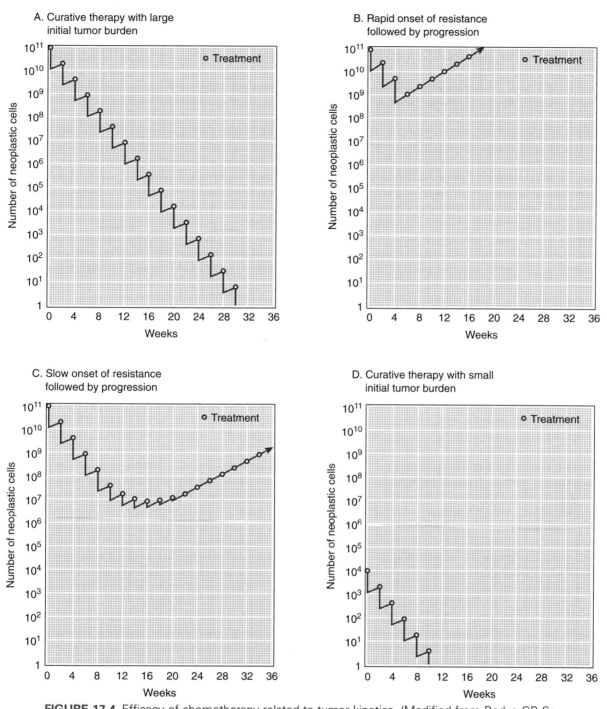

FIGURE 17.4 Efficacy of chemotherapy related to tumor kinetics. (Modified from Bodye GB Sr, Frei E III, Luce JK. The Systemic Approach to Cancer Therapy. *Hosp Pract* 1967;2(10):42.)

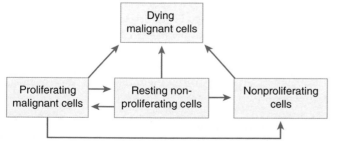

FIGURE 17.5 Dynamics of tumor growth, showing the inter-relationship of cell compartments contributing to the clinical presence of tumor.

although excretion in bile, stool, and respiration may also contribute in some cases. Organ dysfunction may result in increased drug toxicity and may require dose modification.

Drug Interactions

Although patients undergoing chemotherapy treatment may also receive a variety of other drugs for treatment of acute side effects or chronic medical conditions, few drug interactions are clinically significant. **However, a few interactions are noteworthy. In particular, whereas doxorubicin and taxane agents are known to exert increased toxicity in the setting of impaired** biliary excretion, the platinum compounds and methotrexate may cause increased toxicity in the setting of decreased renal function. Aspirin and sulfonamides are known to displace methotrexate from plasma proteins, and direct chemical interactions are noted between cisplatin and mannitol and mitoxantrone and heparin.

Drug Resistance

The effectiveness of any cancer treatment is limited by drug resistance, which may be intrinsic or acquired and may develop to one drug or to multiple drugs (pleiotropic resistance). It has been suggested that spontaneous mutation is a basis for drug resistance. This spontaneous mutation occurs rapidly in malignant tumors. **This concept, the Goldie–Coldman hypothesis, has been applied to the growth of malignant tumors and has important clinical implications.** The theory suggests that most malignant cells begin with intrinsic sensitivity to chemotherapeutic agents but develop spontaneous resistance at variable rates. Goldie and Coldman have developed a mathematic model that relates curability to the time of recurrence of the singly or doubly resistant cells. Assuming that there is a natural mutation rate, the model predicts a variation in the size of the resistant fraction in tumors of the same size and type, which depends on that mutation rate and the point at which the mutation develops. Thus, the proportion of resistant cells in any untreated tumor is likely to be small, and the initial response to treatment would not be influenced by the number of resistant cells. In clinical practice, this means that a complete remission could be obtained even if the resistant cell line were present. The failure to cure such a patient, however, would depend directly on the presence of these resistant cells. This model of spontaneous drug resistance implies that minimizing the emergence of drug-resistant clones requires that multiple effective drugs or therapies be applied as early as possible in the course of the patient's malignant disease process.

In cell lines and animal models, resistance to specific drugs likely occurs via a wide variety of mechanisms, although only a few have been confirmed to be of clinical significance in human cancers. These include increase in proficiency of DNA repair, decrease in drug uptake or increase in efflux by cells, increased levels of or alterations in target enzymes, alterations in drug activation or degradation, gene amplification, and defective drug metabolism. These mechanisms are reviewed in Table 17.4.

Multidrug resistance also occurs via various mechanisms. Some experimental evidence in murine tumors suggests that one form of multiple-drug resistance relates to the ability of drug-resistant tumor cells to limit drug accumulation of structurally unrelated agents. This cross-resistance is seen most often with natural products (eg, doxorubicin, etoposide, paclitaxel, and vinca alkaloids); resistance to a single drug may confer a cross-resistance to structurally dissimilar drugs with different modes of action. This is the best studied mechanism for multidrug resistance and has been characterized involving the p-170 glycoprotein and its gene *MDR1*. Ling initially demonstrated the appearance of a P-glycoprotein with a molecular weight of 170 kD on the cell membrane. The appearance of pleiotropic

TABLE 17.4 Probable Mechanisms Associated With Resistance to Some Commonly Used Anticancer Drugs	
Mechanism	**Drugs**
Increase in proficiency of repair of DNA	Alkylating agents, cisplatin
Decrease in cellular uptake or increase in efflux of drugs	Cisplatin, doxorubicin, etoposide, melphalan, 6-mercaptopurine, methotrexate, nitrogen mustard, vinblastine, vincristine
Increase in levels of "target" enzyme	Methotrexate
Alterations in target enzyme	5-Fluorouracil, 6-mercaptopurine, methotrexate, 6-thioguanine
Decrease in drug activation	Cytosine arabinoside, doxorubicin, 5-fluorouracil, 6-mercaptopurine, 6-thioguanine
Increase in drug degradation	Bleomycin, cytosine arabinoside, 6-mercaptopurine
Alternative biochemical pathways	Cytosine arabinoside
Inactivation of active metabolites by binding to	Alkylating agents, cisplatin, doxorubicin sulfhydryl compounds
Decreased activity of topoisomerase	Camptothecins, doxorubicin, etoposide
Alteration of tubulin-binding sites	Vincristine, paclitaxel, ixabepilone
Increased damage tolerance	Alkylating agents, cisplatin

Modified from Tannock IF, Hill RT, eds. *The Basic Science of Oncology*, 3rd ed. New York, 1988, McGraw-Hill. Reproduced by permission of The McGraw-Hill Companies.)

drug resistance is associated with permeability of the cell to accumulate and retain antineoplastic drugs. It has been demonstrated that this P-glycoprotein is directly related to the expression of resistance, and cells that revert to the drug-sensitive state lose this membrane glycoprotein. DNA can be transferred from resistant cells to the sensitive cells, producing a transfer of pleiotropic resistance to unexposed cells.

Although best characterized, *MDR1* is unlikely to be the most common mechanism for chemotherapy resistance among ovarian cancers, given that most do not express the *MDR1* gene. Another mechanism for the multiple-drug resistance phenotype is seen among alkylating agents, cisplatin, and irradiation. Resistance in this group of agents has been linked to elevations in intracellular glutathione levels and is not associated with an overall measurable decrease in drug accumulation. Other transport proteins, including multidrug resistance–associated protein, have been identified that do not involve the p-170 glycoprotein pump. Furthermore, alterations in genes controlling apoptosis and growth arrest have also been cited. Although the relative importance of these separate mechanisms in ovarian cancer remains to be established, it seems most likely that in clinical situations various combinations of mechanisms are at work.

Calculation of Dosage

Dosages of chemotherapeutic agents are usually discussed in terms of mg/kg of body weight or mg/m^2 of total body surface area (Table 17.5). Dosage based on surface area is preferable to

TABLE 17.5 Equations for Calculation of Body Surface Area

	Equation*
Mostellar (m²)	$\sqrt{Weight \times Height/3600}$
DuBois and DuBois (m²)	$(Weight^{0.425}) \times (Height^{0.725}) \times 71.84$
Haycock (m²)	$(Weight^{0.5378}) \times (Height^{0.3964}) \times 0.024265$

*Weight in kilograms; height in centimeters.

FIGURE 17.6 Nomogram for calculating the body surface area of adults.

that based on weight, because surface area changes much less during the course of therapy, allowing a more consistent absolute amount of drug to be given throughout therapy. Dosages per unit are also more comparable in adults and children (Figs. 17.6 and 17.7), and the variation in total dose between very obese and very thin people is minimized. Dosage in experimental

animals expressed as mg/m² is more easily related to that in humans. In adults, mg/kg can be converted with reasonable accuracy to mg/m² by multiplying by 40.

Dose adjustments should be made for patients who are likely to have a compromised bone marrow reserve—that is, those older than 70 years of age, those who have received previous pelvic or abdominal irradiation, and those who have had previous chemotherapy. In these subsets of patients, the physician should consider beginning with a dose reduced by 35% to 50% and escalate up to a full dose with subsequent courses if initial doses are well tolerated. In a similar manner, any moderate to severe toxicity during the patient's course of therapy should direct a reduction in future doses. The adverse effects criteria table used by the Gynecologic Oncology Group is included as Appendix B.

Dose adjustments are often required in patients receiving anticancer agents that are eliminated by the kidneys. These adjustments reduce the likelihood of overly high plasma drug concentrations and the attendant risk of serious renal toxicity. Several techniques have been used to assess renal function (glomerular filtration rate [GFR]) in individuals with cancer. The calculated creatinine clearance (Cr Cl) using serum creatinine is the most commonly used. The elimination of creatinine is primarily via glomerular filtration, although a small amount may be secreted in the renal tubules. Several studies have compared the different methods of estimating Cr Cl using a serum creatinine value. These methods are based on correlations of Cr Cl with age, body weight, serum creatinine, and creatinine metabolism. The most utilized methods follow.

Jelliffe Method

The Jelliffe method was used originally as a simple estimate of Cr Cl using serum creatinine, making minor adjustments in the calculation for female patients. The current Jelliffe formula takes into consideration age and renal function, and is as follows:

$$Cr\ Cl\ (mL/min) = (98 - (0.8 \times (age - 20)))/$$
$$(serum\ creatinine\ in\ mg/dL)) \times Patient's\ BSA/1.73\ m^2$$

(For female patients, use 90% of predicted Cr Cl.)

Cockroft–Gault Method

This equation includes factors for lean body weight, which is especially important for obese patients, and correlation for female patients (the obtained value is multiplied by 0.85 for women). This method is similar to the Jelliffe calculation and is as follows:

$$Cr\ Cl = (140 - Age) \times (Lean\ body\ weight\ [in\ kg])/$$
$$(Serum\ creatinine) \times 72$$

Calvert Formula

The use of the Cr Cl has also been incorporated into the so-called Calvert formula. Based on good data, there is evidence showing that there is an inverse linear correlation between the GFR and the AUC of drugs such as carboplatin (Table 17.6).

FIGURE 17.7 Nomogram for calculating the body surface area of children.

TABLE 17.6   Recommended Individualized Dosing of Carboplatin

Carboplatin dose (mg) = Target AUC × (GFR+ 25)*
AUC is selected for appropriate clinical situation:
AUC 6 in untreated patients, when used in combination with taxanes
AUC 5 in previously treated patients
AUC 7 in previously untreated patients

*Glomerular filtration rate (GFR) is equivalent to creatinine clearance, which can be measured or can be estimated from the patient's age, weight, and serum creatinine.
AUC, Area under the curve.

This finding suggests that to obtain the desired AUC, the dose must not only be decreased in patients with low renal function but also higher than standard doses may be required for patients with high renal clearance values. The Calvert formula is as follows:

$$\text{Dose (mg)} = \text{Target AUC} \times (\text{GFR} + 25)$$

The original Calvert calculations were derived from GFR as measured by the chromium-51–EDTA (ethylenediaminetetraacetic acid) method. Although calculated GFR is not the same as one that is measured and Cr Cl can exceed GFR by 10% to 40%, the majority of physicians calculate rather than measure the GFR by using formulas such as Jelliffe or Cockcroft–Gault formula and then insert these numbers into the Calvert formula.

CATEGORIES OF DRUGS IN CURRENT USE (TABLE 17.7)

Alkylating Agents

Alkylating agents prevent cell division primarily by cross-linking strands of DNA. Because of continued synthesis of other cell constituents, such as RNA and protein, growth is

Text continued on p. 463

TABLE 17.7 Chemotherapy Agents Used in the Treatment of Gynecologic Cancer

Drug	Dosage and Route of Administration	Acute Side Effects	Toxicity	Precautions	Major Indications
ALKYLATING AGENTS					
Cisplatin (CDDP or Platinol)	50–100 mg/m² IV every 3 wk; 40 mg/m² IV every week with radiation therapy; 75–100 mg/m² IP in 2 L over 30 min every 3 wk	Nausea and vomiting, often severe	Renal damage, moderate myelosuppression, neurotoxicity; severe renal damage can be minimized by not exceeding a total dose of 500 mg/m² in any treatment course	Infuse at a rate not to exceed 1 mg/min and only after 10–12 hr of hydration; avoid nephrotoxic antibodies; watch renal function and discontinue if BUN exceeds 30 mg/dL or creatinine exceeds 2 mg/dL	Carcinoma of the ovary, endometrium, or cervix
Carboplatin (Paraplatin)	250–400 mg/m² IV bolus or by 24-hr continuous infusion every 2–4 wk (most authorities recommend dosing to AUC values of 5.0–8.0); may be given IP at AUC 6 every 3 wk	Mild nausea and vomiting	Bone marrow suppression, especially thrombocytopenia	Decreased dose in patients who have had previous chemotherapy	Carcinoma of the cervix, ovary, and endometrium
Cyclophosphamide (Cytoxan)	50–1500 mg/m² as a single dose IV or 1–5 mg/kg/day (usually 50 mg PO per day); dose decreased if severe leukopenia develops; 50 mg PO daily	Nausea and vomiting	Bone marrow depression, alopecia, cystitis	Maintain adequate fluid intake to avoid cystitis	Carcinoma of the cervix, ovary, endometrium, and fallopian tube
Chlorambucil (Leukeran)	0.1–0.2 mg/kg per day PO; dose decreased if severe bone marrow depression develops	Nausea, vomiting (with high doses)	Bone marrow depression	None	—
Ifosfamide (Ifex)	7–10 g/m² IV over 3–5 days every 3–4 wk	Nausea, vomiting	Bone marrow depression, alopecia, cystitis	Uroprotectant to prevent hemorrhagic cystitis	Carcinoma and sarcoma of ovary, cervix, and endometrium
Oxaliplatin	59–130 mg/m² IV as a 20-min or 2-hr infusion every 3 wk	Nausea, vomiting, diarrhea, mucositis	Mild to moderate myelosuppression; transaminase elevation; peripheral neuropathy	Should not be given to patient with significant renal or hepatic dysfunction	Ovarian carcinoma
Altretamine (Hexalen)	4–12 mg/kg per day PO in divided doses for 14–21 days, repeated every 6 wk	Nausea and vomiting	Bone marrow depression; neurotoxicity, both central and peripheral	None	Ovarian carcinoma
ANTIMETABOLITES					
5-Fluorouracil (5-FU)	12 mg/kg per day IV for 4 days; then alternate days at 6 mg/kg for 4 days or until toxicity; repeat course monthly or give weekly IV dose of 12–15 mg/kg; maximal dose, 1 g for either regimen; often used as one drug in combination regimens at a dose of 500 mg/m² IV	Bone marrow depression, diarrhea, stomatitis, alopecia	Occasional nausea and vomiting	Decrease dose in patients with diminished liver, renal, or bone marrow function or after adrenalectomy	Carcinoma of the ovary and endometrium
Methotrexate	Choriocarcinoma: 10–30 mg/day IV for 5 days; ovarian or cervical carcinoma: 200–2000 mg/m² IV with concomitant or sequential systematic antidote ("leucovorin rescue")	None	Bone marrow depression, megaloblastic anemia, diarrhea, stomatitis, vomiting; alopecia less common; occasional hepatic fibroids, vasculitis, pulmonary fibrosis	Adequate renal function must be present, and urine output must be maintained	Choriocarcinoma, carcinoma of the ovary and cervix

Continued

TABLE 17.7 Chemotherapy Agents Used in the Treatment of Gynecologic Cancer—cont'd

Drug	Dosage and Route of Administration	Acute Side Effects	Toxicity	Precautions	Major Indications
Gemcitabine (Gemzar)	800–1000 mg/m² IV days 1, 8, 15 every 28 days; 800–1000 mg/m² IV days 1, 8 every 21 days; 900 mg/m² IV days 1, 8 every 21 days for patients with leiomyosarcoma	Mild nausea, vomiting, malaise (usually mild); transient febrile episodes, maculopapular rash	Bone marrow suppression	None	Carcinoma of the breast and ovary; leiomyosarcoma of the uterus
Capecitabine (Xeloda)	1500–2000 mg/m² PO daily in two divided doses for 2 wk with a 1-week rest period; repeat every 3 wk	Hand and foot syndrome (palmar–plantar syndrome); nausea, vomiting, diarrhea; abdominal pain; constipation	Myelosuppression; hyperbilirubinemia	Should be taken in divided doses 12 hr apart, administered with water 30 min after a meal	Ovarian carcinoma
ANTITUMOR ANTIBIOTICS					
Dactinomycin (actinomycin D, Cosmegen)	15 µg/kg per day IV or 0.5 mg/day for 5 days	Pain on local infiltration with skin necrosis; nausea and vomiting in many patients 2 hr after the dose; occasional cramps and diarrhea	Bone marrow depression, stomatitis, diarrhea, erythema, hyperpigmentation with occasional desquamation in areas of previous irradiation	Administer through running IV infusion; use with care in patients with liver disease and in the presence of inadequate marrow function; prophylactic antiemetics are helpful	Embryonal rhabdomyosarcoma, choriocarcinoma, ovarian germ cell tumors
Bleomycin	10–20 mg/m² IV or IM one or two times a week	Fever, chills, nausea, vomiting; local pain and phlebitis less frequent	Skin: hyperpigmentation, thickening, nail changes, ulceration, rash, peeling, alopecia; pulmonary: pneumonitis with dyspnea, rales, infiltrate can progress to fibrosis; more common in patients older than 70 years of age and with more than a 400-mg total dose but unpredictable	Watch for hypersensitivity in lymphoma with first one or two doses; use with extreme caution in presence of renal or pulmonary disease; start in hospital under observation; do not exceed a total dose of 400 mg	Squamous cell carcinoma of the skin, vulva, and cervix; choriocarcinoma; germ cell and sex cord–stromal tumors
Doxorubicin (Adriamycin)	60–100 mg/m² IV every 3 wk	Nausea, vomiting, fever, local phlebitis, necrosis if extravasated, red urine (not blood)	Bone marrow depression, alopecia, cardiac toxicity related to the cumulative dose, stomatitis; atrophy of the myocardia can occur, especially if a total dose of 450–500 mg/m² is exceeded	Administer through running IV infusion; avoid giving to patients with significant heart disease; observe for ECG abnormalities and signs of heart failure	Adenocarcinoma of the endometrium, fallopian tube, ovary, and vagina; uterine sarcoma
Liposomal doxorubicin hydrochloride (Doxil)	40–50 mg/m² IV every 4 wk	Hand and foot syndrome (palmar–plantar erythrodysesthesia syndrome); mild nausea or vomiting, mucositis, stomatitis	Mild myelosuppression; cardiomyopathy is less common compared with standard doxorubicin	Hypersensitivity reported in approximately seven patients	Ovarian carcinoma
Vinca Alkaloids					
Vinblastine (Velban)	0.10–0.15 mg/kg per week IV	Severe, prolonged inflammation if extravasated; occasional nausea, vomiting, headache, and paresthesias	Bone marrow depression, particularly neutropenia; alopecia, muscle weakness, occasional mild peripheral neuropathy, mental depression 2–3 days after treatment, rarely stomatitis	Administer through running IV infusion or inject with great care to prevent extravasation; decrease dose in liver disease	Choriocarcinoma

Drug	Dose	Acute Toxicity	Delayed Toxicity	Special Precautions	Major Indications
Vincristine (Oncovin)	0.4–1.4 mg/m² IV weekly in adults; 2 mg/m² weekly in children	Local inflammation if extravasated	Paresthesias, weakness, loss of reflexes, constipation; abdominal, chest, and jaw pain, hoarseness, foot drop, mental depression; marrow toxicity generally mild, anemia and reticulocytopenia most prominent; alopecia	Administer through running IV infusion or inject with great care to prevent extravasation; decrease dose in patients with liver disease; patients with underlying neurologic problems may be more susceptible to neurotoxicity; alopecia may be prevented by use of a scalp tourniquet for 5 min during and after administration	Uterine sarcoma, germ cell tumor of the ovary
Vinorelbine (Navelbine)	30 mg/m² weekly IV	Mild nausea, 10% alopecia	Bone marrow depression, mild to moderate peripheral neuropathy	Local irritant, dose modification with hepatic dysfunction	Ovarian carcinoma
Epipodophyllotoxins					
Etoposide (VP-16)	100 mg/m² IV days 1, 3, and 5; repeat in 4 wk	Nausea and vomiting	Leukopenia, thrombocytopenia, alopecia, headache, fever, occasional hypotension	Reduce dose by 25%–50% for hematologic toxicity	Trophoblastic disease, germ cell tumors
Taxanes					
Paclitaxel (Taxol)	135-175 mg/m² IV over 3 hr every 3 wk; as part of **IP dosing** with a platinum, may give 135 mg/m² IV on day 1 with 60 mg/m² IP on day 8 every 3 wk; as part of **dose-dense therapy,** may give 80 mg/m² IV weekly with carboplatin AUC on 6 day 1 every 3 wk	Allergic reaction, nausea, vomiting	Bone marrow depression, severe allergic-like reactions with facial erythema, dyspnea, tachycardia, and hypotension cardiotoxicity with bradycardia, alopecia, stomatitis, fatigue	Cardiac monitoring may be necessary	Ovarian carcinoma; endometrial cancer; cervical cancer
Protein-bound paclitaxel (Abraxane)	80–200 m²/m² IV over 30 min weekly; 175–260 mg/m² IV over 30 min every 3 wk	Nausea, vomiting, diarrhea	Bone marrow depression, 1% hypersensitivity; abnormal ECG; neuropathy	Dose adjustment in hepatic impairment	Ovarian carcinoma
Docetaxel (Taxotere)	60–100 mg/m² IV over 1 h every 3 wk	Hypersensitivity	Myelosuppression; mucositis; alopecia; fluid retention	Requires premedication with steroids	Ovarian carcinoma
Epothilones					
Ixabepilone	20 mg/m² IV day 1, 8, 15 of 28-day cycle	Nausea, vomiting, diarrhea	Myelosuppression; neuropathy; fatigue; mucositis	Avoid concomitant use of CYP3A4 inhibitors; avoid grapefruit juice	Ovarian carcinoma
CAMPTOTHECIN ANALOGS					
Topotecan	1.5 mg/m² daily for 5 days; 4 mg/m² IV on day 1 and day 8; repeat every 21 days	Maculopapular pruritic exanthema	Bone marrow depression	Watch for neutropenic fever	Ovarian carcinoma, cervical carcinoma
Irinotecan (CPT-11)	300 mg/m² IV every 3 wk; 100 mg/m² IV weekly for 4 wk every 6 wk	Nausea and vomiting, diarrhea	Myelosuppression, alopecia, rash	None	Ovarian carcinoma
PARP INHIBITORS					
Olaparib (Lynparza)	400 mg PO BID	Abdominal pain, decreased appetite, nausea, diarrhea, fatigue, arthralgia, myalgia	Anemia, neutropenia, thrombocytopenia, creatinine elevation	Swallow capsules whole, do not chew, dissolve or open capsules; avoid concomitant use with CYP3A inhibitors	Ovarian cancer (germline or tumor *BRCA* mutation positive)

Continued

TABLE 17.7   Chemotherapy Agents Used in the Treatment of Gynecologic Cancer—cont'd

Drug	Dosage and Route of Administration	Acute Side Effects	Toxicity	Precautions	Major Indications
ANTIANGIOGENESIS AGENTS					
Bevacizumab (Avastin)	15 mg/kg IV every 3 wk; 10 mg/kg IV every 2 wk	Pain, abdominal pain, epistaxis, voice alteration, vomiting, constipation, anorexia	Hemorrhage, bowel perforation, delayed wound healing, wound dehiscence, hypertension, arterial and venous thromboembolism; proteinuria	Use with caution in patients with symptoms of bowel obstruction or ileus given risk of bowel perforation; discontinue at least 28 days before elective surgery because of risks of delayed wound healing and dehiscence	Ovarian cancer, cervical cancer
HORMONAL AGENTS					
Progestational Agents					
Medroxyprogesterone acetate	400–800 mg/wk IM or PO	None	Occasional liver function abnormalities, occasional alopecia and hypersensitivity reactions	Use with care when liver dysfunction present	Carcinoma of the endometrium
Hydroxyprogesterone caproate	1000 mg IM twice weekly				
Megestrol acetate (Megace)	20–80 mg PO twice a day				
Antiestrogens					
Tamoxifen	10–20 mg PO twice daily	Nausea, usually mild	Caused by antiestrogenic action (eg, hot flashes, pruritus vulvae, and occasionally vaginal bleeding)	None	Breast cancer, possibly useful in endometrial carcinoma (metastatic)
AROMATASE INHIBITORS					
Anastrozole (Arimidex)	1 mg PO daily	Hot flashes, asthenia, arthritis, arthralgia depression, nausea, vomiting, rash	Liver enzyme elevation, osteoporosis, fracture, depression	Estrogen-containing therapies and tamoxifen should not be used in conjunction with anastrozole	Breast cancer; ovarian and endometrial carcinoma
Letrozole (Femara)	2.5 mg PO daily	Arthralgia, arthritis, hot flashes, night sweats, fatigue, depression, headache	Bone effects, fracture, myocardial infarction, increase in cholesterol		Breast cancer; ovarian and endometrial carcinoma
Exemestane (Aromasin)	25 mg PO daily after a meal	Hot flashes, fatigue, arthralgia, headache, insomnia, increased sweating, nausea	Cardiac ischemic events, hypertension	Co-medications that induce CYP 3A4 may decrease exposure to exemestane	Breast cancer; ovarian and endometrial carcinoma
MISCELLANEOUS					
Hydroxyurea (Hydrea)	80 mg/kg PO every 3 days or 20–30 mg/kg per day	Anorexia and nausea	Bone marrow depression, megaloblastic anemia; stomatitis, diarrhea, and alopecia less common	Decrease dose in patients with marrow and renal dysfunction	Carcinoma of the cervix (with radiotherapy)

AUC, Area under the curve; *BID,* twice a day; *BUN,* blood urea nitrogen; *CDDP,* cisplatin; *ECG,* electrocardiogram; *IM,* intramuscular; *IP,* intraperitoneal; *IV,* intravenous; *PO,* oral.

unbalanced, and the cell dies. Activity of alkylating agents does not depend on DNA synthesis in the target cells. Cyclophosphamide, however, also inhibits DNA synthesis, which makes it distinctive among the alkylating agents in its mode and spectrum of activity. Alkylating agents now used in gynecologic oncology are as follows:

- Carboplatin
- Cisplatin
- Oxaliplatin
- Cyclophosphamide
- Ifosfamide
- Altretamine (hexamethylmelamine)

Antimetabolites

Antimetabolites act by inhibiting essential metabolic processes that are required for synthesis of purines, pyrimidines, and nucleic acids. These agents are typically S phase specific. The currently used drugs in this category are as follows:

- 5-FU
- Methotrexate
- Capecitabine
- Gemcitabine
- Pemetrexed

Antitumor Antibiotics

Antitumor antibiotics have generally been derived from fermentation products of various fungi, and most work via DNA intercalation. Several cytotoxic antibiotics have come into use for chemotherapy of certain neoplasms. Those used in gynecologic oncology are as follows:

- Dactinomycin (actinomycin D)
- Bleomycin
- Doxorubicin and liposomal doxorubicin hydrochloride

Agents Derived From Plants

Several chemotherapeutic agents have been developed from plants. The vinca alkaloids, the epipodophyllotoxins, the epothilones, and the taxanes act to disturb the normal assembly, disassembly, and stabilization of microtubules. The camptothecin analogs serve to inhibit topoisomerase I, thereby inducing single-stranded DNA breaks. Inhibitors of topoisomerase II include etoposide (VP16) and mitoxantrone. These drugs are as follows:

- Vinca alkaloids:
  - Vinblastine
  - Vincristine
  - Vinorelbine
- Taxanes:
  - Paclitaxel
  - Protein-bound paclitaxel
  - Docetaxel
- Epipodophyllotoxin:
  - Etoposide
- Camptothecin analogs:
  - Topotecan
  - Irinotecan
- Epothilone:
  - Ixabepilone

Hormonal Agents

These agents are often used in the treatment of endometrial, breast, and ovarian cancers and are classified in two broad categories: antiestrogens and progestational agents. Megestrol acetate may both downregulate estrogen-responsive genes and reduce the number of available cell surface estrogen receptors. Examples of these agents are as follows:

- Antiestrogen:
  - Tamoxifen
- Progestational agents:
  - Megestrol acetate
  - Medroxyprogesterone acetate
- Aromatase inhibitors:
  - Anastrazole
  - Letrozole
  - Exemestane

Targeted Therapies and Immunotherapy

To date, traditional chemotherapy has predominantly focused on killing rapidly dividing cells. Unfortunately, normal cells may also be affected, causing significant toxicity. Targeted therapies have attempted to focus anticancer treatment on particular pathways and mechanisms that cause cancer to both increase efficacy and decrease toxicity in comparison with traditional chemotherapies. These therapies may aim to affect pathways for angiogenesis, cell cycle, and apoptosis in tumor cells. Several broad categories of targeted therapies exist. Monoclonal antibodies target receptors on the surface of tumor cells. As part of anticancer therapy, monoclonal antibodies have been used in two fashions. First, infusion of the antibody has allowed binding to target cells, which in turn triggers normal effector mechanisms of the body. Second, monoclonal antibodies have been conjugated to a strongly radioactive atom, such as iodine-131, to aid in killing the target. Monoclonal antibodies, such as bevacizumab, directed against vascular endothelial growth factor (VEGF) to block angiogenesis are among the most common used in gynecologic cancer therapy.

Other targeted therapies focus on the internal components and function of the cancer cell, using small molecules to disrupt the function of the cells, triggering apoptosis. Poly(ADP-ribose) polymerase (PARP) inhibitors are a newer class of targeted agent available for treatment of breast and ovarian cancers. PARP is important in repair of single-strand DNA breaks (SSBs). Inhibition of PARP allow SSBs to persist, leading to eventual double-strand breaks (DSBs) as the replication fork progresses. Patients with mutations in BRCA are unable to repair these DSBs, resulting in cell death. Immunotherapies include vaccines (which may be dendritic cell, protein/peptide, DNA, or RNA based) and adoptive immunotherapy. Although many agents are in clinical trial, none are currently approved by the US Food and Drug Administration (FDA) except for bevacizumab and the PARP inhibitor olaparib. Some examples, along with their targets, are as follows:

- Monoclonal antibodies:
  - Oregovomab (CA-125)
  - Cetuximab (EGFR)
  - Bevacizumab (VEGF)
  - Trastuzumab (HER-2/neu)

- Small molecules:
  - Cediranib (VEGFR)
  - Gefitinib (EGFR)
  - Erlotinib (EGFR)
  - Bortezomib (proteosome)
  - Imatinib (Bcr-Abl protein tyrosine kinase, c-kit receptor tyrosine kinase)Pazopanib (VEGFR, platelet-derived growth factor receptor [PDGFR]-α, -β, ckit)
  - Sorafenib (Raf/Mek/Erk, VEGFR)
  - Sunitinib (VEGFR, PDGFR-α, -β)
- PARP inhibitors:
  - Olaparib
  - Rucaparib
  - Veliparib

DRUG TOXICITY

Unfortunately, traditional chemotherapeutic agents are indiscriminate in their effects: Both malignant and normal tissues are affected. Although their goal is to kill more cancerous than normal cells, many side effects, particularly those to organ systems with rapidly proliferating cell populations, are inevitable. Usually, the mechanism of toxicity is similar to the one producing the desired cytotoxic effect. Even organs with limited cell proliferation can be damaged by chemotherapeutic agents, especially if the agents are used at high doses. Chemotherapeutic agents must be used at doses that produce some degree of toxicity to normal tissue in order to be effective. The incidence of severe side effects of chemotherapeutic agents is greatly influenced by states such as severe disability, advancing age, poor nutrition, or direct organ involvement by primary or metastatic lesions. The physician must monitor these patients with extreme care, and appropriate dose modifications must be made (Table 17.8).

Hematologic Toxicity

Hematologic effects are the most frequently observed toxicity. Acute granulocytopenia occurs 6 to 12 days after the

TABLE 17.8 Drug Dose Modification Based on Common Hematologic Toxicity

Count Before Next Course (per mm³)	Dose Modification*
Leukocytes	
>4000	100% of dose
3000–3999	100% of nonmyelotoxic agents
	50% of myelotoxic agents
2000–2999	100% of nonmyelotoxic agents
	25% of myelotoxic agents
1000–1999	25% of myelotoxic agents
≤999	No drug
PLATELETS	
>100,000	100% of dose
50,000–100,000	100% of nonmyelotoxic agents
<50,000	No drug

*Based on myelosuppression.

administration of most myelosuppressive chemotherapeutic agents. Recovery occurs in 10 to 14 days. The megakaryocyte series is affected later, such that platelet suppression usually occurs 4 or 5 days after granulocytopenia and recovers several days after the white blood cell count.

Most clinicians consider patients with absolute granulocyte counts less than 500/mm³ for 5 days or longer to be at a higher risk for sepsis. The practice of using prophylactic broad-spectrum antibiotics in febrile granulocytopenic cancer patients has significantly decreased the incidence of life-threatening infections in this group of patients. Granulocytopenic patients should have their temperatures checked every 4 hours, and they should be examined frequently for evidence of infection. Thrombocytopenic patients with platelet counts less than 20,000/mm³ are at increased risk for spontaneous hemorrhage, particularly from the GI tract. Routine platelet transfusions for platelets under 10,000 to 20,000/mm³ have been used by some clinicians. Others wait and watch until patients manifest some evidence of bleeding. Repeat transfusions of platelets at 2- to 3-day intervals may be necessary in patients with severe thrombocytopenia. Patients with active peptic ulcer disease and patients needing surgical procedures need to be transfused with counts lower than 50,000/mm³.

Growth Factor Therapy

Granulocyte-stimulating therapy. The application of hematopoietic factors to supportive care has been dramatic. Rapid advances in unraveling the molecular biology and biochemistry of these glycoprotein hormones that regulate hematopoiesis have led to their routine clinical use. Since their emergence in 1989, their use has allowed amelioration of therapy-related myelosuppression, modulation of disease-related myelosuppression, and enhanced host defense to infection. This class of agents includes molecules such as granulocyte-colony stimulating factor (G-CSF) and granulocyte macrophage colony–stimulating factor (GM-CSF). The biologic activities of these proteins are complex and multifunctional, stimulating potent changes in the growth, differentiation, distribution, and functional status of mature cells and their precursors (Table 17.9).

Initial studies with G-CSF and GM-CSF focused on their administration via the intravenous (IV) route. Since then, numerous studies have shown that subcutaneous administration once or twice a day is even more myelostimulatory than 2- to 4-hour IV infusions. The recommended dose of GM-CSF is 250 μg/m² or 3to 5 μg/kg. It is interesting that, at least in some cases, a fairly low dose of GM-CSF may be more myelostimulatory than a higher dose. The enhancement of neutrophil function in terms of adherence, phagocytosis, and chemotaxis has also been noted in clinical studies, and GM-CSF may also function to activate lymphocytes. Two types of G-CSF are available: filgrastim and a long-acting pegfilgrastim. The recommended dose of filgrastim is 5 μg/kg, given subcutaneously. Treatment should begin at least 24 hours after completion of chemotherapy and should continue daily until the absolute neutrophil count exceeds 10,000/mm³. Subsequent chemotherapy should not begin until at least 48 hours have elapsed since the last dose. The recommended dose of pegfilgrastim is 6 mg. A

TABLE 17.9 Characteristics of the Hematopoietic Growth Factor Family of Cytokines

Cytokine	Source	Function
Granulocyte-macrophage colony stimulating factor (GM-CSF)	T cells, endothelial cells, stromal cells	Stimulates hematopoiesis of granulocyte and macrophage lineage; activates granulocytes and macrophages
Granulocyte-colony stimulating factor (G-CSF)	Endothelial cells, monocytes, stromal cells	Stimulates hematopoiesis of granulocyte lineage; activates granulocytes
Erythropoietin	Kidney	Stimulates erythroid growth and development
Interleukin-1	Monocytes and macrophages, B and T cells, endothelial cells	Co-stimulates early stages of hematopoiesis; T- and B-cell activation
Interleukin-3	T cells	Stimulates early stages of hematopoiesis
Interleukin-6	T cells, monocytes and macrophages, fibroblasts	Co-stimulates early stages of hematopoiesis; T- and B-cell activation

Modified from Kouides PA. The hematopoietic growth factors. In Haskell CM, ed. *Principles of Cancer Treatment,* 4th ed. Philadelphia, 1995, Saunders.)

subcutaneous injection is recommended at least 24 hours after the completion of chemotherapy infusion and should not be given within 14 days of any subsequent chemotherapy. Bone pain is the most common side effect of G-CSF. Other rarer effects include:

- A cutaneous eruption of macules and papules
- Exacerbation of underlying autoimmune disease
- Anaphylaxis, which is rare
- Mild increased risk of thrombosis
- A theoretic possibility of the exacerbation of the underlying malignancy

Unquestionably, the administration of G-CSF or GM-CSF accelerates neutrophil recovery to a significant degree after standard-dose chemotherapy. G-CSF is indicated to decrease the incidence of febrile neutropenia with regimens associated with a significant incidence of neutropenia with fever.

Erythrocyte-stimulating therapy. The existence of a hormone that regulates erythropoiesis (Epo) has been proposed for 100 years. In 1985, two independent groups cloned the gene responsible for this growth factor. This gene was labeled the Epo gene. The kidney appears to be the major site of production of erythropoietin. Erythropoietin stimulates the division and differentiation of committed erythroid progenitors in the bone marrow. Epoetin alpha is a glycoprotein manufactured by recombinant DNA technology that contains the exact amino acid sequence of the natural Epo.

Epoetin has the potential to reduce the transfusion requirement in anemic patients and may enhance the overall quality of life. Administration may be indicated when hemoglobin levels have decreased below 10 mg/dL during chemotherapy treatment or when a significant chance for blood transfusion exists. However, iron deficiency must be corrected before starting epoetin. Epoetin injected at a dose of 150 U/kg subcutaneously three times a week for 12 weeks has been used by many clinicians. The dose may be increased up to 300 U/kg. Others use a daily dose of 60 U/kg, progressing to a maximum dose of 90 U/kg per day. Another commonly used approach is to inject 40,000 U/week, with escalation to 60,000 U for nonresponders. Darbepoetin alfa is a long-acting form that may be administered at doses of 3.0 μg/kg every 3 weeks. Adverse effects are uncommon but include worsening hypertension in patients with end-stage renal disease. Other effects include edema and diarrhea.

Erythropoiesis-stimulating agents must be used with caution. In 2007, the FDA issued a black box warning regarding the use of both epoetin alfa and darbepoetin alfa. Indeed, two large randomized trials have reported significantly worse tumor control and survival rates in patients receiving epoetin. Research also indicates that the erythropoietin receptor is expressed in several cancer cell lines, raising the concern of possible stimulation of tumor cell growth by these drugs. Epoetin has also been implicated in possible thromboembolic complications, possibly related to elevated hemoglobin levels. Currently, physicians who wish to use these agents for chemotherapy-related anemia must register with the Risk Evaluation and Mitigation Strategy (REMS) program. Manufacturers have implemented the Erythropoiesis Stimulating Agents (ESA) Assisting Providers and cancer Patients with Risk Information for the Safe use of ESAs (APPRISE) Oncology Program as part of a REMS designed for health care providers treating patients with cancer.

Platelet-stimulating Therapy

Oprelvekin is produced in *Escherichia coli* by recombinant DNA methods. The protein is very similar to interleukin (IL)-11, which is a thrombopoietic growth factor that directly stimulates the proliferation of hematopoietic stem cells and megakaryocyte maturation, which in turn increase platelet production. IL-11 is produced by bone marrow stromal cells and is part of the cytokine family. The usual dose is 50 μg/kg, which is given once daily subcutaneously as a single injection in the abdomen, thigh, or hip. Treatment should begin 6 to 24 hours after completion of chemotherapy and continued until the nadir platelet count is 50,000 cells/μL. Potential side effects include mild to moderate fluid retention, and IL-11 should be used with caution in patients with a history of atrial arrhythmia, transient mild visual blurring, and transient rashes at the injection site. Anaphylactic reactions have been reported.

Gastrointestinal Toxicity

Gastrointestinal toxicity is another frequent manifestation of chemotherapeutic agents. Mucositis may be caused by direct effects on the rapidly dividing epithelial mucosa. Concomitant granulocytopenia allows the injured mucosa to become infected and serve as a portal of entry for bacteria and fungi.

The onset of mucositis is frequently 3 to 5 days earlier than myelosuppression. The nasopharyngeal lesions are difficult to distinguish from viral lesions. Candidiasis is often seen and is difficult to distinguish from stomatitis secondary to chemotherapy; antifungal agents have been very effective in treating this condition. Necrotizing enterocolitis is another condition that is seen in patients receiving chemotherapy. Symptoms of this condition are watery or bloody diarrhea, abdominal pain, nausea, vomiting, and fever. Patients usually have abdominal tenderness and distention. They also have a history of broad-spectrum antibiotic use. Most necrotizing enterocolitis is caused by anaerobic bacteria such as *Clostridium difficile.* The treatment of choice for *C. difficile* infection is oral vancomycin, 125 mg four times daily for 10 to 14 days.

The most common side effect of chemotherapy that patients experience is nausea and vomiting. Although the exact mechanisms are not clearly defined, most agents appear to stimulate the chemoreceptor trigger zone in the area postrema of the brain to secrete neurotransmitters such as dopamine, serotonin, and histamine. These neurotransmitters may activate the neighboring vomiting center to induce nausea and emesis. Direct stimulation of serotonin receptors in the GI tract, direct cerebral action, and psychogenic effects may also play a role. Different patterns of emesis include acute emesis (within 24 hours of chemotherapy infusion), delayed emesis (typically beginning 16–24 hours after chemotherapy but persisting up to 72–96 hours), and anticipatory emesis. Common antiemetic regimens are detailed in Table 17.10. The choice of agents should be governed by knowledge of the emetogenic potential of the chemotherapies administered (Table 17.11).

Highly emetogenic chemotherapies include cisplatin (>50 mg/m^2) and high-dose cyclophosphamide (>1500 mg/m^2). Cisplatin may induce both acute and delayed vomiting. A premedication regimen should consist of a combination of antiemetics given 30 minutes before chemotherapy infusion. Common regimens include use of a 5-HT3 receptor antagonist with dexamethasone. Lorazepam and oral aprepitant may also be used. Moderately emetogenic chemotherapies include lower doses of cisplatin (<50 mg/m^2) and cyclophosphamide (750–1500 mg/m^2) and carboplatin, doxorubicin, methotrexate (>1000 mg/m^2), ifosfamide, and high-dose 5-FU. These agents may be premedicated with 5-HT3 receptor antagonists in combination with dexamethasone. Mildly emetogenic chemotherapies include methotrexate, paclitaxel, docetaxel, liposomal doxorubicin, gemcitabine, bleomycin, and etoposide. These agents may be premedicated with single-agent antiemetics.

Delayed emesis requires special consideration. Prophylaxis may include use of single-agent 5-HT3 receptor antagonist therapy or a brief pulse of dexamethasone in combination with metoclopramide, a 5-HT3 receptor antagonist, or aprepitant, a substance P/NK1 antagonist. Long-acting drugs such as palonosetron, a 5-HT3 receptor antagonist, and fosaprepitant, a substance P/NK1 antagonist, are now available and may be administered intravenously on the day of chemotherapy. These drugs are noninferior to standard 3-day oral dosing and may provide advantages in convenience for the patient.

TABLE 17.10   Common Antiemetic Regimens

	Drug	Dosage
PREMEDICATION		
5-HT3 receptor antagonists	Ondansetron	8–24 mg IV/PO
	Granisetron	10 µg/kg IV; 2 mg PO
	Dolasetron	1.8 mg/kg IV; 100 mg IV; 100 mg PO
	Palonosetron (long acting)	0.25 mg IV
Substance P/NK1 receptor antagonist	Aprepitant	125 mg PO
	fosAprepitant (long acting)	150 mg IV
Motility agent	Metoclopramide	2–3 mg/kg IV; 20–40 mg PO
Phenothiazine	Prochlorperazine	10 mg IV/IM/PO; 25 mg PR; 15-mg spansule
Benzodiazepine	Lorazepam	0.5-2 mg IV, PO, or SL
Corticosteroid	Dexamethasone	8-20 mg IV or PO
Acute-phase emesis	Dexamethasone	20 mg IV
	Ondansetron	8–24 mg IV
	Metoclopramide	3 mg/kg IV (repeat every 2 hr prn)
	Diphenhydramine	25–50 mg IV (repeat every 2 hr prn)
	Lorazepam	1–2 mg IV
Prophylaxis of delayed emesis	Dexamethasone	8 mg PO bid × 2 days; then 4 mg PO bid × 2 days
	plus metoclopramide	40 mg PO qid × 2–3 days*
	or 5-HT3 antagonist	Ondansetron 8 mg PO bid or tid × 2–3 days or granisetron 1 mg PO bid or 2 mg PO qid × 2–3 days
	5-HT3 antagonist	PO × 2-3 days alone or plus aprepitant 80 mg PO and dexamethasone 8 mg PO qid × 3 days

*Patients should be advised to take 50 mg of diphenhydramine PO at the first sign of dystonic reaction.
Bid, Twice a day; *IM,* intramuscular; *IV,* intravenous; *PO,* oral; *prn,* as needed; *qid,* four times a day; *tid,* three times a day;

Skin Reactions

Skin reactions, including alopecia and allergic hypersensitivity reactions, are also often seen with chemotherapeutic agents. **Skin necrosis and sloughing at the site of IV extravasation is associated particularly with agents such as doxorubicin, actinomycin D, mitomycin C, vinblastine, vincristine, and nitrogen mustard.** The extent of the necrosis is determined by the amount of extravasated drug. **Management includes removal of the IV line and local infiltration of the area with corticosteroids and ice pack therapy four or five times a day for 3 days.** Long-term monitoring of these patients is essential. **Palmar–plantar erythrodysesthesia, or hand and foot**

TABLE 17.11 Emetogenic Potential of Cancer Chemotherapeutic Agents Used in Gynecologic Oncology

Emetogenic Potential (Frequency, %)	Agent
<10	Bleomycin
	Hydroxyurea
	Melphalan (PO)
	Methotrexate (<50 mg/m^2)
10–30	Docetaxel
	Doxorubicin (<20 mg/m^2)
	Etoposide
	Fluorouracil (<1000 mg/m^2)
	Gemcitabine
	Methotrexate (50–250 mg/m^2)
	Paclitaxel
	Topotecan
30–60	Cyclophosphamide (<750 mg/m^2)
	Dactinomycin (<1.5 mg/m^2)
	Doxorubicin (20–60 mg/m^2)
	Ifosfamide
	Methotrexate (250–1000 mg/m^2)
60–90	Carboplatin
	Cisplatin (<50 mg/m^2)
	Cyclophosphamide (750–1500 mg/m^2)
	Dactinomycin (>1.5 mg/m^2)
	Doxorubicin (>60 mg/m^2)
	Irinotecan
	Melphalan (IV)
	Methotrexate (>1000 mg/m^2)
>90	Cisplatin (>50 mg/m^2)
	Cyclophosphamide (>1500 mg/m^2)

Modified from Hesketh PJ, Kris MG, Grunberg SM, et al. Proposal for classifying the acute emetogenicity of cancer chemotherapy. *J Clin Oncol* 1997;15:103-109.

TABLE 17.12 Prophylaxis for Taxane Hypersensitivity

Agent	Prophylaxis Regimen
Docetaxel	Starting 1 day before infusion: dexamethasone 8 mg PO bid × 3 days
Paclitaxel	Night before and morning of infusion: dexamethasone 20 mg PO*
	30 min before infusion†: diphenhydramine 25–50 mg IV *plus* H2 antagonist IV (cimetidine 300 mg or ranitidine 50 mg)

*May be repeated orally or intravenously 30 minutes before infusion.
†If the first cycle of treatment is well tolerated, subsequent cycles may be premedicated using oral doses.
IV, Intravenous; *PO,* oral.

syndrome, may be a dose-limiting toxicity of liposomal doxorubicin and is characterized by painful edema and erythema. Alopecia is a common side effect of many chemotherapeutic agents. Therapies designed to reduce alopecia have not been successful. Hair growth resumes 10 to 20 days after treatment is completed.

Hypersensitivity

Many chemotherapeutic agents may be associated with hypersensitivity reactions, although only a few agents elicit these responses in more than 5% of patients. Of the agents commonly used in gynecologic oncology, the taxanes and platinum compounds are the most likely culprits, although occasional reactions may also be seen with bleomycin, doxorubicin, etoposide, cyclophosphamide, ifosfamide, and methotrexate.

In phase I trials, the incidence of severe hypersensitivity to paclitaxel was approximately 30%; however, with adequate prophylaxis (Table 17.12), the incidence is now less than 10%. Although hypersensitivity associated with paclitaxel is often attributed to its formulation in Cremophor EL, a polyoxyethylated castor oil, docetaxel has also been associated with a similar incidence of hypersensitivity despite its formulation in Tween 80. With appropriate premedication, hypersensitivity to docetaxel has been reduced to 2% to 3%. The occurrence of hypersensitivity does not preclude further treatment with the drug. If additional diphenhydramine or corticosteroids do not allow the infusion to be completed after a delay, patients may undergo successful systematic desensitization.

The incidence of hypersensitivity to platinum analogs varies from 5% to 20%. Unlike reactions to taxanes, which typically occur within minutes of starting the initial dose, reactions to platinum agents typically do not manifest until several cycles have already been administered. In one series, a median of eight platinum courses was administered before hypersensitivity occurred. Routine premedication for hypersensitivity is not recommended, and patients who experience mild reactions may respond well to the addition of appropriate premedications. Patients with severe reactions may attempt systematic desensitization if indicated, although success is variable.

Hepatic Toxicity

Hepatic toxicity is uncommon. Mild elevations in transaminase, alkaline phosphatase, and bilirubin are seen with many agents, but rarely is the condition severe. Psoriasis and drug-induced hepatitis can affect the amount of the chemotherapeutic agent given, as can preexisting liver disease or exposure to other hepatic toxins.

Pulmonary Toxicity

Interstitial pneumonitis with pulmonary fibrosis is seen with certain chemotherapeutic agents. The agents most likely to produce this are doxorubicin, alkylating agents, and nitrosoureas. Treatment of patients with drug-induced interstitial pneumonitis involves discontinuation of the cytotoxic agent and supportive care. Steroids may be of some benefit.

Cardiac Toxicity

The risk of cardiac toxicity is seen primarily with doxorubicin. The risk increases dramatically when the cumulative dose exceeds 500 mg/m² of ideal body surface area. In recent years, this limit has rarely been exceeded; thus, cardiomyopathy has diminished greatly in incidence. Acute arrhythmias may often be seen, but these disappear with a few days of supportive care. On rare occasions, cyclophosphamide has been reported to produce cardiotoxicity, particularly when it is used in massive doses. Mitomycin C has been reported to cause endocardial fibrosis and myocardial fibrosis, but again these events occur rarely.

Renal Toxicity

Nephrotoxicity may be dose limiting in up to 35% of patients receiving cisplatin. Proximal and distal tubule damage leads to electrolyte wasting and increase in serum creatinine with concomitant decrease in Cr Cl. Renal toxicity may be reduced with adequate IV hydration and mannitol- or furosemide-induced diuresis. Antibiotic therapy with aminoglycosides potentiates the nephrotoxicity of drugs such as cisplatin and should be avoided if possible.

Genitourinary Toxicity

Metabolites of cyclophosphamide are irritants to the bladder mucosa and can cause chronic hemorrhagic cystitis. The toxic metabolite of cyclophosphamide that causes bladder toxicity is known as acrolein. Vigorous hydration and diuresis during administration of cyclophosphamide are essential. Cisplatin produces renal tubular toxicity associated with azotemia and magnesium wasting. Again, this complication can be minimized with diuresis during administration of cisplatin. Other agents known to cause genitourinary toxicity are methotrexate, nitrosoureas, and mitomycin C. Mesna or N-acetylcysteine has been used in recent times in conjunction with cyclophosphamide to prevent bladder toxicity. This agent acts by inactivating the toxic metabolite acrolein.

Neurologic Toxicity

In general, most antineoplastic drugs are associated with mild neurologic side effects. There are some exceptions, however. Vinca alkaloids are commonly associated with peripheral motor sensory and autonomic neuropathies. Agents such as vincristine, vinblastine, paclitaxel, and vinorelbine can produce loss of deep tendon reflexes with distal paresthesias. Paclitaxel may also cause peripheral neuropathy. In most cases, these neurologic toxicities are reversible after cessation of the drug. Cisplatin produces ototoxicity and peripheral neuropathy and occasionally retrobulbar neuritis. **High doses of cisplatin, which are often used in ovarian cancer therapy, are particularly likely to produce progressive and somewhat delayed peripheral neuropathy.** 5-FU has been associated with acute cerebellar toxicity. Hexamethylmelamine is reported to produce peripheral neuropathy and encephalopathy. Ifosfamide has also been associated with encephalopathy, particularly in patients with low serum albumin levels.

Gonadal Dysfunction

Many chemotherapeutic agents have lasting effects on testicular and ovarian functions. This is particularly true of alkylating agents, which can cause azoospermia and amenorrhea. The onset of amenorrhea and ovarian failure is accompanied by an elevation of the serum follicle-stimulating hormone and a fall in serum estradiol. Indeed, these patients often end up with premature menopause. The younger the patient at the onset of therapy, the less likely it is that chemotherapy would eventuate in permanent gonadal dysfunction. **In women older than 30 years of age, most chemotherapeutic regimens are associated with a high incidence of premature ovarian failure.**

Supportive Care

Supportive social workers, chaplains, and psychiatrists in a concentrated total care setting are of great value in enabling a patient to cope with the emotionally and financially shattering experience of having cancer. Home health care services have improved in most areas of the United States, so that IV fluids, antibiotics, IV alimentation, and even chemotherapy can be administered in the home if the situation allows. Although treatment of many patients must be conducted at large medical centers where new agents and multidisciplinary facilities are available, continuing collaboration between the medical center and the patient's primary physician is essential. Problems caused by the disease or its treatment often arise when the patient returns to her community. An informed local physician can rapidly evaluate these crises and take appropriate action. The performance status of the patient should be watched carefully (Table 17.13).

EVALUATION OF NEW AGENTS

The development of new, promising agents is a long, complicated, and expensive process. After identification of potential drugs in in vitro and animal models, all anticancer therapeutic agents must undergo rigorous clinical testing. Several levels of clinical trials are necessary to demonstrate that a newly developed agent should be allowed in regular medical practice. Such trials have been defined as follows.

Phase I

These initial trials are designed to test new drugs at various doses to evaluate toxicity and determine the tolerance to a particular agent. The primary endpoint to these trials is safety evaluation. A dose escalation design is often used in order to define the maximum tolerated dose and to characterize the dose-limiting toxicities of the drug. Some therapeutic effects may be observed, even though the intent of these trials is not response measurement.

Phase II

Phase II studies attempt to determine the response rate of the particular agent at the dose and schedule defined by phase I trials. Secondary endpoints include determination of progression-free interval, determination of toxicity, and overall survival. Most phase II trials are single-arm nonrandomized studies.

TABLE 17.13   Performance Status

GOG/ECOG Group Score	Zubrod Description	Scale (%)	Karnofsky Description	Scale (%)
0	Fully active, able to carry on all predisease performance without restriction	90–100	Normal, no complaints, no evidence of disease	100
			Able to carry on normal activity; minor symptoms or signs of disease	90
1	Restricted in physically strenuous activity but ambulatory and able to carry out work of a light or sedentary nature (eg, light housework, office work)	70–80	Normal activity with effort; some signs and symptoms of disease	80
			Cares for self; unable to perform normal activity or to do active work	70
2	Ambulatory and capable of all self-care but unable to carry out any work activities; up and about more than 50% of waking hours	50–60	Requires occasional assistance but is able to care for most of own needs	60
			Requires considerable assistance and frequent medical care	60
3	Capable of only limited self-care; confined to bed or chair more than 50% of waking hours	30–40	Requires special care and assistance; disabled	40
			Severely disabled; hospitalization indicated, although death not imminent	30
4	Completely disabled; cannot carry on any self-care; totally confined to bed or chair	10–20	Very sick, hospitalization indicated	20
			Fatal processes progressing rapidly; moribund	10
5	Dead	0	Dead	0

ECOG, European Cooperative Oncology; *GOG*, Gynecologic Oncology Group.

Phase III

Phase III trials are designed to compare a drug identified as promising in phase II trials with current standard treatment regimens. Commonly, a new drug is tested against the accepted gold-standard drug therapy for a particular disease site and histology. These trials are typically large in order to provide sufficient power to detect a difference between the treatment arms. Whereas the primary endpoint in phase III trials is usually progression-free survival, secondary endpoints usually include response rate and overall survival.

For the bibliography list, log onto www.expertconsult.com ⟨http://www.expertconsult.com⟩.

18

Targeted Therapy and Molecular Genetics

Shannon N. Westin, MD, MPH, Anil K. Sood, MD, Robert L. Coleman, MD

OUTLINE

KEY POINTS

1. The development of new and effective therapies should be rooted in a clear understanding of tumor biology.
2. Bevacizumab, a humanized monoclonal antibody to human vascular endothelial growth factor, was the first US Food and Drug Administration–approved drug targeting angiogenesis
3. Reverse protein leukoencephalopathy is a rare complication of antiangiogenic agents, including bevacizumab, sorafenib, and sunitinib.

4. As knowledge regarding tumor biology and pathogenesis continues to expand, the number of targeted agents will no doubt increase exponentially. These agents have the potential to have a profound impact on the treatment of patients with gynecologic malignancies.

TARGETED THERAPY

The use of site-specific combinations of surgery, chemotherapy, and radiation therapy in gynecologic malignancies has led to marked initial improvements in patient survival. Unfortunately, over the past 30 years, there has been little improvement in disease-specific mortality rates from the three major gynecologic malignancies (Table 18.1). Furthermore, the incidence of these cancers has remained fairly stable since 1985, especially among endometrial cancers (Table 18.2). The addition of traditional cytotoxic chemotherapies to current treatment regimens is likely to offer only increased toxicities in the absence of further survival benefit. To critically affect patient outcome and improve quality of life, the therapeutic armamentarium of modern oncologists must be expanded. **The search for novel therapeutic options has led to an exploration of therapies targeting molecular pathways critical to the survival of cancer cells.**

FOUNDATION OF TARGETED THERAPY

The development of new and effective therapies should be rooted in a clear understanding of tumor biology. In a pair of seminal papers in 2000 and 2011, Hanahan and Weinberg described the key capabilities acquired by normal cells that lead to the development of cancer. Fig. 18.1 represents the 10 "hallmarks of cancer" implicated in the tumorigenic process. Sustained proliferative signaling and evading growth suppressors relate to the development of cellular autonomy, which is essential for uncontrolled proliferation. Enabling replicative immortality indicates that the cell is unencumbered by two typical processes of senescence: (1) the cessation of growth upon reaching a set number of cellular doublings and (2) crisis, which involves massive cellular death. Resisting cell death is a feature seen in most cancer types, allowing the cells to continue to grow and replicate in the setting of damage that would lead to attrition in a normal cell. The ability to activate invasion of tissues and metastasis is crucial to the continued expansion of tumor

when space and nutrients become limited. Inducing sustained angiogenesis describes uncontrolled growth of new blood vessels, which supply oxygen and nutrients to the tumor. Evading immune destruction allows the tumor to avoid detection by immune cells and limit the extent of immunologic killing. Finally, the ability to reprogram energy metabolism allows adjustment of energy use and creation to prioritize tumor growth and survival. Two additional enabling characteristics allow the cancer to leverage the above mechanisms into cellular growth and survival. Genomic instability hampers the cell's ability to detect and repair DNA errors and damage. Thus, mutations accumulate, and genomic integrity is lost. The presence of rich immune infiltrates in the tumor microenvironment can support tumorigenesis by growth and prosurvival factors. Collectively, these steps enable tumor initiation, growth, and progression.

Acquisition of survival capabilities by cancer cells is theorized to be directly related to dysfunction of the normal molecular mechanisms and pathways within the cell and surrounding microenvironment. Because these pathways drive the progression of cancer, identifying and targeting the changes in the pathways to treat malignancy is a rational strategy. Thus, the field of targeted therapy has flourished in modern cancer treatment, especially among common gynecologic malignancies.

Cytotoxic chemotherapy typically acts primarily on any rapidly dividing cells. Although this may have the desired effects on tumor cells, these drugs do not discriminate between tumor cells and normal host cells, resulting in undesirable side effects in the gastrointestinal (GI) tract, bone marrow, and integumentary and other systems. Ideal targeted therapies provide a more

TABLE 18.1 Mortality Rates* of Major Gynecologic Malignancies Over 30 Years

	1975	1985	1995	2005	2008–2012
Cervical	5.55	3.82	3.24	2.42	2.3
Endometrial	5.28	4.61	4.15	4.12	4.4
Ovarian	9.84	9.08	9.12	8.66	7.7

*Mortality rates presented as per 100,000 women.

TABLE 18.2 Incidence Rates* of Major Gynecologic Malignancies Over 30 Years

	1975	1985	1995	2005	2008–2012
Cervical	14.79	10.23	8.91	6.86	7.7
Endometrial	35.47	25.23	25.33	24.97	25.1
Ovarian	16.32	16.55	14.59	12.96	12.1

*Incidence rates presented as per 100,000 women.

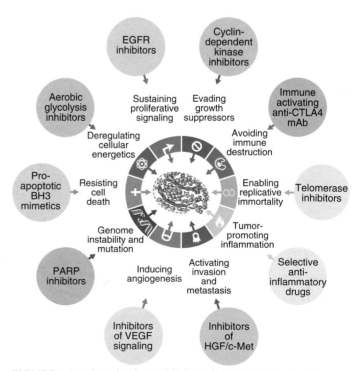

FIGURE 18.1 Acquired capabilities of cancer. (Used with permission from Hanahan D, Weinberg RA. Hallmarks of cancer: the next generation. *Cell* 2011;144(5):646-651.)

directed approach by acting on targets selectively leveraged in tumor cells or in the tumor microenvironment. These targets are typically members of the pathways involved in tumorigenesis, supporting growth, proliferation, metastasis, and angiogenesis. By honing in on those pathways rather than broad-based activity, normal tissues could be spared, and adverse events are minimized.

These therapies hold the potential to reduce mortality rates from gynecologic malignancies while concurrently reducing the morbidity associated with cancer treatment by targeting abnormal rather than normal tissue. This chapter provides a broad overview of the pertinent molecular pathways in gynecologic cancer and the targeted agents that are currently being explored as treatment options. In addition, the unique toxicities of these targeted agents are reviewed. As our knowledge continues to expand, there will no doubt be myriad other pathways to exploit along with agents used to treat gynecologic malignancies.

TARGETED AGENTS

Targeting molecular pathways that drive tumor progression can be accomplished through a variety of mechanisms. The first is a humanized monoclonal antibody (mAb), which is created to bind cancer-associated antigens or molecules for cancer therapy. mAbs may be directed toward ligands or cell surface molecules that participate in pathways of tumorigenesis. Table 18.3 describes the standard nomenclature of the mAb classes. These agents are classified based on the origin of the antibody. By definition, mAbs have affinity for a single target, which allows for minimal non–tumor-related effects. These agents are administered systemically and have long clearance times, allowing biweekly to monthly administration. One such

agent is bevacizumab, which is an mAb to vascular endothelial growth factor A (VEGF-A), a key active ligand in angiogenesis, to be discussed later in the chapter. Engineered antibodies are also being developed that can interact with more than one ligand or binding domain.

Small molecule inhibitors are primarily oral agents that inhibit the function of molecular receptors through the blockage tyrosine kinase activity. Tyrosine kinases are enzymes involved in an array of normal and abnormal cellular functions. Their activity causes the transfer of a phosphate group from adenosine triphosphate (ATP) to a downstream protein tyrosine residue, resulting in changes in protein conformation and association, affecting innumerable biologic processes. Two types of tyrosine kinases exist: receptor and nonreceptor tyrosine kinases. Fig. 18.2 demonstrates the typical structure of a receptor tyrosine kinase, exhibiting three major domains: extracellular ligand binding, transmembrane, and cytoplasmic. Currently, approximately 100 receptor tyrosine kinases have been identified and classified. Nonreceptor tyrosine kinases are typically present in the cytoplasm or nucleus and interact with

TABLE 18.3 Biologically Targeted Monoclonal Antibody Class and Nomenclature

Suffix	Antibody Class	HAMA Potential	Example
"-omab"	Murine	+++	
"-ximab"	Chimeric	+/++	Cetuximab
"-zumab"	Humanized	+	Bevacizumab
"-mumab"	Fully human	–	Panitumumab

HAMA, Human anti-mouse antibody.

FIGURE 18.2 Schematic of two types of tyrosine kinases: receptor (**A**) and nonreceptor (**B**).

transmembrane receptors to phosphorylate downstream substrates. They may also be activated through signals derived from extracellular processes such as ion exchange. Erlotinib is one small molecule inhibitor that targets the epidermal growth factor receptor (EGFR) pathway affecting cellular division and proliferation.

Small molecule inhibitors typically block tyrosine kinase phosphorylation through interaction with the ATP-binding site on the intracellular domain of the tyrosine kinase. Binding to this site may be reversible or irreversible, depending on the agent. These molecules often have short half-lives, which necessitates frequent administration. Secondary to the high degree of homology found at the ATP-binding domain of the various tyrosine kinases, many of these molecules may inhibit one or more receptors within the cellular mechanism. Depending on the pathways affected, this can improve antitumor activity or lead to undesired adverse effects related to "off-target" inhibition.

To reduce off-target associations, unique structural features of a given target are being identified. Then agents that are chemically altered to maximize interaction with these specific components can be introduced. One example is the development of wrapping technology. This involves targeting a defect that is inherently specific to a given region in a protein called a dehydron. Dehydrons are hydrogen bonds of the protein that are poorly protected from water. Drugs designed to protect a given dehydron from water will selectively direct ligands to the receptor with that specific defect. Additional methods of introducing selectivity are being explored, including the disruption of protein–protein interactions.

The use of RNA interference technology has great promise for expanding targeted therapy through knockdown of expression of specific genes involved in tumorigenesis. RNA silencing pathways are mechanisms within the cell that directly control gene expression. In general, short interfering RNAs (siRNAs) are generated from double-stranded RNA (dsRNA) within the cell by an endonuclease called Dicer. The antisense strands of the siRNA then associate with an RNA-induced silencing complex (RISC) that targets a specific messenger RNA (mRNA) for cleavage by Argonaute 2. Cleavage of the mRNA can silence genes involved in cellular survival, proliferation, invasion, and metastasis. Of note, the level of expression of the components of RNA silencing pathways correlates with survival in a variety of cancers.

The delivery of siRNA in vivo has been challenging. However, local delivery (intranasal or intravitreal) approaches have been advanced into clinical trials in nonmalignant diseases such as macular degeneration. Recent methods of delivery using biodegradable lipids and polymers have shown safety and efficacy in cancer models. Furthermore, an ongoing first-in-human phase I trial has demonstrated successful delivery of siRNA through nanoparticles. Early results from this trial revealed induction of RNA interference mechanisms at specific targeted sites. Nanodelivery vehicles for selective delivery can further enhance tumor specificity. This approach to targeted therapy has the potential to greatly expand the possible targets while reducing undesirable adverse effects.

Other unique agents have also been explored as prospective biologic options to disrupt carcinogenic pathways. Decoy receptors that bind key ligands of carcinogenic pathways have been developed. An example of this is VEGF-Trap (aflibercept), which binds VEGF to negatively affect angiogenesis. Antibody–drug conjugates (ADCs) combine a highly toxic cytotoxic agent with a specific immunoglobulin meant to create a targeted therapy that spares normal tissues that lack expression of the selected target. Current ADCs in development use targets including CD30, mesothelin, and folate receptor α. There is no doubt that as our knowledge of cellular signaling mechanisms grows, so will the variety of agents for targeted therapy.

ANGIOGENESIS

Arguably, the most successful examples of targeted therapy in gynecologic cancer are found in the arena of angiogenesis. Angiogenesis is a key process for the supply of nutrients, oxygen, growth factors, and dissemination of a tumor. Thus, the development of new vasculature is an essential process for a tumor to grow beyond 1 mm in size. There are two primary mechanisms for the growth of new blood vessels in both the normal and tumor microenvironment. Sprouting, the dominant means of vessel formation, is the branching of a new vessel from an established blood vessel. The other major mechanism is nonsprouting, which occurs when an existing blood vessel enlarges and splits into two separate vessels. Aggressive tumor cells may also develop microvascular channels to support neovascularization in a process known as vasculogenic mimicry. Finally, existing vasculature in the host tissue may be coopted by the tumors to increase vascular supply.

In normal tissues, the vasculature is organized and uniform in size and shape. Angiogenesis in the tumor microenvironment results in vessels that are more irregular, appearing tortuous, dilated, and leaky. The regulation of angiogenic mechanisms is provided by a complex set of growth factors that stimulate and inhibit vascular growth in response to internal and external stimuli. In general, these factors act on the cells lining the blood vessel (the endothelial cells) to regulate activity within the cellular microenvironment. In the normal cellular microenvironment, the endothelial cells are stable, dividing rarely. Pathologic angiogenesis secondary to an increase in proangiogenic factors results in endothelial cells that demonstrate unregulated division and growth. In fact, high expression of proangiogenic molecules and increased microvessel density (a marker of increased tumor vascularization) are poor prognostic factors in many solid malignancies.

VASCULAR ENDOTHELIAL GROWTH FACTORS AND VASCULAR ENDOTHELIAL GROWTH FACTOR RECEPTORS

Fig. 18.3 demonstrates a schematic of the VEGF pathway, a key contributor to the regulation of angiogenesis. Activation of this pathway promotes the proliferation, survival, and migration of endothelial cells leading to vascular growth. In addition, VEGF

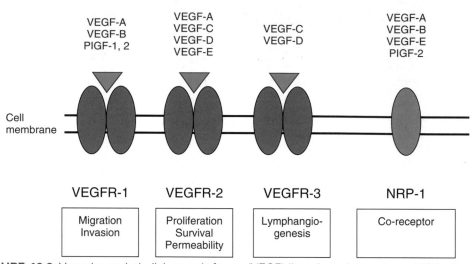

FIGURE 18.3 Vascular endothelial growth factor (VEGF) ligands and receptors. *PIGF*, placental growth factor; *VEGFR*, vascular endothelial growth factor receptor.

stimulation increases cell fenestration and vascular permeability, which has been associated with the development of malignant effusions in the lungs and peritoneal cavity. VEGF overexpression has been found in a majority of solid tumors, including all three major gynecologic cancers, and is associated with poor prognosis and tumor progression.

As demonstrated in Fig. 18.3, the VEGF pathway includes seven different ligands: VEGF-A, VEGF-B, VEGF-C, VEGF-D, VEGF-E, placental growth factor (PlGF)-1, and PlGF-2. The mediation of the angiogenic effects for each VEGF ligand is accomplished through one of three receptors (VEGFRs), including VEGFR-1, VEGFR-2, and VEGFR-3. These receptors belong to the class III family of tyrosine kinase receptors and are typically expressed on the vascular and lymphatic endothelium. However, these receptors may also be expressed by tumor tissue. The overexpression of VEGF in tumor cells is associated with increased tumor growth and metastasis in several solid malignancies, including ovarian and endometrial cancer. Recent studies revealed that ovarian cancers expressing VEGF receptors have higher mortality rates compared with tumors lacking VEGF receptor expression. In cervical cancer, human papilloma virus infection can lead to degradation of p53 and subsequent upregulation of hypoxia inducible factor (HIF-1). This factor can lead to increased neovascularization, supporting the rationale for antiangiogenic therapy in cervical cancer.

Activation of a given VEGFR results in subsequent downstream activation of a variety of known survival, proliferation, and migration pathways in the cell. These downstream pathways include phosphoinositide-3-kinase/akt (PI3K-AKT), Ras and Raf superfamily-MAPK (Ras-Raf-MAPK), focal adhesion kinase (FAK), and v-src sarcoma viral oncogene homolog (SRC). The activity of the VEGFR2 appears to be potentiated by the binding of co-receptors, neuropilin-1 (NRP-1) on arteries, and NRP-2 on venous and lymphatic vessels. NRP-1 and NRP-2 may have intrinsic activity through the binding of small G proteins and regulation of the cytoskeleton also.

Given the importance of the VEGF pathway, the majority of angiogenesis-related targeted therapies are focused on the VEGF family of ligands and receptors. Current options for therapy include drugs that directly target VEGF and its receptors and vascular disrupting agents that damage existing tumor related blood vessels.

Agents Targeting the Vascular Endothelial Growth Factor Pathway

Bevacizumab

Ovarian cancer. Bevacizumab, a humanized mAb to human VEGF, was the first US Food and Drug Administration (FDA)–approved drug targeting angiogenesis. In ovarian cancer, bevacizumab has been evaluated both as a single agent and in combination therapy for primary and recurrent disease. After encouraging preclinical studies and multiple case studies, the Gynecologic Oncology Group (GOG) instituted a phase II trial of single-agent bevacizumab (15 mg/kg every 3 weeks) in persistent or recurrent refractory epithelial ovarian cancer. Despite a heavily pretreated cohort, the authors reported 13 of 62 patients (21%) experienced a clinical response, including 11 patients with partial response and two patients with a complete response. The median number of cycles was seven, and 25 patients (40.3%) had a progression-free survival (PFS) time of at least 6 months. Overall, toxicity was low, and there were no reports of bowel perforation. Another phase II trial of bevacizumab (15 mg/kg every 3 weeks) in 44 patients with ovarian cancer receiving third- or fourth-line chemotherapy demonstrated a partial response rate of 16%. The median PFS time was 4.4 months, and the median overall survival (OS) period was 10.7 months at study closure. This study was terminated early secondary to five patients (11.4%) experiencing spontaneous bowel perforation. The risk of bowel perforation appeared to be higher in patients with a higher median number of prior treatments and in whom impending bowel obstruction was suspected. Further studies are ongoing to elucidate a clear list of risk factors for perforation in the setting of bevacizumab therapy.

In the setting of relapsed disease, bevacizumab has been evaluated in combination with both cytotoxic and biologic therapies. A phase II study of bevacizumab (10 mg/kg every 2 weeks) combined with oral cyclophosphamide (50 mg/day) demonstrated a partial response rate of 24% (17 of 70 patients) at a median follow-up period of 23.2 months. The probability of being progression free at 6 months was 56% in this study. Overall toxicity was acceptable in this study. This combination has also been evaluated retrospectively at several institutions with similar encouraging results (objective response rates, 44%–53.3%). A phase II trial combining bevacizumab (15 mg/kg every 21 days) and oral erlotinib (150 mg/day) in 13 patients with recurrent Müllerian cancer showed an objective response rate of 15% and a stable disease (SD) rate of 54%. However, this trial was stopped early secondary to lack of clear benefit of the combination over single-agent bevacizumab and a higher than expected rate of bowel perforation (15%).

Success in the platinum-resistant recurrent setting as well as in several phase II trials in the upfront setting led to five major phase III trials in ovarian cancer. In the upfront setting, GOG 218 and International Collaborative Ovarian Neoplasm (ICON) 7 both include bevacizumab in combination with standard cytotoxics followed by maintenance bevacizumab. Key characteristics of these studies are summarized in Table 18.4. Preliminary data from GOG 218 revealed a PFS benefit of 3 months in the arm that included bevacizumab treatment up front and continued as single-agent maintenance (14.1 vs. 11.2 months; hazards ratio [HR], 0.72; P <0.001). It is interesting that there was no PFS benefit in the patients who only received adjuvant bevacizumab compared with standard therapy alone. No OS benefit was noted in the arms containing bevacizumab, although this was not a primary endpoint of the study. Although different in design, ICON7 reached similar conclusions. In the arm receiving paclitaxel, carboplatin, and bevacizumab followed by bevacizumab maintenance, the PFS time was improved by 1.7 months (24.1 vs. 22.4 months; HR, 0.87; P = 0.04). OS, albeit immature, was similar between the arms.

More promising results for bevacizumab have been observed in the phase III trials in the recurrent setting. GOG 213 is a bifactorial randomized study to evaluate the effect of the addition of bevacizumab to standard carboplatin and paclitaxel or gemcitabine on OS in platinum-sensitive patients (Fig. 18.4). Preliminary results of this study demonstrated a significant improvement in PFS as well as a trend toward improved OS in the arm containing bevacizumab. This study is also addressing the benefit of secondary cytoreductive surgery by randomly assigning a subset of patients who meet criteria for cytoreduction to surgery versus no surgery before initiation of chemotherapy.

TABLE 18.4   Comparison of Trial Design of Gynecologic Oncology Group (GOG) 218 and International Collaborative Ovarian Neoplasm (ICON) 7

	GOG 218	ICON 7
Patients (n)	2000	1520
Type	Randomized	Randomized
	Placebo-controlled	Open Label
Primary endpoints	Overall survival	Progression-free survival
	Progression-free survival	
Secondary endpoints	Toxicity	Overall survival
	Quality of life	Response rate
	Translational research	Biologic progression-free survival
		Toxicity
		Quality of life
		Economics
Strata	Stage (III ≤1 cm vs. >1 cm vs. IV)	Stage (I–III ≤1 cm vs. >1 cm vs. IV)
	PS: (0 vs. 1–2)	Chemo start (≤4 wk vs. > 4)
		Enrolling center
Sites	490	142
Opened	September 2005	April 2006
Closed	June 2009	February 2009

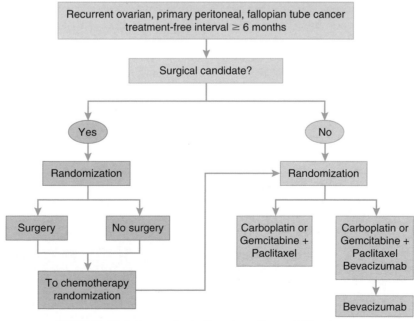

FIGURE 18.4 Gynecologic Oncology Group 213 schema.

In the OCEANS trial, patients with platinum-sensitive ovarian cancer were treated with gemcitabine and carboplatin with or without bevacizumab. This trial aimed to evaluate PFS and potential GI toxicity of this combination. Similar to GOG 213, the arm containing bevacizumab demonstrated a significant improvement in PFS of 4 months. This did not, however, yield a difference in OS. In the platinum-resistant setting, the AURELIA trial compared bevacizumab with a physician choice standard agent, including paclitaxel, liposomal doxorubicin, or topotecan, with the standard agent alone. Bevacizumab provided a statistically significant improvement in response rate and PFS when added to standard chemotherapy. Interestingly, when a subanalysis stratified by each chemotherapy cohort was performed, the greatest PFS benefit (6 months) was found in the cohort that combined weekly paclitaxel with bevacizumab. The high crossover to bevacizumab after trial participation likely influenced the lack of OS difference noted in this trial. The results of this trial yielded an FDA approval for bevacizumab in combination with chemotherapy in platinum-resistant ovarian cancer receiving one or two prior regimens.

Bevacizumab has also shown promise in nonepithelial ovarian cancer. A retrospective review of eight patients with recurrent granulosa cell tumors demonstrated a partial response rate of 38% and SD rate of 25%. This study has encouraged the development of a phase II trial by the GOG evaluating bevacizumab for women with recurrent ovarian sex cord–stromal tumors. Among 36 patients treated, 16.7% had a partial response, and 77.8% achieved SD. Certainly, these results are promising in this notoriously chemoresistant disease.

Uterine cancer. Vascular endothelial growth factor expression has been correlated with adverse outcomes in endometrial cancer, and bevacizumab has demonstrated encouraging results in early phase clinical settings. The GOG initiated a phase II study of single-agent bevacizumab (15 mg/kg every 21 days) for advanced endometrial cancer demonstrating a 13.5% response rate and 40.4% surviving progression free at 6 months. The median OS time was 10.5 months in this trial. A subsequent trial attempted to maximize this benefit by combining bevacizumab with temsirolimus, an mTORC1 inhibitor described later in this chapter. The combination was deemed active based on reasonable response rate (24.5%) and 47% of patients surviving

progression free at 6 months; however, its development has been limited by increased toxicity. In the upfront setting, the addition of bevacizumab to Intensity Modulated Radiation Therapy (IMRT) with cisplatin was evaluated in high-risk endometrial cancer. Overall, toxicity was reasonable, and the OS rate for the cohort was 96.7% at 2 years.

Cervical cancer. Bevacizumab is the first targeted agent that has demonstrated activity in recurrent cervical cancer. A phase II trial of single-agent bevacizumab (15 mg/kg every 21 days) had promising results in a cohort of patients with fewer than three prior regimens, achieving a median OS period of 7.29 months and acceptable toxicity. Five patients (10.9%) had a partial response, and an additional 11 patients were progression free for a minimum of 6 months. Furthermore, an analysis of six patients treated with bevacizumab in combination with 5-fluorouracil or capecitabine demonstrated a clinical benefit rate of 67%. There are several trials with bevacizumab in cervical cancer actively accruing or completed in the upfront and recurrent settings. GOG 240 combined bevacizumab with standard chemotherapy in four regimens, described in Fig. 18.5. This study found a significantly significant improvement in OS among the arms that received bevacizumab (17.0 vs. 13.3 months, 0,71; *P* = 0.004), which led to an FDA approval for bevacizumab in combination with chemotherapy for advanced and recurrent cervical cancer.

VEGF-Trap (Aflibercept)

Aflibercept is a manufactured protein that acts as a decoy receptor for all VEGF-A isoforms and placental growth factor. This agent was engineered through fusion of the ligand-binding domains from two VEGF receptors with the constant region of IgG1, resulting in high-affinity VEGF binding and prevention of VEGF pathway activation. In the in vivo setting, aflibercept was found to improve ascites and reduce tumor growth.

Initial phase I trials of aflibercept for advanced solid malignancy demonstrated acceptable toxicity with clinical benefit approaching 50%. Several partial responses were observed in ovarian cancer. This led to a randomized phase II trial of aflibercept (2 mg/kg vs. 4 mg/kg) in platinum-resistant recurrent ovarian cancer. A response rate of 11% was reported with five partial responses and no mention of SD. Aflibercept has

FIGURE 18.5 Gynecologic Oncology Group 240 schema.

also been studied for the treatment of malignant ascites in ovarian cancer. Colombo and colleagues treated 12 patients with aflibercept (4 mg/kg) every 2 weeks and found successful prolongation in time to repeat paracentesis with minimal adverse advents. A phase I/II, multi-institutional trial reported the activity and toxicity of aflibercept in combination with docetaxel in women with recurrent ovarian cancer. Overall response in the phase II component was 54%, including 11 of 25 responders being complete. Median PFS and OS periods were 6.4 and 26.6 month, respectively. As expected, the most frequent aflibercept-associated toxicity was hypertension (11% grade 1 or 2). In endometrial cancer, the GOG performed a phase II study of aflibercept in the recurrent setting. This agent achieved a 7% response rate, and 23% of patients survived progression free for 6 months.

Agents Targeting Vascular Endothelial Growth Factor Receptors
AZD2171 (Cediranib)

Cediranib is a small molecule inhibitor of VEGFR-2, platelet-derived growth factor receptor (PDGFR), and c-kit, which has shown promise in several phase II trials. In a study of 46 patients with recurrent ovarian cancer, the clinical benefit rate of single-agent cediranib was 30%. Eight patients achieved partial response, and six patients had SD, and median PFS for the group was 5.2 months. Hirte and colleagues reported a response rate of 41% in platinum-sensitive and 29% in platinum-resistant ovarian malignancy. Toxicities in both studies included diarrhea, hypertension, mucositis, fatigue, and anorexia. Cediranib was evaluated in the upfront setting in combination with standard paclitaxel and carboplatin as part of ICON6 (Fig. 18.6). Toxicity of the combination was well tolerated and yielded a PFS benefit of 3 months. Importantly, the use of cediranib in the maintenance setting was not associated with a significant improvement in OS. This combination of paclitaxel and carboplatin with cediranib was studied in cervical cancer as well, yielding 2 months of increased PFS at the expense of increased toxicity. Single-agent cediranib in endometrial cancer had promising activity, with a 12% response rate and 30% of patients progression free at 6 months, leading to the development of an ongoing combination trial with standard of care chemotherapy.

IMC-1121B (Ramucirumab)

IMC-1121B is the most developed fully humanized mAb to VEGFR-2. A phase I trial in 12 patients with advanced solid malignancies demonstrated a clinical benefit in nine patients (two partial responses, seven with SD). These promising results led to a phase II trial of ramucirumab in recurrent ovarian cancer. This study revealed that single-agent ramucirumab (8 mg/kg) only achieved a response rate of 6% with 56.7% of patients having SD. Thus, there has been minimal effort to explore this agent further in gynecologic malignancies. Several other mAbs to VEGF receptors are still in development, including IMC-18F1 and IMC-1C11.

Agents Targeting Multiple Vascular Endothelial Growth Factor–Related Molecules
Sunitinib

Sunitinib is an oral receptor tyrosine kinase inhibitor whose targets include VEGFR, PDGFR, epidermal growth factor (EGF), and the stem cell factor (KIT) receptor. This drug has been evaluated in the treatment of recurrent ovarian cancer in several phase II trials and one phase III trial. A phase II trial of sunitinib (50 mg/day intermittent dosing, 4 of 6 weeks vs. 37.5 mg/day) in recurrent platinum-sensitive and platinum-resistant ovarian cancer demonstrated a 66% clinical benefit with partial response in one patient, CA125 responses in three patients, and SD in 16 patients. Of note, responses were only seen in patients in the intermittent cohort. Common side effects were hand and foot reaction, fatigue, hypertension, and mucositis. Mackay and colleagues reported the results from a phase II trial of sunitinib (50 mg/day) in 19 patients with advanced or metastatic cervical cancer. Although they achieved no objective responses, 16 patients achieved SD with a median duration of 4.4 months. There are several ongoing active phase II trials of single-agent sunitinib in endometrial and cervical cancer and clear cell ovarian cancer (GOG 254).

Pazopanib

Pazopanib inhibits all of the VEGF receptors (VEGFR1, VEGFR2, and VEGFR3) and PDGFR-α and -β and the KIT receptor. This small molecule inhibitor (800 mg/day) has been evaluated in a phase II study of 36 patients with recurrent ovarian cancer by CA-125 and nonbulky disease. This study

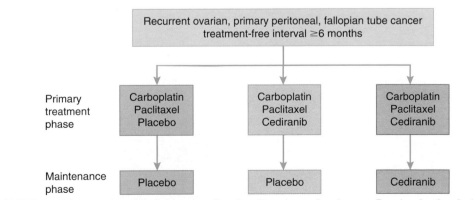

FIGURE 18.6 International Collaborative Ovarian Neoplasm 6 schema. Randomization is 2:3:3 in this trial.

revealed a 31% response by CA-125 level and a 56% SD rate. Among the 17 patients with measurable disease, 18% had a partial response. Ongoing ovarian cancer studies of pazopanib include combination with liposomal doxorubicin in the recurrent setting and in combination with paclitaxel and carboplatin in the upfront setting. A phase III, placebo-controlled study of pazopanib for consolidation after completion of primary chemotherapy in ovarian cancer was recently published. Use of pazopanib as maintenance therapy prolonged PFS by 5.6 months when compared to placebo. Adverse events were increased in the pazopanib arm, with 33% of patients terminating this agent early. Interim results did not yield a subsequent benefit in OS. Interestingly, a subset analysis of East Asian women included in this study revealed a negative impact of pazopanib on PFS among this cohort. Further studies are ongoing to understand the mechanism underlying this difference. Pazopanib has also been combined with chemotherapy in the recurrent ovarian cancer setting. One randomized phase II trial comparing weekly paclitaxel with or without pazopanib revealed a 3-month PFS benefit in the setting of moderately increased adverse events, including neutropenia and fatigue. However, another placebo-controlled trial failed to demonstrate a benefit with the addition of pazopanib to weekly paclitaxel in recurrent ovarian cancer. In cervical cancer, pazopanib was explored alone and in combination with lapatinib (a small molecule EGFR inhibitor to be discussed later) in the treatment of advanced and recurrent disease (Fig. 18.7). The combination pazopanib and lapatinib arm was closed early after a futility analysis, leaving the randomized phase II trial to compare pazopanib with single-agent lapatinib. Both progression-free (HR, 0.66; 90% CI 0.48–0.91) and OS (HR, 0.67; 90% CI 0.49–0.99) were superior in the monotherapy pazopanib arm. Median OS was 50.7 weeks versus 39.1 weeks for pazopanib and lapatinib, respectively.

Brivanib

Brivanib alaninate is a prodrug of brivanib, a dual inhibitor of VEGFR2 and FGFR. This compound has demonstrated acceptable toxicity and activity when given alone or in combination, in multiple solid tumors, including hepatocellular carcinoma refractory to other antiangiogenic therapies. Brivanib was evaluated in a phase II study for recurrent or persistent endometrial cancer and found worthy to pursue further based on a response rate of 19% (one complete response and seven partial responses) and 30% of patients surviving progression free at 6 months. Similar favorable activity was found in the first stage of a phase II trial of brivanib in recurrent cervical cancer; however, the trial was closed early because of drug availability.

Nintedanib

Nintedanib is a multikinase inhibitor targeting three key angiogenic receptors: VEGFR, PDGFR, and FGFR. A phase I trial of this agent in patients with gynecologic malignancies revealed a promising response rate, with five of seven patients with measurable disease demonstrating response and two achieving SD. Nintedanib (250 mg/day) was evaluated as a maintenance therapy compared with placebo in recurrent ovarian cancer after response to standard therapy. Although the trial was not powered to compare the two arms, PFS was less in the placebo arm (2.8 months) compared with the nintedanib arm (4.8 months). A randomized phase III placebo-controlled trial compared standard paclitaxel and carboplatin with or without nintedanib in previously untreated primary ovarian cancer patients. The combination arm was associated with significantly prolonged PFS, although clinically, this was a median increase of approximately 2 weeks. Furthermore, there was significant toxicity in the combination arm, including GI and hematologic adverse events. A phase II study of this agent in recurrent endometrial cancer did not provide sufficient activity to warrant further study as a single agent.

Vascular Disrupting Agents

This broad group of antiangiogenic drugs acts to occlude preexisting vasculature in the tumor rather than prevent neovascularization. The disturbance of existing vessels leads to ischemia; hemorrhagic necrosis; and ultimately, cellular death.

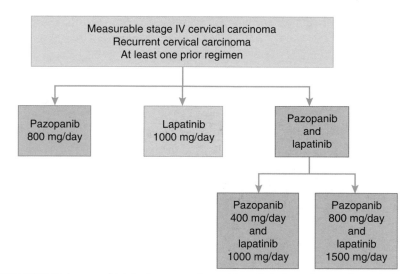

FIGURE 18.7 Schema of trial of pazopanib and lapatinib for advanced cervical cancer.

Of note, these agents are able to selectively target tumor blood vessels by taking advantage of the differences between normal and tumor endothelial cells. Two major types of vascular disrupting agents exist: small molecule based and ligand based. The majority of vascular disrupting agents under evaluation in gynecologic cancers target small molecules.

Vadimezan (ASA404/DMXAA)

Vadimezan, 5,6-dimethylxanthenone-4-acetic acid, is a flavone acetic acid analog that increases production and release of tumor necrosis factor α. This leads to endothelial cell apoptosis and decreased perfusion of the tumor. Gabra and colleagues evaluated this drug in combination with paclitaxel and carboplatin for the treatment of recurrent ovarian cancer. **The arm that received vadimezan conferred significant improvement in response rate compared with the control arm (64% vs. 49%) without additional adverse effects.**

Fosbretabulin (Combretastatin A4); Ombrabulin (AVE8062)

Fosbretablin is a tubulin-binding agent that causes vascular congestion and decreased tumor blood flow by changing endothelial cell shape. This effect is very rapid, occurring within 1 hour of drug administration. This agent has been evaluated primarily for the treatment of platinum-resistant ovarian cancer. Treatment with combretastatin A4 (63 mg/m^2) in addition to paclitaxel (175 mg/m^2) and carboplatin (area under the curve [AUC] 5) resulted in a 13.5% response rate by Response Evaluation Criteria for Solid Tumors (RECIST) and a 34% response rate by Gynecologic Cancer Inter Group (GCIG) criteria without additional observed toxicity. A randomized phase II trial of bevacizumab with or without fosbretabulin demonstrated higher response rate as well as improved PFS in the combination arm among patients with platinum-resistant ovarian cancer. OS data from this study have not yet been presented. Ombrabulin is a combrestatin derivative that has shown excellent efficacy in preclinical ovarian cancer models. This agent appears to have a similar toxicity profile to combretastatin A4 and is undergoing evaluation in a phase II trial in combination with paclitaxel and carboplatin in platinum-sensitive recurrent ovarian cancer (OPSALIN).

Other Antiangiogenic Agents
Thalidomide

Thalidomide is a legacy agent that has found recent renewed interest as an antiangiogenic agent. Thalidomide inhibits FGF-2 by interacting with the FGF-2 receptor. In addition, this agent acts as an immune modulator by inducing production of interferon-γ, interleukin-2 (IL-2), and IL-10. Thalidomide (200 mg/day) added 4 months to OS when added to topotecan (1.25 mg/m^2) for the treatment of recurrent ovarian cancer. A phase II of thalidomide (200–1000 mg/day) in persistent or recurrent endometrial cancer demonstrated a 25% clinical benefit with two partial responses and four patients with disease stabilization. The GOG reported randomized phase III trial results comparing thalidomide (200 mg/day) with tamoxifen (20 mg/day) for biochemically recurrent ovarian carcinoma. In this study, there was essentially no difference in PFS, with

thalidomide achieving 3.2 months compared with 4.5 months for tamoxifen. Patients on the thalidomide arm had an increased risk of death (HR, 1.76; 95% CI 1.16–2.68). Furthermore, patients receiving thalidomide had a higher incidence of grade III and IV toxicity. Common toxicities of thalidomide include hematologic, GI, and cardiovascular complications. Lenalidomide (Revlimid) is a thalidomide derivative that demonstrated modest activity in platinum resistant ovarian cancer, yielding a clinical benefit rate of 38% at 4 months, including four partial responses by RECIST.

PHOSPHATIDYLINOSITOL-3-KINASE/AKT PATHWAY

The PI3K/AKT pathway plays a central role in cell survival, growth, and avoidance of apoptosis. Fig. 18.8 demonstrates a simple schematic of this complex pathway that is known to interact with many other cellular growth and survival pathways. This pathway may be activated by a large number of receptor tyrosine kinases, including the EGFR family and the insulin-like growth factor receptors (IGFRs). Thus a variety of mitogenic substances are involved in its activation.

Activation of the pathway starts with the PI3K family, which consists lipid and serine/threonine kinases composed of heterodimers, including a catalytic and regulatory subunit. Activation of PI3K leads to phosphorylation of phosphatidylionositol-4,5-bisphospate (PIP2) to phosphatidylinositol-3,4,5-triphosphate (PIP3). PIP3 acts as a second messenger to bind a variety of targets and recruit them to the plasma membrane, leading to their activation. One critical downstream mediator of PIP3 is AKT, which on activation acts on a number of different targets that directly affect cellular survival, proliferation through activation of transcription and translation, evasion of apoptosis, and resistance to chemotherapy. One key downstream target of AKT is the mammalian target of rapamycin (mTOR), a serine/threonine kinase. The upregulation of mTOR by AKT leads to activation of downstream regulator protein S6 kinase, which directly affects protein translation and the progression of growth through the cell cycle.

The PI3K/AKT pathway is known to be activated in a variety of cancers, especially in gynecologic malignancies. The phosphatase and tensin homolog on chromosome 10 (PTEN) is a tumor suppressor that encodes for a serine/threonine kinase, which acts directly to dephosphorylate PIP3 to PIP2. In patients with PTEN mutation and loss of function, there is an overaccumulation of PIP3, leading to constitutive activation of the AKT pathway. The PI3K/AKT pathway is also frequently activated through mutations in PIK3CA, which encodes for the activating subunit (110α) of PI3K or through mutations in AKT.

As described in Chapter 19, the aforementioned mutations are commonly found in endometrial cancer and less frequently in the other gynecologic malignancies. Furthermore, this pathway is thought to be targeted more frequently in cancer than any other pathway aside from p53. Thus, PI3K/AKT signaling provides a promising target for the treatment of malignancy and is under active exploration. Currently, the drugs

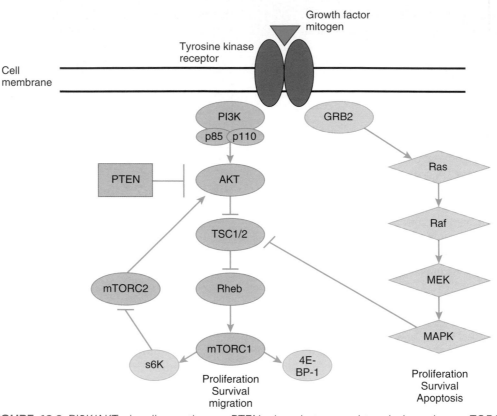

FIGURE 18.8 PI3K/AKT signaling pathway. *PTEN*, phosphatase and tensin homolog; *mTORC*, mammalian target of rapamycin complex; *PI3K*, Phosphatidylinositol-3-kinase; *AKT*, protein kinase B; *TSC*, tuberous sclerosis complex; *Rheb*, Ras homolog enriched in brain; *GRB*, growth factor receptor-bound protein; *Ras*, human rat sarcoma protein; *Raf*, Rapidly accelerated fibrosarcoma protein; *MEK*, mitogen-activated protein kinase kinase.

targeting this pathway consist primarily of small molecule inhibitors of key pathway components. The inhibition of only one member of the pathway may not be sufficient to affect tumor growth given the significant pathway cross-talk and feedback loops. For example, mTOR is known to regulate cellular growth and proliferation through activation of several downstream proteins. These proteins also participate in a feedback loop that can lead to subsequent upregulation of AKT phosphorylation. Thus, the exploration of combination therapies in this pathway is paramount.

Agents Targeting mTOR

mTOR is a key downstream protein of the PI3K/AKT pathway, consisting of two major complexes (mTORC1 and mTORC2). Initial attempts at targeting this pathway node were directed at mTORC1 (rapalogs). Overall, trials in gynecologic cancer with rapalogs have demonstrated only modest success. Thus, there are newer agents in development that compete with ATP on the mTOR catalytic site and inhibit mTORC1 and mTORC2.

Temsirolimus (CC1-779)

Temsirolimus (25 mg intravenously weekly), a water-soluble ester of rapamycin, had a favorable response rate in a phase II trial of patients with recurrent or metastatic endometrial cancer treated with a maximum of one prior regimen. Among the chemotherapy naïve cohort, 14% of 29 evaluable patients had

a partial response, and an additional 69% achieved SD. However, among patients treated with prior chemotherapy, only 4% had partial responses, and 48% had SD of median 4 months' duration. A study of temsirolimus in 54 heavily pretreated patients with recurrent endometrial cancer yielded 9% partial responses and 24% progression free at 6 months. Temkin and colleagues reported on a phase I trial of temsirolimus combined with topotecan to treat a variety of advanced and recurrent gynecologic malignancies. The drug combination was well tolerated in patients without a history of radiotherapy and achieved SD in 9 of 11 patients at 8 weeks. Trials incorporating temsirolimus have shown manageable toxicities, including hypertriglyceridemia, hyperglycemia, electrolyte abnormalities, and rash. This agent has been combined with a variety of combination chemotherapies and targeted therapies in endometrial cancer. As noted earlier, the combination of temsirolimus with bevacizumab did not yield a significant increase in response or PFS at 6 months to warrant further exploration. Results of this combination in ovarian cancer were similar as well. To improve on the current standard of care for advanced and recurrent chemotherapy-naïve endometrial cancer, the GOG performed a randomized phase II trial with three arms: (1) temsirolimus in combination with paclitaxel and carboplatin; (2) bevacizumab, paclitaxel, carboplatin; and (3) ixabepilone, paclitaxel, and carboplatin. This trial did not demonstrate a significant increase in PFS in any of the arms compared to historical controls. Interestingly, the secondary endpoint of OS was increased in the bevacizumab arm (HR, 0.71; 92% CI 0.55–0.91 compared with historical controls). In recurrent cervical cancer, single-agent temsirolimus had similar modest effects, achieving only one (3%) partial response and a 6-month PFS rate of 28%. A phase II trial combining temsirolimus with carboplatin and paclitaxel was recently completed in advanced clear cell carcinoma of the ovary; results are anticipated soon.

Everolimus (RAD001)

Everolimus is an orally bioavailable ester that is a potent inhibitor of mTOR. Two phase II studies of everolimus (10 mg/day) as a single agent in recurrent endometrial cancer have been reported, with only modest activity. Slomovitz and colleagues demonstrate a short- and long-term clinical benefit rate with 43% and 21% of patients achieving SD at 8 weeks and 20 weeks, respectively. The ENDORAD study of 54 metastatic endometrial cancer patients reported five partial responders and a median PFS period of only 2.8 months. Given these results, attempts have been made to maximize the success of this drug in combination with other targeted agents, traditional cytotoxic chemotherapy, and hormones. The latter combination has gained keen interest in breast and endometrial cancers because endocrine resistance may be mediated by activation of the PI3K pathway. A phase II study of the combination of everolimus and letrozole markedly improved on the single-agent efficacy, with confirmed objective response rate of 32%, including nine complete responders. Furthermore, the clinical benefit rate was 40%, and the combination was well tolerated.

Ridaforolimus (AP23573; MK-8669)

Ridaforolimus, previously known as deforolimus, is an mTOR inhibitor that may be given orally or intravenously. In a phase II study of ridaforolimus (12.5 mg intravenously daily for 5 days every other week) for patients with advanced or recurrent endometrial cancer, 13 of 45 patients achieved clinical benefit, including five with partial response. The oral formulation (40 mg orally daily for 5 days every 3 weeks) was evaluated in recurrent endometrial cancer as well. Similar to the intravenous (IV) formulation, ridaforolimus yielded a response rate of 8.8% and disease stabilization of 53%. Final results of a multi-institutional randomized phase II trial of ridaforolimus (40 mg orally for 5 days every 28 days) in women with recurrent, previously treated endometrial cancer were reported in 2015. The control arm of the trial was the physician's choice of either hormones or chemotherapy. Overall, 130 patients (114 evaluable) were enrolled—64 to ridaforolimus, 52 to hormonal therapy, and 13 to chemotherapy. The response rates in each arm were similar (0% vs. 4% for ridaforolimus and control participant, respectively). However, PFS was significantly longer in the ridaforolimus arm (1.7 months) when assessed by either the investigators or by independent radiologic review. OS has not been reported.

Agents Targeting AKT

Given the modest activity of targeting downstream regulators of the PI3K/AKT pathway, there is interest in targeting higher level nodes of the pathway. There are several AKT-inhibiting agents in development and the majority are undergoing evaluation in phase I trials. MK-2206 is a highly selective non-ATP competitive allosteric Akt inhibitor that is equally potent against Akt1 and Akt2 and demonstrated efficacy in vitro and in vivo in several tumor models. A phase I dose escalation study in patients with solid tumors has been completed to identify tolerance of the compound at 60 mg orally every other day. Dose-limiting toxicities were skin rash, mucosal inflammation, and hyperglycemia. Three ovarian cancer patients treated in this study had reducing CA-125 values. A single-agent study of MK-2206 in recurrent endometrial cancer stratified by presence of PI3KCA mutation had only modest response rates (6%) and little overall clinical benefit.

Agents Targeting PI3K

Although several companies are exploring the inhibition of PI3Kinase in solid tumors, there are only two PI3K inhibitors in phase II trials. Pilaralisib is a highly selective oral inhibitor of PI3K and successfully inhibits tumor growth in vivo. A phase I trial revealed acceptable toxicity and durable clinical benefit. A phase I trial combining pilaralisib with carboplatin and paclitaxel incorporated a dose expansion for ovarian and endometrial cancer patients secondary to favorable responses in those tumor types, although final results have not yet been reported. In recurrent endometrial cancer, pilaralisib as a single agent yielded only a 6% response, and the rate of PFS at 6 months was only 12%.

Enzastaurin is an oral multikinase inhibitor that primarily acts to suppress tumor growth through the inhibition of PI3K. A phase I study of enzastaurin combined with bevacizumab revealed promising responses in advanced solid tumors, especially among ovarian cancer (29% partial response or complete response). Furthermore, 51% of 21 ovarian cancer patients remained in the study for greater than 6 months. A phase II study of enzastaurin alone in recurrent ovarian cancer had limited activity, with a response rate of only 7.4% (D. Armstrong, personal communication). These results led to the development of several phase II trials of enzastaurin in combination with standard chemotherapy for advanced ovarian cancer. Vergote and colleagues reported that the combination was well tolerated, however, did not yield a statistically significant improvement in progression free survival.

Combination Agents

In addition to the agents targeting specific aspects of the PI3K/AKT pathway noted previously, there are a large number of combination drugs in development and in early clinical trials. These include combination PI3K/mTOR, PI3K/AKT, and PI3K/MEK inhibitors. Given the extensive cross-talk and feedback loops involved in this pathway, the inhibition of two major nodes in one or more pathways is rational and may lead to improved outcomes. Unfortunately, early reports from single-agent studies of PI3K/mTOR inhibitors have not yielded increased efficacy over the single node agents reported earlier. Furthermore, the majority of published studies combining PI3K/AKT pathway inhibitors with MEK inhibitors have reported limited activity

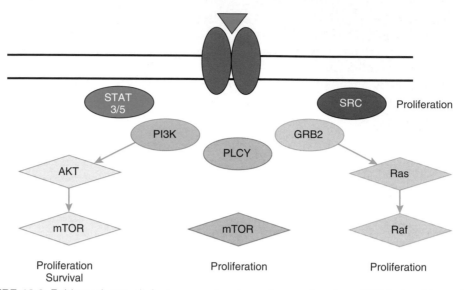

FIGURE 18.9 Epidermal growth factor receptor downstream signaling. *STAT,* signal transducer and activator of transcription; *AKT,* protein kinase B; *PI3K,* Phosphatidylinositol-3-kinase; *mTORC,* mammalian target of rapamycin complex; *PLCY,* phospholipace C gamma; *GRB2,* growth factor receptor-bound protein 2; *SRC,* proto-oncogene tyrosine-protein kinase; *Ras,* human rat sarcoma protein; *Raf,* Rapidly accelerated fibrosarcoma protein.

secondary to significant toxicities found with the combinations. A large study of the combination of SAR245409 (PI3K/mTOR inhibitor) with pimasertib (MEK inhibitor) is ongoing in low-grade serous ovarian cancer.

RAS/RAF PATHWAY

The Ras/Raf pathway is an essential regulator of tumorigenesis, including regulation of cell growth, survival, death, and motility (Fig. 18.9). This pathway is tightly linked to the PI3K/AKT pathway, creating series of feedback loops that can lead to chemotherapy and targeted therapy resistance. Furthermore, this pathway is often activated in tandem with the PI3K/AKT pathway because it shares activating mitogens and receptors, including the EGFR family. Ras is a GTPase that is activated by cell surface signaling and subsequently phosphorylates downstream extracellular signal-related kinases (ERKs). Two essential pathway kinases are Raf and MEK, which ultimately serve to activate numerous downstream regulators and drive tumorigenic processes. Activation of the Ras/Raf pathway can occur through activating mutations in *KRAS, HRAS, BRAF,* and *MEK.* Ras mutations are the most common across solid tumors; however, targeting these proteins has been difficult. Thus, agents directed at downstream targets such as MEK and ERK are the most well developed.

Agents Targeting MEK

The highest rates of Ras/Raf pathway aberrations are found in low-grade serous and mucinous ovarian cancer as well as endometrial cancer. The rarity of mucinous cancer has limited the exploration of targeted agents for this indication. However, MEK inhibitors have been quite successful for the treatment of low-grade ovarian cancer. Selumetinib was explored in a phase II trial by the GOG, yielding a 15% objective response rate and

a 65% SD rate in this notoriously chemo-insensitive disease. Based on the results of this trial, two large phase III studies are ongoing to compare MEK inhibition therapy with physician choice chemotherapy in recurrent low-grade serous ovarian cancer. In recurrent endometrial cancer, single-agent results for MEK inhibition have been limited. A phase II GOG trial of selumetinib reported a 6% objective response ($n = 3$) and an event-free survival rate at 6 months of 12%. As noted earlier, these modest results have led to exploration of MEK inhibitor combinations for endometrial cancer.

POLY-ADP-RIBOSE POLYMERASE PATHWAY

DNA damage can be repaired through a variety of pathways in the cell, including base excision, direct repair, mismatch repair, and nucleotide excision repair. High activity of DNA damage repair pathways is a known mechanism of resistance to cytotoxic chemotherapy. Poly-ADP-ribose polymerase (PARP) is a nuclear enzyme that contributes to the repair of single-stranded breaks in DNA along the base excision repair pathway (Fig. 18.10). There are several key mechanisms of action of this therapy. When PARP is inhibited, accumulation of single-stranded breaks can lead to double-stranded breaks and ultimately, cellular death. The use of PARP inhibitors in carriers of *BRCA* mutations is effective because tumor cells in these patients have dysfunctional homologous recombination repair, a primary double-stranded break repair mechanism. Furthermore, PARP inhibitors also stimulate a separate DNA repair mechanism, the nonhomologous end joining (NHEJ) pathway, which is error prone and yields cell death. Finally, PARP inhibitors appear to gain antitumor function through PARP "trapping" in which the PARP protein is trapped on the DNA complex, interfering with further DNA repair and replication. Of note, some *BRCA* mutation carriers appear resistant

FIGURE 18.10 Single-stranded DNA repair. *PAR,* Poly-ADP-ribose; *PARP,* poly-ADP-ribose polymerase.

to PARP inhibition. Proposed mechanisms of PARP inhibitor resistance include the presence of secondary *BRCA2* mutations that restore *BRCA* function, activation of Rad51, loss of 53BP1 leading to suppression of the NHEJ pathway, and increased activity of drug efflux pumps. A better understanding of these mechanisms will no doubt lead to expansion of the use of PARP inhibitors alone and in combination for the treatment of gynecologic malignancies.

PARP inhibitors have been primarily explored in ovarian cancer given the strong correlation between *BRCA* mutations and this disease. The potential indication of PARP inhibitor use is actively expanding to tumors with homologous recombination deficiency, including those with *BRCA1* promotor methylation, aberrations in ataxia telangiectasia mutated (ATM), ataxia telangiectasia and Rad3-related (ATR) and the Fanconi anemia pathway. Certainly, preclinical data supporting the consideration of PARP inhibition in other gynecologic malignancies exist, including the similar genomic landscape found in a subset of endometrial cancers based on molecular data generated from The Cancer Genome Atlas, indicating genomic instability and homologous recombination deficiency. In addition, the presence of PTEN alterations in endometrial cancer may increase sensitivity to PARP inhibition, based on work in cell lines as well as a case report. Similarly, preclinical data have supported potential synergy between PARPs in combination with chemotherapy or with radiation in cervical cancer cell lines. Thus, early-stage trials to evaluate PARP inhibition in both of these tumor types have been initiated.

Olaparib

Olaparib is the most studied PARP inhibitor to date in ovarian cancer. Preclinically, this orally active PARP inhibitor induces synthetic lethality in cells deficient in *BRCA*. In a study of two doses of olaparib in *BRCA*-mutant patients with advanced ovarian cancer, both doses were well tolerated and demonstrated modest effect. Olaparib at 100 mg twice a day (bid) achieved a

response rate of 12.5% and a clinical benefit rate of 16.7% among 24 patients. The 400-mg bid dose had higher levels of response and clinical benefit among 33 patients, 33% and 57.6%, respectively. Additional phase II studies of olaparib in recurrent high serous ovarian cancer have confirmed favorable response in patients with and without *BRCA* mutations. Olaparib also appears to reintroduce chemosensitivity to carboplatin and paclitaxel in heavily pretreated patients.

Although olaparib has been well tolerated as a single agent with primarily adverse events consisting of fatigue, nausea, and vomiting, early studies have indicated that there may be increased toxicity in combination with cytotoxic chemotherapy, necessitating dose reduction. Oza and colleagues compared the combination of olaparib with paclitaxel and carboplatin versus paclitaxel and carboplatin alone in platinum-sensitive recurrent ovarian cancer. This study included a maintenance arm of olaparib alone. Although there was no significant difference in response rate, there was improvement in PFS in the olaparib arm, which became clear during the maintenance phase of the trial. An additional study confirmed that olaparib monotherapy as maintenance after platinum-based chemotherapy for platinum-sensitive recurrence significantly increased PFS, especially in women with *BRCA* mutations.

Whether this class of compounds outperforms chemotherapy in selected germline *BRCA* mutation carries is unclear. A randomized phase II trial compared olaparib (200 mg bid and 400 mg bid) with pegylated liposomal doxorubicin (50 mg/m^2) in *BRCA* patients progressing within 12 months of platinum. The primary endpoint was PFS. Although response rates were numerically higher for the olaparib arms, PFS was no different between the arms. This may be due to higher than expected efficacy of liposomal doxorubicin in *BRCA*-mutant ovarian cancer patients.

Activity as a single agent in a platinum-resistant setting led to the FDA approval of olaparib in a tight niche, including those treated for ovarian cancer with more than three prior chemotherapies for recurrent disease. The approval of olaparib for *BRCA*-related ovarian cancer marks the first therapy approved for gynecologic malignancies with an associated biomarker. Olaparib has also achieved registration in Europe as a maintenance therapy after response to platinum-therapy after platinum-sensitive recurrence. Additional phase III trials to evaluate the role of olaparib as maintenance therapy in *BRCA*-mutant ovarian cancer in the upfront or platinum-sensitive recurrent setting have either completed accrual or are ongoing.

Veliparib

Veliparib, an oral inhibitor of PARP-1 and PARP-2, has also demonstrated encouraging activity in recurrent ovarian cancer. A phase 2 study of veliparib as a single agent yielded a response rate of 26% in women with *BRCA*-mutant ovarian cancer. Adverse events were modest and expected, consisting primarily of hematologic toxicities. Thus far, compared with other PARP inhibitors, this agent has been the most successfully combined with cytotoxic agents. However, it is unclear what benefit the addition of veliparib may add to cytotoxic chemotherapy. A randomized phase II trial of oral cyclophosphamide with veliparib did not find additional benefit in terms of response rate when compared with cyclophosphamide alone. A subsequent large scale phase 1 trial identified a tolerable recommended phase II dose of veliparib in combination with paclitaxel, carboplatin, and bevacizumab therapy in upfront advanced ovarian cancer. The combination including maintenance veliparib is now under study as part of a phase III clinical trial of the NRG Oncology group (GOG 3005).

Rucaparib

Preclinical studies of rucaparib have revealed that this agent is a potent inhibitor of PARP-1 and -2 with significant activity in ovarian cancer. The phase 1 trial of the single agent discovered a phase II dose that is well tolerated, with toxicities primarily including neutropenia, anemia, and elevated liver enzymes. A subset analysis of four patients with ovarian and primary peritoneal cancer reported 80% with objective response leading to the ongoing ARIEL2 study in women with platinum-sensitive recurrent ovarian cancer. An objective of this trial is to evaluate a genomic signature to predict response to PARP inhibition in pretreatment tumor tissue. *BRCA*-mutant tumors had impressive overall response rate of 69% and median PFS of 9.4 months. Conversely, BRCA negative tumors had the lowest evidence of activity with response rate and median PFS of 13% and 3.7 months, respectively. BRCA-like tumors included those with evidence of genome-wide loss of heterozygosity in the absence of BRCA mutation. Interestingly, these tumors had evidence of efficacy with response rates of 30% and median PFS of 7.1 months. Rucaparib is currently under evaluation as a switch maintenance therapy in the platinum-sensitive recurrent setting after response to chemotherapy in the ARIEL3 trial.

Niraparib

Similar to the aforementioned agents, niraparib inhibits PARP-1 and PARP-2 across a variety of advanced solid tumors. The phase 1 trial identified a recommended phase II dose of 300 mg/day, with the most common adverse events including myelosuppression, fatigue, and GI toxicity. The trials included *BRCA*-mutant and proficient tumors, achieving objective response rates of 40% and 16%, respectively. After these promising results, niraparib is undergoing evaluation in similar setting to rucaparib (ARIEL3) and olaparib (SOLO-2). A single-agent study of niraparib (QUADRA) in women who have received at least three prior lines of chemotherapy is ongoing for *BRCA*-mutant ovarian cancer. This agent is also under evaluation in the maintenance setting as well as in combination with immune therapies.

EPIDERMAL GROWTH FACTOR RECEPTOR PATHWAY

The EGFR pathway was identified as an anticancer therapy target secondary to myriad genetic alterations found in a variety of solid tumor types, including ovarian, endometrial, and cervical carcinomas. The pathway consists of four tyrosine kinase cell-surface receptors, including EGFR (ErbB-1), HER2/neu (ErbB-2), Her-3 (ErbB-3), and Her-4 (ErbB-4).

TABLE 18.5 Epidermal Growth Factor Ligands and Receptor	
EGF Receptor	**Ligands**
EGFR (ErbB-1)	EGF
	Transforming growth factor α
	Amphiregulin
	Epigen
	Betacellulin
	Heparin-binding growth factor
	Epiregulin
HER2/neu (ErbB-2)	None
HER-3 (ErbB-3)	Neuregulin 1
	Neuregulin 2
HER-4 (ErbB-4)	Betacellulin
	Heparin-binding growth factor
	Epiregulin
	Neuregulin 1
	Neuregulin 2
	Neuregulin 3
	Neuregulin 4
	Tomoregulin

EGF, Epidermal growth factor; *EGFR,* epidermal growth factor receptor.

Each receptor is specific for a variety of ligands, including EGF, transforming growth factor α (TGF-α), and neuregulins (NRGs) (Table 18.5). Although the receptors are activated through a traditional tyrosine kinase receptor mechanism, they also require the union between two identical receptors (homodimerization) or two different receptors within the same family (heterodimerization) for downstream activation.

Upon activation, the EGFRs induce activation of a variety of cell survival pathways, including the Ras/Raf/MEK and PI3K pathways (see Fig. 18.9). In addition, EGFRs are known to negatively affect apoptosis and induce invasion. EGFRs are also present on endothelial cells within the tumor microenvironment. EGF ligands demonstrate a direct effect on the endothelial cells, leading to increase in endothelial cell proliferation and angiogenesis. Thus, targeting this pathway has been an area of significant research for the treatment of gynecologic malignancies. Unfortunately, recent studies of drugs affecting the EGFR pathway have only demonstrated modest success in gynecologic cancer. This may be explained, in part, by research that demonstrates that EGFR has a role in glucose transport in cancer cells. EGFR associates with the sodium/glucose cotransporter (SGLT1) to promote the uptake of glucose into cancer cells. Of note, the action appears to be kinase independent. Thus, the blockage of kinase activity with antibodies or small molecules may not be sufficient to make a significant impact on tumorigenesis. Furthermore, based on data in multiple tumor types, response to EGFR inhibitors appears to be correlated with mutation status rather than expression. The rate of EGFR mutations in gynecologic malignancies is quite low; thus, the potential for success of these compounds as a single agent is unclear.

Small Molecule Inhibitors Targeting Epidermal Growth Factor Receptor

Gefitinib

Gefitinib is a small molecule inhibitor that prevents EGFR activation through binding the ATP-binding site of the receptor. This agent has been evaluated extensively in ovarian cancer with unsatisfactory results. Gefitinib (500 mg/day) was evaluated in a phase II trial in 30 patients with recurrent or persistent ovarian cancer treated with up to two prior regimens. Of 27 evaluable patients, four had SD for more than 6 months, and only one patient had an objective response. Of note, patients with EGFR expression in their tumors had longer median PFS periods, and the one objective response was found in a patient with a mutation in EGFR. This suggests that the use of mutation status to guide targeted therapies may provide better response rates.

Gefitinib (500 mg/day) has also been evaluated in combination with carboplatin (AUC 5) and paclitaxel (175 mg/m^2) for platinum-sensitive and platinum-resistant recurrent ovarian cancer. Nineteen percent of platinum-resistant and 62% of platinum-sensitive patients had responses to this combination therapy. OS was also acceptable, reaching 17 months for the resistant group and 26 months for the sensitive group. However, there appeared to be more hematologic toxicity compared with the standard regimen. The combination of gefitinib (500 mg/day) with tamoxifen (40 mg/day) in recurrent ovarian cancer required dose reduction secondary to diarrhea in 10 of 56 patients and resulted in no objective responses. However, 16 patients achieved SD, and the median survival period was 253 days.

The only published trial of gefitinib (500 mg/day) in cervical cancer reported minimal activity. Of 28 evaluable patients, there were no objective responses, and 20% achieved SD for a median duration of 112 days. It is interesting that disease control was not associated with the expression of EGFR in tumor specimens. Similarly, a study of gefitinib as a single agent in recurrent endometrial cancer achieved only one responder (4%), and four patients were progression free at 6 months (15%). EGFR mutation, EGFR expression, and hormonal expression were not associated with survival in this study.

Erlotinib

Erlotinib (150 mg/day) is reversible inhibitor of EGFR, acting to block autophosphorylation of the tyrosine kinase portion of the receptor. Based on overexpression of EGFR and preclinical results that indicated that the combination of EGFR-directed therapies and chemotherapy would potentially be synergistic, a phase II trial of erlotinib in combination with standard paclitaxel (175 mg/m^2) and carboplatin (AUC 6) for first-line treatment in ovarian cancer was performed. The primary endpoint was pathologic complete response rate with a plan to compare with historical control participants. Of a total of 56 patients treated, erlotinib in combination with standard chemotherapy achieved a pathologic complete response rate in 11 patients, which was not a significant improvement over historical control participants. Erlotinib was also explored as a maintenance therapy in patients with no sign of progression after frontline treatment for ovarian cancer in a large randomized control trial. After

2 years of therapy, there was no difference in PFS or OS between the erlotinib and observation arms.

In the setting of recurrent ovarian cancer, erlotinib has been primarily evaluated in combination with other therapies, although a solo trial is ongoing. Erlotinib in combination with carboplatin (AUC 5) achieved a response rate of 57% in the platinum-sensitive arm and 7% in the platinum-resistant arm with no unexpected toxicities. As noted previously, a trial of erlotinib with bevacizumab (15 mg/kg) was terminated early secondary to a high level of bowel perforation. The use of erlotinib as a single agent in chemotherapy-naïve endometrial cancer was well tolerated, and four of 32 patients had an objective response. In addition, 15 patients had SD lasting a median of 4 months. EGFR mutations were evaluated and did not correlate with response.

Schilder and colleagues reported disappointing results of erlotinib as a single agent in cervical cancer, with only one of 25 patients achieving objective response and four with SD. Only one patient in this trial had PFS period longer than 6 months. The combination of erlotinib with cisplatin (40 mg/m^2 weekly) with radiotherapy in locally advanced cervical cancer was found to be feasible, with acceptable toxicity and a complete response rate of 91%.

Monoclonal Antibodies Targeting Epidermal Growth Factor Receptor

Cetuximab

Cetuximab (250 mg/m^2) is a chimerized mAb to the ligand-binding domain EGFR, which has been evaluated as a treatment for primary and recurrent ovarian cancer as a single agent and in combination with traditional cytotoxics. As a single agent in 25 patients, cetuximab achieved only one partial response and nine patients with SD. The median PFS period was only 2.1 months. Cetuximab in combination with carboplatin (AUC 6) in 28 patients with recurrent platinum-sensitive ovarian cancer also had disappointing results, with only nine objective responses and eight patients with SD. Although cetuximab in combination with paclitaxel (175 mg/m^2) and carboplatin (AUC 6) was well tolerated, it offered no increased benefit in terms of PFS compared with traditional cytotoxic agents alone.

Cetuximab was given as a single agent in a phase II trial of cervical cancer performed by the GOG. There were no clinical responses, and only five patients (14%) were progression free at 6 months. The combination of cetuximab with topotecan (0.75 mg/m^2) and cisplatin (50 mg/m^2) for advanced cervical cancer induced a high rate of serious adverse events, including myelosuppression, infection, and skin reaction. Furthermore, five patients died, with three deaths attributable to toxicity. Cetuximab and cisplatin (30 mg/m^2) for recurrent cervical cancer was better tolerated but did not show any additional benefit compared with historical rates of cisplatin alone. A recent study of single-agent cetuximab for recurrent endometrial cancer has completed accrual, and preliminary results are pending.

Trastuzumab

The overexpression of HER2 in gynecologic cancers has been associated with prognosis in endometrial cancer and other gynecologic malignancies. Trastuzumab is a humanized mAb to the extracellular domain of HER2, which prevents ligand binding. Although this drug has found great success in the treatment of Her-2/neu–positive breast cancer, its use in gynecologic oncology has been limited. Bookman and colleagues performed a phase II trial of trastuzumab in HER-2–positive recurrent ovarian cancer. Of 837 patients screened, only 11.4% were found to have high expression of HER-2. The low prevalence of this abnormality combined with a modest objective response rate of 7.3% has limited further exploration of this agent in ovarian cancer. Similarly, a phase II trial of trastuzumab (2 mg/kg) for patients with advanced or recurrent HER-2–positive endometrial cancer demonstrated no responses. Of 30 patients, 12 had SD, and the trial was closed early secondary to poor accrual. Recent data have supported the selection of only uterine serous tumors; thus, a phase II randomized trial is ongoing examining standard chemotherapy with or without trastuzumab.

Pertuzumab

The humanized mAb pertuzumab prevents the linkage of HER2 to other receptors by binding a protein site in the dimerization domain. To date, pertuzumab has only been evaluated in recurrent ovarian cancer. In a trial of two dosing regimens of pertuzumab (840 mg loading with 420 mg every 21 days vs. 1050 mg every 21 days), five patients achieved partial response, and eight patients had SD. This study found a trend toward improved median PFS and expression of phospho-HER2. The GOG evaluated pertuzumab as a monotherapy in recurrent ovarian cancer and achieved an overall response rate of 4.3%. An additional 6.8% of patients had SD for longer than 6 months. A large randomized trial comparing gemcitabine (800 mg/m^2) alone with gemcitabine with pertuzumab (420 mg every 21 days) found that the addition of pertuzumab resulted in improved response rates (4.6% vs. 13.8%, respectively) and a trend toward improved PFS. The greatest treatment benefit was found in patients with low HER3 mRNA expression.

Seribantumab

HER3 has also been identified as a potential target of interest in gynecologic malignancies, specifically ovarian cancer. Seribantumab is a mAb that targets HER3 to block heregulin-mediated ErbB3 signaling and chemotherapy resistance. After identification of a recommended phase II dose, seribantumab has been primarily evaluated in combination with cytotoxic and targeted therapies to treat advanced solid tumors. A randomized phase II trial of seribantumab in combination with paclitaxel revealed no difference in PFS compared with paclitaxel alone in recurrent ovarian cancer. A specific panel of biomarkers, including heregulin mRNA expression and low HER2, were associated with benefit from the addition of seribantumab to paclitaxel.

Combination Agents
Lapatinib

Lapatinib is an oral tyrosine kinase inhibitor of EGFR and HER2. It acts through binding of the ATP-binding domain and

prevents pathway activation downstream. A single-agent study in recurrent ovarian cancer conducted by the GOG revealed no objective responses and only two patients progression free at 6 months (8%). As a combination, lapatinib (1000 mg/day) with metronomic carboplatin (AUC 2 weekly) and paclitaxel (60 mg/m^2 weekly) achieved response rates of 50% and SD in 30% of patients with recurrent ovarian cancer. These results were encouraging given the high number of median prior therapies in this group of patients. Other combinations with lapatinib including carboplatin and topotecan have not been as successful and have demonstrated unacceptable toxicity.

The use of lapatinib in combination with pazopanib in cervical cancer was discussed earlier in the chapter. The GOG also performed a phase II trial of lapatinib as monotherapy in recurrent or advanced endometrial cancer. Similar to the results in ovarian cancer, there was only one objective response, and seven patients achieved a best response of SD.

MULTIPATHWAY TARGETED AGENTS
Sorafenib

Sorafenib is an interesting small molecule inhibitor that effectively blocks several angiogenesis-related receptors (VEGFR, PDGFR, and KIT) and Raf, a key component of the Raf-MAPK kinase (MEK)-MAPK proliferation pathway. Sorafenib is of considerable interest in ovarian cancer that has been shown to harbor alterations in this pathway. Consequently, several trials are ongoing to evaluate the efficacy of sorafenib in the upfront, recurrent, and consolidation setting. Matei and colleagues reported the results of a phase II trial of sorafenib (400 mg bid) in recurrent ovarian cancer treated with fewer than two prior therapies. Of 73 patients, 22 achieved partial response or SD with toxicities, including rash and metabolic abnormalities. Of note, among the 59 patients with measurable disease, 12 were progression free for at least 6 months. The combination of sorafenib (200 mg twice daily) with bevacizumab (5 mg/kg) for the treatment of solid tumors was explored in a phase I study. Although the combination appeared to have significant activity in 13 patients with ovarian cancer (43% response rate), toxicity was common, leading to sorafenib dose reductions in 74% of patients. The most prevalent toxicities were diarrhea, elevated liver transaminases, hypertension, hand and foot syndrome, and fatigue.

In combination with traditional cytotoxic chemotherapy, including topotecan and gemcitabine, sorafenib has shown similar clinical benefit rates in recurrent ovarian cancer with minimal additional toxicity. A current phase III trial in newly diagnosed ovarian cancer after cytoreductive surgery seeks to determine if the addition of sorafenib (400 mg bid) to standard paclitaxel (175 mg/m^2) and carboplatin (AUC 6) provides any additional PFS benefit. Sorafenib is also being explored as a maintenance agent in ovarian cancer and an additional chemosensitizer in the upfront treatment of advanced cervical cancer with radiotherapy.

Vandetanib

Vandetanib inhibits the tyrosine kinase activity of two parallel pathways through action on VEGFR-2 and EGFR. This leads to suppression of angiogenesis, cell proliferation, migration, and survival mechanisms. A phase II trial of vandetanib alone to treat recurrent ovarian cancer was terminated after the first stage of accrual because no patients achieved response or SD. Of note, molecular testing in this study revealed evidence of blockage of the EGFR pathway but no activity against VEGFR. Although single-agent activity has been disappointing, this agent underwent exploration in combination with docetaxel and liposomal doxorubicin for the treatment of ovarian cancer. A randomized phase I/II study of liposomal doxorubicin alone or in combination with vandetanib was limited by significant toxicity, which led to cessation in a high number of patients treated with the combination. Conversely, in a separate randomized phase II study, vandetanib in combination with docetaxel was tolerable; however, there was no improvement in PFS compared with docetaxel alone.

Imatinib

Imatinib mesylate is an example of a small molecule that inhibits multiple pathways, including c-kit, bcr-abl, and PDGFR. Although imatinib has been quite successful for the treatment of chronic myelogenous leukemia, in which the tyrosine kinase bcr-abl is constitutively activated, the success in gynecologic malignancies as a single agent has been limited. This may result in part from the impact of the PDGF axis on pericytes, which are mesenchymal cells that support endothelial cells and newly developing blood vessels. PDGF activity recruits pericytes, which produce VEGF to stimulate angiogenesis and survival. Research on pericytes has indicated that blocking the PDGF axis in addition to the VEGF axis may be necessary to achieve improved response rates. Thus far, imatinib has only been explored as a single agent or in combination with cytotoxic chemotherapy for gynecologic malignancies.

Several phase II trials for recurrent ovarian cancer, both high and low grade, have been performed using imatinib (400 mg/day) as a single agent. Unfortunately, rates of response have been low, with only one objective responder among all trials. Rates of SD ranged from 9% to 33%. Similar disappointing results have been seen in cervical cancer. In a trial of 12 patients with recurrent cervical cancer treated with imatinib, there were no responses and only one patient with SD. In all trials, expression of drug-related targets has not been associated with response. The use of imatinib in combination with docetaxel (30 mg/m^2 weekly) in 23 patients with recurrent ovarian cancer achieved five responses, including one complete response. Three additional patients had SD lasting longer than 4 months. Further evaluations of this drug in combination with other cytotoxic chemotherapy for recurrent ovarian cancer have yielded minimal success.

Dasatinib

Dasatinib is a strong inhibitor of the Src family of kinases, which participate in the regulation of cellular growth, adhesion, invasion, and migration. At higher concentrations, dasatinib has effects on a variety of different targets relevant to tumor progression, including bcr-abl, c-kit, and PDGF. In addition, dasatinib targets the EphA2 receptor, which modulates cell migration, survival, proliferation, and angiogenesis. EphA2 overexpression correlates with poor outcome in ovarian cancer. Dasatinib (150 mg/day) has been explored in multiple solid tumors in early-phase trials with promising response rates. A phase I trial of this agent in combination with paclitaxel (175 mg/m^2) and carboplatin (AUC 6) was tolerable with reasonable activity. This combination has also been evaluated in advanced endometrial cancer with results pending.

Cabozantinib (XL-184)

Exploration into mechanisms of resistance to anti-VEGF therapies has suggested pathways responsive to the observed upregulation of HIF-1α. One pathway of interest is c-Met, which is also implicated in tumor growth, survival, and metastases. Cabozantinib is a small molecule inhibitor of VEGFR-2 and c-Met, which has been evaluated in a number of solid tumors including, recently, ovarian cancer. In a phase II randomized discontinuation trial, cabozantinib was administered to 68 platinum-sensitive and -resistant patients. Overall response was 24% with 35% of patients also exhibiting prolonged SD. Response rates were similar between the platinum-sensitive and -resistant cohorts. Because of better-than-expected results, the trial was terminated early. A subsequent GOG study compared this agent with weekly paclitaxel in recurrent ovarian cancer. Cabozantinib failed to meet prespecified endpoints of interest, demonstrating lower levels of response than weekly paclitaxel.

OTHER TARGETS OF INTEREST

Angiopoietin (Ang)/Tie-2

In addition to the classic VEGF pathways of angiogenesis, other pathways involved in later stages of neovascularization hold promise for targeted therapy. Ang-1 and Ang-2 bind the receptor Tie-2 to activate pathways that stimulate endothelial cell proliferation, motility, and survival. In addition, the angiopoietins recruit pericytes to support vascular maturation. Trebananib (AMG-386) is a peptibody, a peptide fusion protein, that selectively binds Ang-1 and Ang-2, preventing interaction with Tie-2. In phase I studies of solid tumors, this compound was well tolerated, without many of the classic toxicities associated with antiangiogenic agents. A phase II study comparing two different dose levels of trebananib (3 mg/kg, 10 mg/kg) versus placebo in combination with weekly paclitaxel (80 mg/m^2) demonstrated a trend toward improved PFS in patients who achieved higher steady-state concentrations of trebananib. These results lead to the dose selection for TRINOVA-1, a study comparing trebananib versus placebo plus weekly paclitaxel in recurrent ovarian cancer. The addition of trebananib yielded a significant improvement in PFS period of 2 months. A phase Ib study of trebananib in combination with paclitaxel and carboplatin was found to be tolerable in women with advanced ovarian cancer. This led to development of TRINOVA-3, a randomized phase III study in upfront ovarian cancer. Results have not yet been reported. AMG-386 (10 mg/kg) has been explored in combination with liposomal doxorubicin (50 mg/m^2) or topotecan (4 mg/m^2) for recurrent ovarian cancer in a phase Ib trial. Interim results have demonstrated acceptable toxicity; however, efficacy data are not yet mature. In recurrent endometrial cancer, trebananib as a single agent did not have sufficient efficacy to pursue further evaluation, with only one objective response of 32 patients treated.

Aurora Kinase

Three members of the aurora kinase family (Aurora kinase, A, B, and C) play large roles in the phases of mitosis. These proteins are serine/threonine kinases that act to control cell division through regulation of spindle assembly, chromosome separation, and centrosome maturation. Overexpression of Aurora A and Aurora B is associated with tumorigenesis in multiple solid tumor types. Currently, there are 14 agents targeting Aurora kinase activity, which are under investigation in phase I and II trials. One agent targeting Aurora kinase A, alisertib (MLN8237), demonstrated significant activity in recurrent ovarian cancer and was evaluated as a single agent in a phase II study. Ten percent of patients treated with alisertib achieved a partial response, and 20% had SD for more than 3 months. A subsequent randomized phase II study of weekly paclitaxel alone or in combination with alisertib yielded improved PFS in the combination arm (6.7 vs. 4.7 months; HR, 0.75; 95% CI 0.58–0.96). Objective responses by RECIST were higher as well in the combination arm. An interesting new Aurora kinase A inhibitor, ENMD-2076, has additional activity against VEGFR, Flt-3, and FGFR3 kinases and has demonstrated activity in a phase I expansion cohort study of refractory ovarian cancer patients. Based on RECIST (defined later) or GCIG CA-125 response criteria, two of 20 patients and six of 20 patients, respectively, responded to single-agent therapy. This encouraged pursuit of additional phase II studies in ovarian cancer patients, which are ongoing.

Delta-Like 4 (Dll4)/Notch

The Notch signaling pathway participates in the regulation of angiogenesis, proliferation, and apoptosis, making it an attractive potential target for anticancer therapy. One major avenue of Notch activation is through one of its ligands, Dll4, which creates a negative feedback loop to block cellular proliferation stimulated through VEGFR2. In addition, Notch signaling through Dll4 appears to activate cell cycle arrest through a variety of mechanisms. Notch overexpression has been demonstrated in multiple tumor types, including ovarian carcinoma. Two major therapeutic avenues exist that block signaling through the Notch pathway. The gamma secretase complex acts as a mediator of Notch signaling. Gamma secretase inhibitors are nonspecific agents that are currently in multiple phase I trials for solid tumors. Their lack of specificity has led to significant toxicity in the GI tract. Thus, antibodies that target the Dll4 ligand have been developed to reduce toxicity. These compounds have demonstrated significant activity in in vivo models and are undergoing evaluation in early-phase clinical trials. Demcizumab, an anti-Dll4 antibody, achieved reasonable dose levels with adverse events, including hypertension, fatigue, anemia, and headache. This agent is undergoing evaluation in combination with weekly paclitaxel in recurrent ovarian cancer. Other agents, including tarextumab, MK-0752, R04929097, and PF63084014, are under study in early-phase clinical trials.

Folate Receptor α

Folate receptor α binds folic acid with high affinity and is involved in folate transport. This is quite relevant in gynecologic malignancy because this receptor is overexpressed in more than 90% of ovarian cancers. Furthermore, there is minimal expression of this target in normal tissues, making this an attractive target for anticancer therapy. Farletuzumab (MORAb-003), a humanized mAb to folate receptor α, demonstrated inhibition of cellular proliferation and stimulation of cell death in preclinical models. A phase II trial of this agent (100 mg/m^2) in platinum-sensitive ovarian cancer was designed as a single-agent study with subsequent addition of traditional chemotherapy (carboplatin and paclitaxel) at the time of disease progression. In the single-agent arm, 24 of 28 patients remained on therapy at least 9 weeks. With combination therapy, 80% of patients achieved normalization of their CA-125, and 75% had complete or partial response. Unfortunately, farletuzumab in combination with carboplatin and paclitaxel did not yield superior outcomes compared with chemotherapy alone. Of note, a planned subset analysis found that lower pretreatment CA125 and higher exposure to farletuzumab yielded improved PFS compared with placebo.

Mirvetuximab soravtansine (IMGN853) is an antibody–drug conjugate targeting folate receptor α. The folate receptor antibody is attached to maytansinoid, a highly toxic agent that targets microtubules to induce cellular death. This agent is quite potent against cells that are folate receptor positive and even to nearby folate receptor–negative cells. A phase I trial of mirvetuximab soravtansine revealed that the agent was well tolerated, and in a small expansion cohort of ovarian cancer ($n = 17$), 53% had an objective response despite platinum-resistant disease. This agent may undergo further development, alone and in combination with bevacizumab, in ovarian and endometrial cancer.

Vintafolide (EC-145)

Another agent leveraging the folate receptor α is vintafolide. This novel ligand drug conjugate combines folic acid with desacetylvinblastine hydrazide, a chemotherapeutic agent difficult to deliver systemically. In a randomized phase II trial, vintafolide combined with pegylated liposomal doxorubicin (PLD) was associated with a significantly longer PFS than PLD alone (5 vs. 2.7 months; HR, 0.63; $P = 0.031$). Of interest, and in support of the target selectivity, there were few differences in the observed toxicities between the two arms. Furthermore, patients with global tumor expression of folate receptor α as measured by EC-20, a tracer conjugated to folic acid, had a PFS that was similar to that of the overall population but substantially better than the control arm, suggesting that high receptor expression is associated with poor prognosis. Unfortunately, a subsequent phase III trial was stopped early because of futility, although final results have not yet been reported.

Antimesothelin Antibodies

Mesothelin is an antigen that is highly expressed in several advanced solid tumors, including ovarian cancer. Growing data indicate that this protein may have a role in the peritoneal spread of ovarian cancer. Thus, a number of antibody–drug conjugates containing an antimesothelin antibody are in development. DMOT4039A was studied in the phase I setting for unresectable pancreatic and platinum-resistant ovarian cancer. Toxicities included GI and constitutional, and many were cumulative over time. Objective activity was seen, and this agent is under further evaluation. There are several other agents in development, although no results have been reported.

Histone Acetyltransferases and Histone Deacetylases

The epigenetic modulation of gene expression is a promising target for the treatment of gynecologic malignancies. The post-translational modification of histones is a key mechanism to regulate the expression of certain genes and has been implicated in tumorigenesis. Histones may be modified through acetylation, methylation, phosphorylation, and ubiquitination. Two enzymes, histone acetyltransferase and histone deacetylases (HDAC), mediate the addition and removal of acetyl groups, respectively. HDAC activity leads to a change in the histone structure, which leads to a change in transcription activity. Through activation of oncogenes or inactivation of tumor suppressors, cell growth, proliferation, and evasion of apoptosis may occur. HDAC inhibitors have been explored in a variety of solid tumor types. Suberoylanilide hydroxamic acid (Vorinostat) is FDA approved for the treatment of refractory cutaneous T-cell lymphoma and has been explored in recurrent ovarian cancer. A phase II study of single-agent vorinostat (400 mg/day) in 27 patients had limited success with only one partial response (4%) and two patients with SD for 6 months (7%). The HDAC inhibitor belinostat was evaluated as a single agent in platinum resistant ovary and micropapillary low malignant potential tumors. This study of 32 patients demonstrated modest activity with only one partial response and 19 patients with SD. There is evidence to suggest that the combination of HDAC inhibitors with traditional cytotoxic chemotherapy may yield improved results; thus, these agents have been explored in combination with traditional chemotherapy regimens. The combination of vorinostat with gemcitabine and carboplatin was quite toxic, although some activity was achieved. The study was terminated early secondary to overall poor tolerance. Conversely, belinostat was successfully combined with carboplatin as well as with carboplatin and paclitaxel. Although both combinations were tolerable, only belinostat in combination with carboplatin and paclitaxel yielded response rates worthy of further study.

Platelet-derived Growth Factor

In addition to the combination agents noted previously, there are agents in development that solely target the PDGFR. This is supported by recent research indicating that the v-sis oncogene is derived from the PDGF gene. Furthermore, the PDGF pathway is involved not only in angiogenesis but also in stimulation of cancer growth and regulation of fibroblasts. The use

of a mAb to target this pathway promises to improve efficacy and reduce off-target effects. Olaratumab (IMG-3G3) is a mAb to PDGF-α that has demonstrated significant antitumor activity in preclinical studies in ovarian cancer cell lines. Phase I trials in advanced solid malignancy toxicity have led to the development of a current phase II study of this agent (20 mg/kg) in combination with liposomal doxorubicin (40 mg/m^2) for platinum-resistant recurrent ovarian cancer. As noted previously, as a result of the effects on pericytes, the use of this agent in combination with other therapies promises to improve efficacy over it as a single agent.

P53

Given its high prevalence across a number of gynecologic malignancies and advanced solid tumors, there is great interest to leverage targeted agents against p53 mutations. **By far, Wee1 inhibitors are the furthest developed against this important target. Tumors with mutations in p53 are dependent on the G2 cell cycle checkpoint, which is regulated by Wee1, to repair damaged DNA.** Inhibition of Wee1 creates a situation of synthetic lethality among p53 mutant tumors. AZD1775 is a Wee1 inhibitor that has been combined with carboplatin and paclitaxel in the platinum-sensitive recurrent setting of ovarian cancer. The combination of chemotherapy with a Wee1 inhibitor yielded an improved response rate and PFS compared with chemotherapy alone. This agent is now under evaluation alone and in combination with several targeted agents for ovarian cancer. In addition to Wee1 inhibitors, several molecules are in early development that appear to restore the function of p53 across a number of p53 mutant tumors in the preclinical setting.

Immune Therapy

As noted earlier, immune escape is an essential contribution to successful tumorigenesis. Over the past 5 years, the number of successful immune therapy agents has skyrocketed. Early studies have focused on notoriously immune-driven cancers, including melanoma and non–small cell lung cancer. Single-agent studies of agents targeting PD-1 and PD-L1, including avelumab, nivolumab, and pembrolizumab, have been less successful in ovarian cancer, yielding modest response rates approaching 15% in an unselected platinum-resistant setting, primarily among patients with clear cell histology. Responses among high-grade serous ovarian cancer have been limited. However, growing data indicate that activity of immune therapy may be related to common features of gynecologic malignancies, such as mutations in BRCA, POLE, or the presence of microsatellite instability. This has led to development of immune therapy trials in ovarian, endometrial, and cervical cancer both alone and in combination with chemotherapy or targeted therapy. In addition to the checkpoint inhibitor trials described earlier, the use of tumor-directed T cells (adoptive T-cell therapy) has been explored in cervical malignancies. A small study of this therapy in nine women with metastatic cervical cancer yielded three objective responses, including two durable complete responses. Certainly, these therapies are promising and results from larger clinical trials are eagerly anticipated. In addition, approaches to enhance cytotoxic T lymphocytes (CTL) entry into tumor islets will be important for improving the efficacy of immune therapies.

UNIQUE TOXICITIES OF TARGETED THERAPY

In addition to survival benefit, a major goal of targeting tumor-specific pathways is to reduce the incidence of adverse events caused by "nonspecific" cytotoxic agents. Targeted agents may have similar toxicities to the traditional agents such as myelosuppression, fatigue, and diarrhea. As our experience with novel targeted agents grows, it is apparent that there exist toxicities unique to these compounds. Side effects may be secondary to the inherent mechanism of the agent or unintended "off-target" effects. This section of the chapter serves as a brief review of the most commonly encountered toxicities and methods of prevention and treatment.

Hypertension

Hypertension is one of the most commonly experienced side effects related to targeted agents, with a prevalence that approaches 40%. This adverse event is most commonly related to the use of antiangiogenic agents, including bevacizumab, and combination agents such as sorafenib. The mechanism of hypertension is currently hypothesized to be twofold. First, the inhibition of VEGF results in the reduction of production of nitric oxide by endothelial cells. Resultant vasoconstriction and endothelial cell dysfunction are compounded by the occurrence of microvascular rarefaction. Microvascular rarefaction is a process found in a majority of patients with hypertension, regardless of etiology, and consists of the loss of the arterioles and capillaries that make up the microcirculation. Vasoconstriction from loss of nitric oxide serves to exacerbate nonperfusion and elevate peripheral vascular resistance, which can result in permanent microvessel extinction.

Hypertension appears to be dose dependent for several of the antiangiogenic agents. Bevacizumab at the typical doses given for gynecologic malignancies (10–15 mg/kg) has an incidence of hypertension between 18% and 36% compared with an incidence of 3% to 30% in patients treated with low-dose bevacizumab (3–7.5 mg/kg). This incidence may be further increased when bevacizumab is combined with cytotoxic agents known to have antiangiogenic activity such as topotecan or paclitaxel. Agents affecting the HIF-1α pathway reduce nitric acid synthesis and metabolism, leading to exacerbation of antiangiogenic drug-induced hypertension. Of note, small molecular inhibitors to VEGF have reduced incidence and severity of hypertension compared with mAbs targeting the receptor.

Hypertension induced by antiangiogenic agents is most commonly found in patients with preexisting hypertension. Thus, active management of blood pressure and cardiac risk factors such as elevated lipids is paramount. The use of several antihypertensive agents is often necessary to control hypertension in this setting. Acceptable treatments for angiogenesis inhibitor–induced hypertension include angiotensin-converting enzyme inhibitors, beta-blockers, and dihydropyridine calcium channel blockers (amlodipine, felodipine). Nondihydropyridine calcium channel blockers should be avoided given their inhibition of the P450 CYP3A4, which can affect the metabolism of tyrosine kinase inhibitors. Nifedipine is also not an optimal therapeutic choice secondary to the increase in VEGF levels associated with chronic use.

Reverse Protein Leukoencephalopathy

Reverse protein leukoencephalopathy (RPLS) is a rare complication of antiangiogenic agents, including bevacizumab, sorafenib, and sunitinib. Occurring in fewer than 1% of all patients treated with these agents, this syndrome is characterized by finding of diffuse, hyperintense T2-weighted signaling secondary to leaking of the capillaries in the brain. Symptoms of RPLS include change in mental status, headache, seizures, and lethargy. Aggressive antihypertensive management and supportive care typically lead to full recovery; however, in rare cases, this syndrome may be fatal. Typically, further use of anti-VEGF therapy in these patients is contraindicated.

Cardiotoxicity

Other effects of targeted agents on the cardiovascular system can include left ventricular dysfunction, congestive heart failure, and myocardial infarction. Uncontrolled hypertension can lead to left ventricular hypertrophy and cardiac musculature that outgrows its vascular supply. This results in traumatic cardiovascular events, which may be seen in any of the anti-VEGF agents. Furthermore, any tyrosine kinase inhibitor may have off-target effects that damage cardiac muscle cells and impair their survival. For example, sorafenib and sunitinib have been associated with decreased left ventricular ejection fraction in up to 30% of patients. Of note, this damage appears to be reversible secondary to mitochondrial dysfunction rather than the permanent free radical–induced cardiac damage found after anthracycline cardiac toxicity.

Thus far, prediction of the development of cardiac toxicity from targeted agents has been difficult. It does appear more common in patients with preexisting cardiac disease and prior treatment with anthracyclines. Again, aggressive medical management of preexisting conditions and careful monitoring of cardiac function are essential to maximize outcomes.

Renal Toxicity

Renal adverse effects may be found in response to a variety of targeted agents as a result of the expression of key targets along the nephron. The most common toxicity is proteinuria, especially among the antiangiogenic agents. This is thought to originate secondary to damage of endothelial cells, which depend on VEGF for integrity and regulation of permeability. In addition, thrombotic microangiopathy that leads to further damage of the glomerular capillaries may compound the loss of protein from the vasculature. Proteinuria is typically low grade, is asymptomatic, and may be monitored through assessment of albumin levels by urine dipstick. If protein readings exceed 2+ protein, collection of 24-hour urine protein is indicated for treatment decision making. Urine protein levels exceeding 2 g require treatment interruption and possible dose reduction depending on protocol requirements. Spot urine protein to creatinine ratios may also be used to monitor renal effect of targeted agents. Renal failure caused by targeted agents is rare and appears to be primarily related to glomerulonephritis, interstitial nephritis, and acute tubular necrosis. Prevention and management of renal toxicity is based on thorough assessment of renal risk factors before therapy institution and optimization of any preexisting conditions.

Thromboembolic Events

The risk of venous thromboembolism (VTE) is increased at baseline among patients with active malignancy receiving chemotherapy. Antiangiogenic agents also appear to increase the propensity for thrombosis, especially arterial thromboembolism (ATE), including myocardial, cardiovascular, cerebral, and peripheral vascular events. In a large meta-analysis of patients treated as part of a randomized trial for a variety of solid tumors, patients treated with bevacizumab in addition to chemotherapy had two times greater incidence of ATE. Multivariate analysis revealed that bevacizumab remained a significant risk factor for ATE, in addition to age 65 years or older and prior history of ATE. Of note, the rate of thromboembolic complications appears low for VEGF-Trap and VEGF tyrosine kinase inhibitors. This may be secondary to formation of complexes by anti-VEGF antibodies that create a nidus for the formation of thromboses in the vasculature. Further study of this complication in large randomized controlled trials is necessary to determine the true incidence rates. At this point, patients with a history of VTE warrant the careful assessment and aggressive use of anticoagulation therapy. Anti-VEGF therapy should be avoided in patients with a history of prior ATE. Support for the use of routine thromboprophylaxis has not been established.

Gastrointestinal Perforation and Fistula

Gastrointestinal toxicity is a life-threatening complication that has been primarily associated with anti-VEGF therapy. Risk of intestinal perforation or fistula in any tumor type is associated with prior GI surgery, acute diverticulitis or active abdominal infection, obstruction, carcinomatosis, or history of prior radiotherapy. Rates of bowel perforation are highest among patients with ovarian cancer, ranging as high as 11% in one study of bevacizumab in the recurrent setting. In this study, a higher risk of perforation was associated with a history of more than two prior chemotherapy regimens. Furthermore, the high perforation rate in a trial combining bevacizumab and erlotinib in ovarian cancer led to early closure. Of note, frontline treatment does not appear to lead to increased GI toxicities, as evidenced by equivalent rates of perforation in the control and experimental arms of GOG 218 (reviewed in Table 18.4). Proposed mechanisms for bowel injury include the negative effect on wound healing secondary to damage of normal endothelial cells. Anti-VEGF therapies may induce microangiopathic events in the intestinal lining that cause edema and hemorrhage, making the wall more susceptible to bacterial dissemination and infection. In addition, rapid tumor shrinkage may cause the bowel wall to become weak, leading to perforation.

The management of anti-VEGF therapy-induced GI perforation must be individualized based on patient history, amount of disease, and status. In general, surgical exploration with intestinal diversion is the standard of care for patients with acceptable performance status; however, consideration should be made for risk of further poor wound healing. If a patient cannot undergo surgical exploration, conservative management with decompression, bowel rest, drainage, antibiotics, and nutritional support may be indicated.

Diarrhea and mucositis are common among patients treated with a majority of the small molecule inhibitors regardless of target. These adverse events may be the dose-limiting toxicity for a patient, requiring admission for IV hydration and drug discontinuation. Prevention with antimotility agents or neutralizing mouthwashes may be helpful to reduce incidence of these off-target effects. Esophagitis or gastritis may be an issue in patients treated with sorafenib or sunitinib; therefore, prevention with a proton pump inhibitor is reasonable.

Cutaneous Complications

Skin toxicities are quite common in patients treated with anti-EGFR agents (50%–100%), are dose dependent, and appear to be indicative of drug efficacy. Typically, an acneiform rash consisting of pruritic papules and pustules presents within 3 weeks of treatment on skin areas that have sebaceous glands. A similar rash may be seen in patients treated with mTOR inhibitors. The mechanism is thought to be related to follicular hyperkeratosis that causes glands blockage and inflammatory eruption.

This rash may be managed with topical antiseptics and antiinflammatory agents. Oral antibiotics such as doxycycline or minocycline may be used daily for a short course to improve rash severity and symptoms. In addition to this rash, patients may experience significant xerosis, which may be managed with over-the-counter emollients. Changes to the nail bed may be seen, including fragility, paronychia (inflammation of nail folds), and fissures. The hair may also be affected by the use of these agents. Most commonly, hypertrichosis, including growth of the eyelashes and scalp hair, has been reported.

Hand and foot skin reaction or acral erythema is a classic skin toxicity of sorafenib and sunitinib. Occurring in 20% to 25% of patients, it may consist of erythema, hyperkeratosis, xerosis, and dysesthesias and paresthesia in the bilateral hands, feet, or both. Patients can develop callous-like blisters and desquamation in both pressure- and non–pressure-bearing areas. Treatment for hand and foot skin reaction is primarily supportive, consisting of elevation, compresses, avoidance of trauma, and topical application of corticosteroid cream. Symptoms usually resolve during the course of therapy, but some patients may require dose reduction or complete cessation of therapy. In addition to hand and foot skin reaction, patients treated with sorafenib or sunitinib can develop stomatitis, scalp dysesthesias, perianal rash, and a skin rash that resembles seborrheic dermatitis.

Metabolic Abnormalities

The nonspecific nature of some of the targeted agents has led to a variety of unique metabolic side effects, requiring careful monitoring and action. Endocrine effects of tyrosine kinase inhibitors may include altered thyroid function, glucose metabolism, and bone metabolism. For example, sunitinib and sorafenib have been associated with onset of hypothyroidism in previous euthyroid patients. mTOR inhibitors, including temsirolimus and everolimus, have been associated with incidence of any hyperglycemia as high as 50%. Of note, alterations in glucose metabolism can occur in either direction in patients treated with sunitinib or imatinib. Glucose levels must be monitored closely because these changes may necessitate change in dosing of antihyperglycemic agents among patients with diabetes. Glycemic control should be maximized before treatment with these agents. Lipid abnormalities, including elevated triglycerides and cholesterol, are common toxicities experienced by patients treated with mTOR inhibitors. These levels should be followed during treatment and, depending on patient cardiac risk factors, lipid-lowering agents may be instituted. Electrolytes should be monitored during treatment with targeted agents because many tyrosine kinase inhibitors have caused profound hypophosphatemia manifested as muscle weakness and fatigue.

SPECIAL CONSIDERATIONS FOR TARGETED THERAPIES

The unique nature of the targeted agents has led to several areas of controversy in the clinical management of patients receiving these drugs. Specifically, the design of clinical trials incorporating such agents is receiving scrutiny. The traditional method of determining the efficacy of a given drug by RECIST is based on the mechanism of action of cytotoxic chemotherapy (Table 18.6). These drugs are expected to shrink tumor cells, and thus a "successful" response as defined by RECIST would include a complete response or partial response. Typically, SD would be considered a failure of the agent. However, as noted earlier, targeted agents are generally cytostatic. Given that these agents may simply inhibit tumor growth, SD may actually indicate an efficacious targeted agent. In fact, some authors have advocated the inclusion of SD into the endpoints of early clinical trials of targeted agents to ensure that potentially beneficial treatments are not eliminated from further study.

For patients with ovarian cancer, response to treatment may be monitored using CA-125 levels. However, it is unclear if this method is reliable for patients being treated with a targeted agent. In the aforementioned study of patients with recurrent ovarian cancer treated with bevacizumab and sorafenib, Azad and colleagues noted that changes in the concentration of CA-125 did not correspond to response based on RECIST measurements in all patients. Of note, three patients with partial response by RECIST had elevations in their CA-125 level that would have required removal from the study if strict CA-125 criteria had been used. Conversely, of eight patients with response by CA-125, only five had responses confirmed by computed tomography results.

It is clear that the expression of the receptors and proteins targeted by these agents varies across each tumor and histology type. The use of a targeted agent in an unselected patient population may lead to lower response rates and lack of further exploration of a potentially useful drug. It is clear that determination of which patients are more likely to benefit from a given targeted therapy is necessary. As molecular testing continues to advance, we anticipate that pretreatment determination of mutation status, gene and protein expression levels, or target function will result in patients being treated with appropriately selected targeted agents. Such predictive biomarkers will be increasingly expected to be included in clinical trials and for drug approvals.

The cytostatic nature of the targeted agents may also limit their effectiveness as a single-agent therapy. As seen in the text, many of these agents may control disease but not eliminate the disease entirely. Thus, the combination of targeted agents with other treatment modalities such as cytotoxic chemotherapy, surgery, and radiation is rational and currently being explored. As the use of targeted agents continues to increase, the considerations noted previously will need to be addressed and consensus achieved to ensure appropriate trial design and patient management.

CONCLUSIONS

As knowledge regarding tumor biology and pathogenesis continues to expand, the number of targeted agents will no doubt increase exponentially. These agents have the potential to have a profound impact on the treatment of patients with gynecologic malignancies. Future considerations will include determining the appropriate combination of targeted agents with other modalities to optimize survival outcomes and quality of life. Furthermore, directly targeting genes with RNA interference technology and assigning therapies based on the molecular or cellular profile of the tumor hold the promise to personalize the care of each gynecologic cancer patient.

ACKNOWLEDGMENTS

The authors would like to acknowledge support from the National Institutes of Health (CA 110793, CA 109298, K12 CA088084, P50 CA083639, P50 CA098258, U54 CA151668), the Andrew Sabin Fellows Fund, the Ovarian Cancer Research Fund, Inc. (Program Project Development Grant), CPRIT 120214, Jimmy V Foundation, Judy Reis Ovarian Cancer Fund, the Frank McGraw Memorial Chair, the Anne Rife Cox Chair in Gynecology, the Gynecologic Cancer Foundation, and the Meyer and Ida Gordon Foundation.

For the bibliography list, log onto www.expertconsult.com ⟨http://www.expertconsult.com⟩.

TABLE 18.6	Response Evaluation Criteria for Solid Tumors (RECIST) Response Definitions	
Response	**Definition**
Complete response (CR)	Disappearance of all target and nontarget lesions
Partial response (PR)	30% decrease in the sum of the diameters of the target lesions; stable nontarget lesions
Stable disease (SD)	Neither sufficient decrease or increase in the sum of the diameters of target lesions to qualify for CR or PD
Progressive disease (PD)	20% increase in sum of the diameters of the target lesions; progressive nontarget lesions; new lesions

19

Genes and Cancer: Genetic Counseling and Clinical Management

David G. Mutch, MD, Sheri A. Babb, MS, CGC, Philip J. Di Saia, MD

OUTLINE

KEY POINTS

1. Cancer is not always inherited, but it is always genetic.
2. The inherited aspect of cancer always needs to be considered and appropriate counseling and testing arranged.
3. Genetic counseling and testing needs to be an integral part of all cancer management.
4. Genetic counselors are necessary for management and treatment of inherited disease.
5. Management is continuously changing, and communication among patients, their families, and the health care team is important.

Cancer is always genetic at the cellular level, but it is not always due to inherited risk. Overall, approximately 5% to 10% of cancers are clearly caused by inherited (germline) mutations. More recent data suggest that 10% to 25% of epithelial ovarian cancers are due to inherited risk. Mutations, if they occur in a gene or genes critical for cell growth, may allow a cell to reproduce in an uncontrolled fashion. This uncontrolled growth of a cell or tissue is known as a cancer. Cancer is seldom the result of a single mutation but is more commonly caused by a multitude of acquired mutations in many different genes, allowing uncontrolled cell division. The concept that cancer is the result solely

of genetic or epigenetic changes is relatively new and comes from the past 4 decades of cancer research. Before the 1970s, the cause of cancer was essentially a black box, and its etiology was largely unknown. To some extent, it is still unclear, but we no longer believe that defective immunity, viruses, or metabolic errors directly cause cancer. These factors may contribute to the development of this disease, but the basis of cancer lies in an individual organism's DNA and in that individual organism's ability to express the genetic material in a normal fashion. This is simply related to the DNA sequences that make up that individual's genome that has been inherited and altered

FIGURE 19.1 Disease-associated mutations that alter protein function.

FIGURE 19.2 A depiction of a polymorphism.

through the course of normal living. Thus, cancer is a disease of abnormal DNA expression. Alterations or differences in the DNA sequences are known as mutations (changes in DNA such that a protein alteration occurs) or polymorphisms (changes in DNA that results in a subtle change in gene function and protein structure that do not cause disease). Polymorphisms are one of the factors responsible for normal population differences. There is a fine line between a mutation and polymorphism (Figs. 19.1 and 19.2) (<1% but protein function remains).

An individual may inherit a genetic mutation or may be exposed to an environmental insult that predisposes to the development of a cancer. Such insults can occur from everyday living or as the result of repetitive exposure to an agent that can cause DNA damage such as known carcinogens or other environmental factors that cause DNA damage. In addition, any process that causes cells to divide, such as ovulation, can allow an opportunity for an error in DNA replication to be made. For instance, an individual prone to the development of ovarian cancer can reduce her risk of developing this disease by taking

oral contraceptives. This will inhibit ovulation and decrease the damage to the surface of the ovary that could allow a mutation to occur. **Recent hypotheses suggest that ovarian cancer may arise from the epithelium of the tubal epithelium. If this circumstance is true, then the etiology of oral contractive protection is not known.**

Cancers, unlike many other inherited diseases, become apparent after there is an accumulation of several genetic injuries or mutations. In this respect, cancer is different from most inborn errors of metabolism because more than one genetic event is required to allow expression of the disease. One does not inherit cancers as one would inherit cystic fibrosis or sickle cell disease. One may inherit a mutation in a gene that predisposes one to the development of cancer, but most cancers are the result of the accumulation of somatic mutations that result from the process of normal living. Viruses, smoking, eating charcoal-broiled steak, or simply random mistakes made during DNA replication may cause these mutations. After all, a replicating cell must copy 3 billion base pairs—with each division, mistakes will occur.

FIGURE 19.3 A model for colorectal tumorigenesis. This shows the molecular progression of normal colon epithelium to frank cancer.

Progression from a normal cell to a malignant cell is the result of the accumulation of a series of mutations. This progression has probably best been demonstrated in colon cancer by Burt Vogelstein and colleagues (Fig. 19.3). In this model, a series of mutations must occur that involve tumor suppressor genes and oncogenes; a benign tumor progresses to a malignant tumor as the necessary mutations occur during a prolonged and somewhat erratic interval.

Three broad classes of genes are involved in the development of cancer. These are tumor suppressor genes, oncogenes, and mismatch repair (MMR) genes. Tumor suppressor genes are responsible for making a product that inhibits cell growth. These types of genes are expressed in a recessive manner, and therefore both alleles need to be defective before the phenotype becomes apparent. Oncogenes are expressed dominantly and are usually responsible for a product that promotes cell growth. Overexpression of an oncogene protein results in uncontrolled cell growth. MMR genes are responsible for repairing DNA damage that results from loss of fidelity in normal DNA replication. If one of these genes does not function properly, errors in DNA can accumulate, and ultimately, some of these errors will occur in genes critical for cell control, resulting in uncontrolled cell growth. The development of cancers is therefore not the result of a single error or insult but rather the accumulation of genetic errors over time.

Mutations are a means of evolution. The paradox of life is that mutations can be responsible for an individual organism's death in the form of cancer or metabolic error, but other mutations can account for the evolution of the species. Therefore, mutations can be good, bad, or even neutral.

GENETIC ALTERATIONS IN CANCER

Genetics is not a new field and has been a study for several centuries from Mendel in 1865 to the present. Johannsen first coined the term *gene* in 1911 as it applied to the unit of a hereditary characteristic. This was further refined to the one gene–one enzyme concept in the 1940s and put forth by Tatum and Beadle. These concepts have been clearly defined in *Drosophila* but apply equally to humans and other organisms; after all, all living things are defined by their DNA. Humans have more DNA than other organisms and are therefore more complex, but the DNA behaves the same way in all organisms.

The one gene–one enzyme concept that developed from the ideas expressed by Tatum and Beadle can be summarized as follows:

1. All biologic processes are under genetic control.
2. These biochemical processes are expressed as a series of stepwise reactions.
3. Each biochemical reaction is ultimately under the control of different single genes.
4. Mutation of a single gene results in an alteration of the cell to carry out a single chemical reaction.

The one gene–one enzyme concept has since been refined and extended to cover proteins that are not enzymes. Now further information suggests that some genes combine with others to form unique proteins, indicating that a few genes may interact to form more than one protein per gene. The human genome is estimated to contain about 3 billion base pairs and was thought to have between 50,000 and 100,000 genes. Now that the human genome has been sequenced, we have discovered that there are only about 30,000 genes. These genes are stored on linear strands of DNA and interact much more than we previously believed. The genes are not continuous sequences of DNA but consist of coding sequences called exons interrupted by noncoding sequences called introns. Most of the DNA is composed of intronic DNA that is usually not expressed in any form. An approximation of the size of the human genome and its organization can be seen in Fig. 19.4. The functional length of the human chromosome is expressed in centimorgans (cM). A cM is the distance over which there is a 1% chance of crossover during meiosis and is really a measure of "genetic distance." Linkage studies indicate that the human genome is about 3000 cM. The average chromosome contains about 1500 genes in 130 million base pairs. Fig. 19.4 shows the estimated physical and functional size of the genome. Whereas the physical size is estimated in base pairs, the functional size is estimated in centimorgans. Much, if not most, of the human genome is composed of noncoded DNA and is therefore not expressed.

DNA is transcribed into RNA that is translated into protein. Therefore, the sequence of DNA base pairs ultimately determines the sequence of the functional proteins within the cell. All cellular functions are expressed in this manner (Fig. 19.5):

$$DNA \rightarrow RNA \rightarrow Protein$$

Humans and other mammals may be more complex than some other organisms in that pieces of genes may combine with parts of other genes to make a totally new protein. Hence, we

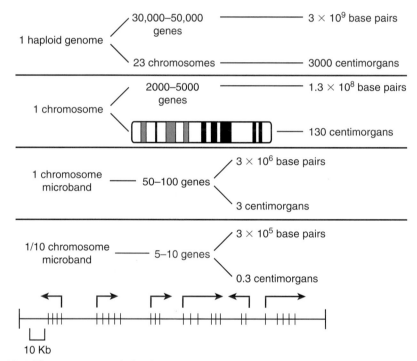

FIGURE 19.4 The structure of the human chromosome demonstrated in terms of functional units (centimorgans) and physical units (base pairs).

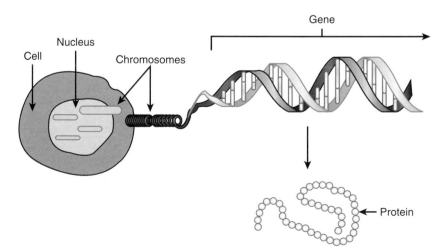

FIGURE 19.5 The progression of protein synthesis from DNA to RNA to protein. (From National Cancer Institute. *Understanding Gene Testing.* Rockville, MD, 1995, National Cancer Institute.)

may essentially increase the number of genes expressed without really increasing the amount of functional DNA or the number of actual genes. Overall, less than 30% of our genetic material is expressed.

MECHANISMS OF HUMAN GENE MUTATION

All cancers result from alterations in DNA structure, leading to changes in the proteins responsible for cellular function. All living organisms use the same 20 amino acids as building blocks for proteins. The translation of a nucleotide sequence from DNA to protein is dependent on a triplet code of nucleotides. Each of these triplet codes is called a *codon*. Some codons have very special functions. The code AUG codes for methionine, and this starts the initiation of synthesis (translation) of every protein. The code UAA is a stop codon and ends translation of a protein (Fig. 19.6). Much of the data available about genetic alterations in cancers come from studies other than of gynecologic malignant neoplasms. These studies often involve hematologic malignant neoplasms such as lymphomas and leukemia because pure subsets of cells are easily obtained. More recently, we have been able to improve our study of solid carcinomas because of our ability to study pure tumor preparations, single out cells, and isolate the DNA with microdissection and laser capture techniques. Using this technique and techniques like it, we can dissect out a single cancer cell, replicate its DNA, and evaluate the mutations that occur in this single cell or group of cells. Fig. 19.7 demonstrates the heterogeneity of cancer and why there is a need for these special techniques. Cancer is the result of clonal expansion, but as the various cells replicate in an uncontrolled manner, they continue to mutate. Initially, cancers usually have a single clonal origin. As the cancer progresses, mutations occur, and therefore some cells may become genetically different from the original cancer. **Hence, the term *mutator phenotype* is often applied to cancers.**

A wide number of and various types of mutations have been described. These mutations are fundamental to the understanding of cancer and of human evolution. Although many types of mutations can occur, some common ones are listed in Table 19.1.

A codon is made of three base pairs
64 codons total

| 1 codon (AUG) encodes methionine *and* starts translation of all proteins | 61 codons encode 20 amino acids (redundant code) | 3 codons stop protein translation |

A U G
Met

G C A
Ala

U A A
STOP

FIGURE 19.6 Stop codons.

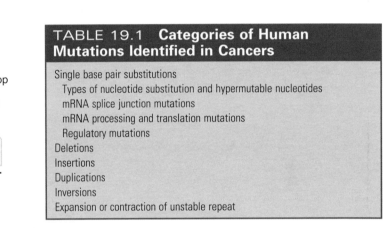

TABLE 19.1 **Categories of Human Mutations Identified in Cancers**
Single base pair substitutions
Types of nucleotide substitution and hypermutable nucleotides
mRNA splice junction mutations
mRNA processing and translation mutations
Regulatory mutations
Deletions
Insertions
Duplications
Inversions
Expansion or contraction of unstable repeat

Biopsy enriched for cancer cells

Biopsy with modest neoplastic cell content

Biopsy containing few neoplastic cells

○ Nonneoplastic cell
● Neoplastic cell

FIGURE 19.7 Heterogeneity within tumors often prevents accurate evaluation of tumor because of normal contamination.

Multiple searchable databases are publicly available that provide a comprehensive listing of gene specific mutations reported in the somatic cancer tissue as well as germline (inherited) mutations. Examples of these databases include The Human Gene Mutation Database (HGMD) (http://www.hgmd.cf.ac.uk/ac/index.php), Clinvar (http://www.ncbi.nlm.nih.gov/clincar), and COSMIC (Catalogue of Somatic Mutations in Cancer; http://www.cancer.sanger.ac.uk/cosmic). These databases are periodically updated as most researchers and commercial laboratories publicly share their data. Illustrations of some common mutations can be seen in Figs. 19.8 to 19.13.

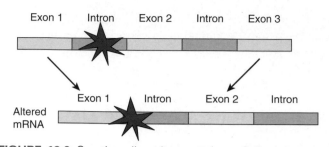

FIGURE 19.9 Cryptic splice site mutations. Splice site mutation, a change that results in altered RNA sequence.

FIGURE 19.8 Example of how a point mutation (a change in a single base pair) can result in changing the meaning of a gene sequence using a common phrase.

FIGURE 19.10 Exon skipping splice site mutations. Splice site mutation, a change that results in altered RNA sequence.

FIGURE 19.11 Missense mutation, changes to a codon for another amino acid (can be a harmful mutation or neutral polymorphism).

FIGURE 19.12 Nonsense mutation, change from an amino acid codon to a stop codon, producing a shortened protein.

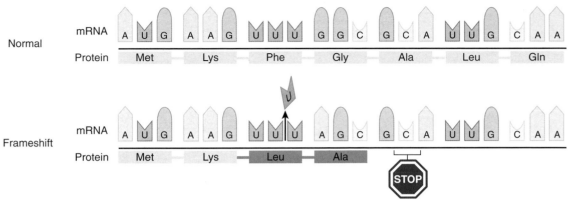

FIGURE 19.13 Frame shift mutation in which insertion or deletion of base pairs produces a stop codon downstream and (usually) a shortened protein.

Single Base Pair Substitutions and Point Mutations

DNA replication is the result of an accurate yet accident-prone process. The final accuracy of DNA replication depends on the fidelity of the initial process and the ability of subsequent repair processes to correct any mistakes. Point mutations lead to single changes in the DNA sequence. These single mutations can have very different effects on the reading of a protein, as demonstrated in Figs. 19.10 and 19.11. If this mutation is in a regulatory portion of a gene, loss or alteration of regulation of gene expression can occur. If the mutation is in a coding portion of the gene, an altered protein can be formed. HGMD is one of several catalogs of reported point mutations that can be obtained from the Internet.

One of the most common mutations as the result of substitution occurs in CpG dinucleotides (3′ cytosine-guanine 5′). Data show that these transversions account for about 30% of point mutations. The fidelity of this process is related to the efficiency and accuracy of the DNA polymerase responsible for replication. Other types of these small nucleotide substitutions that can also occur are messenger ribonucleic acid (mRNA) splice junction mutations, translational mutations, and single deletions. Alternatively, mismatches can occur by slipped mispairing, which leads to single base pair mutagenesis and deletion.

Deletion or insertion of a single nucleotide may be secondary to DNA mispairing during replication. This type of mutation often occurs in runs of identical base pairs and is the result of slippage of a single base pair (Fig. 19.14). This mechanism is similar to larger deletions caused by this same mechanism. The significance of this type of mutation to human malignant neoplasia is as yet undefined. As more information becomes available about mismatch repair, we should have a better estimate of the significance of this type of mutation to cancer formation. However, this slippage is common and similar to the errors found in individuals who have an inherited cancer syndrome, hereditary nonpolyposis colon cancer (HNPCC), or Lynch syndrome.

CpG dinucleotides are very susceptible to mutations. Methylation of cytosine results in a high level of mutation because

FIGURE 19.14 DNA mispairing that results in a single base deletion of a T. This causes a complete change of sequence. Attempt at correction adds a G or C to the sequence.

of its propensity to undergo deamination. This then forms thymidine and therefore can result in a change of gene expression. The evolution of the human genome seems to indicate a progressive loss of CpG islands because of this transition. The frequency of these islands is about 20% to 30% of the predicted frequency, probably because of the progressive loss of CpG dinucleotides. This excess of transition from cytosine to thymine (C to T) transitions was first reported by Vogel and Rohrborn in a study of the mutations responsible for variants of hemoglobin. Others now also have shown that CpG islands are associated with a high rate of transition, supporting the thought that these mutations play a significant role in human disease (Fig. 19.15).

Larger Deletions

Gene deletions are responsible for more than 150 inherited diseases. Deletions can range from a few base pairs to several

FIGURE 19.15 Cytosine to thymine transition from methylation. (From Korf B, ed. *Human Genetics: A Problem-Based Approach,* 2nd ed. 2000, Blackwell Publishers.)

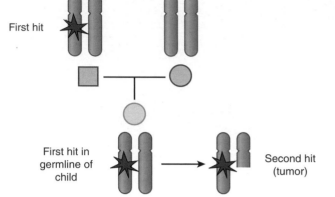

FIGURE 19.16 Knudsen's two-hit theory that is essential to the concept of tumor suppressor genes.

hundred kilobases and are often classified by size. These are also nonrandom in that certain sequences appear to be more prone to deletion than others are. This nonrandomness is apparent when one evaluates genetic disease. Spontaneous deletions often occur in the same sequences of various genes, indicating that some sequences of DNA are more prone to deletion than others.

Deletions occur when there is homologous but unequal recombination between gene sequences. Similar sequences in the human genome can cross over during mitosis or meiosis, resulting in a shortened portion of the gene sequence. Long areas of homology (homology boxes) are thought to be the most likely to have this type of mutation. Repetitive DNA sequences are particularly susceptible to deletions because this can allow slippage. This mechanism is called homolog or unequal recombination between repetitive sequence elements. The most common repetitive sequence is the Alu repeat (up to 106 Alu sequences are in the human genome). Alu repeats are characterized by an average spacing of 4 kilobases and 300–base pair length separated by a short A-rich region. The Alu element is 70% to 90% homologous to the consensus sequence. The 3′ homology (homology boxes) is thought to be the most likely to have this type of mutation. Repetitive DNA sequences are particularly prone to mutation.

There are more than 400 gross gene deletions recorded in the HGMD and 3000 or so smaller gene deletions. Almost 2500 gene deletions of 20 base pairs or fewer have been identified. These can be the result of deletion of repeats or a part of the excision repair process. Deletion is not random; particular sequences are more prone to deletion and often contain regions involving guanine or other repeats. The application of the techniques of molecular biology, such as gene cloning, in situ hybridization, restriction endonuclease mapping of genetic sequences, and polymerase chain reaction analysis of gene transcription, has led to the conclusion that a given chromosome abnormality may be associated with a variety of neoplasms and that a given oncogene may be activated in a variety of human cancers. The most common defects in solid tumors are deletions in specific gene sequences, observed as a loss of part of a banding region or the loss of heterozygosity of a specific genetic allele. Deletion of genetic material in a cancer cell suggests loss of function that regulates cell proliferation and differentiation. Many human solid tumors have been shown to

have some type of chromosome deletion. The Tp53 tumor suppressor gene–containing region of chromosome 17p is deleted or mutated in a wide variety of human cancers. The fact that there is such commonality among cancer cell types in the loss of chromosome material suggests that these regions contain genes coding for regulating functions of a wide variety of cell types. Induction of the malignant neoplastic process must involve at least two hits when a tumor suppressor gene is involved. This implies that two mutations or deletions in each of the two alleles are necessary before the effect can be expressed. This is the two-hit theory proposed by Knudson. The possibilities for the two hits necessary to express a recessive gene can be seen in Fig. 19.16. This explained why some people could inherit a predisposition for a malignant disease and also raised the question of whether sporadic cancers could have a genetic basis. In a genetically predisposed cell, the remaining single normal allele may be sufficient to maintain normal growth and regulation; a second deletion or mutation is required to inactivate the remaining normal allele.

Insertions

Most insertions appear to be small, between one and a few base pairs. This phenomenon has been studied extensively, and these insertions often appear to be nonrandom in character. Predisposing factors lead to these insertions. These insertions can be due to slipped mispairings, or they may be mediated by inverted repeat sequences or by symmetric elements. These sorts of DNA sequences are particularly prone to mutation.

Less common are large insertions. The largest insertion known is the 220-kilobase segment inserted into the DMD gene. Alu and LINE (long interspersed nucleotide elements) sequences are especially susceptible to insertion and deletion. Mutations are nonrandom, and some DNA segments are more susceptible to mutation than others are. For example, the myc gene is especially susceptible to insertions; a 50–base pair LINE element has been noted to be inserted in this gene in breast cancer cell lines. The fact that insertional mutations may not be random is underscored by the finding of Fearon and Vogelstein, who reported 10 independent examples of insertions within the same 170–base pair intronic region of the DCC gene involved in the progression of colorectal cancers.

Duplications

Duplication of small parts of whole exons, or even of whole chromosomes, has played a large part in the development of cancer. This phenomenon also has a large role in the evolution of the human genome. Again, the paradox is that mutations are sometimes good and sometimes bad. Duplication of larger segments of DNA may lead to gene amplification. Gene amplifications can occur in many ways. A gene that is usually present in a single copy in the normal cell may be duplicated or may undergo a small increase in the copy number. Another type of amplification may involve a 10- to 100-fold increase in copies of a genetic locus containing key regulatory genes. A third type of amplification can result in the duplication of whole chromosomes. One can envision how amplification has been important over the course of evolution. We have 23 pairs of chromosomes, and all other organisms have fewer chromosomes. This is due to millions of years of evolution resulting from innumerable insertions and duplications.

Inversions

Inversions are perhaps the least common type of mutation. In this mutation, a long segment of DNA forms a loop and alters its direction; the 3′ end now becomes the 5′ end. These segments can obviously be large or quite small. The most important inversion event in human disease involves the factor VIII gene, causing severe hemophilia A. An MSH2 inversion has been reported in exons 1 to 7 in Lynch syndrome and is one of the few cancer-associated inversions.

Translocations

More than 100 common translocations have been observed in malignant cells. Many of these occur consistently in certain specific cancer types, which argues that these areas are involved in the malignant process of the cell. Some of the translocations may be secondary events in the evolution of more aggressive phenotypic changes. The inherent genetic instability of malignant cells leads to further karyotypic abnormalities as the disease progresses, reflecting additional genetic alterations that increase growth potential. Evidence that malignant transformation does not usually result from a single translocation event comes from the study of patients with ataxia-telangiectasia, who are at high risk for leukemia. These patients have lymphocytes with a characteristic translocation present for many years before a malignant change develops.

A common finding in cancers is some form of genetic instability. This is most clearly manifested in Lynch syndrome (or HNPCC). Lynch syndrome is characterized by genetic instability at microsatellite sequences and has been linked to several MMR genes. Mutation rates in cells that are positive for MMR defects are orders of magnitude higher than MMR intact cells.

Cancers in patients with hereditary cancer syndromes may serve as a model for sporadic disease because mutations that occur in the sporadic tumors are often very similar. The same genes and sequences seem to be targeted. For instance, Krawczak

and Cooper demonstrated that the bulk of single base substitutions in the Tp53 gene in sporadic cancers strongly resemble those found in inherited cancers.

CANCER EPIGENETICS

Epigenetics refers to modification of gene expression not specifically related to changes in the DNA sequence of a gene. This is a concept of differential expression of the genotype based on factors outside of the genome. It is interesting that these differences can be inherited and appear to be quite stable. Epigenetic changes can involve chromatin structure; histone modification; changes in transcriptional activity; and, most easily measured in mammals, changes in methylation of CpG loci.

Methylation is the only known covalent modification of DNA in normal mammalian cells. This change occurs at the fifth position of cytosine at 5CG-3′ dinucleotides. About 80% of these types of dinucleotides are methylated and therefore are probably important in cell control and gene expression. Generalized hypomethylation is present in colorectal cancers and endometrial cancers early on in the development of these diseases, but the exact cause and effect of this observation is unclear. Presumably, hypomethylation allows some genes to be overexpressed. Alternatively, some regions on some genes, particularly the promoter region of MMR genes, can cause gene silencing (Fig. 19.17). This allows a tumor suppressor gene to be silenced, thus promoting the development of that cancer. Changes in methylation status are not clonal. Hence, some cancers can have different gene expression in the same cancer because of differential methylation. Changes in methylation

FIGURE 19.17 Methylation can cause gene silencing. (From Korf B, ed. *Human Genetics: A Problem-Based Approach*, 2nd ed. 2000, Blackwell Publishers.)

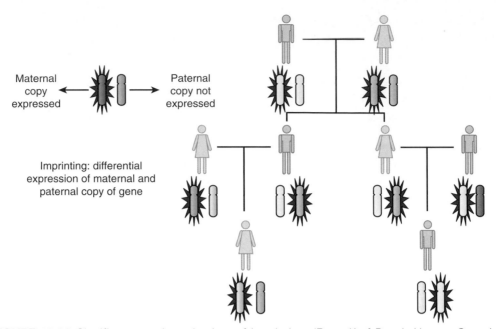

Maternal copy expressed ← → Paternal copy not expressed

Imprinting: differential expression of maternal and paternal copy of gene

FIGURE 19.18 Significance and mechanism of imprinting. (From Korf B, ed. *Human Genetics: A Problem-Based Approach,* 2nd ed. 2000, Blackwell Publishers.)

status could also cause aberrant chromosome condensation during division and result in abnormal chromosome segregation. Therefore, epigenetics can affect tumor behavior in several ways.

GENOMIC IMPRINTING AND CANCER

Genomic imprinting is a modification of DNA that leads to a different expression of the gene depending on the parent of origin. This may be passed from generation to generation. However, the specific expression of these modifications may increase, decrease, or remain stable from generation to generation (Fig. 19.18). These epigenetic alterations appear to occur commonly in human malignancies and because of their unique properties may lead to novel forms of therapy.

Assumptions are made in Mendelian genetics, which we apply to human disease, that the maternal and paternal alleles are equivalent. We also assume that both copies of the gene are necessary for normal function. This is not true with respect to genomic imprinting. An example of imprinting is the differences noted between the mule and the hinny. The mule is the cross between a maternal horse and a paternal donkey. It is much larger than the hinny, which is a cross between a maternal mule and a paternal horse. Although these two have the same genomic equivalent, they are distinctly different, indicating differential expression of maternal and paternal genes.

Examples of genomic imprinting and cancer are the hydatidiform mole and the teratoma. The hydatidiform mole is composed of paternal chromosomes, and the teratoma is composed of only maternal chromosomes. These examples demonstrate that not only does it take 46 chromosomes to make a human being, but there must also be a balance between maternal and paternal elements.

GENETIC ALTERATIONS THAT CAUSE CANCER

Oncogenes

The past 25 years have contributed significantly to our understanding of the molecular mechanism of cancer and have identified three types of molecular aberrations that can lead to cancer: dominant transforming genes called oncogenes, recessive transforming genes called tumor suppressor genes, and genes responsible for repairing DNA errors (MMR genes). Many oncogenes have been isolated as forms of proto-oncogenes acquired by RNA tumor viruses. We have known for many years that viruses can cause malignant tumors in animals. The link noted in animals spurred a great deal of research aimed at identifying the cancer-causing genes carried by the viruses and finding the human genes that were affected. These investigations surprisingly revealed that the genes implicated in malignant disease were often altered forms of viral genes. These were probably acquired when the virus infected the animal and then moved on to other animals. At other times, the viruses activated host genes that were normally quiescent. The normal versions of these pirated and activated genes, now termed *proto-oncogenes*, carried codes specifying the composition of proteins that encourage and stimulate cell replication. These growth-promoting genes come in various forms. Some specify the amino acid sequences of receptors that are found on the cell surface and bind to molecules known as growth factors. When bound by such factors, the receptor issues an intracellular signal that ultimately causes cells to replicate. Other growth-promoting genes code for proteins that lie inside the cell and govern the propagation of intracellular growth signals. A third group encodes proteins that control cell division and are under nuclear control. These oncogenes can be activated via several mechanisms. The oncogene can be amplified, and many copies of the

Normal genes
(regulate cell growth)

1st mutation
(leads to accelerated
cell division)

FIGURE 19.19 Schematic of oncogene function.

gene can become activated. Occasionally, the gene may be translocated to another chromosome, where, under the influence of another promoter, it promotes uncontrolled growth.

The three classes of oncogenes are controlled differently. The first comprises a group of peptide growth factors and their receptors. Included in this group are the peptide growth factors and their receptors such as epidermal growth factor receptor (EDGFR) and platelet-derived growth factor (PDGFR). These peptide growth factor receptors likely serve as stimulatory cofactors rather than the actual force that drives the malignant process. Targeted therapy is becoming a reality as our understanding of these cancer-promoting entities increases. Unique molecules are aimed at gene products or proteins activated by these factors. **Another class of oncogenes comes from non–membrane-traversing extranuclear growth factors. These include G-proteins and the ras gene family. Finally, there are oncogenes of the nuclear regulatory variety such as myc.** A schematic of oncogenes representing their function can be seen in Fig. 19.19. A more detailed description of targeted therapy can be found in Chapter 18.

The discovery that viral genes had human counterparts introduced the intriguing possibility that human cancers, including the majority not caused by viruses, might originate from mutations that convert useful proto-oncogenes into harmful genes—that is, oncogenes. Consistent with this notion, studies indicated that alteration of just one copy, or allele, of these proto-oncogenes was enough to transform and render cancerous some types of cells growing in culture. Such dominant mutations cause cells to overproduce a normal protein or make an aberrant form that is overactive. In either case, the result is that stimulatory signals increase within the cell even when no such signals come from the outside.

It is ironic that research on animal RNA tumor viruses (retroviruses) having no ability to cause human cancer provided the first key to uncovering the identity of some oncogenes and the verification that they actually exist. These retroviruses, which infected chickens, rodents, cats, and monkeys, were extremely tumorigenic in that infected animals often showed tumors on initial exposure to the virus. One of these viruses, the Rous sarcoma virus of a chicken, was found to carry a specific gene that it used to transform infected cells to a malignant state. This type of transforming oncogene was termed a

viral oncogene. A single oncogene carried onto a chicken cell by a Rous sarcoma virus was able to derail and redirect the entire metabolism of the cell, forcing it to grow in a malignant fashion.

In 1976, Varmus and Bishop found that the oncogene in the Rous sarcoma virus was not a viral gene at all; instead, it arose directly from a preexisting cellular gene that had been captured by an ancestor of the Rous sarcoma virus. After it was captured, this gene was used by the Rous sarcoma virus to transform mammalian cells. The early ancestor of the Rous sarcoma virus was capable of replicating in infected cells but was unable to transform them; it instantly gained tumorigenic potency by kidnapping this normal cellular gene, the proto-oncogene. In the end, this work by Varmus and Bishop revealed much more about the cell than it did about the Rous sarcoma virus because it pointed to the existence of a gene residing in a normal mammalian genome that possessed potent transforming ability when appropriately activated, in this case by a retrovirus. Here was clear proof of the presence of at least one gene in the normal cellular DNA that might serve as one of the target genes activated by nonviral carcinogens of the retrovirus; such nonviral agents might also activate this proto-oncogene, converting it to a powerful oncogene. A cell carrying such a mutant gene might, in turn, respond to this damage by launching a program of deregulated growth and thus become a cancer cell.

The information uncovered concerning retroviruses and oncogenes provided little immediate comfort to investigators interested in the origins of human cancer. Retroviruses, similar to Rous sarcoma virus, never infected humans and therefore could not act to mobilize human proto-oncogenes. The possible connection came from a notion that many such proto-oncogenes could be activated through an alternative route. Changes in the DNA sequence created by chemical or physical rearrangement might substitute for the virus. Mutations induced by these chemical or physical conditions in the genomes of target cells in one or another tissue might be as effective as retroviruses in activating latent carcinogenic potential in the proto-oncogenes. By the early 1980s, these suspicions were validated: mutated genes (proto-oncogenes) were found in human tumor genomes. In each case, a change in the sequence of the gene was identified as being responsible for converting a proto-oncogene into an active oncogene. For example, a ras oncogene in one human bladder carcinoma was found to have arisen through a single base change that altered the DNA sequence of a precursor proto-oncogene; myc oncogenes arose through gene amplification in various malignant neoplasms.

Next, researchers tried to ascertain how these genes succeeded in transforming cells. A simple theme emerged that makes it possible to understand and explain the mechanism of action of most, if not all, of the oncogenes. This comes through the understanding of how cells regulate their own growth. The growth and division of a normal cell residing in a particular tissue is controlled largely by its surroundings. A normal cell rarely, if ever, decides its own rate of proliferation; rather, it responds to the signals or messages from surrounding cells. These messages, which may carry growth-stimulatory or growth-inhibitory information, are conveyed by growth factors released by surrounding cells, traverse the intercellular space, and bind to the cell surfaces. These cells then respond to these growth signals by activating their synthetic machinery, copying their DNA, and dividing. A normal cell will never commit itself to such a growth program without having been simulated by these external signals. Each cell possesses complex machinery that enables it to receive these signals, process them, and launch a growth program. The machinery consists of an array of proteins that function to acquire growth-activating signals and transmit them throughout the cell. These proteins include the following:

1. Cell surface receptors that recognize the presence of growth factors in the extracellular space and transmit signals into the cell's interior
2. Cytoplasmic signal transducers that become activated by these receptors and then pass signals farther into the cell
3. Nuclear transcription factors that are activated by the cytoplasmic signal transducers and in turn respond by activating entire banks of cellular genes

These activated gene banks together orchestrate the cell's growth program; they detail events that, acting in concert, enable the cell to grow and divide. Proto-oncogenes encode many of the proteins in this complex signaling circuitry that enable a normal cell to respond to exogenous growth factors. Oncogenes participate in this signaling circuitry by selecting aberrantly functioning versions of the components of this circuitry. Oncogene proteins succeed in activating these signal circuits even in the absence of stimulation by extracellular growth factors. In doing so, they force a cell to grow even when its surroundings do not contain some of the clues that are normally required to provoke growth.

Other researchers suggest that mutations in at least two proto-oncogenes have to be present and that only certain combinations of mutations lead to malignant change. These findings suggest that individual oncogenes, although powerful controllers of cell metabolism, are not capable of causing malignant neoplasms by themselves. Thus, oncogenes cannot explain most cancers by themselves. This view was strengthened by the discovery of more than a dozen different oncogenes in human tumors (Table 19.2). However, on careful evaluation, only about 20% of tumors turned out to carry expected alterations. None of the tumors had pairs of cooperative alterations sometimes found in cultured cells. It also appeared that the inherited mutations responsible for predisposing people to cancer were not oncogenes. The concept of a recessive-type antioncogene was conceived. This type of gene is called a tumor suppressor gene. This class of gene appears to be equally important in the development of cancer.

Tumor Suppressor Genes

The direct identification of tumor suppressor genes has been more difficult than the identification of oncogenes. Tumor suppressor genes were first conceived of in a theoretical sense long before any were actually identified. Harris was the first to demonstrate that the malignant characteristics of a cell could be suppressed when malignant cells were fused with nonmalignant cells. Furthermore, loss of portions of chromosomes can be associated with malignant transformation, and transfer of a

TABLE 19.2	Functional Classification of Selected Oncogenes and Associated Human Tumors
Oncogene	**Associated Tumors**
hst	Gastric cancer
Neu-erB-B2	Breast, ovary, and gastric cancers
trk	Papillary thyroid and colon cancers
Ha-ras	Bladder cancer
Ki-ras	Lung and colon cancers
N-ras	Leukemias
gsp	Pituitary tumors
raf	Gastric cancer
met	Osteosarcoma
abl	Leukemia and lymphoma
myc	Lymphomas and carcinomas
N-myc	Neuroblastoma
L-myc	Small cell lung cancer
bcl-2	Follicular and undifferentiated lymphoma
mas	Breast cancer
ret	Papillary thyroid cancer

From Mastrangelo MJ, Berd D, Nathan FE, Lattime EC. Gene therapy for human cancer: an essay for clinicians. *Semin Oncol* 1996;23:4.

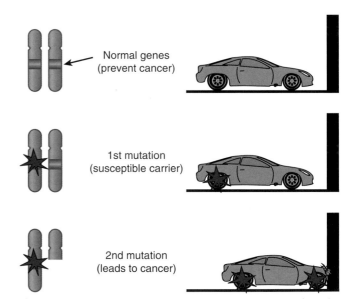

FIGURE 19.20 Schematic of tumor suppressor gene function.

normal chromosome can reverse these traits into the malignant cells. These data suggested a recessive type of control in normal cells. A schematic of a tumor suppressor gene can be seen in Fig. 19.20.

The first tumor suppressor gene cloned was the *RB* gene; it is the defective gene in retinoblastoma. Knudson extensively studied the epidemiology of retinoblastoma. Most cases of retinoblastoma are sporadic, but some cases appear to be clustered around families. He noted that cases of familial retinoblastoma were more likely to be bilateral or multifocal. On the basis of these data, he developed the two-hit hypothesis that bears his name (see Fig. 19.16). That is to say that two mutagenic events are required for retinoblastoma to develop. In patients with inherited disease, the first hit was inherited in one allele of the *RB* gene in the germline. Although one abnormality was not enough for development of the disease, there was an increased likelihood that the second allele would be damaged during eye development. The hypothesis of two mutational events developed by Knudson applies specifically to tumor suppressor genes. This is the basis of most inherited gene models.

Tumor suppressor genes have proved difficult to identify, and many techniques have been used to locate such genes within the human genome. Cytogenetic studies provide some clues to the location of tumor suppressor genes. A significant percentage of patients with retinoblastoma or some patients with Wilms tumor have large deletions in 13q14 or 11p13, respectively. These are the regions of the respective tumor suppressor genes responsible for each malignant neoplasm. Significant loss on 5q is associated with adenomatous polyps of the colon. This can be measured on a gel during electrophoresis and is called loss of heterozygosity. Although recurrent loss of a chromosome region associated with a specific malignant neoplasm is highly suggestive that this region is important in the development of the cancer, it is not sufficient to prove that there is a tumor suppressor gene in this region. Fig. 19.16 shows the possible combinations of loss that would lead to the expression of a tumor suppressor gene. Use of genome-wide linkage scans can further localize the presence of such a gene. Much smaller areas of deletion can be detected by molecular techniques such as pulsed-field electrophoresis. Now we can also easily and cheaply sequence long segments of the genome as these technologies improve.

When scientists were first trying to identify the regions of loss, they used DNA probes for specific regions of chromosomes. If allelic loss is noted, this is called loss of heterozygosity; if this loss is disproportionate relative to the general population, this suggests a tumor suppressor gene in the region specific for the probe. An example of loss of heterozygosity can be seen in Fig. 19.16. Here, a region on 10q in endometrial cancers indicates the existence of a possible tumor suppressor gene. By use of various markers, a precise location of the tumor suppressor gene can be identified. A contig of the region must then be built and the region sequenced to look for specific genes. Many regions of loss have been identified by this technique. There are many more candidate regions than actual tumor suppressor genes.

The tumor suppressor gene Tp53 is a gene associated with many cancers that was identified by searching for loss of heterozygosity. Several other tumor suppressor genes have been identified since. This is almost certainly only the tip of the iceberg, and many more tumor suppressor genes are likely to be discovered as investigators learn more about cancer cell genetics and as the potential of the Human Genome Project is realized and new genetic testing technologies continue to bring genetic testing to the forefront of medicine. Several generalizations can be made, and a comparison with the activation of oncogenes is constructive. Mutations in oncogenes are gain of

TABLE 19.3 Comparison of Oncogenes and Tumor Suppressor Genes

Characteristic	Oncogene	Tumor Suppressor Gene
Number of mutational events in cancer	One	Two
Role of mutation	Gain of function ("dominant")	Loss of function ("recessive")
Germline inheritance	No	Yes
Somatic mutations	Yes	Yes
Genetic alterations	Point mutations, amplifications, gene rearrangements	Point mutations, deletions
Effect on growth control	Activates cell proliferation	Negatively regulates growth-promoting genes
Result of gene transfection	Transforms cells to a partly malignant behavior	Suppresses malignant phenotype

function events and lead to increased cell proliferation and decreased cell differentiation. Oncogene mutations do not appear to be inherited through the germline. In contrast, tumor suppressor gene inactivations are loss of function events, usually requiring a mutational event in one allele followed by a loss or inactivation of the other allele. This loss of gene function leads to loss of cellular control and unchecked growth. Tumor suppressor genes are recessive, and mutations may be inherited as a germline mutation. Somatic mutations may occur in both types of genes and accumulate throughout life. Comparison of oncogenes and tumor suppressor genes is made in Table 19.3. Common tumor suppressor genes are listed in Table 19.4.

Apoptosis

Apoptosis means programmed cell death and refers to the "intentional" induction of cell death. Apoptosis is important in the growth and development of an organism because as an organism matures and differentiates, cells must die to give way to more differentiated and specialized cells. If a cell does not die and becomes immortal, a tumor or cancer can result. Apoptosis was first described in the 1970s, but only recently have scientists begun to realize the importance of this phenomenon in organism development, differentiation, and cancer formation. Excitement about this process has been driven by the finding that apoptosis is controlled at the molecular level by genes associated with malignant change (ie, oncogenes, proto-oncogenes, and tumor suppressor genes). It is also clear that many of these same controlling elements and pathways are active during development. Many believe that understanding the control of the apoptotic process is essential to understanding the control of the developing organism and control of senescence. Loss of these aspects of cellular control could lead to cancer.

Apoptosis is a distinct mode of cell death that is responsible for the deletion of cells in normal tissues; of note, it also occurs in pathologic conditions. The process of apoptosis is

TABLE 19.4 Tumor Suppressor Genes

Gene	Gene Product	Tumor Associations
RB1 (13q)*	110-kDa nuclear hypophosphorylated protein, negative cell cycle regulator	Retinoblastoma Osteosarcoma Small cell lung cancer Soft tissue sarcoma Breast cancer Bladder cancer
p53 (17p)	53-kDa sequence-specific DNA-binding protein and transcriptional activator	Li-Fraumeni syndrome Most common alteration in human cancer
DCC (18q)	1447–amino acid transmembrane protein with homology to known adhesion molecules; role in terminal cell differentiation	Colorectal cancer
APC (5q21)	2843–amino acid protein that interacts with membrane-associated cadherin-catenin complexes and with microtubules	Familial adenomatous polyposis Gardner syndrome
MTSI (9q21)	148–amino acid protein inhibitor of cyclin-dependent kinase-4	Familial melanoma Bladder cancer
BRCA1 (17q)	1863–amino acid protein with zinc finger–like domains suggesting function as a transcriptional factor	Breast cancer Ovarian cancer
BRCA2 (13q)	Possibly BRUSH I	Familial breast cancer
VHL (3p)	Protein with short homology to a glycan-anchored membrane protein of *Trypanosoma brucei*; no function assigned	Pheochromocytoma Renal cell cancer Pancreatic cancer Hemangioblastomas of CNS and retina
WT1 (11q)	50-kDa gene, related to the early growth response gene; encodes four 46- to 49-kDa proteins, which appear to function as DNA-binding transcriptional repressors	Wilms tumor
NF1 (17q11.2)	Neurofibromin (~2500 amino acids); probably negative regulator for p21 ras	von Recklinghausen neurofibromatosis
NF2 (22q12)	Schwannomin (~600 amino acids), regulator of cellular response to external environment	Neurofibromatosis type 2

*Chromosome location.
CNS, central nervous system.
From Mastrangelo MJ, Berd D, Nathan FE, Lattime EC. Gene therapy for human cancer: an essay for clinicians. *Semin Oncol* 1996;23:4.

characterized histologically by cell contraction, blebbing of the cell membrane, and condensation of the nucleus. Apoptotic bodies are formed that contain intact organelles; surrounding cells eventually phagocytose these. There is no associated inflammatory response. Cell swelling and disintegration of the cell components characterize necrotic cell death, and there is a marked inflammatory response. On a molecular level, apoptotic death causes cellular enzymes to autodigest the genome into

little fragments, and this can be identified on polyacrylamide gels by multiple regular fragments seen as a DNA ladder.

Apoptosis is important in the development of the normal organism, and it is important in the development and growth of cancers. It occurs spontaneously in malignant tumors, often markedly retarding their growth, and it is increased in tumors responding to radiation, chemotherapy, heat, and hormone damage. In cancer, apoptosis appears to be a mechanism for deleting cells from the population that have sustained carcinogenic DNA damage; however, when apoptosis of such cells is blocked or inhibited by mutations in genes that help control this process, such as *BCL2* or *Tp53*, these cells are suddenly free to continue replicating and propagating their mutations. This genetic instability may be an early step in the development of cancers. Many of the current cancer treatments, such as radiotherapy and chemotherapy, kill cells by the production of DNA damage. Mutations in BCL2 and Tp53 may then influence the effectiveness of these therapies through their ability to inhibit cell death.

The primary importance of apoptosis related to cancer and cancer treatment lies in its being a regulated phenomenon subject to stimulation and inhibition. Although little is known about how to establish therapeutic agents to affect its initiation, it seems reasonable to suggest that greater understanding of the process of apoptosis might lead to the development of improved treatment possibilities. Inhibitory mechanisms such as *BCL2* proto-oncogene expression may be implicated in the development of resistance to therapeutic agents and may contribute to tumor growth and perhaps to oncogenesis by allowing the inappropriate survival of cells with DNA abnormalities. It is likely that other inhibitory mechanisms will be identified, and a better understanding of the apoptotic process may lead to novel treatment regimens by allowing us to control cell death. Apoptosis is not simply a description of cell death, nor is it a spurious trend in the biology literature. It is a fundamental process and is controlled at the molecular level; as such, it can be understood and manipulated. Fig. 19.21 demonstrates how apoptosis may occur.

Mismatch Repair Defects

A number of mechanisms are involved in the correction of DNA changes that result from exogenous or endogenous mutagenic agents. These mechanisms include base excision repair, nucleotide excision repair, and DNA mismatch repair. The MMR system repairs mistakes that are made in the course of normal cellular division. These mutations often occur in regions of multiple repeats because these regions appear to be particularly prone to DNA slippage. One can intuitively see how this can happen by looking at Fig. 19.22. Six genes must work in concert to repair DNA damage. These genes and an example of how we think they work can be seen in Fig. 19.23.

A paradox of human tumor genesis is that the rates of mutation in normal cells are too low to account for the transformation of benign to malignant. The instability of some colon cancers was the first strong evidence for the so-called mutator phenotype. If a cell cannot repair DNA damage that occurs during the course of normal cell division, mutations can

FIGURE 19.21 Possible pathways and possible factors controlling apoptosis. A signal from outside the cell initiates a cascade of events involving *BCL2*, *BCL-xL*, and *BAX*. This results in the programmed death of the cell. This pathway can be blocked at a number of points, resulting in cell immortality. *ICE*, Interleukin-1βA signal fleukin-1id. (From Rudin CM, Thompson CB. Apoptosis and disease: regulation and clinical relevance of programmed cell death. *Annu Rev Med* 1997;48:267.)

1. 5′AGCTTGGCTGCAGGTG **CACA** GTGTCACGGTCAGGTAC3′
    TCGAACCGACGTCCAC **GTGT** CACAGTGCCAGTCCATG

                        Replication

2. 5′AGCTTGGCTGCAGGTG **CACA** GTGTCACGGTCAGGTAC3′
        GT CACAGTGCCAGTCCATG

  Mismatch Repair
  susceptible intermediate   **CA**   **Slippage**
3. 5′AGCTTGGCTGCAGGTG   **CA** GTGTCACGGTCAGGTAC3′
        C   **GT** CACAGTGCCAGTCCATG

  −2Frameshift   **Replication**
4. 5′AGCTTGGCTGCAGGTG **CA** GTGTCACGGTCAGGTAC3′
    TCGAACCGACGTCCAC **GT** CACAGTGCCAGTCCATG

FIGURE 19.22 Mismatch repair occurs by slippage of CA within a CA repeat. This results in the deletion of a CA. This is the exact kind of deletion that the mismatch repair (MMR) system is designed to correct. If the MMR system is not working properly, errors cannot be corrected, and mutations accumulate.

continue to accumulate; eventually, enough mutations occur in genes critical for cell control, and cancer results. Many studies have shown that tumors, which have microsatellite instability (MSI), have defects in mismatch repair. Key metabolic genes usually do not have large areas of microsatellite repeats that are particularly prone to mismatch problems. The mutation rate in nonrepetitive sequences is also elevated 100 to 10,000 times above that in normal cells with normal mismatch repair. Although microsatellite sequences are largely absent from functional genes, mononuclear repeats in some key genes can lead to their inactivation. Examples of such genes include

$TGF\text{-}BR2H$ (A_{10}), $hMSH3$ (A_8), $hMSH6/GTBP$ (C_8), $IGF2R$ (G_8), and BAX (G_8). Paradoxically, instability of chromosome numbers is often observed in tumors without MMR defects; tumors with MMR defects often have stability of chromosome number.

Mismatch repair proteins interact to form complexes that recognize mismatched DNA base pairs and abnormal loops of DNA. The repair complexes initiated by MMR genes trigger excision and repair of DNA mutations. This system is critically important in ensuring the fidelity of the replicative process and is highly conserved throughout all living organisms. Areas in the genome that contain simple repetitive DNA base sequences called microsatellites (eg, CACACACA or AAAAAAA) are especially prone to mutation. If the MMR system does not function normally, these errors will go unrecognized and continue to accumulate. Cells in which both copies of one of the MMR genes have been inactivated exhibit the so-called mutator phenotype; this allows cells to accumulate mutations as they divide. These random mutations eventually accumulate in a series of genes that are important in controlling cellular growth; the result is loss of growth control and transformation to cancer.

Cells with a defective MMR system exhibit a phenomenon called MSI. This phenomenon occurs as DNA mismatches cause shortening or lengthening of repetitive DNA sequences and these mismatches go unchecked. This results in generation of alleles in the cancer that contain a greater or lesser number of repeats than are present in normal cells from that individual. Laboratory testing for MSI uses an established consensus panel of five microsatellite markers (D2S123, D5S346, D17S250, Bat 25, and Bat 26). Fig. 19.24 shows an example of MSI detection when mismatch prone regions are compared in blood and tumor.

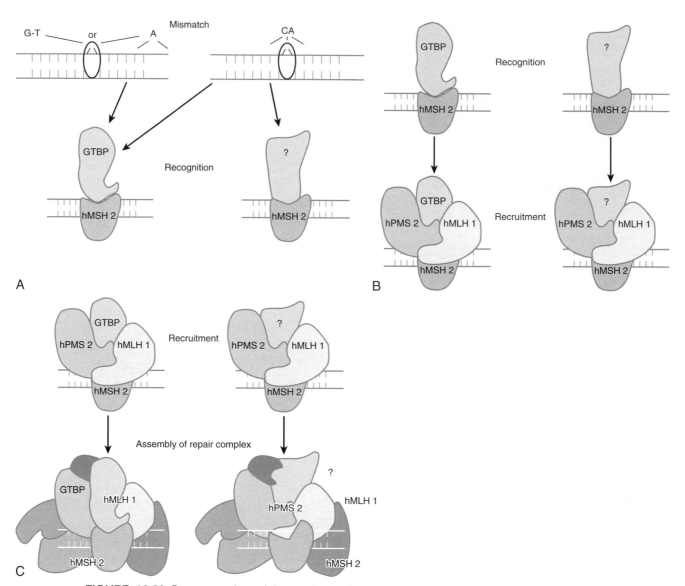

FIGURE 19.23 Demonstration of how mismatch repair is accomplished by the six proteins required for correction. There must be the following: recognition of slippage (**A**); recruitment of repair complex (**B**); and, finally, repair (**C**). (From Karran P. Microsatellite instability and DNA mismatch repair in human cancer. *Semin Cancer Biol* 1996;7:15.)

Germline mutations in MMR genes (MLH1, MSH2, MSH6, PMS2) are present in many families and is known as Lynch syndrome. This syndrome is associated with increased risk for colon cancer, endometrial cancer, ovarian cancer, stomach cancer, small bowel, stomach, renal pelvis, biliary tract, and brain cancer. Mutations in one of the Lynch syndrome genes accounts for about 5% of all colon cancers and approximately 2% of all newly diagnosed endometrial cancers.

The Amsterdam II criteria, used to identify Lynch syndrome based on the pattern of cancer in a family is defined as follows:
1. Three or more relatives with Lynch syndrome–associated cancer; one must be a first-degree relative to the other two.
2. At least two successive generations must be involved.
3. At least one of the cancers must have been diagnosed before the age of 50 years.

Seventy percent of patients with that meet Amsterdam II criteria have a germline mutation segregated around an MMR gene: *hMLH1* (49%), *hMLH2* (45%), and *hPMS2* (6%). Approximately 25% of endometrial cancers have an MMR defect; approximately one-fourth of these are germline mutations, and the rest are largely the result of somatic *MLH1* inactivation resulting from hypermethylation of the promoter region. MMR will be increasingly investigated and more clearly defined during the next decade.

Telomerase

Normal cells divide; this process is repeated many times as an organism grows and matures. Normal cells stop dividing and terminally differentiate, but cancer cells continue to divide. Cells from younger animals divide more times than do cells

FIGURE 19.24 Karyotype of the human genome showing location of the *BRCA1* and *BRCA2* genes.

Disease	Genetic Abnormality
Hereditary breast–ovarian	*BRCA-FA* pathway genes, including *BRCA1*, *BRCA2*, *RAD51C*, *RAD51D*, *PALB2*, *BARD1*, and *BRIP1*
Lynch syndrome	*MLH1*, *MSH2*, *MSH6*, *PMS2*, *EPCAM*
Cowden syndrome	*PTEN*
Li-Fraumeni syndrome	*TP53*
Ovarian cancer: small cell hypercalcemic	*SMARCA4*
PPB	*DICER1*

from older animals. One difference between normal cells and tumor cells is at the end of their chromosomes. Telomeres, specialized structures at the ends of chromosomes, act as protective caps. In humans, telomeres are made up of 5000 to 15,000 base pairs of TTAGGG repeats. These terminal structures protect the chromosome ends from exonuclease digestion, prevent aberrant chromosome recombination, and form specific complexes that bind proteins.

Normal cells lose about 50 to 100 base pairs from the end of each chromosome every time the cell divides. When a telomere loses a critical number of base pairs, it triggers a signal for the cell to stop dividing and for senescence. Cells have developed several mechanisms to get around this terminal trigger. Some of these are uncommon, such as complex recombination and retrotransport techniques. The most common mechanism is the development of an enzyme complex called telomerase, which adds back telomere sequences lost during replication. Cells that have significant telomerase activity are often immortal cells such as cancer cells and germ cells.

Normal cells lack telomerase activity. Telomerase becomes reactivated in most cancer cells. It is the most prevalent cancer marker known. Therefore, telomerase may be used as a generic cancer marker and as a possible treatment.

HEREDITARY CANCER RISK ASSESSMENT: GENETIC COUNSELING AND GENETIC TESTING

Clinically Relevant Hereditary Syndromes

The advent of linkage analysis and the rapidity of DNA sequencing with other molecular technologies have made it possible to identify many inherited disorders that we could not identify a few short decades ago. Gynecologic malignancies associated with autosomal dominant inherited cancer predisposition that have been identified thus far are as follows:

Ovarian cancer
  Epithelial
    Hereditary breast and ovarian cancer (HBOC): all epithelial histologies; rarely mucinous; most commonly high-grade serous
    Lynch syndrome: all epithelial histologies typically endometrioid
  Epithelial: borderline tumors
    Rarely associated with hereditary cancer syndromes
  Germ cell
    Not believed to be a part of HBOC
  Sex cord–stomal tumors
    Granulosa cell tumors
      Peutz-Jeghers syndrome (PJS)
    Sex cord tumors with annular tubules
      PJS
  Sertoli-Leydig and juvenile granulosa cell tumors
    Pleuropulmonary blastoma (PPB) syndrome
Fallopian tube or primary peritoneal cancer
  HBOC
  Lynch syndrome
Uterine cancer
  Epithelial (majority of uterine cancers)
    Lynch syndrome (typically endometrioid, less commonly clear cell; rarely uterine papillary serous (UPSC): not typically thought to be associated with HBOC (reports of UPSC associated with HBOC)
    Mesenchymal (endometrial stromal sarcoma, leiomyosarcoma, other nonspecific sarcomas) (rare)
    Rarely associated with hereditary cancer syndromes
    Uterine soft tissue sarcoma
    Li-Fraumeni syndrome
  Mixed: Malignant mixed Mullerian tumor (MMMT) or carcinosarcoma, adenosarcoma
    Rarely associated with hereditary cancer syndromes; seen in some cases of Lynch syndrome
Cervix
  Rarely associated with hereditary cancer syndromes
  Cervix adenoma malignum associated with PJS
Vaginal or vulvar cancer
  No known association with hereditary cancer syndromes
Gestational trophoblastic disease
  No known association with hereditary cancer syndromes
Hereditary cancer syndromes that include increased risk for developing gynecologic cancers.

Commercial clinical genetic testing is available for hereditary cancer risk and has undergone rapid changes in the last several years. Massively parallel sequencing, also called next-generation sequencing (NGS), technology allows for rapid testing of large amounts of DNA sequence. NGS is quicker and less expensive than previous genetic testing tools. It is becoming routine to order a single test that simultaneously evaluates multiple genes thus testing for multiple hereditary cancer syndromes at once. The Supreme Court Decision in June 2013, overturning the ruling on allowing gene patents, particularly *BRCA1* and *BRCA2*, brought an immediate change in the availability of multigene panel testing through multiple different commercial laboratories.

Our understanding of the tumor spectrum associated with the different hereditary cancer predisposition genes, the risks for cancer, and targeted therapy options is growing exponentially. An increasing number of individuals are seeking the advice of physicians and genetic counselors regarding options for genetic testing hereditary risk for cancer. It is important to have an understanding of hereditary cancer syndromes associated with an increased risk for developing gynecologic cancers.

Hereditary Breast and Ovarian Cancer (*BRCA1* and *BRCA2*; Other DNA Repair Pathway Genes)

Hereditary breast and ovarian cancer syndrome is the best known and most well characterized of the hereditary cancer syndromes. *BRCA1* and *BRCA2* and were identified in the early 1990s (1994 for *BRCA1* and 1995 for *BRCA2*). Genetic testing for the predisposition to breast and ovarian cancer by testing for mutations in the *BRCA1* or *BRCA2* genes became clinically available in 1996. The *BRCA1* and *BRCA2* genes are located on chromosomes 17q and 13q, respectively (Figs. 19.25 and 19.26). Both of these genes are quite large, containing at least 20 exons (coding regions) and are of at least 7000 base pairs (see Fig. 19.26). Genetic testing for *BRCA1* and *BRCA2* has changed significantly since 1996; the initial testing in 1996 only included sequencing for *BRCA1* and *BRCA2*. This testing was later updated to include five specific *BRCA1* rearrangements; deletions or duplications not detected through gene sequencing. In 2006, the addition of deletion and duplication (also called large rearrangement testing) for both *BRCA1* and *BRCA2* was automatically run for individuals from high-risk families who met certain family history criteria or as an optional add-on for additional cost. Current testing includes

sequencing and deletion and duplication analysis automatically for both genes in every test, regardless of personal or family history. Individuals who had genetic testing for *BRCA1* and *BRCA2* previously may benefit from updated genetic testing, especially if no mutations were identified.

Founder mutations are mutations that are common or even unique to a specific patient population and occur in populations of patients that have been genetically isolated for many generations. The population may have shrunk as a result of a disaster, but the mutation was preserved in a few individuals. When the population reexpands, the frequency of that specific mutation can be quite high within a population (Fig. 19.27). One example of founder mutations occurs in *BRCA1* and *BRCA2*. (Fig. 19.28). Approximately 2% of individuals of Ashkenazi (Eastern European) Jewish ancestry have one of three founder BRCA mutation: 187delAG (*BRCA1*), 5385insC (*BRCA1*), and 6174delT (*BRCA2*). Historically, targeted testing for the specific found mutations was initiated first with reflex testing to full *BRCA1* and *BRCA2* gene testing if none of the three mutations were identified. The adoption of NGS tools for genetic testing is changing this process and the specific testing founder mutation testing is skipped and in favor of proceeding directly to multigene testing. These founder mutations are identified with the NGS technology.

Cancer risks for individuals with *BRCA1* or *BRCA2* mutation are presented as lifetime risk ranges. These are typically

BRCA1

BRCA2

BRCA1
- Tumor suppressor gene on chromosome 17
- Coding region: 5589 nucleotides
- Span 81-kb genomic DNA
- ~1200 different mutations reported

BRCA2
- Tumor suppressor gene on chromosome 13
- Coding region: 10,254 nucleotides
- Span 84-kb genomic DNA
- ~1380 different mutations reported

FIGURE 19.25 Representation of the *BRCA1* and *BRCA2* genes with characteristics of each.

7%–10%

Other genes (16%)

BRCA1 (52%)

BRCA2 (32%)

■ Sporadic
■ Hereditary

FIGURE 19.26 Hereditary breast and ovarian cancer. Representation of the percent contribution of inherited disease and the percent contribution by each of the known genes predisposing patients to cancer. (Modified from Ford D, Easton DF, Stratton M, et al. Genetic heterogeneity and penetrance analysis of the BRCA1 and BRCA2 genes in breast cancer families. The Breast Cancer Linkage Consortium. *Am J Hum Genet* 1998;62:676.)

FIGURE 19.27 Cumulative incidence of cancer over time in individuals with *BRCA* mutations. Summary analysis of 22 studies. (Modified from Antoniou A, Pharoah PD, Narod S, et al. Average risks of breast and ovarian cancer associated with BRCA1 or BRCA2 mutations detected in case Series unselected for family history: a combined analysis of 22 studies. *Am J Hum Genet* 2003;72:1117.)

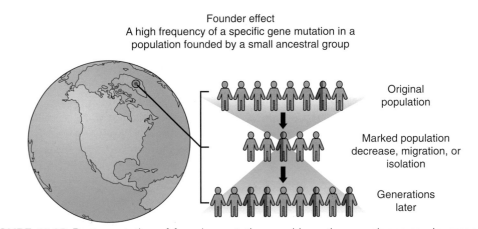

FIGURE 19.28 Representation of founder mutations and how the prevalence can increase in a population over time. *With permission from SGO.*

broad risk ranges because the actual reported risk varies depending on the population studied in any given report. Reports of lifetime risk for ovarian cancer ranges from 8% to 62%. The age of onset for ovarian cancer is not necessarily an indication of hereditary risk. Reported lifetime risk for breast cancer range from 41% to 90%. There is limited data to provide individualized risks or mutation specific risks. Unlike ovarian cancer, early age of onset for breast cancer is a hallmark of hereditary risk, but later ages of onset for breast cancer should not be discounted. This should be considered in the context of the cancer family history when determining concern for inherited risk. Additionally, triple-negative breast cancer seems to have a greater association with *BRCA1* mutations.

Additional genes in the DNA repair BRCA-FA (Fanconi anemia) pathway were reported to confer increased risk for breast and ovarian cancer beginning around 2010. Genes in the DNA repair *BRCA-FA* (Fanconi anemia) pathway include *BRCA1, BRCA2, CHEK2, BRIP1, RAD50, RAD51C, RAD51D, PALB2, BARD1, MRE11,* and *NBN*. Current information

suggests a moderately increased risk for cancer for individuals with mutations in these genes as compared with the higher risks reported with mutations in *BRCA1* or *BRCA2*. Some of these genes within the *BRCA-FA* DNA repair pathway may turn out to be associated with a more significant risk for developing cancer than others, and clinical availability of testing this genes will also change over time.

A 2011 study of 360 women with primary ovarian, peritoneal, or fallopian tube carcinoma not selected for age or family history found 24% carried pathogenic mutations in 12 different genes, including *BRCA1, BRCA2 BARD1, BRIP1, CHEK2, MRE11A,MSH6, NBN, PALB2, RAD50, RAD51C,* and *TP53*. The majority were attributed to mutation in *BRCA1* or *BRCA2*. The remaining portion of inherited risk is due to mutations in one of the Lynch syndrome genes or one of the newly identified *BRCA-FA* DNA repair pathway genes. The overall contribution of each gene to the risk of ovarian cancer can be seen in Fig. 19.29. A 2015 study of 1915 women with primary ovarian, peritoneal, or fallopian tube carcinoma not selected for age

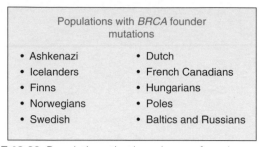

FIGURE 19.29 Populations that have known founder mutations.

or family history found 18% carried a pathogenic germline mutation and suggests that 11 genes comprise the majority of hereditary risk for ovarian cancer: *BRCA1, BRCA2, BRIP1, RAD51C, RAD51D, PALB2, BARD1, MLH1, MSH2, MSH6,* and *PMS2.* Mutations in these genes are rare and in some studies not significantly more frequent in ovarian cancer patients compared with control populations so the data continue to emerge to sort out the significance of these and other *BRCA/FA* pathway genes. National Comprehensive Cancer Network (NCCN) guidelines suggest the following genes to recommend or consider risk-reducing salpingo-oophorectomy (RRSO) if there is a mutation: *BRCA1 or BRCA2* and any of the Lynch syndrome genes, *BRIP1, RAD51C,* and *RAD51D.* Research continues, and data are quickly evolving regarding the frequency of these mutations associated with specific cancer types, the cumulative risk for cancer, and the most appropriate medical management recommendations for cancer detection or prevention for women with hereditary mutations in these genes.

Cumulative risk is the concept of total risk over time. For individuals with a mutation in a gene involved in a DNA repair pathway, mistakes cannot be adequately repaired that occur with normal DNA replication in cellular division as well as with environmental damage. Therefore, there is a greater risk for developing cancer over time compared with an individual at average risk and the development of cancer tends to occur at earlier ages. Cumulative risks of breast and ovarian cancer associated with mutations in *BRCA1* and *BRCA2* are shown in Fig. 19.30.

Pathologic characteristics of tumors have been studied as a method of determining which patients should be referred for hereditary cancer risk assessment. For example, there is a preponderance of triple-negative (ER-/PR-/her2-) breast cancers associated with *BRCA1.* High-grade serous ovarian cancer is most commonly associated with mutations in *BRCA1* or *BRCA2.* However, there are reports of mutations identified in individuals with most of the histologic subtypes. Mucinous ovarian cancers are rarely associated with mutations in *BRCA1* or *BRCA2.* Current recommendations by the Society of Gynecologic Oncologists and NCCN suggest referral of all patients with epithelial ovarian cancer for genetic counseling and genetic testing.

Identification of germline *BRCA* mutations, and possibly the other *BRCA-FA* DNA repair genes, is also becoming more important in treatment decisions. Patients with *BRCA1* or *BRCA2* mutation–associated cancers tend to have longer survival periods compared with patients with no identifiable germline mutations. These cancers have been found to be more susceptible to chemotherapeutic agents that cause DNA damage. The addition of a poly-ADP-ribose polymerase I (PARP) inhibitor exploits the breakdown of this DNA repair pathway, and these tumors may become even more sensitive to the traditional chemotherapeutic agents. PARP inhibitor Olaparib made by Astra Zeneca is now available for clinical use in patients with DNA repair defects.

Management Guidelines for Hereditary Breast and Ovarian Cancer (*BRCA1* and *BRCA2*)

Multiple organizations have published guidelines for genetic risk assessment and management guidelines for individuals with HBOC caused by *BRCA1* and *BRCA2* with small variances among the different groups. These organizations include the US Preventive Services Task Force (USPSTF), NCCN, American Society of Clinical Oncology (ASCO), European Society for Medical Oncology (ESMO), American College of Obstetricians and Gynecologists (ACOG), and Society of Gynecologic Oncologists (SGO). These guidelines are readily available. The NCCN guidelines are reviewed an updated at least annually. The current recommendations (version 1.2016) suggest clinical breast examination every 6 to 12 months and annual breast magnetic resonance imaging (MRI) beginning at age 25 years. Beginning at age 30 to 75 years, annual mammography and annual breast MRI are recommended, often at staggered 6-month intervals. Women with a *BRCA* mutation and a personal history of breast cancer should continue with annual mammography and breast MRI. A discussion of the option of risk-reducing mastectomy is also recommended. Data do not support routine ovarian cancer screening. RRSO is recommended between the ages of 35 and 40 years or when childbearing is complete. The option of delaying RRSO until age 40 to 45 years in women with *BRCA2* mutations may be considered because there appears to be a later average age of onset of approximately 8 to 10 years compared with *BRCA1* mutation carriers. It is important to review a multigeneration family history and take note of the ages of onset of ovarian cancer in the family and adjust this recommendation if there are women with early onset disease. NCCN guidelines also review cancer risks and recommendations for men relative to prostate cancer and mention no specific screening guidelines for pancreatic cancer or melanoma.

Women with *BRCA2* mutations of reproductive age should be made aware of options for prenatal diagnosis and preimplantation genetic diagnosis. Cancer family history should be obtained for their partners and consider genetic testing for *BRCA2*, especially if there is Ashkenazi Jewish ancestry or family history of breast and ovarian cancer. If both parents carry a *BRCA2* mutation, there is risk for a rare autosomal recessive disorder called Fanconi anemia.

As survival improves for patients with ovarian cancer, identification of a mutation can guide cancer screening or prevention recommendations to hopefully keep patients from developing another primary cancer or at least detect the cancer early.

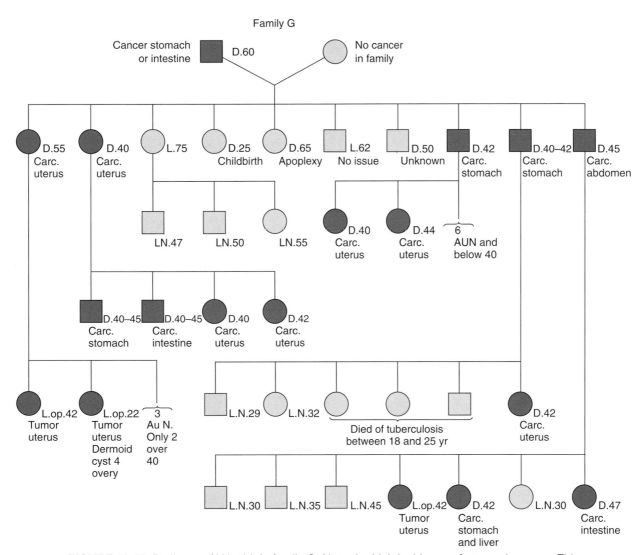

FIGURE 19.30 Pedigree of Warthin's family G. Note the high incidence of stomach cancer. This transitioned to colon cancer through the 1900s.

Lynch Syndrome (Hereditary Nonpolyposis Colon Cancer)

In 1895, a pathologist at the University of Michigan, Aldred Scott Warthin, had a seamstress who had a family with a preponderance of gastric and endometrial cancers. This family became known as family G and is part of the basis for the discovery of Lynch syndrome or HNPCC. Warthin described this family in a report in the *Archives of Internal Medicine* in 1913 (Fig. 19.31). The family pedigree was updated in 1925 but was largely forgotten until Henry Lynch and colleagues discovered two other families with similar pedigrees in Iowa and Nebraska, which they reported in the 1970s. This was proposed as the "cancer family syndrome" (CFS) in 1971, later changed to HNPCC. The current terminology refers to this syndrome as Lynch syndrome, believing that HNPCC fails to adequately acknowledge the importance of extracolonic malignancies such

as endometrial, ovarian, upper gastrointestinal (GI) tract, and urinary tract cancers.

Lynch syndrome is inherited in an autosomal dominant pattern and results from a mutation in one of the DNA MMR genes, *MLH1, MSH2, EPCAM, MSH6,* or *PMS2*. These genes code for proteins that proofread DNA and correct mistakes that are made during the normal process of replication. MMR is covered in detail earlier in this chapter.

Mutations in *MSH2* and *MLH1* account for the majority of cases of Lynch syndrome. Mutations in *MSH6, EPCAM,* and *PMS2* account for a smaller percentage. *EPCAM* and *MSH2* are located on 2p21, *MSH6* on chromosome 2p16, *MLH1* on chromosome 3p22, and *PMS2* on chromosome 7p22 (Fig. 19.32). Large germline deletions of the last exon of *EPCAM*, located upstream from *MSH2*, were reported in 2009 in 5 of 27 families suspected of having Lynch syndrome who previously

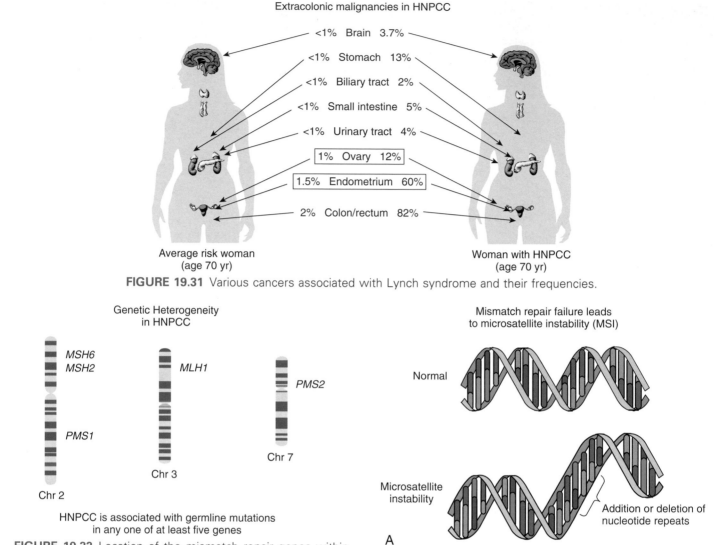

Extracolonic malignancies in HNPCC

<1%	Brain	3.7%
<1%	Stomach	13%
<1%	Biliary tract	2%
<1%	Small intestine	5%
<1%	Urinary tract	4%
1%	Ovary	12%
1.5%	Endometrium	60%
2%	Colon/rectum	82%

Average risk woman
(age 70 yr)

Woman with HNPCC
(age 70 yr)

FIGURE 19.31 Various cancers associated with Lynch syndrome and their frequencies.

Genetic Heterogeneity
in HNPCC

MSH6
MSH2

MLH1

PMS2

PMS1

Chr 7

Chr 3

Chr 2

HNPCC is associated with germline mutations
in any one of at least five genes

FIGURE 19.32 Location of the mismatch repair genes within the human genome.

Mismatch repair failure leads
to microsatellite instability (MSI)

Normal

Microsatellite
instability

Addition or deletion of
nucleotide repeats

A

Example of MSI analysis
(RER)

1044   1061   1062
N   T   N   T   N   T

B

FIGURE 19.33 A, Representation of how mismatch repair occurs and how a DNA segment is lengthened or shortened. **B,** Gel showing microsatellite instability. N stands for normal tissue. Note two bands. T stands for tumor and not the smearing of the bands, indicating that there are fragments of different sizes of that DNA segment.

tested negative for *MLH1* or *MSH2*. Analysis of the 3′ region of *EPCAM* is now standard in genetic testing for Lynch syndrome.

Endometrial cancer is the most common gynecologic cancer in the United States and accounts for 6% of all gynecologic cancers in women. This accounts for around 50,000 cancers per year. Approximately 5% of endometrial cancers are caused by inherited risk, with the majority of this 5% caused by Lynch syndrome. A list of cancer types associated with Lynch syndrome and a comparison of the increased risk with to average risk are depicted in Fig. 19.33 and Table 19.5. The cumulative lifetime risk of endometrial cancer is between 40% and 60%, and the ovarian cancer risk is approximately 12%. The cumulative risk of colon cancer is 40% to 80%. There appears to be lower cumulative risks associated with *MSH6* and *PMS2* perhaps with later ages of onset. Up to 5% of all cases of endometrial cancer and colon cancer are caused by inherited mutations in one of the Lynch syndrome genes. The most common histologic subtype of endometrial cancer associated with Lynch syndrome is endometrioid; uterine papillary serous carcinoma is the least

TABLE 19.5 Risk of Lynch Syndrome

Condition	Risk (%)
Endometrial cancer at any age	1.8
Endometrial cancer diagnosed before 50 years of age	9
Endometrial and colon cancer at any age	18
Endometrial and colon cancer before 50 years of age	43
Endometrial and ovarian cancer	7

TABLE 19.6 Amsterdam Criteria: Three Two One Rule

Three or more relatives with verified Lynch-associated cancer within the family
  Colorectal, endometrial, small bowel, ureter, or renal pelvis
  Any combination of histologies in three different generations
  One case is a first-degree relative of the other two
At least two successive generations affected
One or more cases by 50 years of age
Exclude familial adenomatous polyposis

TABLE 19.7 Criteria for Referral to a Genetic Counselor for Suspected Lynch Syndrome

Bethesda guidelines
Amsterdam Criteria fulfilled
Persons with two relatives with Lynch syndrome
Colorectal cancer and first-degree relative with a Lynch cancer before 45 years or a first-degree relative with an adenoma before 40 years of age
Colorectal cancer or endometrial cancer before 45 years of age
Right-sided, undifferentiated colon cancer before 45 years of age
Signet ring colon cancer before 45 years of age
Adenoma before 40 years of age

TABLE 19.8 Revised Bethesda Guidelines for Testing Colorectal Tumors for Microsatellite Instability

Tumors from individuals should be tested for MSI in the following situations:
1. Colorectal cancer diagnosed in a patient who is younger than 50 years of age
2. Presence of synchronous, metachronous colorectal, or other HNPCC-associated tumors* regardless of age
3. Colorectal cancer with the MSI-H histology diagnosed in a patient who is younger than 60 years of age
4. Colorectal cancer diagnosed in one or more first-degree relatives with an HNPCC-related tumor, with one of the cancers being diagnosed before age 50 years
5. Colorectal cancer diagnosed in two or more first- or second-degree relatives with HNPCC-related tumors, regardless of age

*Hereditary nonpolyposis colorectal cancer (HNPCC)–related tumors
MSI, Microsatellite instability.

likely subtype type to be associated with Lynch syndrome. Approximately 2% to 3% of cases of epithelial ovarian cancer are caused by inherited mutations in one of the Lynch syndrome genes. Lynch syndrome associated ovarian cancers tend to be nonserous types.

Family history criteria used to classify a family as having Lynch syndrome are the Amsterdam I and Amsterdam II criteria. Amsterdam I criteria only included colon cancer. Amsterdam II criteria shown in Table 19.6 include other Lynch syndrome–associated cancers. Colon cancers associated with Lynch syndrome have a propensity to occur in the ascending colon, relative to sporadic cases, which are more often distal. Individuals with Lynch syndrome tend to have shorter intervals in formation of adenomatous polyps and transformation to malignancy, as well as earlier ages of diagnosis.

Genetic Testing for Lynch Syndrome

Historically, the recommendation for genetic testing for Lynch syndrome was determined by cancer family history (Table 19.7). In families that fulfill the Amsterdam II criteria, the likelihood that a mutation will be found is quite high; the chance of identifying a mutation in one of the *MMR* genes is between 50% and 92%. The Bethesda criteria were developed to provide guidelines to order MSI for colon tumors (Table 19.8). There are no similar guidelines for endometrial cancer for guidance on when to order tumor genetic screening.

Recent collaborative efforts have focused on the adoption of universal tumor screening (UTS) for all newly diagnosed endometrial and colon cancers to include immunohistochemistry (IHC) and MSI. The Lynch Syndrome Screening Network (http://www.lynchscreening.net) was formed in 2011 to enable ongoing cooperative efforts toward UTS for all patients with newly diagnosed colon and endometrial tumors. Updated information regarding implementation of a universal screening program is available on their website. A 2014 consensus statement from US Multi-Society Task Force recommends that all newly diagnosed colorectal cancers should be tested for MMR deficiency either by IHC testing for *MLH1, MSH2, MSH6,* and *PMS2* and/or MSI testing. Colon tumors that have absent staining of *MLH1* or *MSI-high* should undergo *BRAF* testing of *MLH1* promoter hypermethylation to determine if the abnormal MMR screen is most likely attributable to somatic inactivation of *MLH1*. Similar guidelines have been proposed for all endometrial cancers. However, *BRAF* mutations are not commonly seen in endometrial cancers, so reflex testing should be for *MLH1* promoter hypermethylation if IHC shows absent staining for *MLH1*. Approximately 20% to 25% of all endometrial exhibit MSI as a result of epigenetic inactivation of *MLH1* caused by hypermethylation of the promoter.

NCCN guidelines version 2.2015 for Lynch syndrome provide a detailed grid of tumor testing results and additional

Pedigree of Lynch family kindred

FIGURE 19.34 Typical pedigree of a family with Lynch syndrome.

testing strategies based on those results. A typical screening algorithm is seen in Fig. 19.34.

Data suggest that approximately 2% of all endometrial cancers are caused by Lynch syndrome. As many as 7 of 10 individuals with Lynch syndrome who develop endometrial cancer do not meet any published criteria for Lynch syndrome, and many of these cancers are diagnosed after age 50 years. Multiple studies evaluating the feasibility of implementing an IHC-based screening protocol for lynch syndrome in endometrial cancer show this detects Lynch syndrome that would have been previously missed and increases the referral and uptake for genetic counseling and genetic testing.

If there is no tumor tissue available, then personal and family history of cancer can guide recommendations for genetic testing. Referral of the endometrial cancer patient is discussed below.

With the increased adoption of NGS, genetic testing usually includes multiple genes tested simultaneously. This is true for Lynch syndrome as well. Genetic testing based on cancer family history consistent with Amsterdam II should include all five Lynch syndrome genes. Given the overlap of hereditary cancer syndromes, including colon cancer and other cancer types, testing may include multiple hereditary cancer syndromes, including Lynch syndrome. Genetic testing based on abnormal IHC findings typically involves two or three of the Lynch syndrome genes because of the formation of heterodimers. Reports of IHC showing loss of a single protein yet the germline mutation is in the companion genes.

A typical pedigree of a family meeting the criteria for a Lynch syndrome family can be seen in Fig. 19.35. An example of a pedigree of a family that does not raise suspicion for Lynch syndrome but was identified through abnormal IHC and subsequent genetic testing is shown in Fig. 19.24.

Management Guidelines for Lynch Syndrome (Fig. 19.36)

As noted earlier for HBOC, multiple organizations published guidelines for genetic risk assessment and management guidelines for individuals Lynch with small variances between the different groups. These organizations include the USPSTF, NCCN, ASCO, ESMO, ACOG, and SGO. These guidelines are readily available. The NCCN evaluates current data and updates recommendations at least annually and is freely accessible at NCCN.org. The most recent version for Lynch syndrome, version 2.2015, outlines the following: Colonoscopy initiated between the ages of 20 to 25 years and repeated every 1 to 2 years. For families with a case of colon cancer diagnosed before age 25 years, screening should begin 2 to 5 years younger than the youngest diagnosis. Prophylactic colectomy is not routine but may be recommended for individuals with significant repeat adenomatous polyp formation or for individuals who are unable to undergo regular surveillance. Incidence of and mortality from colorectal cancers in this group have been shown to be reduced by colonoscopy screening (Figs. 19.37 and 19.38). Chemoprevention using aspirin to reduce the risk of colon cancer has been suggested, but data are still forthcoming, and it is not standard of care at this time. There is no clear evidence to support screening for endometrial cancer by annual pelvic examination and pelvic ultrasonography, but annual endometrial sampling is an option. Similarly, screening for ovarian cancer by pelvic ultrasonography and serum CA-125 are options but also lack sensitivity and specificity for the diagnosis of ovarian cancer. Therefore, risk-reducing surgery to include

FIGURE 19.35 Screening algorithm used by the Ohio State group. (From Backes, Leon ME, Ivanov I, et al. Prospective evaluation of DNA mismatch repair protein expression in primary endometrial cancer. *Gynecol Oncol* 2009;114:486.)

Surveillance options for carriers of HNPCC-associated mutations		
Malignancy	Intervention	Recommendation
Colorectal cancer	Colonoscopy	Begin at age 20–25, repeat every 1–2 years
Endometrial cancer	• Transvaginal ultrasonography • Endometrial aspirate	• Annually, starting at age 25–35 • Consider urine cytology yearly

FIGURE 19.36 Recommended screening in families with Lynch syndrome. (From Cancer Genetics Studies Consortium Task Force Recommendations. Modified from Burke W, Petersen G, Lynch P, et al., Recommendations for follow-up care of individuals with an inherited predisposition to cancer. I. Hereditary nonpolyposis colon cancer. Cancer Genetics Studies Consortium. *JAMA* 1997;277:915.)

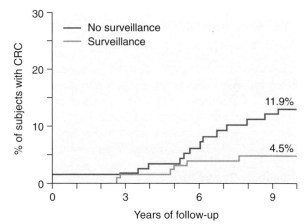

FIGURE 19.37 Effect of recommended colon screening on incidence of colon cancer in families with Lynch syndrome. Regular recommended screening decreases the incidence. (Modified from Järvinen HJ, Mecklin JP, Sistonen P. Screening reduces colorectal cancer rate in families with hereditary nonpolyposis colorectal cancer. *Gastroenterology* 1995;108:1405.)

hysterectomy and bilateral salpingo-oophorectomy is an option that should be considered for women who are age 40 years or after childbearing is completed. Research continues to evolve in developing better screening tools and chemoprevention options for ovarian cancer and endometrial cancer. If the patient is being explored for another reason, consideration should be given to counseling regarding possible risks and benefits of a total hysterectomy with bilateral salpingo-oophorectomy. Data are also limited, suggesting efficacy regarding screening and prevention for the other Lynch syndrome–associated cancers such as gastric, small bowel, pancreatic, kidney, and brain tumors. Breast cancer is not typically considered a Lynch syndrome–associated cancer, but there are reports of increased risks in some Lynch syndrome families. There are not enough data to suggest increased breast cancer screening in individuals with Lynch syndrome at this time.

Guidelines for management of individuals with inherited cancer risk are updated regularly and across multiple professional organizations and should be consulted when counseling high-risk individuals regarding cancer screening and prevention. In our era of medical specialties, it is reasonable to arrange for referral to high-risk specialists for each cancer type for an initial consult to discuss the risks, benefits, and limitations of screening and prevention for the various cancer types. The pattern of cancer types and ages of diagnosis of cancer in the family may impact the medical management recommendations.

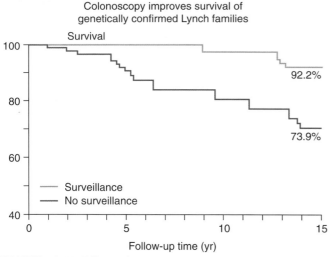

FIGURE 19.38 Effect of colon screening on mortality caused by colon cancer in families with Lynch syndrome. Regular recommended screening decreases mortality from Lynch syndrome. (From Järvinen HJ, Aarnio M, Mustonen H, et al. Controlled 15-year trial on screening for colorectal cancer in families with hereditary nonpolyposis colorectal cancer. *Gastroenterology* 2000;118:829.)

Less Common Inherited Cancer Syndromes Relevant to Gynecologic Oncology

Other less common hereditary cancer syndromes that include gynecologic malignancies as part of the tumor spectrum include PJS, Cowden syndrome, and Li-Fraumeni syndrome. Two additional genes recently described and available clinically that are associated with hereditary cancer risk and gynecologic cancer are *DICER1* (PPB) and *SMARCA4*.

Peutz-Jeghers Syndrome

Peutz-Jeghers syndrome is characterized by hamartomatous polyps of the GI tract, particularly the small intestine. Intussusception and bleeding are the usual symptoms. PJS is also characterized by flat pigmented lesions that look like dark bluish freckles visible on the mucosal surfaces such as the mouth and lips, buccal mucosa, soles of the feet, palms of the hands, and perianal area. These hyperpigmented lesions occur in about 95% of cases and are seen on very characteristic surfaces; the most easily seen are those on the lips and buccal mucosa. The pigmented lesions tend to present within the first 2 years of life. After puberty, the external lesions can fade, often making the diagnosis difficult later in life. However, the buccal lesions tend to persist, so this is always an important area to examine.

The clinical diagnosis of PJS occurs in an individual has two or more of the following: (1) two or more PJS type hamartomatous polyps of the small intestine; (2) mucocutaneous hyperpigmentation of the mouth, lips, nose, eyes, genitalia, or fingers; or (3) family history of PJS. PJS is named after Dr. Johannes Laurentius Augustinus Peutz, who first described the syndrome in 1921, and Dr. Harold Joseph Jeghers, who subsequently described this syndrome in 1949.

The PJS susceptibility gene, *STK11,* was identified in 1998. *STK11* maps to chromosome 19p13. *STK11,* a tumor suppressor gene, is a serine/threonine kinase that regulates energy metabolism and cell polarity. A mutation in *STK11* is identified in 80% to 94% of individuals who meet clinical criteria for PJS.

The cancer types associated with PJS include breast, colon, stomach, small intestine, pancreas, gynecologic, testicle, and lung. The cumulative risk for colon cancer is approximately 40% and for breast cancer is 45% to 50%. Pancreatic cancer risk is estimated to be 11% to 36%, and screening is recommended to be initiated between ages 30 and 35 years.

The gynecologic cancers associated with PJS include specific types of ovarian and cervical cancer. A very unusual ovarian stoma tumor known as sex cord–stromal tumors with annular tubules have the distinction of almost always being associated with PJS and are fortunately usually benign and are usually found incidentally. Other ovarian tumors that are associated with PJS are tumors of low malignant potential, granulosa cell tumors, Sertoli-Leydig cell tumors, and mucinous tumors. The overall risk for ovarian cancer in individuals with PJS is approximately 18% to 21%. Another gynecologic tumor associated with PJS is a rare cervical cancer known as adenoma malignum. This tumor appears to be histologically benign but can behave quite aggressively. Therefore, patients with PJS should have annual cervical examinations with this in mind, and any abnormality should be evaluated aggressively.

Patients with PJS have a significantly elevated risk of developing a malignancy. One meta-analysis suggested that the risk could be as high as 93%. However, most studies put the risk at 50% or below.

Management guidelines for Peutz-Jeghers syndrome. Surveillance for cancers associated with PJS is outlined in current NCCN guidelines and the practice guideline published in 2015 by the American College of Gastroenterology. Increased breast cancer screening to include annual mammography and breast MRI and clinical breast examination every 6 months is recommended beginning at approximately age 25 years. There are insufficient data to recommend risk-reducing mastectomy or risk-reducing oophorectomy for women with *STK11* mutations. Annual testicular examination should begin around age 10 years. No specific recommendations have been made for screening for lung cancer beyond education regarding symptoms and smoking cessation. Screening of the small intestine should begin by age 8 to 10 years and screening of the colon at 2- to 3-year intervals. Upper endoscopy should be considered starting in the late teens and continued every year or two to screen for stomach cancer. Annual pelvic examination and Pap smears should be initiated at age 18 to 20 years with consideration of annual transvaginal ultrasonography. Magnetic resonance cholangiopancreatography or endoscopic ultrasonography beginning at age 30 to 35 years can be considered. The greatest morbidity from the GI tract occurs in the 20s from large GI hamartomas; endoscopic resection of these may be helpful early in life. Finally, genetic counseling is critically important to help the patient and family assess risks of this disease, make future reproductive choices, and undergo testing.

Cowden Syndrome

Cowden syndrome was first described in the family of Rachel Cowden in 1963. This is a multiple hamartoma syndrome and is characterized by individuals with multiple hamartomas and a predisposition to a variety of cancers. The criteria for genetic testing for Cowden can be seen in Table 19.9 and can be found on the NCCN's website for Cowden syndrome. Patients who meet the criteria for Cowden syndrome should be offered counseling and, if indicated, subsequent genetic testing. Management guidelines for Cowden syndrome include initiating clinical breast examination at age 25 years and mammography and breast MRI at age 30 years consideration of annual endometrial biopsy and prophylactic hysterectomy at completion of childbearing. Men and women should initiate thyroid examination at age 18 years, colonoscopy at age 35 years, and renal ultrasonography at age 40 years as well as dermatologic examination. These recommendations are regularly reevaluated and updated, and one must check current sources before making recommendations.

Li-Fraumeni Syndrome

Li-Fraumeni syndrome was first described in 1969. This was noted as a familial clustering of soft tissue sarcomas and a clustering of diverse neoplasms, including early-onset breast cancer. In 1988, Li-Fraumeni published the follow-up of 24 families. This established what is now known as the classic criteria for diagnosing this syndrome (Table 19.10). Approximately 70% of individuals who meet the classic criteria are found to have a *TP53* mutation. Approximately 20% of individuals who meet other criteria for Li-Fraumeni syndrome called the Chompret criteria are found to have a mutation in *TP53*. Any woman with personal history of early-onset breast cancer and no *BRCA* mutation should be considered for *TP53* testing. In 1990, deleterious germline mutations were discovered in the tumor suppressor gene *p53*, establishing a molecular diagnosis for Li-Fraumeni syndrome.

Gynecologic cancers are not a one of the major cancers associated with Li-Fraumeni syndrome, although the overall cumulative risk for cancer with Li-Fraumeni syndrome is

TABLE 19.9 Criteria for Genetic Testing for Cowden Syndrome

Testing criteria	Known PTEN mutation in the family
	Individual meeting clinical criteria for Cowden syndrome
	Individual with personal history of adult Lhermitte-Duclos disease *or* ASD and microcephaly *or* trichilemmomas (two or more biopsy proven)
	Individuals meeting two or more major criteria below (one must be macrocephaly)
	Individuals meeting three major criteria without macrocephaly
	Individuals meeting one major criteria and three or more minor criteria
	Individuals meeting four or more minor criteria
Major criteria	Breast cancer
	Follicular thyroid cancer
	Macrocephaly
	Endometrial cancer
	Macular pigmentation of the glans penis
	Multiple GI hamartomas or ganglioneuromas
	Specific mucocutaneous lesions: biopsy-proven trichilemmoma, multiple palmoplantar keratoses, multifocal oral mucosal papillomatosis, multiple cutaneous facial papules
Minor criteria	Thyroid lesions (adenomas or goiter)
	Intellectual disability (IQ ≤75) or ASD
	Colon cancer or papillary thyroid cancer or follicular variant of papillary thyroid cancer or renal cell carcinoma
	GI hamartomas or testicular lipomatosis or lipoma
	Vascular anomalies such as multiple intracranial developmental venous anomalies
Diagnosis in an individual	Any single pathognomonic criterion but mucocutaneous lesions if meeting specific criteria one major and at least three criteria or at least four minor criteria alone
Diagnosis in a family in which one individual has characteristics diagnostic for Cowden syndrome	Individuals must have at least one of the following: Pathognomonic criteria Any one major criteria with or without minor criteria
Two minor criteria or history of Bannayan-Riley-Ruvalcaba syndrome	

ASD, Autism spectrum disorder; *GI*, gastrointestinal.

TABLE 19.10 Diagnostic Criteria for Li-Fraumeni Syndrome

Classic Criteria (Must Meet All Conditions)
Proband of younger than 45 years of age with a sarcoma
Plus
First-degree relative younger than 45 years of age with any cancer
Plus
Additional first- or second-degree relative in the same lineage with any cancer or sarcoma

Chompret Criteria
Proband with a tumor belonging to the LFS tumor spectrum (eg, soft tissue sarcoma, osteosarcoma, brain tumor, premenopausal breast cancer, adrenocortical carcinoma, leukemia, lung bronchoalveolar cancer) before age 46 years *and* at least one first- or second-degree relative with a LFS tumor (except breast cancer if the proband has breast cancer) before age 56 years or with multiple tumors *or*
Proband with multiple tumors (except multiple breast tumors), two of which belong to the LFS tumor spectrum and the first of which occurred before age 46 years *or*
Proband with adrenocortical carcinoma or choroid plexus tumor, regardless of family history

LFS, Li-Fraumeni syndrome.

approximately 90%, and this includes multiple cancer types as well as gynecologic cancers. The screening recommendations have typically focused on early and more frequent breast cancer screening, consideration of risk-reducing mastectomy, colonoscopy beginning at age 25 years and repeating every 2 to 5 years, annual dermatologic examination, an awareness by pediatrician of the risk for childhood cancers, and avoidance of therapeutic radiation therapy whenever possible given the hypersensitivity to radiation-induced DNA damage. Recent publications include consideration of annual whole-body MRI. There are no specific screening or prevention recommendations for gynecologic malignancies at this time given the lower incidence of these cancer compared with the other cancer types in individuals with this syndrome.

GENETIC COUNSELING AND GENETIC TESTING FOR HEREDITARY CANCERS

The National Society of Genetic Counselors redefined genetic counseling in 2006 as the process of helping people understand and adapt to the medical, psychological, and familial implications of genetic contributions to disease. This process integrates interpretation of family and medical histories to assess the chance of disease occurrence or recurrence; education about inheritance, testing, management, prevention, resources, and research; and counseling to promote informed choices and adaptation to the risk or condition. A searchable directory of board-certified genetic counselors has been developed to assist physicians, patients, and other genetic counselors in locating genetic counseling services. Genetic counselors can be searched by state, city, counselor's name, work setting, and type of specialist such as inherited cancer risk assessment. This directory can be found on the National Society of Genetic Counselors' website (http://www.NSGC.org).

The ASCO published an expert statement on the collection and use of a cancer family history for oncology providers in 2014. ASCO recommends minimum cancer family history intake by physicians should include documentation of family history of cancer in first-degree relatives (parents, children, and siblings) and second-degree relatives (grandparents, aunts, uncles, nieces, nephews, half siblings). This should include the primary cancer, age of diagnosis for each cancer, and notation of maternal or paternal lineage. Additionally, patients should be asked if anyone in the family had genetic testing for hereditary cancer risk and obtain a copy of these results. Ethnicity should be noted, particularly Ashkenazi Jewish ancestry. This level of detail may be necessary to determine the appropriateness for referral for hereditary cancer risk assessment.

Formal hereditary cancer risk assessment should include review of at least a three-generation pedigree, including first-, second-, and third-degree (cousins) relatives from both maternal and paternal families. Occasionally, expansion of the pedigree beyond these relatives may reveal important information that will guide recommendations for genetic testing and medical management. The choice of genetic tests since the adoption of multigene panels that cover multiple hereditary cancer

syndromes relies less on family history than prior methods of gene-specific testing or syndrome-specific testing. The cancer family history is still of great importance when interpreting results and providing follow-up recommendations based on the pattern of cancer and ages of diagnosis in the family.

Information to document for each family member, if available, to document a detailed cancer family history includes the following:

- Current age or age at death
- History of benign tumors and specific diagnosis
- History of colon polyps, including the total number and types of polyps
- Cancer history; verify by obtaining pathology report or other medical records if possible; age of diagnosis; primary cancer site and treatment; prior genetic testing (if so, obtain a copy of the result)
- Reproductive history, including menarche, age first birth, menopause, and hormone use
- History of cancer prevention surgeries or cancer screening history
- Environmental exposures such as smoking

This level of detail may not be available for all relatives. It is not unusual for the cancer family history to be different from that initially reported to the physician after the patient initiates this conversation with family members. Limitations of obtaining cancer family history, as outlined in the ASCO expert opinion piece, include limited patient knowledge of family history, small families, or families with limited communication. Families with few at-risk women may also mask the presence of hereditary risk for breast and ovarian cancer. It is also important to inquire about updated cancer family history information at follow-up visits and to encourage the patient to call when the cancer family history information changes. Updated cancer family history information may change the risk assessment and recommendations.

Verification of the reported cancer diagnoses in a family is important because the risk assessment and subsequent recommendations are based on this verbal family history. Gynecologic cancers are notoriously misreported within a cancer family history. Data show that the accuracy of verbal family history deceases with increasing degrees of relatedness. It is also important to obtain medical records to confirm any cancer diagnosis in the patient presenting for genetic counseling for accurate tumor type and histology information. Verification of the total number and types of colon polyps is also important because many patients may not have accurate recall of this history for themselves and are unlikely to know this information about family members. The pathology report is the most reliable source for verification of both the age of diagnosis and histology and should be obtained whenever possible. The pathology report provides minimal personal information, so family members may be more willing to share these reports if they are reluctant to share their medical information with family members. It is still appropriate to proceed with hereditary cancer risk assessment and genetic testing if the family history cannot be verified. Patients need to understand that the both the risk assessment and recommendations are based on the family history as presented, and accurate information provides the best base for these recommendations.

Patients should be encouraged to gather the medical family history even if they decline referral for genetic counseling. This is a gift of information to the next generation because the family history may significantly impact future medical recommendations for that family, and as the older generations passes, this information may not be easy to accumulate.

A formal genetic counseling assessment should include discussion of the psychosocial issues some experience living with a personal history of cancer or cancer family history. The patient may experience recall of emotions and memories of family members diagnosed with cancer in the process of gathering and reviewing the cancer family history and should have an opportunity to address these emotions. This is especially true for a genetic counseling client who was young when his or her family member was diagnosed or died or if the individual was a primary caregiver for the relative with cancer. The genetic counseling appointment should also include discussion of the potential emotional impact of undergoing genetic testing and learning that one is at significant increased risk for cancer. Survivor guilt is also a common response for individuals who undergo testing and learn they did not inherit the familial mutation previously identified in other family members. Referral for psychological support for any patient undergoing hereditary cancer risk assessment is appropriate. Finally, the genetic counselor can be available to schedule annual follow-up visits to review and update family history and review updated genetic testing options or updates to the recommendations for follow-up based on family history or genetic testing results.

REFERRAL OF GYNECOLOGIC CANCER PATIENTS FOR HEREDITARY CANCER RISK ASSESSMENT

Ovarian Cancer

Although the hallmark for hereditary cancer is early age of onset, this is not necessarily the case for ovarian cancer. All patients with epithelial ovarian cancer, fallopian tube cancer, and primary peritoneal cancer should be offered genetic counseling and genetic testing for hereditary cancer risk regardless of their age of onset or cancer family history. Current data suggests that 10% to 20% of all epithelial ovarian cancers are associated with a mutation in a hereditary cancer predisposition gene. This is sufficient to recommend genetic testing regardless of family history of cancer. Current SGO guidelines note that nearly one third of women with hereditary ovarian cancer have no close relatives with cancer, and 35% of women with hereditary ovarian cancer are diagnosed after age 60 years.

It is appropriate to refer an unaffected woman for hereditary cancer risk assessment who has a close relative, especially a mother or sister, with ovarian cancer. Ideally, the relative with ovarian cancer should initiate genetic testing. If the relative with ovarian cancer is either unwilling to proceed with genetic testing or is deceased and never had genetic testing, it is appropriate to refer the unaffected woman for genetic counseling

for hereditary cancer risk assessment and consideration of genetic testing.

Timing of Referral for Patients With Ovarian Cancer

We support providing referral information very near the time of diagnosis for all ovarian cancer patients for several reasons beyond the high mortality rate for ovarian cancer:

1. Patients with ovarian cancer often express concern regarding risk for their daughters and granddaughters very early in their ovarian cancer journey, so they are already thinking about it.
2. Providing referral near the time of diagnosis gives the patient a choice. Patients who are not ready to proceed will tell their physicians. The option can be revisited after treatment is complete if the patient has not revisited during her treatment process.
3. Many patients with ovarian cancer are proceeding with counseling and testing at some point during the initial treatment phase, especially in the past few years with greater public awareness of cancer genetics. This is also a great time because many patients with ovarian cancer have family members with them during the treatment phase.
4. The daughters and sisters of patients with ovarian cancer are often offered genetic testing by their gynecologists at the first visit they mention their mother or sister has ovarian cancer. Ideally, the patient with ovarian cancer should initiate testing first.
5. Hereditary ovarian cancer also includes risks for cancers that are not gender specific, so it is equally important for the male relatives to undergo testing.
6. Identification of a mutation in one of the hereditary genes may impact reproductive decisions for at-risk relatives still of childbearing age.
7. We can offer DNA banking for patients who decline testing upfront.

Borderline ovarian tumors and nonepithelial ovarian tumors are not commonly associated with hereditary cancer syndromes.

Endometrial Cancer

Approximately 3% of all endometrial cancers are caused by inherited risk related to Lynch syndrome. Referral of patients with endometrial cancer for hereditary cancer risk assessment is based on the cancer family history or personal history of endometrial cancer and the results of tumor genetic screening studies that may be performed as part of the pathologic diagnosis of the cancer after surgery. A 2015 joint practice guideline from the American College of Medical Genetics and Genomics and the National Society of Genetic Counselors suggests referral of the endometrial cancer patient for genetic counseling that meets the following:

1. Diagnosis of endometrial cancer before 50 years of age
2. Endometrial cancer at any age if there is a first-degree relatives with colon or endometrial cancer at any age
3. Synchronous or metachronous colorectal or endometrial cancer
4. Endometrial cancer showing MMR deficiency on tumor screening

5. Endometrial cancer and two additional cases of any of the Lynch syndrome–associated cancers in the same person or close relatives
6. Epithelial endometrial cancer and two additional Cowden syndrome criteria in the same person

A significant cancer family history warrants referral for hereditary cancer risk assessment even in patients with endometrial cancer with normal tumor screening results. It is always possible that the tumor screening results represent a false-negative result or the individual developed endometrial cancer by chance but still has a hereditary risk for cancer in the family.

Referral of the Patient for Genetic Counseling Based on Personal History of Breast Cancer or Family History of Cancer

Other criteria for referral for hereditary cancer risk assessment for HBOC as outlined by the NCCN guidelines include:
- Women with a personal history of breast cancer and ovarian cancer at any age
- Women with a personal history of ovarian cancer and a close relative with breast cancer at younger than 50 years of age or ovarian cancer at any age

Given the stringency of these criteria, many inherited cancers may be missed. Other features that may be useful in deciding whether a patient should be referred to a genetic counselor for counseling and possible testing are outlined in Table 19.11.

GENETIC TESTING

General Guidelines for Genetic Testing for Hereditary Cancer Risk

Genetic testing should always be initiated in an affected relative, if possible, to determine if there is an identifiable mutation in one of the hereditary cancer genes. If the relative with cancer does not have a mutation, it may be appropriate to test another affected relative in the event there is a mutation in the family and the first person tested is a phenocopy and developed cancer by chance. If no mutation is identified in the affected relative, it is not appropriate to pursue genetic testing in the unaffected relative. The cancer family history should be used to guide recommendations for increased cancer screening and prevention because genetic testing is not informative. If an affected relative is found to have a mutation, targeted mutation-specific testing can be offered to unaffected relatives. It is important to always obtain both maternal and paternal cancer family history for any patient undergoing genetic testing to determine if there may be additional cancer risk from the other side of the family. It is important to confirm the parental origin of a mutation and not just assume the mutation explains the family history. It is possible that more than one mutation may be traveling in a family. Without confirmation of the lineage or presence of the mutation in other affected relatives, a multigene test may still be appropriate.

Criteria for referral for hereditary cancer risk assessment and genetic testing continue to evolve. Referral to a genetic counselor for risk counseling and possible testing should not be

TABLE 19.11 **Testing Criteria for Breast Ovarian Cancer Syndrome***
Individual from a family with a known deleterious *BRCA1* or *BRCA2* gene mutation
Personal history of breast cancer plus one or more of the following:
Diagnosed before or at 45 years of age
Diagnosed before or at 50 years of age with
An additional breast cancer primary
At least one close blood relative with breast cancer at any age
At least one close relative with pancreatic cancer
At least one close relative with prostate cancer
An unknown or limited family history
Diagnosed at of age 60 with
Triple-negative breast cancer
Diagnosed at any age with
At least one close blood relative with breast cancer before 50 years of age
At least two close blood relatives with breast cancer at any age
At least one close blood relative with ovarian cancer
At least one close blood relative with pancreatic cancer
At least two close blood relatives with prostate cancer
A close male blood relative with ovarian cancer
An individual of ethnicity associated with a higher mutation frequency
Personal history of ovarian cancer
Personal history of male breast cancer
Personal history of prostate cancer at any age with a close relative with breast, ovarian, or pancreatic cancer at any age
Personal history of pancreatic cancer and Ashkenazi Jewish ancestry
Family history meeting any of the above criteria
See NCCN guidelines for the most up-to-date and detailed description for counseling and testing.

*For more detailed information, see the National Comprehensive Cancer Network (NCCN) guidelines.

limited to those with high-risk criteria. Some features may not be apparent at first glance in the patient's history. Inaccurate histories are common; furthermore, as families become smaller, the accuracy of family history in predicting inherited disease becomes less. Referral to a counselor can occur at any time, but immediately after or during treatment seems like the most practical and common.

Informed Consent

Informed consent is a necessary component of genetic testing. The rapid adoption of multigene panels and the impact on the informed consent process was recently addressed by ASCO. Informed consent should include the following:
- Psychosocial assessment and support
- Purpose of the test and who to test
- Discussion of options of gene specific testing versus multigene testing
- Possible test results
- The implication of those results with particular attention to the implications of a mutation in a less well-characterized gene or in a gene association with a hereditary syndrome not suggested by the personal or family history of cancer
- Likelihood of finding a mutation

- Technical aspects and accuracy of the test including possibility that test will not be informative, paying particular attention to the current high rate of variants of uncertain significance
- Fees involved in testing and counseling
- Information regarding concerns for genetic discrimination and medical privacy and confidentiality
- Psychosocial aspects, including anticipated reaction to results, timing and readiness for testing, family issues, and preparing for results
- Utilization of test results, including options and limitations of medical surveillance and strategies for prevention
- Options and limitations of medical screening and prevention without genetic testing as well as how genetic testing can impact recommendations
- Importance of sharing genetic test results with at-risk relatives: risks for children, siblings, or other biologic relatives who may inherit an identified mutation
- Laboratory policy on storage of DNA sample and possible use for future research
- Potential reproductive implications to family of mutation in a gene linked to a recessive disorder (ie, ATM, Fanconi anemia, constitutional MMR syndrome)
- Option of DNA banking to allow for genetic testing in the future for the patient's family

Most health insurance plans provide coverage for the majority of the cost of genetic testing, and many have published criteria for coverage that are easily accessible on the Internet.

Ordering Genetic Testing

Genetic testing is usually performed on a blood sample with DNA extraction from the lymphocytes. Some laboratories offer the option of buccal swabs or buccal spit kits as an alternative to a blood draw. Before 2013, *BRCA1* and *BRCA2* were only available through a single laboratory. This changed after the Supreme Court ruling overturning gene patents. Multigene testing, including *BRCA1* and *BRCA2*, is available through a multitude of laboratories. The cost of genetic testing for the multigene panels varies significantly among laboratories. Most medical insurance plans cover the cost of genetic testing for hereditary cancer risk if the patient or family is suggestive of hereditary cancer risk. Many of the commercial laboratories have financial assistance programs, and some offer a set out-of-pocket cost for those without insurance coverage. ASCO's 2015 Policy Statement Update for Genetic and Genomic Testing for Cancer Susceptibility notes a commitment to ensure access to high-quality cancer genetic services and supports continued expansion of third-party reimbursement. There seems to be a push to reduce the cost and increase accessibility to genetic testing for hereditary cancer risk. The costs and options for multigene testing are changing rapidly, and it is best to obtain up-to-date information directly from the laboratory of choice. A listing of laboratories providing genetic testing for hereditary cancer risk can be found on GeneTests (http://www.genetests.org). GeneTests, funded by the National Institutes of Health, provides an updated listing of laboratories offering clinical and research genetic testing and information on genetic testing and its use in diagnosis, management, and genetic counseling.

Interpreting the Test Results

Regardless of the number of genes included on a multigene panel, each gene has four possible results.

1. **Positive:** Deleterious mutation identified. This is a true positive, meaning the mutation is known to be significantly alter the function of the gene and is associated with increased risks of developing cancer.
2. **Negative for mutation-specific testing in the context of a known mutation identified in a family member:** This is a true negative and typically indicates that this individual is at general population risk to develop cancer. However, it is still important to assess the detailed cancer family history for both the maternal and paternal families. One cannot always assume parental origin based on the reported cancer family history because there are cases of more than one hereditary mutation in a given family.
3. **Negative:** No mutation identified in an individual for whom no mutation has been identified in other family members. This is not a true negative. In this case, the negative genetic testing result does not necessarily rule out hereditary risk. Testing another relative in the family diagnosed with cancer may be recommended. Recommendations for cancer screening and prevention should be based on personal medical history and cancer family history, not negative genetic testing results. Possible explanations for a negative result include:
   a. There could be a hereditary mutation in one of the genes listed earlier that is not detectable by the current technology.
   b. There could be a hereditary mutation in a gene not tested.
   c. There could be a hereditary mutation in the family that she did not inherit and developed cancer for other reasons.
   d. There may not be inherited cancer risk in the family.
4. **Variant of uncertain significance (VUS):** This is an inconclusive result. This means an alteration in the gene has been identified, but it is unknown whether the alteration will affect gene function. The rate of VUS findings varies from 10% to 41% in the multigene panels depending on the number of genes tested and the number of newly characterized genes and differs among laboratories. No recommendations for cancer screening or prevention should be made based on a VUS. Testing unaffected relatives for the VUS is not appropriate because medical recommendations cannot be made based on the presence or absence of a VUS. Appropriate medical management should be based on family history and personal medical history. The laboratory that identified the VUS may offer family research testing to the parents or other close relatives who have had cancer because these data can be helpful in attempting to establish the clinical significance of a variant.

An algorithm for the various possible test results can be seen in Figs. 19.39 and 19.40.

LEGAL ASPECTS OF GENETIC TESTING

Concern over the legal consequences of genetic evaluation remains a barrier for patients and health care providers when considering genetic testing for hereditary risk. There is fear over genetic discrimination in health insurance, life insurance, and disability insurance procurement and even discrimination with regard to employment. Both state and federal legislation has been passed preventing discrimination on the basis of genetic information. Current efforts for health care reform focus on reducing "preexisting" conditions being used by insurance companies to determine coverage and rates for health care insurance. There is also some increased protection to individuals under the Health Insurance Portability and Accountability Act (HIPAA). This law offers protection of those who are members of group insurance plans, including the federal group plans Medicare and Medicaid.

The Genetic Information Nondiscrimination Act (GINA) of 2008 offers expanded protection of individuals and groups. GINA expands on the protection offered by HIPAA to further limit the ability of insurance carriers to raise rates or deny coverage to individuals and groups. Again, the actual impact of these laws need to be tested in court, and it is therefore difficult to predict exactly what effect these laws will ultimately have on genetic discrimination. Several important points should be considered here: (1) the actual incidence of genetic discrimination is exceedingly small, with few cases nationwide that address this issue; (2) genetic testing is becoming routine in many areas of medicine, and most insurance companies have guidelines for coverage for genetic testing; and (3) national sympathy clearly sides with those with the possibility of genetic disease. Nonetheless, part of counseling should include the possibility of discrimination with information gained from the test.

It is the duty and obligation of the physician to inform the patient of the risks of a positive genetic test result. However, there is also a duty of the physician to inform other family members who are at risk for the disease. Case law at this time generally falls on the side of favoring the individual's right to privacy over the physician's obligation to inform other family members. However, there is a case litigated in 1996, *Safer v Estate of Pack*, in which an individual with familial adenomatous polyposis died from colon cancer. He requested that his family not be informed. His daughter developed colon cancer at the age of 36 years and sued her father's physician's estate, claiming that he had an obligation to warn those at risk and that he had failed to fulfill these obligations. The case was dismissed, but this was later reversed by the New Jersey Court of Appeals, which ruled that a physician's obligation may extend beyond that of the immediate family and that the physician had an obligation to tell the patient that he had an obligation toward the health of his children.

Genetic tests are unique compared with many other medical tests in that they affect not only the individual but may also affect immediate and extended family. We can encourage our patients to share this information with their family members by providing them with tools and written communication to assist them in sharing this information. The best recommendation is to have family members schedule genetic counseling appointments to review the information and discuss options for genetic testing and cancer screening and prevention based on family history and genetic testing results.

FIGURE 19.39 Algorithm for testing and management of an affected individual.

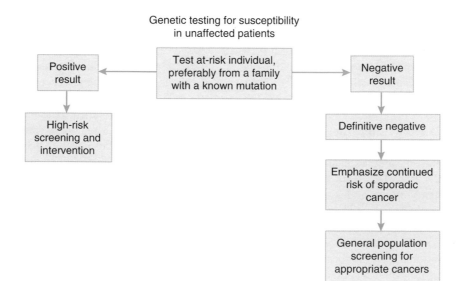

FIGURE 19.40 Algorithm for testing and management in individuals who are not affected but have a family history.

Finally, there is a duty by physicians to meet the standard of care. This is defined as what is reasonable or what a reasonable physician should do for his or her patient. Genetic testing and counseling are quite new, so clear standards have not been established. However, it is clear that it is important to take a family history and inform patients of diseases for which they may be at risk and offer testing for these diseases when available. Although there are no universally established standards, most specialties, such as the ASCO and the American Medical Association, have their own guidelines. This information provides a reasonable template for clinicians to follow.

LONG-TERM CONTACT FOR PATIENTS AND FAMILIES WITH HEREDITARY RISK FOR CANCER

Health care providers caring for families with hereditary risk for cancer should encourage patients to maintain annual contact with their high-risk specialists and genetic counselor to discuss updates to cancer family history and any updates to the cancer screening and prevention recommendations. Additionally, the popular media continues to provide more coverage regarding celebrities with hereditary risk and new scientific discoveries. Patients should be encouraged to schedule follow-up appointment to review new information in context with their personal history. Patients should also be provided resources for support both through mental health providers as well as local and national support groups for the specific hereditary cancer syndromes or cancer types. Different patients have different needs, and providing them with a variety of resources allows them to find information that fulfills individual needs.

Significant technologic advances are bringing about rapid changes in the availability of genetic testing as well as in follow-up recommendations. Changes in family history may significantly impact the risk assessment and subsequent recommendations. Additionally, the future generations need to be made aware of the cancer family history and known mutation in the family (if identified) and encouraged to seek genetic counseling for hereditary cancer risk to understand the risks and options for genetic testing.

A number of Internet support organizations are available for specific hereditary cancer syndromes and specific hereditary cancer types. Examples include FORCE: Facing Our Risk of Cancer Empowered (http://www.facingourrisk.org). FORCE is a nonprofit organization with an advisory board of cancer genetic specialists that provides updated information and support for individuals concerned with HBOC. Be Bright Pink (https://www.brightpink.org) focuses on prevention and early detection of breast and ovarian cancer in young women. Two examples of organizations that focus on the different syndromes associated with hereditary risk for colon cancer include Hereditary Colon Cancer Takes Guts (http://www.hcctakesguts.org) and Colon Cancer Alliance for Research & Education for Lynch Syndrome (CCARE Lynch Syndrome; http://www.fightlynch.org).

Other valuable websites include national cancer organization such as the National Cancer Institute (http://www.cancer.gov) and American Cancer Society (http://www.cancer.org).

Because this information is changing rapidly, detailed chart documentation, scans of tables, charts, and articles discussed can become a part of a patient's medical record for reference to compare current recommendations or scientific information with what was discussed with a patient in past appointments.

DNA BANKING

DNA banking is an option for all cancer patients even if a mutation is identified. Advances in technology and genetic testing and research will likely bring about significant changes in genetic testing and in our understanding of the roles of genes. DNA banking is also an important option for terminally ill cancer patients, when the patient or family does not have the time for traditional genetic risk assessment or are simply overwhelmed by planning for the end of life and cannot process additional medical information. There is no guarantee a family will use the stored DNA, and costs for future genetic testing are uncertain. However, DNA storage is reasonable cost ranging from less than $100 to more than $300 with storage times from 5 years to 25 years or more. This allows for the option for genetic testing in the future for the family.

CONCLUSION

The field of hereditary cancer risk assessment and management of these high-risk families continues to evolve. Our understanding of the spectrum of cancer and risk of cancer is changing as new technologies are used for broader genetic testing and the criteria for who to test change. Referral to health care professionals with expertise in cancer genetics and management of high-risk patients is essential.

Focused cancer family history should be part of the initial evaluation of all patients. Maternal and paternal pedigrees should be constructed to include at least three generations (the patient, her parents, and her grandparents) if hereditary risk is suspected. Information regarding the family member's age at diagnosis and additional details such as bilaterality of breast cancer are very helpful. Updates of the family history should be asked about at annual examinations because additions and new diagnoses may alter the initial recommendation regarding genetic testing.

Guidelines for offering genetic testing continue to evolve. All patients with epithelial ovarian cancer should be offered genetic testing. Other indicators of a possible hereditary cancer syndrome include early age at diagnosis, multiple primary cancers (eg, breast and ovarian cancer, colon and endometrial cancer, or bilateral breast cancer), cancer in two or more close relatives on the same side of the family, or rare cancers such as male breast cancer or ureteral cancer. If after review of the patients' pedigree a hereditary cancer syndrome is suspected, the patient should be referred for genetic counseling and possibly testing. The counselor may expand on the pedigree and request documents to verify cancer diagnoses. These documents include pathology reports, operative reports, and death certificates.

The ASCO and NCCN offer guidelines for cancer predisposition testing that are followed by most cancer geneticists.

Genetic testing is recommended when the individual has a personal history or family history suggestive of a cancer susceptibility syndrome, when the test can be adequately interpreted, and when the test result will influence medical management.

It is critically important that counseling be done both before and after testing. Appropriate counseling will provide the following:

1. Informed consent
2. Psychological assessment and support
3. Purpose of the test and who should be tested
4. General information about the genes and the mutations to be tested for
5. Possible test results and implications of these results
6. Accuracy of the tests and the likelihood of finding a mutation
7. Cost of testing
8. Possible consequences of testing (ie, genetic discrimination)
9. Importance of sharing results with family members
10. Banking DNA for future testing
11. Options for treatment if testing is declined
12. Management strategies if the test result is positive. These include surveillance, prevention, and prophylaxis

GLOSSARY

Allele   Alternative forms of the same gene. Because of the paired nature of chromosomes, every gene exists in two copies. Each is an allele.

Antioncogene   See tumor suppressor gene.

***c-erb-b2* proto-oncogene**   Also referred to as HER-2 or neu, this gene encodes a protein that is structurally similar to the receptor for epidermal growth factor. When it is amplified, the gene is of prognostic significance in breast and ovarian neoplasms.

Capping   The addition of 7-methylguanosine residues to the 5′ end of most eukaryotic mRNA.

Chromosome   One mechanism for activating oncogenes.

Chromosome translocation   Exchange of genes or a portion of genes between different chromosomes.

Cloning   An in vivo method to produce unlimited quantities of specific DNA fragments from as little as a single DNA molecule. Also, the process by which a DNA molecule is joined to another DNA molecule that can replicate autonomously in a specially designed host, usually a bacterium or yeast.

Codon   A group of three nucleotides forming a base-coding message in the gene sequence. In ras genes, for example, the 12th, 13th, or 61st codon is often mutated, leading to oncogene activation.

Complementary DNA (cDNA)   DNA synthesized from mRNA template such that the DNA sequence is complementary to the mRNA.

Contig   The sequence of DNA created by use of Yeast artificial chromosomes (YACs), Bacterial artificial chromosomes (BACs), and cosmids to fill an unknown region of DNA suspected of having a candidate gene.

Cosmid   Used for large-scale analysis of the human genome when large DNA fragments of known sequence are needed (40 kb).

Cytoplasmic signal transduction molecules   Proteins within the cytoplasm of cells responsible for transmitting signals from one event to the next event.

DNA probe   A short segment of DNA in which the base sequence is specifically complementary to a particular gene segment. The probe is used, for example, on the Southern blot assay to determine whether a certain gene is present in a tumor sample undergoing DNA analysis.

Exons   The coding portion of genes.

Gel electrophoresis   A molecular biology laboratory technique in which DNA, RNA, or proteins are separated according to molecular weight, charge, and spatial characteristics in an electric field applied to a gel. For example, because DNA is negatively charged, it migrates toward the positively charged electrode.

Gene amplification   The presence of multiple copies of a gene within a cell that is normally present in only two copies per somatic cell. An increased number of copies of an individual gene, usually a proto-oncogene, per cell.

Gene deletion   The deletion of part or all of a gene through removal of DNA sequences by any of several mechanisms.

Gene expression   The active transcription of a gene into an RNA molecule followed by translation of the protein product.

Gene rearrangement   The process by which part or all of a gene is moved from its normal location in the genome to another site within the genome.

Genomic imprinting   An epigenetic modification of a parental allele of a gene that leads to differential expression of that allele.

Growth factor   Protein that acts on cells to promote cell growth.

Growth factor receptors   Proteins that interact with growth factors and transmit the growth signal to the cell.

HER-2   See *c-erb-b2* proto-oncogene.

Heteronuclear RNA   A form of RNA, a pre-mRNA, that exists before splicing and consists of both introns and exons.

Heterozygosity   Two different forms of the same gene in a cell. An oncogene is generally heterozygous. For example, one allele may be mutated while the other copy remains normal. In addition, different forms of a gene may be normal variants. Variations in the exact base sequence within DNA are common in the genome among humans. These are called polymorphisms and are often responsible for the heterozygous state.

Informative   A term used to describe the situation in which two homologous chromosomes from an individual can be distinguished from one another at a given locus; *heterozygous* is an alternative term.

Insertion   The addition of a DNA sequence into the genome.

Introns   Portions of genomic DNA that are interspersed between exons and are transcribed along with the exons into heteronuclear RNA.

Locus   A general term to describe a defined chromosome region.

Loss of heterozygosity   Losses of specific regions of DNA from one copy of a given chromosome that can be distinguished from the region retained on the other chromosome.

Messenger RNA (mRNA)   The mature form of processed RNA used as a template for directing translation of proteins.

Myc proto-oncogenes   The proto-oncogene family that includes *c-myc*, *N-myc*, *L-myc*, and *R-myc*. They encode nuclear-associated DNA-binding proteins that affect DNA replication and transcription.

Neu   See *c-erb-b2* proto-oncogene.

Nonsense mutation   A nucleotide substitution that results in a truncated protein product by generating a stop codon specifying premature cessation of translation within an open reading frame.

Nuclear transcription factors   Proteins involved in regulating the expression of genes by controlling transcription. Some factors enhance and others repress gene expression, and others do both, depending on the intracellular environment.

Oncogenes   Genes that regulate cell growth in a positive fashion (ie, promote cell growth). Oncogenes include transforming genes of viruses and normal cellular genes (proto-oncogenes) that are activated by mutations to promote cell growth.

Open reading frame   A sequence of DNA representing at least some of the coding portion of a gene that is transcribed and subsequently translated into a protein because it does not contain any internal translation termination codons.

Palindrome (inverted repeats)   Sequences that look the same if read forward or backward. This allows the sequence to fold back on itself, and it is particularly susceptible to mutation.

Point mutation   The replacement of one nucleotide in the DNA sequence of the wild type with another nucleotide.

Polymorphism   Variation in the exact base sequence of DNA that makes up the genome. These occurrences are normal and common in humans. Polymorphisms are used in the study of molecular genetics because they are inherited. Ones found near or within disease genes can be used to study linkage in genetics.

Primers   Short DNA pieces that are complementary to portions of specific DNA sequences.

Promoter The DNA sequence of a gene to which RNA polymerase binds and initiates transcription.

Proto-oncogenes Any of a number of genes that encode various proteins involved in normal cell growth and proliferation, including growth factors, growth factor receptors, regulators of DNA synthesis, and phosphorylating modifiers of protein function. These are cellular genes that are the normal counterparts of transforming viral oncogenes.

ras **gene** A family of genes that encode similar cell membrane-bound proteins involved in signal transduction. Three types, *K-ras, N-ras,* and *H-ras,* are the widely studied ras genes in human tumors. Their proto-oncogene becomes activated by point mutations, most often in specific codons, of the gene sequence.

RB The first tumor suppressor gene to be discovered. It is a 4.7-kilobase gene, located on chromosome 13q14, and encodes a 110,000-dalton nuclear phosphoprotein that suppresses the cell cycle. Absence of *RB* is the cause of retinoblastoma, and research is revealing that it is involved in the pathogenesis of many other neoplasms.

Reverse transcriptase An enzyme discovered in retroviruses that has the unique ability to transcribe DNA from an RNA template. This is the reverse of the normal physiologic process.

Tp53 **gene** A tumor suppressor gene that encodes a nuclear phosphoprotein that arrests cells from entering the S-phase of the cell cycle. Located on chromosome 17(p13), *Tp53* is postulated to contribute to diverse tumorigenesis.

Transcription The process of converting the DNA code into a complementary mRNA segment.

Translation The process by which specific amino acids are incorporated into a protein as dictated by the sequence of the mRNA template.

Translocation Nonhomologous recombination.

Tumor suppressor gene A gene that suppresses cellular growth and proliferation. Therefore, when its protein products are absent, it contributes to tumor development or progression. Also known as antioncogenes, these normal cellular genes encode proteins that are thought to normally regulate growth in a negative fashion.

Uninformative The term used to describe the situation when the two homologous chromosomes from an individual cannot be distinguished from one another at a given locus; *homozygous* is an alternative term.

Vector A DNA vehicle that can be propagated in living cells (eg, bacteria and yeast) into which foreign DNA can be inserted and propagated with the vector DNA. Examples of vectors include bacterial plasmids; cosmids; bacteriophages; and, most recently, yeast artificial chromosomes.

Wild type The term used to describe the normal gene or gene product. In contrast, a gene that has had its DNA sequence altered is referred to as a mutant gene, and its resultant product is a mutant protein. A gene that encodes a proto-oncogene, for example, is a wild-type gene because it is unaltered.

For the bibliography list, log onto www.expertconsult.com ⟨http://www.expertconsult.com⟩.

20

Palliative Care and Quality of Life

Dana M. Chase, MD, Siu-Fun Wong, PharmD, FASHP, FCSHP,
Lari B. Wenzel, PhD, Bradley J. Monk, MD

OUTLINE

KEY POINTS

1. Palliative care is interdisciplinary care that seeks to prevent, relieve, or reduce the symptoms of a disease without affecting a cure.
2. Certain treatments may not result in improved survival but may result in decreased symptoms. Clinical trials have therefore begun measuring quality of life (QoL).
3. Other QoL measures include survivorship. That is the process of helping the patient have the highest QoL after treatment.
4. Often pain associated with cancer is undertreated. Other symptoms, especially psychological ones, are often ignored or not recognized.
5. A multidisciplinary team is required to recognize and care for this aspect of cancer care and includes social workers, pastoral care, nutritionists, oncologists, pain specialists, psychologists, physical therapists, and caseworkers.
6. Palliative care is an important emerging field in cancer care.

EVOLUTION OF PALLIATIVE CARE

Once viewed as limited and focused care during the final days of life, the scope of palliative medical care and quality of life (QoL) research has evolved since the 1990s. **Although several definitions of palliative care exist, it is broadly defined as interdisciplinary care that seeks to prevent, relieve, or reduce the symptoms of a disease or disorder without affecting a cure.** "Palliative care" and the related term "palliative medicine" are being used with increasing frequency in the United States and have become the labels of choice throughout the world to describe programs based on the hospice philosophy. When approaching death, including care at the end of life, the Institute of Medicine (IOM) recommends: "Palliative care should

become, if not a medical specialty, at least a defined area of expertise, education and research."

Palliative care overlaps with "terminal care," "death and dying," "hospice," "end-of-life care," "comfort care," and "supportive care." The term "supportive care," which is often used by oncologists, is particularly ill defined and sometimes refers to comfort care or palliative support of critically ill patients, particularly those suffering from the adverse effects of cancer treatment. All of these terms have a number of meanings and are often unfamiliar to clinicians. They outline the relationships of health care professionals with patients and family members during the terminal stages of life and the treatment of advanced malignancies (Table 20.1)

TABLE 20.1 Issues in Palliative and End-of-Life Care

Emphasis on the trajectory
Symptom control and psychological support
Comprehensive assessment
Cancer pain management
Communicating effectively
Diagnosis and prognosis
Symptoms
Negotiating goals of care
Clinical trials
Withdrawing and withholding therapy
Advanced care planning
Cancer doctors and burnout

TABLE 20.2 Improving End-of-Life Care: Recommendations of the Institute of Medicine

1. Reliable and skilful supportive care
2. Effective use of knowledge to prevent and relieve pain and other symptoms
3. Policymakers, consumers, health practitioners, and organizations:
   - Measure quality of life (QoL) and other outcomes.
   - Develop tools for improving QoL and hold health care organizations accountable.
   - Revise payment mechanisms to encourage good end-of-life care.
   - Reform laws and regulations that impede effective use of opioids.
4. Change medical education to ensure relevant attitudes, knowledge, and skills.
5. Recognition of palliative care as a defined area of expertise, education, and research
6. Research establishment to strengthen knowledge base.
7. Promote public education.

Barriers to Optimal End-of-Life Care Identified by the American Society of Clinical Oncology

1. Inappropriate attitudes of health care professionals and patients (eg, reluctance to discuss death and dying)
2. Ineffective communication about the prognosis
3. Unrealistic expectations and treatment options
4. Failure of physicians to recognize and emphasize the importance of symptom management and psychosocial support
5. Social attitudes (eg, fear of opioid addiction)
6. Economic barriers, including lack of universal access to care and underfunding of end-of-life care
7. Fear of the attending physician losing control of the patient's care; hospice teams to work more closely with attending physicians
8. Lack of systematic education for physicians about clinical and psychosocial aspects of care

Modified from the Institute of Medicine's Report and ASCO Task Force.

QoL is a concern in all areas of medicine and of primary importance in the palliative care setting. Within the clinical setting, assessment of a patient's QoL begins with an understanding of a patient's knowledge about his or her condition and potential management strategies, his or her values, and his or her personal cost–benefit calculations. **Certain therapies have no chance of improving survival endpoints but may have an acceptable therapeutic index based on a reasonable balance between the toxicity of the intervention and the resolution of symptoms secondary to the condition being treated. With this concept in mind, investigators and clinicians have begun to collectively measure QoL in clinical trials and community-based practices in an attempt to define alterations in QoL and to prospectively ascertain interventions that might improve "survivorship."** It is no longer appropriate to simply survive one's illness; rather, one must avoid the "killing cure," allowing patients to enjoy life and function productively while interacting with their environment during multimodality cancer treatment.

The gynecologic oncologist is in a unique position to function collectively as a primary care provider, surgeon, radiation oncologist, and chemotherapist, allowing comprehensive transfer of treatment with an emphasis on the patient's QoL. Reports from the Institute of Medicine's Committee on Care at the End of Life and the American Society of Clinical Oncology (ASCO) Task Force on Cancer Care at the End of Life, both published in 1998, clearly acknowledge the physician's responsibility in caring for patients throughout the continuum of their illness (Table 20.2). The ASCO document asserts: "In addition to appropriate anti-cancer treatment, comprehensive care includes symptom control and psychosocial support during all phases of life."

In addition, in 2015, the Society of Gynecologic Oncology has published recommendations regarding improving the quality and cost of gynecologic oncology practice. These recommendations include prompt referral to palliative care services for advanced and recurrent gynecologic cancer patients. In addition, the recommendations discourage the use of unnecessary chemotherapy and surgery close to the end of life in these patients because research has shown an alarmingly high percentage of patients receiving these procedures within the last 6 months of life. Furthermore, multiple studies have indicated that trainees are not adequately prepared in the realm of palliative care support for gynecologic cancer patients.

Gynecologic oncologists are not only faced with the challenge of providing end-of-life care, but they must also explore ways to integrate palliative care throughout the continuum of illness. Indeed, recent literature suggests that gynecologic oncologists recognize the growing importance of their role as the patient's disease progresses. It is in this role, when the challenges of effective, compassionate care and communication are heightened, that an understanding of the principles and the clinical practice of palliative medicine are critical. A review of the recommendations for and barriers to effective palliative and end-of-life care as outlined by the Institute of Medicine and ASCO is listed in Table 20.2.

Palliative care is differentiated from other medical specialties by its fundamental philosophy of care delivery; care is collaboratively provided by an interdisciplinary team prompted by issues and concerns of the patient and family. "Family" as defined by the patient and staff may include friends as well as relatives.

Palliative care is, by definition, care delivered through the coordinated efforts of the team that is collectively confident and skilled when assessing and addressing the physical, psychosocial, and spiritual needs of the patient and family. It differs from more traditional "multidisciplinary" care that is directed by a physician, which allows team members to simply focus on their own areas of expertise. In contrast, the palliative care "intradisciplinary" team recognizes that all information about the patient and family is relevant. Thus, the home health aide or the pharmacist may have a point of view that would be helpful for the care plan. **Common members of these multidisciplinary teams include medical social workers, pastoral care, nutritionists, radiation oncologist, medical oncologist, pain specialists, psychologists, physical therapists, and caseworkers.** Early in the treatment of a gynecologic cancer, side effects of therapy should be anticipated and treated prophylactically. Later, some symptoms may be dealt with without the extensive evaluation associated with the assessment of tumor response or disease status. However, the development of symptoms often indicates disease progression, and appropriate laboratory or radiographic studies may lead to an alteration of treatment. As the cancer progresses, making cytotoxic therapy less likely to be effective, the workup of new symptoms must be tailored to the individual patient based on the prognosis as well as on the desires expressed by the patient and family. In end-of-life care, there is no room for long-term evaluation or a "wait and see" attitude. In fact, within even just 1 day of referral to palliative care services, symptom burden improves for patients. **Data have indicated that the triad of younger age (<50 years), a history of pain, and depression or anxiety can perhaps capture patients that will have higher symptom burden and should perhaps be either watched carefully for palliative care needs or referred early to palliative care services.** Furthermore, QoL improves, depression decreases, and the use of chemotherapy close to death is reduced when patients are introduced at least once to palliative care services during their treatment experience. As a result, control of annoying symptoms may be pursued more aggressively, and management may resemble that given in an intensive care situation but without an extensive diagnostic evaluation. Control of symptoms is not an end in itself, but it should be sought to allow the patient time to optimize QoL and to support the patient in reaching peace with self and closure with important people in the patient's life.

QUALITY OF LIFE IN GYNECOLOGIC CANCERS

QoL varies depending on the gynecologic cancer disease site, stage, and treatment. In ovarian cancer, for example, the majority of patients present in their 60s with advanced metastatic disease. These patients experience a decline of QoL before diagnosis. However, many respond well to treatment, which creates symptomatic improvement, easing the disease burden and therefore improving QoL. Unfortunately, most patients with advanced ovarian cancer have recurrences, and despite poor outcomes, patients are often treated with multiple rounds of chemotherapy. In contrast, patients with cervical cancer overall present at a younger age with minimal symptoms in the

earlier stages of disease. However, whether it is fertility-terminating surgery or chemotherapy and radiation, the therapy can be life-altering or toxic. Despite its initial expectation of lower toxicity index, the use of targeted therapy has not yet demonstrated a significant alleviation of the adverse drug event burden as originally intended. These side effects suffered, however, may be acceptable in the event of likely cure. However, in the advanced cases, when these women have recurrences, their already low QoL, combined with new symptoms related to recurrence, makes further treatment difficult in the setting of often ineffective therapy. Furthermore, patients with cervical cancer are often of lower socioeconomic status and present with unique social and emotional challenges, especially in the setting of cancer diagnosis, treatment, and follow-up care. Patients with endometrial cancer are perhaps the most favorable in terms of QoL in that they frequently present in early stage and are often treated with surgery alone. However, their medical comorbidities, including obesity and diabetes, are challenging to address in survivorship.

Quality of Life in Ovarian Cancer

Because the majority of patients with ovarian cancer present in advanced stages, most women enter treatment with some QoL dysfunction likely related to symptom severity at presentation. The study of QoL in ovarian cancer therefore must take into consideration this baseline level of dysfunction and monitor the effect of surgery or chemotherapy. Because the prognosis is generally poor for those with advanced ovarian cancer, the goal of therapy is perhaps to extend life without greatly compromising the patient's QoL. In clinical trials, great attention is now paid to measuring QoL throughout the study of cancer therapeutics. QoL has also been monitored posttherapy to document the needs and deficiencies of these women. In the measurement of QoL, a standardized and validated measure, the Functional Assessment of Cancer Therapy-Ovarian (FACT-O), is frequently used in clinical trials. The FACT-O is a combination of the FACT-G (General) plus additional questions related specifically to ovarian cancer (Tables 20.3 and 20.4). The FACT-G is composed of four subscales: the physical, social/family, emotional, and functional well-being. Patients can answer on a scale of 0 to 4, with 0 being not at all and 4 being very much. In the physical well-being subscale, the patient is asked to elaborate on pain, nausea, and lack of energy and how these physical symptoms affect their life and how bothered by these symptoms the patient is. The social/family well-being subscale addresses the amount of emotional support the patient has from her friends, family, and partner. The emotional well-being subscale targets the patient's feelings and emotions regarding her illness and how anxious she is about dying from this disease. Finally, the functional well-being subscale concerns the patient's ability to function in society, such as her ability to work, sleep, and enjoy life. This subscale looks at the patient's ability to accept illness and move on to live a "normal" life again. In the final section of the FACT-O, there is an additional concerns scale that targets specific symptoms, life-altering changes, and chemotherapy in ovarian cancer. In 2011, Donovan et al. performed a comprehensive review of the QoL literature related to ovarian

TABLE 20.3 TABLE 1 The FACT-G Versus the EORTC QLQ-CS

FACT-G	QLQ-C30
Physical Well-Being	1. Short of breath
1. Lack of energy	2. Pain
2. Nausea	3. Need to rest
3. Trouble meeting the needs of family	4. Trouble sleeping
4. Pain	5. Felt weak
5. Side effects of treatment	6. Lacked appetite
6. Ill feeling	7. Felt nauseated
7. Forced to spend time in bed	8. Vomited
	9. Constipation
Social/Family Well-Being	10. Diarrhea
1. Close to friends	11. Fatigue
2. Emotional support from family	12. Staying in bed or chair
3. Support from friends	13. Strenuous activity
4. Family acceptance of illness	14. Long walk
5. Satisfaction with family communication about illness	15. Short walk
	16. Help with daily functions
6. Feeling close to partner	17. Limited in work or daily activities
7. Satisfaction with sex life	
	18. Limited in leisure activities
Emotional Well-Being	19. Difficulty concentrating
1. Sadness	20. Feeling tense
2. Satisfaction with coping with illness	21. Worry
3. Losing hope in the fight against illness	22. Irritable
4. Feeling nervous	23. Depressed
5. Worry about dying	24. Difficulty with memory
6. Worry that condition will get worse	25. Physical condition affecting family life
	26. Physical condition affecting social life
Functional Well-Being	27. Physical condition affecting financial status
1. Ability to work	
2. Work is fulfilling	
3. Enjoying life	
4. Accepting illness	
5. Sleeping well	
6. Enjoying the things I usually do for fun	
7. Content with quality of life	

FACT-G, Functional Assessment of Cancer Therapy-General; *QLQ-C30,* Quality of Life Questionnaire Module C30.

TABLE 20.4 Additional Concerns Scales

	Cervical	Ovarian	Endometrial
Bleeding or discharge	X		X
Odor	X		
Fear of sex	X		
Sexually attractive	X		
Narrow or short vagina	X		
Fertility concerns	X	X	
Fear of harms of treatment	X		
Interest in sex	X	X	
Body appearance	X	X	X
Constipation	X		X
Appetite	X		
Urinary incontinence, dysuria, discomfort with urination, frequency	X		X
Ability to eat foods that are liked	X		
Swelling in stomach		X	X
Weight loss		X	
Control of bowels		X	
Vomiting		X	
Hair loss		X	
Appetite		X	
Ability to get around		X	
Feel like a woman		X	
Stomach cramping		X	X
Discomfort of pain in stomach			X
Hot flashes			X
Cold sweats			X
Fatigue			X
Pain with intercourse			X
Trouble with digestion			X
Shortness of breath			X
Discomfort or pain in pelvis			X

cancer between the years 2000 and 2011. They sought to find the most important symptoms that should be recorded to measure QoL in ovarian cancer trials. **The panel of experts identified the following "core" ovarian cancer symptoms: abdominal pain, bloating, cramping, fear of recurrence or disease progression, indigestion, sexual dysfunction, vomiting, weight gain, and weight loss.** In addition, ovarian cancer–specific symptoms were suggested to be of value in the design of future QoL endpoints: abdominal pain, bloating, cramping, fear of recurrence, indigestion, sexual dysfunction, vomiting, weight gain, and weight loss.

Several prospective randomized trials in the United States have used the FACT-O measure to assess QoL. The Gynecologic Oncology Group (GOG) has used the FACT-O in prospective phase III randomized trials to monitor QoL during various experimental treatment protocols (Table 20.5). The first ovarian cancer GOG trial using the FACT-O was published by Wenzel

et al. in 2005. They published the QoL results for a randomized trial of interval secondary cytoreduction in advanced ovarian cancer patients. In this trial (GOG protocol 152), 424 patients were enrolled, and 380 (90%) of these women completed the initial and midtreatment questionnaires. Roughly 80% of the patients continued to complete the measures at the second though fourth assessment points. In this study, a better QoL as measured by the FACT-O was associated with improved overall survival (OS). Although the FACT-O results did not differ between the groups receiving this surgical intervention or not, this trial did emphasize that improvements in QoL existed for women in both arms at 6 and 12 months after therapy.

Notably, an effective treatment regimen demonstrated for women with stage III ovarian cancer that has been optimally surgically debulked is a combination of intraperitoneal (IP) and intravenous (IV) chemotherapy. GOG 172, a phase III trial comparing IP cisplatin and paclitaxel plus IV paclitaxel with IV cisplatin and IV paclitaxel, demonstrated that the IP/IV regimen was associated with the longest median survival time (65.6 months for IP/IV vs. 49.7 months for IV) that has yet been reported in women with optimally debulked stage III ovarian

TABLE 20.5 Prospective Gynecologic Oncology Group (GOG) Trials Including Quality of Life Measurements

Cancer Site	GOG Protocol Number	Study Title
Ovarian	GOG 152 (2005)	A randomized trial of interval secondary cytoreduction in advanced ovarian carcinoma
	GOG 172 (2007)	A randomized trial intravenous paclitaxel and cisplatin versus intravenous paclitaxel, intraperitoneal cisplatin and intraperitoneal paclitaxel in patients with optimal stage III epithelial ovarian carcinoma or primary peritoneal carcinoma
	GOG 218 (2013)	A randomized trial of intravenous carboplatin and paclitaxel with or without bevacizumab
Cervical	GOG 169 (2006)	A randomized trial of cisplatin versus cisplatin plus paclitaxel in advanced cervical cancer
	GOG 179 (2005)	A randomized trial of cisplatin with or without topotecan in advanced carcinoma of the cervix
	GOG 204	A randomized trial of paclitaxel plus cisplatin versus vinorelbine plus cisplatin versus gemcitabine plus cisplatin versus topotecan plus cisplatin in stage IVB, recurrent, or persistent carcinoma of the cervix
	GOG 240	A randomized trial of chemotherapy with or without bevacizumab for advanced or recurrent cervical cancer
Endometrial	GOG 122 (2007)	A randomized trial of whole abdominal irradiation and combination chemotherapy in advanced endometrial carcinoma
	LAP-2	A randomized clinical trial of laparoscopy (scope) versus open laparotomy (open) for the surgical resection and staging of uterine cancer

LAP, long-acting release.

cancer. This statistically significant and clinically meaningful difference between IP and IV chemotherapy prompted a National Cancer Institute (NCI) Clinical Announcement (2006) alerting the public and health professionals to the superiority of IP chemotherapy in the optimal disease setting. However, the superior survival outcomes, demonstrated with the IP regimen in GOG 172, was associated with considerable toxicity, and patients randomized to IP therapy reported significantly worse QoL before cycle 4 (P <0.0001) and at 3 to 6 weeks after treatment (P = 0.0035). However, there were no significant overall QoL differences between regimens 1 year posttreatment. Despite the reported benefits of IP therapy for progression-free survival (PFS) and OS, this study demonstrated physical and functional well-being deficits both during and after therapy in the IP arm. Neurotoxicity and abdominal discomfort were also more prevalent in the IP arm. Although the QoL scores improved over time, specifically at 12 months from initial treatment, this manuscript perhaps prompted physicians to reconsider this

treatment modality secondary to toxicity concerns. In addition, IP is a more difficult treatment for the treatment team to administer as well as potentially more toxic. However, ultimately, the QoL differences between regimens were not significant long term. In 2015, Wright et al. looked at the use and effectiveness of IP chemotherapy in 823 women at six different institutions. These authors demonstrate a relatively poor acceptance of IP chemotherapy (<50%) despite published survival advantages. They cite certain factors as potential barriers to IP/IV chemotherapy usage including toxicities, patients' preferences, the inconvenience of administration, potentially higher rates of extraabdominal cancer recurrences, and beliefs that other chemotherapy regimens may be comparable with fewer toxicities. This study did demonstrate improved survival advantages, but IP chemotherapy usage is associated with younger age and fewer medical comorbidities, thus perhaps explaining the less than 50% adoption of this route of treatment.

In 2009, von Gruenigan et al. combined the results from the above described trials and reported the specific line items in the FACT-O that were reported between cycles. For example, the authors report significant differences in concerns such as pain, nausea, feeling ill, and side effects of treatment. Because significant functional well-being deficits were also reported, they suggest interventions aimed at specific side effects as a means to improve patients' functional status. Social well-being went relatively unharmed except for satisfaction with one's sex life. Emotional deficits were also noted across all items except for acceptance of illness. This study demonstrated that when broken down into individual line items, perhaps interventions can be designed to target improvement in these various areas. In 2013, Monk et al. reported on the QoL outcomes of a randomized trial incorporating bevacizumab into the carboplatin and paclitaxel IV chemotherapy. This study included a maintenance of bevacizumab versus placebo for a total of 22 cycles (treatment given every 3 weeks). During the initial chemotherapy phase of six cycles of carboplatin and paclitaxel, the patients on bevacizumab experienced significantly lower QoL scores (worse QoL) than those on chemotherapy alone. It was curious that bevacizumab compromised QoL during the chemotherapy phase only of treatment. Most striking, though, is perhaps the idea that extending PFS did not translate into enhanced QoL according to the authors. However, although QoL was not improved, the authors use the QoL data to conclude that this new regimen is an acceptable alternative to standard care.

Several European studies have also evaluated QoL in prospective trials. Although these studies use different QoL tools, it is important to comment on some of these studies in which QoL data in the United States are lacking. First, in 2010, Vergote et al. published the results of a randomized trial of neoadjuvant chemotherapy followed by interval surgical cytoreduction versus primary surgical debulking followed by chemotherapy. The QoL results were then published in 2013. Per the authors, QoL was assessed by the European Organization for Research and Treatment of Cancer (EORTC) Quality of Life Questionnaire Module-C30 (QLQ-C30) core questionnaire version 3, which consists of a global health status and QoL scale, multi-item functional scales and symptom scales, and a scale regarding financial difficulties. The trial results demonstrated similar OS outcomes between the two groups. The authors chose to limit inclusion to the QoL analysis to institutions with at least 50% compliance and more than at least 35% during the follow-up period. There were no statistically significant differences between the two groups, although those with the primary debulking group at baseline had more pain but less dyspnea.

In addition, the AURELIA trial studies the use of physician's choice chemotherapy with or without bevacizumab in platinum-resistant recurrent ovarian cancer. Using the EORTC Quality of Life Questionnaire–Ovarian Cancer Module 28 (EORTC QLQ-OV28) and Functional Assessment of Cancer Therapy–Ovarian Cancer symptom index (FOSI), the investigators demonstrated that with the use of bevacizumab, there was greater than 15% improvement in QoL and abdominal or gastrointestinal (GI) symptoms specifically. The CALYPSO trial was another European trial that randomized patients with platinum-sensitive ovarian cancer to carboplatin and pegylated liposomal doxorubicin versus carboplatin and paclitaxel. The QoL results, published in 2012, were generated by the EORTC QoL-QC30 questionnaire and OV28 ovarian cancer module. In this trial, patients treated with carboplatin and pegylated liposomal doxorubicin had improved QoL scores and fewer cancer- and chemotherapy-related symptoms. This study, although designed as a noninferiority trial, did suggest that improved outcomes with the experimental arm were not at the expense of decreased QoL

Quality of Life in Cervical Cancer

Although patients with cervical cancer may present with pelvic pain or bleeding (or both) in more advanced stages, cervical cancer may also be detected based on screening tests alone. The usual treatment involves surgery for early stage followed by possible radiation, chemotherapy, or both for high-risk cases versus chemotherapy and radiation alone for more advanced stages. **Patients with cervical cancer present with a unique set of symptoms, side effects from treatment, and socioeconomic issues not seen in patients with ovarian cancer. For example, these women have a lower median age at presentation; this group also has a larger percentage of Latina or nonwhite patients and a larger percentage of lower income patients. Furthermore, the chemotherapy and specifically the radiation received by these women produce such symptoms as sexual dysfunction and urinary and bowel dysfunction that perhaps affect women in unique ways.**

In the measurement of QoL for cervical cancer, there are, similar to ovarian cancer, two tools that are most widely used, the FACT-Cx and the QLQ-CX24. The FACT-Cx is composed of the same physical, social, functional, and emotional well-being subscales as the FACT-G but in addition it has a seven-item scale for concerns related specifically to cervical cancer. These concerns involve vaginal discharge, bleeding, odor, narrowing or shortening, constipation, and dysuria. The GOG has published studies in advanced cervical cancer that have used the FACT-Cx. These patients have a poor median survival time, typically less than 6 months, and therefore it is still of debate whether

or not treatment is futile in this setting. This is especially of concern in such advanced cancer when symptomatology can be debilitating and further aggressive treatment perhaps does more harm than good. This is an ideal patient population to study QoL because if QoL decreases with treatment, then one might argue against treatment in a disease in which OS is so poor.

In 2006, GOG protocol 169 was published by McQuellon et al. and reported QoL endpoints in a randomized trial that compared cisplatin versus cisplatin plus paclitaxel in advanced cervical cancer (see Table 20.5). Despite the impressive deficits in QoL compared with the general population, these two treatment regimens did not differ with regards to QoL. The cisplatin and paclitaxel arms did demonstrate improvements in response rate and PFS; therefore, the QoL data help to promote this regimen. In 2005, the QoL data from GOG 179 were published by Monk et al. This randomized trial studied cisplatin as compared with cisplatin and topotecan in advanced or recurrent cervical cancer cases. The FACT-Cx was used to document QoL between these two regimens in addition to exploring its relation to prognosis. There were statistical differences in QoL between the two regimens, but of interest was the relationship of the FACT-Cx to OS. As the FACT-Cx score increased, so did OS, and this was statistically significant. Finally, in GOG protocol 204, which studied multiple platinum-doublets in this population, it demonstrated again no difference in QoL scores between these regimens. The QoL data were published in 2010, and there were no reported differences among the four regimens. In 2015, Penson et al. reported the QoL results of GOG protocol 240, which introduced bevacizumab into the standard chemotherapy treatment of advanced or recurrent cervical cancer. Using the Functional Assessment of Cancer Therapy—Cervix Trial Outcome Index (FACT-Cx TOI), there were no significant differences in QoL. Thus, despite improved PFS and OS, this did not necessarily translate into improved QoL. The FACT-Cx TOI in this analysis was associated with survival in that for every increment of 10 on the QoL score, hazard of progression or death was also incrementally affected. This same concept of QoL scores at baseline predicting outcomes in QoL analyses has been demonstrated in multiple investigations. In fact, Chase et al. did demonstrate that on several GOG cervical cancer trials, QoL measurement alone at baseline could predict the development of toxicity, including leukopenia, anemia, and GI toxicity. This association remained significant despite controlling for important patient characteristics such as performance status, age, and treatment type. Finally, in a randomized Japanese GOG study of carboplatin and paclitaxel versus cisplatin and paclitaxel in advanced or recurrent cervical cancer, the investigators used hospitalizations as an objective measurement of QoL. The carboplatin arm demonstrated less hospitalization time, which the authors suggest might equal improved QoL of that regimen.

Several other areas within the trajectory of cervical cancer have been explored in relation to QoL. These include preinvasive disease, surgery, radiation therapy, and survivorship. In 2013, a multicenter observational and cross-sectional study of 842 women in the United Kingdom was published. This study included women without dysplasia and genital warts as well as a spectrum of preinvasive cervical and vulvar disease. QoL assessment indicated a significant negative impact of these diseases on psychosocial well-being, including sexual functioning. Of note, anxiety and depression as well as pain were particularly noteworthy in women with genital warts. These effects on QoL not only persist throughout treatment but are also demonstrated in survivorship. For example, several studies have indicated that long-term effects can include worsening lymphedema and bowel, genitourinary, and sexual function after completion of multimodality treatment including chemotherapy or radiation. In addition, psychosocial functioning is affected in the long term. This prompted researchers to evaluate a program of telephone counseling for cervical cancer survivors. A total of 204 patients were randomized to telephone counseling versus usual care. This study not only demonstrated improvements in depression, gynecologic, and cancer-specific concerns in the intervention group but also demonstrated positive effects on biomarkers for psychosocial stress, with decreased levels of cytokines such as various interleukins. The hope is that research will continue to demonstrate improvements in patient-reported outcomes that can be objectively measured by biomarkers of stress and that ultimately this can link to clinical outcomes.

Quality of Life in Endometrial Cancer

Endometrial cancer usually presents with vaginal bleeding and at an early stage. Treatment is surgical and occasionally involves postoperative chemotherapy, radiation, or both. **Likely because of the less invasive or aggressive treatment, with the majority of patients presenting at an early stage, there are not as many studies that focused exclusively on QoL in patients with endometrial cancer. A Cochrane review published in 2012 but edited in 2015 included trials in advanced or recurrent endometrial cancer. Of the 14 randomized trials reported, no QoL results were identified and thus analyzed.** In fact, in the GOG, there are only two published reports of QoL in patients with endometrial cancer, and there has yet to be an endometrial cancer–specific subscale incorporated into this research. In 2007, Bruner et al. published the results of the QoL components of GOG protocol 122, which compared whole-abdominal irradiation (WAI) and combination chemotherapy in advanced patients with endometrial cancer (see Table 20.5). In this study using the FACT-G in addition to the Fatigue Scale (FS), Assessment of Peripheral Neuropathy (APN), and Functional Alterations due to Changes in Elimination (FACE), QoL was measured before and after therapy. The WAI arm suffered greater deficits in the FS and FACE scores, but these scores somewhat improved over the varying time points. Conversely, the neuropathy scores were worse in the chemotherapy arm. Interestingly, the FACT-G scores did not differ between the two arms at any time point. The data generated in this study provide patients with the risks and benefits of each therapy and can perhaps shed light on whether QoL concerns in patients can overshadow the potential survival benefits of one modality.

In 2009, the QoL data were published from Europe's Post Operative Radiation Therapy in Endometrial Cancer

(PORTEC-2) trial, in which patients received external-beam versus vaginal brachytherapy. This study used the QLQ-C30 measure in addition to subscales from the prostate cancer and ovarian cancer module, which included both bowel and bladder symptoms and sexual functioning symptoms from those scales. Despite the lack of significant differences between groups, there was a low level of sexual functioning in the two groups. The vaginal brachytherapy group overall reported better social functioning, fewer bowel symptoms, and less limitation in activity because of these side effects compared with external-beam radiation therapy. These results suggest the use of a treatment modality potentially as effective with less impact on QoL. In another GOG trial, Kornblith et al. published the results of the QoL component of the LAP-2 protocol, which compared patients undergoing laparoscopic staging versus laparotomy. The measures used included the FACT-G as well as a six-item scale consisting of items related to surgical side effects. In addition, they used the Physical Functioning Subscale of the Medical Outcome Study-Short Form (MOS-SF36. PF), which was developed to assess activities of daily living. The differences in QoL between these two groups favored the laparoscopy group, but this difference was modest. The authors very eloquently describe that to spare one patient the short-term QoL decline with laparotomy, 10 patients would have to be offered laparoscopy. In fact, only better body image persisted in the laparoscopy group at 6 months; all other measurements became comparable by that time point. QoL data can be complex in analysis and interpretation but can shed light on misconceptions regarding the benefits of one therapy or intervention over another.

More recently, several endometrial trials have focused on diet and exercise interventions focused on the prevalence of obesity in these patients. A systematic review and meta-analysis of body mass index and QoL in endometrial cancer included four studies with a total of 1362 patients. Indeed, obese endometrial cancer survivors demonstrate poorer physical, social, and role functioning compared with nonobese patients. One hundred patients with posttherapy endometrial cancer stage I to IIIA participated in a 6-month study of a home-based exercise intervention. In this study, the nonobese women demonstrated higher baseline QoL. Although the obese women had fewer improvements in QoL, both the obese and nonobese groups demonstrated some improvements in QoL with this exercise intervention over the period of 6 months.

The SUCCEED trial looked at an intervention of self-efficacy, weight loss, and QoL in obese endometrial cancer survivors. This study included 75 women randomized to usual care versus an intervention. The intervention group demonstrated significant improvements in the Weight Efficacy Life-style questionnaire. Essentially, this questionnaire measures a patient's ability to resist weight gain and maintain healthy lifestyle behaviors. However, the FACT-G differences (QoL measurement tool) between the groups were reported as minimal except perhaps in the fatigue domain. Future trials such as the feMMe or the REWARD trial will look at the incorporation of the intrauterine device, weight loss interventions, and/or metformin in low-risk endometrial cancer patients.

MANAGEMENT OF COMMON PHYSICAL SYMPTOMS

Even when cancer can be treated effectively and a cure or life prolongation achieved, there are always physical, psychosocial, or spiritual concerns that must be addressed to maintain function and to optimize the QoL. Symptoms are a reminder to the patient and caregivers of the cancer and the potentially devastating effects of treatment. **Symptoms related to cancer and its treatment have not attracted much notice in the past when patients and physicians alike felt that pursuing them might detract from the "real" goal of controlling the tumor.** Consequently, symptoms have been taken for granted by the medical profession. Successful and appropriate management of physical symptoms can allow the care team to focus on the psychosocial closure of life and provide the patient an opportunity to participate more fully in the decisions of care and to rebuild or establish stronger relationships with family, friends, and coworkers.

Many physicians and nurses find symptom management in patients with advanced disease to be a frustrating experience because the symptoms may persist or progress. **Although the symptoms are not always completely controlled, acknowledgment of the problem and working toward its relief offer invaluable support to the patient.** Reliance on medical and drug therapies has been the traditional method to control symptoms. There is increasing recognition that nonpharmacologic approaches have significant benefits for individual patients. **Nontraditional approaches such as acupuncture, biofeedback, aromatherapy, massage, and herbal medicine may have a role in the management of symptoms. Each of the following four physical symptoms is addressed in detail: fatigue, pain, nausea and vomiting, and diarrhea and constipation.**

Fatigue

Fatigue is perhaps the most common symptom experienced by patients with gynecologic cancers. Fatigue is the most prevalent (60%–96%) and one of the least understood symptoms that affect cancer patients. Several factors are implicated in the causes of fatigue, for example, anemia, pain, nutrition, insomnia, cognitive dysfunction, and psychological distress. Fatigue has been reported by gynecologic patients as severe, distressing, and uncontrollable. Unfortunately, cancer-related fatigue is not relieved by rest and might not improve posttherapy. **Patients have identified fatigue with cancer as the major obstacle to normal functioning and good QoL.** Although almost a universal symptom of patients undergoing primary antineoplastic therapy or treatment with biologic response modifiers, it is also extremely common in populations with persistent or advanced cancer. Perhaps this is the result of inadequate attention on the part of health care professionals coupled with patients' reluctance to discuss their fatigue.

Given the prevalence and impact of cancer-related fatigue, there have been remarkably few studies of the phenomenon. Its epidemiology has been poorly defined, and the variety of clinical presentations remains anecdotal. Perhaps this is secondary to the inability of fatigue to be measured in any way other

than subjectively. The existence of discrete fatigue syndromes linked with predisposing factors or potential etiologies has not been confirmed, and clinical trials to evaluate putative therapies for specific types of cancer-related fatigue are almost entirely lacking.

Patients and practitioners can generally differentiate the "normal" fatigue experienced by the general population from the clinical fatigue associated with cancer or its treatment. The term "asthenia" has been used to describe fatigue in oncology patients but has no specific meaning apart from the more common term. This condition is inherently subjective and multidimensional. Typically, it develops over time and is characterized by diminishing energy, mental capacity, and the psychological condition of cancer patients (Table 20.6). It is also linked with lethargy and malaise in the revised National Cancer Institute Common Toxicity Criteria. These classifications may enhance awareness of fatigue and improve reporting of the condition.

When fatigue is primarily related to a treatment, there is generally a clear temporal relationship between the condition and the intervention. In patients receiving cytotoxic chemotherapy, for example, it often peaks within a few days and declines into the next treatment cycle. **During the course of fractionated radiotherapy, it is often cumulative and may peak over a period of weeks.** Occasionally, it persists for a prolonged period beyond the end of chemotherapy or radiation treatment. The relationship between fatigue and demographic characteristics, physiologic factors, and psychosocial factors is

TABLE 20.6 Proposed Criteria for Cancer-Related Fatigue

The following symptoms commonly present almost daily during the same 2-week period in the past month:
- Significant fatigue, diminished energy, or increased need to rest disproportionate to any recent change in activity level

Plus five (or more) of the following:
- Complaints of generalized weakness or limb heaviness
- Diminished concentration of attention
- Decreased motivation or interest in engaging in usual activities
- Insomnia or hypersomnia
- Experience of sleep as unrefreshing or nonrestorative
- Perceived need to struggle to overcome inactivity
- Marked emotional reactivity (eg, sadness, frustration, or irritability) when feeling fatigued
- Difficulty completing daily tasks attributed to feeling fatigued
- Perceived problems with short-term memory
- Postexertional malaise lasting several hours
- The symptoms cause clinically significant distress or impairment in social, occupational, or other important areas of functioning
- There is evidence from the history, physical examination, or laboratory findings that the symptoms are a consequence of cancer or cancer-related therapy
- The symptoms are not primarily a consequence of a comorbid psychiatric disorders, such as major depression, somatization disorder, or delirium

Adapted from Cella D, Peterman A, Passik S, et al. Progress toward guidelines for the management of fatigue. *Oncology* 1998;12: 369-377.

TABLE 20.7 Potential Predisposing Factors With Cancer-Related Fatigue

Physiologic
- Underlying disease
- Treatment for the disease
  - Chemotherapy
  - Radiotherapy
  - Surgery
  - Biologic response modifiers (eg, interferon)
- Intercurrent systemic disorders
  - Anemia
  - Infection
  - Pulmonary disorders
  - Hepatic failure
  - Heart failure
  - Renal insufficiency
  - Malnutrition
  - Neuromuscular disorders
  - Dehydration or electrolyte disturbances
- Sleep disorders
- Immobility and lack of exercise
- Chronic pain
- Use of centrally acting drugs (eg, opioids)

Psychosocial
- Anxiety disorders
- Depressive disorders
  - Stress related
  - Environmental reinforcers

Adapted from Portenoy RK. *Principles and Practice of Supportive Oncology.* Philadelphia, 1998, Lippincott-Raven, pp 109-118.

not well defined. The specific mechanisms that precipitate or sustain the syndrome are unknown. **Fatigue may present a final common pathway to which many predisposing or etiologic factors contribute** (Table 20.7). The pathophysiology in any individual may be multifactorial. Proposed mechanisms include abnormalities in energy metabolism related to increased nutritional requirements (eg, caused by tumor growth, infection, fever, or surgery), decreased availability of metabolic substrate (eg, caused by anemia, hypoxemia, or poor nutrition), or the abnormal production of substances that impair metabolism or normal function of muscles (eg, cytokines or antibodies). Other proposed mechanisms link fatigue to the pathophysiology of sleep disorders and major depression. Further research is necessary to determine mediating mechanisms and optimal interventions.

A detailed characterization of fatigue combined with an understanding of the most likely etiologic factors is necessary to develop a therapeutic strategy (Fig. 20.1). The initial approach to fatigue should involve a screening tool. The recommended screen for cancer-related fatigue begins with a simple question: How would you rate your fatigue on a scale of 0 to 10 over the past 7 days? The score generated from this scale can drive the approach to treatment. A score of 0 to 3 is considered mild, 4 to 6 moderate, and greater than 6 severe. Those in the moderate to severe range should be evaluated immediately, but mild

fatigue may be reevaluated. Evaluation of fatigue can then be approached differently depending on the patient's being in active treatment, remission, or the end of life. Patients screening positive for moderate to severe fatigue should undergo a comprehensive assessment includes the description of fatigue-related phenomena, a physical examination, and a review of laboratory and imaging studies that may allow a possible hypothesis concerning pathogenesis, which, in turn, may suggest appropriate treatment strategies. Patients may describe fatigue in terms of decreased vitality or lack of energy, muscular weakness, dysphoric mood, insomnia, impaired cognitive functioning, or some combination of these disturbances. Although this variability suggests the existence of fatigue subtypes, this has not yet been confirmed. Regardless, the patient's history should clarify the spectrum of complaints and attempt to characterize features associated with each component. This information may suggest specific causes (eg, depression) and influence the choice of therapy. Neurologic and psychological evaluation may also help further clarify potential causes of fatigue in some patients. Other characteristics are similarly important. Onset and duration, for example, distinguish acute and chronic fatigue. Acute fatigue of recent onset is anticipated to end in the near future. Chronic fatigue is persistent for a prolonged period (weeks to months or longer), and it is not expected to remit in a short time. Patients perceived to have chronic fatigue typically require more intensive evaluation as well as a management approach focused on both short- and long-term goals. Other important descriptors of fatigue include the severity, daily pattern, course over time, exacerbating and palliative factors, and associated distress. An assessment of cancer-related fatigue should also include consideration of broader concerns, including global QoL, other symptoms, and disease status. Fatigue may be only one of numerous factors that influence QoL. Among these factors are progressive physical decline, psychological disorders, social isolation, financial concerns, and spiritual distress. Optimal care of the cancer patient includes a broader assessment of these factors and should be directed toward maintaining or enhancing QoL. Successful strategies should ameliorate fatigue within a broader approach of patient care. Evaluation of the patient regarding the nature of fatigue, options for therapy, and anticipated outcomes is an essential aspect of the therapy. **Unfortunately, results of a patient survey indicate that patients and their oncologists seldom discuss fatigue.**

An initial approach to cancer-related fatigue includes efforts to correct potential etiologies, if possible and appropriate. This may include elimination of nonessential centrally acting drugs, treatment of a sleep disorder, reversal of anemia or metabolic abnormalities, or management of major depression. Referring to the National Comprehensive Cancer Network (NCCN) guidelines for the approach to pain, emotional distress, anemia, and nutrition may prove helpful. Perhaps sleep disturbances, interventions aimed at increasing activity levels, and the management of comorbidities may be more straightforward. Many of these initial interventions are relatively simple and pose minimal burdens to the patient, health care provider, and caregiver.

PATIENT WITH CANCER-RELATED FATIGUE

FIGURE 20.1 Evaluation and approach to management of a patient with cancer-related fatigue. *Hgb,* Hemoglobin; *TIBC,* Total iron-binding capacity. (Adapted from Portenoy RK, Itri LM: Cancer-related fatigue: guidelines for evaluation and management. *Oncologist* 1999;4(1):1-10. Copyright 1999 AlphaMed Press. All rights reserved.)

In general, education and counselling are advised in the initial treatment of cancer-related fatigue. Patients and family may be requested to document fatigue levels in a diary or on a scale and to describe associations or exacerbations and timing of the symptom. Similar to the approach to urinary incontinence, patients may be counseled toward behavior modifications or adjustments to help avoid this symptom such as eliminating nonessential potentially "tiring" behaviors that may call for unnecessary expenditure of energy. Conversely, increasing physical activity has been proposed as a treatment for cancer-related fatigue. A Cochrane analysis demonstrated improvements in fatigue with an exercise intervention. Adherence to the US Surgeon General's recommendations for 30 minutes of exercise on most days of the week may thus be advisable for cancer patients in recovery. Physical therapy referrals should be made in certain patients, and caution with activity should be obvious in certain patients such as those with bone metastasis, neutropenia, anemia, thrombocytopenia, or active infection. Therapies such as massage, acupuncture, or psychosocial interventions are also described in the NCCN guidelines.

In patients with fatigue-associated major depression, treatment with an antidepressant is strongly indicated. As many as 25% of cancer patients develop major depression at some point during their illnesses. Patients at greatest risk are those with advanced disease, uncontrolled physical symptoms (eg, pain), or a previous history of a psychiatric disorder. Although the relationship between depression and fatigue is not well understood, they often occur together and both adversely affect QoL. **Despite the high prevalence in the cancer population, depression is often underdiagnosed and consequently undertreated.** A trial with an antidepressant is usually warranted in a patient with fatigue associated with any significant degree of depressed mood and similarly can be therapeutic when concurrent anxiety or pain exists. In addition, brief, focused psychological counseling can be helpful for several reasons when a mood disorder (eg, depression or anxiety) and a physical symptom (eg, pain or fatigue) co-occur. First, counseling offers the patient an opportunity to identify and express her fears, which are often driving the depressed or anxious mood. Second, the depressed or anxious mood can exacerbate existing physical symptoms such as pain. Therefore, provision of counseling has the dual benefit of reducing the mood disorder, which by extension reduces fatigue and pain. Third, brief, focused counseling can offer the patient important behavioral modifications such as time and energy management strategies that permit and teach the patient to conserve energy physically and emotionally for the priorities in their life. This is useful to address the practical challenges associated with fatigue and pain management.

Anemia may be a major factor in the development of cancer-related fatigue. Anecdotally, transfusion therapy for severe anemia has often been associated with substantial improvement in fatigue. Compared to other cancers, gynecologic cancers are especially known for being associated with severe anemia, with hemoglobin levels less than 9.9 g/dL in many cases. Not only does anemia have a significant correlation

with poor performance status, but it may also be implicated in tumor sensitivity to radiation and chemotherapy. It has been suggested that an optimal oxygen level for tumors to respond to therapy is reflected by a hemoglobin level between 12 and 14 g/dL. However, recent data of increased risk of thrombotic event associated with hemoglobin level higher than 12 g/dL should be taken into consideration.

New data demonstrate the association between chemotherapy-induced mild to moderate anemia and both fatigue and QoL impairment. For example, combined data from 413 patients and three randomized placebo controlled trials of epoetin alfa, the recombinant form of human erythropoietin (EPO), reveal that treated patients experienced a significant increase in hematocrit, a reduced need for transfusion, and a significant improvement in overall QoL. Patients with an increase in hematocrit of greater than 6% also demonstrated significant improvement in energy level and daily activities. Additional studies in patients treated with chemotherapy and radiation therapy for various gynecologic tumors confirm that epoetin alfa has positive effects on hemoglobin levels. Two large, prospective, randomized, multicenter community trials have demonstrated that patients experience significant improvement in energy levels, activity level, functional status, and overall QoL when epoetin alfa is administered as an adjunct to cytotoxic chemotherapy.

Blood transfusion is an option for the treatment of cancer-related anemia; however, transfusions are associated with poor outcomes and QoL caused by infections, allergies, or dependence on medical centers. For those reasons, many practitioners rely on growth factors, including epoetin alfa (rHuEPO—Epogen or Procrit) or darbepoetin alfa (Aranesp), to treat anemia. Kurz et al. concluded that rHuEPO increases hemoglobin levels and decreases transfusions in patients with gynecologic malignancies undergoing polychemotherapy without compromising QoL. It has even been suggested that rHuEPO may be given prophylactically in older patients (>65 years) and those with baseline hemoglobin levels of less than 10.5 g/dL who are going to be given chemotherapy consisting of carboplatin and paclitaxel. Although Aranesp has a longer half-life and therefore may be given less frequently, there are few clear advantages compared with Procrit. Unfortunately, this therapy is not without risks, and there are concerns that the risk of venous thromboembolism (VTE) is increased for these patients. Results from meta-analyses from 2008 to 2013 indicated an association between increased risk of thrombotic events and erythropoiesis-stimulating agents (ESA) usage with statistically significant risk and odds ratios ranging from 1.48 to 1.69. The increased risk for thromboembolism in patients with cancer became a black box warning in the updated Food and Drug Administration (FDA) labels and subsequently as part of the Risk Evaluation and Mitigation Strategy (REMS). The increase FDA restrictions stemmed from eight randomized studies showing a decrease in OS or decreased locoregional disease control with EPO usage, including a cervical cancer study. More recently, research has shown that survival may be decreased in women receiving rHuEPO for correction of anemia for hemoglobin levels over 12 g/dL. Therefore, currently, patients with cancer may be counseled about the risks and benefits of the use of growth factors for the correction of anemia.

The NCCN and ASCO guidelines recommends that EPO should not be recommended to patients who are receiving myelosuppressive chemotherapy with curative intent. Patients who are undergoing palliative treatment may receive EPO under REMS guidelines and with the informed consent of the patient. Many of the pharmacologic therapies for fatigue associated with medical illness have not been rigorously evaluated in controlled trials. Nonetheless, there is evidence to support the use of several drug classes. Psychostimulants, such as methylphenidate and dextroamphetamine, have been well studied for the treatment of opioid-related somnolence and cognitive impairment and depression in elderly and medically ill patients. There are no controlled studies of these drugs for cancer-related fatigue, but empiric administration may yield favorable results in some patients. The national guidelines, however, are cautious in their suggestion of these interventions.

A clinical response to one drug does not necessarily predict a response to the others, and sequential trials may be needed to identify the most beneficial therapy. Methylphenidate has been more extensively evaluated in the cancer population than other stimulant drugs and is often the first drug to be administered. It is available in a chewable formulation that can be absorbed through the buccal mucosa for patients who are unable to swallow or take oral medications.

Adverse effects associated with the psychostimulants include anorexia, insomnia, tremulousness, anxiety, delirium, and tachycardia. To ensure safety, slow and careful dose escalation should be undertaken to minimize potential adverse effects. A regimen of methylphenidate, for example, usually begins with a dose of 5 to 10 mg once or twice daily (morning and, if needed, midday). If the drug is tolerated, the dose is increased. Most patients appear to require less than 60 mg/day, but some require much higher doses.

Extensive anecdotal observations and very limited data from controlled trials support the use of low-dose corticosteroid therapy in fatigued patients with advanced disease and multiple symptoms. Dexamethasone and prednisone are most commonly used. There have been no comparative trials.

The selective serotonin reuptake inhibitors, secondary amine tricyclics (eg, nortriptyline and desipramine), and bupropion are sometimes associated with the experience of increased energy that appears disproportionate to any change in mood. For this reason, these agents have also been tried empirically in nondepressed patients with fatigue. Given the limited experience in the use of these drugs for this indication, an empirical trial should be considered only in severe and refractory cases.

Amantadine has been used to treat fatigue in patients with multiple sclerosis, but it has not been studied in other patient populations. This drug is usually well tolerated, and an empirical trial may be warranted in selected patients with severe refractory cancer-related fatigue.

Nonpharmacologic approaches for the management of cancer-related fatigue are supported mainly by favorable anecdotal experience (Table 20.8). Patient preferences should be

TABLE 20.8 Nonpharmacologic Interventions for the Management of Cancer-Related Fatigue
Patient Education
Consider the patient's preferences, education level, and readiness to learn
Use of a patient's diary
Exercise
Individualize exercise program
Use of rhythmic and repetitive types of exercise
Initiate gradually
Modification of Activity and Rest Patterns
Assess sleep hygiene
Establish routine sleep patterns
Avoid use of stimulants before sleep
Regular exercise
Stress Management and Cognitive Therapies
Use of stress reduction techniques or cognitive therapies
Use of relaxation therapy, hypnosis, or distraction
Adequate nutrition and hydration
Proper diet
Monitor weight and hydration status regularly
Referral to a dietitian

Adapted from Portenoy RK. *Principles and Practice of Supportive Oncology.* Philadelphia, 1998, Lippincott-Raven, pp 109-118.

considered in the selection of one or more of these approaches. In particular, sleep hygiene principles should be tailored to the individual patients and might include the establishment of a specific bedtime, awake time, and routine procedures before sleep. Patients should also be instructed to avoid stimulants and central nervous system (CNS) depressants before going to sleep. Whereas regular exercise performed at least 6 hours before bedtime may improve sleep, napping in the late afternoon or evening may worsen it.

Cancer and its treatment can also interfere with dietary intake. With aggressive approaches to management, the patient's weight, hydration status, and electrolyte balance should be monitored and maintained to every extent possible. Regular exercise may improve appetite and increase nutritional appetite. Referral to a dietitian for nutritional guidance and suggestions for nutritional supplements may be useful.

The NCCN cancer-related fatigue guidelines were recently updated. This update includes further emphasizing the incorporation of fatigue as a cancer patient's "vital sign." Specific attention should now be paid toward improving sleep hygiene and enhancing the education of family members on cancer-related fatigue. In summary, the strategy aimed at combating fatigue should include physical activity, psychosocial interventions (ie, mindfulness-based therapy), nutrition counselling, and sleep interventions. Pharmacologic interventions such as psychostimulants can be used, but particular attention toward medications to address comorbidities, sleep, pain, anemia and mood is considered important.

Pain

Cancer pain can be managed effectively through relatively simple means in up to 90% of the 8 million Americans who have cancer or a history of cancer. Unfortunately, pain associated with cancer is often undertreated. Although cancer pain or associated symptoms cannot always be eliminated, proper use of available therapies can effectively relieve pain for most patients. Management of pain extends beyond pain relief and encompasses the patient's QoL and the ability to work productively, to enjoy recreation, and to function normally in the family and society.

State and local laws often restrict the medical use of opioids to relieve cancer pain, and third-party payers may not reimburse for noninvasive pain control treatments. Thus, clinicians should work with regulators, state cancer pain initiatives, and other groups to eliminate these health care system barriers to effective pain management (Table 20.9).

Flexibility is the key to management of cancer pain. Thorough discussions with the patient and their families encouraging them to be active in pain management are critical (Table 20.10). Patients often need reassurance to report pain because effective treatment strategies exist. Failure to assess pain is a critical factor leading to undertreatment. Thus, a simple screening tool should be used to inquire about the patient's pain level. This is described as "universal screening" by the NCCN. The goal of the initial assessment of pain is to characterize the pain by location, intensity, and etiology. This can be accomplished through a detailed history, physical examination, social assessment, and diagnostic evaluation. The mainstay of pain assessment is patient self-reporting. To enhance pain management across all settings, clinicians should teach patients to use pain assessment tools in their homes. Clinicians should listen to the patient's descriptive words about the quality of the pain, inquiring about its location, severity, and aggravating or relieving factors and the patient's cognitive response to the discomfort. Finally, goals for pain control should be clear with active engagement of the patient in the decision process. Continued assessment of cancer pain is crucial. Changes in pain patterns and the development of new pain should trigger diagnostic evaluation and modification of the treatment plan. Persistent pain indicates the need to consider other etiologies (eg, related to disease progression or treatment, and alternative—perhaps more invasive—treatment; Fig. 20.2). Pain related to an oncologic emergency should be addressed immediately. This includes pain resulting from a bone fracture or impending fracture, brain or epidural metastases, infection, or obstructed or perforated viscous.

Drug therapy is the cornerstone of cancer pain management. It is effective, relatively low risk, and inexpensive and usually works quickly. Even within the same family of analgesic drugs, individual variations in tolerability and side effects are well recognized. Recommendations for pharmacologic therapy begin with the World Health Organization (WHO) ladder (Fig. 20.3), a three-step hierarchy for analgesic pain management. Substitution of drugs within a category should be tried before switching therapy. The simplest dosage and schedule as well as the least invasive pain management modality should be attempted first. For mild to moderate pain, nonsteroidal antiinflammatory drugs (NSAIDs) (WHO ladder step 1) are often effective (see Table 20.10). When pain persists or increases (Table 20.11), opioids can be added (WHO ladder step 2). Moderate to severe pain requires opioids of higher potency and dose (WHO ladder step 3) (Table 20.12). Dosing should be on a regular schedule (ie, "by the clock") to maintain a level of drugs that would help prevent the recurrence of pain. Ask for patient and family cooperation in establishing the effective level when administering medications to prevent long-term cancer pain on an around-the-clock basis with additional doses ("as needed" and usually required).

TABLE 20.9   Barriers to Cancer Pain Management

Problems related to health care professionals
Inadequate knowledge of pain management
Poor assessment of pain
Concern about regulation of controlled substances
Fear of patient addiction
Concern about side effects of analgesics
Concern about patients becoming tolerant to analgesics
Problems related to patients
Lack of cultural competency and communication
Reluctance to report pain
- Concern about distracting physicians from treatment of underlying disease
- Fear that pain means disease is worse
- Concern about not being a "good" patient
Reluctance to take pain medications
- Fear of addiction or of being thought of as an addict
- Worries about unmanageable side effects
- Concern about becoming tolerant to pain medications
Problems related to the health care system
Low priority given to cancer pain treatment
Inadequate reimbursement
- The most appropriate treatment may not be reimbursed or may be too costly for patients and families.
Restrictive regulation of controlled substances
- Problems of availability of treatment or access to it

Adapted from U.S. Department of Health and Human Services. *Management of Cancer Pain: Adults.* Washington, DC, 1994, Author.

TABLE 20.10   Recommended Clinical Approach

A Ask about pain regularly.
Assess pain systematically.
B Believe the patient and family in their reports of pain and what relieves it.
C Choose pain control options appropriate for the patient, family, and setting.
D Deliver interventions in a timely, logical, coordinated fashion.
E Empower patients and their families.
Enable patients to control their course to the greatest extent possible.

Adapted from U.S. Department of Health and Human Services. *Management of Cancer Pain: Adults.* Washington, DC, 1994, Author.

FIGURE 20.2 Continuing pain management. *IV,* Intravenous; *NSAID,* nonsteroidal antiinflammatory drug; *PCA,* patient-controlled analgesia; *SC,* subcutaneous. (Adapted from U.S. Department of Health and Human Services. *Management of Cancer Pain: Adults.* Washington, DC, 1994, Author.)

Oral administration is preferred because it is convenient and usually cost effective. When patients cannot take oral medications, other less invasive (eg, rectal or transdermal) routes should be offered. Parenteral methods should be used only when simpler, less demanding, less costly methods are inappropriate or ineffective. An assessment of the patient's response to several different oral opioids is usually advisable before abandoning the oral route in favor of parenteral, neurosurgical, or other invasive approaches. Rectal administration is a safe, inexpensive, and effective route for the delivery of opioids as well as nonopioids when patients have nausea or vomiting. Rectal administration is inappropriate for patients who have

diarrhea, anal or rectal involvement, or mucositis; are neutropenic or thrombocytopenic; are physically unable to place the suppository in the rectum; or who prefer other routes. Transdermal administration is also feasible but does not allow rapid dose titration. Patient-controlled analgesia (PCA) devices can be used both on an inpatient or outpatient basis. The opioid may be administered orally or via a dedicated portable pump to deliver the drug intravenously, subcutaneously, or epidurally (intraspinally). Intraspinal administration should be considered for patients who develop intractable pain or intolerable side effects from other routes of administration. Use of this route requires skill and expertise that may not be available in certain

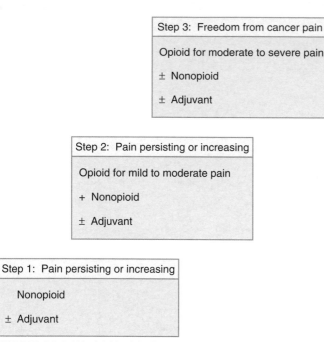

Step 3: Freedom from cancer pain

Opioid for moderate to severe pain

± Nonopioid

± Adjuvant

Step 2: Pain persisting or increasing

Opioid for mild to moderate pain

+ Nonopioid

± Adjuvant

Step 1: Pain persisting or increasing

Nonopioid

± Adjuvant

FIGURE 20.3 World Health Organization three-step analgesic ladder. (Adapted from World Health Organization. *Cancer Pain Relief and Palliative Care.* Geneva, Switzerland, 1990, Author.)

settings. Table 20.13 presents the advantages and disadvantages of regional administration. This route is often efficacious because gynecologic tumors often affect the pelvis, making profound analgesia frequently possible without motor or sympathetic blockade. Drugs and routes of administration that are not recommended for the management of cancer pain are summarized in Table 20.14.

The general principles to pain management are described by the NCCN and were updated in 2015. This includes a dose of medication that sustains pain relief for the full time period before the next dose. The dose should be calculated based on the patient's requirements for the previous 24 hours. A sustained dose with an around-the-clock medication should be started in addition to an as needed medication. The around the clock and as needed doses are increased based on the severity of the uncontrolled pain. Of note, noncombination opioid preparations are preferred to eliminate the risk of overdosing acetaminophen or ibuprofen. The "as needed" medication should be about 10% to 20% of the sustained total 24-hour dose. Before converting to a transdermal approach, the pain should be relatively well-controlled by an around-the-clock opioid pain regimen. The maximum fentanyl transdermal dose is 100 mcg/h, but if a patient requires a higher dose, multiple patches may be used. An IV dose of 0.67 mg/day of IV morphine or 2 mg/day of oral morphine is equivalent to 1 mcg/h of transdermal fentanyl. Although the patch lasts typically for 72 hours, cachectic patients, fever, or heat from external sources such as electric blankets may increase the absorption of the transdermal fentanyl and thus may be contraindications to patch use. Some patients may require a new patch every 48 hours. The idea of opioid rotating to decrease cost, intolerance, or a change in the patient's condition is suggested.

Clinicians who follow patients during long-term opioid treatment should watch for potential side effects and administer agents to manage them, and, in some cases, prophylactically. Constipation, as well as nausea and vomiting, both common side effects to opioid analgesics, are discussed later. Drug-induced sedation is common and can be treated by a reduction in opioid dose or use of low-dose CNS stimulants such as caffeine, methylphenidate, dextroamphetamine, or modafinil in the morning or early afternoon may be considered. Patients should also be assured that tolerance may develop over time, especially after an opioid dose escalation. Patients receiving long-term opioid therapy generally develop tolerance to the respiratory depressant effects of these agents. When indicated for reversal of opioid-induced respiratory depression, administration of naloxone is recommended with titration in small increments to improve respiratory function without reversing analgesia. Careful monitoring is mandatory until the episode of respiratory depression resolves. For more subacute respiratory depression, simply withholding one or two doses until the symptoms resolve followed by restarting at 25% of the total dose is often effective. A combination of opioids and NSAIDs is frequently used to optimize cancer pain management, especially in patients with bone and lymphatic involvements. Dry mouth, urinary retention, pruritus, myoclonus, altered cognitive function, dysphoria, euphoria, sleep disturbances, sexual dysfunction, physiologic dependence, tolerance, and inappropriate secretion of antidiuretic hormone are also reported side effects of opioid agents.

Adjuvant drugs are valuable during all phases of pain management to enhance the analgesic efficacy, treat concurrent symptoms, and provide independent analgesia for specific types of pain. These adjuvants include corticosteroids, anticonvulsants, antidepressants, neuroleptics, local analgesics, hydroxyzine, and psychostimulants. Corticosteroids provide a range of effects, including mood elevation, antiinflammatory activity, antiemetic activity, and appetite stimulation, and may be beneficial in the management of cachexia and anorexia. They also reduce cerebral and spinal cord edema and are essential in the emergency management of elevated intracranial pressure and epidural spinal cord compression. Anticonvulsant agents are used to manage neuropathic pain, especially lancinating or burning pain. They should be used with caution when administered to patients undergoing marrow suppressant therapy such as chemotherapy and radiation. Tricyclic antidepressants (TCAs) are useful in the pharmacologic management of neuropathic pain. These drugs have innate analgesic properties and may potentiate the analgesic effects of opioids. Perhaps the most widely reported experience has been with amitriptyline, a tertiary amine, which may be more efficacious but secondary amines (ie, nortriptyline, imipramine) are usually better tolerated. The use of serotonin–norepinephrine reuptake inhibitors such as duloxetine and venlafaxine have increased because of better tolerance. More frequently, anticonvulsants have become more popular, especially with the availability of pregabalin, which has a more desirable side effect profile than the antidepressants and less dizziness than its parent drug, gabapentin.

Text continued on p. 547

TABLE 20.11 Dosing Regimens for Acetaminophen and Nonsteroidal Antiinflammatory Drugs*

Medications	Common Proprietary (Trade) Name	Usual Daily Dose (Adults) Dosage and Route	Frequency	Usual Daily Dose or Maximum Dose (Adults)
Acetaminophen	Tylenol, others	325–650 mg PO	q4h	Immediate release: 3250 mg
		650–1000 mg PO	qid	ER: 3900 mg
		650 mg PR	q4h	
SALICYLATES				
Aspirin (acetylsalicylic acid)	Others	600–1000 mg PO	qid	4000 mg
Same for buffered and enteric-coated oral formulations		300–600 mg PR	q4h	
Magnesium salicylates	Doan's, others	650 mg PO	qid	4000 mg
Choline magnesium trisalicylate	Trilisate	500–1000 mg PO	tid	4000 mg
		750–1500 mg	bid	
Diflunisal	Others	500–750 mg PO	bid	1500 mg
Salsalate	Disalcid	750–1500 mg PO	bid	3000 mg
PROPIONIC ACID DERIVATIVES				
Fenoprofen	Nalfon, others	200–600 mg PO	qid	3200 mg
Flurbiprofen	others	50–75 mg PO	qid	300 mg
Ibuprofen (OTC and Rx)	Motrin, Advil, Midol, others	200–000 mg PO	qid	3200 mg
Ketoprofen	Others	25–75 mg PO	tid–qid	300 mg
		200 mg ER PO	daily	200 mg XR
Naproxen	Aleve, Anaprox Naprosyn, EC-Naprosyn, Midol, Pamprin, others	220–500 mg PO	bid–tid	1500 mg
		750–1000 mg ER PO	daily	1000 mg ER
Oxaprozin	Daypro, others	600–1200 mg PO	Daily	1800 mg
ACETIC ACID DERIVATIVES				
Diclofenac	Voltaren, Voltaren-XR, Cataflam, Flector (transdermal), others	50–75 mg PO	bid-tid	200 mg (PO)
		100 mg–XR	Daily–bid	32 g/day total to affected area(s)
		1%–3% patch, Gel, cream, solution (TDS)	bid	
Indomethacin	Indocin, Indomethacin ER	25–50 mg PO	tid–qid	200 mg (both PO and PR)
		75 mg ER PO	bid	150 mg ER
		50 mg PR	bid–tid	
Sulindac	Others	150–200 mg PO	bid	400 mg
Tolmetin	Others	400–600 mg PO	tid	1800 mg
PYRANOCARBOXYLIC ACID				
Etodolac	Others	200–400 mg PO	tid–qid	1000 mg
		400–600 mg ER PO	Daily–bid	1200 mg ER
PYRROLIZINE CARBOXYLIC ACID				
Ketorolac	Sprix (intranasal), Others	10 mg PO	qid	40 mg
		15.75 mg/nostril	tid–qid	126 mg (intranasal)
		15–30 mg IM/IV	qid	120 mg–IM/IV
FENAMATES (ANTHRANILIC ACIDS)				
Meclofenamate	Others	50–100 mg PO	tid–qid	400 mg
Mefenamic acid	Ponstel, others	250 mg PO	qid	not established
ENOLIC ACID DERIVATIVES				
Meloxicam	Mobic, others	7.5–15 mg PO	daily	15 mg
Piroxicam	Feldene, others	10-20 mg PO	daily	20 mg
NAPHTHALAKANONE				
Nabumetone	Others	1000–2000 mg PO	daily	2000 mg
COX-2 SELECTIVE AGENT				
Celecoxib	Celebrex, others	50–200 mg	daily-bid	Not established

*Most nonsteroidal antiinflammatory drugs have negligible hepatic metabolism, except for etodolac, ketorolac, nabumetone, oxaprozin, and meloxicam. Celecoxib and mefenamic acid undergo metabolism via cytochrome P450 2C9 isoenzymes. Excretion is via the kidney, primarily as metabolites. Sulindac and nabumetone are inactive prodrugs converted by the liver to active metabolites

bid, Twice a day; *ER*, extended release; *IM*, intramuscular; *IV*, intravenous; *OTC*, over the counter; *PO*, oral; *PR*, rectal; *q*, every; *qid*; four times a day; *Rx*, prescription; *SR*, sustained release; *TDS*, transdermal; *tid*, three times a day; *XR*, extended release.
Data from Pain Management for Primary Care Clinicians. Arthur G. Lipman, editor. 2004; Guideline for the Management of Cancer Pain in Adults and Children. American Pain Society 2005 and Facts and Comparisions® E Answers, 2015 Wolters Kluwer Health.

TABLE 20.12 Dosing of Opioid Analgesics for the Management of Persistent Cancer Pain

Medication	Proprietary (Trade) Name	Usual Starting Dose for Moderate to Severe Cancer Pain in Adults ≥50 kg of Body Weight			Usual Starting Dose for Moderate to Severe Cancer Pain in Adults <50 kg of Body Weight			Approximate Equianalgesic Dosing of Opioid Analgesics in Adults[s]		
		Oral	Parenteral	Rectal	Oral	Parenteral	Rectal	Oral	Parenteral	Rectal
Codeine		15–60 mg q4h	NA	NA	0.5–1 mg/kg q4h	NA	NA	NA	NA	NA
Codeine combination products	Tylenol #2, #3, #4; others	1–2 tablets q4h (maximum, acetaminophen 4000 mg/day)	NA	NA	Codeine: 0.5–1 mg/kg q4h Acetaminophen: 10–15 mg/kg q4h	NA	NA	Per codeine recommendations above		NA
Hydrocodone	Hysingla ER (24 h) Zohydro ER (12 h)	20 mg/day or 10 mg bid	NA	NA	NA	NA	NA	20 mg	NA	NA
Hydrocodone–acetaminophen combination products	Vicodin, Lorcet, Lortab, Norco others	1–2 tablets q4h (maximum, acetaminophen 4000 mg/day)	NA	NA	Hydrocodone: 0.135 mg/kg q4h; acetaminophen: 10–15 mg/kg q4h	NA	NA	20 mg	NA	NA
Hydrocodone–ibuprofen (200-mg) combination products	Vicoprofen, Xylon, others	1 tablet q4h (maximum, ibuprofen 3200/day)	NA	NA	NA	NA	NA	20 mg	NA	NA
Fentanyl	Duragesic (TDS); Sublimaze, others (IV); (Fentora [buccal]; Actiq [lozenge]; Lazanda [intranasal]; and Abstral, Subsys [SL]—for breakthrough pain only)	Buccal: 100 mcg/dose, MRx1 Lozenge: 200 mcg/dose, MRx1 SL: 100 mcg/dose, MRX1	TDS: 25 mcg/h q 72h mcg/kg Intranasal: 100 mcg/spray, MRX1 in 2 h IV: 20–50 mcg/h	NA	NA	TDS: 12 mcg/h q72h for opioid-tolerant patients IV: 0.5 mcg/kg/h	NA	NA	0.1 mg TDS and IV	NA
Hydromorphone	Dilaudid; Exalgo. other (ER tablet)	2–4 mg q4h; 8 mg: ER daily	0.2–0.6 mg q2h	3 mg 6h	0.03–0.08 mg/kg/dose q 4 hr (maximum, 5 mg/dose)	1 mcg/kg/h	NA	7.5 mg	1.5 mg	3 mg
Levorphanol	Others	2 mg q6h	NA	NA	NA	NA	NA	4 mg	2 mg	NA
Meperidine	Demerol, others	50–150 mg q3h	50–150 mg q3h 10 mg/h	NA	1.1–1.5 mg/kg q 3 hr	1.1–1.8 mg/kg q3h	NA	300 mg	75 mg	NA
Methadone	Dolophine, others	2.5 mg q8h	2.5 mg q8h	NA	0.7 mg/kg q 4 hr	0.7 mg/kg q4h	NA	20 mg	10 mg	NA
Morphine immediate release	Others	5 mg q4h (tablet) 10 mg q4h (solution)	10 mg q4hr; 1 mg/h	10–20 mg q 4 hr	0.02–0.5 mg/kg/dose q 4 hr	0.05–0.1 mg/kg/dose q4; 0.005 mg/kg/h	NA	60 mg	10 mg	60 mg

Drug	Products/Other names	Dose	Dose	Dose (children/<50 kg)	‡				
Morphine ER	Kadian (ER); Avinza (ER); MS Contin (CR); others	MS Contin: 15 mg q12h; Kadian: 30 mg/day; Avinza: 30 mg/day	MS Contin: 15–30 mg q 12 hr	0.3–0.6 mg/kg/dose q 12 hr	NA	NA	30 mg	NA	30 mg
Oxycodone	Others	10 mg q4h	NA	0.1–0.2 mg/kg q4h	NA	NA	60 mg	NA	NA
Oxycodone ER	OxyContin, others	10 mg q12h	10 mg q 12 h	NA	NA	NA	20 mg	NA	13 mg
Oxycodone combination products	Percocet, Xartemis XR (with acetaminophen 32 5 mg); oxycodone–ibuprofen 400 mg	5 mg q6h (maximum, APAP, 4000 mg/day; ibuprofen 3200 mg/day)	NA	0.1–0.2 mg/kg q 4 hr	NA	NA	NA	NA	NA
	Others	1 tablet q 2h (XR)							
Oxymorphone immediate release	Opana, others	10 mg q4h	0.5 mg q4h	NA	NA	NA	6.6	1	NA
Oxymorphone ER	Opana ER, others	5 mg q12h	NA	NA	NA	NA	3.3	NA	NA
Tapentadol	Nucynta	50 mg q4h	NA	NA	NA	NA	NA	NA	NA
Tapentadol ER	Nucynta ER	100 mg q12 h	NA	NA	NA	NA	NA	NA	NA
Tramadol	Ultram, Ultram ER, others	25–50 mg q6 h (maximum, 400 mg/day); ER: 100 mg/day (maximum, 300 mg/day)	NA	NA	NA	NA	NA	NA	NA
Tramadol 37.5 mg + acetaminophen 325 mg	Ultracet, others	2 tablets q6h	NA	NA	NA	NA	NA	NA	NA

*Caution: Recommended doses do not apply to patients with renal or hepatic insufficiency or other conditions affecting drug metabolism and kinetics.

†Fentanyl TDS: Doses above 25 µ/h should not be used in opioid-naive patients.

‡Recommended doses do not apply to patients with renal or hepatic insufficiency or other conditions affecting drug metabolism and kinetics. Starting doses should be lower for elderly patients.

§Published tables vary in the suggested doses that are equianalgesic to morphine. Clinical response is the criterion that must be applied for each patient; titration to clinical responses is necessary. Because there is not complete cross-tolerance among these drugs, it is usually necessary to use a lower than equianalgesic dose when changing drugs and to retitrate to response.

APAP, acetaminophen; bid, twice a day; CR, controlled-release; ER, extended release; IM, intramuscular; MRX1, may repeat one time as needed; NA, not available; q, every; SC, subcutaneous; SL, sublingual; TDS, transdermal; XR, extended release.

Modified from Management of Cancer Pain: Adults. Washington, D.C., U.S. Dept of Health and Human Services, March 1994.

Data from Facts and Comparisions® E Answers, 2015 Wolters Kluwer Health.

TABLE 20.13 Advantages and Disadvantages of Intraspinal Drug Administration

System	Advantages	Disadvantages
Percutaneous temporary catheter	Used extensively both intraoperatively and postoperatively Useful when the prognosis is limited (<1 mo)	Mechanical problems include dislodgment, kinking, and catheter migration
Permanent silicone-rubber epidural	Catheter implantation is a minor procedure Dislodgment and infection are less common than with temporary catheters Bolus injections, continuous infusions, or PCA (with or without continuous delivery) can be given	
Subcutaneous implanted injection	Increased stability; less risk of dislodgment Can deliver bolus injections or continuous infusions (with or without PCA) Useful when the prognosis is limited (<1 mo)	Implantation more invasive than external port Approved only for epidural catheter in the United States Potential for infection increases with frequent injections Need for more extensive procedure
Subcutaneous reservoir	Potentially reduced infection in comparison with external system	Difficult to access, and fibrosis may occur after repeated injection
Implanted pumps (continuous and programmable)		Potentially decreased risk of infection Need for more extensive operative procedure; need for equipment with programmable systems

PCA, Patient-controlled analgesia.
Adapted from U.S. Department of Health and Human Services. *Management of Cancer Pain: Adults.* Washington, DC, 1994, Author.

TABLE 20.14 Drugs and Routes of Administration Not Recommended for Treatment of Cancer Pain

Class	Drug	Rationale for Not Recommending
Opioids	Meperidine	Short (2- to 3-h) duration; repeated administration may lead to CNS toxicity (tremor, confusion, or seizures) because of cumulation of neurotoxic active metabolite, normeperidine; high oral doses required to relieve severe pain (especially >800 mg/day and in the presence of renal dysfunction); may further increase the risk of CNS toxicity
Miscellaneous	Cannabinoids	Side effects of dysphoria, drowsiness, hypotension, and bradycardia preclude its routine use as an analgesic
	Cocaine	Has demonstrated no efficacy as an analgesic or co-analgesic in combination with opioids
Opioid agonist–antagonists	Pentazocine Butorphanol Nalbuphine	Risk of precipitating withdrawal in opioid-dependent patients; analgesic ceiling; possible production of unpleasant psychomimetic effects (eg, hallucinations)
Partial agonist	Buprenorphine	Analgesic ceiling; can precipitate withdrawal
Antagonist	Naloxone Naltrexone	May precipitate withdrawal; limit use to treatment of life-threatening respiratory depression
Combination preparations	Brompton's cocktail	No evidence of analgesic benefit to using Brompton's cocktail over single opioid analgesics Painful; absorption unreliable; should not be used for short (2- to 3-h) duration;
	DPT (meperidine, promethazine and chlorpromazine)	Efficacy poor compared with that of other analgesics; high incidence of adverse effects
Anxiolytics	Benzodiazepine (eg, alprazolam)	Analgesic properties not demonstrated except for some cases of neuropathic pain; added sedation from anxiolytics may limit opioid dosing
Sedative–hypnotic drugs	Barbiturates Benzodiazepine	Analgesic properties not demonstrated; added sedation sedative–hypnotic drugs limit opioid dosing

Route of Administration	Rationale for Not Recommending	
Intramuscular	Painful; absorption unreliable; should not be used for children or patients likely to develop dependent edema or in patients with thrombocytopenia	

CNS, Central nervous system.
Adapted from U.S. Department of Health and Human Services. *Management of Cancer Pain: Adults.* Washington, DC, 1994, Author.

Local analgesics have been used to treat neuropathic pain but are limited in their effectiveness without concurrent use of an opioid, antidepressant, and/or anticonvulsant. Psychostimulants, as discussed earlier, may be useful in reducing opioid-induced sedation when opioid dose adjustment (eg, reduced dose and lengthening dosing intervals) is not effective.

Patients should be encouraged to remain active and participate in self-care when possible. Noninvasive physical and psychosocial modalities can be used concurrently with drugs and other interventions to manage pain during all phases of treatment. The effectiveness of these modalities depends on the patient's participation and communication concerning which methods best alleviate pain. **Generalized weakness, deconditioning, and aches and pains associated with cancer diagnosis and therapy may be treated by cutaneous stimulation such as heat or cold, massage, pressure, and vibration.** Unfortunately, these modalities sometimes increase pain before relief occurs. Massage should not be substituted for exercise in ambulatory patients. Exercise is useful for treating subacute and chronic pain because it strengthens weak muscles, mobilizes stiff joints, and helps to restore coordination and balance, thus enhancing patient comfort and providing cardiovascular conditioning. Physical therapists may be consulted to increase weightbearing exercise. Repositioning is also effective to maintain correct body alignment and prevent or alleviate pain and possibly prevent ulcers. Immobilization is only effective to stabilize fractures or otherwise compromised limbs or joints. Finally, acupuncture, which involves inserting small solid needles into the skin, may be an effective alternative to more standard therapies.

Cognitive behavioral interventions are an important part of a multimodal approach to pain management. They help to give the patient a sense of control and to develop appropriate skills to deal with pain. These skills include relaxation and imagery, cognitive distraction and reframing, patient education, psychotherapy, biofeedback, structured support, and support groups and pastoral counseling.

With rare exceptions, a less invasive analgesic approach should precede invasive palliative approaches. However, for a few patients in whom behavioral, physical, and drug therapy do not alleviate pain, invasive therapies are useful. These include radiation therapy to destructive bone metastasis, palliative surgical approaches, and nerve blocks.

Because vulvar cancers and occasionally ovarian or endometrial cancers occur in elderly patients, they especially require comprehensive assessment and aggressive management when cancer pain occurs. **Older patients are at risk for undertreatment of pain because of underestimation of their sensitivity to pain, the expectation that they tolerate pain well, underreporting because of declined cognitive functions, and the misconceptions about their ability to benefit from the use of opioids. Careful consideration should be given to elderly patients who are in pain and who have multiple chronic diseases that increase their risk for drug–drug and drug–disease interactions.** In addition, visual, hearing, motor, and cognitive impairments may require simpler pain assessment scales and more frequent pain assessments. NSAIDs are more likely to

cause gastric and renal toxicity and other drug reactions such as cognitive impairment, constipation, and headaches in older patients. Alternative NSAIDs (eg, choline magnesium trisalicylate) or co-administration of misoprostol should be considered to reduce gastric toxicity. Older persons tend to be more sensitive to the analgesic effects of opioids. In addition, the peak opioid effect is higher, and the duration of pain relief is longer. Drug clearance may also be slower, thus making cautious initial dosing and subsequent titration and monitoring necessary. Elderly patients may not be able to physically place rectal suppositories or activate PCA devices. Because of the addictive property of opioid analgesics, the NCCN and the FDA have incorporated a detailed algorithm, the REMS, for monitoring patients for both safety and abuse. Transdermal, transmucosal, and long-acting opioids are included in this list of highly monitored medications, and health care providers are encouraged to identify patients at risk for abuse or misuse.

Nausea and Vomiting

Nausea and vomiting also have a high prevalence in patients with advanced cancer. **The cause may be divided into physiologic, treatment-related, metabolic, and psychological causes.** As is the case in many symptoms of advanced cancer, the causes of nausea are often multifactorial. **More than 50% of patients receiving opioids experience nausea in the first 10 to 14 days of therapy until they develop tolerance to this side effect.** Many palliative specialists may prescribe antiemetics for the first weeks of opioid therapy. The most successful therapy is given orally and prophylactically. Nausea and vomiting tend to be the most feared symptom related to cancer treatment. Chemotherapy-induced nausea and vomiting (CINV) may occur in 70% to 80% of patients receiving chemotherapy. CINV can be divided into four subcategories. The NCCN defines *acute CINV* as occurring shortly after chemotherapy administration but resolving within the first 24 hours. *Delayed CINV* occurs after 24 hours, peaks 48 to 72 hours, and resolves by 6 to 7 days. *Anticipatory CINV* is described as a learned or conditioned response before chemotherapy, and finally, *breakthrough CINV* can occur when a patient experiences symptoms despite appropriate therapy.

An evaluation and approach to the management of patients with chemotherapy-induced emesis appears in Fig. 20.4. Agents used to control nausea and vomiting have different mechanisms of action and may be used in combination for better control (Table 20.15). There are basically three main classes of drugs for CINV: 5-HT serotonin receptor antagonists, corticosteroids, and the neurokinin-1 (NK$_1$) antagonists. The ASCO recently updated its guidelines for the use of antiemetics in oncology; these recommendations, with some additions, are detailed in Fig. 20.5. All have a high therapeutic index for CINV and should be considered first-line therapy. **The 5-HT3 antagonist blocks serotonin receptors of the peripheral GI tract and the chemoreceptor trigger zone (CTZ) to prevent vomiting. Corticosteroids are often used to enhance the effect of other agents, yet they have an unclear antiemetic action. It has been postulated that corticosteroids overcome the adrenal insufficiency that causes nausea and vomiting in patients with advanced**

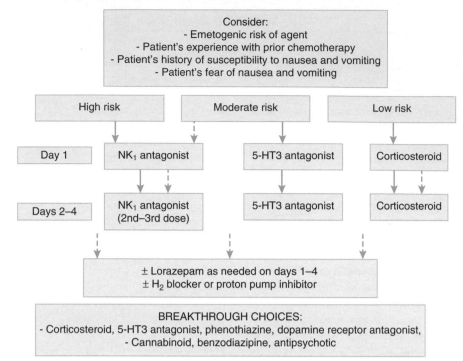

FIGURE 20.4 Evaluation and approach to management of patients with chemotherapy-induced emesis. *NK₁*, Neurokinin-1. (Reproduced with permission from The NCCN I. 2007 *Antiemesis Guidelines: Clinical Practice Guidelines in Oncology.* © 2006 National Comprehensive Cancer Network, Inc. Available at: http://www.nccn.org. To view the most recent and complete version of the guideline, go online to www.nccn.org.)

FIGURE 20.5 Fair process for considering futility cases. (Adapted from Medical futility in end-of-life care: report of the council on ethical and judicial affairs. *JAMA* 1999;281:939.)

TABLE 20.15 Antiemetic Agents (Adult Dosages)

Medications	Common Proprietary (Trade) Name	Usual Daily Dose (Adults)		
		Oral Dose	Parenteral Dose	Rectal Dose
ANTIDOPAMINERGICS*				
PHENOTHIAZINES				
Chlorpromazine	NA	10–25 mg q4hr	25–50 mg IM/slow IV q4h	NA
Perphenazine	NA	2–6 mg q6h	NA	NA
Prochlorperazine	Compazine	5–10 mg q6h	5–10 mg IM/slow IV q3h (maximum, 40 mg/day)	25 mg bid
Promethazine	Phenergan	12.5–25 mg q4h	12.5–25 mg IM/slow IV q h	12.5–25 mg q4h
OTHERS				
Metoclopramide	Reglan, Metozolv ODT	0.5 mg/kg q6h 20–40 mg bid–qid (delayed CINV)	1–2 mg/kg q2h up to five doses	NA
Olanzapine	Zyprexa	2.5–5 mg bid	NA	NA
ANTICHOLINGERICS				
Scopolamine	Transderm Scop	NA	NA	TDS: 1 patch (1 mg) q72h, starts 4 h prior
Trimethobenzamide	Tigan	300 mg q6h	200 mg IM q6h	NA
ANTIHISTAMINE				
Diphenhydramine	Benadryl	25–50 mg q6h	25–50 mg q6h	NA
BENZODIAZEPINE				
Lorazepam	Ativan	0.5–2 mg PO/SL q4h	0.5–2 mg IV q4 hr	NA
BUTYROPHENONE				
Droperidol	NA	NA	2.5 mg; then 1.25 mg	NA
CORTICOSTEROID				
Dexamethasone	Decadron	10 mg/day or bid (short term)	10–20 mg × 1	NA
5-HT3 (SEROTONIN) RECEPTOR ANTAGONISTS				
Dolasetron	Anzemet	100 mg/day	1.8 mg/kg or 100 mg/day	NA
Granisetron	Kytril, Sancuso (TDS)	2 mg/day or 1 mg bid	10 mcg/kg/dose or 1 mg/day or bid	TDS: 1 patch (3.1 mg/day) up to 7 day per application, start 24–48 h prior
Ondansetron	Zofran, Zofran ODT	24 mg/day or 8 mg bid Radiation treatment: 8 mg tid	0.15 mg/kg q 4 hr × 3 or 16 mg/day	NA
Palonosetron	Aloxi		0.25 mg IV × 1	NA
Netupitant–palonosetron (300 mg/0.5 mg capsule)	Akynzeo	1 capsule 1 h before chemotherapy	NA	NA
SUBSTANCE P/NEUROKININ 1 RECEPTOR ANTAGONIST				
Aprepitant (PO) or fosaprepitant (IV)	Emend	125 mg day 1; then 80 mg/day on days 2 and 3	150 mg day 1	NA
CANNABINOIDS				
Dronabinol	Marinol	2.5–10 mg qid	NA	NA
Nabilone	Cesamet	1–2 mg tid	NA	NA

*Antidopaminergics: If extrapyramidal symptoms occur, administer 50 mg of diphenhydramine IM or IV.
bid, Twice a day; *CINV,* chemotherapy-induced nausea and vomiting; *IM,* intramuscular; *IV,* intravenous; *NA,* not available; *PO,* oral; *q,* every; *qid,* four times a day; *SL,* sublingual; *TDS,* transdermal; *tid,* three times a day.
Data from Facts and Comparisions® E Answers, 2015 Wolters Kluwer Health.

cancer. **Dexamethasone (20 mg IV) is most effective when administered with a 5-HT3 antagonist.** There are several 5-HT serotonin receptor antagonists that all have similar therapeutic and side effect profiles. Several large, multicenter, double-blind, randomized phase III trials have shown that palonosetron performs superior to other agents in this class in preventing emesis associated with both moderate and high emetic risk chemotherapy regimens, particularly for delayed emesis. The three-drug combination of 5-HT receptor antagonists in addition to dexamethasone and receptor antagonists are indicated for the control of CINV in high-dose chemotherapy regimens. NK_1 receptor antagonist plays a significant role as an adjunct for acute CINV control and single agent for delayed CINV control. For breakthrough CINV, the following agents may be considered as a replacement or adjunct agent when first-line therapeutics fail: metoclopramide, phenothiazines, butyrophenones, and cannabinoids. Metoclopramide has its effect locally in the gut and is excellent to control vomiting because of gastric stasis. In chemotherapy prophylaxis, it can be combined safely with steroids or benzodiazepines. Phenothiazines partially inhibit the CTZ and are the drugs of choice for mild CINV. Ondansetron is the drug of choice for radiation-induced nausea and vomiting. Benzodiazepines are indicated for anticipatory vomiting and can be used in patient with nausea caused by high anxiety. The amnesic effects of benzodiazepines are helpful to many patients. Olanzapine, an atypical antipsychotic, has been found to be effective for CINV, especially for patients with high rates of nausea. However, olanzapine should be used with caution in elderly patients because of its boxed warning and precautions. Patients who describe around-the-clock nausea, not just intermittent with meals, may have a CNS lesion or a proximal small bowel obstruction that must be evaluated. Cannabinoids are best used in younger patients and have equivalent or superior activity compared with the phenothiazine agents. Specifically, the cannabinoids dronabinol and nabilone, both approved by the FDA, are indicated for refractory CINV and despite dysphoric side effects hindering their prescription, patients have been shown to prefer the use of these agents for subsequent chemotherapy cycles. In anticipatory CINV, the most important concept is the prevention of acute and delayed emesis with the above drugs. However, ultimately when one is faced with controlling anticipatory CINV, benzodiazepines and behavioral therapy are suggested. Finally, when CINV proves to be refractory, one must consider other causes of nausea and vomiting. With the change of legislature, the use of medical marijuana may be sought by patients. Although the route of administration (inhalation, nasal, and edible) may all be effective. Physicians must become familiar with state and federal requirements before prescribing to assure patient safety and to honor professional oath.

Last, an important concept in CINV is the selection of therapy based on the risk assessment of the chemotherapeutic agents used, a concept highlighted in the recent ASCO guidelines. The emetogenicity of these antineoplastic drugs is separated into four categories: high, moderate, low, and minimal risk. For example, a high-risk drug such as cisplatin requires combination treatment with 5-HT receptor blockers, NK_1 receptor antagonist, and corticosteroids followed by corticosteroid and NK_1 receptor antagonist for delayed CINV. Low emetogenic drugs (eg, paclitaxel) may only require dexamethasone without additional agents for acute CINV.

Diarrhea and Constipation

Diarrhea is a common complication of pelvic radiation and systemic chemotherapy. It can generally be managed with intestinal opioid receptor agonist such as loperamide. Rarely, tinctures of opium or octreotide are required for refractory or secretory diarrhea (Table 20.16). **Patients who have been previously treated with antibacterial therapy or are immunocompromised should be tested for** *Clostridium difficile* (eg, enzyme-linked immunosorbent assay [ELISA] for enterotoxin)

before antidiarrheal therapy. When detected, metronidazole or vancomycin therapy is usually effective. Rarely, cholestyramine is needed to control the symptoms of *C. difficile* infectious diarrhea. A search for more unusual infectious etiologies such as salmonella, shigella, *Escherichia coli,* and parasites has not been cost effective among gynecologic oncology patients in the absence of foreign travel or other data, which might suggest these etiologic agents.

Constipation is highly prevalent in patients with advanced cancer. Close to 90% of patients receiving opioids have difficulty passing stool or pass stool infrequently. **One cardinal rule of palliative care is "the hand that writes the opioids writes the laxative at the same time."** Other causes of constipation are advanced disease, other medications such as anticholinergic agents, inability to eat a high-fiber diet, insufficient fluid intake, and lack of activity.

A specific discussion regarding opioid-induced constipation is warranted here. Of note, a tolerance to the opioid used with regards to constipation does not occur. In general, a mild stimulant laxative and a stool softener should be used prophylactically, for example, senna with docusate. Adequate fluid intake and physical activity should be encouraged. Such agents as Metamucil that increase fiber content in the stool are not recommended. If constipation persists, secondary etiologies, such as bowel obstruction, should be considered. Impaction should be ruled out, and then secondary anticonstipation agents should be considered. These agents include magnesium hydroxide or citrate, bisacodyl, lactulose, sorbitol, polyethylene glycol, naloxegol, and methylnaltrexone. Various enemas or agents such as metoclopramide may also be added. A general approach should be to begin patient on a stool softener and stimulant; if in 48 hours no bowel movement results, then additional agents should be started such as Milk of Magnesia or lactulose. If no bowel movement in 72 hours, then fecal impaction should be assessed and treated. If no impaction is present, then such interventions as an enema, mineral oil, or magnesium citrate should be tried. If impacted, a glycerine suppository or oil retention enema should be used.

Metabolic causes of constipation include hypercalcemia and hypokalemia. **Evaluation of complaints of constipation should include consideration of bowel obstruction and spinal cord compression.** A manual rectal examination is critical when evaluating this complaint.

Several treatment options are now available for nonsurgical candidates with bowel obstructions secondary to advanced cancer. A discussion of these treatments follows.

Cachexia and Malnutrition

Cachexia is defined by Femia and Goyette as loss of over 5% of body weight over 2 to 6 months. Clearly, cachexia is related to nutritional status because the cancer itself causes metabolic alterations such as increased muscle protein breakdown and glucose metabolism, and the treatment of cancer affects appetite and food intake. The literature supports the fact that the patient's body habitus, and therefore QoL, is altered by these changes. Furthermore, it is evident that malnutrition contributes to poor outcome in gynecologic oncology patients. Clearly,

TABLE 20.16 Antidiarrheal Agents (Adult Dosages)

Medications	Common Proprietary (Trade) Name	Dosing Regimen	Comments
ANTISECRETORY			
Bismuth subsalicylate	Kaopectate, Pepto-Bismol, Kao-Tin, Maalox Total Stomach Relief Liquid	2 tablets or 30 mL q1h up to 8 doses per day (regular strength) or four doses/day (maximum strength)	Contains aspirin. Watch for maximum daily dose of aspirin; may cause Reye syndrome. Interferes with radiologic examinations of GI tract (bismuth is radiopaque); stool may appear gray-black in color.
Octreotide	Sandostatin, others	0.1–0.5 mg SC 2–3 times per day (maximum, 2.4 mg/day) LAR: 10–40 mg IM per month	50% dose reduction in patients requiring dialysis or with liver cirrhosis
ANTIPERISTALTIC			
Loperamide	Imodium A-D, others	4 mg; then 2 mg after each stool (maximum, 8 mg/day OTC; 16 mg/day Rx) Maintenance: 2–4 mg q6h	
Diphenoxylate 2.5 mg/ atropine 0.025 mg	Lomotil, Lonox, others	2 tablet or 10 mL (5 mg diphenoxylate) qid (maximum, 20 mg/day)	Use with extreme caution in patients with hepatorenal disease or abnormal liver function; may cause hepatic coma.
Difenoxin 1 mg/atropine 0.025 mg	Motofen	2 tablets; then 1 tablet after each loose stool Maintenance: 1 tablet q3–4h (maximum, 8 tabs per day)	Use with extreme caution in patients with hepatorenal disease or abnormal liver function; may cause hepatic coma.
Opium	Opium Tincture (C-II), Paregoric (C-III)	Opium tincture: 0.6 mL qid Paregoric: 5–10 mL qid	
Codeine	Codeine sulfate	15–60 mg q4h	

GI, gastrointestinal;

IM, intramuscular; *LAR*, long acting depot formulation; *OTC*, over the counter; *qid*; four times a day; *Rx*, prescription; *SC*, subcutaneous.
Data from Facts and Comparisions® E Answers, 2015 Wolters Kluwer Health.

oncologists need to be aware of the implications of malnutrition in patients receiving therapy because poor nutritional status may negatively affect a patient's response to therapy as well as her QoL during therapy.

Nutritional support using dietary supplements and shakes (e.g., Ensure) along with the oncologist's attention to this issue may improve the response to treatment for some patients. Nutritional counseling, oral nutritional supplementation, and home parenteral nutrition (TPN) have also been linked to improved QoL. Finally, although appetite stimulants such as megestrol acetate (Megace) are thought to improve cancer-related anorexia and cachexia, they have not been shown to affect survival or global QoL. However, of note, Megace is thought to be more effective than either eicosapentaenoic acid (α-3-omega fatty acid) or marijuana derivatives, and only corticosteroids may perform as effective as Megace. Unfortunately, Megace carries the risk of VTE perhaps as high as a sixfold increase, and this might limit its use in the gynecologic oncology patient population.

On the contrary, oncologists and patients may differ when it comes to nutrition and hydration in the supportive or palliative care setting. Brown et al found that the majority (63%) of patients would like nutrition and hydration to be continued even though the use of respiratory supports, such as oxygen or ventilators, might be limited. The authors state that patients may not consider nutritional support "heroic." Even though patients might not agree with discontinuation of nutritional support, the management of malnutrition in the palliative

setting remains controversial. For example, although TPN or home parenteral nutrition is considered by many to be unnecessary in terminally ill patients, there is some evidence that it has a positive impact in certain patient populations, including patients with a life expectancy of longer than 3 months. TPN carries its own risks and discomfort, so strong QoL studies need to address this issue.

PSYCHOSOCIAL AND SPIRITUAL NEEDS OF PATIENTS AND FAMILIES

Management of only the physical symptoms of cancer is now considered to be an inadequate approach to oncologic care. It is well recognized that physical and psychological symptoms are intertwined and can benefit from a multidisciplinary approach to care. **A growing body of literature suggests that tailored psychosocial interventions can enhance not only QoL for cancer survivors but may have the additional benefit of improving neuroendocrine and immune functioning, which could positively affect disease states. If proven effective, this complementary and cost-efficient approach could significantly improve patient care, QoL, and aspects of survival.** The effect of cancer on the family and patient is profound and touches every area of their lives. Effective care of the patient requires that these needs be addressed. A team of professionals is needed to foster effective communication in the patient–physician relationship, to assess the effect of disease and its treatment on the patient's psychosocial and spiritual well-being, and to achieve optimal care for the patient and family.

Strategies for Breaking Bad News and Preserving Hope

Perhaps the most important tool in caring for patients and their families is effective communication. Transferring information about the diagnosis, prognosis, risks, and benefits of treatment and progression of disease is a difficult and unavoidable responsibility. **Sharing bad news and responding to the questions presented by the patient and family require compassion, empathy, and skill.** Unfortunately, development of these skills has not historically been emphasized in medical training even though powerful medical institutions and societies (eg, ASCO, IOM, American Cancer Society, NCI) demand excellence and vigilance when caring for people with progressing cancer. The absence of an integrated formal palliative care curriculum throughout medical training continues to promote a skill set gap.

Identification of cancer progression, or progressive cancer-related symptoms, is often the catalyst for planning alterations in care and readdressing issues about the patient's and family's goals and objectives. Breaking bad news is a difficult and emotionally laden task for the physician. Thoughtful planning and delivery of such information, however, can shape the patient's subjective experience of the physician and perception of his or her degree of support and caring. The individual's response to news is often determined by the adequacy of information given and whether the person delivering the information showed and responded to the patient's concerns.

Although wishes vary from one individual to another, most patients (80%) want to know their diagnosis, their chance of cure, and the adverse effects of any treatments. Significantly, patients do vary in the degree of information that they are able to assimilate at one time. Traditionally, men with advanced disease, older patients, and individuals from lower socioeconomic backgrounds are likely to want to hear fewer details and may comfortably defer to the physician or family with regard to decision making. In most cases, patients want to hear the diagnosis from the physician who will be responsible for their care.

When breaking bad news, it is critical to project reasonable hope and confidence. Despite the most sensitive and effective communication style, patients are left with major concerns about their situation as it relates to their physical, social, psychological, and spiritual well-being. **Open communication should be maintained, and these concerns should be explored throughout the continuum of care using expertise and support from other team members. Excessive concern about the need to preserve hope can lead to false optimism or less than full disclosure over time. This approach leads to poor coping skills and failed expectations. Lending strength does not require that the physician be less than honest but that the truth be disclosed over a period of time in a setting where the patient has the support required and with repetition so that information can be assimilated and understood in small amounts.** Patients should be encouraged and nurtured to develop their own coping strategies and defense mechanisms in dealing with their illness. This strategy brings hope against all odds. For example, if asked, "Doctor, I know I am dying, but can there still be a miracle?" The answer is, "Yes, there can be." This suggests that the medical information is clearly understood but demonstrates confidence to overcome suffering and despair. However, it is unusual for patients to so clearly articulate their inevitable demise; more likely, they would ask, "Is there still hope?" **The physician's capacity to appropriately convey hope through articulation of a comprehensive care plan will help the patient to recognize that quality time is a reasonable expectation.** Forcing a patient to adopt the physician's view of the odds (chance of a cure) does not take into consideration what can generally harm the personal framework that patients must deal with. It also corrodes the patient–physician relationship that must endure through the palliative therapy or future care. **Thus, maintaining hope is best achieved through honesty, cautious optimism, compassion, and acceptance of the vulnerability experienced by all cancer patients.**

Timing is critical to breaking bad news. Judging what portion of the information should be disclosed is an art. Conveying a balance of honesty and maintaining hope can sometimes seem impossible, often because physicians tend to project their own concerns onto patients and assume that they will give up hope. In reality, hope is an innate characteristic that is rarely abandoned by open and compassionate discussion of the prognosis and treatment options. When there are no remaining viable cytotoxic treatment options, there are still many palliative options that can achieve meaningful therapeutic ends, thus preserving hope and avoiding a sense of helplessness. It is useful for patients to hear such optimism in the face of a generally poor prognosis. As the patient's illness advances, feelings of helplessness because of a loss of control and fear of dying may resurface. At this point, the physician can openly recognize the patient's fear and grief and externally acknowledge his or her own attitudes toward death. **Unfortunately, doctors and other staff tend to spend less time with patients as the disease progresses and patients deteriorate into a terminal condition.** This is presumably because the health care professionals feel helpless (and perhaps even threatened) when confronted with the imminence of death. Many health care professionals fail to realize the importance of compassion and active palliative care. Actively participating in symptom management and compassionate listening helps to ease the patient's mind, thus allowing the patient to ask questions that help plan realistically for the future and maintain a sense of control. Although most patients know when they are dying and can verbalize this realization, they also retain hope. **The physician is uniquely poised to encourage and reinforce the patient's hope without giving false or insincere reassurance.** One study that focused on end-of-life preferences of gynecologic cancer patients reported that only 5% of 108 patients would stop fighting after receiving a poor prognosis with no medically recommended treatment options left. Most (70%) of these patients expressed their resolve to continue fighting against their disease, even under the poorest prognostic circumstances. Proper management involves directing resources to assist with this fight and fostering this hope

TABLE 20.17 Psychosocial Challenges Experienced by Cancer Patients

Threat of or Actual:

Loss of ability to engage in employment because of side effects or symptoms

Loss of ability to participate in all social activities previously enjoyed because of symptoms of side effects or infection concerns

Guilt feeling about the impact of the diagnosis on people about whom the patient cares

Diminished sense of self-esteem and self-worth

Changes in body image

Discrimination or stigmatization by others

Role conflicts (eg, meeting the demands of multiple responsibilities, including those of being a patient)

Loss of comfort with sexual intimacy with a significant other

Fear of the dying process and concerns about symptoms that conjure up images of physical suffering (eg, pain, cachexia, and shortness of breath)

Adapted from Portenoy RK. *Principles and Practice of Supportive Oncology.* Philadelphia, 1998, Lippincott Raven, pp 100-110.

TABLE 20.18 Tasks of Dying Patients

Practical

Complete a family trust.

Put affairs in order.

Complete advanced directives.

Communicate wishes regarding funeral and burial arrangements.

Plan for the future of surviving family members.

Psychosocial

Grieve the loss of dreams for the future.

Accept the reality of the prognosis and impending death.

Use medical intervention and own internal resources to cope with physical deterioration.

Express thanks and love to family and friends.

Find closure around interpersonal conflicts ("I forgive you; please forgive me").

Say goodbye to family and friends.

Spiritual

Engage in life review, reflect on the past and present.

Make meaning of one's life.

Resolve existential or spiritual conflict.

Adapted from Loscalzo M, Zabora J. Care of the cancer patient: responses of family and staff. In Bruera E, Portenoy R, eds. *Topics in Palliative Care,* vol 2. New York, 1998, Oxford University Press. © Oxford University Press. Reproduced by permission of Oxford University Press, Inc., www.oup.com.

among dying patients. The involvement of other professionals familiar with care for the dying can relieve the physician of being the sole provider of hope with sensitive attention to incurable problems.

MANAGEMENT OF PSYCHOSOCIAL AND SPIRITUAL DISTRESS

Approaching "the person, not the disease" is a prerequisite to understanding the patient's experience and providing appropriate physical, psychosocial, and spiritual care. A cancer diagnosis creates a profound sense of loss of control and fear for many individuals. Changes in physical function and the effect on psychosocial issues may further compound this sense. Stressors commonly experienced by patients undergoing cancer treatment may be as problematic for the patient as the physical decline. Table 20.17 highlights the complex challenges faced by patients.

Patients are often reluctant to disclose struggles, including feelings of depression and anxiety, if they do not perceive this disclosure to be relevant to their physical care. Recent research has shown that many individuals are fearful of burdening their family members emotionally, physically, and financially during their final days. A recent prospective study examining the prevalence of depressed mood and request for euthanasia among terminally ill cancer patients noted that of 138 patients, 32 patients (22%) had depressed mood and made an explicit request for euthanasia. The risk to request euthanasia for patients with depressed mood was 4.1 times higher than that of patients without depressed mood at inclusion (95% confidence interval, 2.0–8.5). This information heightens our awareness to formally evaluate depression in terminally ill cancer patients and provide timely intervention as indicated.

Discussions about resources available to assist patients and families, including the role and function of community agencies, support groups, and hospice programs, are critical. There

are many tasks that a patient should have the opportunity to accomplish in the time before death. These tasks are summarized in Table 20.18.

Identification and treatment of psychosocial problems, including depression and anxiety, should involve interventions and expertise that will offer optimal care to the patient and family. As noted earlier, pharmacologic interventions are often necessary but should be considered in combination with psychological counseling, supportive interventions, and education for the patient and family. Determination of the appropriate referral depends in large part on the type and magnitude of the psychosocial or psychological disruption, as well as the extent to which this diagnosis interfaces with physical symptomatology such as pain or fatigue. Optimal programs include a team consisting of psychiatry, psychology, social work, and chaplain services. In addition, **novel programs are acknowledging, if not incorporating, aspects of complementary and alternative medicine (CAM) based on recognition that a substantial proportion of cancer patients seek out various CAM methodologies.**

Psychosocial care must continue to address the needs of the family as death imminently approaches and after death occurs. The health care team has an opportunity through the period of anticipatory grieving to assess and monitor the family and to identify risk factors indicating the need for more intensive intervention. **An understanding of the spectrum of grief and the nature of "normal" grief is essential for providers to effectively support grieving families, identify abnormal reactions, and intervene.** Table 20.19 illustrates the range of bereavement services that may be available for family members.

TABLE 20.19 Interventions for Bereaved Individuals*

Provision of information or education: offers education to surviving family members about grief response, explaining death to children, practical information to facilitate problem solving and arranging for disposition of the body (eg, funeral and burial arrangements), and future memorial activities

Bereavement follow-up: offers formalized contracts by the staff or volunteers at identified intervals to provide support, monitor for difficulties, and arrange for intervention as needed

Individual or family grief counseling: offers counseling for bereaved individuals experiencing grief; some individuals may require long-term psychotherapy or psychiatric care if bereavement-related depression or risk of suicide exists

Bereavement support groups: offers a forum for the mutual support among bereaved individuals; may have a special purpose (eg, for parents who have lost a child) or have a particular religious affiliation

Memorial or remembrance services: offered by the hospital or hospice to acknowledge the grief process

*Families of patients who die in hospitals would not necessarily have knowledge of or access to any follow-up if a bereavement program is not in place at the institution. Bereavement follow-up is typically a part of hospice services, and institutions may successfully partner with local hospices to make this service accessible for these families.
Adapted from Portenoy RK. *Principles and Practice of Supportive Oncology.* Philadelphia, 1998, Lippincott-Raven, pp 109-118.

QUALITY OF LIFE ISSUES IN ADVANCED AND RECURRENT OVARIAN CANCER

Pleural Effusions

Dyspnea is the subjective feeling of respiratory distress and thus is often an interplay between anxiety and hypoxia from tumor burden. Some have suggested that supportive care of this symptom should include the provider's ability to address the patient's subjective breathlessness. Because dyspnea may indicate a poorer prognosis and shorter interval to death, addressing this symptom is paramount to enhancing QoL in the time period near death.

Dyspnea may result from a combination of three different complications: (1) obstructive pathology such as pleural effusions, (2) cancer cachexia or malnutrition and weakness, and (3) an increase in ventilator requirements such as metabolic acidosis or anemia. Perhaps gynecologic oncologists most frequently encounter this tumor effect in the ovarian cancer patients because the dyspnea may be secondary to pleural effusions. It is suggested that thoracocentesis and chemical pleurodesis be reserved for palliative situations in which chemotherapy or other treatments are not likely to reverse the effusions. For symptomatic control or when mechanical control of the pleural effusion is not an option, most advocate opioids, oxygen therapy, or both. Benzodiazepines as well as oxygen therapy may also have a role in control of dyspnea, although evidence is lacking. Finally, some have advocated activity modifications to prevent the onset of dyspnea, which may involve caregiver instruction to tailor activities of daily living.

Small Bowel Obstruction

Although epithelial ovarian cancer is a surface-spreading disease that rarely invades vital organs, partial or complete bowel obstruction is often seen at the time of initial diagnosis or, more frequently, in association with recurrent disease. **Obstruction may be secondary to extrinsic compression of the small bowel or hypoperistalsis caused by mesenteric and bowel surface implants.** The symptoms, which are almost always present, are intestinal colic, continuous abdominal pain, nausea, and vomiting. In most cases, nausea and vomiting can be relieved by conservative measures, and intestinal symptoms usually resolve after primary cytoreductive surgery and multiagent cisplatin-based cytotoxic chemotherapy. Despite the high objective response rate of primary epithelial ovarian cancer to several platinum-based combination chemotherapeutic regimens, most patients with advanced disease often develop IP recurrences and require a salvage regimen for palliation of symptoms. Several therapeutic strategies have been used in these patients, such as including retreatment with cisplatin or carboplatin or the use of paclitaxel, hexamethylmelamine, oral etoposide, tamoxifen, gemcitabine, liposomal doxorubicin, vinorelbine, or topotecan. Multiple clinical factors must be considered when selecting the most appropriate salvage therapy. Unfortunately, in patients previously treated with cisplatin, other therapeutic agents are not likely to be effective in relieving symptoms of bowel obstruction or ascites.

For most patients who present with bowel obstruction secondary to recurrent IP cancer, initial management should include proper radiographic documentation of the obstruction, hydration, correction of any electrolyte abnormalities, parenteral alimentation, and intestinal intubation and decompression. There is a fair representation of various treatment options in the literature. A recent retrospective study found that surgery carries a higher morbidity, although chemotherapy and surgery had similar outcomes in terms of reobstruction. Of note, conservative management alone has much earlier reobstruction rates. In some patients, the obstruction may be relieved with this conservative approach. However, palliative surgery is usually considered in almost every patient at some time before disease progression and death. When surgery is indicated, the type of surgery depends on the extent of the disease as well as on the number and location of obstructions. If the obstruction is mainly contained in one area, this area can be either resected (if secondary cytoreduction is indicated) or bypassed. Because the success of secondary cytoreduction depends on the chemosensitivity of the residual disease present after debulking surgery, intestinal bypass is generally preferable rather than resection because most patients present after multiple failed attempts at cytotoxic therapy resulting in chemotherapy-resistant cancer. In addition, intestinal bypass surgeries such as enterocolostomy are usually associated with reduced morbidity compared with a radical resection. At the time of operation, the balloon at the end of a long intestinal tube can often be palpated and used to identify the small bowel proximal to the obstruction. This small bowel can then be anastomosed in a side-to-side fashion to the most appropriate area of colon, thus bypassing the site of obstruction. Obviously, it is critical to obtain a preoperative

Gastrografin enema to ensure that there is no obstruction of the lower colon beyond the bypass site. In rare cases, the colon may be encased in tumor, necessitating a colostomy with or without bypass surgery. Sadly, multiple sites of obstruction are common in patients with recurrent epithelial ovarian cancer. **When multiple sites of obstruction are present, resection of several segments of intestine is usually not indicated.** In inoperable cases or situations when the patient or oncologist decides to proceed with medical or conservative management, several options exist. A percutaneous endoscopic gastrostomy allows patients to hydrate themselves by mouth. By decreasing intestinal secretions, octreotide has improved QoL and lessens hospitalization. Moretti et al. used temporary nasogastric drainage with the simultaneous use of octreotide and anti-emetic and analgesics in a terminal patient. Critical in their algorithm is fluid management because they stress keeping daily water intake to between 0.5 and 1.5 L. In the last month of life, this combined medical and conservative approach decreased pain, nausea, dry mouth, thirst, dyspnea, feelings of abdominal distention, and drowsiness in the palliative setting. **In such cases, an ileostomy or even a proximal jejunostomy may be necessary to provide adequate intestinal diversion. On the contrary, if the extent of disease is so great that the morbidity of intestinal surgery seems excessive, stomach decompression with a gastrostomy may be effective in palliating symptoms** of obstruction and ascites such as pressure, nausea, vomiting, and pain. When the stomach and anterior abdominal wall are not involved with tumor, drainage tubes can often be placed percutaneously, thus avoiding the morbidity of a laparotomy.

With careful attention to nutrition, chemosensitivity or resistance of disease, and the sites of intestinal obstruction, some degree of palliation can generally be obtained with surgery, chemotherapy, or gastric decompression. Careful attention to each of these factors is necessary to avoid unnecessary morbidity and unindicated surgery in these debilitated terminal patients with recurrent or refractory ovarian cancer.

Many have attempted to define the prognostic factors which predict benefit after surgery and some of the key factors include age older than 65 years, nutritional status, tumor burden, rapidly reaccumulating ascites, poor nutritional status, carcinomatosis, previous chemotherapy for recurrence, and radiation therapy to the whole intestine. Krebs and Gopelrud used a predictive index by scoring patients with a value of 0, 1, or 2 in six of these categories and found that patients who scored higher than six had worse outcomes with surgery. However, if surgery is chosen, the patient must understand the possibility of living with an ileostomy in roughly 50% of cases with potential complications of fistula(s) for the balance of the patient's life. In a study by Mangili et al., only surgical treatment was a prognostic factor for improved survival; however, it is likely that patients who were offered surgery had other qualities that predisposed them to improved survival.

Ascites

Because malignant ascites is almost always the result of IP cancer, treatment of these effusions generally involves therapy directed against the associated malignant neoplasm. However,

treatments are occasionally directed specifically toward the palliation of symptoms related to malignant ascites, particularly when the IP cancer is refractory to all known treatments. **The traditional treatment with diuretics and salt and fluid restriction is rarely effective. Therefore, patients usually undergo therapeutic paracentesis, resulting in an imbalance of protein and electrolytes.** For this reason, novel therapies such as IP immunotherapy and drainage using a Denver peritoneal venous shunt have been proposed to palliate symptoms associated with malignant ascites. One series involved 42 patients who were treated over a 5-year period with a peritoneal venous shunt, which diverted peritoneal fluid into the vascular space. This treatment relieved symptoms with neither hematogenous metastasis nor evidence of disseminated intravascular coagulation. Interestingly, the median survival time of patients with breast and gynecologic cancer after surgery was significantly longer than that of patients with primarily gastric and intestinal neoplasms resulting in an improvement in QoL.

Management approaches with diuretics with or without serial paracentesis versus permanent indwelling catheters are case dependent. A recent phase I/II trial using monoclonal antibodies against ascites-specific malignant cells, specifically epithelial cell adhesion molecule (EpCAM) on the surface of ascitic tumor cells, in the control of ascites, but randomized controlled studies are still lacking. Other approaches suggested include the use of vascular endothelial growth factor (VEGF) antagonists to reduce ascites because VEGF may be implicated in the formation of ascites by increasing vascular permeability. A hope for cure is no longer possible when a woman develops recurrent disease associated with symptomatic bowel obstruction and ascites. However, a sense of optimism and hope are still common, not for a cure but toward a goal of symptom relief and palliation with chemotherapy, surgery, tube drainage, or supportive care. Only through careful patient selection and insight into the toxicity associated with these therapies can hope for acceptable QoL be realized. A Cochrane review published in 2010 failed to support or refute the use of drains for ascites because it did not find any eligible trials to review.

Role of Palliative Surgical Procedures

The role of surgery to palliate bowel obstruction was discussed earlier. Surgery can be useful in the palliation of pain or fistula during the terminal phase of ovarian cancer progression. The advantages and disadvantages of these procedures must be continually weighed. Cytoreductive surgery for debulking as a means to palliate pain is indicated when effective chemotherapy exists to treat unresected residua.

QUALITY OF LIFE ISSUES IN ADVANCED AND RECURRENT UTERINE AND CERVICAL CANCER

Ureteral Obstruction

A patient with bilateral ureteral obstruction and uremia secondary to the extension of cervical or uterine cancer presents a serious dilemma for the clinician. **Management should be divided into two subsets of patients: (1) those who have not** received prior radiation therapy and (2) those who have recurrent disease after pelvic radiation.

Ureteral obstruction resulting from endometrial cancer differs from obstruction secondary to cervical cancer in that it is more frequently associated with disease outside of the pelvis and because it is more difficult to cure. In addition, adequate doses of radiation are more difficult to deliver to the corpus than to the cervix using standard brachytherapy techniques, thus contributing to the lower rate of pelvic control among patients with endometrial cancer after radiation therapy.

Patients with bilateral ureteral obstruction from untreated cancer or from recurrent pelvic disease after surgical therapy should be seriously considered for urinary diversion followed by appropriate radiation therapy. However, because the salvage rate in this clinical situation is low, supportive care alone allowing progressive uremia and demise must be considered as an alternative to more aggressive therapy. Placement of retrograde ureteral stands using cystoscopy should be attempted first if supportive care alone is declined. When this is not possible, a percutaneous nephrostomy should be placed followed by an attempt at antegrade stent placement. A third option is surgical urinary diversion such as a urinary conduit and anastomosing both ureters into an isolated loop of ileum (Bricker procedure) or creating a continent pouch from a segment of bowel. When necessary, urinary diversion is usually performed before the radiation has begun, thus allowing for surgical assessment of the extent of the disease. If extrapelvic disease is discovered at laparotomy, therapy is altered because the chance of a cure is greatly diminished.

The patient with a bilateral ureteral obstruction after a full dose of pelvic radiation therapy presents a more complicated problem. Fewer than 5% of these patients will have obstruction caused by radiation fibrosis, and often this group is difficult to identify. To identify patients whose obstruction is a result of recurrent disease, an examination under anesthesia, cystoscopy, and proctoscopy with multiple biopsies is recommended. When recurrent cancer is absent, simple diversion of the urinary stream can be lifesaving; therefore, all patients must be considered to belong to this category until the recurrent malignancy is found.

When the presence of recurrent disease is established as the cause of bilateral ureteral obstruction, the decision process becomes difficult and somewhat philosophical. Numerous studies suggest that "useful life" is not achieved by urinary diversion in this subset of patients. Brin and colleagues reported on 47 patients (five with cervical cancer) with ureteral obstruction secondary to advanced pelvic malignancy undergoing diversion. The results of this report are discouraging. The average survival time was 5.3 months; only 50% of the patients were alive at 3 months, and only 20% were alive at 6 months. After the diversion, 63.8% of the survival time was spent in the hospital. Delgado also reported on a group of patients with recurrent pelvic cancer and renal failure who were treated with urinary conduit diversion. Delgado's results show an insignificant increase in survival time, and he suggests that these patients should never undergo urinary diversion because a more preferable method of expiration (uremia) is then eliminated from the

patient's future. Obviously, this decision should be made in consultation with the family and even with the patient, if possible. When urinary diversion is performed, accentuation of the other clinical manifestations of recurrent pelvic cancer (ie, severe pelvic pain, repetitive infections, and hemorrhage) is generally observed, leading to increased suffering. Pain control and progressive cachexia burden the physician and the patient. Episodes of massive pelvic hemorrhage are associated with difficult decisions concerning transfusion. An extension of the inpatient hospital stay is inevitable, and the financial impact of the patient on her family is often considerable.

Fistula

Urinary or colon fistulas are common sequelae of progressive cervical cancer and uterine corpus cancer. Because both urinary and intestinal fistulas have a great impact on QoL, consideration should always be given to diversion of either the urinary or fecal stream to reduce symptomatology. Bladder drainage can often sufficiently reduce the incontinence associated with a urinary fistula without the need for surgical urinary diversion. Ureteral ligation with percutaneous nephrostomy drainage is another option. However, urinary conduit or other surgical procedures are often necessary to adequately divert the urinary stream. Surgical repair of a urinary fistula secondary to recurrent cancer or radiation is rarely successful with existing surgical techniques.

Colovaginal fistulas can generally be palliated with a colostomy. Although controversial, a loop colostomy often provides adequate fecal stream interruption to prevent further fistula drainage. However, some surgeons argue that an end colostomy with a Hartmann pouch is necessary to completely interrupt the fecal stream. In either situation, a mini-laparotomy is generally all that is required to adequately accomplish the palliative goal.

Sexual Dysfunction

The treatment of women with gynecologic malignancies may result in vaginal abnormalities that interfere with sexual function. Disturbances in sexuality are more common after the treatment of vulvar, vaginal, and cervical carcinoma compared with corpus and ovarian cancer. This is a result of the frequent use of radical surgery and radiotherapy to treat the three former malignancies. The reported frequency of sexual dysfunction after surgery, radiotherapy, or both varies considerably. A total of 4% to 100% of women report a shortened vagina after a radical hysterectomy, and 17% to 58% have reduced lubrication. However, until recently, there were no reliable data on reductions in vaginal elasticity or genital swelling during sexual stimulation after radical hysterectomy. A report from Sweden published in the *New England Journal of Medicine* in 1999 demonstrated a statistically significant decrease in vaginal elasticity (23%) among women treated for early cervical cancer compared with a control group (4%). In addition, this study of 256 patients with cervical cancer, who were retrospectively surveyed and compared with 350 control participants, also showed a decrease in lubrication during arousal and a reduction in perceived vaginal length after treatment. Furthermore, a large number of women indicated that these changes and their effects on sexual intercourse distressed them. Interestingly, the frequency of orgasms and orgasmic pleasure were similar in the two groups, although dyspareunia was more common in the women who had cervical cancer. Finally, **this study did not show any significant difference among those women treated with radical surgery versus radiotherapy,** although other retrospective comparisons have documented a significant increase in sexual dysfunction among those patients treated with radiation versus surgery. A direct comparison between radiation and surgery in the treatment of cervical cancer emphasizing not only outcome but also QoL and sexual function is needed. **Regular vaginal dilatation is widely recommended to those women treated with radiation as a way to maintain vaginal length and elasticity.** Again, this intervention has never been tested in a prospective fashion. **The appropriate use of hormone replacement therapy and lubricants may also improve coital function.**

Dyspareunia resulting from gynecologic cancer therapy should be evaluated and treated, because dyspareunia can lead to loss of desire and can cause women to become sexually avoidant. This often leads to difficult interpersonal relationships between the woman and her partner. Loss of sexual desire in the postcancer population is common and represents a challenging problem. Long after ordinary physical health has been regained, women may describe feeling little or no sexual desire. Counseling and support groups may be helpful in overcoming this frustration.

Anxiety and Depression

The prevalence of depressive and anxiety disorders among women with gynecologic cancers approaches 50%. In a study by Fowler et al., depressive and anxiety symptoms were high in women who had sought consult by a gynecologic oncologist, 42% and 30%, respectively. The severity and prevalence of these psychological symptoms correlated highly with the number of gynecologic symptoms. Of note, older women and those women without a partner were more likely to suffer from depression and anxiety.

The prevalence and severity of symptoms may fluctuate during the patient's treatment course. Chan and Woodruff tracked the psychosocial state in patients with gynecologic cancer to identify risk factors for maladjustment during treatment. Although most patients adjusted well in their sample of 74 women, those with lower socioeconomic status and those without family support or religious belief suffered greater from adjustment disorders. Furthermore, pain, health-related QoL, and poor performance status have been shown to affect these psychological disorders.

There is limited evidence reporting the optimal pharmacologic and psychosocial interventions in depressive disorders among cancer patients. Four classes of drugs have been used: TCAs, serotonin reuptake inhibitors (SSRIs), neuroleptics, and benzodiazepines. It has been suggested that TCAs may be particularly helpful in patients with insomnia and cachexia and that SSRIs may be indicated for patients with low energy, although the evidence regarding dosages and drug choice are heterogeneous. The neuroleptics, such as haloperidol, and the benzodiazepines are not only indicated in patients with anxiety but can ameliorate nausea and vomiting simultaneously. Apart from medical therapy, it has been shown that actively seeking support for psychological concerns enhances QoL and mood. It is not surprising that treatment of depressive and anxiety disorders in these patients might require medical therapy combined with such psychosocial therapy as can be found in cancer support groups.

END-OF-LIFE DECISION MAKING

As summarized in the American College of Obstetrics and Gynecology Committee Opinion published in May 1995, **the moral character of medicine is based on three values central to the human relationship:**
1. **Patient benefit;**
2. **Patient self-determination; and**
3. **The ethical integrity of the health care professional.**

Patient Benefit

The obligation to promote the good of the patient is a basic presumption of medical care and the defining feature of a physician's ethical responsibility. To promote the patient's good is to provide care in which benefits outweigh burdens or harms. Benefits, in turn, are understood only relative to the goals that the patient and physician hope to achieve through medical care.

Patient Self-determination

The inherent value of individual autonomy or self-determination is one of the fundamental bases of democracy in the United States and provides certain protection during end-of-life decision making. In health care, the value of individual autonomy is as firm in the ethical and legal doctrines as in informed consent. Under this doctrine, the patient has a right to control what happens to her body. This means that:
1. **no treatment may be given to the patient without her consent (or if she lacks decision-making capacity, the consent of her surrogate)**
2. **the patient (or her surrogate) has the right to refuse unwanted medical treatment. This right is not contingent on the presence or absence of a terminal illness, on the agreement of family members, or on the approval of physicians or hospital administrators.**

In the medical context, physician respect for patient self-determination consists of an active inclusion of the patient in decisions regarding her own care. This involves frank discussion of the diagnosis and prognosis; the relative risks and benefits of alternative treatments; and, based on these discussions, the identification or the operative goals of care.

Legal Developments That Have a Bearing on End-of-Life Decision Making

In the 1990s, several developments in the law influenced end-of-life decision making. First, in June 1990, in a decision on the *Cruzan* case, **the United States Supreme Court affirmed** that patients have a constitutionally protected right to refuse unwanted medical treatments. The ruling reaffirms states' authority to adopt procedural requirements for the withdrawal and withholding of life-prolonging medical interventions. A second legal development was the passage of the federal Patient Self-Determination Act (PSDA), which took effect on December 1, 1991. The PSDA requires Medicaid- and Medicare-participating health care institutions to inform all adult patients of their rights "to make decisions concerning medical care, including the right to accept or refuse medical or surgical treatment and the right to formulate an advance directive." Under the PSDA, institutions are legally required to provide this information to patients upon admission for care or upon enrollment in health maintenance organizations (HMOs). The institution must note in the chart the existence of an advance directive and must respect such a directive to the fullest extent under state law.

An advance directive is the formal mechanism by which a patient may express her values regarding her future health status. It may take the form of a proxy directive, an instructional directive, or both. Proxy directives, such as the durable power of attorney for health care, designate a surrogate to make medical decisions on behalf of the patient who is no longer competent to express her choices. Instructional directives, such as "living wills," focus on the types of life-sustaining treatments that a person would or would not choose in various clinical circumstances.

A patient's goals of care are very likely to change with time in different clinical circumstances. As a static expression of the patient's wishes, an instructional directive may thus be a limited tool that could conceivably undermine a patient's most current desires. With this in mind, the patient's appointment of a proxy who knows her interest and accepts the role of surrogate decision maker may be the best way of ensuring that her wishes will be carried out (proxy directive).

Surrogate Decision Making

If the patient who lacks decision-making capacity has not designated a health care proxy, state law may dictate the order in which relatives should be asked to serve as surrogates. The person selected should be one who knows the patient's values and wishes and will respect them in his or her role as a surrogate decision maker. If there is conflict regarding the decision of a surrogate, it may be appropriate to seek the advice of an ethics committee or consultant or, possibly, the courts.

In proxy decision making for a dying patient, surrogates and health care providers should be aware that there is documentation and gender disparity in clinical medicine and research in court decisions surrounding the right to refuse life-sustaining treatment. In review of "right to die" cases, it was found that courts honored the previously stated treatment decisions of men in 75% of cases, but they respected the prior choices of female patients in only 14% of cases. Given the persistence and pervasiveness of social attitudes to take women's moral choices less seriously than those of men, gynecologists and patient surrogates must prevent these vices from undermining their

advocacy for female patients. Likewise, this evidence should further motivate women to make a treatment decision as explicit as possible.

Futility

Treatments that offer no benefit to patients are clearly not obligatory. However, there is no single point at which all patients will conclude that they have completed a certain number of therapeutic interventions, thus making further control of their disease impossible. Although the cancer is increasingly less likely to respond to second-, third-, or fourth-line agents, this is not necessarily an indication of their potential efficacy in the individual patient. Ovarian cancer, in particular, is a disease entity that requires treatment individualized to the needs and presentations of each patient in ways that other disease practices do not.

The American Medical Association (AMA) Council On Ethical and Judicial Affairs to date has not defined an approach to determine what treatment is and is not medically futile, although the council has discussed related issues concerning end-of-life care in many reports. For example, it has affirmed the ethical standing of withdrawing and withholding unwanted interventions, noted the constructive role that advanced care planning can play in preempting difficult and conflicting situations, and advised the use of a range of orders not to intervene. The council has also opposed physician-assisted suicide out of concern that recent calls from citizens and professionals for physician-assisted suicides are a response to experiences of excessive and futile interventions at the end of life. Because definitions of futile care are value laden, universal consensus on futile care is unlikely to be achieved. Rather, a process-based approach has been proposed that includes four distinguishable steps aimed at deliberation and resolution, two steps aimed at securing alternatives in case of irresolvable differences, and a final step aimed at closure when all alternatives have been exhausted (see Fig. 21.5). This has been outlined by the report of the Council on Ethical and Judicial Affairs of the AMA published in its journal in March 1999.

First, earnest attempts should be made to deliberate over and negotiate a prior understanding among the patient, proxy, and physician about what constitutes futile care for the patient and what falls within acceptable limits for the physicians, family, and possibly also the institution. This prior understanding is best achieved before critical illness occurs. If serious disagreement is irresolvable, provisions can be made for a sensitive and orderly transfer of care at such a time that it can preempt later conflicts.

Second, joint decision making should also be made at the bedside between the patient or proxy and physician. This joint decision making should:

- make use of outcome data whenever possible
- incorporate the physician's and patient's or proxy's intent or goals for treatment
- abide by established standards of deliberation and informed consent

Third, the assistance of an individual consultant or a patient representative is a further step and is often helpful to reach a resolution within all parties' acceptable limits. The role of this individual consultant is not to singlehandedly resolve the conflict but rather to facilitate discussions that help to reach that end.

Fourth, an institutional committee, such as an ethics committee, may be involved if disagreements are irresolvable. A final step may occur if the outcome of the institutional process coincides with the patient's desire but the physician remains unpersuaded. In such a case, arrangements may be needed for transfer to another physician within the institution.

Alternatively, arrangements for transfers to another institution may be sought if the physician's position does not agree with that of the patient. Finally, if transfer is not possible because no physician and no institution can be found to follow the patient's or the proxy's wishes, it may be because the request is considered offensive to medical ethics and professional standards in the eyes of a majority of the health care profession. In such cases, by ethics standards, the intervention in question need not be provided, although the legal ramifications of this course of action are uncertain.

Because of the complicated nature of these proceedings, the AMA Council recommends that all health care institutions, whether large or small, adopt the policy of medical futility and those policies on medical futility follow their process approach presented earlier.

Hospice

Palliative care programs often foster identification with hospice, and some have integrated hospice home care or inpatient programs. **In the United States, hospice has come to mean primarily a government-regulated organization or program for dying persons and their families that typically focuses on home care and is limited to the following patients and situations:**

1. Life expectancy of 6 months or less
2. A focus on comfort measures. This is sometimes (but not always) defined by hospice programs as a desire to forgo various "aggressive" and often expensive management approaches. These approaches may usually include cardiopulmonary resuscitation; blood product replacement; and some forms of radiotherapy, surgery, chemotherapy, and acute care hospitalization, at least insofar as these treatment modalities are used to try to cure or prolong life rather than to palliate symptoms
3. A general preference for care at home (except where inpatient hospice is available and specifically sought)

4. A willingness to sign a form acknowledging the desire to enter a hospice program and to focus on comfort care
5. Health insurance that covers hospice

Many hospice programs also require a primary caregiver to be either in the home or regularly available. Another requirement reported by patients or family members is that they had to agree to forgo cardiopulmonary resuscitation, calls for emergency services, and future hospitalization. This requirement is not embodied in federal hospice regulations or the PSDA.

Although hospice staff may be perceived as more knowledgeable and empathic than conventional home care workers, hospice may actually provide much fewer hours of formal care, particularly home health aide time. This finding was recently documented for home care patients with amyotrophic lateral sclerosis. Thus, patients and families are often forced to choose between hospice care with insufficient home health aide support and a conventional home care approach that includes significantly more hours of home health aide time. Hospice programs in the United States are increasingly constricted by the eligibility requirements created by Medicare and other insurers and by the limits of reimbursement, thus making it difficult to cover expensive treatments or provide as much home health aide time as conventional programs. Many programs have become extremely cautious about admission or recertification in the face of the threat posed by an unsympathetic and perhaps ill-conceived government audit that scrutinizes long-stay patients and those with diagnoses other than cancer. At the same time, HMOs and insurers have attempted to "unbundle" hospice services, providing and paying for only part of the hospice package (eg, home nurses without social service, chaplains, volunteers, or bereavement care).

Throughout the world, palliative care is developing as an area of special clinical expertise. It is a recognized specialty in Great Britain and Australia and has been the subject of national attention in the Canadian undergraduate medical curriculum. Although a fledging field, it can boast of multiple clinical centers and training programs; various fine textbooks, journals, and educational conferences; and a small body of research expertise. **The challenge that palliative care faces today is to avoid orthodoxy while moving toward greater unanimity about the nature of the field, with improved standards for palliative care professionals and programs.**

For the bibliography list, log onto www.expertconsult.com ⟨http://www.expertconsult.com⟩.

21

Role of Minimally Invasive Surgery in Gynecologic Malignancies

Floor J. Backes, MD, David E. Cohn, MD, Robert S. Mannel, MD, Jeffrey M. Fowler, MD

OUTLINE

KEY POINTS

1. Minimally invasive surgery (MIS) is practiced by more than 90% of gynecologic oncologists.
2. Knowledge of anatomy, the disease process, and surgical technique is key during these complicated surgical procedures.
3. Several studies have shown that 10 to 20 cases are needed to gain proficiency with a certain procedure.
4. MIS reduces blood loss, transfusions, length of hospital stay, and wound complications without compromising adequacy of the procedure or staging even in (extremely) morbidly obese patients.
5. Survival outcomes for endometrial and cervical cancer are similar after MIS and laparotomy.
6. Several safe methods exist to extract an enlarged uterus after MIS. Morcellation is not recommended when there is suspicion or proven preinvasive or invasive disease.
7. Laparoscopy can be used in ovarian cancer to assess the extent of disease and chance of complete debulking surgery. MIS in advanced or recurrent ovarian cancer is still under investigation, and prospective trials are ongoing.

LAPAROSCOPIC SURGERY IN GYNECOLOGIC ONCOLOGY

Recent advances in the techniques of minimally invasive surgery (MIS) have greatly expanded its role in the management of gynecologic malignancies. Before the 1990s, MIS was mostly limited to laparoscopy for diagnosis of pelvic disease and for tubal sterilization procedures. The great majority of gynecologic oncology procedures for definitive surgical management were performed via large midline abdominal incisions to accomplish appropriate extirpation of the malignancy and surgical staging. Laparotomy causes significant trauma to the patient with many potential associated morbidities, which are increased in incidence and severity in patients with comorbid conditions. The potential applications for MIS in patients diagnosed with gynecologic malignancies have gradually expanded over the past 20 years with improvements in video-laparoscopic

instrumentation and surgical training. Since 2005, advances in robotic surgery have led to the increased use of MIS for comprehensive surgical management of patients with gynecologic cancers. Most gynecologic oncologists now offer MIS as an option for surgical management of patients diagnosed with cervical, endometrial, and ovarian neoplasia.

Advanced laparoscopic procedures have been an option for a subpopulation of gynecologic oncology patients in the 1990s. The goal of MIS is to decrease patient discomfort, hospital stay, and short- and long-term morbidity while at the same time providing an overall improvement in quality of life (QoL) and allowing for earlier implementation of other adjuvant therapies if necessary. Incorporating laparoscopic procedures into the comprehensive management of gynecologic oncology patients has been only moderately successful secondary to limitations of the available technology; a difficult and long learning curve; variability in surgeon training and experience; longer operative times; and patient factors limiting the use of MIS such as prior surgeries, extent of disease, and obesity. Technologic limitations to rapid implementation of complicated laparoscopic surgery in gynecologic oncology include a limited two-dimensional field of vision, counterintuitive motions often required for the surgeon and assistant, limited degrees of freedom of the instruments, and ergonomic disadvantages for the surgeon. Advanced robotic technologies have improved most of these limitations, allowing for expansion of the role of MIS in patients with gynecologic cancer.

As illustrated in other chapters in this textbook, there is a long history in the evolution of surgery in patients with gynecologic cancers. These include incorporation of modifications to radical surgical procedures that reduce the toxicities of treatment with the goal of obtaining the optimal oncologic outcome while improving overall patient QoL. It is important that the goals of cancer control and patient safety are not compromised by a given surgical approach. In other words, MIS serves as another tool to achieve these goals rather than a separate end itself. The historical advantages of laparotomy compared to laparoscopy include maximal surgical exposure, three-dimensional (3D) vision, direct tissue palpation and manipulation, and ease of suturing and other instrument use. Improvements in MIS technology, such as the robotic platform and 3D laparoscopy, have allowed MIS to get a step closer to the surgical experience with laparotomy. The previously mentioned disadvantages of MIS are balanced by potential patient outcome–related improvements. Regardless of surgical approach, it is still imperative that the surgeon adheres to the primary surgical principles of optimal exposure, meticulous tissue dissection, expert knowledge of anatomy, and an understanding of the natural history of the diseases being treated to overcome any potential compromise.

LAPAROSCOPIC SURGICAL STAGING OF GYNECOLOGIC MALIGNANCIES

The cornerstone of appropriate surgical staging is an accurate pelvic and paraaortic lymph node dissection. Incorporation of MIS into the surgical management of patients with gynecologic cancer was not feasible until a technique for adequate laparoscopic lymph node dissection was made possible. Pioneering descriptions of laparoscopic procedures for pelvic lymph node (PLN) dissection came from Europe in the late 1980s by Dargent and Querleu and coworkers. Although exciting in terms of the prospects of MIS, there were concerns regarding the adequacy of lymph node dissection, operative risks, and ability to access the paraaortic nodes. Since that time, laparoscopic skills evolved, and this approach has been demonstrated to be feasible with many descriptions of the surgical technique and outcomes of the laparoscopic pelvic and paraaortic lymph node dissections now reported. Data concerning the laparoscopic approach in the surgical treatment of gynecologic oncology patients are primarily nonrandomized and retrospective, aiming to establish the feasibility of MIS lymphadenectomy in highly selected patients. Only a few multicenter prospective randomized clinical trials have been completed regarding the feasibility of comprehensive

laparoscopic management in patients with gynecologic cancer. These trials have demonstrated that laparoscopy does not have inferior outcomes compared with laparotomy in terms of surgical procedures, adequacy of staging, complications, and survival.

ROBOTIC SURGERY IN GYNECOLOGIC MALIGNANCIES

Robotic surgery overcomes many of the technologic limitations of laparoscopy. The robotic platform provides the surgeon with superior high-definition 3D vision, magnification, wristed instruments, and motion scaling. The surgeon has much more ability to directly control the operative field compared with traditional laparoscopy, thus eliminating many important disadvantages of laparoscopy. The operator of the robotic platform not only has improved vision but also controls the direction and distance of the camera from the operative field without relying on the assistant. In addition, the surgeon has three other port sites to use for a dissector, cutting instrument, and another retracting instrument. Loss of haptic feedback is a potential disadvantage; however, the experienced surgeon is able to overcome loss of this sense with heightened visual feedback and meticulous surgical technique. In addition, there are no significant ergonomic disadvantages and a reduced risk of injury to the surgeon and much less risk of fatigue has been demonstrated in some studies. These significant technological improvements have allowed the gynecologic surgeon to perform much more complicated surgeries via MIS on a heterogeneous group of patients. Ten years after Food and Drug Administration approval of robotic surgery for gynecologic surgery (2005), many publications have confirmed the safety and feasibility of robotic surgery compared with traditional laparoscopy and laparotomy. Initial series focused mostly on staging procedures for endometrial cancer; however, the experience has evolved to more advanced procedures such as radical hysterectomy, radical trachelectomy, and even ovarian cancer debulking surgery and pelvic exenteration. It is now the dominant MIS surgical approach in gynecologic oncology

MINIMALLY INVASIVE SURGERY LEARNING CURVE

Recent advances in the techniques of MIS have greatly expanded its role in the management of gynecologic malignancies. Several recent studies have shown an increasing use of laparoscopy as a treatment modality in gynecologic malignancies. Although advanced laparoscopic technology has been available for more than 2 decades, the incorporation of MIS into surgical management of the gynecologic oncology patient has been relatively slow. Whether this relative lack of mainstream adaptation of LS into the practice is a result of technology or training limitations is unclear, although strong biases support both potential causes. Although difficult to quantify, there is a long and difficult learning curve related to laparoscopy and advanced pelvic operations. The availability of the robotic surgery platform is rapidly expanding the role and adaptation of MIS in the surgical management of women with gynecologic cancer. Nevertheless, these procedures remain major surgeries performed through small incisions and therefore offer unique challenges to the surgeon. Appropriate patient selection, along with a comprehensive understanding of surgical techniques and contraindications, allows for optimal utilization of MIS in the gynecologic oncology patient population.

Little information exists to define the learning curve for laparoscopy and gynecologic oncology surgical procedures. Eltabbakh reported on 75 consecutive patients for laparoscopic management of women with endometrial cancer undergoing laparoscopic-assisted vaginal hysterectomy (LAVH), bilateral salpingo-oophorectomy (BSO), and PLN sampling. There was both a significant decrease in operating time and a significant increase in the number of PLNs harvested with increasing surgeon experience. The experience of the operative assistant has also been shown to be important in major laparoscopic procedures for gynecologic malignancies. Scribner and associates reported a significant difference in successful completion of laparoscopic lymphadenectomies when the first assistant was a skilled attending surgeon compared with a resident or fellow in training. The primary surgeon's experience is the most important factor in improving outcomes in gynecologic oncology laparoscopic surgery. Melendez and colleagues noted improvements in operating room time and a decrease in complications over time in patients with endometrial cancer; however, it required 12 years to gain this experience in 124 patients with endometrial cancer, which reflects a highly selected population of patients. Based on this report and others, it likely requires roughly 20 to 25 laparoscopic endometrial cancer cases to gain proficiency in this procedure, but individual surgeon experience and outcomes are quite heterogeneous. In the largest single-institution report on transperitoneal laparoscopic pelvic and paraaortic lymph node dissection, Schneider and colleagues estimated 20 operations were required to gain the needed experience for laparoscopic pelvic lymphadenectomy and up to 100 for paraaortic lymphadenectomy.

The robotic platform is being more rapidly adapted by gynecologic oncologists to perform extrafascial and radical hysterectomies with pelvic and paraaortic lymph node dissections and is similarly associated with a learning curve. Seamon and colleagues determined that proficiency for hysterectomy with pelvic and paraaortic lymph node dissection in women with endometrial cancer is achieved at 20 cases, and further efficiency continues to improve over time. Holloway and colleagues demonstrated improved operating room times and ability to perform aortic node dissections in a similar group of patients with improvement in patient safety over time. The learning curve for the robotic radical hysterectomy has not been defined but likely is longer than the extrafascial hysterectomy because this is a more complicated surgical procedure. Patient selection based on previous surgical history and, most important, level of obesity significantly influence the learning curve (in addition to surgeon experience in both laparoscopic and robotic MIS.)

The laparoscopic surgical technique is principally different from open laparotomy in the loss of 3D vision, counterintuitive

movements, subtle tactile sensation, limitations of instrumentation, and a heavy reliance on skilled surgical assistance. The surgeon needs to compensate for these losses with a thorough understanding of abdominal and pelvic anatomy when operating laparoscopically. In a prospective, randomized trial, Coleman and Muller reported significant improvement in laparoscopic proficiency in residents exposed to a laboratory-based skills curriculum. Training specifically geared toward laparoscopic surgery using models, cadavers, and animal laboratories is important in gaining proficiency in advanced laparoscopic surgery. The learning curve for robotics does appear to be distinctly different from that for laparoscopy as investigators have demonstrated that surgical drills and suturing are performed with enhanced precision and dexterity when comparing robotic technologies with laparoscopy in a training laboratory. In a 2002 survey of laparoscopy training among Society of Gynecologic Oncology (SGO) members, 85% reported receiving no or limited laparoscopic training during their fellowship. A follow-up survey in 2009 among members of the SGO demonstrated that 91% performed laparoscopic surgery in their practices even though 76% reported that they had limited or no exposure to laparoscopic training during fellowship. Ninety-seven percent of gynecologic oncologists now perform robotic surgery. The introduction of simulators, formal resident and fellow training, and the dual-console da Vinci system (Intuitive Surgical) in 2009 allow for a safe training environment and similar patient outcomes compared with traditional laparoscopic surgery. A recent survey of gynecologic oncology fellows showed that most fellows considered even advanced pelvic procedures such as radical hysterectomy and trachelectomy appropriate for MIS. Sixty percent of fellows performed at least 11 procedures per month, an increase compared with 2007. The transition from laparoscopy to robotic surgery for the MIS management of gynecologic cancers will likely further diminish experience in laparoscopic surgery in this population. There may be an advantage to the robotic platform for novice minimally invasive surgeons given the ability for higher magnification and 3D vision. However, any novel technology does not obviate the need for sound surgical principles and technique, knowledge of anatomy, and understanding of the natural history of the diseases being treated.

MINIMALLY INVASIVE SURGICAL TECHNIQUE

Positioning of the Patient

Positioning of the patient is critical in advanced MIS. For most gynecologic procedures, the appropriate position is in a dorsal lithotomy position with adjustable Allen stirrups to allow for manipulation of the uterus and LAVH as indicated. In patients who do not have a uterus or in whom the uterus is not anticipated to be removed, placement in a supine position may be appropriate. The patient's arms should be tucked by her side to allow mobility and ergonomic comfort for the operating surgeon and assistant. Care should be used in protecting both the upper and lower extremities with appropriate padding to prevent pressure points and nerve injuries. For laparoscopic surgery, video monitors should be placed on each side of the

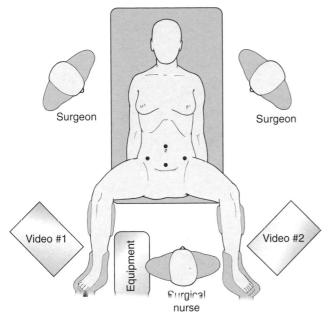

FIGURE 21.1 Operating room setup for laparoscopic surgery. Positioning of patient for laparoscopic gynecologic surgery. Note: Arms tucked (*1*), two video monitors toward foot of table (*2*), and modified dorsal lithotomy position with adjustable stirrups (*3*).

FIGURE 21.2 Anterior abdominal wall. *LUL,* Lateral umbilical ligament; *MUL,* medial umbilical ligament; *RL,* round ligament.

table across from the operating surgeon and the assistant and located toward the foot of the table. This allows for comfortable positioning of the surgeon in a natural angle of viewing the video monitor and minimizing of counterintuitive surgical movement. Placement of the monitors toward the patient's head can be considered when extensive upper abdominal surgery will be undertaken (Fig. 21.1).

Port Sites and Setup

The number, position, and size of trocars for laparoscopic surgery depend on the surgery anticipated. In cases that require removal of an adnexal mass or lymph nodes, a 10- to 12-mm accessory port will be needed for extraction of the specimen. Most laparoscopy (LS) can be accomplished successfully with the placement of a 5- or 10-mm port at the level of the umbilicus for camera placement, a 10- to 12-mm port suprapubically, and a 5-mm port in each of the lateral lower quadrants. Gynecologic oncologists usually use a total of four to six ports to obtain adequate exposure and accomplish advanced pelvic procedures. Safe placement of the primary port, or camera port, is the most critical part of the procedure in terms of minimizing major surgical complications. A number of surgical approaches have been described and accepted for placement of the primary port. An oropharyngeal tube should be used to achieve gastric decompression before placement of the Veress needle or primary trochar. Lateral ports can safely be placed in a line one-third of the distance from the anterior superior iliac spine to the umbilicus. Care should be taken when placing the lateral port and to do so under direct visualization with inspection of the deep inferior epigastric vessels lying along the lateral boundary of the

rectus abdominis muscles. These can be directly identified lateral to the obliterated umbilical ligaments (Fig. 21.2). Transillumination will not reliably reveal the location of these vessels.

The port-site setup for robotic surgery is different from that for laparoscopic procedures because ports are generally placed above the umbilicus (Fig. 21.3). Various port setups have been described for robotic gynecologic oncology surgery. Most gynecologic oncologists use one or two laparoscopic port and two additional laparoscopy ports to be controlled by the bedside assistant. In addition, the robot must be "docked" or attached to the ports, which is accomplished between the legs or from the side of the patient. When the surgical procedure commences, the experienced robotic surgeon can efficiently alternate (swap) control of the various robotic ports through a unique clutching system using both hand and foot controls, can operate all instruments in real time, and has direct control of both monopolar and bipolar electrosurgical energy sources. Although there is less reliance on the bedside assistant, that person is still instrumental in facilitating the case through robotic instrument changes, manipulation of vaginal instruments, suction irrigation, and use of an additional grasping instrument for retraction.

In addition to multiport surgery the options have expanded to single-port surgery or laparoendoscopic single-site surgery (LESS) and robotic single-site surgery. Single-port surgery uses a GelPort or Single Incision Laparoscopic Surgery (SILS) port in a 2- to 3-cm (umbilical) incision. Through this port, the camera port and usually two or three additional trocars are placed. Possible advantages include better cosmesis and decreased postoperative pain. Disadvantages such as port crowding, crossing of instruments, and need for advanced laparoscopic skills have limited the uptake for advanced and complicated pelvic surgeries. Robotic single site surgery allowed for computerized optical reversal of crossing instruments and hands with improved ergonomics and 3D visualization. Recently, an articulated needle driver has been added to the

FIGURE 21.3 An example of a robotic port set up for endometrial cancer staging (many variations exist depending on surgeon preference and experience). Trocar placement for hysterectomy, pelvic and aortic lymphadenectomy. Note the robotic ports (RP) are 8 mm, assistant arm (AA) #1 is 5 to 12 mm, and AA#2 is a 5-mm port. Although the placement of RP#1 and 3 corresponds to approximately the midclavicular line, AA#1 and RP#4 are at the midaxillary line. (From Seamon LG, Cohn DE, Valmadre S,, et al. Robotic hysterectomy and lymphadenectomy for endometrial cancer: technical aspects and details of success: the Ohio State University method. *J Robotic Surg* 2008;2:71.)

single-port platform, further improving surgeon comfort and easier applicability or single-site surgery. Cases have to be carefully selected because single ports will not allow for use in very obese patients with thick subcutaneous tissues, and the use of adequate uterine manipulators is imperative without the availability of ports to provide retraction and manipulation.

Surgical Procedure and Technique

After the ports are placed, actual surgical technique varies little except for the surgical steps required to complete various aspects of the procedure. After successful insufflation and placement of the trocars are accomplished, visual inspection of the abdominal cavity is undertaken, and the patient is placed in a steep Trendelenburg position. **As in any surgical procedure, excellent exposure should be accomplished initially and maintained throughout the case.** Use of steep Trendelenburg position is necessary, in lieu of packing the bowel, to achieve adequate visualization of the pelvis and lower abdominal region. Lysis of any adhesions holding the small bowel or omentum into the pelvis or lower abdomen should occur before beginning the pelvic and upper abdominal dissection. The small bowel is carefully placed in the upper abdomen by flipping the bowel from a caudad to a cranial position, exposing the mesentery of the small bowel and the aortic bifurcation (Fig. 21.4). Care should be taken with this maneuver by using blunt instruments and gentle technique. In obese patients, body habitus may not allow a steep Trendelenburg position because of unacceptably high peak inspiratory pressure. Surgery may be able to be completed by decreasing the amount of Trendelenburg positioning

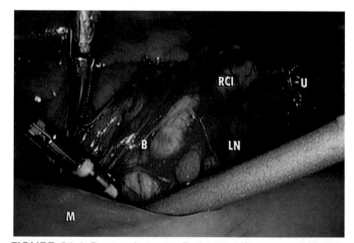

FIGURE 21.4 Paraaortic area. *B*, Aortic bifurcation; *LN*, right paraaortic lymph nodes; *M*, bowel mesentery; *RCI*, right common iliac artery; *U*, ureter.

(while the robot is undocked) or by decreasing the insufflation pressure slightly. Adjusting the respiratory frequency and tidal volume may further improve ventilation. In addition, obesity may prevent adequate mobilization of the small bowel out of the pelvis and upper abdomen to allow for retroperitoneal dissection. Some authors have advocated the use of additional port sites to help circumvent this problem; laparoscopic paddle or fan retractors may also improve exposure.

The key to successful advanced MIS is the same as that for open laparotomy: access to the retroperitoneum. In the pelvis,

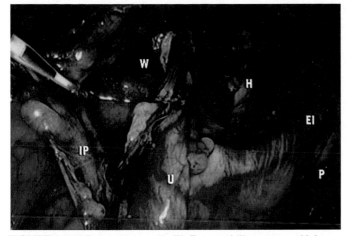

FIGURE 21.5 Pelvic sidewall. *EI*, External iliac artery; *H*, hypogastric artery; *IP*, infundibulopelvic ligament; *P*, psoas muscle; *U*, ureter; *W*, peritoneal window.

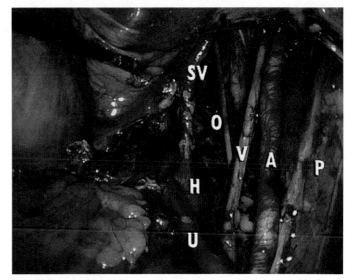

FIGURE 21.6 Pelvic sidewall retroperitoneal anatomy. *A*, External iliac artery; *H*, hypogastric artery; *O*, obturator nerve; *P*, psoas muscle; *SV*, superior vesicle artery; *U*, ureter; *V*, external iliac vein.

FIGURE 21.7 Paraaortic retroperitoneal anatomy. *A*, Aorta; *B*, aortic bifurcation; *IMA*, inferior mesenteric artery; *LCI*, left common iliac artery; *M*, bowel mesentery; *N*, sympathetic nerve; *P*, psoas muscle; *RCI*, right common iliac artery; *U*, right ureter; *V*, inferior vena cava.

this is accomplished by dividing the round ligament laterally or opening the pelvic peritoneum lateral and parallel to the infundibulopelvic ligament. Some surgeons prefer to keep the round ligament intact so they can retract against it to keep the paravesical space open while dissecting tissue. Dissection is then carried down to the level of the external iliac artery, which is then followed in a cephalad and medial direction to the common iliac artery. At this point, the ureter can be found crossing the pelvic brim, and a window can be created between the ovarian vessels and the ureter (Fig. 21.5). Development of the pararectal space is under direct visualization after identification of the bifurcation of the common iliac vessel and the ureter. The surgeon places traction on the ureter, medially developing the pararectal space between the hypogastric artery laterally and the ureter and rectum medially. Care must be taken during this dissection to avoid disrupting the cardinal web deep in the retroperitoneum. Because of the positive pressure environment of MIS resulting from the pneumoperitoneum, the boundaries of the paravesical space can be identified visually during laparoscopic surgery. The superior vesicle artery and umbilical artery are clearly visible as the medial umbilical ligament (see Fig. 21.2). Dissection is carried along the external iliac artery to the level of the superior vesicle artery. At this point, the superior vesicle artery is retracted in a medial direction, and the paravesical space is easily developed with the bladder and superior vesicle artery medially and external artery and obturator node bundle laterally. After this is accomplished, the uterine artery can be clearly identified at the origin of the superior vesicle artery from the hypogastric artery. This retroperitoneal pelvic dissection is the cornerstone of any laparoscopic surgery performed in the pelvis, including removal of an adnexal mass, LAVH, laparoscopic radical hysterectomy (LRH), and PLN dissection (Fig. 21.6). Dissection can be facilitated with a variety of energy sources and clip appliers, each with its own advocates.

Extension of the incision along the peritoneum overlying the right common iliac artery and then along the aorta to the level of the duodenum allows for exposure of the paraaortic retroperitoneum (Fig. 21.7). During this dissection, the peritoneum attached to the base of the cecum can be elevated in an anterior-cephalad direction, providing excellent exposure to the right paraaortic lymph node region. Margins of resection are identical to an open approach and can be extended to the level of the renal vessels. The left-sided paraaortic lymph node dissection requires dissection underneath the inferior mesenteric artery, mobilizing the descending colon and rectosigmoid off the left common iliac artery and retracting the inferior mesenteric artery and ureter laterally and cephalad. This gives excellent exposure to the left paraaortic lymph nodes inferior to the inferior mesenteric artery. Dissection can be continued above the inferior mesenteric artery in a similar manner. Some authors have advocated sacrificing the inferior mesenteric artery to get enhanced exposure to the upper left paraaortic nodes.

Unfortunately, the potential limitations previously described for MIS compared with laparotomy lead to the potential for inherent compromises in surgical technique. Therefore, the surgeon needs to obtain experience over time to optimize patient outcomes and emphasize excellent surgical technique. Knowledge of anatomy, the disease process, and surgical technique is key during these complicated surgical procedures. To minimize complications that are possible with any major surgical procedure, vigilance and meticulous surgical technique are required.

APPLICATIONS OF MINIMALLY INVASIVE SURGERY IN GYNECOLOGIC ONCOLOGY

Cervical Cancer

The pioneering reports describing the use of advanced laparoscopic techniques in gynecologic oncology were initially described in patients with cervical cancer in which laparoscopy was used for PLN dissection in patients with early-stage disease to assess the feasibility for abdominal radical hysterectomy. One of the initial concerns about MIS in cervical cancer was that the laparoscopic approach would not be as thorough as laparotomy in assessing metastatic cancer and performing a comprehensive lymphadenectomy. Early studies in patients undergoing initial laparoscopic lymphadenectomy before laparotomy confirmed that a thorough pelvic and paraaortic lymphadenectomy is possible via LS, with no positive nodes discovered at laparotomy performed after laparoscopic lymphadenectomy. Nevertheless, the completeness of laparoscopic dissection was dependent on the experience of the surgeon, and the most common area for missed lymph nodes was lateral to the common iliac bifurcation. After the feasibility of laparoscopic lymphadenectomy was established, the use of MIS for radical surgery in patients with early-stage cervical cancer and for preradiation surgical assessment in patients with advanced disease was made possible.

Early-stage Cervical Cancer: Radical Hysterectomy

The establishment of the feasibility of laparoscopic lymphadenectomy led to the renewed interest in radical vaginal hysterectomy with laparoscopic lymphadenectomy and the development of novel minimally invasive radical hysterectomy techniques. Several groups worldwide have demonstrated the feasibility of the Schauta radical vaginal hysterectomy, laparoscopic-assisted radical vaginal hysterectomy (LAVRH), and total LRH with the goals of maintaining a high level of cancer control with improved patient outcomes in women with early-stage cervical cancer. The Schauta radical vaginal hysterectomy, described more than 100 years ago, and its subsequent modifications are performed completely vaginally; however, the surgeon does not have the opportunity to perform a retroperitoneal lymph node dissection. The LAVRH has many descriptions but usually involves a laparoscopic phase that includes the lymphadenectomy followed by developing the pararectal and paravesical spaces, dividing the parametria and paravaginal pedicles, and completing the remainder of the procedure vaginally. For the LRH, the entire radical pelvic operation is completed with MIS techniques. One advantage of the LAVRH over the LRH is the ability to precisely define the vaginal incision. Additionally, the performance of LAVRH allows for the development of the MIS skills required to perform a fertility-sparing radical vaginal trachelectomy. Currently, the favored laparoscopic approach is the LRH or robotic-assisted radical hysterectomy (RARH) because there is no need for a perineal phase for the performance of a vaginal incision, exposure is improved, visualization of critical anatomy and surgical planes is better, and anatomic limitations are fewer as a result of a narrow pelvis or lack of uterine descensus. Most important, however, is the fact that LRH mimics the well-established steps of an abdominal radical hysterectomy, thereby making LHR easier to adopt. Certainly, LRH is a technically challenging procedure. Most surgeons who use robotic techniques feel that the superior vision and wristed instruments provide optimal MIS capacity to perform the meticulous dissection required for the radical hysterectomy. Thus, the availability of the robotic platform allows for a significant shortening of the learning curve for MIS radical pelvic procedures and increased uptake of radical hysterectomy via the minimally invasive approach.

There is no doubt that the LARVH, LRH, and RARH are feasible for patients with early-stage cervical cancer. It has been demonstrated that these techniques can accomplish the oncologic goals of the surgery, allowing for the identification of critical anatomy, performance of a thorough lymph node dissection, and completion of the radical resection of the primary tumor with adequate margins. Most reports on LARVH and LRH demonstrate rates of complications comparable to those seen with the traditional open approach. A number of single-institution series reveal that the operative time is longer for LRH and RARH but associated with a decreased length of hospital stay (Tables 21.1 and 21.2). More recent series are larger and also report recurrence and survival data, which compare favorably with matched historical patients undergoing a traditional radical hysterectomy for cervical cancer. A recent meta-analysis comparing abdominal radical hysterectomy with laparoscopic or robotic radical hysterectomy demonstrated less estimated blood loss, shorter length of stay (LOS), fewer wound-related complications, and febrile morbidity in patients undergoing minimally invasive radical hysterectomy. A large multi-institutional retrospective comparison reported similar findings with increased operating time for robotic radical hysterectomy compared with open radical hysterectomy but with lower blood loss and transfusion rates. Overall complication types were similar but occurred less frequently in the robotic radical hysterectomy group; intraoperative complications occurred in 4% versus 11%, and postoperative complications were seen in 30% versus 27% of patients undergoing robotic and open radical hysterectomy, respectively. Of note, recurrence and survival rates were similar. The traditional abdominal radical hysterectomy and the LRH/LARVH procedures are now being

TABLE 21.1   Representative Sample of Single-Institutional Series on Laparoscopic Radical Hysterectomies

Study	Patients (n)	Operating Room Time (h)	Blood Transfusion (%)	Intraoperative Complications (%)	Postoperative Complications (%)	Chronic Genitourinary (%)	Length of Stay (days)
Argentina, 1999	56	4.5	NR	2	6	2	4
Quebec, 2000	54	4.5	4	7	10	0	5
France, 2002	50	4.5	2	4	16	4	8
France 2, 2002	95	4.0	NR	NR	12	2	NR
WCC, 2002	78	3.5	1.3	9	9	1.3	3
Germany, 2003	200	5.5	19	13	15	3.5	NR
MSKCC, 2003	19	6.0	5	11	5	0	4.5
Toronto, 2004	71	3.5	7	13	14	3	1
MDA, 2007	35	5.75	11.0	11	>20	0	2
China, 2007	90	4.5	NR	9	40	3	NR
Italy, 2009	65	3.25	0	5	10	1.5	4

MDA, MD Anderson Cancer Center; *MSKCC,* Memorial Sloan Kettering Cancer Center; *NR,* not reported; *WCC,* Palo Alto Women's Cancer Center.

TABLE 21.2   Comparison of Radical Hysterectomy With *N* >40 Patients Via the Laparoscopic, Robotic, or Abdominal Approach

A. Laparoscopic

Reference (year)	Patients (n)	EBL (mL)	Operative Time (min)	LN Count	Intraoperative Complications (n)	Postoperative Complications (n)	Length of Stay (days)
Kim et al. (2014)	69	350	236	19	1	n/a	9
Yim et al. (2014)	42	145	216	20	1	n/a	10
Gortchev et al. (2012)	46		232	11	0	1	4.8
Chong et al. (2013)	50	202	211	23	4	n/a	8.7
Tinelli et al. (2011)	76	95	255	38	2	n/a	4

B. Robotic

Reference (year)	Patients (n)	EBL (mL)	Operative Time (min)	LN Count	Intraoperative Complications (n)	Postoperative Complications (n)	Length of Stay (days)
Yim et al. (2014)	60	100	n/a	18	0	n/a	11
Gortchev et al. (2012)	73	n/a	152	11	0	3	4.1
Chong et al. (2013)	50	55	n/a	25	0	n/a	9.6
Cantrell et al. (2010)	63	50	213	29	1	2	1
Maggioni et al. (2009)	40	78	272	20	2	n/a	3.7
Boggess et al. (2008a,b)	51	96.5	248	34	n/a	4	1

C. Abdominal

Reference (year)	Patients (n)	EBL (mL)	Operative Time (min)	LN Count	Intraoperative Complications (n)	Postoperative Complications (n)	Length of Stay (days)
Gortchev et al. (2012)	176	n/a	168	16	1	9	9.6
Cantrell et al. (2010)	64	400	240	24	1	3	4
Maggioni et al. (2009)	40	222	200	26	5	n/a	5
Boggess (2008)	49	417	211	23	n/a	8	3.2

EBL, Estimated blood loss; *LN,* lymph node; *n/a,* not reliably able to be assessed from manuscript.

compared in a prospective randomized study, and recruitment is ongoing.

Most authors stress that there is a lengthy learning curve for LRH and that complications decrease and overall operative efficiency improves as the surgeon gains experience. Therefore, these procedures should be performed by highly skilled and experienced surgeons in selected patients to obtain optimal outcomes. Of note, improvements in subspecialty training, collective and individual experience in performing the traditional abdominal radical hysterectomy, better perioperative care, and a general trend toward decreased hospital stay have demonstrated an overall improvement in the outcomes of patients undergoing the open abdominal approach. In fact, the shortest average length of hospital stay reported in many of the LRH series is similar to that reported in contemporaneous series of open radical hysterectomy. There is a lack of prospective data to compare cost and morbidity between the two approaches, and retrospective data do not definitively establish a significant advantage or disadvantage for the laparoscopic approach. **Currently, it appears that with appropriate training and experience, minimally invasive radical hysterectomy is at least comparable to the open technique with regard to cost, morbidity, other perioperative outcomes, and survival.**

Early-Stage Cervical Cancer: Fertility-Sparing Surgery

The ability to perform an adequate laparoscopic lymphadenectomy combined with the revival of the radical vaginal hysterectomy have led to the development of novel techniques for fertility preservation in young patients with early-stage cervical cancer. The laparoscopic vaginal radical trachelectomy (LVRT) is one of the most exciting applications of MIS in gynecologic oncology. In an effort to define the potential number of patients in whom this procedure would be considered, Sonoda and coworkers reported on 435 patients undergoing radical hysterectomy. Eighty-nine of these patients were younger than 40 years of age and had tumors that met the criteria for fertility-sparing radical trachelectomy (which represented 20% of their early-stage population) (Table 21.3). This study clearly shows that there is a substantial population of patients who may benefit from this approach.

The LVRT technique combines laparoscopic pelvic and common iliac lymph node dissection with a radical vaginal trachelectomy (with preservation of the uterine fundus and creation of a neocervix). This procedure was initially described by Dargent in 1987; since then, several centers have reported preliminary results on fertility-sparing radical trachelectomy with laparoscopic lymphadenectomy. Survival and fertility follow-up reports have been encouraging. To date, more than 300 cases have been reported with a recurrence rate of 4.1% and a death rate of 2.5%, which falls well within the range of survival seen with traditional radical hysterectomy

in similar populations. Randomized prospective comparisons are not available, but case-control studies in matched patients reveal equivalent oncologic outcomes when comparing radical hysterectomy with radical trachelectomy. Plante et al. reported on the obstetric outcomes of 72 patients undergoing the surgery over a 12-year time span. A total of 50 pregnancies occurred in 31 women. Infertility rates and first and second trimester pregnancy loss did not appear to be increased. Of the patients reaching the third trimester, 22% had preterm delivery (although only 8% were delivered before 32 weeks). **There appear to be enough data now published to consider fertility-sparing radical trachelectomy a viable option for select and motivated patients. Chuang and colleagues first reported robotic fertility-sparing radical trachelectomy in which the entire procedure is performed minimally invasively without a perineal or vaginal phase. Subsequent reports, limited by a small number of patients enrolled, have demonstrated the feasibility of robotic radical trachelectomy with decreased blood loss and LOS compared with open radical trachelectomy and without compromise of histopathologic or cancer outcomes. Approximately half of the patients who attempted pregnancy were able to conceive, and pregnancy rates were higher in the open surgery group. Whether this is due to shorter follow-up times in the MIS group or a true difference will have to be determined in future studies.**

Advanced-Stage Cervical Cancer: Surgical Staging

Patients with advanced-stage disease or bulky early-stage cervical cancers are generally treated with definitive radiotherapy and concurrent chemotherapy. For this group of patients, laparoscopy has been used for surgical staging and to assist radiation oncologists in the safe placement of interstitial brachytherapy implants. Even positron emission tomography or computed tomography scans will not identify all patients with extrapelvic disease. Although controversial, surgical staging has been advocated to accurately define the extent of disease and guide the subsequent radiation fields. In patients with gross evidence of lymph node metastasis, their removal has been demonstrated in retrospective studies to improve survival compared with radiation of these nodes without debulking.

Before advanced MIS techniques, retroperitoneal lymphadenectomy for surgical staging of cervical cancer was performed at the time of extraperitoneal laparotomy. This approach afforded the surgeon excellent exposure to both the pelvic and paraaortic nodes with the ability to debulk grossly positive nodes. A transperitoneal laparotomy approach is not recommended because it is associated with a significant increase in the rate of severe postirradiation enteric morbidity compared with extraperitoneal laparotomy, presumably secondary to adhesion formation. Both transperitoneal and extraperitoneal laparoscopic approaches have been described for surgical staging of cervical cancer. Initially, there was concern that transperitoneal laparoscopic lymph node dissection would be associated with increased adhesion formation as experienced with transperitoneal laparotomy for lymphadenectomy. The extraperitoneal laparoscopic approach avoids this risk, but the surgeon only has access to the common iliac and paraaortic

---

TABLE 21.3 Suggested Clinical Eligibility Criteria for Laparoscopic Radical Vaginal Trachelectomy or Robotic Radical Trachelectomy

1. Confirmed invasive cervical cancer: squamous, adenocarcinoma, or adenosquamous
2. FIGO stage Ia1 with lymphovascular space involvement, FIGO Ia2 to Ib1
3. Desire to preserve fertility
4. No clinical evidence of impaired fertility
5. Lesion size <2 cm
6. Patient is a candidate for a vaginal hysterectomy
7. Estimated cervical length ≥2 cm clinically
8. Adequate resolution of acute inflammation postcone
9. No evidence of extracervical or metastatic disease

FIGO, Federation of International Gynecologists and Obstetricians.

lymph nodes and is unable to perform a PLN dissection. However, transperitoneal laparoscopy, in general, is associated with fewer intraperitoneal adhesions compared with laparotomy. Blinded studies in animal models reveal a similar rate and severity of adhesions between transperitoneal laparoscopic lymph node dissection and extraperitoneal laparotomy; however, transperitoneal laparoscopic lymphadenectomy is associated with significantly fewer adhesions compared with transperitoneal laparotomy.

Multiple single-institutional series exist describing laparoscopy for pretreatment lymphadenectomy for advanced cervical cancer. The procedure is feasible with acceptable morbidity compared with laparotomy. A significant advantage for the laparoscopic approach is avoiding potential complications of a large abdominal incision and quicker postoperative recovery, allowing the patient to proceed to definitive radiation therapy more quickly. Although laparoscopic resection of nodes grossly involved with metastatic disease is technically feasible, it is definitely more difficult compared with laparotomy, especially when the nodes are fixed to vessels. Therefore, some surgeons prefer extraperitoneal laparotomy in case they encounter nodes that require debulking. The robotic platform obviates many of the inherent disadvantages of laparoscopy. As in laparoscopy, the robotic approach can be used for pelvic and paraaortic lymph node dissection. In addition, advantages of robotic surgery enable the surgeon to perform the more complicated debulking surgeries if necessary.

Endometrial Cancer
Laparoscopy

In the population of patients diagnosed with a gynecologic malignancy, MIS is most often applied for those diagnosed with endometrial cancer. Before the availability of advanced laparoscopic procedures, vaginal hysterectomy was a less invasive option for definitive surgical therapy, especially in patients with severe comorbidities and an increased risk of complications secondary to laparotomy. In fact, assuming the disease is confined to the uterus, the curative potential of the hysterectomy should be equivalent regardless of the surgical approach. The disadvantages of the vaginal hysterectomy in endometrial cancer include the inability to fully inspect the peritoneal cavity and retroperitoneum (lymph nodes) for metastatic disease and potential inability to complete BSO. The addition of laparoscopy to the vaginal hysterectomy essentially eliminates these disadvantages. Most patients with endometrial cancer present with apparent early-stage disease. Approximately 15% to 25% will be upstaged as a result of surgical staging. The majority of patients with extrauterine disease have occult (without gross evidence) spread. Current disease assessment modalities such as preoperative imaging, intraoperative palpation, gross inspection, and frozen section of the uterus all are inaccurate compared with comprehensive surgical staging that includes bilateral pelvic and paraaortic lymph node dissection. Comprehensive surgical staging with lymphadenectomy provides the best definition of the biologic nature of the disease and allows the oncologist to make informed postoperative treatment decisions.

Laparoscopic-assisted vaginal hysterectomy bilateral salpingo-oophorectomy (LAVH-BSO) or total laparoscopic hysterectomy (TLH) can be substituted for total abdominal hysterectomy bilateral salpingo-oophorectomy (TAH-BSO) in the algorithm presented earlier in this book for the management of endometrial cancer.

The overall management of patients with apparent early-stage endometrial cancer continues to evolve. Endometrial cancer remains the least uniformly managed gynecologic malignancy, even among gynecologic oncologists. It remains controversial whether all patients should have surgical lymph node assessment and, in those undergoing lymphadenectomy, the extent to which lymph node dissection should be performed. Nevertheless, until laparoscopic lymph node dissection was described, comprehensive surgical staging of endometrial cancer by MIS was not feasible. The earliest series published on MIS management of endometrial cancer primarily described pelvic lymphadenectomy with a minimum of patients undergoing a paraaortic lymph node dissection. The ability to perform laparoscopic lymphadenectomy evolved from pelvic nodes to right-sided paraaortic nodes to a bilateral paraaortic lymph node dissection to the level of the inferior mesenteric artery. Although controversial, recent reports on surgical staging of endometrial cancer recommend that selected patients at high risk for extrauterine disease have a bilateral paraaortic dissection to the level of the renal vessels. This technique has been described laparoscopically but is technically difficult and likely currently applied to a small minority of patients undergoing MIS management of endometrial cancer.

Until recently, most data describing the experience of laparoscopy in management of endometrial cancer came from single institutions and are primarily retrospective studies. It is clear that advances in MIS technology, training, and experience allow the surgeon the opportunity to ensure removal of the uterus and adnexae, inspect the peritoneal cavity, define the retroperitoneal anatomy, and perform a thorough pelvic and paraaortic lymph node dissection. The reported benefits of a laparoscopic approach in endometrial cancer are lower blood loss and transfusion rates, shorter hospital stay, faster postoperative recovery, and superior short-term QoL, albeit at the expense of longer operative times. However, these studies are biased by the fact that they represent only selected patients (eg, those with low body mass indexes [BMIs]) compared with an institution's entire population of patients with endometrial cancer. Additionally, these series vary as to whether comprehensive surgical staging was performed and, if so, as to the extent of lymph node dissection (Table 21.4). Surgeon experience and patient factors such as obesity or previous abdominal surgery contribute to the many disadvantages of the laparoscopic approach in endometrial cancer, especially if the goal is comprehensive surgical staging. In a study of two California databases from 1997 to 2001, only 7.7% of patients diagnosed with endometrial cancer underwent surgery via a laparoscopic approach. A recent survey of members of the Society of Gynecologic Oncologists (29% responding) revealed that use of MIS as a surgical treatment option for endometrial cancer has continued to increase, with almost 70% of gynecologic oncologists

TABLE 21.4 Large Retrospective Cohort or Comparison Studies of Robotic Surgery (*N* >100) for Endometrial Staging Versus Laparotomy and/or Laparoscopy

A. Robotic

Reference (year)	Patients (*n*)	EBL (mL)	BMI (kg/m^2)	Conversion to Laparotomy (%)	LN Count	Intraoperative Complications (%)	Postoperative Complications (%)	Length of Stay (days)
Paley et al. (2011)	377	47	n/a	3.5	15.5	0.5	5.9	1.4
Backes et al. (2012)	503	90	32	6.4		1.6	7.6	1
Boggess et al. (2008a,b)	103	75	33	3	33	1	5	1
Cardenas-Goicoechea et al. (2010)	102	109	n/a	1	n/a	2	8.8	1.9
Lowe et al. (2009a,b)	405	88	32	6.7	15.5	3.5	14.6	1.8
Seamon et al. (2009a,b,c,d)	105	100	34	12	31	n/a	n/a	1
Seamon et al. (2009a,b,c,d)	109	109	40	15.	25	2.2	11	1

B. Abdominal

Reference (year)	Patients (*n*)	EBL (mL)	BMI (kg/m^2)	LN Count	Intraoperative Complications (%)	Postoperative Complications (%)	Length of Stay (days)
Paley et al. (2011)	131	198	NR	12.1	3	21	5.3
Boggess et al. (2008a,b)	138	266	35	14.9	0.7	29	4.4
Veljovich et al. (2008)	131	13	32	13.1	n/a	20.6	5
Seamon et al. (2009a,b,c,d)	191	394	40	24	2.5	27	3

C. Laparoscopic

Reference (year)	Patients (*n*)	EBL (mL)	BMI (kg/m^2)	Conversion to Laparotomy	LN Count	Intraoperative Complications (%)	Postoperative Complications (%)	Length of Stay (days)
Boggess et al. (2008a,b)	81	146	29	5%	23.1	3.7	10	1.2
Cardenas-Goicoechea et al. (2010)	173	187	n/a	5.2%	n/a	3.5	7.5	2.3
Seamon et al. (2009a,b,c,d)	76	250	29	26%	33	2.6	n/a	2

EBL, Estimated blood loss; *LN,* lymph node; *n/a,* not reliably able to be assessed from manuscript.

stating that this is the procedure they perform most via the MIS approach.

Several prospective randomized trials comparing laparoscopic and open surgery for endometrial cancer staging have been conducted. In 2009, the Gynecologic Oncology Group (GOG) reported the results of the LAP-2 (Laparoscopy compared with laparotomy for comprehensive surgical staging of uterine cancer: Gynecologic Oncology Group Study) trial, which enrolled 2531 patients with apparent early-stage endometrial cancer. All patients in this study were to undergo complete surgical staging and were randomly assigned in a 2:1 ratio of laparoscopy to laparotomy. Of the 1678 patients on the laparoscopy arm, 25.8% required conversion to laparotomy (of note, conversion to laparotomy was mandatory if lymph node dissection could not be completed laparoscopically). More than half of these conversions were a result of poor visualization (exposure), 16% were from metastasis, and 11% were from bleeding. Fig. 21.8 graphs the likelihood of converting from laparoscopy to laparotomy as a function of BMI, age, and evidence of metastatic disease. In this landmark study, there was no significant difference in rate of node positivity between the two groups; however, significantly fewer patients in the laparoscopy arm (78.5%) compared with the laparotomy arm (86.4%) had lymph nodes histologically identified from all four primary nodal regions (which include the right and left periaortic and bilateral PLNs). The incidence of intraoperative complications, reoperations,

and readmissions was similar, but significantly fewer Common Toxicity Criteria grade II or greater postoperative complications (P <0.0001) occurred on the laparoscopy arm (14.3%) compared with the laparotomy arm (21.1%). Similar transfusion rates were seen between the groups (7% to 9%). Consistent with other studies in the literature, operative time was significantly longer for the laparoscopic arm (203 minutes) versus the laparotomy arm (136 minutes). For patients successfully completing laparoscopic surgery, the average length of hospital stay was 2 days versus 4 days for laparotomy (P <0.0001). During the perioperative period, the LAP-2 study revealed significantly better overall QoL, pain scores, resumption of normal activities, and time until return to work in the laparoscopy arm. By 6 months after surgery, no significant QoL differences were found except in that of body image. Previously reported but small single-institution studies reveal no differences in survival between laparoscopy and laparotomy for the surgical management of endometrial cancer. **LAP-2 also examined this most important survival endpoint. The estimated 3-year overall survival rates from this study are 89.8% for laparoscopy and 89.9% for laparotomy, with similar rates of recurrence and death from disease. Other international studies such as the Dutch study by Mourits et al. in which patients were randomized to TLH versus abdominal hysterectomy (without lymph node staging) and the Australian study (Laparoscopic Approach to Cancer of the Endometrium [LACE] trial) by Janda and**

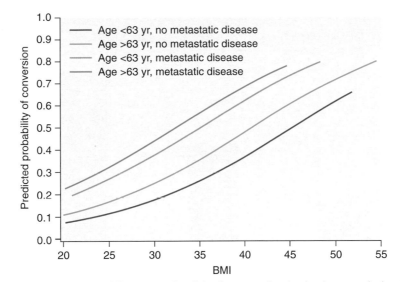

FIGURE 21.8 Predicted probability curve for risk of conversion by body mass index (BMI), age, and metastatic disease. (From Walker JL, Piedmonte MR, Spirtos NM, et al. Laparoscopy compared with laparotomy for comprehensive surgical staging of uterine cancer: gynecologic Oncology Group Study LAP2. *J Clin Oncol* 2009;27:5331.)

coworkers, which also included pelvic lymphadenectomy reported similar findings. The latter also found better QoL up to 6 months after TLH and with fewer complications.

Laparoscopy offers selected patients with endometrial cancer the potential benefits of shorter hospital stay, less need for blood transfusion, and decreased postoperative complications with a similar risk of intraoperative complications. Nevertheless, laparoscopic hysterectomy with pelvic and paraaortic lymph node dissection remains difficult to learn and is least likely to be offered or successful in patients with obesity, the group of patients most likely to benefit from MIS. Although morbid obesity is the most common risk factor for developing endometrial cancer, it is also the major limitation to successful laparoscopic surgical management. Most studies reporting the use of MIS for the treatment of endometrial cancer describe a population of patients with a mean BMI lower than that typically seen in the overall population of patients with endometrial cancer. Even the LAP-2 study represents a selected group of patients because the median BMI was 28 kg/m^2 in both arms. The rate of conversion from laparoscopy to laparotomy ranges quite widely between single-institution reports. Variables such as intent to perform comprehensive staging, adhesions, intraoperative complications, discovery of metastatic disease, and surgeon experience have all been reported as important factors. In the LAP-2 study, the overall conversion rate was 25.8% and strongly influenced by BMI (with a rate of 17.5% in patients with a BMI of 25 kg/m^2 and a rate of 57% in patients with a BMI greater than 40 kg/m^2).

Robotics

As previously mentioned, recent developments in robotic technology have allowed the surgeon to gain advantages compared with laparoscopy, and this technology has rapidly been adopted by gynecologic oncologists independent of their prior laparoscopic experience. Relatively large single-institution and pooled reports reveal that the robotic surgical staging of patients with endometrial cancer is feasible and that the patient experiences the typical benefits of MIS compared with laparotomy. Furthermore, these reports have shown that robotic surgery is likely applicable to a larger portion of patients diagnosed with endometrial cancer compared with laparoscopy, including patients who are morbidly obese (see Table 21.4). Seamon and colleagues demonstrated that comprehensive surgical staging is feasible in a relatively heavy group of patients (mean BMI, 34 kg/m^2), as robotic pelvic and paraaortic dissection was performed in 85% of the patients overall and in 67% of the patients with BMI more than 45 kg/m^2. Gehrig and coworkers compared their robotic and laparoscopic experience in obese patients (BMI >30 kg/m^2) with endometrial cancer and demonstrated a significant difference in hospital stay, blood loss, and operating room time in favor of the robotic group. Seamon and colleagues compared 105 patients with endometrial cancer undergoing robotic surgery with 76 patients managed laparoscopically and revealed a similar ability to complete surgical staging. However, comprehensive surgical staging was able to be performed in heavier patients compared with laparoscopy (BMI, 34 kg/m^2 vs. 29 kg/m^2), and with significantly shorter LOS, lower conversion to laparotomy, and shorter operating room time in favor of the robotic group. Compared with laparotomy, the advantages of the robotic approach are more dramatic in obese patients with endometrial cancer. In a matched cohort study in patients with a median BMI of 40 kg/m^2 and multiple comorbidities, patients managed robotically experienced a decreased LOS (1 vs. 3 days) and significantly lower rates of overall complications (odds ratio [OR], 0.29), blood transfusion (OR, 0.22), and wound complications (OR, 0.10) compared with laparoscopy (Fig. 21.9). Even in extreme morbid obese patients (mean BMIs, 48, 51, and 54 for laparoscopic, robotic, and open hysterectomy, respectively), MIS (laparoscopic and robotic) was associated

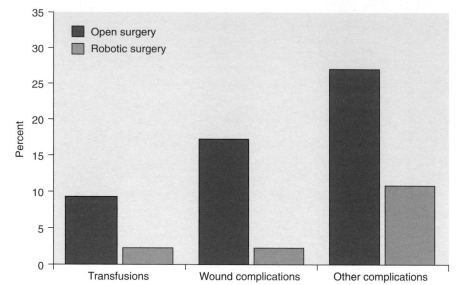

FIGURE 21.9 Transfusion rates, postoperative complications, and wound complications for laparotomy compared with robotic hysterectomy lymphadenectomy for endometrial cancer. The blood transfusion rate (9% compared with 2%; odds ratio [OR], 0.22; 95% confidence interval [CI] 0.05–0.97; $P = 0.046$), wound problems (17% compared with 2%; OR, 0.10; 95% CI 0.02–0.43; $P = 0.002$), and complications (27% compared with 11%; OR, 0.29; 95% CI 0.13–0.65; $P = 0.003$) were reduced for robotic surgery. (From Seamon LG, Fowler JM, Richardson DL, et al. A detailed analysis of the learning curve: robotic hysterectomy and pelvic-aortic lymphadenectomy for endometrial cancer. *Obstet Gynecol* 2009;114:16.)

with lower rates of blood loss and shorter hospital stays despite longer operative times. Similarly, comorbidities, not weight and BMI, were predictive of an increased risk of perioperative complications.

In addition, recurrence rates and survival appear similar to open surgery in retrospective reviews. Although it is most critical that the surgeon have expertise in the management of patients with endometrial cancer, it appears that the learning curve for comprehensive robotic staging of endometrial cancer is not as difficult as laparoscopy. Experiences from several institutions have shown that 10 to 20 cases are needed to gain proficiency with the procedure. Operative times improve as the surgeon and the surgical team become more familiar with the setup and techniques. The robotic platform is now the dominant surgical approach in the management of women with apparent early-stage uterine cancer.

Single-Site Surgery

In 2009, Fader and Escobar reported their initial experience with LESS for gynecologic cancer surgery. Larger series have since been published and have demonstrated safety and feasibility of the single-site approach for endometrial cancer. Although single-site surgery has been reported in moderately obese patients (median BMI, 32–33), abdominal wall thickness remains a limiting factor for the single port in extreme morbidly obese patients.

Minimally Invasive Sentinel Lymph Node Assessment

In an attempt to reduce the risk of side effects and complications (bleeding, lymphocele, lymphedema, longer operating time) seen with comprehensive lymph node dissection, sentinel lymph node (SLN) assessment has been developed and has been part of standard of care in breast cancer, melanoma and vulvar cancer for several years. SLN assessment is now also an acceptable part of standard of care in women with endometrial cancer and cervical cancer and has been incorporated in the National Comprehensive Cancer Network's guidelines (version 2.2015). SLN assessment can be performed using open and minimally invasive techniques, and equipment is available for laparotomy, laparoscopic, and robotic approaches. Blue dye (isosulfan blue, patent blue, methylene blue) has been studied most extensively. Other available methods include radiolabeled technetium-99 with lymphoscintigraphy, indocyanine green dye (ICG) with immunofluorescence detection, and a combination of the various methods. Some studies advocate for using ICG only given the high detection rates and ease of administration as well as a low risk of allergic reaction (1:40,000). For cervical cancer, peritumoral injection is intuitive and relatively easy. In contrast, the best location of injection is not as clear for endometrial cancer. Investigators have studied hysteroscopic tumor injection, fundal or subserosal injection, cervical injection, or a combination of multiple injection sites. Although combined location injection methods have improved SLN detection rates, the overall accuracy of intracervical injection alone is high. Certainly, some surgeons have expressed concern about missing aortic SLNs, but staging studies have demonstrated that the risk of isolated positive aortic lymph nodes in the setting of negative PLNs is rare (1%–2%). However, it is important to keep in mind that in high-risk patients (high-grade histology or deep myometrial invasion), the risk of paraaortic lymph node involvement increases to 4%, and as such, the safety of intracervical injection for SLN assessment in high-risk patients has not yet been confirmed. Most surgeons prefer to perform cervical injections only, and injection protocols vary. In general, 1 mL of dye is injected at the 3 and 9 o'clock position. Some believe dye should be injected superficially (submucosal) and deep (intrastromal), but others inject superficially only. Next, ports are placed, and the retroperitoneal spaces are developed. Care should be taken to maintain excellent hemostasis because blood can obscure visualization of the various types of dye. SLNs are dissected, labeled for location, and sent separately. Detection rates (any detection) vary from 80% to 95% in endometrial cancer and 84% to 99% in cervical cancer depending on the study and methods used, and best detection in cervical cancer is seen in tumors smaller than 2 cm. Bilateral detection varies between 60% and 85% for cervical cancer and 52% and 79% in endometrial cancer. Adherence to an SLN algorithm is critical for successful application of SLN assessment; all suspicious or enlarged lymph nodes should be removed, and a site-specific complete lymphadenectomy is performed when SLNs are not identified. When adhering to these principles, the negative predictive value is high (95%–100%), and false-negative rates are low. Most institutions use ultrastaging (serial sectioning of the SLNs with immunohistochemistry in addition to standard hematoxylin and eosin stain) to assess for metastatic disease; however, the clinical significance of micrometastases detected with ultrastaging has not been defined at this time.

Removal of a Large Uterus

If the uterus is too large or the vaginal opening is too small to remove the uterus through the vagina, the surgeon can place the uterus in a laparoscopic bag (through the vagina or a port site). Sometimes this allows for removal of the uterus through the vagina, providing a smoother outer surface and more equal distribution of pulling forces. If still unsuccessful, the midline camera port can be slightly extended to allow for uterine removal in the laparoscopic bag (mini-laparotomy). Some surgeons bivalve or morcellate the uterus in the bag; however, removing the uterus intact for complete pathologic assessment is preferred. Certainly, power morcellation is not recommended when operating on patients with invasive or preinvasive disease.

Uterine Manipulation for Minimally Invasive Surgery

Adequate uterine and vaginal manipulation is a requirement for successful completion of MIS to identify the correct planes of dissection and to avoid additional ports to retract and move the uterus. Early studies reported increased incidence of positive peritoneal cytology after laparoscopic hysterectomy (10%) compared with open hysterectomy (2.8%). However, more recently, two prospective studies comparing pelvic washings before and after insertion of the uterine manipulator found no significant increase (0%–4%) in positive cytology after insertion of the manipulator. Tubal contamination was reported to be higher after robotic compared with laparoscopic hysterectomy, and avoiding manipulation of the tubes but rather retracting using the round ligaments may be considered. There has been no evidence that true lymphovascular invasion is more common

with the use of uterine manipulators in endometrial or cervical cancer. Most important, there is no evidence that the use of a uterine manipulator leads to increased risk of recurrence or worse prognosis, although randomized studies have not been performed.

Adnexal Mass

One of the most common clinical scenarios presented to gynecologic surgeons is that of the suspicious adnexal mass. Because most masses are asymptomatic, the major reason for surgical removal is to determine if a malignancy is present. The finding of a persistent ovarian mass represents a major reason for surgery in gynecology. Killackey and Neuwirth reported that 17% of laparotomies in gynecology are performed primarily for this indication. It has been reported that 5% of persistent premenopausal ovarian masses and 20% to 50% of those in postmenopausal women are malignant. This risk of malignancy (and potential need for surgical staging or cytoreduction) has led to the recommendation that suspicious ovarian masses be removed through a vertical midline incision. This recommendation, however, is made with the assumption that a gynecologic oncologist or other trained surgeon will be available to provide surgical support if required. This surgery may include radical pelvic or upper abdominal dissection, retroperitoneal lymphadenectomy or lymph node debulking, or bowel resection. Most gynecologists do not have such assistance on standby for every surgery performed for a pelvic mass. Potential advantages of minimally invasive approaches to the pelvic masses are cost savings and decreased morbidity in those women without cancer and early diagnosis and referral for appropriate surgical management in those who are found to have malignancies.

Postmenopausal women undergoing laparotomy for ovarian masses have a much greater likelihood of malignancy than premenopausal women. Postmenopausal patients with ovarian masses differ from premenopausal patients with respect to the predictive value of CA-125. An elevated CA-125 level has a positive predictive value for malignancy of 80% to 98% in this population. Postmenopausal patients with an adnexal mass and an elevated CA-125 level are presumed to have a malignancy and should have surgery by an ovarian cancer specialist regardless of the ultrasound findings. The ability to identify patients preoperatively at highest risk for cancer (with the appropriate selection of surgical approach and consultation or referral for surgical management of this potential cancer) is often challenging. Although pelvic ultrasonography, tumor markers, and clinical presentation all contribute to risk stratification for ovarian cancer, the definitive evaluation of a mass is determined during surgery. However, multiple scoring systems have been devised to provide the surgeon with a preoperative probability of a mass being malignant. The SGO and the American College of Obstetrics and Gynecology jointly published referral guidelines and management recommendations for patients who present with a pelvic mass. Chapter 10 includes a comprehensive discussion of risk assessment of an adnexal mass in both premenopausal and postmenopausal women. In general, if a surgeon stratifies the risk of an adnexal mass into low-, medium-, and high-risk categories for malignancy, then the risk of finding an "unexpected" ovarian cancer at the time of surgery should be extremely low.

Minimally Invasive Surgery Management

Several authors have reported on the LS management of suspected benign ovarian masses. In 1992, Nezhat et al. reported 1209 adnexal masses managed laparoscopically. The majority of patients had endometriosis or functional cysts. However, 64 patients had benign ovarian tumors, and four were malignant. There were no reported major complications in removing masses up to 25 cm in diameter, clearly demonstrating the technical feasibility of managing ovarian masses laparoscopically. Since then, multiple authors have reported on the use of laparoscopic oophorectomy in both premenopausal and postmenopausal women. The complication rates in these nonrandomized reviews of laparoscopic surgery vary from 0% to 18% and include bowel injury, ureteral injury, wound infection, hematoma, and hemorrhage. **A consensus of these retrospective reviews and small randomized trials is that laparoscopic management of adnexal masses is associated with decreased or similar operating time and decreased perioperative morbidity, including pain, infection, and blood loss compared with laparotomy.** These studies also show a decreased LOS and potential cost savings; however, major complications are still possible.

More recently, authors have reported on using laparoscopy in the initial management of ovarian masses suspicious for malignancy. Dottino and coworkers reported on 160 patients with suspicious adnexal masses who had no evidence of gross metastases or extension above the umbilicus. No distinction was made based on other risk factors for malignancy; however, all of these patients were referred for gynecologic oncology consultation. A total of 141 patients were successfully managed laparoscopically. Invasive ovarian cancer was discovered in nine patients, borderline ovarian tumors in eight, and nongynecologic cancer in four. Dottino and associates reported a 3% incidence of intraoperative complications requiring conversion to laparotomy and only one incidence of intraoperative spillage of tumor. This was a sex cord–stromal tumor, which did recur locally. Canis et al. reported on 230 adnexal masses suspicious or solid at ultrasound examination evaluated initially by laparoscopy. Twenty percent of the invasive cancers and 50% of the borderline tumors had cyst puncture or rupture at the time of diagnosis. One case of tumor dissemination occurred with morcellation of an immature teratoma. **These studies highlight the need to prevent tumor spill and morcellation for all suspicious masses.** There is concern that the positive-pressure carbon dioxide environment established during pneumoperitoneum may predispose patients to intraperitoneal seeding. Animal studies have shown an increased seeding rate in the pneumoperitoneum group compared with control participants. This may be explained by peritoneal damage and exposure of the underlying basal lamina, which could facilitate implantation. No clear conclusions can be drawn regarding the risk to humans, but **these studies suggest cyst rupture or spillage should be avoided in all ovarian masses that could possibly be malignant.**

The algorithm presented in Fig. 21.10 is based on a strategy of maximal use of MIS combined with minimal risk of

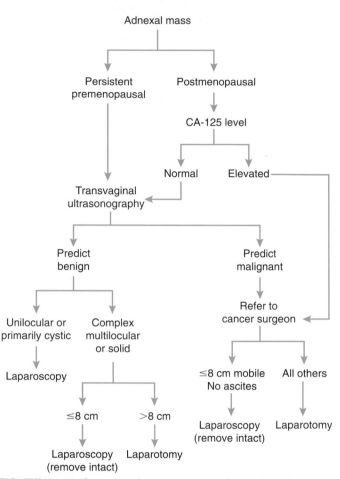

FIGURE 21.10 Suggested management of an adnexal mass.

unexpected finding of ovarian cancer or intraabdominal tumor spill. **The presence of a unilocular cystic mass in premenopausal women is rarely malignant regardless of size.** This fact is important because most of these patients are candidates for ovarian conservation with cystectomy. The same criteria for conservative management can be used with MIS as is already being done with laparotomy. Cystectomy has been described using a variety of techniques using MIS. Equipment such as needle aspirators and intraabdominal bagging devices can allow for cyst decompression without spillage. Techniques have been described for either transabdominal or transvaginal cyst aspiration and removal. Large cysts can be aspirated transvaginally and removed via a posterior colpotomy with no intraabdominal spillage. Size limits for removal of unilocular cysts seem to be related to safety of trocar insertion, surgical exposure, and experience of the surgeon. If oophorectomy is to be performed, the aspiration of the unilocular cyst will allow most of these to be removed through the anterior abdominal wall trocar site. More complex cysts that are believed to be benign can be removed in a bag through a colpotomy or by extending the midline port-site incision at the end of the case. Some multilocular ovarian neoplasms larger than 8 cm in size that are thought to be benign based on ultrasonography have a large dominant cyst. These can be managed through a posterior colpotomy with transvaginal drainage of the dominant cyst and subsequent removal of the ovary through the colpotomy. Suspicious masses should not be intentionally aspirated or morcellated outside of a controlled situation that prevents tumor spill and intraperitoneal dissemination.

If known ultrasound criteria are used, the negative predictive value for ovarian malignancy in premenopausal women should be greater than 95%. If the schema is adhered to, the few women with malignancies should have their tumors removed with no intraabdominal spillage (see Fig. 21.10). The rare finding of malignancy will still allow for appropriate timely referral, surgical staging, and treatment. Because the majority of premenopausal women have masses with benign characteristics, this approach could substantially reduce the number of laparotomies performed for ovarian masses.

When the transvaginal ultrasound examination is consistent with probable malignancy, a different approach is recommended (see Fig. 21.10). The positive predictive value of ultrasonogarphy alone ranges from 30% to 80%. Patients should have primary therapy by a physician trained to deal with ovarian cancer surgery and staging. These tumors can be managed with MIS if they are 8 cm or smaller and can be removed intact (and in a bag) through a colpotomy or mini-laparotomy. If malignancy is documented, these patients should have further surgery by appropriately trained physicians as soon as possible. Patients with ovarian masses larger than 8 cm that are suspicious for malignancy or those that cannot be removed without controlled rupture by laparoscopy should undergo laparotomy by ovarian cancer specialists. Patients who are found to have disease spread beyond the ovary at time of MIS should have a confirmatory biopsy of the extraovarian disease (higher yield than biopsy of a cyst) and referral for definitive therapy and staging as soon as possible.

Ovarian Cancer
Diagnosis of Ovarian Cancer

As a result of the relatively poor ability to predict malignancy with existing preoperative technology, a number of studies have looked at using laparoscopy to assess the presence or absence of ovarian cancer. Aspiration cytology of ovarian cyst fluid has a poor negative predictive value in the range of 58% to 80%. Case reports have raised the possibility that aspiration or biopsy of malignant ovarian cysts may lead to peritoneal tumor implantation, limiting its application for diagnostic purposes. Also, use of therapeutic aspiration is ineffective for resolution of an ovarian cyst, with a recurrence rate as high as 67%. Therefore, routine or intentional cyst aspiration is not recommended, especially in the presence of a suspicious mass. Reports of success are likely to include functional cysts because aspiration does nothing to interrupt the pathologic process of an ovarian neoplasm or endometrioma. When laparoscopic biopsy is highly suspicious for malignancy, definitive surgery should be performed if a trained ovarian cancer surgeon is available; otherwise, the surgery should be aborted, and the patient should be referred immediately to such a specialist.

Ovarian Cyst Rupture

The main concern about managing a suspicious adnexal mass with MIS, especially when a cancer is apparently confined to the ovary, is that rupture may cause dissemination of malignant cells into the peritoneal cavity and adversely affect surgical stage and thus survival. MIS is more likely than laparotomy to result in capsular rupture because it potentially includes more tumor manipulation, and masses often must be drained before removal from the peritoneal cavity. In an assessment of outcomes in the laparoscopic management for adnexal masses, both benign and malignant, mass rupture occurred in 25% of the cases. Therefore, use of laparoscopy has been discouraged because of the potential for rupture of a malignant ovarian cyst. However, the prognostic impact of cyst rupture in an encapsulated stage I ovarian cancer remains controversial. Any spillage should be managed with copious irrigation, as is the case with open surgery.

Another concern regarding MIS for ovarian cancer has been the possible effects of a delay in referral for subsequent definitive surgery and staging after an initial diagnosis of cancer. In an early report by Maiman et al. of 42 patients referred for malignant ovarian neoplasms excised laparoscopically, the mean interval to laparotomy was 5 weeks, and more than 10% of these patients did not undergo subsequent exploratory surgery. The impact of this delay on survival is not known. In a review of 48 cases of surgical staging after laparoscopic removal of malignant ovarian masses, Lehner and associates reported that a delay of more than 17 days was associated with an increased risk of advanced-stage disease for malignant and low-malignant-potential tumors on univariate analysis. These concerns are heightened by Kindermann et al.'s retrospective survey of 192 cases of ovarian malignancy initially diagnosed laparoscopically. Patients with a delay of more than 8 days between laparoscopic biopsy and definitive surgery had an increased risk of port-site metastasis and progression to stage III disease. In this report, only 7% of the apparent stage I tumors were removed intact as a result of biopsy, capsule rupture, and morcellation, making interpretation of these data difficult. These findings suggest that all efforts should be made to avoid intraoperative spillage from the ovary and to limit delay until definitive surgery. If patients are managed according to Fig. 21.10, the unexpected finding of ovarian malignancy should be less than 5%. The few malignant masses that are managed with MIS should be removed without intraabdominal rupture, and survival is unlikely to be negatively affected. Managing patients according to this schema allows for appropriate and timely referral of patients with ovarian malignancy to physicians appropriately trained to manage these patients.

Early-stage Ovarian Cancer

The location and frequency of subclinical metastasis in patients with presumed early-stage ovarian cancer have encouraged investigation of the use of laparoscopic surgery for this patient population. Many areas traditionally evaluated during open laparotomy can be adequately assessed via MIS, including peritoneal cytology, the diaphragm, the omentum, the pelvic and paraaortic lymph nodes, and the pelvic peritoneum. Areas that are less likely to be fully visualized laparoscopically include the abdominal peritoneum and the bowel mesentery and serosa secondary to less ability to "run the bowel" and the inability to palpate. Review of the literature indicates that the most common sites of subclinical metastasis in ovarian cancer include peritoneal cytology, the pelvic and paraaortic lymph nodes, the diaphragm, and the pelvic peritoneum, all of which can be adequately evaluated laparoscopically or robotically (see Table 11.16). The inability to thoroughly evaluate the abdominal peritoneum and bowel mesentery could potentially lead to a 3% to 5% risk of understaging. Laparoscopic staging may be particularly helpful in patients who have undergone a recent exploratory laparotomy for removal of an adnexal mass found to be malignant who did not have appropriate staging. In 1995, Childers et al. reported on the technical feasibility of laparoscopic staging of presumed stage I ovarian cancer. They found metastatic disease in eight of 14 patients, including three with positive paraaortic nodes, three with pelvic disease, and two with positive cytology. Following this report, several small series of laparoscopic staging in this patient population have been published. In a case-controlled series, Chi and coworkers demonstrated equivalent node counts and omental size removed in patients undergoing laparoscopic versus open procedures. There was no significant difference in the rate of metastatic disease between the groups, although the numbers are too small to provide adequate power.

To date, there are no randomized trials looking at surgical staging or survival outcomes in early-stage ovarian cancer managed laparoscopically. An attempted Cochrane meta-analysis in 2009 was unsuccessful because of the low number of studies in the literature. In 2013, Park and associates conducted a meta-analysis of laparoscopic staging in early ovarian cancer and were able to include 11 observational studies. Operative outcomes were similar to those of laparotomy. The overall rates of upstaging and conversion to laparotomy were 22.6% and 3%, respectively, and the tumor rupture was reported at 25.4%. One port-site metastasis was found. A large multi-institutional retrospective review included 300 patients with apparent early-stage ovarian cancer. It compared 150 patients who underwent laparoscopic staging at initial diagnosis with 150 patients who had delayed staging after incidental diagnosis. Patients in the delayed staging group were younger and more likely to be premenopausal with a possible desire for fertility-sparing surgery. Conversion to laparotomy and tumor spillage was higher in the group with immediate staging (16% and 12% vs. 2% and 2%) and upstaging was three times more common (24.9% vs. 7.4%) in the immediate staging group, which also included more poorly differentiated tumors. There were no differences in complication rates, disease-free survival, or recurrence, although the follow-up time was short. No port-site recurrences were identified. These studies and other small studies demonstrate that laparoscopic staging is feasible and safe for apparent early-stage ovarian cancer. Peritoneal surface metastases are the most challenging to identify with limited ability to manipulate tissues during laparoscopic surgery.

Advanced Ovarian Cancer

Minimally invasive surgery has had a limited role in the management of advanced ovarian cancer. However, more recently, there has been a renewed interest in incorporating MIS as part of the initial evaluation of patients with suspected advanced ovarian cancer. Since the early 1980s, authors have reported its role in second-look laparotomy. Initial studies from the early 1980s using laparoscopy followed by immediate laparotomy indicated a false-negative predictive value of 29% to 55% for laparoscopic surgery. With advances in video equipment and surgical technology, there was a brief resurgence of use of laparoscopic surgery in the second look setting. Even using more modern minimally invasive technology, the negative predictive value was 86%, indicating continued deficiencies in the technique. In addition, complete intraperitoneal investigation was only successful in 41% of patients because of adhesions from prior surgery. This information, in combination with the fact that second-look surgery has been determined to be of no therapeutic value, caused laparoscopy for second look to fall out of favor.

Several studies have emphasized the importance of a complete cytoreduction to no gross residual disease for optimal cancer outcomes and survival. However, if optimal or complete cytoreduction is not feasible because of disease distribution or patient factors, neoadjuvant chemotherapy can be considered. To determine the extent of disease in and the feasibility of primary cytoreductive surgery, laparoscopy can be useful. Several algorithms have been developed, some including just findings at laparoscopy and some using radiologic and serologic markers. Using laparoscopy, exact tumor location, extent of tumor spread, and invasion in surrounding structures are assessed, and each parameter receives a score. Findings at laparoscopy have been demonstrated to correlate well with findings at laparotomy, and the total score provides the surgeon with an estimated chance of successful primary debulking surgery to no gross residual disease. Prospective trials are currently ongoing to evaluate the safety, feasibility, and predictive values of laparoscopy to determine resectability at the time of ovarian cancer diagnosis, as well as surgical and survival outcomes (SCORPION [Surgical Complications Related to Primary or Interval debulking in Ovarian Neoplasm] trial NCT01461850, MD Anderson Moon Shot trial, LapOvCa-trial NTR2644).

Laparoscopy has also been used for interval debulking surgery after neoadjuvant therapy. A recent small study comparing 10 patients who underwent laparoscopy and 11 who underwent laparotomy found that laparoscopic interval cytoreduction was feasible with similar recurrence rates. However, the authors recommended that endoscopic surgery for advanced ovarian cancer should be used cautiously because the disease-related mortality rate was higher, and disease-free intervals were shorter in those undergoing endoscopic surgery. Larger prospective trials are needed to determine the safety of endoscopic surgery for advanced ovarian cancer and are currently ongoing (Minimally Invasive Interval Debulking Surgery in Ovarian Neoplasm: a Feasibility Study [MISSION] Trial NCT02324595; Feasibility of Interval Debulking Surgery by Laparoscopy for Peritoneal Carcinosis in Chemosensitive Patients [CILOVE] trial NCT01905163).

In addition, ports for intraperitoneal chemotherapy can be placed with laparoscopic guidance in patients without such access before initiating primary chemotherapy. Last, some investigators have reported on the use of (hand-assisted) laparoscopy as well as robotic surgery for radical intraperitoneal tumor debulking at the time of primary or secondary cytoreductive surgery. These studies lack conclusive data for adequacy of surgery or prospective (randomized) comparison with open technique for morbidity and survival. MIS debulking may be most appropriate for patients requiring a limited number of advanced procedures.

COMPLICATIONS OF LAPAROSCOPIC SURGERY

An evaluation of MIS indicates that adverse events can be categorized into two broad groups—complications that are part of laparoscopic abdominal surgery in general and those that are related to a specific surgical procedure or disease process. Advantages to a MIS technique include smaller incisions, less tissue manipulation and damage, and decreased adhesion formation. Many postoperative complications associated with laparotomy also are decreased. Nevertheless, these are still major surgical procedures performed via minimized access, and therefore major surgical complications are possible, some unique to MIS. Many complications related to the specific surgical procedures will occur at least at a minimum rate and can vary with complexity of the procedure and surgeon experience. General complications such as trocar insertion, injuries to bowel or vessels, CO_2 pneumoperitoneum extravasation, and port-site herniations are unique to MIS. Major intraoperative complications during MIS are fortunately uncommon. Approximately 50% of serious intraoperative complications in laparoscopy occur with trochar insertion. In general, gynecology major vascular injuries are almost exclusively related to trochar insertion; however, in gynecologic oncology, such injuries may also occur during retroperitoneal dissection. Gastrointestinal (GI) and urologic injuries are more common than major vascular injuries. Most GI injuries will be related to placement of ports, mobilization of the bowel to gain exposure, adhesiolysis, thermal damage, port-site hernias, and occasionally secondary directly to the surgical dissection. Prevention of GI injuries is most important because these types of complications often go unrecognized and may be more difficult to identify during an MIS case. Vigilance is required in addressing serious and subtle signs or symptoms that may indicate an occult GI injury resulting from MIS. There should be a high index of suspicion and the expectation should be continuous improvement in the patient's status postoperatively. In gynecologic MIS, most urologic complications result from adnexectomy or hysterectomy. A marked increase in major genitourinary complications was noted after the advent of advanced gynecology MIS procedures. Genitourinary complications are prevented by meticulous dissection, wide mobilization of the bladder off the lower uterine segment and cervix, and skeletonization of the uterine vessels.

As noted previously in this chapter, a number of studies have reported on complications associated with laparoscopic pelvic and paraaortic lymphadenectomy and radical pelvic dissection. Most series of MIS in gynecologic oncology report a decrease in perioperative and postoperative complications compared

with laparotomy. In early series, there appeared to be an increased number of ureteral, bladder, and vascular injuries compared with open techniques. Prevention of complications begins long before the actual operative procedure with appropriate treatment selection and preoperative counseling. Selection of a surgical route is often based on a surgeon's formal training and experience. It is recommended that surgeons develop a careful accumulated experience of increasingly complex MIS procedures. Further analysis almost uniformly indicates that there is a learning curve associated with advanced MIS, and larger, more mature series have intraoperative complication rates comparable to an open approach.

The overall incidence of MIS complications is difficult to quantitatively define because it is primarily based on retrospective reports and very likely to be underreported. The data on MIS complications are mostly anecdotal, based on single institutional experience and even less commonly based on meta-analysis and rarely prospective or randomized studies. This is not unique to MIS because most data on surgical complications are retrospective and therefore biased and imprecise. Various series on MIS in gynecology and gynecologic oncology report the incidence to be less than 1% to greater than 10%. The actual rate of surgical complications that occur in MIS depends on institutional and surgeon experience, types and mix of surgical procedures, and associated patient comorbidities. Chi and associates reported on the risk factors for complications and conversion to laparotomy in 1451 patients undergoing a wide variety of laparoscopic procedures by a gynecologic oncology division over a 10-year time frame. Significant complications occurred in 2.5% of the patients and were associated with increased age, previous radiation, and malignancy. The complication rates reported in this series fall within the accepted range using an open technique. Likewise, the need to convert to laparotomy has been associated with prior abdominal surgeries, obesity, bleeding, and adhesive disease. Conversion rates decrease with increased surgeon experience and should not be considered a complication but rather sound intraoperative judgment. Similar conclusions can be drawn from the experience with LAVH compared with abdominal or vaginal hysterectomy.

In general, MIS offers many potential advantages and disadvantages to the surgeon (and therefore the patient) but introduces additional layers of technological, human, and procedural complexity for any given surgical procedure traditionally performed via laparotomy. There is no substitution for knowledge of anatomy, the steps in the surgical procedure itself, and the natural history of the patient's disease or condition. Counterintuitive movement, depth perception, and blind aspects to the surgical field are all unique potential compromises to MIS, especially laparoscopy. Major complications in MIS can often be attributed to misperception rather than a pure technical error. These are all obviated, especially earlier in the surgeon's experience, by deliberate camera work and meticulous dissection, which eventually become more instinctual and automatic as the surgeon gains experience. There is no substitute for continued practice and accumulated experience, which allows for development of innate skills in avoiding potential problems. Knowledge of energy sources used is critical in preventing MIS surgical complications. Meticulous skeletonization of pedicles and mobilization of adjacent structures away from the field of dissection reduce the chance of unintended thermal damage. Laparoscopy gives partial loss of haptic feedback and loss of 3D vision, but the current robotic technology gives no haptic or touch feedback but allows for high-definition 3D vision. Both limitations in sensory feedback can be overcome with practice and experience while maintaining rigorous surgical discipline.

Port-site Recurrences

Since 1978, port-site recurrences have been reported in multiple carcinomas, including gynecologic malignancies. Concern has been expressed that incisional seeding may be increased in laparoscopic surgery, potentially leading to a reduction in overall survival. A review of the literature by Ramirez et al. in 2003 found 31 articles describing port-site metastases in 58 patients with gynecologic cancer. These included 33 invasive ovarian cancers, seven low-malignant-potential tumors of the ovary, 12 cervical cancers, four endometrial cancers, and one each of fallopian tube and vaginal cancer. In the ovarian cancer patients, 83% had advanced-stage disease with most reporting carcinomatosis and ascites. The median time to diagnosis was 17 days, and it is unclear how this affected survival. Reports of abdominal wall metastasis after paracentesis in a similar population are common. It appears that proper preoperative assessment may have spared many of these patients a laparoscopic procedure. The 12 patients with cervical cancer reported with port-site metastasis are cause for concern given that there are only a few isolated reports of metastases to an abdominal scar. Of these 12 patients, 75% had laparoscopic lymphadenectomy, and the majority had positive nodes. Half of the patients had recurrence in the port used for placement of the laparoscope. The median time to port-site recurrence was 5 months, and of the 11 patients for whom data were given, only 27% were without evidence of disease with a median 12-month follow-up. Of the four patients reported to have port-site recurrences in endometrial cancer, only one had disease limited to the uterus. The small number of port-site recurrences makes it difficult to document any benefit to clipping the fallopian tubes or minimizing uterine manipulation as a way to prevent these complications. Analysis of a large prospective database identified 1694 patients who underwent laparoscopy for a malignant intraabdominal condition. Twenty (1.2%) of patients were diagnosed with a port-site metastasis at a median time from laparoscopy of 7 months (range, 0.1–26.2 months). Fifteen patients had ovarian cancer, two cervical cancer, and one uterine cancer, and 95% had synchronous metastases at the time of port-site metastasis.

A number of factors have been proposed to explain the etiology of port-site metastasis. Studies have suggested that the risk may be increased with the use of carbon dioxide compared with other insufflating agents. The positive pressure associated with a pneumoperitoneum has been associated with increased tumor growth and a high incidence of port-site metastasis when compared with gasless laparoscopy. Some investigations have shown the potential aerosolization of viable tumor cells and efflux with gas through the trocar sites. Also theorized is a diminution of inflammatory response using minimally invasive versus open laparotomy incisions. Childers et al. reported port-site metastasis to be 0.3% per trocar site, which is comparable with the 0.1% risk of abdominal wall seeding with percutaneous biopsy of abdominal malignancies. As a result of the advanced stage of most of the reported cases, it is not clear whether port-site metastases occur because of the aggressive nature of the disease or because of risk factors uniquely associated with laparoscopic surgery. To date, use of laparoscopy has not been associated with a decrease in survival rates for patients with cancer.

CONCLUSIONS

Laparotomy causes significant trauma to the patient with many potential associated morbidities, which are increased in incidence and severity in patients with comorbid conditions. In an attempt to reduce surgical morbidity, minimally invasive procedures have been developed and have been shown to be feasible and safe alternatives to open surgery with shorter LOS, decreased blood loss, and similar or decreased postoperative complications. Uptake of traditional laparoscopy was slow and only moderately successful secondary to a difficult and long learning curve, variability in surgical experience, longer operative times, and patient factors such as surgical history and obesity. However, now almost 10 years after the introduction of the robotic platform in gynecologic surgery, the majority of procedures for endometrial and cervical cancer in the United States are performed using a minimally invasive approach.

The technological improvements offered by robotic surgery have allowed gynecologic surgeons to perform much more complicated surgeries via MIS on a heterogeneous group of patients. Surgeons at the beginning of their learning curve will need to build their case complexity appropriately and consider operating room duration along with other potential surgical risks. Previous laparoscopic experience is very helpful, at least in the initial phase of adapting to robotics; however, the robotic platform translates quite nicely from laparotomy because surgeons are able to mimic the procedure robotically from their laparotomy experience. As technology continues to improve and surgeons gain more experience, a higher proportion of patients diagnosed with a gynecologic malignancy is eligible for MIS, and benefits are especially also seen in extremely morbidly obese patients. Technology advances do not substitute for subspecialty training, surgical experience and judgment, and knowledge of disease and anatomy. It is also a certainty that the technology will continue to change and improve and hopefully will become less expensive.

For the bibliography list, log onto www.expertconsult.com <http://www.expertconsult.com>

22

Epidemiology of Commonly Used Statistical Terms and Analysis of Clinical Studies

Wendy R. Brewster, MD, PhD

KEY POINTS

1. Epidemiology is the study of distribution of disease and factors the determine disease occurrence in populations.
2. As much as possible, medical decisions should be based on quality evidence. The best evidence is a properly designed randomized controlled trial. Evidence from nonrandomized but well-designed control trials is of lesser quality. Next in reliability is well-designed cohort or case-control studies, which have been repeated by several investigators. Opinions of respected authorities and extensive clinical experience are least reliable.

EPIDEMIOLOGY

Epidemiology is the study of distribution of disease and the factors that determine disease occurrence in populations. The focus is on groups rather than the individual. Persons within a population do not have equal risk for disease occurrence, and the risk of a disease is a function of personal characteristics and environmental exposures. Patterns of disease occurrence within specific populations can be evaluated to determine why certain groups develop illness when others do not. The impact of epidemiology on gynecologic oncology is evidenced by the significance of studies such as the association with infection of oncogenic human papillomavirus and cervical cancer, obesity and the risk of endometrial cancer, and the risk factors for gestational trophoblastic neoplasia. Epidemiologic studies are unique in their focus on human populations and their reliance on nonexperimental observations. Epidemiologic methods are used in searching for causes of disease, disease surveillance, determining the cause of disease, diagnostic testing, searching for prognostic factors, and testing new treatments.

Because the quality of epidemiologic evidence varies greatly among studies, the scientific community endorses the principles of Sir Austin Bradford Hill, an eminent British statistician, when attempting to identify causal associations. A cause of a specific disease is an antecedent event or characteristic that is necessary for the occurrence of the disease (Box 22.1).

EVIDENCE-BASED MEDICINE

As much as possible, medical decisions should be based on quality evidence. The best evidence is a properly designed randomized controlled trial. Evidence from nonrandomized but well-designed control trials is of lesser quality. Next in reliability is a well-designed cohort or case-control studies, which have been repeated by several investigators. Opinions of respected authorities and extensive clinical experience are least reliable.

Physicians are currently encouraged to practice evidence-based medicine. This means that clinical trial evidence must pass statistically valid tests for conclusions to have meaning. Good science depends on accurate (ie, statistically significant and meaningful) data from clinical trials. The best trials are usually experimental, powered, randomized, and blinded. Patients randomly assigned to a treatment group or a control group must have an equal probability of being assigned to either group. This prevents selection bias (eg, putting healthier or better prognosis patients in one group and those with a poor prognosis or high likelihood of disease risk in another group). Blinding prevents patients, investigators, or statisticians from knowing who is in the control group and experimental group; thus, biased actions are avoided.

Whereas retrospective and observational studies are descriptive and do not involve either an intervention or a manipulation, an experimental study does. A prospective trial poses the

TABLE 22.1 Mathematical Definitions of Statistical Terms

Terminology	Mathematical Definition
Prevalence rate	Number of persons with disease/Total number in the group
Incidence rate	Number of new cases/Total number at risk per unit of time
Kappa	$(P_{obs} - P_{chance})/(1 - P_{chance})$
Sensitivity	True positive/(True positive + False negative)
Specificity	True negative/(True negative + False positive)
Predictive value positive	True positive/(True positive + False positive)
Predictive value negative	True negative/(True negative + False negative)

question before the data are collected, thus allowing better control of confounding variables, unlike a retrospective study, which poses the question after the data are collected.

MEASURES IN EPIDEMIOLOGY

To describe and compare groups in a meaningful manner, it is important to find and enumerate appropriate denominators and statistical terms (Table 22.1).

- **Incidence rate:** Measures the new cases of a specific disease that develop during a defined period of time and the approximation of the risk for developing the disease. The incidence rate focuses on events. Incidence measures the probability of developing a disease.
- **Kappa coefficient:** Kappa indicates how much observers agree beyond the level of agreement that could be expected by chance. Kappa is estimated as $(P_{obs} - P_{chance})/(1 - P_{chance})$. Thus, the kappa coefficient is the observed agreement, corrected for chance as a fraction of the maximum obtainable agreement, also corrected for chance. Landis and Koch have suggested useful categorizations. Kappa = 0.00 should be taken as representing "poor" agreement, 0.00 ± 0.20 as "slight" agreement, 0.21 ± 0.40 as "fair" agreement, 0.41 ± 0.60 as "moderate" agreement, 0.61 ± 0.80 as "substantial" agreement, and 0.81 ± 0.99 as "almost perfect" agreement. A kappa coefficient of 1 represents perfect agreement.
- **Mean:** The average of a sample of observations
- **Median:** The middle value when the values are arranged in order from the smallest to the largest

- **Meta-analysis:** The statistical process of pooling the results from separate studies concerned with the same treatment or issue is frequently used in the context of medical statistics and provides the quantitative backbone of the evidence-based medicine program. A large number of meta-analyses are undertaken with the broad aim of combining divergent outcomes into a single estimate of treatment effect. For example, the Cochrane Collaboration endeavors to collate and synthesize high-quality evidence on the effects of important health care interventions for a worldwide, multidisciplinary audience and publishes them in the *Cochrane Database of Systematic* Reviews. Meta-analyses increase the statistical power by increasing the sample size, resolve uncertainty when reports do not agree, and improve the estimates of effect size. The bias of publication only of positive results is a concern for those using results of meta-analyses because, if statistically significant or "positive" results are more likely to be published, a meta-analysis based on the resulting literature will be biased. The quality of the studies included is important to the quality of the final result.
- **Pearson's correlation r:** The degree to which two variables are related is called correlation. Pearson's correlation is represented by the value *r* and varies between −1 and +1. It is usually presented as a scatter point graph. A value of −1 suggests a perfect negative linear relationship, a value of 0 reflects no linear relationship, and a value of 1 reflects a perfect linear relationship. Values of −1, 0, and +1 are rare.
- **Person time:** The sum of the observation period of risk for the persons in a group being studied.
- **Predictive value positive:** The proportion of positive test results that is truly positive (ie, the probability that someone classified as exposed is truly exposed). This value only refers to positive tests.
- **Predictive value negative:** The proportion of negative test results that is truly negative. The predictive value of a negative test result refers to the proportion of patients with a negative test result who are free of disease.

These values, unlike sensitivity and specificity, indicate the reliability of the test in the determination of presence or absence of disease.

- **Prevalence rate:** The amount of disease in a population. Prevalence measures the proportion of diseased individuals at a particular time and represents a snapshot of the disease. Other commonly used terms are *prevalence proportion* and *point prevalence*. It is a measure of status and includes individuals with newly diagnosed disease and those surviving with disease. The numerator is the number of affected individuals in a specific time period. The denominator is the total number of persons in the group. Prevalence rates range between 0 and 1.
- **Quality-adjusted life year (QALY):** The QALY was developed as an attempt to combine the value length of life and quality of life into a single index number. One year of perfect health is given a value of 1. Death is given a value less than 0. A year of less than perfect health will have a value less than 1. States of health considered worse than death can be argued to have a negative value. The QALY value is

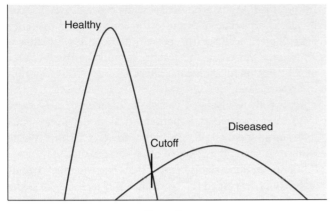

FIGURE 22.1 Effects of shifting cutoff point on sensitivity and specificity.

determined by multiplying the utility value associated with that state of health by the years lived in that state. QALY is a metric used to compare the benefit of health care interventions. Combination of QALYs with the cost of an intervention (Cost/QALY) can provided an economic framework for comparisons of therapies. QALYs have several limitations and should not be used alone in decision making.

- **Sensitivity:** The proportion of truly diseased persons who are classified as diseased by the test. The sensitivity of a test is therefore the probability of a test being positive when the disease is present. The sensitivity of test may also be called the true-positive rate. In Fig. 22.1, it is evident that the cutoff point of a test can affect the sensitivity. If the cutoff point is moved to the left, more diseased persons will be identified. At the same time, more healthy persons will be erroneously classified as sick. However, as the cutoff value for normal is moved to the right, the test will become less sensitive because fewer diseased persons will be classified as such.
- **Specificity:** The proportion of a population of disease-free individuals who are classified as undiseased by a test. In contrast to the sensitivity of a test, the specificity of a test is the probability that a test result will be negative when the disease is absent. The cutoff point of a test for normality influences the specificity. As the value of normality or cutoff moves to the left, the test becomes less specific because fewer health individuals are recognized as such. In contrast, moving the cutoff values to the right increases the specificity (see Fig. 22.1). In the best scenario, a test would be able to discriminate between diseased and healthy individuals without any overlap. **More often, the scenario is as presented in Fig. 22.1, in which there is significant overlap and whatever the cutoff value healthy persons may be classified as diseased and sick persons classified as healthy.** When we set the cutoff point for a test, we must be attentive to the purpose of the test. If the disease is treatable and missing the disease has serious ramifications, then we must favor sensitivity over specificity. Alternatively, if it is more important to correctly identify healthy individuals, then specificity is prioritized. Published reports of the performance of tests usually just

provide sensitivity and specificity results. Variations of these measures occur under many conditions and will also produce variations in predictive values.

- **Standard deviation (SD):** A measure of the variability within each group. If there is a normal (bell-shaped curve) distribution, approximately 95% of the values are within 2 SDs on both sides of the average.
- **Tests of heterogeneity:** Before performing a meta-analysis, it is customary to assess evidence of variation in the underlying effects. This variation, termed "heterogeneity," arises because of differences across studies in populations, exposures *or* interventions, outcomes, design, or conduct. A forest plot is useful for visual assessment of consistency of results across studies. A statistic that measures the consistency of findings as the proportion of total variation in point estimates attributable to heterogeneity is now widely used.

ANALYSIS OF CLINICAL TRIALS

- **Null hypothesis:** This hypothesis, symbolized by H0, is a statement claiming that there is no difference between the experimental and population means. The alternative hypothesis (H1) is the opposite of the null hypothesis. Often in research, we need to be able to test for both the positive and adverse outcomes; therefore, a two-tailed hypothesis is chosen even though the expectation of the experiment is in a particular direction.
- **Significance level:** A level of significance termed the alpha value is determined before the study has begun. The alpha value is the likelihood that a difference as large or larger that occurred between the study groups could be determined by chance alone. The alpha level is established by those designing the study and becomes the level of statistical significance. The most typical alpha level is 0.05.
- **One-tail test:** A test to determine a difference in only one direction (eg, to determine if drug A is better than drug B)
- **Two-tail test:** A test to determine any difference between the variable (eg, if either drug A or drug B is superior to the other). It is usually considered that in a two-tailed test, more trust can be placed in the statistically significant results than with a one-tailed test. When in doubt, the two-tailed test is preferred.
- **Confidence interval (CI):** The range of values that is believed to contain the true value within a specific level of certainty.
- **Alpha error:** The rejection of the null hypothesis when it is, in fact, correct; also called a type I error.
- **Beta error:** Failure to reject the null hypothesis when it is, in fact, incorrect; also called a type II error.
- **Power:** The probability that a study will be able to correctly detect a true effect of a specific magnitude. The statistical power refers to the probability of finding a difference when one truly exists or how well the null hypothesis will be rejected. The power is usually specified beforehand in prospective studies. The values of 0.8 (80%) or 0.9 (90%) are typical. The higher the value, the less chance there is of a type II error. A 0.9 value means that a type II error would be avoided 90% of the time.

- **Risk:** The proportion of unaffected individuals who, on average, will contract the disease of interest over a specified period of time. Results of a trial are often expressed as absolute or relative risk reductions. The absolute difference is the actual difference between the units of the difference. In relative risk, the differences are the percentage change. Relative risk reductions often sound much more dramatic than do the absolute values. One must consider the prevalence of a disease when evaluating risk reductions. When there is a low prevalence of a disease process, small risk reductions become unimpressive and must be evaluated in terms of the benefits of a particular mode of therapy.

- **Incremental cost-effectiveness ratio:** The additional cost divided by the incremental benefit compared with an alternate strategy. A strategy was strongly dominated if it was more costly and less effective than another or cost effective if it had an incremental cost-effectiveness ratio of $50,000 to 100,000 per year of life gained relative to an alternate strategy.

- **Odds ratio (OR):** The ratio of the odds that an event will occur in one group compared with the odds that the event will occur in the other group. In an osteoporosis study, if 14 of 22 people who are thin, have fractures, the odds of having a fracture are 14 in 22 or 0.64. If 5 of the 33 nonthin people fracture bone, the odds are 5 in 33 or 0.15. The OR is 0.64 divided by 0.15 or 4.2, meaning that thin people are 4.2 times more likely to receive fractures. An OR of 1 means that both groups have a similar likelihood of having an event.

- **Overall survival (OS):** The interval from the completion of treatment to censoring or death from any cause.

- **Progression-free survival (PFS):** The interval from the date of randomization to the documentation of progression of the illness or death from any cause.

- **Actuarial (life table) survival:** This technique uses grouped information to estimate the survival curve. The data are grouped into fixed time periods (eg, months, years) that include the maximum follow-up. The survival curve is estimated as a continuous curve and gives an estimate of the proportions of a group of patients who will be alive at different times after the initial observation. The group includes patients with incomplete follow-up.

- **Chi square ($\chi 2$):** The primary statistical test used for studying the relationship between variables. This is a test used to compare proportions of categorical variables.

- **Cox proportional hazard regression analysis:** Cox regression analysis is a technique for assessing the association between variables and survival rate. The measure of risk provided for each variable is the risk ratio (RR). An RR of 1 means that the risk is the same for each participant. An RR greater than 1 indicates increased risk; a ratio less than 1 indicates less risk. A ratio of 5.4 means that the patients with a variable are 5.4 times more likely to have the outcome being studied. CIs can also be provided with RRs. This type of analysis is usually presented in a table.

- **Efficacy:** The possibility that an intervention will result in a change (eg, in vaccine trials).

- **Imputation:** In many analytical scenarios, a case is discarded if it is missing data relevant to the analysis. This may introduce a bias, decrease the power of the study, or alter the representativeness of the results. Imputation is the process of substituting missing data. There are numerous techniques to impute data.

- **Multivariate analysis:** A technique of analysis of data that factors many variables. A mathematical model is constructed that simultaneously determines the effect of one variable while evaluating the effect of other factors that may have an influence on the variable being tested. The two most common algorithms developed to accomplish this task are the step-up and step-down procedures. Variables are added to an initial small set or deleted from an initial large set while testing repeatedly to see which new factor makes a statistical contribution to the overall model.

- **Propensity score:** In studies in which randomization is not possible, investigators use this score to adjust for the bias due to confounding variables inherent in treatment selection for groups being compared (eg, in observational trials when the treatment of the participants is not random). Assignment to intervention does not occur by chance but depends on patient characteristics that can influence the effect of the intervention on the outcome. The propensity score is the probability that a patient would receive the treatment of interest based on the characteristics of the patient, clinician, and clinical environment. Several different techniques can be used to balance the groups being compared. The most common strategy is propensity score matching. Propensity score methods are usually better than matching on specific characteristics or stratification because it adjusts for confounding better than other strategies. This is a valuable approach when completion of a randomized trial is not feasible.

- **Receiver operator characteristics (ROCs):** These curves are the best way to demonstrate the relationships between sensitivity and specificity. The curves plot sensitivity (true-positive rate) against the false-positive rate (1 − Specificity) (Fig. 22.2). The closer the curve is to the upper lefthand corner, the more accurate it is because the true-positive rate is closer to 1 and the false-positive rate is closer to 0. Along any particular ROC curve one can observe the impact of compromising the true-positive and false-positive rates. As the requirement that a test has a high true-positive rate increases, the false-positive rate will also increase. The closer the curve is to the 45-degree diagonal of the ROC area under the curve, the less accurate the test (see Fig. 22.2).

- **Sensitivity analysis:** Modeling is a tool that permits the incorporation of data from different sources to predict outcomes that may be likely. This tool allows for various interventions and numerous scenarios. Interpretation of the findings depends on the confidence the operator has in various factors of the model. Sensitivity analysis involves examination of the variation in the outcome as the variables change.

- **One-way sensitivity analysis:** This is the simplest form of sensitivity analysis in which the effectiveness of only one

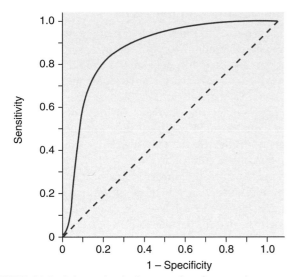

FIGURE 22.2 A hypothetical example of a receiver operating characteristic curve. The *solid line* represents the performance of the diagnostic test of interest; the *dashed diagonal line* serves as a reference of a test with no diagnostic value. (From Greenberg RS, Daniels SR, Flanders WD, et al: *Medical Epidemiology,* 3rd ed. Lange Medical Books/McGraw-Hill, 2001 Reproduced by permission of The McGraw-Hill Companies.)

BOX 22.2 Types of Clinical Trials

Single-patient clinical trials
Multicenter trials
National clinical trials
Continuation trials
Compassionate plea trials
Pharmacoeconomic trials
Trials to evaluate medical devices
Pharmacokinetic trials

variable in the model is analyzed to assess the range of impact of that variable on the outcome.

- **Univariate analysis:** Analyses may be univariate or multivariate because they examine one or more variables at a time, respectively.

TYPES OF CLINICAL TRIALS

Clinical trials are experiments in which the investigator intervenes rather than observes and is the best test of a cause-and-effect relationship. A properly conducted experiment requires that when the intervention is applied to one group, there is a control group or some other suitable standard by which participants of the clinical experiment or their guardians must give informed consent. The gold standard of clinical trials is the randomized experiment. With randomization, each participant has an equal chance of being in either of the arms of the trials. Randomization is important because it equalizes baseline characteristics of the participants so that the comparison of the treatments is fair. If randomization is not feasible, possible nonrandom standards of comparison must include patients similar to the treated group. Randomization is the current norm for demonstrating efficacy and safety of investigational methods. The advantages of randomization are numerous:

- Decreases investigator's bias in assigning patients to treatment groups
- Permits certain statistical methods to be used in the resulting data
- Allows for blinding of the patient and investigator
- Is the current norm for demonstrating efficacy and safety of investigational medicines

Unacceptable methods of randomization include the following:

- Alternate assignments
- Alternate day assignments
- Birthday assignments
- Coin tosses
- Initials of a patient

Single-patient clinical trials are indicated only in specific situations. They are generally used to evaluate rare diseases when other types of trials are inappropriate or when only a small percentage of patients respond to a specific treatment. Single-patient clinical trials are useful to determine the response of a particular patient is a result of placebo or if an adverse reaction is related to a specific medication. The disease should be chronic, and the disease severity must be stable during the clinical trial duration. It should be expected that the effect of the treatment should be measurable in a short time, and the effect should be rapidly reversible after the treatment has stopped. The investigator and patient should be blinded, and the patient's condition should return preexisting baselines between treatment legs.

Multicenter trials are advantageous because they offer more rapid patient accrual and allow for greater protocol complexity. Multicenter trials reduce the opportunity for an individual's bias to influence the conduct of the trial; they increase the likelihood for the inclusion of a more representative study population and facilitate a higher standard for data processing and analysis. Disadvantages of multicenter trials are the administrative considerations that underlie the management and administrative arrangements (eg, institutional review board, ethics committees). Considerations must be delineated for criteria for patient enrollment, diagnostic classification, and assessment of treatment outcome. These trials are inherently more costly (Box 22.2).

EVALUATION OF CLINICAL TRIALS

Many factors must be considered when evaluating a clinical trial. The most important is the clinical trial objective or aim. Whether the objectives of the trial are adequately assessed depends on the presence and extent of bias and confounding factors. Bias is a nonrandom error in a study that can alter the outcome. Types of bias to consider when evaluating a manuscript are listed in Table 22.2.

TABLE 22.2 Bias and Confounding Factors: Examination of the Literature in the Field

- Specifying and selecting the clinical trial sample
  - Popularity bias
  - Referral filter bias
  - Diagnostic or access bias
  - Wrong sample size
  - Migrator, nonrespondent, or volunteer bias
- Executing the exposure
- Contamination, withdrawal, or compliance/therapeutic bias
- Information bias
- Observer bias
- Interviewer bias
- Use of nonvalidated instruments
- Active control bias
- Analyzing the data
  - Post hoc significance bias
  - Fishing expeditions
- Interpreting the analysis
- Publishing the results

Specifying the sample size or number of participants in the study needed to detect a difference or an effect of a given magnitude depends on many variables. The most important is the magnitude of the effect desired or expected. Other important considerations are the desired probability of the study to identify the correct outcome (power), the variability of the variables being analyzed, the number of parts of the clinical trial, the magnitude of the placebo effect, and the number of dependent parts of the clinical trials. When determining the sample size, one must consider if the size of the treatment groups will be equal or nonequal (eg, 2:1 ratio). **An advantage of using groups of unequal size is that more information will be gained about patient responses in the larger arm. A disadvantage is the loss in study power; however, this detraction is not usually substantial if the ratios are kept under 3:1.**

Placebo Treatment Groups

Placebo treatment groups control for the psychological aspects of being in a treatment trial. They also control for adverse events being attributed to a medicine when they result from spontaneous changes in the disease or from other causes and allow a stronger interpretation of the data. Placebo treatment groups are considered ethical if the following occur:

- No standard treatment exists.
- The standard treatment has been proven ineffective.
- Standard treatment is inappropriate for the particular clinical trial.
- Placebo has been reported to be effective in treating the condition.
- The disease is mild and lack of treatment is not considered to be medically important.
- The disease process is characterized by frequent spontaneous exacerbations and remissions.

Controls Used in Clinical Trials

Control groups in clinical trials may be obtained by many different methods. Randomized control groups are the most traditional and accepted and only chance should determine who enters any of the study arms. Nonrandom control groups may also be used. Participants in these nonrandom control groups should have similar characteristics to those of the "treatment arm" and may include historical data obtained on the same patients on no therapy, the same therapy, or different therapy. Participants in the control arm may be assigned to a placebo, an active medication, or concurrent use of nontreatment; use a different dose of the same medication; or receive usual care.

Dropouts from clinical trials are inevitable. The simplest reasons may be that the participants declined to participate after enrollment or that the clinical course during the trial required a change in therapy. Whatever the reason for noncompliance or dropout, these participants should be followed because it is essential to analyze the outcomes of the groups as intent to treat. Inclusion of these data provides a conservative estimate of the differences in treatment.

Studies of Therapy

There are many different types of clinical trials; in general, they are categorized into categories or phases. Phase I trials are usually to screen the safety of the intervention or drug. These trials can be inclusive of multiple doses of a new medicine or evaluation of an old medicine in a new therapeutic area. These trials usually consist of 10 to 100 participants.

Phase II trials clarify and establish the protocol and elucidate the experimental conditions that will allow the most important phase of the trial to give a definitive result. These trials are valuable because they establish protocols and the experimental conditions that will allow the final phase of the trial to give a definitive result. They allow for the following:

- The evaluation of a variable related to the clinical pharmacology of a medicine
- Development of clinical experience by research personnel under open-label conditions before initiation of a double-blind trial

Aims of phase II trials are to assess how many people should be included in the final phase of testing, determine the endpoints of the trial, and provide preliminary estimates of effective dose and duration of treatment.

Phase III trials are for comparison to standard therapy or placebo if ethically justifiable. These trials are more commonly randomized and are regarded as the best way to obtain unbiased data.

Blinding

Blind refers to the lack of knowledge of the investigational agent by the patients, investigators, ancillary personnel, data review committees, and statisticians. Blinding is used to decrease the biases that may occur during a clinical trial. An open-label trial indicates that no blind is used. Examples of open-label trials are as follows:

- Pilot trials
- Case studies in life-threatening situations

- Unusual studies in which definitive data may be obtained (eg, coma patients)
- Clinical trials in which ethical considerations do not permit blinding

In single-blind clinical trials, either the patient or investigator is unaware of the treatment received. Single-blind trials provide a degree of control when a double-blind trial is impossible or impractical and provides a degree of assurance of the data's validity compared with open-label trials. In double-blind trials, neither the investigator nor the patient is aware of what treatment the patient is receiving. This allows for strong data interpretation if all other aspects of the trial were properly designed and conducted, the blind remained intact, the protocol was not seriously breached, the power of the trial was adequate, and the patients were compliant. Triple-blind trials are situations in which anyone who interacts with either the patient of physician is blinded. These studies allow for the strongest interpretation of data if the conditions can be met.

If blinding is to be used, then the study should be designed so that it is very difficult to break the blind. Unblinding may occur based on any of the following:

- Adverse reactions
- Lack of efficacy
- Efficacy
- Changes in laboratory values
- Errors in labeling
- Comments from unblinded study personnel
- Information presented in correspondence or reports
- Intentionally looking for clues (Box 22.3)

When to Stop a Clinical Trial

The decision to stop a clinical trial has many important ramifications. The ethical dilemmas include the needs of the next eligible patient insomuch that a participant should never be randomly assigned to an established inferior treatment. This must be balanced by the collective needs of society that terminating a trial will still result in the correct policy for the future and the need for sufficient data to change clinical practice for the better.

Early termination of a trial has its disadvantages. If the trial is stopped after recruitment of a small number of participants, the results may lack credibility. The assumed treatment difference may be the result of chance and a false-positive result. The early stopping of trials can result in imprecision and wide CIs for treatment effect. Finally, the treatment recommendation that results from stopping a trial early may be unduly enthusiastic.

Statistical stopping guidelines should be determined before the clinical trial begins. A sufficiently small P value for treatment difference on a trial's primary endpoint can be a guideline for when it is ethically desirable to stop a trial. It is most acceptable to have a limited number of preplanned interim analyses. Multiple repeated looks at the data can guard against the risk of a false-positive result.

For the bibliography list, log onto www.expertconsult.com ⟨http://www.expertconsult.com⟩.

BOX 22.3 **Types of Blinds**

Open label
Single blind
Double blind
Full double blind: keeping blind everyone who interacts with the patient
Full triple blind: keeping blind anyone who interacts with the patients and the investigators

23

Basic Principles in Gynecologic Radiotherapy

Catheryn M. Yashar, MD, FACR, FACRO

KEY POINTS

1. Radiation therapy is used for the treatment of primary and metastatic gynecologic carcinomas.
2. Radiation therapy depends on the differential susceptibility of tumors to irradiation compared with normal tissues, and research attempts to maximize the therapeutic ratio are ongoing.
3. Photons, a nonparticulate form of radiation, are the primary modality of therapeutic irradiation used in gynecologic carcinomas.
4. Particulate irradiation with electrons and protons are also used in many centers but have specialized indications.
5. Radiation is measured in international system (SI) unit of centigray and Gray. A typical dose for therapeutic irradiation for adjuvant therapy is 45 to 50 Gy and for gross disease, as in cervical carcinoma, is 80 to 85 Gy.
6. Radiation is primarily generated from human-made sources, as in a linear accelerator, called x-rays, or from naturally radioactive decay, termed gamma rays. Therapeutically, these are indistinguishable, although photons or electrons may be the therapeutic source.
7. A variety of DNA lesions are produced by radiation including base damage, DNA–protein crosslinking, single-strand breaks, and double-strand breaks.

8. In general, radiation is delivered in two basic manners. External-beam radiation therapy delivers radiation to the body from an external source. Brachytherapy, a crucial component to the safest and most effective treatment of many gynecologic cancers, delivers radiation from sources that are placed within the body.
9. An important concept, crucial to the delivery of brachytherapy, is that the dose of radiation at a given point is inversely proportional to the square of the distance from the source of radiation (dose $\propto 1/$ Distance^2). This forms the basis of high therapeutic dose directly to the tumor and safe doses to adjacent critical organs. External methods of delivery cannot duplicate this delivery. A level of expertise is absolutely crucial to the delivery of this modality.
10. Low-dose-rate brachytherapy is being replaced in most centers by high-dose-rate brachytherapy or pulse-dose-rate brachytherapy.
11. Image guidance with computed tomography, magnetic resonance imaging, or positron emission computed tomography scans, in all aspects of radiation therapy (planning, external and brachytherapy), appears to increase the therapeutic ratio.

12. Concurrent therapies (radiosensitizers and protectors) seek to increase this therapeutic ratio, each with its own mechanism of action to be exploited.

13. The short- and long-term effects of irradiation are not trivial, and a risk-to-benefit discussion is crucial to the patient and multidisciplinary oncology team. During and after therapy, a team approach best serves the patient.

14. Intensity-modulated radiation therapy, image-guided radiation therapy, and stereotactic radiation therapy are all tools in an ever increasingly complex toolbox for the radiation oncologist to use for increased local control, survival, and palliation. Ongoing studies evaluate the risk-to-benefit ratio and cost effectiveness of these new and expensive technologies.

A basic understanding of the principles of radiation oncology is essential to gynecologic oncologists. Radiation therapy is used in the curative treatment of locoregionally advanced cervical and vaginal carcinoma. It is often an adjuvant therapy prescribed for uterine or vulvar carcinoma and in inoperable patients may be the only definitive therapy available. Last, it can be used for the palliative treatment of gynecologic carcinomas.

INTRODUCTION TO ELECTROMAGNETIC RADIATION

Radiant energy or radiation is an essential component of life on earth. For example, sunlight provides heat, light, and energy for plant photosynthesis, and radio waves provide a method of communication. This electromagnetic radiation physically consists of photons, or "packets" of energy without mass or charge. The primary difference between the radiations is the energy of the photons. The energy is proportional to frequency ($E = h\nu$, where h is Planck's constant and ν is frequency) and inversely proportional to wavelength (Table 23.1). A common analogy is to compare wavelength to the length of a person's stride when walking; the number of strides per minute is the frequency of the wave.

Photons, a nonparticulate radiation, are only one form of radiation. Another form of radiation is particulate radiation. Particulate radiation consists of subatomic particles such as electrons, protons, α particles, and neutrons.

Radiation is not harmful in ordinary quantities and is actually helpful to life processes. In fact, exposure to radiation is a constant phenomenon (Tables 23.2 and 23.3). However, high-energy, or "ionizing," radiation is not entirely harmless, although it is commonly used for both diagnostic and therapeutic purposes. High-energy radiation can be injurious to biologic material, and its use in oncology depends on the ability of normal tissue to recover from the effects more effectively

or efficiently than malignant tissue. Radiation causes both reversible and irreversible changes in normal tissue, and these effects are placed into two categories: acute effects (apparent during or shortly after the radiation course) and long-term effects (apparent from 6 months to years after completion of therapy). Radiation effects may not be initially apparent except by careful chemical or microscopic study. Indeed, the effects may not be apparent for many years or may manifest only in the offspring of the irradiated organism. The accepted position regarding radiation exposure is that incidental environmental radiation, diagnostic tests, and therapeutic radiation can all be detrimental. Although in many cases the chance of injury from diagnostic or environmental radiation is slight, the possibility of damage from a known exposure must always be weighed against the importance of the information to be gained or the effect desired. Incidental exposure must be avoided through control of environmental hazards whenever possible by following the ALARA (as low as reasonably achievable) principle.

There are many forms and sources of radiation, including natural isotopes and human-made radiations. The natural radiation emissions (gamma and beta rays) of isotopes such as iridium, iodine, and cesium are used for therapeutic purposes in many human malignancies (Table 23.4). In addition, during the past 4 decades, increasingly sophisticated machines have been manufactured to produce high-intensity, directed radiation to treat both malignant and benign conditions. Modern machines emit energies greater than 1 million electron volts (1 MeV) and are termed *supervoltage* or *megavoltage machines* (Table 23.5). The most commonly available are called linear accelerators (linacs). Even these have recently become more sophisticated to allow increasingly precise delivery of radiation in the form of intensity-modulated radiation therapy (IMRT). The newest generation models allow for real-time computed tomography (CT) for position verification, termed image-guided radiation therapy, or IGRT. Image guidance is also more

TABLE 23.1	**Electromagnetic Spectrum**		
	Wavelength (M)	**Frequency (Hz)**	**Energy (J)**
Radio	$>1 \times 10^{-1}$	$<3 \times 10^{9}$	$<2 \times 10^{-24}$
Microwave	$1 \times 10^{-3} - 1 \times 10^{-1}$	$3 \times 10^{9} - 3 \times 10^{11}$	$2 \times 10^{-24} - 2 \times 10^{-22}$
Infrared	$7 \times 10^{-7} - 1 \times 10^{-3}$	$3 \times 10^{11} - 4 \times 10^{14}$	$2 \times 10^{-22} - 3 \times 10^{-19}$
Visible	$4 \times 10^{-7} - 7 \times 10^{-7}$	$4 \times 10^{14} - 7.5 \times 10^{14}$	$3 \times 10^{-19} - 5 \times 10^{-19}$
Ultraviolet	$1 \times 10^{-8} - 4 \times 10^{-7}$	$7.5 \times 10^{14} - 3 \times 10^{16}$	$5 \times 10^{-19} - 2 \times 10^{-17}$
X-ray	$1 \times 10^{-11} - 1 \times 10^{-8}$	$3 \times 10^{16} - 3 \times 10^{19}$	$2 \times 10^{-17} - 2 \times 10^{-14}$
Gamma ray	$<1 \times 10^{-11}$	$>3 \times 10^{19}$	$>2 \times 10^{-14}$

TABLE 23.2   General Population Radiation Exposure

Radiation Source	Average Annual Whole-Body Dose (millirem/yr)
Natural: cosmic	29
Terrestrial	29
Radon	200
Internal (eg, ^{40}K, ^{14}C)	40
Human made (diagnostic radiography, nuclear medicine, consumer products such as smoke detectors)	64
All others (fallout, air travel, occupational)	2
Average annual total	360\
Tobacco smokers: add ~280 mrem	

TABLE 23.3   Radiation Associated With Common Activities

Activity	Typical Radiation Dose
Smoking	280 mrem/yr
Chest radiography	8 mrem/single radiograph
Drinking water	5 mrem/yr
Cross-country airplane trip	5 mrem/yr

TABLE 23.4   Radioactive Isotopes Used in Radiation Oncology

Element	Isotope	E_{max} (MeV)	$T_{1/2}$	Clinical Use
Radium	^{236}Ra	3.26	1600 yr	Historical
Cesium	^{137}Cs	0.514, 1.17	30 yr	Temporary intracavitary implants
Iridium	^{192}Ir	0.38_{ave}	74.2 d	Temporary interstitial implants and source for high dose rate machine
Iodine	^{125}I	0.028_{ave}	60.2 d	Permanent interstitial implants
Phosphorus	^{32}P	None	14.3 d	Permanent intracavitary placement
Palladium	^{103}Pd	20KV	17 d	Permanent prostate seed implant

TABLE 23.5   Radiation Delivery by Energy

Modality	Voltage	Source
Low voltage (superficial)	85–150 keV	X-ray
Medium voltage (orthovotage)	180–400 keV	X-ray
Supervoltage	500 keV–8 MeV	Linear accelerator, ^{60}Co machine
Megavoltage	Above supervoltage energy	Betatron, linear accelerator

TABLE 23.6   Historical and International System (SI) Units of Radiation

Quantity	Historical Unit	SI Unit	Conversion Factor
Exposure	R	C/kg	2.58×10^{-4} C/kg/R
Absorbed dose	Rad	Gray (Gy)	10^{-2} Gy/rad
Dose equivalent (used in radiation protection)	Rem	Seivert (Sv)	10^{-2} Sv/rem
Activity	Curie (Ci)	Becquerel (Bq)	3.7×10^{10} Bq/Ci

commonly used in brachytherapy, which historically used only two-dimensional imaging. With the advent of CT- and magnetic resonance imaging (MRI)–compatible brachytherapy applicators, imaging modalities are used to more precisely direct the radiation to the tissues at risk while simultaneously avoiding normal, uninvolved tissues. The acceleration in technology has paralleled the advances in computer technology. In addition, simulations that combine radiation delivery planning with positron emission tomography (PET) and MRI are currently being used at several centers.

RADIATION UNITS

Those in training and in practice must familiarize themselves with the international system (SI) of weights and measures used today. The SI units and appropriate conversions are shown in Table 23.6.

When a radiation exposure occurs, the resultant ionizations deposit energy in the air. **If a patient lies in the path of the beam, energy will be deposited in the patient. This deposition of energy by radiation exposure is called *r*adiation-*a*bsorbed *d*ose, measured in the acronym rad. One rad is equivalent to the deposition of 100 ergs of energy into each gram of the irradiated object. The SI unit of radiation absorbed dose is the gray (Gy), and 1 Gy = 1 cGy =100 rads = 1 joule/kg. The erg and joule are units of energy.**

RADIATION PHYSICS

Energy Deposition

Radiation energy is deposited into the tissue in one of two ways: direct or indirect ionization. Ionization is when an outer shell electron is stripped from an atom, leaving a positive charge. Direct ionization is the predominant mechanism of action of particles that possess charge, but photons can also cause direct ionization. Examples of directly ionizing particles include particulate radiation such as protons and neutrons. Indirect ionization produces free radicals of other molecules, namely water, which diffuse and damage critical targets (Fig. 23.1). A free radical has an unpaired outer shell electron that is chemically unstable and very reactive. The hydroxyl free radical (made by the lysis of H_2O) diffuses only about 1 nm and breaks the chemical bonds in cellular proteins and other key substances such as DNA. Either form of energy deposition results in ionization of

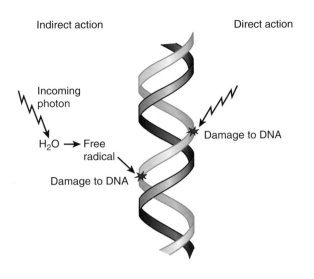

Indirect action   Direct action

Incoming
photon

$H_2O \rightarrow$ Free
radical

Damage to DNA

Damage to DNA

DNA

FIGURE 23.1 Direct and indirect actions of radiation. DNA, the most lethal target of radiation is schematically shown in the center. In direct action, the incident photon displaces an electron from the target (DNA) molecule. In indirect action, another molecule, such as water, is ionized, and the displaced electron diffuses to the target and damages the DNA.

target molecules. Scientists estimate that about two-thirds of cell biologic damage is from indirect action by ionizing radiation, from sources such as x-rays and gamma rays.

The electrons generated by penetrating photons lose their energy slowly, resulting in a low energy deposition along the electron track, or low linear energy transfer (LET; defined as energy transferred per unit length of track, or keV/μm). High LET radiations (neutrons, negative p mesons, or alpha particles) deposit more energy per unit length, are more commonly directly ionizing, and are less susceptible to perturbations such as oxygen tension. This means that for the same reaction produced in healthy cells by all radiation modalities, high LET radiation has a higher probability (1.5 to 2.5 times that of x-rays) of killing those cells in less than ideal circumstances (ie, hypoxic tumor cells, cells in a resistant part of the cell cycle).

Sources of Radiation

Gamma rays are the photons emitted from the atomic nuclear decay of radioactive isotopes—for example, ^{137}Cs (cesium) or ^{60}Co (cobalt). *X-rays* are photons electrically generated by bombarding a target such as tungsten with electrons (how a linear accelerator works). When these fast-moving electrons approach the tungsten nuclear field, they are attracted to the nucleus and thus veer from their original path. This change in direction causes deceleration and kinetic energy is converted to x-rays in the form of bremsstrahlung photons. These emitted x-rays, or photons, vary in energy from zero to a maximum determined by the kinetic energy of the bombarding electrons. Machines such as the betatron and linear accelerator generate electrons with high kinetic energy and thus produce high-energy x-rays. In addition to bremsstrahlung photons, characteristic photons are also produced as atoms seek to fill electron

orbital vacancies (see later discussion). Gamma rays and x-rays can be collectively called *photons*, and what is of medical importance is the energy and delivery of the photon, not the source.

Photon Interactions

The interaction of photons with matter is accomplished through six mechanisms: **(1) Compton scattering, (2) photoelectric absorption, (3) pair production, (4) triplet production, (5) photodisintegration, and (6) coherent scattering (no energy transfer).** The Compton effect is the major interaction of photons in tissue used in modern radiotherapy (Fig. 23.2). When the photon from the linear accelerator interacts with outer orbital atomic electrons, part of the photon energy transfers to the electron as kinetic energy. The photon is deflected with reduced energy. The ejected electron is propelled forward and sets up a cascade of increasing energy deposition by displacing more electrons. As a result of this initiation and subsequent *buildup effect*, megavoltage photon beams have a skin-sparing effect not seen in older machines and therefore produce less superficial tissue change.

The photoelectric effect is seen at lower energies. This effect is the most important in diagnostic radiology. In this interaction, the incident photon is absorbed completely by an inner shell electron. The inner shell electron is ejected with kinetic energy equal to the incident photon energy less the electron-binding energy. An outer shell electron then drops into the vacancy. As this electron changes orbit, its energy is reduced, and the excess energy is given off in the form of a photon, called a "characteristic photon."

In pair production, photon energies greater than 1.02 MeV interact with the strong electric field of the nucleus and lose all incident energy. The incident photon energy is converted into matter in the form of a positron–electron pair. If this happens in the field of an orbital electron, three particles are produced in the interaction, and the interaction is called triplet production.

Last, in photodisintegration, the high-energy photon enters the nucleus and ejects a neutron, proton, or alpha particle. This is important for shielding considerations in linear accelerators that operate at energies above 15 MeV.

Radioactive Decay

Naturally radioactive substances decay to more stable substances by several methods: (1) beta decay (^{32}P, ^{18}F), (2) electron capture (^{125}I), (3) alpha decay (^{226}Ra), and (4) isomeric transition (gamma emission and internal conversion). "Decay" is the manner in which an isotope releases, or gains, matter, or energy to become a more stable substance. The rate of decay of a radionuclide is exponential and is termed the "activity." The old unit for activity was the Curie (Ci). The SI unit is the becquerel (Bq) defined by 1 Bq = 1 dps (disintegration per second). The half-life ($T^{1/2}$) is the time required to disintegrate to half the original activity. $T^{1/2}$ of commonly used radioactive substances is in Table 23.4.

^{137}Cs (Cesium-137), used in low dose rate (LDR) applications, is a byproduct of the fission process in a nuclear reactor and decays via beta and gamma emission. In beta decay, a neutron from the nucleus converts into a proton (positively

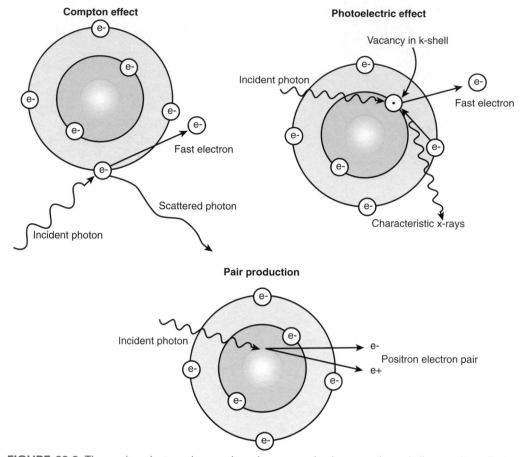

FIGURE 23.2 The major photons interactions important in therapeutic and diagnostic radiation oncology.

charged) and an electron. Again, to increase stability, a photon is released, and the ^{127}Cs becomes the more stable ^{137}Ba (Fig. 23.3). ^{137}Cs decays approximately 2%/year.

^{192}Ir (iridium 192) is also produced in a nuclear reactor and decays via beta decay (see earlier) and electron capture. In electron capture, the nucleus "captures" an orbital electron and converts a proton into a neutron. ^{192}Ir then becomes the excitable ^{192m}Pt and ^{192m}Os, which release gamma rays to stabilize. ^{192}Ir is the primary isotope used for high dose rate (HDR) applications and interstitial implants. It decays approximately 1%/day.

Inverse Square Law

Another important physics concept in radiotherapy is the inverse square law. This law states that the dose of radiation at a given point is inversely proportional to the square of the distance from the source of radiation (dose ∝ 1/distance²). This rapid decrease in dose is very important in brachytherapy. It underscores why the bladder and rectum can be relatively protected from the high intracavitary doses of radiation, especially with good vaginal packing to maximize the distance from the source to the normal organ. It also underscores why good geometry is critical when performing implants. Last, it explains the reasoning behind standing at the door (increasing the distance) while conversing with a brachytherapy patient. As a

Cesium

Iridium

FIGURE 23.3 Decay diagram of ^{137}Cs and ^{192}Ir.

simplistic example, consider the following. The dose at point A is 4. Two feet away the dose would be 4 divided by the square of the distance (2^2) or $4/4 = 1$. Another 2 feet away, the dose would be 1/4 ($4/4^2 = 4/16 = 1/4$).

Depth Dose Characteristics of Radiation

The last physics concept to master is variation in radiation beam characteristics based on energy. **To that end, it is important to realize that the energy and penetrating power of ionizing radiation increase as the photon frequency increases and wavelength decreases.** In addition, as energy increases, the depth of maximum dose increases (D_{max}; remember the *buildup effect* discussed earlier). For low energies, such as 250 keV, the maximum dose is at the skin surface. For a 4-MeV (4 million electron volts) accelerator, the D_{max} is approximately 1 cm; for 6 MeV, D_{max} is at 1.5 cm; for 22 MeV, D_{max} is at 3.5 cm; and so on. Knowing this, one can see why higher energy beams are more suited to treat deeply seated tumors, such as in the uterine or cervix. These higher energy beams differentially spare more superficial tissues. Depths of maximum dose curves and isodose distributions (areas receiving similar dose) for various energies are shown in Fig. 23.4.

The reduced effect on skin of supervoltage radiation, compared with orthovoltage (keV range) radiation, is based on a physical characteristic of radiation. With higher energy, forward movement of the energy cascade (in the direction of the primary beam) is greater with reduced lateral scattering. As the energy increases, it becomes more penetrating, and the photons and resultant liberated electrons travel a greater distance into the absorbing material. Therefore, the percentage of radiation at any specific depth, compared with the surface dose, increases as the energy increases.

In summary, above the energy of 400 to 800 keV, the advantages to higher energy photons are less damage to the skin at the portal of entry, greater radiation at depth relative to the surface, and reduced lateral scatter of radiation in the tissues. In addition, there is less photoelectric effect at higher energies and therefore less absorption in bone.

RADIOBIOLOGY

The selective destruction of tissues forms the basis of therapeutic radiation. Neoplastic cells are preferentially killed by radiation compared with the surrounding normal tissues, primarily as a result of differences in repair capabilities. This differential radiosensitivity between normal and cancerous tissues determines in large part whether a radiated neoplasm is eradicated. **The ratio that defines the dose necessary to effect tumor kill**

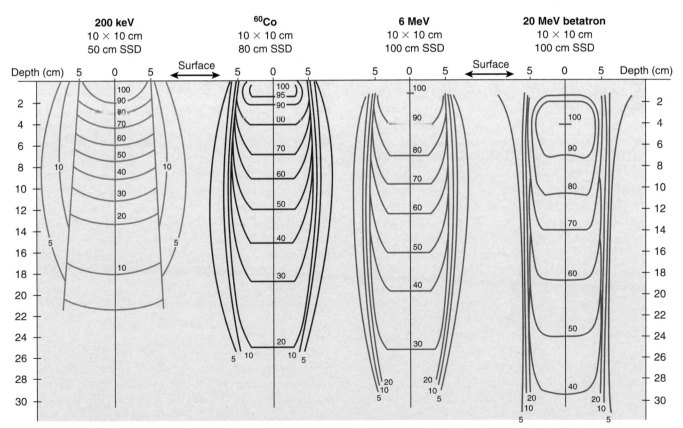

FIGURE 23.4 Comparison isodose curves and depth-dose distribution through a single field. Each machine is delivering photons of different energies. Note that higher energy machines deliver radiation to a greater depth for the same surface dose. Note also the skin sparing with 6- and 20-MV equipment. Last, note the difference in lateral scattering—higher energy photons are more "forward moving" with less lateral scatter.

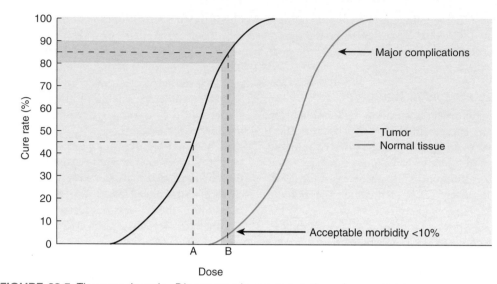

FIGURE 23.5 Therapeutic ratio. Diagrammatic representation of a parallel tumor response and normal tissue tolerance curve demonstrating the relationship between increasing dose, increasing cure rate, and increasing morbidity. Under ideal circumstances *(B)*, an 80% to 90% cure rate can be achieved with 5% to 10% morbidity. Pushing the cure rate carries with it an increase in morbidity. However, attempts to avoid all morbidity *(A)* significantly reduce the ability to cure. Although the shape of these curves varies for various tumor types and dose rates, general concepts are valid whenever radiotherapy is used to treat malignant lesions.

with the dose likely to cause normal tissue damage is the therapeutic ratio, and modern radiotherapy is striving to maximize this ratio (Fig. 23.5).

Structural Changes

Deposition of radiation energy in the cell can lead to a variety of changes that alter normal function. Degradation, or breaking into smaller units, and cross-linking are examples of structural damage that can affect proteins, enzymes, and nucleic acids. The initial chemical change occurs in a fraction of a second and is rarely detected directly. Some changes are repaired almost immediately, but others can never be repaired. Although various morphologic and functional changes occur in irradiated cells, the bulk of direct and indirect evidence suggests that the biologic effects of radiation result principally from DNA damage. For example, it has been calculated that 1 million cGy is required to inactivate cell cytoplasmic enzyme systems, and doses of 1000 cGy are required to damage cell membranes. In contrast, chromosomal aberrations and mutations can be produced by very low doses of radiation. Because only a few hundred cGy are needed to produce a high degree of lethality in cell tissue culture, it seems logical that nuclear changes are responsible for cell death.

Radiation-induced DNA damage destroys the cell by one of several mechanisms. It may stimulate cell apoptosis, called interphase death, which is visible by several methods, including light microscopy and Western blot. Radiation may also cause mitotic death. In this form of damage, the cell outwardly appears normal but is sufficiently damaged so that cell division is not possible. Actual death of the cell does not occur, however, until cell division is attempted. This is why tumors may continue to regress after completion of radiation.

A variety of DNA lesions are produced by radiation including base damage, DNA–protein crosslinking, single-strand breaks, and double-strand breaks (DSBs). Repairing even a single nucleotide requires many genes and a series of steps. The most toxic cellular lesion inflicted by ionizing radiation is the DSB. In fact, the proficiency of repair of DSB correlates well with radiation-induced lethality. The repair of DSB can occur by several mechanisms. Religation of complementary DSB ends, homologous recombination (HR), is efficient, and cells can usually survive. The Mre11 protein is attracted when a DSB occurs and may be the first sensor of the break and primarily involved in repair through nuclease activity, unwinding DNA, or removing hairpin loops. When the ends are not complementary, nonhomologous end joining (NHEJ) is used and can be complicated by small DNA deletions or insertions. These errors in turn can lead to cell death or mutation. Some of the necessary proteins for NHEJ are Ku70, Ku80, DNA ligase IV, and XRCC4. The Ku70/Ku80 complex binds to the DSB and unwinds the strand while the DNA ligase IV/XRCC4 complex repairs DSBs. Mammalian cells seem to repair more by NHEJ than HR.

Radiosensitivity

Radiosensitivity is the response of the tumor to irradiation that can be measured by the extent of regression, rapidity of response, and response durability. Radiosensitivity depends on several factors. These factors include the ability to repair damage, hypoxia, cell cycle position, and growth fraction. In addition, the volume of the initial tumor has been demonstrated to influence the ability to eradicate tumors.

Understanding that radiosensitivity and radiocurability are not identical in meaning is essential. Relatively radioresistant tumors accessible to high-dose local radiation therapy can be

cured, but radiosensitive tumors that are widely metastatic can only be controlled locally. An excellent example of a relatively radioresistant tumor is squamous cell carcinoma of the cervix; however, this malignancy remains one of the most curable tumors in humans because of its accessibility to high-dose irradiation and the relatively radioresistant nature of the hosting normal tissues (eg, cervix and vagina). The ability to place radium or cesium in juxtaposition to the malignancy within dose ranges tolerable to the surrounding normal tissue is the key to success.

Many attempts have been made to develop an assay to predict tumor radiosensitivity. However, no assay yet developed accurately predicts the outcome in a given tumor. **This is likely secondary to tumors containing mixed cell populations with differing sensitivities to chemotherapy and radiation. Sensitive cells are eliminated, but resistant cells continue to grow. This explains why many tumors initially respond to therapy but are ultimately incurable.**

In vitro models have been developed to predict and study tumor cell radiosensitivity. Cellular radiosensitivity is generally quantified by measuring the loss of reproductive capacity, which can be plotted in a survival curve. Survival curves are characterized by an initial slope, α, and the terminal slope, β. α represents irreparable damage to the cell, and β represents the repairable damage (Fig. 23.6). The α/β ratio is the dose at which the contribution from alpha equals the contribution from beta and is a measure of radiosensitivity. Large ratios are seen with rapidly dividing cells and help predict the response of tumors and the early effects of radiation. Low ratios characterize late responding tissues.

In addition, the size of the shoulder (Dq) on a survival curve relays valuable information because it represents the magnitude of repair of sublethal damage (SLD). Broad shoulders have small α/β ratios and good repair of SLD. This repair of sublethal damage takes several hours (2–6 hours) to complete. The ability of cells to repair SLD forms the basis for the use of fractionated doses in clinical radiation therapy, in which differential capacities between normal tissue and tumor to repair a sublethal injury can be exploited (Fig. 23.7). This differential repair capacity also forms the basis for accelerated fractionation or hyperfractionation in which the dose is given twice a day. This approach works very well with rapidly growing tumors. Treated twice a day, the normal tissues have sufficient time to repair, but the tumor tissues, which are less organized, efficient, and accurate, are differentially killed. Some cells have almost no shoulder, indicating a limited ability to repair sublethal damage, and these cells can be eradicated with relatively low doses of radiation. For example, dysgerminomas are highly curable with relatively low doses of radiation (20–30 Gy) compared with cervical cancer tumors, which may require more than 70 Gy to obtain cure.

The availability of oxygen is of vital importance to the radiosensitivity of the cell also. As radiation enters the cell, it interacts with organic molecules (DNA). This molecule may repair itself unless an oxygen molecule becomes attached, thereby "fixing" the damage. The addition of O_2 will enhance low LET radiation (photons) but does not similarly affect high LET radiation. The ability of oxygen to enhance radiation is measured by the oxygen enhancement ratio, or oxygen enhancement ratio (OER) (OER = Dose of XRT without O_2 for a given effect/Dose of XRT with O_2 for the same effect). It takes at least 2% (17 mm Hg) tissue O_2 to see the full oxygen effect.

Tumor cells with potentially unlimited capacity for growth are limited as they outgrow the blood supply. In fact, tumors above 200 μm have necrotic cores secondary to a limited diffusion distance for oxygen. Oxygen may effectively penetrate approximately 70 μm from the blood vessel (Fig. 23.8). Outside this distance, tumor cells become deficient and enter a noncycling phase. They may become hypoxic or even anoxic and necrotic.

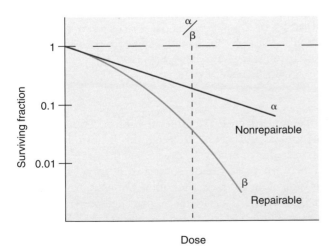

FIGURE 23.6 Cell survival curve. The initial slope, α, represents irreparable damage, and the terminal slope, β, represents reparable damage. The α/β ratio is the point on the curve where the two are equal.

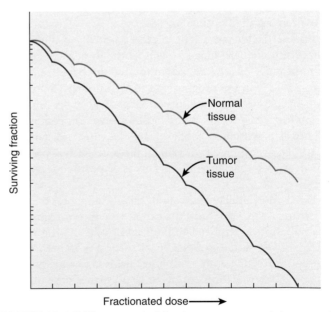

FIGURE 23.7 Different capacities between normal tissue and tumor to accumulate and repair sublethal injury from fractionated doses result in differential survival. The normal tissue is able to repair more efficiently and effectively.

FIGURE 23.8 As the distance from the blood supply increases, cells become hypoxic and even anoxic. Hypoxic cells are more radioresistant and therefore harder to sterilize. Oxygen diffuses about 70 μm from the capillary.

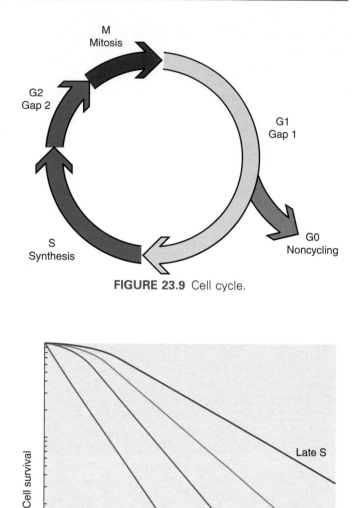

FIGURE 23.9 Cell cycle.

This is important from a radiobiologic standpoint because noncycling cells exhibit a greater capacity to repair radiation injury. Hypoxic cells are more resistant to the effects of radiation than are cells with normal oxygen tension. Thus large tumors can be difficult to control with radiation therapy, not only because there is a greater number of cells to sterilize but also because a proportion of these cells are hypoxic, noncycling, and radioresistant. As a clinical example, experience notes that exophytic friable cervical lesions that hemorrhage easily on contact respond better and more quickly than infiltrative lesions. The blood supply and oxygenation vary considerably between these two lesions, with the friable lesion better vascularized and oxygenated and therefore more radiosensitive. Unfortunately, attempts to overcome this differential sensitivity by mechanisms such as hyperbaric oxygen and radiosensitizers have been less than optimal to date.

Another factor important in radiosensitivity is the proportion of mitotic or clonogenic cells in the tumor. Cycling cells are more radiosensitive. In fact, mitotic counts have been shown to correlate with the prognosis in many tumors. The position in the cell cycle is also important (Fig. 23.9). Cells in late G2 and mitosis (M-phase) are the most sensitive to radiation, and cells in late synthesis (S-phase) are the most resistant (Fig. 23.10). This is exploited with chemotherapies such as paclitaxel, which arrests cells in mitosis and is a profound radiation sensitizer.

Finally, the initial tumor volume greatly influences the ability to sterilize a site. **Generally, the smaller the tumor volume, the less radiation is required to destroy all cells. As the volume increases, the dose to obtain local control is increased.** The concept of treating with "shrinking" fields is to serially reduce the size of the radiation portals to give a higher dose of radiation therapy to the central portion of the tumor, where presumably more hypoxic, radioresistant cells are present.

Historically, clinicians attempted to correlate radiation tumor response and local tumor control. Generally, the faster and more complete the tumor response at the completion of

FIGURE 23.10 The survival curve for cells in mitosis, and G2 is steep and has no shoulder. The curve for cells late in S phase is shallower and has a large shoulder. G1 and early S are intermediate in sensitivity.

the therapy, the greater long-term control, assuming that no distant metastasis occurs. Although this is not uniformly true, it has been shown in cervical cancer that there is a good correlation between local tumor control and complete or partial regression of the cancer at the completion of radiation. In addition, Grigsby and associates have correlated posttreatment PET tumor response (which measures glucose metabolism) with survival.

Another factor limiting radiocurability is the normal tissue toxicity with increasing radiation doses. Normal tissue effects depend on total dose, dose fraction size, volume, and inherent tissue radiosensitivity. The ultimate goal is to obtain maximal curability with minimal side effects. Combining radiation therapy with surgery or chemotherapy decreases normal tissue tolerance to a given dose. Well-established port size, total dose, and fractionation schemes have been identified but cannot remain static. Variations are being investigated to increase curability and decrease complications, including new chemotherapeutic radiosensitizers, technological advances in the delivery of radiation such as IMRT, and radioprotectors such as Ethyol.

RADIOSENSITIZERS, HYPOXIC CELL SENSITIZERS, AND RADIOPROTECTORS

Radiation sensitizers and protectors are being actively investigated to increase the effectiveness of radiation or allow dose escalation while minimizing side effects. **Radiation sensitizers increase the ability of radiation to cause permanent, lethal damage.** This therapeutic gain may be from a variety of mechanisms, including selective uptake, targeting, or activation. To be effective, sensitizers must have acceptable normal tissue side effects. Known radiation sensitizers include chemotherapeutic agents such as cisplatin, 5-fluorouracil, paclitaxel, Adriamycin, and gemcitabine. Hypoxic cell sensitizers include the imidazole drugs such as misonidazole and bioreductive agents such as tirapazamine. Endogenous sulfhydryl compounds and Ethyol afford radioprotection to normal tissues.

The advantages afforded by chemoradiation can be by several mechanisms. Some agents (eg, cisplatin) inhibit the repair of radiation damage, but others (eg, paclitaxel) block cells in a radiosensitive cell cycle phase. Adriamycin, docetaxel, and paclitaxel have unique effects when combined serially with radiation because "radiation recall" is an uncommon but distressing phenomenon. After a course of radiation, the normal tissue sensitization can be "recalled" when the chemotherapy is initiated—this phenomenon is a reemergence of a prior radiation burn that conforms exactly to the prior radiation portal. The mechanism of this is unknown but well described for these chemotherapies.

The nitroimidazoles such as metronidazole, misonidazole, etanidazole, and nimorazole are electron affinic and increase the sensitivity of radioresistant hypoxic cells to XRT. They mimic oxygen and can diffuse into hypoxic areas. Unfortunately, clinical studies to date have demonstrated significant toxicity and little clinical utility with these drugs.

Tirapazamine is entering clinical trials as an adjunct to radiotherapy. Gynecologic Oncology Group (GOG) trial 219 randomized chemoradiation for cervical cancer with and without tirapazamine. Tirapazamine is bioactivated intracellularly to a cytotoxic, active free radical that causes extensive chromosomal breaks and inhibits DNA repair. The reaction is driven by low tissue oxygen tension and when combined with radiation may allow more effective destruction of tumors with hypoxic cores. The GOG published a phase II trial for advanced or recurrent cervical carcinoma using tirapazamine and cisplatin and concluded that the combination was fairly well tolerated. A subsequent phase III trial randomizing stages Ib2 to IVa between standard cisplatin and radiation versus cisplatin, radiation, and tirapazamine was opened but closed for accrual in 2009.

Radioprotection has been proved in several sites with the use of Ethyol. Amifostine (Ethyol; WR-2721) is an organic thiophosphate extensively studied by the Walter Reed Army Institute of Research. Normal tissues noted to be protected included the salivary glands, bone marrow, immune system, skin, oral mucosa, esophagus, intestinal mucosa, kidney, and testes. It is dephosphorylated to the active metabolite (WR-1065) in the tissues.

It is believed that tissue versus tumor alkaline phosphatase concentration variations provide the differential protective effect. In addition, tissue pH differences afford selective tissue versus tumor uptake of Ethyol. When given intravenously, the plasma half-life is less than 10 minutes, but there is prolonged retention of the drug in normal tissue. In the first 30 minutes, drug uptake into normal tissues has been shown to be 100 times that of tumor tissues. When inside the cell, the metabolite scavenges oxygen free radicals and provides an alternative target for alkylating agents, such as cisplatin.

There have been numerous studies of the protective effect of Ethyol with no reported decrease in antitumor efficacy. A phase III trial in head and neck cancer unequivocally established its role in salivary gland protection, confirming earlier studies. Other clinical trials have shown Ethyol protects from cisplatin-induced renal, neurologic, and bone marrow toxicity. Liu published a phase III randomized trial in rectal cancer patients treated with pelvic radiation with and without Ethyol (340 mg/m²). The toxicity in the mucous membranes and genitourinary (GU) and gastrointestinal (GI) tracts was reduced by 50% in the Ethyol arm. Moderate to severe late toxicities were seen in 14% of those treated without Ethyol compared with zero in the Ethyol-treated patients.

Athanassiou and colleagues randomly assigned 205 patients with pelvic radiation plus or minus Ethyol and demonstrated a significant decrease in bladder and GI toxicity. Complete responses to therapy and median survival were not significantly different between the arms. The RTOG (Radiation Therapy Oncology Group 0116) completed a two-arm trial using Ethyol with chemoradiation for pelvic and paraaortic radiation with concomitant cisplatin in cervical carcinoma. Arm 1 consisted of cisplatin chemotherapy concomitant with paraaortic radiation and demonstrated significant acute and late toxicity. Arm 2 again demonstrated significant acute and long-term toxicity, with no significant benefit demonstrated with the addition of Ethyol, although compliance to the medication was disappointing. Ethyol has been found to be useful in reducing early and late toxicity with hypofractionated accelerated conformal radiation by Koukourakis. Toxicities with intravenous administration include hypotension and nausea. Data on subcutaneous administration demonstrate less hypotension but treatable nausea and skin effects persist. There have been rare reports of Stevens-Johnson syndrome.

Genetic Effects

It is not possible to generalize and assign a specific mutation rate to a given radiation dose. Gene loci differ greatly in their

mutability, and the random damage exerted by irradiation on any particular chromosome makes predictability impossible. The mitotic stage, cell type, sex, species, and dose rate influence the mutation rate as studied in lower animals and bacteria. Data from lower animals are difficult to extrapolate to humans, and therefore prediction of mutation rates cannot be expected from the evidence that has been accumulated from various types of radiation exposure. Direct evidence of radiation-induced mutation in humans is lacking, although there is strong anecdotal evidence for carcinogenesis in those exposed to radiation. A few examples are excess skin cancers seen in those exposed to x-rays before safety standards were established, lung cancer in pitchblende miners, bone tumors in radium dial painters, and liver tumors in those exposed to Thorotrast contrast. The largest groups of humans available for study are survivors and descendants of those exposed in Hiroshima and Nagasaki. Although there has been no detectable effect on the frequency of prenatal or neonatal deaths or on the frequency of malformations in subsequent generations, this does not mean that no hereditary effects were produced. The number of exposed parents was small, and dosages were so low that it would have been surprising if an increase in mutation had been detected in such a brief period. There has not been sufficient time for the several generations needed to reveal recessive damage.

Radiation does not produce new and unique mutations but increases the incidence of spontaneous mutations. Based largely on experiments in mice, it is estimated that the doubling dose (ie, the dose that will double the spontaneous mutation rate) for humans is probably 100 cGy. Between 1% and 6% of spontaneous mutations in humans can be ascribed to background radiation. With the use of image intensifiers, improved radiographic film, and appropriate shielding to prevent scatter, it is possible to attain satisfactory radiographic visualization of internal structures with reduced exposure. The average dose of irradiation to the gonads of some common diagnostic techniques is given in Table 23.7. The use of diagnostic radiographs and CT scans has increased and fueled concerns that toxic radiation effects may emerge, especially among children exposed to increased diagnostic medical irradiation. Current recommendations stress the use of ionizing radiation only when necessary and substitution of alternate sources of imaging, such as MRI, which relies on magnetic fields, when possible.

In general, most mutations are harmful, and there is no known threshold dose for the genetic effect. Permanent sterility in females is estimated to have a threshold of 250 to 600 cGy to acute exposure and 0.2 Gy/year for protracted exposure. The threshold dose for sterility varies based on the age of the patient, with younger patients being more resistant to the deleterious effect.

Fetal Effects

The classic effects of radiation on the mammalian embryo are as follows: (1) intrauterine and extrauterine growth restriction; (2) embryonic, fetal, or neonatal death; and (3) gross congenital malformations. Dose, gestational age, and dose rate are all important factors influencing radiation damage. The recommendation for fetal dose during the entire gestation is 0.5 rem

TABLE 23.7 Radiation Doses to Low Pelvis From Diagnostic Scans

Examination	Dose to Fetus (First Trimester) and Maternal Gonads (mcGy)
Lower extremity radiography	1
Cervical spine radiography	2
Chest radiography	8
Chest fluoroscopy	70
Lumbar spine radiography	275
Hip radiography	100
IVP	585
Upper GI	330
Lower GI	465
Chest CT	8
Abdominal CT	800
Pelvic CT	2300

CT, Computed tomography; *GI*, gastrointestinal; *IVP*, intravenous pyelography.
Modified from DiSaia PJ. In Scott JR, DiSaia PJ, Hammond CB, Spellacy WN, eds. *Danforth's Obstetrics and Gynecology*, 8th ed. Philadelphia, 1999, JB Lippincott.

or less (roughly 0.5 cGy). Monthly exposures should not exceed 0.05 rem. If a pregnant patient receives 10 cGy in the sensitive period of 10 days to 26 weeks, therapeutic abortion should be considered to avoid radiation effects, including malformations, microcephaly, and mental retardation.

The peak incidence of gross malformations occurs during early organogenesis (10–40 days of gestation in humans), although cellular, tissue, and organ hypoplasia can be produced by radiation throughout the fetal and neonatal period with sufficient dose. Diagnostic x-ray procedures should be avoided in the pregnant woman unless there is overwhelming urgency. In women of childbearing age, possible damage to an early conceptus can be prevented by performing tests immediately after the commencement of a menstrual period and obtaining a negative pregnancy test result. Compelling evidence that radiation may be a causative agent in childhood cancer after prenatal exposure comes from several studies in Great Britain and the United States.

Some concrete information is available from the Japanese survivors of the atom bomb attacks in 1945. Examination of children born to survivors demonstrates the primary effect from in utero radiation was microcephaly and mental retardation. The most sensitive phase for mental retardation was from 8 to 15 weeks of gestation. In addition, permanent growth restriction was also observed, especially in embryos exposed less than 1500 m from the center of the explosion. Hall reached the following conclusions:

1. Moderately large doses of radiation (>200 cGy) delivered to human embryos before 2 to 3 weeks of gestation are unlikely to produce severe abnormalities in most children born, although a considerable number of embryos may be reabsorbed or aborted (all-or-none phenomenon).

2. Significant irradiation between 4 and 11 weeks of gestation leads to severe abnormalities in many organs.
3. Irradiation between 11 and 16 weeks of gestation may produce some eye, skeletal, and genital organ abnormalities; however, stunted growth, microcephaly, and mental retardation are often present.
4. Irradiation of fetuses between 16 and 20 weeks of gestation may lead to a mild degree of microcephaly, mental retardation, and stunting of growth.
5. Irradiation after 30 weeks of gestation is unlikely to produce gross structural abnormalities leading to a serious disability but could cause functional disabilities.

PRINCIPLES OF CLINICAL RADIATION THERAPY

The technical modalities used in modern radiation therapy may be divided into two major categories:

1. **External irradiation:** This applies to irradiation from sources at a distance from the body (eg, teletherapy with $_{60}$Co, linear accelerator, betatron, or orthovoltage radiograph machines).
2. **Local irradiation** (brachytherapy): This applies to irradiation from sources in direct proximity to the tissue or tumor. Brachytherapy can be delivered with either an LDR system or an HDR system. LDR systems require hospital admission to a shielded room and dose delivery at roughly 50 to 100 cGy/h. HDR systems are commonly done on an outpatient basis and deliver doses of 120 cGy/h.
   a. **Intracavitary irradiation** is done with applicators loaded with radioactive materials such as cesium or iridium (eg, vaginal ovoids, vaginal cylinder, intrauterine tandem, tandem and ring, or, historically, Heyman capsules).
   b. **Interstitial irradiation** (endocurie therapy) is usually delivered in the form of removable needles containing cesium or iridium. The term also applies to permanent isotope implants, such as ^{125}I (iodine) seeds or ^{103}Pd (palladium).
   c. **Direct therapy** was historically delivered by means of cones from an orthovoltage machine (eg, transvaginal) but is rarely available today.
   d. **Intraperitoneal or intrapleural** instillation of radioactive colloids, such as ^{32}P, is yet another local therapy but is infrequently used.

External-beam Radiation (Teletherapy)

External radiation is radiation therapy that is delivered from outside the body. It is most commonly delivered with photons, electrons, or protons. Machinery to deliver the radiation includes ^{60}Co units, orthovoltage machines, and linear accelerators, although linear accelerators are the overwhelming majority. Except in the developing world, ^{60}Co units are unusual. Typically, a patient will need planning done before initiation of radiation, called simulation. Marks or permanent tattoos are applied to the skin to allow for daily setup and, commonly, a planning CT is performed replacing the traditional fluoroscopic simulation. The use of MRI, CT, or PET images to fuse with treatment planning CT data is widely available to better delineate tumor targets and normal tissue and in many centers is part of the standard simulator machine. Three areas must be targeted. The gross tumor volume requires the highest radiation dose. Microscopic extensions into surrounding tissues must be targeted but generally require a lesser dose for sterilization. Subclinical disease presumed to be present in postoperative beds or regional nodes must also be treated to prevent marginal failures.

Local Radiation (Brachytherapy)

Local application of radiation (also known as brachytherapy) permits very high doses to restricted tissue volumes. In this situation, the physical principle (inverse square law) that the intensity of irradiation rapidly decreases with distance from the radiation source is used to advantage. Brachytherapy is well suited to treat small tumors with well-defined limits and a clinical situation in which it is desirable to restrict the volume of tissue irradiated. Larger volumes of tissue that need radiation therapy are best treated with external irradiation. Historically, radium (^{226}Ra) had been the most common isotope used for local application, but because of storage, risk of leaks, and extremely long half-life, it is rarely used in the United State. Sources used today are often converted to mg-Ra-equivalents. Brachytherapy sources such as ^{125}I, ^{137}Cs, ^{192}Ir, and ^{103}Pd are more commonly used today (see Table 23.4).

Although conventional LDR intracavitary brachytherapy has produced very good results in cervical cancer, remote afterloading HDR intracavitary brachytherapy is becoming more widespread. The treatment results of LDR and HDR appear to be similar both for local control and survival, although there are no large American randomized trials. Retrospective studies, however, mirror the results of the randomized studies. There remain concerns over potential differences in late complications resulting from the different biologic mechanisms between the continuous low dose rate of LDR and the intermittent high dose rate of HDR. The increased interest in HDR arises from cost of inpatient hospitalization, the risks of prolonged bed rest, and radiation exposure to medical personnel with LDR systems. In both LDR and HDR, it is very important to keep the doses to normal tissues as low as possible by proper placement of radiation carriers and the use of shielding and packing or retraction techniques. HDR units use computer technology to "optimize" the dwell time of a single source to give the required distribution. The American Brachytherapy Society has published consensus guidelines on the administration of HDR for both cervical and uterine carcinomas. Also in use as an alternative to LDR or HDR is pulsed dose rate (PDR), although randomized trials on this method are lacking, and published reports are few but increasing.

The term *dosimetry* is applied to the measurement and calculation of dose that the patient receives. In brachytherapy, as radiation intensity rapidly decreases with increasing distance from the source, tissue adjacent to the radiation source is treated to a high dose while relatively sparing surrounding tissue. The effectiveness of this distribution of irradiation depends on meticulous application of these sources. Interstitial application of radioactive sources is more difficult than intracavitary application. It is essential that the gynecologic oncologist be able to critically assess the placement of tandem and ovoids, cylinder, and ring to assess the optimal placement of brachytherapy sources (Figs. 23.11 and 23.12). Increased use of computer planning to optimize the dose to the tumor and minimize the dose to the normal tissues is under active clinical investigation and is likely to replace the current two-dimensional dosing guidelines and restrictions based on calculated doses to points (eg, points A, B, and bladder and rectal points) with three-dimensional, volume-directed, image-guided brachytherapy (IGBT). The European collaborative group Groupe Européen de Curiethérapie and the European Society for Therapeutic Radiology and Oncology (GEC-ESTRO) have published extensive work on this subject and an international trial. EMBRACE (Mri-guided BRachytherapy in CErvical cancer) is open to test the utility and applicability of the new guidelines.

Normal Tissue Tolerance

The tolerance of any tissue (normal or tumor) to irradiation therapy depends on several characteristics of radiation, including (1) fractionation technique, (2) field arrangement, (3) total dose, (4) dose rate, and (5) volume irradiated.

Fractionation is the number of treatments needed to deliver the total dose. Pelvic radiation delivered to a patient for a total dose of 5000 cGy given in five daily fractions of 200 cGy each week for 5 weeks is well tolerated in most cases. However, if that same total dose of 5000 cGy were given in five fractions of 1000 cGy every Monday for 5 consecutive weeks, tolerance would be low.

In addition, multiple fields are used to minimize toxicity by dividing the exposure of normal tissue into multiple different regions. Three-dimensional conformal therapy (3DCF), IMRT, and IGRT are areas of active investigation to further maximize dose to tumor and minimize toxicity to the surrounding normal tissues (Fig. 23.13). With external irradiation, the patient is treated to all fields 5 days/week.

As is seen in LDR brachytherapy versus HDR brachytherapy, dose rate affects tolerance. The final dose in HDR is necessarily lower to compensate for normal tissue tolerance concerns with the markedly higher dose rate in HDR. Conversion of doses to a 2-Gy dose equivalent is recommended by the Groupe Euro-Péen de Curiethérapie-European for Radiotherapy and Oncology (GECT-ESTRO) guidelines and is becoming more common (see later).

Finally, the volume of tissue irradiated is also an integral factor in tolerance. For example, a 1-cm circular field of skin would easily tolerate the fractionation and dose rate of 1000 cGy each Monday for 5 consecutive weeks. However, for a larger volume, such as whole-pelvis radiation, such a treatment plan is intolerable.

Patient factors also affect normal tissue tolerance. Previous surgery affects the morbidity of radiation therapy. In both cervical and uterine cancer, surgery identifies adverse surgical pathologic findings that direct radiation therapy. In cervical cancer, surgical evaluation of possible lymph node metastases, particularly in advanced cancers, may be done, or a radical hysterectomy may be aborted because on inspection, the tumor

is more advanced than originally indicated. Transperitoneal lymph node dissection followed by pelvic and possibly para-aortic radiation increases radiation-induced complications, particularly to the bowel. Radiation complications can be severe, including fistula formation, bowel obstruction, and perforation. The retroperitoneal approach to lymph node dissection has a decreased complication rate and is the preferred method of surgically evaluating lymph node status in cervical cancer. Medical conditions that affect blood flow such as diabetes, hypertension, and peripheral vascular disease can also decrease normal tissue tolerance.

Pelvic Organ Tolerance

Irradiation tolerance of the normal organs of the pelvis varies from one patient to another and is subject to the factors previously mentioned, such as volume, fractionation, and total dose of irradiation. As is illustrated in many areas of oncology, the more advanced lesions require higher doses for tumor eradication, and hence the possibility of morbidity increases. This, combined with the fact that advanced cancer often already compromises the integrity of the bladder and rectum, means that serious sequelae can develop in patients with advanced cervical, vaginal, and corpus lesions when curative therapy is sought. New advances in radiation delivery will, hopefully, decrease these adverse effects.

The normal tissues of the cervix and the corpus of the uterus can tolerate very high doses of radiation. In fact, they withstand higher doses better than any other comparable volume of tissue in the body; surface doses of 20,000 to 30,000 cGy in about 2 weeks are tolerated. This remarkable tolerance level permits a large tumor dose and allows a very high percentage of central control of cervical cancer. **The unusual radiation tolerance of the uterus and the vagina, stemming from an unusual ability to recover from radiation injury, accounts for the success of brachytherapy in the treatment of cervical lesions.**

In contrast, the sigmoid, rectosigmoid, and rectum are more susceptible to radiation injury than are other pelvic organs. The frequency of injury to the large bowel often depends on the total dose administered by both the external beam and the intracavitary system. With external-beam radiation alone, the large bowel is the most sensitive of the pelvic structures. The bladder tolerates slightly more radiation than does the rectosigmoid, according to most authorities. Acceptable maximal point doses are 75 Gy and 70 Gy to the bladder and rectum, respectively. Fletcher proposed a rule that gives the upper limits of pelvic irradiation and indirectly gives the tolerance of the bladder and rectum. The guidelines limit the sum of the central dose, stating that external-beam radiation dose plus the number of milligram-hours of cesium administered by brachytherapy should never exceed 10,000. There is a parallel time guideline also critical to this limit. This is a necessary safety to prevent compact systems from exceeding vaginal or cervical tolerance. This guideline is valid only when the Fletcher-Suit brachytherapy systems are used. Most of this is applicable to therapy for the uterus, cervix, and vagina. In general, if a large dose of intracavitary irradiation is applied centrally for a small lesion, the amount of external beam applied centrally

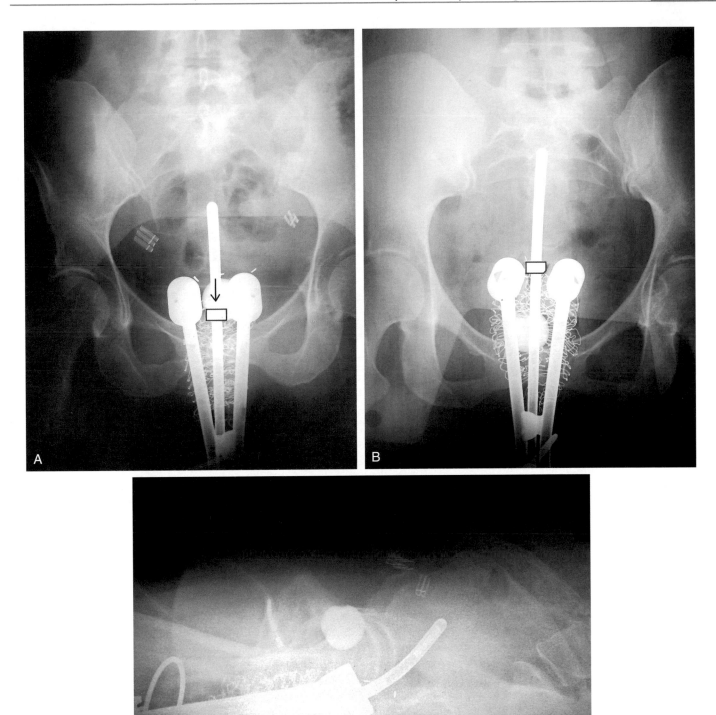

FIGURE 23.11 Assessing proper placement of tandem and ovoids. In both photos, small interstitial silver seeds mark the cervix. Note that in **A,** the cervical stop, outlined in *red,* has dropped away from the cervix, compromising the dose delivery to the tumor and increasing the complications. In **B,** this has been corrected. Also note that the vaginal packing (delineated by radiopaque string) lies below the ovoids and that the tandem is midline and bisects the ovoids. In **C,** a lateral radiograph, the tandem again bisects the ovoids and lies beneath the bladder (the Foley balloon is filled with contrast material) and does not lie too close to the sacrum.

FIGURE 23.12 Isodose curves surrounding a typical Fletcher-Suit intracavitary application (tandem plus ovoids) for cervical cancer. Note the location of points *A* and *B* and the relative dose rates at distances from the system.

must be reduced. Conversely, if a lesion is large and the vaginal geometry is poor, a smaller intracavitary dose can be given and the dose administered by external beam may be raised (6000–7000 cGy).

GEC-ESTRO dose/volume guidelines limit the bladder to 90 Gy$_{EQD2}$ and rectum/sigmoid to 70 to 75 Gy$_{EQD2}$ for a calculated 2-cc volume combining doses from both external-beam irradiation and brachytherapy. In this system, doses from HDR brachytherapy are converted by a formula to a 2-Gy equivalent to allow the doses to be added (EQD2, or equivalent dose at 2 Gy). The formula for conversion is EQD2 = D X [(d + α/β)/2 + α/β], where D is total dose, d is dose/fraction, and α/β is 3 for late-responding tissues and 10 for tumor/acute-responding tissues. Certain assumptions are made in this model, such as the same 2 cc of bladder, rectum, and sigmoid receive the maximal amount of irradiation with each fraction of brachytherapy. Especially in the mobile sigmoid colon, this assumption may be erroneous but models the worst-case scenario. A recent paper by Georg and colleagues demonstrated that the 5-year actuarial rectal toxicity rate was 20% if the dose exceeded 75 Gy$_{EQD2}$ and 5% if the 2-cc dose remained below 75 Gy$_{EQD2}$. For the bladder, the 5-year actuarial toxicity rate was 13% versus 9% if a value of 100 Gy$_{EQD2}$ was used. Insufficient events occurred in the sigmoid colon in this study for definitive analysis, but recommendations remain to keep the sigmoid less than 70 to 75 Gy$_{EQD2}$. It is hoped that further study will refine these guidelines.

Pelvic radiation spares a significant portion of the small bowel because bowel is normally in episodic motion. This tends to prevent any one segment from receiving an excessive dose. However, if loops of small bowel are immobilized as a result of adhesions caused by previous surgery, they may be held directly in the path of the radiation beam and thus injured (Fig. 23.14). The result of such an injury is usually not manifested for at least 6 months or longer after completion of radiation. Studies demonstrate that the use of IMRT in the postoperative setting can decrease the acute effects of irradiation on the bladder and

bowel, but definitive randomized studies are not available to date (see later).

Long-term Effects

Finally, it is important to understand the permanent nature of radiation injury. When any area of the body is subjected to tumoricidal doses of radiation, the normal tissues of that area sustain an injury that is only partially repaired. The tumor tissue disappears, but the normal tissue bed remains, and residual radiation changes must be seriously considered if other disease processes ensue. Radiobiologists estimate that in the case of injury to normal tissues, only 5% to 20% of the damage is repaired. If a second malignant neoplasm arises in that same area many years later, additional tumoricidal radiation is frequently impossible because of permanent radiation changes. In addition, any surgical procedures performed within a previously irradiated field are at higher risk for poor healing, fistula formation, and so forth.

Radiation-induced soft tissue necrosis can be a significant complication. This is usually a result of a progressive obliterative endarteritis that leads to decreased blood flow and a resultant hypoxic tissue bed. This causes increased fibrosis, poor healing, and chronic ulceration. Local conservative management (eg, hydrogen peroxide douche, estrogen therapy) resolves the problem in many cases. A small group of patients has significant tissue breakdown that may be painful and may lead to fistula formation. The use of hyperbaric oxygen has been shown to enhance healing in these radiation-induced injuries. Treatment with hyperbaric oxygen requires entering a tank where one breathes 100% oxygen at an increased atmospheric pressure. This increases the oxygen concentration in all body tissues up to 20 times normal. This treatment is done daily for 6 to 8 weeks. Side effects include nausea, claustrophobia, painful pressure on the ears—similar to the changes experienced with airline pressure changes—pneumothorax, and oxygen toxicity.

Permanent changes to the GU and GI tract can cause signs and symptoms such as decreased bladder capacity, hematuria, ureteral or urethral stricture, hematochezia, bowel obstruction, chronic diarrhea, tenesmus, fecal incontinence, and fistula formation. Gynecologic changes include dryness and shortening of the vagina, dyspareunia, and decreased orgasm. All of these long-term effects should be addressed by the oncology team to maximize the patient's quality of life.

NEW RADIATION MODALITIES

Protons

Protons result in an excellent physical dose distribution. The dose increases slowly with depth and reaches a sharp maximum near the end of the particle's range called the Bragg peak. This sharp dose peak allows for extremely precise, circumscribed delivery. Other than the physical distribution advantage, protons have biologic properties similar to x-rays. Protons are ideal for specific clinical situations, such as spinal cord tumors and eye melanomas, in which a sharp dose delivery is critical to avoid normal tissue damage. Reports also describe the utility in more common tumors, such as prostate cancer. Although useful in

FIGURE 23.13 Comparison of normal tissue irradiated with four field box technique (**A**), three-dimensional conformal therapy (**B**), and intensity-modulated radiation therapy (**C**). The *red* represents areas that receive 100% of the prescription dose, *yellow* 90%, *green* 50%, and *blue* 40%. Notice how the normal tissue volume receives less dose as the treatment is delivered more conformally.

FIGURE 23.14 Small bowel in the pelvis demonstrated by small bowel contrast.

several clinical situations, the cost of delivery from a cyclotron or special linear accelerator makes it currently available in a few cities, although interest is mounting and new centers are being built or contemplated in other areas.

Electrons

Most modern linear accelerators can produce high-energy electron beams. Electrons lose energy rapidly as they travel in tissue and interact with tissue atoms, and ultimately their kinetic energy is reduced to zero. Therefore, unlike photons, electrons have a specific range dependent on energy and the tissue traversed. Transvaginal electron irradiation can be used for a copiously bleeding exophytic cervical lesion to induce hemostasis. The dosimetry is such that most of the energy delivered transvaginally is absorbed into the malignant lesions itself. Lesions of the vulva and inguinofemoral lymph nodes are also treated with electron beams in many institutions. The limitations of electron therapy are related to the strengths. Because it loses energy rapidly, it cannot be used for deep-seated tumors, and the applicator must rest very close to the tumor itself, so only fairly superficial, shallow lesions are appropriately treated with electrons.

Fast Neutrons

Neutrons interact in tissue to produce recoil protons, α particles, and other nuclear particles. Their potential usefulness stems from a reduced OER (this translates into decreased hypoxic cell resistance), reduced differential killing by cell cycle, reduced ability for cells to repair sublethal damage, and higher effectiveness for slowly cycling tumors.

Although randomized controlled trials demonstrated that neutron therapy provided improved local control in some tumors, its utility was limited by higher morbidity and cost. Overall, use is limited by the cost of the cyclotron, limited depth penetrations, high surface entrance dose, lack of sharp beam boundaries, and variable intensity modulation.

Negative Pi Mesons and Other Heavy Ions

Negative pi mesons, or pions, are negatively charged particles that have a mass 273 times that of an electron. These are produced in a cyclotron or linear accelerator using 400 to 800 MeV protons that bombard a beryllium target. Pions exhibit a Bragg peak produced by elicited protons, neutrons, and α particles. Other heavy ions such as neon, argon, and carbon have been studied, but equipment to produce these special particles is expensive and not widely available. Use is limited to experimental therapy only. As with neutrons, these forms of radiation have a high biologic effectiveness and a low dependence on oxygen.

NEW RADIATION DELIVERY TECHNOLOGY

Intraoperative Radiation

Several centers throughout the world are investigating the utility of large-fraction intraoperative external irradiation. Patients are subjected to operative procedures in which the area of involvement is carefully defined, and radiation fractions of 1500 to 2500 cGy are delivered directly to the area identified. Applications of this technique in gynecologic oncology have been in the treatment of biopsy-proven positive paraaortic or pelvic nodes and marginally resectable recurrences. Electron beam radiation is delivered with one high-dose fraction with the bowel and other sensitive normal tissues packed to the side, thus minimizing the probability of visceral injuries. For best results, external-beam radiation is often combined with intraoperative therapy. Because the intraoperative accelerators only deliver electrons, it is subject to the same limitations as all electron beams (see previous discussion). Experience in both primary and recurrent tumors has been reported. The results are limited but have shown increased local control when used selectively. The role of intraoperative radiation in gynecology is not widespread and is limited to a few institutions that are capable of providing this specialized therapy. New techniques involving intraoperative low-energy radiation sources in the kV range are being investigated in other sites such as breast, but there are no reports of use in gynecologic cancers as yet.

Hyperthermia

As discussed previously, solid tumor masses often have hypovascular centers, which are poorly penetrated by antineoplastic drugs and have hypoxic, radioresistant cell fractions. Hyperthermia is another method used to overcome these relatively radioresistant tumors. Although several anecdotal clinical observations have been made, current interest in hyperthermia is based mainly on careful biologic studies on cells and transplantable tumors performed in the 1980s. Although there is no evidence that tumor cells are consistently more sensitive to heat than normal cells, several factors may contribute to a therapeutic gain. Tumor hypoxic cell populations have an acidic pH and are nutritionally deprived. These factors increase sensitivity to heat. Therapeutic gain is also derived from selective heat retention in the tumor. The hypoxic core is maintained at a higher temperature than the normal tissues, which more efficiently remove heat secondary to better-organized vasculature. Ultimately, cell death is dependent on the temperature achieved and is time dependent. Hyperthermia is combined with radiation as each modality preferentially kills a separate part of the tumor; in addition, heat increases the cell kill of external radiation by inhibiting sublethal and potentially lethal damage repair. Late S phase is the most sensitive phase to hyperthermia but the most resistant to low LET (photon) radiation, and thus the two modalities complement one another. The first notable use of hyperthermia in gynecologic oncology has been with interstitial hyperthermia for deep tumors of the pelvis. Increased survival has been demonstrated, although reports are mixed and the therapy is not commonly available.

Three-dimensional Conformal Radiation Therapy

Three-dimensional conformal radiation therapy is linked to a multiplicity of imaging modalities, especially CT. Beam placement using a CT simulator replaces the conventional simulator (fluoroscopic planning machine) for plan design to the extent that the term "virtual simulation" is used to describe it. The digitally reconstructed radiographs link the plan to the treatment unit in a manner that is rapidly replacing the conventional simulator. Three dimensional conformal therapy (3DCF) entails shaping of the beam to conform to the target as seen by CT imaging. The physician arranges the beams to maximize dose to the tumor and minimize dose to normal tissues. Patient, tumor, and normal target movement demand patient immobilization and that adequate margin be placed around the targets to prevent a "marginal miss."

Intensity-modulated Radiation Therapy

Intensity-modulated radiation therapy, compared with 3DCF therapy, uses the power of computers to perform hundreds to thousands of iterations of planning to maximize and shape tumor dose and minimize normal tissue dose (Fig. 23.15). This form of planning, called forward planning, gives the computer instructions on what dose to deliver to the targets and sets limitations on normal structures. Both 3DCF therapy and IMRT use small collimator "leaves" to finely shape the beam. These "leaves" are mobile and block portions of the generated x-rays. If the collimator "leaves" move while the radiation beam is on and vary the beam intensity, areas of tumor and normal tissue can receive a spectrum of doses, hence the term *intensity modulated*. These collimator "leaves" also allow for irregular shapes to be treated. This technology has demonstrated similar local control with reduced complications in several sites such as prostate and head and neck. In gynecologic cancer, decreased radiation to normal tissues, including bowel, bladder, and bone

marrow, has been demonstrated, especially in the postoperative setting. Papers have been published on the use of IMRT in postoperative uterine and cervical carcinoma, vulvar carcinoma, whole abdominal radiotherapy, vaginal carcinoma, and intact cervical carcinoma. Because of the daily variation in bladder and rectal filling, the mobility of the upper vagina and cervix, and the change in cervical volume over the span of treatment in intact cervical cancer, use of IMRT should be undertaken with extreme caution and special attention should be given to assure that the target is accurately delineated and treated with each fraction. Randomized, prospective trials evaluating IMRT are anticipated, and consensus guidelines for clinical target volume delineation have been recently published by Lim and colleagues. Introduction of new technology such as tomotherapy (a linear accelerator linked to an online CT scanner), CyberKnife (a linear accelerator capable of fiducial imaging to target radiation), and cone-beam CT (CT scan mounted to the linear accelerator) for image-guided radiotherapy assists in daily target and normal tissue localization but in gynecologic cancer is still investigational. Other concerns regarding this technology include the enormous physician and physics time used for planning, increased cost, and the unknown long-term consequences of lower dose but increased volume of tissue exposed to radiation.

Stereotactic Radiotherapy

Stereotactic radiation and gamma knife radiation are similar to IMRT and 3DCF radiation because they allow precise, high-dose delivery of external radiation. It is commonly used for both primary and metastatic brain tumors, small lung tumors, and an increasing number of other sites. Whereas stereotactic radiation uses a modification of the linear accelerator, gamma knife is a separate machine with 201 separate ^{60}Co sources used to focus on the target.

Immune-tagged Radiation Therapy

Recently, several products that tag a radioisotope to a monoclonal antibody have entered the market. This modality of radiation allows delivery of the radioactive isotope to the unique antibody target. It has been used successfully in lymphomas and awaits the identification of a unique target before development for a gynecologic use.

GLOSSARY

absorbed dose The energy imparted to matter by ionizing radiation per unit mass of irradiated material. The unit is the gray (Gy), defined to be an energy absorption of 1 joule/kg. The old unit was the rad, which was defined as an energy absorption of 100 ergs/g.

brachytherapy Treatment of malignant tumors by radioactive sources that are implanted close to (intracavitary) or within (interstitial) the tumor.

dosimetry The term applied to the measurement and calculation of dose that the patient receives.

electron volt (eV) The energy of motion acquired by an electron accelerated through a potential difference of 1 volt.

excitation The moving of an electron to a more distant orbit within the same atom.

gamma rays Electromagnetic irradiation (originating inside the nucleus) emitted by excited nuclei. The gamma rays from an isotope will have one or several sharply defined energies.

FIGURE 23.15 In **A** and **B,** note how little normal tissue is treated to accomplish the sidewall nodal boost. In **C,** note how the renal parenchyma and spinal cord are relatively spared in treating the paraaortic recurrence.

Gray (Gy) The special name for the unit of absorbed dose and specific energy impacted; 1 Gy = 1 joule/kg = 100 rads.

half-life The time in which half the atoms of a radioactive species disintegrate.

image-guided brachytherapy (IGBT) The use of imaging for three-dimensional, volume directed planning.

image-guided radiation therapy (IGRT) The use of images taken before, during, or after treatment while in the treatment room to allow visualization of target, fiducial markers, or organs at risk.

intensity modulated radiation therapy (IMRT) Computer technology that allows variable fluence across the beam and increased conformance to target relative to normal tissues.

inverse square law The intensity of radiation from a point varies inversely as the square of the distance from the source. Thus, the dose rate at 2 cm from a source is one fourth that at 1 cm. At 3 cm, the dose rate is one-ninth that at 1 cm.

ionization The removal of an electron from an atom, leaving a positively charged ion.

ionizing radiation Radiation capable of causing ionization.

isotope Nuclides having an equal number of protons but a different number of neutrons (excitable situation).

keV 1000 eV.

linear energy transfer (LET) The energy lost by the particle or photon per micron of path depth. High LET radiations are more effective against hypoxic cells.

meV 1,000,000 eV.

oxygen enhancement ratio (OER) The ratio of the dose required for a given level of cell killing under hypoxic conditions compared with the dose needed in air.

penumbra The radiation outside the full beam, which is often caused by scatter or incomplete collimation.

rad A unit-absorbed dose of ionizing radiation equivalent to the absorption of 100 erg per gram of irradiated material.

relative biologic effectiveness (RBE) A ratio of the absorbed dose of a reference radiation to the absorbed dose of a test radiation to produce the same level of biologic effect, other conditions being equal.

rem The old unit of dose equivalent. It is the product of the absorbed dose in rads and modifying factor and is being replaced by the sievert.

roentgen (R) An internationally accepted unit of radiation quantity: It is the quantity of "x-ray or gamma irradiation such that the associated corpuscular emission per 0.001293 g of air produces, in air, ions carrying 1 esu of quantity of electricity of either sign." X-rays originate outside the nucleus.

Sievert (SU): The unit of dose equivalent in the SI system (1 Sv = 100 rem).

x-rays: Rays emitted by a particular generator will emit a spectrum of energies.

For the bibliography list, log onto www.expertconsult.com ⟨http://www.expertconsult.com⟩.

Staging: Staging of Cancer at Gynecologic Sites

ABSTRACT

For complete details of anatomy, staging classification, and rules for classification by sites of malignant tumors of the female pelvis, please, go to expertconsult.com. To access your account, look for your activation instructions on the inside front cover of this book.

CERVIX UTERI, CORPUS UTERI, OVARY, VAGINA, VULVA, GESTATIONAL TROPHOBLASTIC TUMORS, AND FALLOPIAN TUBE

In 1976, the American Joint Committee adopted the classification of the International Federation of Gynecology and Obstetrics (FIGO), which is the format used in the *Annual Report on the Results of Treatment in Carcinoma of the Uterus, Vagina and Ovary*, which is published every 3 years. This report has used the FIGO classification with periodic modifications since 1937, the last being 2009. Numerous institutions throughout the world contribute their statistics for inclusion in this voluntary collaborative presentation of data.

The cervix and corpus uteri were among the first anatomic sites to be classified by the TNM system. This uses extent of primary tumor (T), nodal metastasis (N), and distant metastasis (M) status to stage cancers. This system has been approved by the American Joint Committee on Cancer (AJCC) and the International Union Against Cancer (UICC). FIGO has worked closely for many years with the AJCC and UICC in the classification of cancer at gynecologic sites. Staging of malignant tumors is essentially the same, and stages are comparable in the two (FIGO and TNM) systems regarding categories and details.

Modified From Common Terminology Criteria for Adverse Events (Common Terminology Criteria for Adverse Events)*

(version 4.0)
U.S. Department of Health and Human Services
National Institutes of Health, National Cancer Institute
Published May 28, 2009 (v4.03: June 14, 2010)
For the complete table containing common terminology criteria for adverse events, please go to expertconsult.com. To access your account, look for your activation instructions on the inside front cover of this book.

QUICK REFERENCE

The National Cancer Institute (NCI) Common Terminology Criteria for Adverse Events is a descriptive terminology that can be used for adverse event (AE) reporting. A grading (severity) scale is provided for each AE term.

COMPONENTS AND ORGANIZATION

System Organ Class

System Organ Class (SOC), the highest level of the Medical Dictionary for Regulatory Activities (MedDRA) hierarchy, is identified by anatomic or physiologic system, etiology, or purpose (eg, SOC investigations for laboratory test results).

CTCAE terms are grouped by MedDRA Primary SOCs. Within each SOC, AEs are listed and accompanied by descriptions of severity (grade).

CTCAE Terms

An AE is any unfavorable and unintended sign (including an abnormal laboratory finding), symptom, or disease temporally associated with the use of a medical treatment or procedure that may or may *not* be considered related to the medical treatment or procedure. An AE is a term that is a unique representation of a specific event used for medical documentation and scientific analyses. Each CTCAE v4.0 term is a MedDRA LLT (lowest level term).

Definitions

A brief definition is provided to clarify the meaning of each AE term.

Grades

Grade refers to the severity of the AE. The CTCAE displays grades 1 through 5 with unique clinical descriptions of severity for each AE based on this general guideline.

---

*CTCAE v4.0 incorporates certain elements of the MedDRA terminology. For further details on MedDRA, refer to the MedDRA MSSO website (http://www.meddramsso.com).

CAPPENDIX

Blood Component Therapy

Despite the recent increase in the use of hematopoietic growth factors, transfusion therapy plays an important role in caring for oncology patients, particularly now that more effective treatment regimens have led to longer survival. In many instances, a patient with cancer behaves like a patient with a chronic disease requiring frequent blood components caused by disorders secondary to the disease, treatment, or both. Whole blood is separated into cellular and noncellular components, including red blood cells (RBCs), platelets, and plasma.

1. Blood component: A portion of blood is separated by physical and mechanical means, such as differential centrifugation (Fig. C.1). Cell separation technology, capable of collecting platelets, plasma, granulocytes, peripheral blood stem cells, and RBCs, has an increasingly important role in transfusion medicine. Anticoagulants and other additives used in blood collection containers allow storage of liquid red cells for up to 42 days.
   a. Packed red blood cells (PRBCs): These cells are prepared from whole blood by centrifugation and subsequent removal of plasma.
      (1) Hematocrit: 60% to 80%
      (2) Indications
          (a) Replacement of hemoglobin-containing cells in an anemic patient with heart failure, renal failure, burns, or bone marrow failure
          (b) Debilitated patients
          (c) Elderly patients
          (d) Patients with liver disease
      (3) Recommend to use PRBCs for losses of blood less than 1000 to 1500 mL/70 kg; with greater losses, other blood components should be used
      (4) Therapeutic effect: In a 70-kg adult, each unit should increase the hematocrit by 3% to 4%.
   b. Frozen RBCs: Long-term preservation of frozen RBCs without damage can be accomplished by the addition of glycerol; before transfusion, the RBCs should be thawed and washed to remove glycerol
      (1) Advantages
          (a) Blood of rare types can be stored for long periods.
          (b) 2,3-Diphosphoglycerol and adenosine triphosphate levels remain the same as they were on the day that the blood was frozen.
          (c) Free of plasma protein, platelets, white blood cells, and fibrin

          (d) Has been claimed to reduce the incidence of hepatitis acquired from a blood transfusion
      (2) Disadvantages
          (a) Expensive
          (b) Outdated in 24 hours after thaw
          (c) Takes time to thaw and deglycerolize
   c. Buffy coat: poor erythrocytes; would reduce the incidence of febrile transfusion reaction
      (1) Indications
          (a) Patients with repeated febrile nonhemolytic transfusion reaction caused by leukocyte antibody
          (b) Hematopoietic growth factors applied to oncologies from transfusion therapy is designed to limit the exposure of patients to allogenic blood with its innate risks. The synthesis of erythropoietin (EPO) by recombinant technology was a very important advance in decreasing RBC transfusions. EPO has also been used to increase the yield of autologous donations and to stimulate erythropoiesis after surgery.
   d. Platelet concentrates
      (1) One unit of platelet concentrate contains 5.5×10^{10} platelets suspended in 30 to 50 mL of plasma
      (2) Shelf-life: 72 hours at room temperature
      (3) Thrombocytopenia does not usually produce serious bleeding unless the platelet count is below 20,000, except if there is a platelet function defect, a coagulation defect, or local cause of hemorrhage (e.g., trauma, surgery)
   e. Fresh-frozen plasma (FFP)
      (1) Contains albumin, globulin, active coagulation factors, complement, and electrolytes
      (2) Should be type specific
      (3) Shelf life: 12 months at $-20°$ to $-30°C$; should be used within 2 hours after thawing
      (4) Indications
          (a) Deficiency in coagulation factors
          (b) Situation with plasma loss
          (c) Rapid reversal of oral anticoagulant therapy
   f. Cryoprecipitate: Cold insoluble precipitate remains when FFP is allowed to thaw at 4°C; it contains factor VIII with fibrinogen and factor XIII
      (1) Indications
          (a) von Willebrand disease
          (b) Replacement of fibrinogen, factor XIII

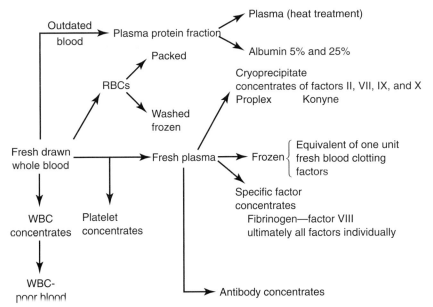

FIGURE C.1 Separation of a unit of whole blood into its various components. *RBC,* Red blood cell; *WBC,* white blood cell.

2. Plasma fraction: derivatives of plasma are obtained by a chemical process such as alcohol precipitation
   a. Coagulation factor concentrates
      (1) Factor VIII concentrates
      (2) Factor IX concentrates
      (3) Prothrombin complex (factor II, VII, IX, X concentrates)
      (4) Fibrinogen concentrates
   b. Immunoglobulin concentrates
   c. Albumin: filtered and pasteurized by heating for 10 hours at 60°C to eliminate the risks of viral hepatitis
      (1) 5% albumin: isosmotic, sodium 145 mEq/L; for rapid expansion of vascular volume
      (2) 25% albumin: sodium 145 mEq/L; given intravenously; one volume of 25% albumin will draw about four volumes of additional fluid from the extravascular space into the circulation; used for treatment of hypoalbuminemia
   d. Plasma protein factor: 5% solution of selected human plasma protein in buffered saline solution; heat treated to eliminate the risk of hepatitis; indicated for rapid expansion of vascular volume
3. Stroma-free hemoglobin solution
   a. Advantages
      (1) No need for blood typing
      (2) Longer storage capacity
      (3) Maintains better microcirculation
      (4) Potentially improved oxygenation of ischemic myocardium
      (5) No antigenicity
4. Autologous blood: The collection and reinfusion of the patient's own blood by preoperative autologous blood donation or intraoperative blood salvage. For autologous blood donation, the blood should be taken at least 2 weeks before

TABLE C.1 **Risk of Infection**	
Agent Risk	**Unit**
Hepatitis B	1:50,000
Hepatitis C	1:100,000
Human immunodeficiency virus	1:150,000–1:1,000,000
Human T cell lymphotropic virus	1:50,000

From ACOG, Technical Bulletin 199, Nov. 1994, and Management of Hepatitis C. NIH Consensus Statement Online 1997;15(3):1.

the surgical procedure, and the patient must maintain a hemoglobin level of 11 g/dL or more. If large amounts of blood are required, frozen cells are another option. Many patients can donate as often as once a week. Intraoperative blood salvage requires the sterile collection and reinfusion of shed blood that is free of infecting agents such as malignant cells. The RBCs are collected in sterile plastic bags, washed, and concentrated before being reinfused into the patient.

5. Complications: infection, transfusion reactions, and alloimmunization are the major complications associated with the transfusion of blood components (Table C.1).

Once in each 6000 units of blood transferred, an acute hemolytic reaction will occur, with a mortality rate of 1 in 17. These reactions are usually due to ABO incompatibility and resultant intracellular hemolysis. Patients develop fever, chills, chest pain, nausea, hypotension, and disseminated intravascular coagulation. Mild reactions to leukocyte and platelet antigens are usually associated with a febrile episode alone. Hemolytic reactions to other blood groups such as Kidd, Duffy, and Kell can be associated with fever, anemia, and hyperbilirubinemia and a positive direct Coombs test result. Some of these milder transfusions reactions manifest themselves 7 to 10 days after the transfusion.

Hematopoietic growth factors are designed to limit the exposure of oncology patients to blood and blood products. RBC substitutes are currently in development, and some are in phase II and III clinical trials. None are currently approved for clinical use in the United States. They consist of artificially derived products that have oxygen-carrying properties and are structurally similar to hemoglobin. Their development has been hampered by relatively short half-life in the circulation.

The isolation and then synthesis of erythropoietin has been very helpful in limiting RBC transfusions. Granulocyte colony-stimulating factor (G-CSF) has been proven to decrease infection rates in neutropenic patients after chemotherapy. The limitations of platelet transfusions have stimulated the research into agents that can stimulate platelet production, and such products are now available. In addition, thrombopoietic growth factors have the potential to stimulate platelet apheresis donors and increase stem cell harvest yields, thus expanding progenitor cells.

For the bibliography list, log onto ⟨www.expertconsult.com⟩.

Suggested Recommendations for Routine Cancer Screening

CERVICAL CANCER

Cervical cancer screening should begin at age 21 years. Cytologic screening is recommended every 2 years for women ages 21 to 29 years with either conventional or liquid-based cytology. Women ages 30 years and older who have had three consecutive cervical cytology test results that are negative for intraepithelial lesions and malignancy may be screened every 3 years. Women with any of the following risk factors may require more frequent cervical cytology:

1. Women who are immunosuppressed
2. Women who are infected with human immunodeficiency virus (HIV)
3. Women who were exposed to diethylstilbestrol in utero
4. Women who were previously treated for cervical intraepithelial neoplasia (CIN) 2 or 3 or cancer

Co-testing using the combination of cytology plus HPV DNA testing is appropriate screening for women older than 30 years. Co-testing in women younger than 30 years is not recommended.

In women who have had a total hysterectomy for benign indications with no history of high-grade CIN, routine cytology testing should be discontinued.

It is reasonable to discontinue cervical cancer screening between 65 and 70 years of age in women who have had three or more negative cytology test results in a row and no abnormal test results in the past 10 years.

Women who have been immunized against HPV-16 and HPV-18 should be screened by the same regimen as nonimmunized women.

BREAST CANCER

Mammography should be performed every year for women 40 years of age and older.

Evidence from several studies indicates that there is a decrease in mortality for all women when appropriate screening by mammography is instituted and performed by qualified personnel. The efficacy of mammography is not in doubt. The question that remains is the optimal screening frequency, and the answer may be provided by data now being compiled. Safety is no longer a concern, but it is recognized that mammography is the most costly of all screening modalities. Dedicated equipment is essential, and considerable skill and experience are required to interpret the films. It is important, therefore, to determine the most prudent utilization of resources. Until the optimal screening frequency is determined, it appears reasonable to follow recommendations of the American College of Obstetricians and Gynecologists, American Cancer Society, and National Cancer Institute.

ENDOMETRIAL CANCER

Total population screening for endometrial cancer and its precursors is neither cost effective nor warranted. High-risk patients may require endometrial sampling.

The cost effectiveness of screening asymptomatic women for endometrial cancer and its precursors is very low; therefore, the practice is unwarranted. On the other hand, perimenopausal and postmenopausal women with a history or evidence of abnormal vaginal hemorrhage are at high risk for endometrial cancer, and their symptoms should be investigated by endometrial biopsy or curettage. Dilatation and curettage are recommended when endometrial hyperplasia or questionable endometrial carcinoma is present and when there is insufficient tissue for diagnosis by endometrial biopsy.

If estrogen and progestin therapy is instituted, endometrial biopsy is not required before treatment is begun unless there are reasons (e.g., abnormal bleeding) to place the patient at high risk for endometrial neoplasia. If unexpected breakthrough bleeding occurs during therapy, endometrial biopsy is recommended to rule out the development of abnormal endometrial histology. Endometrial biopsy by aspiration curettage performed in the office is diagnostically reliable and cost effective in symptomatic patients. The timing of further biopsies, if needed, is a clinical decision that should be based on previous histologic results and the patient's history.

OVARIAN CANCER

No available techniques are currently suitable for routine screening. Many different techniques, including peritoneal fluid profiles, investigation of tumor-associated antigens, and ultrasonography, have been or are being investigated as possible screening tools for ovarian cancer. To date, none of these techniques has proved to be practical or effective.

COLORECTAL CANCER

Beginning at 50 years of age, one of three screening options should be selected: (1) yearly fecal occult blood testing plus flexible sigmoidoscopy every 5 years, (2) colonoscopy every 10 years, or (3) double-contrast barium enema (DCBE) every 5 to 10 years. A digital rectal examination should be performed at the time of each screening sigmoidoscopy, colonoscopy, or DCBE.

Available data do not substantiate the cost-effectiveness of various screening recommendations. Because colorectal cancer is a significant risk to women, the task force suggests that the recommendations of the American Cancer Society (American College of Obstetricians and Gynecology [ACOG]) and the National Cancer Institute be used as a guide.

LUNG CANCER

No available techniques are currently suitable for routine screening. The only effective way to reduce mortality from lung cancer is to promote a "stop smoking" message to the public. Although some support is evolving for annual radiographic screening for those at risk (i.e., women 50 years and older who smoke more than one pack of cigarettes daily), neither the American Cancer Society nor the National Cancer Institute has adopted this guideline. This information is based on the ACOG Committee Opinion, No. 247, December 2000.

Nutritional Therapy

In patients with cancer, malnutrition may appear simultaneously with the disease. Patients with cancer often exhibit anorexia because of decreased nutritional intake with resultant weight loss. There may be an increased nutritional requirement because of the increased demands of the patient and the tumor. Resting metabolic rates can vary greatly, but in as many as 60% of patients, the rate may be elevated. The stage of malnutrition in patients with cancer can lead to cachexia with weakness and tissue wasting. The extent of malnutrition in the patient may be greater than can be explained by decreased nutritional intake. Metabolic abnormalities include an abnormal response to glucose tolerance testing, increased gluconeogenesis (which can result in decreased muscle protein synthesis), and abnormalities in protein and fat metabolism. A patient with a malignancy may need additional nutritional support while undergoing intensive treatment, which can include surgery and chemotherapy. **Parenteral nutrition seems to improve a patient's tolerance of the treatment and improves her nutritional state; however, parenteral nutrition has not been shown to improve survival.**

The malnutrition seen in cancer patients is commonly referred to as *cancer cachexia*. Nutritional depletion is seen as a protein-calorie malnutrition with a loss of body cell mass. The importance of protein-calorie nutrition is its association with increases in postoperative complications, deficiencies in immune function, and poorer tolerance of therapy.

Dietary nutrients required for good health include water, protein, fat, carbohydrates, vitamins, and minerals. Energy is required for normal body function, growth, and repair. Protein is necessary for growth and development to maintain body structures and function. It is the source of the essential amino acids and nitrogen needed for the synthesis of nonessential amino acids. Dietary protein replaces the essential amino acids and nitrogen that are lost through protein turnover and normal body functions. During illness, protein requirements increase. **Nitrogen balance is essential for good health and requires intake of protein and energy.** At higher energy intakes, less protein is needed to achieve nitrogen balance. Nitrogen is lost continuously in the body through normal body functions. Fat is the food substance with the highest concentration of calories.

The visual protein compartment is best measured by assessment of the plasma albumin, transferrin, and total lymphocyte count. Albumin is the major determinant of plasma colloidal osmotic pressure because its large size does not permit it to pass the capillary membrane. The appearance of edema is often a sign of low serum albumin. Serum levels lower than 3.0 g/dL

are reflective of nutritional deficiency. Transferrin is a protein of hepatic origin and transports iron. The level is reflective of the patient's ability to make serum protein. Transferrin levels are more sensitive than albumin levels because of its shorter half-life (8 days compared with 20 days), and it is preferable to evaluate the efficacy of nutritional therapy. The response of a patient's total lymphocyte count to nutritional therapy may also be a favorable prognostic sign during the first 7 to 14 days of therapy (Table E.1).

Linoleic acid is the only essential fatty acid required in the diet; it is necessary for the synthesis of arachidonic acid, which is a major precursor of prostaglandin. Linoleic acid comes mainly from polyunsaturated vegetable oils. **A deficiency of essential fatty acids results in poor wound healing, hair loss, and dermatitis.** Fatty acids and cholesterol make up most of the fat in our diets. Carbohydrates include sugar, starch, and fibers. **When carbohydrates are not included in the diet, ketosis begins to occur, and there is excessive breakdown of protein as amino acids are used for gluconeogenesis.** Water-soluble and fat-soluble vitamins cannot be synthesized in adequate amounts by the body. **Fat-soluble vitamins are required for absorption, transport, metabolism, and storage.** They are not excreted in the urine like the water-soluble vitamins, and an excess accumulation can lead to well-known toxic conditions. Major minerals, as well as trace elements, are important in human nutrition.

Lack of appetite with reduction in food intake is a key factor in cancer cachexia. The role of the neurotransmitter serotonin appears to be central to appetite. Inhibition of serotonin increases appetite and food intake in animals. Cancer patients also report a loss of taste and smell with a resulting loss of appeal of most foods. Weight loss may also be greatly influenced when the location of the tumor affects the ability to take nutrition (eg, a mass causing a partial bowel obstruction). Cytokines produced by the patient in response to a growing neoplasm may result in nutritional derangements. Cytokines can regulate appetite and metabolic rate, so they can be very important factors. Dudrick and coworkers suggest that patients who have a 10-lb weight loss or a 10% decrease in body weight 2 months before assessment, serum albumin of less than 3.4 g/dL, alergy to four of five standard skin test antigens, and a low total lymphocyte count and who cannot or will not eat enough are candidates for nutritional assessment. Nutritional history, with a 24-hour dietary recall, can be used to assess nutritional intake. Anthropometric measurements are useful when assessing the

TABLE E.1   **Indications for Total Parenteral Nutrition***
Severely malnourished patients undergoing surgery
Patients with postoperative complications that require nutritional support
Therapy-induced complications that require nutritional support

*Routine use of total parenteral nutrition (TPN) in patients with cancer is not indicated.

patient's nutritional status. **Relative body weight is probably the most useful of these measurements because rapid weight loss is usually an indication of protein-calorie undernutrition.** The triceps skinfold test assesses fat stores, and midarm circumference tends to assess protein status. **Edema, which is often seen with protein-calorie deficiency, can mask true weight loss and muscle wasting. Serum albumin is probably the single most important test for determining protein calorie undernutrition. Albumin is the main plasma protein needed to maintain plasma osmotic pressure as well as other functions.** In a patient with low albumin, morbidity and mortality are increased. Albumin can be influenced by conditions other than malnutrition and may be affected by hydration status. **Transferrin binds and transports iron in the plasma and is a good indicator of protein nutritional status.** The extent of malnutrition depends on the type and site of the cancer. Cancers such as ovarian cancer, with its potential effect on the gastrointestinal (GI) tract, appear to contribute to malnutrition to a greater degree than does cervical cancer. As expected, malnutrition becomes worse as the cancer progresses. The mechanism of cancer-related malnutrition is unknown. There are probably multiple contributing factors. **Decreased food intake because of anorexia, early satiety, nausea, and vomiting can all play a role. Poor absorption of nutrients can also be a contributing factor. Food aversion, particularly in patients undergoing chemotherapy or irradiation, is well known.** Change of taste and smell can contribute to decreased intake. Generalized weakness may also contribute to decreased food intake. Decrease in total lymphocyte count (<1200 cells/mL) is also suggestive of malnutrition. Creatinine height index (CHI) may be helpful because urinary creatinine excretion is proportional to total body muscle mass. As muscles become depleted, creatinine excretion falls. A CHI of 80% or more usually indicates a normal lean body mass. A CHI between 60% and 80% indicates moderate depletion; a CHI of less than 60% indicates severe depletion.

ENTERNAL NUTRITION

Numerous clinical trials have been published using aggressive enteral nutritional support as a supplement during cancer therapy in patients who would not eat well. The trials are not consistent in demonstrating benefit of enteral nutrition. However, it is a well-accepted concept that enteral therapy is the preferred route for feeding cancer patients when the GI tract is not obstructed. Methods of enteral nutrition vary from frequent snack between meals to the insertion of a comfortable nasogastric feeding tube on a continuous drip of nutritional supplements. Others have used gastrostomy or jejunostomy feeding tubes.

The role of total parenteral nutrition (TPN) in patients with cancer has yet to be determined. TPN can correct nutritional deficits that commonly occur in patients with cancer. TPN can also improve nitrogen balance and decrease catabolism. Glucose turnover and clearance rates are increased, gluconeogenesis is suppressed, and free fatty acid oxidation is increased. TPN can increase body weight and reverse serum markers of malnutrition; however, as an adjuvant to cancer therapy, the results have not been encouraging. TPN has not added to lean body mass or eliminated the GI or hematologic toxicity associated with chemotherapy. **In patients treated with chemotherapy, response rates and survival have not been increased with TPN.** Although irradiation can contribute to poor nutrition (eg, diarrhea, enteritis, and malabsorption), particularly to the GI tract when gynecologic cancers are treated, **TPN has not produced a significant improvement regarding treatment response, tolerance to treatment, local control, survival, or decreased complications of therapy. Nutritional support for patients with cancer requiring surgery is also ill defined.** Malnourished patients undergoing surgery have a higher postoperative morbidity and mortality compared with well-nourished patients. Whether TPN can affect morbidity and mortality in patients with cancer is undetermined, and the concern that TPN may stimulate tumor growth is unfounded. **Although routine use of TPN in patients with cancer is not warranted, it may be indicated in severely malnourished patients undergoing surgery or for those with postoperative complications.**

Nutritional supports are of two main types: enteric and parenteral. For a patient with a functional GI tract, enteric nutrition may be considered through the use of a nasoenteric tube. A gastrostomy or jejunostomy tube may also be used. Obviously, GI dysfunction is a contraindication to this method. Nevertheless, this method appears to be cost effective; it probably maintains the GI mucosa integrity, provides a normal sequence of intestinal and hepatic metabolism before systemic distribution, appears to preserve normal hormonal patterns, and avoids the risk of sepsis. Enteric solutions differ in composition, calorie content, and multiple other factors. These solutions are usually complete because they contain a full supplement of nutrient requirements or incomplete when they are designated to contain a specific macronutrient such as fat, protein, or carbohydrate. **Most solutions contain 1000 calories and 37 to 45 g/L of protein.** Elemental diets consist mainly of amino acids and simple sugars. They are extremely hypertonic and may induce diarrhea, which may be corrected with a formula of lower osmolarity. Electrolyte imbalance and glucose intolerance can also occur.

Many patients with cancer who require nutritional supplementation will need TPN. In some cases, TPN can be administered through a peripheral vein, particularly if TPN is to be given for only a short amount of time. Although adequate protein can usually be infused peripherally, high-caloric supplementation is usually given centrally. Fat solutions, which can account for a high caloric intake, can be given peripherally. **Major complications of peripheral TPN are thrombophlebitis and infiltration. In most cases, TPN is given through a central vein—either the subclavian vein or a major neck vessel.** The catheter can be inserted in the superior vena cava, which allows rapid infusion of hypertonic solutions without difficulty. **Infusion of parenteral solution should be started slowly to prevent hyperglycemia. If glucose intolerance develops, a small amount of insulin is used to control blood sugars.** Meticulous care must be taken of the central catheter because this site can be a major source of infection. Frequent changing of intravenous tubing and filters and the catheter is required routinely. TPN is usually managed as a team endeavor with the attending physician, nutritionist, nurse, pharmacist, and dietitian. Daily requirements must be standardized regarding calories, proteins, fat, minerals, vitamins, and trace elements. These should be varied as the situation demands. **Metabolic**

complications may include hyperglycemia or hypoglycemia, hyperosmolarity, azotemia, hyperchloremic metabolic acidosis, mineral electrolyte disorder, liver enzyme elevations, and anemia. In many hospitals, standard hyperalimentation solutions with appropriate nutrients have been formulated, and adjustments are made for specific needs. Intense metabolic monitoring is required in these patients, and established hospital protocols are now available in many institutions.

Today, both enteric and parenteral nutritional support can be implemented successfully on an outpatient basis. Indications are not uniformly agreed on for this method of nutrition. In patients with cancer, nutritional support may be indicated to help satisfy nutritional needs while toxicity of treatment is abating. Most authorities do not believe that home nutritional support is needed for terminally ill cancer patients.

A typical nutritional guideline for adult patients is shown in Table E.2 (see the Expert Consult website). Many institutions have nutritional protocols in place. Although there may be

---

TABLE E.2 Nutritional Guidelines for Adult Patients

I. Daily protein needs

Maintenance	0.8–1 g/kg
Mild to moderate stress	1–1.5 g/kg
Moderate to severe stress	1.5–2 g/kg
Very high stress or burns	>2 g/kg

II. Daily caloric needs
   (Consider initiating HAL with 50%–75% of estimated patient needs on day 1.)
   - Maintenance, mild stress: 20–25 kcal/kg (15–20 NPC/kg)
   - Mild to moderate stress (routine surgery, minor infection): 25–30 kcal/kg (20–25 NPC/kg)
   - Moderate to severe stress (major surgery, sepsis, tumor treatment): 30–35 kcal/kg (25–30 NPC/kg)

III. Body weight calculations
   - TBW = patient's weight (kg)
   - IBW (male) = 50 kg + (2.3 × no. of inches >5 ft)
   - IBW (female) = 45 kg + (2.3 × no. of inches >5 ft)
   - ABW for an obese patient = IBW + 0.3 × (TBW − IBW)

IV. Suggested laboratory tests
   - Baseline and weekly: Chem 10, Chem 13
   - Daily: Chem 10 × 3 days or until stabilized prealbumin as clinically indicated

V. Formula
   A. Standard formula

	Central	Peripheral (D^{10}A$_{3,6}$)
Amino acids (g)	55 mg/L	30 g/L
Dextrose (kcal)	555 kcal/L	280 kcal/L
Lipids (kcal)	400 kcal/L	350 kcal/L
NPC	955 NPC/L	630 NPC/L
Total kcal	1175 kcal/L	750 kcal/L
Desired total volume/day	_____ mL*	_____ mL*

   B. Modified central formula
   1. Protein:
      Daily protein needs × Body weight calculations = _____ g protein/day
   2. NPC:
      Daily caloric needs × Body weight calculations = _____ NPC/day
   3. Percentages of NPC:
      Usually 50%–70% of daily NPC as CHO + usually 30%–50% of daily NPC as fat = 100%
   4. Infusion rate (see HAL bag for exact infusion rate)
      ☐ Maximally concentrated† or ☐ infusion rate _____ mg/h

Continued

TABLE E.2   Nutritional Guidelines for Adult Patients—cont'd

VI. Electrolytes	□ Standard	□ Modified	Acetate/Chloride
Sodium	80 mEq/L	_____ mEq/L	_____ balance
Potassium	40 mEq/L	_____ mEq/L	_____ maximum acetate
Calcium	5 mEq/L	_____ mEq/L	_____ maximum chloride
Magnesium	8 mEq/L	_____ mEq/L	_____ : _____ chloride : acetate

VII. Vitamins and trace elements

(MV1-12 and standard trace elements will automatically be added unless otherwise specified)

_____ vitamin K 1 mg/day   _____ no vitamin K

A. Content of MV1-12

Vitamin A	3300 IU	Vitamin B$_5$	15 mg
Vitamin D	200 IU	Vitamin B$_6$	4 mg
Vitamin E	10 mg	Vitamin B$_{12}$	5 mcg
Vitamin B$_1$	3 mg	Vitamin C	100 mg
Vitamin B$_2$	3.6 mg	Biotin	60 mcg
Vitamin B$_3$	40 mg	Folic acid	0.4 mg

B. Content of standard trace elements chromium chloride   12 mcg

Copper sulfate   1.2 mg

Manganese sulfate   0.3 mg

Zinc sulfate   3 mg

VIII. Other additives

_____ Humulin regular insulin _____ units/day

_____ H$_2$ antagonist _____ m/day

_____ Other (specify)

IX. Hyperalimentation access

_____ Central   _____ Peripheral

X. Special instructions

*See HAL bag for exact infusion rate.

†Calculation of volume of maximally concentrated HAL:

¹AA: _____ protein/day × 10 mL/g AA = _____ mL 10% AA solution.

²Dextrose: _____ NPC/day × _____% as CHO = _____ kcal CHO ÷ 3.4 kcal/g CHO = _____ g CHO × 1.43 mL/g = _____ mL D70.

³Lipid: _____ NPC/day × _____% as fat = _____ kcal fat ÷ 2 kcal/mL = _____ mL 20% lipids.

⁴Maximally concentrated volume = _____ (from 1 above) mL 10% AA + _____ (from 2 above) mL D70 + _____ (from 3 above) mL 20% lipids = _____ mL/day.

⁵Approximate infusion rate = _____ (from 4 above) mL/day ÷ 24 hr/day = _____ mL/hr. (Actual infusion rate may be altered by volume of additives; see HAL bag for exact infusion rate.)

AA, Amino acid; *ABW,* adjusted body weight; *CHO,* carbohydrate; *HAL,* hyperalimentation; *IBW,* ideal body weight; *MV,* multivitamins; *TBW,* total body weight.

Courtesy of the Nutritional and Pharmacy Divisions of the Medical University of South Carolina.

variations on the theme, these guidelines have become relatively standardized.

Additional therapies can also be considered along with nutritional support to alleviate cancer cachexia. Synthetic progestins (megestrol acetate and medroxyprogesterone acetate) in high doses decrease the production of cytokines and serotonin and thus improve appetite and a sense of well-being. Responses often are seen within 15 to 30 days of therapy, and side effects are minimal. Some authors have reported more thromboembolic events with megestrol acetate but not in placebo-controlled studies.

For the bibliography list, log onto ⟨http://www.expertconsult .com⟩

Page numbers followed by "*f*" indicate figures,
"*t*" indicate tables.